EMERGENCY MEDICINE

A COMPREHENSIVE STUDY GUIDE
FIFTH EDITION

Companion Handbook

Renee Hernandez RN

EDITORS

David Cline, M.D.

*Clinical Associate Professor, Assistant
Residency Director, Department of Emergency
Medicine, University of North Carolina School
of Medicine, Chapel Hill, and Education
Director, WakeMed
Raleigh, North Carolina*

O. John Ma, M.D.

*Assistant Professor and Research Director
Department of Emergency Medicine
Truman Medical Center
University of Missouri–Kansas City School of Medicine
Kansas City, Missouri*

Judith E. Tintinalli, M.D., M.S.

*Professor and Chair
Department of Emergency Medicine
University of North Carolina at Chapel Hill
Chapel Hill, North Carolina*

Gabor D. Kelen, M.D.

*Professor and Chair
Department of Emergency Medicine
Johns Hopkins University
Baltimore, Maryland*

J. Stephan Stapczynski, M.D.

*Professor and Chair
Department of Emergency Medicine
University of Kentucky
Lexington, Kentucky*

EMERGENCY MEDICINE

A COMPREHENSIVE STUDY GUIDE

FIFTH EDITION

Companion Handbook

American
College of
Emergency
Physicians

David M. Cline
O. John Ma
Judith E. Tintinalli
Gabor D. Kelen
J. Stephan Stapczynski

McGraw-Hill
Health Professions Division

*New York   St. Louis   San Francisco   Auckland
Bogotá   Caracas   Lisbon   London   Madrid
Mexico City   Milan   Montreal   New Delhi
San Juan   Singapore   Sydney   Tokyo   Toronto*

McGraw-Hill

*A Division of The **McGraw·Hill** Companies*

EMERGENCY MEDICINE, A Comprehensive Study Guide, 5/e
COMPANION HANDBOOK

Copyright © 2000, 1996, by The McGraw-Hill Companies, Inc. All rights reserved. Printed in the United States of America. Except as permitted under the United States Copyright Act of 1976, no part of this publication may be reproduced or distributed in any form or by any means, or stored in a data base or retrieval system, without the prior written permission of the publisher.

3 4 5 6 7 8 9 0   DOC DOC   0 9 8 7 6 5 4 3 2 1

ISBN 0-07-012039-0

This book was set in Times Roman by The PRD Group, Inc. The editors were John J. Dolan, Mariapaz Ramos Englis, and Lester A. Sheinis. The production supervisor was Richard C. Ruzycka. The indexer was Irving Condé Tullar. The cover designer was Joan O'Connor. R. R. Donnelley & Sons Company was printer and binder.

This book is printed on acid-free paper.

CONTENTS

Section 12 Toxicology   511

Section 13 Environmental Injuries   599

Section 14 Endocrine Emergencies   651

Section 15 Hematologic and Oncologic Emergencies   667

CONTRIBUTORS

Stephanie B. Abbuhl, M.D., Associate Professor, Medical Director, Department of Emergency Medicine, University of Pennsylvania School of Medicine, Hospital of the University of Pennsylvania, Philadelphia, Pennsylvania (Chapter 15)

Amy J. Behrman, M.D., Assistant Professor, Director, Occupational Health Services, Department of Emergency Medicine, University of Pennsylvania School of Medicine, Hospital of the University of Pennsylvania, Philadelphia, Pennsylvania (Chapter 32)

Burton Bentley II, M.D., Attending Physician, Department of Emergency Medicine, Northwest Medical Center, Tucson, Arizona (Chapters 116, 145–148, 180)

William J. Brady, M.D., Assistant Professor, Departments of Emergency Medicine and Internal Medicine, University of Virginia Health Sciences Center, Charlottesville, Virginia (Chapters 149, 150)

David F. M. Brown, M.D., Instructor, Division of Emergency Medicine, Harvard Medical School; Assistant Chief, Department of Emergency Medicine, Massachusetts General Hospital, Boston, Massachusetts (Chapters 31, 34)

Lance Brown, M.D., M.P.H., Clinical Instructor, Department of Emergency Medicine, University of North Carolina School of Medicine, Chapel Hill; Attending Physician, Department of Emergency Medicine, WakeMed, Raleigh, North Carolina (Chapters 28, 29)

Martin J. Carey, M.D., Assistant Professor, Residency Director, Medical Sciences, Department of Emergency Medicine, University of Arkansas, Little Rock, Arkansas (Chapters 16, 17)

Michael E. Chansky, M.D., Associate Professor, Chairman, Department of Emergency Medicine, Cooper Hospital/University Medical Center, Camden, New Jersey (Chapters 18, 30, 49)

David M. Cline, M.D., Clinical Associate Professor, Assistant Residency Director, Department of Emergency Medicine, University of North Carolina School of Medicine, Chapel Hill; Education Director, WakeMed, Raleigh, North Carolina (Chapters 1, 2, 11, 14, 23, 24, 26, 52, 56, 61, 64, 66, 94, 95)

C. James Corrall, M.D., M.P.H., Clinical Associate Professor of Emergency Medicine and Pediatrics, Department of Emergency Medicine, Methodist Hospital of Indiana, Indianapolis, Indiana (Chapters 67, 69, 89)

Jeffrey D. Dixon, M.D., Medical Director, Department of Emergency Medicine, Hillcrest Medical Center, Tulsa, Oklahoma (Chapter 170)

David A. Dubow, M.D., Clinical Instructor, Department of Emergency Medicine, University of North Carolina School of Medicine, Chapel Hill; Attending Physician, Department of Emergency Medicine, WakeMed, Raleigh, North Carolina (Chapter 25)

Sally Fuller, M.D., Clinical Instructor, Department of Emergency Medicine, University of North Carolina School of Medicine, Chapel Hill; Attending Physician, WakeMed, Raleigh, North Carolina (Chapters 58–60)

Gary Gaddis, M.D., Ph.D., Clinical Associate Professor of Emergency Medicine, St. Luke's Hospital, University of Missouri-Kansas City School of Medicine, Kansas City, Missouri (Chapters 171, 172)

Peggy Goodman, M.D., Assistant Professor, Department of Emergency Medicine, East Carolina University School of Medicine, Greenville, North Carolina (Chapters 36, 37, 39, 41)

John E. Gough, M.D., Assistant Professor, Assistant Medical Director, Division of Emergency Medical Services, Department of Emergency Medicine, East Carolina University School of Medicine, Greenville, North Carolina

Charles J. Graham, M.D., Assistant Professor of Pediatrics, Associate Medical Director, Emergency Department, Arkansas Children's Hospital, Little Rock, Arkansas (Chapter 3)

Gregory S. Hall, M.D., Assistant Professor, Department of Emergency Medicine, University of Arkansas for Medical Sciences, Little Rock, Arkansas (Chapters 47, 48, 92)

Kent N. Hall, M.D., Attending Physician, Department of Emergency Medicine, Mercy Hospital-Fairfield, Fairfield, Ohio (Chapters 114, 136, 137, 159)

Charles J. Havel, Jr., M.D., Assistant Professor, Departments of Emergency Medicine and Pediatrics, Medical College of Wisconsin, Milwaukee, WI (Chapters 109, 110, 151, 152, 156, 158, 173, 174)

Marilyn P. Hicks, M.D., Clinical Associate Professor, Department of Emergency Medicine, University of North Carolina School of Medicine, Chapel Hill; Director of Pediatrics, Department of

Emergency Medicine, WakeMed, Raleigh, North Carolina (Chapters 68, 70–72)

Cheryl Jackson, M.D., Clinical Instructor, Department of Emergency Medicine, University of North Carolina School of Medicine, Chapel Hill; Attending Physician, Pediatrics, Department of Emergency Medicine, WakeMed, Raleigh, North Carolina (Chapter 84)

Howard E. Jarvis III, M.D., Emergency Physician, Department of Emergency Medicine, MetroHealth Medical Center, Case Western Reserve University, Cleveland, Ohio (Chapters 113, 122, 142)

Michael P. Kefer, M.D., Associate Professor of Emergency Medicine, Medical College of Wisconsin, Milwaukee, Wisconsin (Chapters 100, 125, 126, 128, 164, 165, 176, 177)

Elicia Sinor Kennedy, M.D., Attending Physician, Baptist Medical Center, Little Rock, Arkansas (Chapter 55)

Judith A. Linden, M.D., Assistant Professor of Emergency Medicine, Associate Residency Director, Boston University School of Medicine, Boston, Massachusetts (Chapters 101, 107, 108, 168, 169)

O. John Ma, M.D., Assistant Professor of Emergency Medicine, Research Director, Truman Medical Center, University of Missouri-Kansas City School of Medicine, Kansas City, Missouri (Chapters 106, 144, 153, 155, 160)

Juan A. March, M.D., Assistant Professor, Department of Emergency Medicine, Chief Medical Director, Division of Emergency Medical Services, East Carolina University School of Medicine, Greenville, North Carolina (Chapters 65, 77, 80, 81)

Keith L. Mausner, M.D., Medical Director, Injury Prevention and EMS Bureau, New Mexico Department of Health; Attending Physician, Espanola Hospital, Espanola, New Mexico (Chapters 97, 99, 102, 117–119, 123, 133, 134)

Cary C. McDonald, M.D., Clinical Associate Professor, Department of Emergency Medicine, University of North Carolina School of Medicine, Chapel Hill; EMS Director, Department of Emergency Medicine, WakeMed, Raleigh, North Carolina (Chapters 38, 44)

Leslie McKinney, M.D., Medical Director, Priority Care, Cary, North Carolina (Chapters 76, 87)

C. Crawford Mechem, M.D., Assistant Professor of Emergency Medicine, University of Pennsylvania School of Medicine; EMS Medical Director, Philadelphia Fire Department, Philadelphia, Pennsylvania (Chapters 98, 104, 138, 139, 141, 154, 157, 162, 163)

Stephen W. Meldon, M.D., Assistant Professor of Emergency Medicine, Case Western Reserve University, MetroHealth Medical Center, Cleveland, Ohio (Chapters 120, 121, 127, 161, 166, 167, 182, 183)

Frantz R. Melio, M.D., Clinical Associate Professor, Department of Emergency Medicine, University of North Carolina School of Medicine, Chapel Hill; Chairman and Medical Director, Department of Emergency Medicine, WakeMed, Raleigh, North Carolina (Chapters 10, 22, 35)

Chris Melton, M.D., Assistant Professor, Department of Emergency Medicine, University of Arkansas, Little Rock, Arkansas (Chapter 93)

Vincent Nacouzi, M.D., Clinical Instructor, Department of Emergency Medicine, University of North Carolina School of Medicine, Chapel Hill; Attending Physician, Department of Emergency Medicine, WakeMed, Raleigh, North Carolina (Chapters 4, 27)

Sandra L. Najarian, M.D., Senior Instructor of Emergency Medicine, Case Western Reserve University, MetroHealth Medical Center, Cleveland, Ohio (Chapters 96, 124, 129, 132)

David A. Peak, M.D., Clinical Instructor of Emergency Medicine, Massachusetts General Hospital, Boston, Massachusetts (Chapter 175)

Debra G. Perina, M.D., Associate Professor, Department of Emergency Medicine; Director, Prehospital Care Division, University of Virginia Health Sciences Center, Charlottesville, Virginia (Chapters 74, 75, 78, 79)

Michael C. Plewa, M.D., Clinical Assistant Professor in Surgery, Medical College of Ohio, Toledo; Director of Research, Emergency Medicine Residency Program, St. Vincent Medical Center, Toledo, Ohio (Chapter 73)

N. Heramba Prasad, M.D., Associate Professor of Emergency Medicine, Residency Director, Department of Emergency Medicine, SUNY Health Sciences Center, Syracuse, New York (Chapters 42, 45, 50)

Thomas A. Rebbecchi, M.D., Assistant Professor, Department of Emergency Medicine, Cooper Hospital/University Medical Center, Camden, New Jersey (Chapter 20)

Rebecca S. Rich, M.D., Attending Physician, Emergency Department, Durham Regional Hospital, Durham, North Carolina (Chapters 57, 62, 63, 82, 83, 85, 86, 90, 91)

Mark B. Rogers, M.D., Attending Physician, Breech Medical Center, Lebanon, Missouri (Chapters 103, 105, 143, 178)

Todd C. Rothenhaus, M.D., Assistant Professor of Emergency Medicine, Boston University School of Medicine, Boston, Massachusetts (Chapters 111, 112, 115)

Eugenia B. Smith, M.D., Clinical Instructor, Department of Emergency Medicine, University of North Carolina School of Medicine, Chapel Hill; Attending Physician, Department of Emergency Medicine, WakeMed, Raleigh, North Carolina (Chapter 19)

Marc D. Squillante, D.O., Program Director, Emergency Medicine Residency, Saint Francis Medical Center, The University of Illinois College of Medicine–Peoria, Peoria, Illinois (Chapter 51)

John Sverha, M.D., Clinical Instructor of Emergency Medicine, University of North Carolina School of Medicine, Chapel Hill, North Carolina (Chapters 130, 131, 135, 179, 181)

Gary L. Swart, M.D., Assistant Professor of Emergency Medicine, Medical College of Wisconsin, Milwaukee, Wisconsin (Chapter 140)

Arthur Tascone, M.D., Clinical Instructor, Department of Emergency Medicine, University of North Carolina School of Medicine, Chapel Hill; Attending Physician, Department of Emergency Medicine, WakeMed, Raleigh, North Carolina (Chapter 88)

Stephen H. Thomas, M.D., Assistant Professor, Massachusetts General Hospital; Instructor, Division of Emergency Medicine, Harvard Medical School; Associate Medical Director, Boston Med-Flight, Boston, Massachusetts (Chapters 53, 54)

Christian A. Tomaszewski, M.D., Clinical Assistant Professor, Department of Emergency Medicine, University of North Carolina School of Medicine, Chapel Hill; Medical Director, Hyperbaric Medicine, Carolinas Medical Center, Charlotte, North Carolina (Chapters 9, 21, 40, 46)

Michael Utecht, M.D., Clinical Instructor, Department of Emergency Medicine, University of North Carolina School of Medicine, Chapel Hill; Attending Physician, Department of Emergency Medicine, WakeMed, Raleigh, North Carolina (Chapters 12, 13)

Gary D. Wright, M.D., Medical Director, Emergency Department, South Baldwin Regional Medical Center, Foley, Alabama (Chapters 33, 43)

PREFACE

The tremendous growth in the specialty of emergency medicine is reflected in the depth and breadth of the fifth edition of *Emergency Medicine: A Comprehensive Study Guide*. In 1996, the *Companion Handbook* was published as a clinical tool to guide in the diagnosis and management of patients in the emergency department. The *Companion Handbook* is now published in English, Spanish, French, and Italian, which further reflects the growing number of emergency medicine practitioners worldwide.

The original goal of the *Handbook* is preserved in this second edition. This text is written by and for health care workers who are engaged in the practice of clinical emergency medicine. Each chapter continues to emphasize the Clinical Features, Diagnosis and Differential, and Emergency Department Care and Disposition of the disease entity. We hope that this text will assist practitioners of emergency medicine in their primary endeavor: the skillful and timely care of their patients in the emergency department. We would like to express our deep appreciation to the *Handbook* chapter authors for their commitment in helping to produce this text. We also are indebted to numerous individuals who assisted us with this project; in particular, we would like to thank John J. Dolan, Lester A. Sheinis, Richard C. Ruzycka, and Mariapaz Ramos Englis at McGraw-Hill. Finally, without the love and encouragement of our families, this book would not have been possible. DMC thanks his family and his secretary, Nell, and OJM thanks his wife, Elizabeth, for her love and support.

David M. Cline, M.D.
O. John Ma, M.D.

EMERGENCY MEDICINE

A COMPREHENSIVE STUDY GUIDE
FIFTH EDITION

Companion Handbook

RESUSCITATIVE PROBLEMS AND TECHNIQUES

1 | Advanced Airway Support

David M. Cline

Control of the airway is the single most important task for emergency resuscitation. If the patient has inadequate oxygenation or ventilation, inability to protect the airway due to altered sensorium from illness or drugs, or external forces compromising the airway (i.e., trauma), he or she may need advanced airway techniques as described in this chapter.

INITIAL APPROACH

The initial approach to airway management is simultaneous assessment and management of the adequacy of airway patency (the *A* of ABCs) and oxygenation and ventilation (the *B* of ABCs).

1. The patient's color and respiratory rate must be assessed; marked hypoventilation with or without cyanosis may be an indication for immediate intubation.
2. The airway should be opened with head tilt–chin lift maneuver (jaw thrust should be used if C-spine injury is suspected). If needed, the patient should be bagged with the bag-valve-mask device, including an O_2 reservoir. For a good seal, the proper size mask should be ensured. This technique may require an oral or nasal airway or two rescuers to both seal the mask (two hands) and bag the patient.
3. The patient should be placed on a cardiac monitor, pulse oximetry, and possibly capnography (end-tidal CO_2), while the remaining vitals, pulse, and blood pressure (temperature is important but can be delayed to assure the ABCs) can be collected.
4. The need for invasive airway management techniques must be determined as described later. It is essential to not wait for arterial blood gas analyses (ABG) if the initial assessment declares the need for invasive airway management. If the patient

does not require immediate airway or ventilation control, he or she should be administered oxygen by face mask, as necessary, to assure an O_2 saturation of 95%. Laboratory studies should be collected as needed. Do not remove a patient from oxygen to draw an ABG unless deemed safe from the initial assessment.

OROTRACHEAL INTUBATION

The most reliable means to ensure a patent airway, prevent aspiration, and provide oxygenation and ventilation is endotracheal (ET) intubation. Many conscious patients require intubation (see the section, "Rapid Sequence Induction" later). Selection of the blade should be considered in advance, if possible. The curved blade rests in the vallecula above the epiglottis and indirectly lifts it off the larynx because of traction on the frenulum. The straight blade is used to lift the epiglottis directly. The curved blade does a better job of clearing the tongue from view and may be less traumatic and reflex-stimulating. The straight blade is mechanically easier to insert in many patients.

Emergency Department Care and Disposition

1. Adequate ventilation must be ensured while the equipment is prepared. The patient should be preoxygenated, with or without a bag-valve-mask device, depending on the clinical need. Vital signs must be monitored and pulse oximetry used throughout the procedure.
2. The blade type and size (usually #3 or #4 curved blade, or #2 or #3 straight blade) should be selected; the blade light should be tested. The tube size (usually 7.5 to 8.0 in women, 8.0 to 8.5 in men) must be selected and the balloon cuff tested. The end of the tube should be lubricated with lidocaine jelly or similar lubricant. The use of a flexible stylet should be considered; the distal end should be bent upward if the patient's anatomy requires it. The tube and tonsillar tip suction should be placed within easy reach. If there is an assistant, he or she should be asked to pass the items when needed.
3. The patient should be positioned with the head extended and neck flexed, possibly with a rolled towel under the occiput. If C-spine injury is suspected, the head or neck should not be moved. Rapid sequence induction with in-line traction, nasotracheal intubation, or cricothyrotomy should be considered.
4. The blade should be inserted on the right and slowly advanced in search of the epiglottis. The patient should be suctioned as necessary. If the curved blade is used, the tip should be slid into the vallecula and lifted (indirectly lifting the epiglottis); if

a straight blade is used, the epiglottis should be lifted directly in the direction the handle points, that is, 90° to the blade. It is important to not rock back on the teeth.

5. Once the vocal cords are visualized, it is important to not lose sight of them. The assistant should be asked to place the tube in the physician's hand. Pass the tube between the cords, avoiding force. The stylet should be removed, the balloon cuff inflated. Ventilate the patient with a bag-valve device and check for bilateral breath sounds. Placement should be confirmed with an end-tidal CO_2 detector (not reliable if the patient is in cardiac arrest) or capnography. Tube length should be checked; the usual distance (marked on the tube) from the corner of the mouth to 2 cm above the carina is 23 cm in men and 21 cm in woman.

6. The tube should be taped in place and a bite block inserted. Correct intubation and tube placement can be verified with a portable chest x-ray.

7. If unsuccessful, reoxygenation should be performed with bag-valve-mask device. The technique can be changed by possibly using a smaller tube, different blade type or size, or repositioning the patient and reattempting intubation.

Short-term complications from orotracheal intubation (trauma to surrounding structures) are unusual, as long as correct position is confirmed. Failure to confirm position immediately can result in hypoxia and neurologic injury. Endobronchial intubation is usually on the right side and is corrected by withdrawing the tube 2 cm and listening for equal breath sounds.

NASOTRACHEAL INTUBATION

Nasotracheal intubation is indicated in situations where laryngoscopy is difficult, neuromuscular blockade is hazardous, or cricothyrotomy unnecessary. Severely dyspneic, awake patients with congestive heart failure, chronic obstructive pulmonary disease, or asthma often cannot remain supine for other airway maneuvers but do tolerate nasotracheal intubation in the sitting position. Relative contraindications for this technique include complex nasal and massive midface fractures and bleeding disorders.

Emergency Department Care and Disposition

1. Both nares should be sprayed with a topical vasoconstrictor and anesthetic. Between 4 to 10% cocaine solution is an appropriate single agent, but may cause unwanted systemic cardiovascular effects. Topical neosynephrine is an effective vasoconstrictor, and tetracaine is a safe effective topical anesthetic.

2. The tube size must be chosen, usually between 7.0 to 7.5 in

women and 7.5 to 8.0 in men. The balloon cuff of the tube should be checked for leaks. The tube should be lubricated with lidocaine jelly or similar lubricant.

3. The largest nares should be used or the right side if the nares are equal. Some operators recommend dilating the nares with a lubricated nasal airway. The patient may be sitting up or supine.

4. An assistant can immobilize the patient's neck. The physician should stand to the patient's side, with one hand on the tube and with the thumb and index finger of the other hand straddling the larynx. The tube should be advanced slowly, with steady gentle pressure. The tube should be twisted to help move past obstructions in the nose and nasopharynx. The tube should be advanced until maximal airflow is heard through the tube; this means the larynx is now close by.

5. The physician should listen carefully to the rhythm of inspiration and expiration. The tube should then be gently but swiftly advanced during the beginning of inspiration. Entrance into the larynx may initiate a cough, and most expired air should exit the tube even though the cuff is uninflated. If the tube is foggy the cuff should be inflated.

6. If intubation is unsuccessful, the physician should carefully look for a bulge lateral to the larynx (usually the tip of the tube is in the pyriform fossa on the same side as the nares used). If found, the tube must be retracted until maximal breath sounds are heard and then intubation should be reattempted by manually displacing the larynx toward the bulge. If no bulge is seen, it is possible that the tube has gone posteriorly into the esophagus. In this case, the tube should be withdrawn until maximal breath sounds are heard. Intubation should again be reattempted after the patient's head is extended and a Sellick's maneuver performed. Another option is to use a directional control tip (Endotrol) or fiberoptic laryngoscope. The head should not be moved if C-spine injury is suspected.

Complications other than local bleeding are rare. Occasionally, marked bleeding will prompt the need for orotracheal intubation or cricothyrotomy.

CRICOTHYROTOMY

Indications for immediate cricothyrotomy include severe, ongoing tracheobronchial hemorrhage, massive midface trauma, and inability to control the airway with the usual less-invasive maneuvers. Cricothyrotomy is relatively contraindicated in patients with acute laryngeal disease due to trauma or infection or recent prolonged intubation and should not be used in children below the age of 12.

Emergency Department Care and Disposition

1. Sterile technique should be used. The cricothyroid membrane should be palpated with digital stabilizion of the larynx (see Fig. 1-1). With a #11 scalpel, a vertical 3 to 4 cm incision should be started at the superior border of the thyroid cartilage and incised caudally toward the suprasternal notch.
2. The membrane should be repalpated and a horizontal stab should be made through its inferior aspect. The blade should be kept temporarily in place.
3. The larynx should be stabilized by inserting the tracheal hook into the cricothyroid space and retracting upon the inferior edge of the thyroid cartilage (an assistant should hold after the hook is placed). Leaving the blade tip in the space, a slightly open hemostat should be inserted straddling the blade and spread open horizontally.
4. The scalpel should be removed and a dilator inserted (LaBorde or Trousseau). The tracheal hook can then be removed.
5. A #4 Shiley tracheostomy tube should be introduced (or the largest tube that will fit). Alternatively, a small cuffed endotrachial tube may be used (#6 or the largest tube that will fit). The balloon should be inflated and the tube secured in place.
6. The physician should check for bilateral breath sounds. Make sure subcutaneous air is not introduced. Placement can be checked with an end-tidal CO_2 detector and chest x-ray.

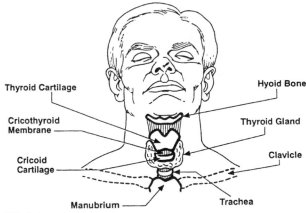

FIG. 1-1   Anatomy of the neck.

RAPID SEQUENCE INDUCTION

Complex airway emergencies in select nonfasted patients may require rapid sequence induction. This technique couples sedation to induce unconsciousness (induction) with muscular paralysis. Intubation follows laryngoscopy while maintaining cricoid pressure to prevent aspiration. The principle contraindication is any condition preventing mask ventilation or intubation.

1. The cardiac monitor, oximetry, and capnography should be set up, if available. Equipment should be checked.
2. The patient should be preoxygenated with 100% oxygen.
3. **Lidocaine** (1.5 mg/kg intravenously) should be considered in a head trauma patient to prevent increased intracranial pressure. Atropine (0.4 mg/kg intravenously) should be considered to prevent reflex bradycardia, but is not essential.
4. Medication for sedation or analgesia should be considered, if such agents are not being used for induction.
5. A defasciculating dose of a nondepolarizing agent (i.e., vecuronium at 0.02 mg/kg) is used if succinylcholine is given for paralysis.
6. The patient should be induced with **thiopental** (3 to 5 mg/kg), **methohexital** (1 to 2 mg/kg), or midazolam (0.1 mg/kg with 5 mg maximum dose). Barbiturates should not be used in a patient with hypotension or reactive airway disease (caution in head injury). Benzodiazepines may be inadequate for induction, however, midazolam is an excellent amnestic agent. **Etomidate,** 0.3 mg/kg, is an excellent alternative in a hypotensive patient. **Ketamine,** 1 to 2 mg/kg, should be considered for the induction of a patient who has active bronchospasm for its bronchodilator properties.
7. In a patient needing analgesia in addition to sedation, opiates should be considered for induction. These agents are reversible with naloxone. **Fentanyl,** 2 to 10 μg/kg, is commonly used.
8. Cricoid pressure should be applied before paralysis and maintained until intubation is accomplished.
9. **Succinylcholine** (1.0 mg/kg) is chosen for paralysis in many cases because of its rapid onset and short duration of action; it should not be used in a patient with preexisting paralysis or > 2 h after severe burns, as hyperkalemia may occur. A nondepolarizing agent such as **vecuronium** (0.2 mg/kg) may be chosen for a patient with increased intracranial pressure, one in status asthmaticus, or at operator discretion.
10. The trachea should be intubated and cricoid pressure released.
11. The physician should be prepared to bag the patient if intubation proves unsuccessful. Invasive airway techniques should be considered as indicated.

Alternative drugs for rapid sequence induction are listed in Chap. 15 of *Emergency Medicine, A Comprehensive Study Guide,* 5th ed. Airway management alternatives to the methods described earlier include retrograde tracheal intubation, translaryngeal ventilation, digital intubation, transillumination, fiberoptic assistance, and formal tracheostomy. Translaryngeal ventilation may be used to temporarily provide ventilation until a more definitive procedure is possible. When oral intubation is indicated but has been unsuccessful, and the patient can be temporarily ventilated with a bag-valve-mask unit, the following assist methods are warranted. Retrograde tracheal intubation, digital intubation, transillumination, or fiberoptic assistance may be helpful. Formal tracheostomy is reserved for those experienced in the technique when less-invasive or more-rapid methods (cricothyrotomy) are unsuccessful. These techniques are described in Chaps. 14, 15, and 16 of *Emergency Medicine: A Comprehensive Study Guide,* 5th ed.

For further reading in *Emergency Medicine: A Comprehensive Study Guide,* 5th ed., see Chap. 14, "Noninvasive Airway Management," by A. Michael Roman; Chap. 15, "Tracheal Intubation and Mechanical Ventilation," by Daniel F. Danzl; and Chap. 16, "Surgical Airway Management," by David R. Gens.

2	Dysrhythmia Management
	David M. Cline

SUPRAVENTRICULAR DYSRHYTHMIAS

Sinus Dysrhythmia

Clinical Features

Some variation in the sinus node discharge rate is common, but if the variation exceeds 0.12 s between the longest and shortest intervals, sinus dysrhythmia is present. The electrocardiogram (ECG) characteristics of sinus dysrhythmia are (*a*) normal sinus

P waves and PR intervals; (*b*) 1:1 atrioventricular (AV) conduction; and (*c*) variation of at least 0.12 s between the shortest and longest P-P interval (Fig. 2-1). Sinus dysrhythmias are primarily affected by respiration and are most commonly found in children and young adults, disappearing with advancing age. No treatment is required.

Sinus Bradycardia

Clinical Features

Sinus bradycardia occurs when the sinus node rate falls below 60. The ECG characteristics of sinus bradycardia are (*a*) normal sinus P waves and PR intervals; (*b*) 1:1 AV conduction; and (*c*) atrial rate below 60 (Fig. 2-2). Sinus bradycardia represents a suppression of the sinus node discharge rate, usually in response to 3 categories of stimuli: (*a*) physiologic; (*b*) pharmacologic; and (*c*) pathologic (acute inferior myocardial infarction (MI), increased intracranial pressure, carotid sinus hypersensitivity, and hypothyroidism).

Emergency Department Care and Disposition

1. Sinus bradycardia usually does not require specific treatment unless the heart rate is below 50 and there is evidence of hypoperfusion.
2. Initial therapy should begin with atropine 0.5 to 1 mg IV intravenously and may be repeated up to 3 mg.
3. External cardiac pacing can be used in the patient refractory to atropine.
    a. The patient should be attached to the monitor leads of the external pacing device.
    b. The pacing pads should be attached to the patient. The anterior pad should be placed over the precordium, which may require retracting a woman's breast superiorly. The posterior pad should be placed at the level of the heart, between the spine and the left scapula. The multifunction pacing defibrillation pads should not be used unless the pa-

FIG. 2-1   Sinus dysrhythmia.

FIG. 2-2   Sinus bradycardia, rate 44.

tient is unconscious, as these pads cause more discomfort with pacing.

c. The pacing rate should be turned from 0 to between 60 and 80.

d. The pacing output should be slowly turned from 0 to the lowest point where continuous pacing is observed, usually in the range of 50 to 80 mA.

e. Electrical capture should be noted on the monitor, which can be recognized by a widened QRS following each pacing spike.

f. The patient may require sedation with lorazepam (1 to 2 mg intravenously) or a similar agent, or pain control with morphine (1 to 2 mg intravenously) or similar agent.

4. Epinephrine or dopamine drips may be used if external pacing is not available.

5. Internal pacing is required in the patient with symptomatic recurrent or persistent sinus bradycardia.

Sinus Tachycardia

Clinical Features

The ECG characteristics of sinus tachycardia are (a) normal sinus P waves and PR intervals; (b) an atrial rate usually between 100 and 160; and, (c) normally, 1:1 conduction between the atria and ventricles (although rapid rates can occur with AV blocks; Fig. 2-3). Sinus tachycardia occurs in response to 3 categories of stimuli:

FIG. 2-3   Sinus tachycardia, rate 176.

(*a*) physiologic, (*b*) pharmacologic, or (*c*) pathologic (fever, hypoxia, anemia, hypovolemia, or pulmonary embolism). In many of these conditions, the increased heart rate occurs in an effort to increase cardiac output to match increased circulatory needs. The underlying condition should be diagnosed and treated.

Premature Atrial Contractions

Clinical Features

The ECG characteristics of premature atrial contractions (PACs) are (*a*) ectopic P wave appearing sooner (premature) than the next expected sinus beat; (*b*) the ectopic P wave has a different shape and direction; and (*c*) the ectopic P wave may or may not be conducted through the AV node (Fig. 2-4). Most PACs are conducted with typical QRS complexes, but some may be conducted aberrantly through the infranodal system. The sinus node is often depolarized and reset so that, while the interval following the PAC is often slightly longer than the previous cycler's length, the pause is less than fully compensatory. PACs are common in all ages and are often seen in the absence of heart disease.

Emergency Department Care and Disposition

1. Any precipitating drugs (alcohol, tobacco, or coffee) or toxins should be discontinued.

FIG. 2-4 Premature atrial contractions (PACs). **A.** Ectopic P′ waves (arrows). **B.** Atrial bigeminy.

2. Underlying disorders should be treated (stress or fatigue).
3. PACs that produce symptoms or initiate sustained tachycardias can be suppressed with various agents such as β-adrenergic antagonist, usually in consultation with a follow-up physician.

Multifocal Atrial Tachycardia

Clinical Features

Multifocal atrial tachycardia (MFAT) is caused by at least two different sites of atrial ectopy. The ECG characteristics of MFAT are (*a*) 3 or more differently shaped P waves; (*b*) varying PP, PR, and RR intervals; and (*c*) atrial rhythm usually between 100 and 180 (Fig. 2-5). MFAT can be confused with atrial flutter or fibrillation. MFAT is most often found in elderly patients with decompensated chronic lung disease, but it also may found in patients with congestive heart failure (CHF) or sepsis or be caused by methylxanthine toxicity.

Emergency Department Care and Disposition

1. Treatment is directed toward the underlying disorder.
2. Specific antidysrhythmic treatment is uncommonly indicated.
3. **Magnesium sulfate,** 2 g intravenously over 60 s, followed by a constant infusion of 1 to 2 g/h, can be used if necessary.
4. The serum potassium levels should be maintained above 4 meq/L. Intravenous verapamil (5 to 10 mg) slows the ventricular response in most patients, decreases atrial ectopy in some patients, and is associated with conversion to sinus rhythm in many patients.
5. Cardioversion has no effect.

Atrial Flutter

Clinical Features

Atrial flutter is a rhythm that originates from a small area within the atria. The exact mechanism—whether reentry, automatic focus, or

FIG. 2-5   Multifocal atrial tachycardia (MFAT).

triggered dysrhythmia—is not yet known. ECG characteristics of atrial flutter are (*a*) regular atrial rate between 250 and 350 (most commonly 280 and 320); (*b*) sawtooth flutter waves directed superiorly and most visible in leads II, III, aV_F; and (*c*) AV block, usually 2:1, but occasionally greater or irregular (Fig. 2-6). Carotid sinus massage is a useful technique to slow the ventricular response, increase the AV block, and unmask flutter waves. Atrial flutter is most commonly seen in patients with ischemic heart disease or acute MI. Less common causes include congestive cardiomyopathy, pulmonary embolus, myocarditis, blunt chest trauma, and, rarely, digoxin toxicity. Atrial flutter may be a transitional dysrhythmia between sinus rhythm and atrial fibrillation. Consider the need for anticoagulation prior to conversion to sinus rhythm.

Emergency Department Care and Disposition

1. Low-energy cardioversion (25 to 50 J) is very successful in converting more than 90 percent of cases of atrial flutter into sinus rhythm.
2. If cardioversion is contraindicated, ventricular rate control can be achieved with **diltiazem,** 0.25 mg/kg intravenously over 2 min; may repeat at 0.35 mg/kg.
3. Intravenous esmolol will convert up to 60 percent of patients with new-onset atrial flutter to sinus rhythm.
4. **Ibutilide,** 0.01 mg/kg intravenously up to 1 mg, over 10 min, has a high success rate for conversion of atrial flutter (and atrial fibrillation) to sinus rhythm. Because of the possibility of provoking torsades de pointes, ibutilide should not be administered to patients with hypokalemia, prolonged QT on the ECG, or CHF.
5. Alternatives include **digoxin** (0.5 mg intravenously), **verapamil** (5 to 10 mg intravenously), or **procainamide** (see ventricular tachycardia management for dosing guidelines).

FIG. 2-6   Atrial flutter.

Atrial Fibrillation

Clinical Features

Atrial fibrillation occurs when there are multiple small areas of atrial myocardium continuously discharging and contracting. The ECG characteristics of atrial fibrillation are (*a*) fibrillatory waves of atrial activity, best seen in leads V_1, V_2, V_3, and V_F; and (*b*) irregular ventricular response, usually around 170 to 180 in patients with a healthy AV node (Fig. 2-7). Disease or drugs (especially digoxin) may reduce AV node conduction and markedly slow ventricular response. Atrial fibrillation can occur in a paroxysmal or sustained manner. Predisposing factors for atrial fibrillation are increased atrial size and mass, increased vagal tone, and variation in refractory periods between different parts of atrial myocardium. Atrial fibrillation is usually found in association with 4 disorders: rheumatic heart disease, hypertension, ischemic heart disease, and thyrotoxicosis.

In patients with left ventricular failure, left atrial contraction makes an important contribution to cardiac output. The loss of effective atrial contraction, as in atrial fibrillation, may produce heart failure in these patients. Conversion from chronic atrial fibrillation to sinus rhythm also carries up to a 1 to 2 percent risk of arterial embolism. Consider anticoagulation with heparin prior to conversion to sinus rhythm.

Emergency Department Care and Disposition

1. Atrial fibrillation with a rapid ventricular response and acute hemodynamic deterioration should be treated with synchronized cardioversion. Over 60 percent can be converted with 100 J, and over 80 percent with 200 J.
2. In more stable patients, the first priority is to achieve ventricular

FIG. 2-7   Atrial fibrillation.

rate control. **Diltiazem** 20 mg (0.25 mg/kg) intravenously over 2 min is extremely effective. An infusion of 10 mg/h is usually started after the initial dose to maintain control and a second dose of 25 mg (0.35 mg/kg) can be given at 15 min if rate control is not achieved. Alternatives include **digoxin** (0.5 mg intravenously), and **verapamil** (5 to 10 mg intravenously).
3. Once ventricular rate control has been achieved, chemical conversion can be considered with **ibutilide** (see earlier comment for atrial flutter), **procainamide,** or verapamil.

Supraventricular Tachycardia

Clinical Features

Supraventricular tachycardia (SVT) is a regular, rapid rhythm that arises from either reentry or an ectopic pacemaker above the bifurcation of the bundle of His. The reentrant variety is clinically the most common (Fig. 2-8). These patients often present with acute, symptomatic episodes termed *paroxysmal supraventricular tachycardia (PSVT)*. Ectopic SVT usually originates in the atria with an atrial rate of 100 to 250 (most commonly 140 to 200) (Fig.

FIG. 2-8 Reentrant supraventricular tachycardia (SVT). **A**. 2d (*) initiates run of PAT. **B**. SVT, rate 286.

FIG. 2-9   Ectopic supraventricular, tachycardia (STV) with 2:1 AV conduction.

2-9). In patients with bypass tracts, reentry can occur in either direction. It usually occurs in a direction that goes down the AV node and up the bypass tract, producing a narrow QRS complex.

Ectopic SVT may be seen in patients with acute MI, chronic lung disease, pneumonia, alcoholic intoxication, and digoxin toxicity. Reentrant SVT can occur in a normal heart, or in association with rheumatic heart disease, acute pericarditis, MI, mitral valve prolapse, or one of the preexcitation syndromes.

Emergency Department Care and Disposition

1. First vagal maneuvers should be attempted. These maneuvers can be done by themselves or after administration of drugs.
    a. Carotid sinus massage attempts to massage the carotid sinus and its baroreceptors against the transverse process of C6. Massage should be done for 10 s at a time, first on the side of the nondominant cerebral hemisphere, and should never be done simultaneously on both sides.
    b. This next maneuver, facial immersion in cold water for 6 to 7 s with the nostrils held closed (diving reflex), is particularly effective in infants.
    c. The Valsalva maneuver done in the supine position appears to be the most effective vagal maneuver for the conversion of reentrant SVT. For maximal effectiveness, the strain phase must be adequate (usually at least 10 s).
2. **Adenosine** can be administered, initially 6 mg of a rapid intravenous bolus. If there is no effect within 2 min, a second dose of 12 mg can be given. Fifty percent of patients experience distressing chest pain or flushing.
3. **Verapamil** can be administered, 0.075 to 0.15 mg/kg (3 to 10 mg) intravenously over 15 to 60 s, with a repeat dose in 30 min, if necessary. Hypotension may occur but can be treated and/or prevented with calcium chloride, 4 mL of a 10% solution.

4. **Diltiazem** can be administered, 20 mg (0.25 mg/kg) intravenously over 2 min.
5. Further alternatives include **esmolol** (300 μg/kg/min), **propranolol** (0.5 to 1 mg intravenously) or **digoxin** (0.5 mg intravenously).
6. Synchronized cardioversion should be done in any unstable patient with hypotension, pulmonary edema, or severe chest pain. The required dose is usually small, less than 50 J.

Junctional Rhythms

Clinical Features

Under normal circumstances, the sinus node discharges at a faster rate than the AV junction, so the pacemaker function of the AV junction is overridden. If sinus node discharge is slow or fails to reach the AV junction, junctional escape beats may occur, usually at a rate between 40 to 60, depending on the level of the pacemaker. Generally, junctional escape beats do not conduct retrograde into the atria, so a QRS complex without a P wave usually is seen (Fig. 2-10). Junctional escape beats may occur whenever there is a long enough pause in the impulses reaching the AV junction, such as in sinus bradycardia, the slow phase of sinus dysrhythmia, AV block, or following premature beats. Sustained junctional escape rhythms may be seen with CHF, myocarditis, hyperkalemia, or digoxin toxicity. If the ventricular rate is too slow, myocardial or cerebral ischemia may develop.

Emergency Department Care and Disposition

1. Isolated, infrequent junctional escape beats usually do not require specific treatment.
2. If sustained junctional escape rhythms are producing symptoms, the underlying cause should be treated. Atropine can be used to accelerate temporarily the sinus node discharge rate and enhance AV nodal conduction.

FIG. 2-10   Junctional escape rhythm, rate 42.

VENTRICULAR DYSRHYTHMIAS

Aberrant Versus Ventricular Tachydysrhythmias

Differentiation between ectopic beats of ventricular origin and those of supraventricular origin that are conducted aberrantly, can be difficult, especially in sustained tachycardias with wide QRS complexes (WCT). In general, the majority of patients with WCT have ventricular tachycardia, which should be approached as ventricular tachycardia, until proved otherwise. Several guidelines follow:

1. A preceding ectopic P wave is good evidence favoring aberrancy, although coincidental atrial and ventricular ectopic beats or retrograde conduction can occur. During a sustained run of tachycardia, AV dissociation favors a ventricular origin of the dysrhythmia.
2. Postectopic pause: A fully compensatory pause is more likely after a ventricular beat, but exceptions occur.
3. Fusion beats are good evidence for ventricular origin but, again, exceptions occur.
4. A varying bundle branch block pattern suggests aberrancy.
5. Coupling intervals are usually constant with ventricular ectopic beats, unless parasystole is present. Varying coupling intervals suggest aberrancy.
6. Response to carotid sinus massage or other vagal maneuvers will slow conduction through the AV node and may abolish reentrant SVT and slow the ventricular response in other supraventricular tachydysrhythmias. These maneuvers have essentially no effect on ventricular dysrhythmias.
7. A QRS duration of longer than 0.14 s is usually found in ventricular ectopy or tachycardia.
8. Historical criteria also have been found to be useful: a patient over 35 years old or a history of MI, CHF, or coronary artery bypass graft strongly suggest ventricular tachycardia in patients with WCT.

Emergency Department Care and Disposition

1. As with ventricular tachycardia **lidocaine** 1 to 1.5 mg/kg intravenously should be started and may be repeated up to 3 mg/kg.
2. **Adenosine** 6 mg intravenously may be tried prior to **procainamide** (see ventricular tachycardia management later for administration guidelines).

Premature Ventricular Contractions

Clinical Features

Premature ventricular contractions (PVCs) are due to impulses originating from single or multiple areas in the ventricles. The

ECG characteristics of PVCs are (*a*) a premature and wide QRS complex; (*b*) no preceding P wave; (*c*) the ST-segment and T wave of the PVC are directed opposite the major QRS deflection; (*d*) most PVCs do not affect the sinus node, so there is usually a fully compensatory postectopic pause, or the PVC may be interpolated between 2 sinus beats; (*e*) many PVCs have a fixed coupling interval (within 0.04 s) from the preceding sinus beat; and (*f*) many PVCs are conducted into the atria, producing a retrograde P wave (Fig. 2-11).

PVCs are common, occur in most patients with ischemic heart disease, and are universally found in patients with acute MI. Other common causes of PVCs include digoxin toxicity, CHF, hypokalemia, alkalosis, hypoxia, and sympathomimetic drugs.

Emergency Department Care and Disposition

1. Most acute patients with PVCs will respond to intravenous **lidocaine** (1 mg/kg intravenously), although some patients may

FIG. 2-11   Premature ventricular contractions (PVCs). **A.** Unifocal PVC. **B.** Interpolated PVC. **C.** Multifocal PVCs.

require procainamide. Although single studies have suggested benefit, pooled data and meta-analysis find no reduction in mortality from either suppressive or prophylactic treatment of PVCs.

Accelerated Idioventricular Rhythm

Clinical Features

The ECG characteristics of accelerated idioventricular rhythm (AIVR) are (a) wide and regular QRS complexes; (b) rate between 40 and 100, often close to the preceding sinus rate; (c) most runs of short duration (3 to 30 beats); and (d) an AIVR often beginning with a fusion beat (Fig. 2-12). This condition is found most commonly with an acute MI.

Emergency Department Care and Disposition

1. Treatment is not necessary. On occasion, AIVR may be the only functioning pacemaker, and suppression with lidocaine can lead to cardiac asystole.

Ventricular Tachycardia

Clinical Features

Ventricular tachycardia is the occurrence of 3 or more beats from a ventricular ectopic pacemaker at a rate greater than 100. The ECG characteristics of ventricular tachycardia are (a) wide QRS complexes; (b) rate greater than 100 (most commonly 150 to 200);

FIG. 2-12   Accelerated idioventricular rhythms (AIVRs).

(*c*) usually regular rhythm, although there may be some beat-to-beat variation; and (*d*) usually constant QRS axis (Fig. 2-13).

Ventricular tachycardia is rare in patients without underlying heart disease. The most common causes of ventricular tachycardia are ischemic heart disease and acute MI. Ventricular tachycardia cannot be differentiated from SVT with aberrancy on the basis of clinical symptoms, blood pressure, or heart rate. Patients who are unstable should be cardioverted, which is effective for both dysrhythmias. In general, it is best to treat all wide complex tachycardias as ventricular tachycardia with lidocaine or procainamide. Adenosine appears to cause little harm in patients with ventricular tachycardia and has potential merit for the treatment of wide QRS complex tachycardias.

Emergency Department Care and Disposition

1. Unstable patients, or those in cardiac arrest, should be treated with synchronized cardioversion. Ventricular tachycardia can be converted with energies as low as 1 J, and over 90 percent can be converted with less than 10 J. ACLS guidelines recommend that pulseless ventricular tachycardia be defibrillated (unsynchronized cardioversion) with 200 J. Another alternative for unstable patients is intravenous amiodarone. (See treatment recommendations under ventricular fibrillation.)
2. Clinically stable patients should be treated with intravenous antidysrhythmics.
   a. **Lidocaine** 75 mg (1.0 to 1.5 mg/kg) intravenously over 60 to 90 s can be administered, followed by a constant infusion at 1 to 4 mg/min (10 to 40 μg/kg/min). A repeat bolus dose of 50 mg lidocaine may be required during the first 20 min to avoid a subtherapeutic dip in serum level due to the early distribution phase.
   b. **Procainamide** can be administered intravenously at less than 30 mg/min until the dysrhythmia converts, the total dose reaches 15 to 17 mg/kg in normals (12 mg/kg in patients with CHF), or early signs of toxicity develop, with hypotension or

FIG. 2-13   Ventricular tachycardia.

QRS prolongation. The loading dose should be followed by a maintenance infusion of 2.8 mg/kg/h in normal subjects.

c. **Bretylium** 500 mg (5 to 10 mg/kg) intravenously over 10 min can be administered, followed by a constant infusion at 1 to 2 mg/min.

Torsades de Pointes

Atypical ventricular tachycardia (torsade de pointes, or twisting of the points) is where the QRS axis swings from a positive to negative direction in a single lead (Fig. 2-14).

Drugs that further prolong repolarization—quinidine, disopyramide, procainamide, phenothiazines, tricyclic antidepressants—exacerbate this dysrhythmia.

1. Reports have revealed that **magnesium sulfate,** 1 to 2 g intravenously over 60 to 90 s followed by an infusion of 1 to 2 g/h, is effective in abolishing torsades de pointes.
2. To date, treatment for torsades de pointes consisted of accelerating the heart rate (thereby shortening ventricular repolarization) with *isoproterenol* (2 to 8 μg/min), while making arrangements for a ventricular pacemaker to overdrive the heart at rates of 90 to 120. Temporary pacing is the most effective and

FIG. 2-14 Two examples of short runs of atypical ventricular tachycardia showing sinusoidal variation in amplitude and direction of the QRS complexes: "Le torsade de pointes" (twisting of the points). Note that the top example is initiated by a late-occurring PVC (lead II).

safest method to treat torsades de pointes and prevent its recurrence.

Ventricular Fibrillation

Clinical Features

Ventricular fibrillation is the totally disorganized depolarization and contraction of small areas of ventricular myocardium—there is no effective ventricular pumping activity. The ECG of ventricular fibrillation shows a fine-to-coarse zigzag pattern without discernible P waves or QRS complexes (Fig. 2-15). Ventricular fibrillation is never accompanied by a pulse or a measurable blood pressure.

Ventricular fibrillation is most commonly seen in patients with severe ischemic heart disease, with or without an acute MI. Primary ventricular fibrillation occurs suddenly, without preceding hemodynamic deterioration, whereas secondary ventricular fibrillation occurs after a prolonged period of left ventricular failure or circulatory shock.

Emergency Department Care and Disposition

1. Current ACLS guidelines recommend immediate electrical defibrillation with 200 J. If ventricular fibrillation persists, defibrillation should be repeated immediately, with 200 to 300 J at the second attempt, increased to 360 J at the third attempt.
2. If the initial 3 attempts at defibrillation are unsuccessful, cardiopulmonary resuscitation and intubation should be initiated.
3. Epinephrine in standard dose should be administered, 1 mg intravenously. If this is not successful, high-dose epinephrine may be subsequently given, 0.1 mg/kg, and repeated every 3 to 5 min.
4. Defibrillation should be attempted after each drug administration, at 360 J, unless lower energy levels have been previously successful.

FIG. 2-15   Ventricular fibrillation.

5. Successive antidysrhythmics should then be administered with defibrillation attempted after each drug. The recommended sequence is **lidocaine,** 1.5 mg/kg, **bretylium,** 5 mg/kg, then possibly **magnesium,** 2 g intravenously, and procainamide (see preceding dosing guidelines).
6. **Amiodarone,** 150 mg over 10 min followed by 1 mg/min for 6 h, may become a preferred treatment for V_F/V_T after lidocaine has failed.

CONDUCTION DISTURBANCES

Atrioventricular Block

First-degree AV block is characterized by a delay in AV conduction, manifested by a prolonged PR interval. First-degree AV block needs no treatment and will not be discussed further. Second-degree AV block is characterized by intermittent AV conduction—some atrial impulses reach the ventricles and others are blocked. Third-degree AV block is characterized by complete interruption in AV conduction.

Second-Degree Mobitz I (Wenckebach) AV Block

Clinical Features

With second-degree Mobitz I (Wenckebach) AV block there is progressive prolongation of AV conduction (and the PR interval) until the atrial impulse is completely blocked. Usually, only a single atrial impulse is blocked. After the dropped beat, the AV conduction returns to normal and the cycle usually repeats itself, with either the same conduction ratio (fixed ratio) or a different conduction ratio (variable ratio).

The Wenckebach phenomenon has a seeming paradox. Even though the PR intervals progressively lengthen prior to the dropped beat, the increments by which they lengthen decrease with successive beats; this produces a progressive shortening of the R-R interval prior to the dropped beat (Fig. 2-16).

FIG. 2-16   Second-degree Mobitz I (Wenckebach) AV block 4:3 AV conduction.

This block is often transient and usually associated with an acute inferior MI, digoxin toxicity, myocarditis, or is seen after cardiac surgery.

Emergency Department Care and Disposition

1. Specific treatment is not necessary unless slow ventricular rates produce signs of hypoperfusion.
2. Atropine, 0.5 mg, can be repeated every 5 min as necessary and titrated to the desired effect or until the total dose reaches 3.0 mg.
3. Although rarely needed, transcutaneous pacing may be used. (See "Sinus Bradycardia" section for technique.)

Second-Degree Mobitz II AV Block

Clinical Features

With second-degree Mobitz II AV block, the PR interval remains constant before and after the nonconducted atrial beats (Fig. 2-17). One or more beats may be nonconducted at a single time.

The QRS complexes are usually wide. When second-degree AV block occurs with a fixed conduction ratio of 2:1, it is not possible to differentiate between a Mobitz type I (Wenckebach) or Mobitz type II block.

FIG. 2-17   A. Second-degree Mobitz II AV block. **B.** Second-degree AV block with 2:1 AV conduction.

Type II blocks imply structural damage to the infranodal conducting system, are usually permanent, and may progress suddenly to complete heart block, especially in the setting of an acute MI.

Emergency Department Care and Disposition

1. **Atropine** (0.5 to 1 mg IVP, may repeat up to 3.0 mg total dose) should be the first drug used.
2. Transcutaneous cardiac pacing is a useful modality in patients unresponsive to atropine. (See "Sinus Bradycardia" section for technique.)
3. Most cases, especially in the setting of acute MI, will require permanent transvenous cardiac pacing.

Third-Degree (Complete) AV Block

Clinical Features

In third-degree AV block, there is no AV conduction. The ventricles are paced by an escape pacemaker at a rate slower than the atrial rate (Fig. 2-18). When third-degree AV block occurs at the AV node, a junctional escape pacemaker takes over with a ventricular rate of 40 to 60 and, since the rhythm originates above the bifurcation of the bundle of His, the QRS complexes are narrow.

When third-degree AV block occurs at the infranodal level, the ventricles are driven by a ventricular escape rhythm at a rate of less than 40. Third-degree AV block located in the bundle branch or Purkinje system invariably have escape rhythms with wide QRS complexes.

Nodal third-degree AV block may develop in up to 8 percent of acute inferior MIs where it is usually transient, although it may last for several days.

Infranodal third-degree AV blocks indicate structural damage to the infranodal conducting system, as seen with an extensive acute anterior MI. The ventricular escape pacemaker is usually

FIG. 2-18   Third-degree AV block.

inadequate to maintain cardiac output and is unstable with periods of ventricular asystole.

Emergency Department Care and Disposition

Third-degree AV blocks should be treated the same as second-degree Mobitz II AV blocks with atropine or ventricular demand pacemaker, as required. External cardiac pacing can be performed before transvenous pacemaker placement.

PRETERMINAL RHYTHMS

Pulseless Electrical Activity

Pulseless electrical activity (PEA) is the presence of electrical complexes without accompanying mechanical contraction of the heart. Potential causes should be diagnosed and treated: severe hypovolemia, cardiac tamponade, tension pneumothorax, massive pulmonary embolus, and rupture of the ventricular well. Stabilizing treatment includes epinephrine 1 mg intravenously, followed by high dose therapy of 0.1 mg/kg if the first dose is not successful. Epinephrine should be repeated every 3 to 5 min. Atropine 1 mg intravenously, up to 3 mg total, is also acceptable therapy if the electrical conduction is slow.

Asystole (Cardiac Standstill)

Asystole is the complete absence of cardiac electrical activity. Treatment is the same as for pulseless electrical activity with the addition of transcutaneous pacing if the preceding measures fail (although this is rarely successful).

PREEXCITATION SYNDROMES

Clinical Features

Preexcitation occurs when some portion of the ventricles are activated by an impulse from the atria sooner than would be expected if the impulse were transmitted down the normal conducting pathway. All forms of preexcitation are felt to be due to accessory tracts that bypass all or part of the normal conducting system, the most common form being Wolff-Parkinson-White syndrome (WPW) (Fig. 2-19).

There is a high incidence of tachydysrhythmias in patients with WPW—atria flutter (about 5 percent), atrial fibrillation (10 to 20 percent), and paroxysmal reentrant SVT (40 to 80 percent).

FIG. 2-19   Type A Wolff-Parkinson-White syndrome.

Emergency Department Care and Disposition

1. Reentrant SVT (orthodromic, narrow QRS complex) in the WPW syndrome can be treated like other cases of reentrant SVT. *Adenosine,* 6 mg intravenously, or **verapamil,** 5 to 10 mg intravenously, are very successful at terminating this dysrhythmia in patients with WPW, but β-adrenergic blockers usually are ineffective.

2. Tachycardia with a wide QRS complex is usually associated with a short refractory period in the bypass tract; patients with this type of tachycardia are at risk for rapid ventricular rates and degeneration into ventricular fibrillation. Stable patients should be treated with intravenous procainamide and unstable patients should be cardioverted. β-adrenergic or calcium channel blockers should be avoided.

3. Atrial flutter or fibrillation with a rapid ventricular response is best treated with cardioversion.

For further reading in *Emergency Medicine: A Comprehensive Study Guide,* 5th ed., see Chap. 24, "Disturbances of Cardiac Rhythm and Conduction," by Edmund Bolton; and Chap. 25, "Pharmacology of Antidysrhythmic and Vasoactive Medications," by Teresa M. Carlin.

3 | Resuscitation of Children and Neonates

Charles J. Graham

Respiratory and cardiac arrest in children is most commonly due to primary respiratory conditions and shock. Because of age and size differences among children, drug dosages, compression and respiratory rates, and equipment sizes vary considerably (Table 3-1).

PEDIATRIC CARDIOPULMONARY RESUSCITATION

Securing the Airway

The airway in infants and children is smaller, more variable in size, and more anterior than in the adult.

Mild extension of the head (sniffing position) opens the airway. Chin lift or jaw thrust maneuvers may relieve obstruction of the airway related to the tongue. Oral airways are not commonly used in pediatrics but may be useful in patients whose airway cannot be maintained manually. Oral airways are inserted with a tongue blade, as in adults.

A bag-valve-mask system is commonly used for ventilation. Minimum volume for ventilation bags for infants and children is 450 mL. The tidal volume necessary to ventilate children is 10 to 15 mL/kg. In emergency situations, however, observation of chest rise and auscultation of breath sounds will ensure adequate ventilation.

Endotracheal intubation is usually performed using a Miller (straight) blade with a properly sized tube. The internal diameter of the tube should be the same size as the end of the patient's little finger. The formula 16 plus age in years divided by 4 gives approximate tube size. Uncuffed tubes are used in children up to 7 to 8 years.

Rapid Sequence Induction

Rapid sequence induction (RSI) is the administration of an intravenous anesthetic with a neuromuscular blocking agent to facilitate endotracheal intubation.

1. Prepare all equipment and supplies. A well functioning intravenous (IV) line must be in place. A cardiac monitor and oximetry should be used. The laryngoscope light source should be

TABLE 3-1 Length-Based Equipment Chart

Item	Patient Length, cm						
	54–70	70–85	85–95	95–107	107–124	124–138	138–155
ET tube size, mm	3.5	4.0	4.5	5.0	5.5	6.0	6.5
Lip-tip length, mm	10.5	12.0	13.5	15.0	16.5	18.0	19.5
Laryngoscope	1 straight	1 straight	2 straight	2 straight or curved	2 straight or curved	2–3 straight or curved	3 straight or curved
Suction catheter	8F	8–10F	10F	10F	10F	10F	12F
Stylet	6F	6F	6F	6F	14F	14F	14F
Oral airway	Infant/small child	Small child	Child	Child	Child/small adult	Child/adult	Medium adult
Bag-valve-mask	Infant	Child	Child	Child	Child	Child/adult	Adult
Oxygen mask	Newborn	Pediatric	Pediatric	Pediatric	Pediatric	Adult	Adult
Vascular access catheter/butterfly	22–24/23–25, intraosseous	20–22/23–25, intraosseous	18–22/21–23, intraosseous	18–22/21–23, intraosseous	18–20/21–23	18–20/21–22	16–20/18–21
Nasogastric tube	5–8F	8–10F	10F	10–12F	12–14F	14–18F	18F
Urinary catheter	5–8F	8–10F	10F	10–12F	10–12F	12F	12F
Chest tube	12–16F	16–20F	20–24F	20–24F	24–32F	28–32F	32–40F
Blood pressure cuff	Newborn/infant	Infant/child	Child	Child	Child	Child/adult	Adult

Note: Directions for use: (1) Measure patient length with centimeter tape; (2) Using measured length in centimeters, access appropriate equipment column.
Source: Adapted from RD Luten, RL Wears, J Broselow, et al: *Ann Emerg Med* 21:900, 1992.

checked. Suction equipment should be on and immediately available.

2. Preoxygenate with 100% oxygen.

3. **Lidocaine** 1 mg/kg IV may be used in head trauma patients to prevent increased intracranial pressure (ICP). Atropine 0.02 mg/kg (minimum dose 0.1 mg) may be used to prevent reflex bradycardia in children under 5 years old.

4. Cricoid pressure should be applied before paralysis and maintained until intubation is accomplished.

5. Induction of anesthesia is accomplished using one of several drug choices, depending on the clinical situation and the experience of the physician. Sodium thiopental 3 to 5 mg/kg is most commonly used. Advantages of **thiopental** include rapid onset of action, safe use with increased ICP, and low cost. Disadvantages include histamine release, possible hypotension, and tissue necrosis if extravasated. **Propofol** 2 to 2.5 mg/kg is a rapid acting induction agent that is safe for increased ICP. Disadvantages include pain on injection and cost. **Ketamine** 0.5 to 2 mg/kg is a dissociative anesthetic that increases heart rate and has bronchodilating effects. It has been used in trauma with hypotension and in patients with asthma. Disadvantages include increased airway secretions, increased ICP, emergence reactions, and possible laryngospasm. **Midazolam** 0.05 to 0.2 mg/kg is a benzodiazepine that can be used for induction. One of the advantages is reversibility. Disadvantages include slower onset of action and possible cardiorespiratory depression.

6. Neuromuscular blockade is accomplished by using succinylcholine, vecuronium, or rocuronium. **Succinylcholine** (1.0 mg/kg if > 12 kg; 2.0 mg/kg if > 12 kg) is a depolarizing blocking agent that has a rapid onset (45 s) but short duration of action (3 to 5 min). Although producing reliable paralysis, it has several disadvantages: (*a*) hyperkalemia, it should not be used in burns, spinal cord injuries, chronic immobilization, crush injuries with significant muscle injury, or conditions predisposing to hyperkalemia; it has been associated with hyperkalemic arrest in children with underlying but undiagnosed myopathies; (*b*) malignant hyperthermia in susceptible individuals; (*c*) elevations in ICP and intraocular pressure; (*d*) bradycardia, particularly in infants (premedicate with atropine in children under 5 years to prevent this effect); (*e*) muscle fasciculations, which may be prevented by a defasciculating dose of a nondepolarizing agent before succinylcholine is given. The short duration of action of succinylcholine may be a particular advantage when a difficult airway is anticipated or when ongoing neurologic assessment

is required. A fast acting nondepolarizing agent, such as vecuronium or rocuronium, may be chosen with the knowledge that the onset of action is slower and the duration of action much longer. **Rocuronium** 0.5 to 1.0 mg/kg is the fastest acting nondepolarizing agent, with onset in 55 to 75 s. The duration of action is 30 to 60 min. **Vecuronium** 0.1 to 0.3 mg/kg has an onset of 60 to 90 s and lasts 90 to 120 min.

7. Intubate the trachea and release cricoid pressure.

Vascular Access

Securing vascular access can be challenging in a critically ill child. Airway management is paramount in pediatric arrest and should not be delayed while obtaining vascular access. Vascular access is obtained in the most rapid, least invasive manner possible; peripheral veins (arm, hand, or scalp) are tried first. Intraosseous access is a quick, safe route for resuscitation medications and may be tried next in the critically ill infant. Percutaneous access of the femoral vein or access of the saphenous vein through cutdown can also be used, but is more time consuming.

The technique for insertion of the intraosseous line is as follows: the bone most commonly used is the proximal tibia. The anterior tibial tuberosity is palpated with the index finger, and the medial aspect of the tibia is grasped with the thumb. An imaginary line is drawn between the two, and the needle is inserted 1 cm distal to the midpoint of this line. A bone marrow needle is most commonly used; if a bone marrow needle is not available, an 18 gauge spinal needle can be used but is prone to bending. With sterile technique, the needle is inserted in a slightly caudal direction until the needle punctures the cortex. The stylet is removed, and marrow is aspirated to confirm placement. Fluids or drugs (including glucose, epinephrine, dopamine, anticonvulsants, and antibiotics) may then be administered as they are through a normal IV line.

Fluids

In shock, IV isotonic fluid (i.e., normal saline solution) boluses of 20 mL/kg should be given as rapidly as possible and should be repeated, depending on the clinical response. If hypovolemia has been corrected and shock or hypotension persist, a pressor agent should be considered.

Drugs

The indications for resuscitation drugs are the same for children as in adults. Drug dose calculations are a problem particular to pediatrics. Using a drug dosage chart or Broselow tape will reduce dosage errors. The Broselow tape is a length based system for estimating the weight of children in emergency situations. The tape has drug dosages, equipment sizes, and fluid volumes displayed according to patient size. A drug dose and equipment size chart or Broselow tape should be readily accessible in emergency care settings. Equipment should be stored so that appropriate sizes are readily accessible.

The rule of sixes may be used to quickly calculate continuous drug infusions (e.g., dopamine, dobutamine, etc.). The calculation is 6 mg times weight in kilograms; fill to 100 mL with D_5W. The infusion rate in milliliters per hour equals the microgram per kilogram per minute rate (i.e., an infusion running at 1 mL/h = 1 μg/kg/min, or 5 mL/h = 5 μg/kg/min).

Epinephrine is the only drug proven effective in cardiac arrest. It is indicated in pulseless arrest and in slow rates that are hypoxia induced and unresponsive to oxygenation and ventilation. If the initial dose of epinephrine (0.01 mg/kg of a 1:10,000 concentration) is not effective, high-dose epinephrine is recommended (0.1 to 0.2 mg/kg of a 1:1000 concentration) subsequently. Primary cardiac causes of bradycardia are rare and may be treated with **atropine** 0.02 mg/kg (minimum dose 0.1 mg) after adequate oxygenation and ventilation are ensured.

Sodium bicarbonate is no longer recommended as a first line resuscitation drug. It is recommended only after epinephrine administration has been ineffective or as guided by arterial blood gas measurements. Calcium is not recommended in routine resuscitation but may be useful in hyperkalemia, hypocalcemia, and calcium channel blocker overdose.

Dysrhythmias

Dysrhythmias in infants and children are most often the result of respiratory insufficiency or arrest, not of primary cardiac causes, as in adults. Careful attention to oxygenation and ventilation are, therefore, cornerstones of dysrhythmia management in pediatrics.

The most common rhythm seen in pediatric arrest situations is bradycardia leading to asystole. Oxygenation and ventilation are often sufficient in this situation; epinephrine may be useful if the condition is unresponsive to ventilation.

After the arrest situation, the most common dysrhythmia is supraventricular tachycardia (SVT). It presents with a narrow-complex tachycardia with rates between 250 and 350 beats per minute. Adenosine 0.1 mg/kg given through a well functioning IV line as close to the central circulation as possible followed by brisk saline flush is the recommended treatment for stable SVT in children. Treatment of the unstable patient with SVT is synchronized cardioversion ($\frac{1}{4}$ to $\frac{1}{2}$ J/kg).

It is sometimes difficult to distinguish between a fast sinus tachycardia and SVT. Small infants may have sinus tachycardia with rates above 200/beats per minute. Patients with sinus tachycardia may have a history of dehydration or shock; examination evidence of dehydration, fever, or pallor; and a normal sized heart on chest x-ray. Infants with SVT often have a nonspecific history, an examination revealing rales and an enlarged liver, and possibly an enlarged heart on x-ray.

Defibrillation and Cardioversion

Ventricular fibrillation is rare in children but may be treated with defibrillation at 2 J/kg. If this attempt is unsuccessful, the energy is doubled to 4 J/kg. If two attempts at defibrillation at 4 J/kg are unsuccessful, epinephrine should be given and oxygenation and acid-base status should be reassessed. Cardioversion is used to treat unstable tachyarrhythmias at a dose of $\frac{1}{4}$ to $\frac{1}{2}$ J/kg.

Use the largest paddles that still allow contact of the entire paddle with the chest wall. Electrode cream or paste is used to prevent burns. One paddle is placed on the right of the sternum at the second intercostal space, and the other is placed at the left midclavicular line at the level of the xiphoid.

NEONATAL RESUSCITATION

Most newborns do not require specific resuscitation after delivery, but about 6 percent of newborns require some form of life support in the delivery room. Emergency departments, therefore, must be prepared to provide neonatal resuscitation in the event of delivery in the emergency department.

1. The first step in neonatal resuscitation is to maintain body temperature. The infant should be dried and placed in a radiant warmer.
2. The airway should be cleared by suctioning the nose and mouth with a bulb syringe or a DeLee trap.
3. Next, a 5- to 10-s examination should assess heart rate, respiratory effort, color, and activity. If the infant is apneic or the heart rate is slow (less than 100 beats per minute), administer positive-pressure ventilation with bag-valve-mask and 100% oxygen. The rate should be 40 breaths per minute. In mildly

depressed infants, a prompt improvement in heart rate and respiratory effort usually occurs.

4. If no improvement is noted after 30 s and the condition deteriorates, endotracheal intubation should be performed.

5. If the heart rate is still below 50 beats per minute after intubation and assisted ventilation, cardiac massage should be started at 120 compressions per minute. Compressions and ventilations should be in a 3:1 ratio.

6. If there is no improvement in heart rate following these efforts, drug therapy may be used. Most neonates respond to appropriate airway management; therefore, drug therapy is rarely needed. Vascular access may be obtained peripherally or via the umbilical vein. The most expedient procedure in the neonate is to place an umbilical catheter in the umbilical vein and advance to 10 to 12 cm.

7. **Epinephrine** 0.01 mg/kg of 1:10,000 solution may be used if the heart rate is still below 100 beats per minute after adequate ventilation.

8. **Naloxone** 0.1 mg/kg IV may be useful to reverse narcotic respiratory depression. Isoproterenol 0.05 to 0.1 μg/min may be infused if epinephrine fails to raise the heart rate.

9. **Sodium bicarbonate** 1 to 2 meq/kg may be given if there is a significant metabolic acidosis; this therapy should be guided by blood gas values.

Prevention of Meconium Aspiration

Aspiration of meconium-stained amniotic fluid is associated with high rates of morbidity and mortality. With proper perinatal management, it is almost entirely preventable. If meconium is noted at the time of delivery, the nose, mouth, and pharynx of the infant should be suctioned with a DeLee trap prior to delivery of the infant's shoulders. Repeat suctioning of the airway should be performed with the infant under the radiant warmer prior to drying and stimulating the infant. This may be accomplished by visualizing the trachea with a laryngoscope and suctioning via an endotracheal tube. After suctioning, the infant should be dried and stimulated.

For further reading in *Emergency Medicine: A Comprehensive Study Guide,* 5th ed., see Chap. 9, "Neonatal Resuscitation and Emergencies," by Eugene E. Cepeda and Seetha Shankaran; Chap. 10, "Pediatric Cardiopulmonary Resuscitation," by William E. Hauda II; and Chap. 11, "Pediatric Airway Management," by Marcie Rubin and Nicholas Sadovnikoff.

4 | Fluids, Electrolytes, and
Acid-Base Disorders

Vincent Nacouzi

FLUIDS

The body's response to fluid and electrolyte abnormalities is stratified. Our first concern, therefore, starts with oxygenation and ventilation, then circulation and, last, acid-base and electrolytes. When altered, fluids and electrolytes should be corrected in the following order: (*a*) volume; (*b*) pH; (*c*) potassium, calcium, magnesium; and (*d*) sodium and chloride. Reestablishing tissue perfusion often reequilibrates the fluid-electrolyte and acid-base balance. Because the osmolarity of normal saline (NS) matches that of the serum, it is an excellent fluid for volume replacement. Hypotonic fluids such as D_5W should never be used to replace volume. Lactated Ringer's (LR) solution is commonly used for surgical patients or trauma patients, however, only NS can be given in the same line with blood components. $D_5.45$ NS, with or without potassium, is given as a maintenance fluid. The more concentrated dextrose solutions, $D_{10}W$ or $D_{20}W$ are used for patients with compromised ability to mobilize glucose stores, such as patients with hepatic failure, or as part of total parental nutrition (TPN) solutions.

Clinical Assessment of Volume Status

Volume loss and dehydration can be inferred by the patient history. Essential historic features to elicit include vomiting, diarrhea, fever, working conditions, fluid intake, chronic disease, level of consciousness, and urine output. Tachycardia and hypotension can be early-to-late signs of dehydration. On physical exam, look for dry mucosa, shrunken tongue (excellent indicator), and decreased skin turgor. In infants and children, sunken fontanelles, decreased capillary refill, lack of tears, and decreased wet diapers are typical signs and symptoms of dehydration. Lethargy and coma are more ominous signs and may indicate a significant comorbid condition. Laboratory values are not reliable indicators of fluid status. Plasma and urine osmolarity are perhaps the most reliable measures of dehydration. Blood urea nitrogen (BUN), creatinine, hematocrit, and other chemistries are insensitive.

Volume overload is a purely clinical diagnosis presenting usually as edema (central or peripheral), respiratory distress (pulmonary edema), jugular venous distention, and pump failure [congestive heart failure (CHF)]. The significant risk factors for volume overload are renal, cardiovascular, and liver disease. Blood pressure does not necessarily correlate with volume status alone; these patients with volume overload can have either hypotension or hypertension.

Maintenance Fluids

Adult: D_5.45 NS at 75 to 125 mL/h + 20 meq/L of potassium chloride for an average adult (approximately 70 kg)

Pediatrics: 100 mL/kg/d for first 10 kg (of body weight), 50 mL/kg/d for second 10 kg, 20 mL/kg/d for every kilogram thereafter

(See Chap. 80 for further discussion of pediatric fluid management including fluid choice.)

ELECTROLYTE DISORDERS

Correcting a single abnormality may not be the only intervention needed as most electrolytes exist in equilibrium with others. Laboratory errors are common. Results should be double-checked when the clinical picture and the laboratory data conflict. Abnormalities should be corrected at the same rate they developed, however, slower correction is usually safe unless the condition warrants rapid and/or early intervention (i.e., hypoglycemia and hyperkalemia). Evaluation of electrolyte disorders frequently requires a comparison of the measured and calculated osmolarity (number of particles per liter of solution). To calculate osmolarity the measured serum values in milliequivalents per liter should be used:

$$Osmolarity \text{ in mosmol/L} = 2Na^+ + \frac{glucose}{18} + \frac{BUN}{2.8} + \frac{ETOH}{4.6}$$

Hyponatremia ($Na^+ < 135$ meq/L)

Clinical Features

The clinical manifestations of hyponatremia occur when the $[Na^+]$ drops below 120 meq/L and include abdominal pain, headache, agitation, hallucinations, cramps, confusion, lethargy, and seizures.

Diagnosis and Differential

First evaluate the volume status and then the measured and calculated osmolarity. True hyponatremia presents with a reduced osmolarity. Factitious hyponatremia presents with a normal-to-high osmolarity. The most common cause is dilutional and may be brought on by trauma, sepsis, cardiac failure, cirrhosis, or renal failure. Hyponatremia may also be factitious (false elevation in the measured sodium) due to hyperglycemia, elevated protein, or hyperlipidemia. Extracellular fluid (ECF) or volume status and urine sodium level can classify true hyponatremia (low osmolarity). Syndrome of inappropriate antidiuretic hormone (SIADH) is a diagnosis made by exclusion. Causes of hyponatremia are listed in Table 4-1.

Emergency Department Care and Disposition

1. First the volume or perfusion deficit, if any, should be corrected using NS.
2. In stable normotensive patients fluids should be restricted (500 to 1500 mL of water daily).
3. In severe hyponatremia ($Na^+ < 120$ meq/L) with central nervous system (CNS) changes, **hypertonic** saline should be given, 3% NS (513 meq/L) at 25 to 100 mL/h. Concomitant use of **furosemide** in small doses of 20 to 40 mg has shown a decrease in the incidence of central pontine myelinolysis (CPM.) The sodium deficit can be calculated by taking the patient's weight in kilograms times 30 percent ($140 -$ measured Na^+). The rate of correction of the $[Na^+]$ should be less than 0.5 meq/L/h. Complications of rapid correction include CHF and CPM, which can cause alterations in consciousness, dysphagia, dysarthria, and paresis.

Hypernatremia ($Na^+ > 150$ meq/L)

Clinical Features

The symptoms of hypernatremia usually begin when the osmolarity is greater than 350. Irritability and ataxia occur with osmolarities above 375. Lethargy, coma, and seizures present with osmolarities above 400. Brain hemorrhage can be seen in neonates after rapid infusion of $NaHCO_3$. An osmolarity increase of 2 percent sets off thirst to prevent hypernatremia. Morbidity and mortality are highest in infants and the elderly who may be unable to respond to increased thirst.

TABLE 4-1 Causes of Hyponatremia

Hypotonic (true) hyponatremia (Posmol < 275)
  Hypovolemic hyponatremia
    Extrarenal losses (urinary Na^+ < 20 meq/L)
      Sweating, vomiting, diarrhea
      Third-space sequestration (burns, peritonitis, pancreatitis)
    Renal losses (urinary Na^+ > 20 meq/L)
      Loop or osmotic diuretics
      Aldosterone deficiency (Addison's disease)
      Ketonuria
      Salt-losing nephropathies; renal tubular acidosis
      Osmotic diuresis (mannitol, hyperglycemia, hyperuricemia)

  Euvolemic hyponatremia (urinary Na^+ > 20 meq/L)
    Inappropriate ADH secretion (CNS, lung, or carcinoma disease)
    Physical and emotional stress or pain
    Myxedema, Addison's disease, Sheehan's syndrome
    Drugs, water intoxication

Hypervolemic hyponatremia
    Urinary Na^+ > 20 meq/L
      Renal failure
    Urinary Na^+ < 20 meq/L
      Cirrhosis
      Cardiac failure
      Renal failure

Isotonic (pseudo) hyponatremia (Posmol 275–295)
  Hyperproteinemia, hyperlipidemia, hyperglycemia

Hypertonic hyponatremia (Posmol > 295)
  Hyperglycemia, mannitol excess and glycerol use

Abbreviations: ADH, antidiuretic hormone; CNS, central nervous system.

Diagnosis and Differential

The most frequent cause of hypernatremia is a decrease in total body water due to decreased intake or excessive loss. Common causes are diarrhea, vomiting, hyperpyrexia, and excessive sweating. An interesting etiology of hypernatremia is *diabetes insipidus* (DI), which results from loss of hypotonic urine. It may be central [no antidiuretic hormone (ADH), secreted] or nephrogenic (unresponsive to ADH.) The causes of hypernatremia are listed in Table 4-2.

Emergency Department Care and Disposition

Any perfusion deficits should be treated with NS or LR. Then, a switch to 0.5 NS should be made after a urine output of 0.5 mL/

TABLE 4-2 Causes of Hypernatremia

Loss of water
  Reduced water intake
    Defective thirst
    Unconsciousness
    Inability to drink water
    Lack of access to water
  Water loss in excess of sodium
    Vomiting, diarrhea
    Sweating, fever
    Dialysis
    Drugs, hyperventilation
    Diabetes insipidus, osmotic diuresis
    Thyrotoxicosis
    Severe burns

Gain of sodium
  Increased intake
    Hypertonic saline ingestion or infusion
    Sodium bicarbonate administration
    Renal salt retention (usually because of poor perfusion)

kg/h is reached. Lowering the Na^+ more than 10 meq/L/d should be avoided. Central venous pressure and pulmonary capillary wedge pressure should be monitored. The following formula should be used to calculate the total body water (TBW) deficit. As a rule, each liter of water deficit causes the Na^+ to increase 3 to 5 meq/L

Water deficit (in liters) = TBW $(1 - $ measured Na^+/desired $Na^+)$

If no urine output is observed after NS/LR rehydration, a rapid switch to 0.5 NS should be made: the body of the extra sodium should be unloaded by using a diuretic (i.e., furosemide, 20 to 40 mg intravenously). Central DI is treated using desmopressin (dDAVP). In children with a serum sodium level greater than 180 meq/L, peritoneal dialysis should be considered by using high glucose–low Na^+ dialysate, which may be life-saving.

Hypokalemia ($K^+ < 3.5$ meq/L)

Clinical Features

The signs and symptoms of hypokalemia usually occur at levels below 2.5 meq/L. They include CNS delete (weakness, cramps, and hyporeflexia), gastrointestinal (GI, ileus), cardiovascular (dysrhythmias, worsening of digoxin toxicity, and hypotension or hypertension, U waves and ST depression, and prolonged QT), and renal disorders (metabolic alkalosis and worsening hepatic encephalopathy), and, last, glucose intolerance can also develop.

Diagnosis and Differential

The most common cause is the use of loop diuretics. Table 4-3 lists the causes.

Emergency Department Care and Disposition

A 20 meq K^+ replacement will raise the K^+ by .25 meq/L. Patients should be monitored continuously for dysrhythmias.

1. Administration of 10 to 15 meq of potassium chloride per hour in 50 to 100 mL of dextrose in water (D_5W) should be made with a piggyback into saline over 3 to 4 h. In general, up to 10 meq/h of KCl can be given through a peripheral intravenous line and up to 20 meq/h can be given through a central line. No more than 40 meq of KCl in a liter of intravenous fluids should be added.
2. Oral replacement (in the awake, asymptomatic patient) is rapid

TABLE 4-3 Causes of Hypokalemia

Shift into the cell
  Raising the pH of blood, β adrenergics
  Administration of insulin and glucose

Reduced intake

Increased loss
  Renal loss
    Primary hyperaldosteronism, osmotic diuresis
    Secondary hyperaldosteronism associated with
    diuretics, malignant hypertension, Bartter's syndrome,
    and renal artery stenosis
    Miscellaneous
      Licorice use
      Use of chewing tobacco
      Hypercalcemia
      Liddle syndrome
      Magnesium deficiency
      Renal tubular acidosis
      Acute myelocytic and monocytic leukemia
      Drugs and toxins (PCN, lithium, L-dopa, theophylline)
  GI loss (vomiting, diarrhea, fistulas)

Abbreviations: PCN, penicillin; GI, gastrointestinal.

and safer than intravenous therapy. In general, 20 to 40 meq/L of KCl or similar agent should be used.

Hyperkalemia ($K^+ > 5.5$ meq/L)

Clinical Features

The most concerning and serious manifestations of hyperkalemia are the cardiac effects. At levels of 6.5 to 7.5 meq/L, the electrocardiogram (ECG) shows peaked T waves (precordial), prolonged PR intervals, and short QT intervals. At levels of 7.5 to 8.0 meq/L, the QRS widens and the P-wave flattens. At levels above 8 meq/L, a sine wave pattern, ventricular fibrillation, and heart blocks occur. Neuromuscular symptoms include weakness and paralysis. GI symptoms include vomiting, colic, and diarrhea.

Diagnosis and Differential

It is important to beware of pseudohyperkalemia, which is caused by hemolysis after blood is drawn. Renal failure with oliguria is the most common cause of true hyperkalemia. Appropriate tests for management include an ECG; electrolytes, calcium, and magnesium levels, arterial blood gas analysis (ABG; check for acidosis), urinalysis, and a digoxin level. Causes of hyperkalemia are listed in Table 4-4.

Emergency Department Care and Disposition

The ECG should always be monitored closely. The treatment of symptomatic patients is a stepwise approach: the cardiac membrane must be stabilized with calcium chloride and then the K^+ must be shifted into the cell using glucose and insulin and/or bicarbonate. Finally, the potassium must be excreted using Kayexalate, diuretics, and dialysis in severe cases.

1. For levels over 7.0 meq/L or if there are any ECG changes, intravenous **calcium chloride,** 5 mL of a 10% solution should be given: caution must be used in a digoxin-toxic patient (risk of dysrhythmias). The presence of digoxin toxicity with hyperkalemia is an indication for Dig-Fab (Digibind) therapy. (See Chap. 104.)
2. For levels above 5.5 meq/L (especially in acidotic patients), 1 to 2 A of sodium bicarbonate should be given.
3. The patient should receive 1 A of **D$_{50}$W,** with 10 U regular **insulin** intravenously (5 U in dialysis patients).
4. Diuresis should be maintained with **furosemide,** 20 to 40 mg intravenously.

TABLE 4-4 Causes of Hyperkalemia

Factitious
  Laboratory error
  Pseudohyperkalemia: hemolysis, thrombocytosis, and
  leukocytosis

Metabolic acidemia (acute)

Increased intake into the plasma
  Exogenous: diet, salt substitutes, low-sodium diet, and
  medications
  Endogenous: hemolysis, GI bleeding, catabolic states,
  crush injury

Inadequate distal delivery of sodium and decreased
distal tubular flow

Oliguric renal failure

Impaired renin-aldosterone axis
  Addison's disease
  Primary hypoaldosteronism
  Other (heparin, β blockers, prostaglandin inhibitors,
  captopril)

Primary renal tubular potassium secretory defect
  Sickle cell disease
  Systemic lupus erythematosus
  Postrenal transplantation
  Obstructive uropathy

Inhibition of renal tubular secretion of potassium
  Spironolactone
  Digitalis

Abnormal potassium distribution
  Insulin deficiency
  Hypertonicity (hyperglycemia)
  β-adrenergic blockers
  Exercise
  Succinylcholine
  Digitalis

Abbreviation: GI, gastrointestinal.

5. **Kayexalate** (orally or PR) 1 g binds 1 meq of K^+ over 10 min. Administration of 15 to 25 g of Kayexalate should be given orally with 50 mL of 20% sorbitol (sorbitol is used because Kayexalate is constipating). Per rectum, 20 g in 200 mL 20% sorbitol over 30 min should be given. Kayexalate can exacerbate CHF.
6. In patients with acute renal failure, consultation should be made for emergent dialysis.

7. Albuterol (by nebulization, 0.5 mL of a 5% solution, 2.5 mg, may also be used to lower K^+ (transient effect).

Hypercalcemia (Ca^{2+} > 10.5 or Ionized Ca^{2+} > 2.7 meq/L)

Several factors affect the serum calcium level: parathyroid hormone (PTH) increases calcium and decreases phosphate; calcitonin and vitamin D metabolites decrease calcium. Decreased $[H^+]$ cause a decrease in ionized Ca^{2+}. Ionized Ca^{2+} is the physiologically active form. Each rise in pH of 0.1 lowers Ca^{2+} by 3 to 8 percent. A decrease in albumin causes a decrease in Ca^{2+} but not in the ionized portion. Most cases of hypercalcemia are due to hyperparathyroidism or malignancies. A third of the patients develop hypokalemia.

Clinical Features

Clinical signs and symptoms develop at levels above 12 mg/dL. A mnemonic to aid recall of common hypercalcemia symptoms is *stones* (renal calculi), *bones* (bone destruction secondary to malignancy), *psychic moans* (lethargy, weakness, fatigue, and confusion) and *abdominal groans* (abdominal pain, constipation, polyuria, and polydipsia). On the ECG one may see depressed ST segments, widened T waves, shortened QT intervals, and heart blocks. Levels above 20 meq/L can cause cardiac arrest. Another mnemonic to aid recall of the common causes is *PAM P. SCHMIDT: P*arathyroid hormone, *A*ddison's disease, *M*ultiple myeloma, *P*aget's disease, *S*arcoidosis, *C*ancer, *H*yperthyroidism, *M*ilk-alkali syndrome, *I*mmobilization, excess Vitamin *D,* and *T*hiazides.

Emergency Department Care and Disposition

Emergency treatment is important in the following conditions: a calcium level above 12 mg/dL, a symptomatic patient, a patient who cannot tolerate oral fluids, or a patient with abnormal renal function.

1. Dehydration should be corrected with NS; 5 to 10 L may be required. Invasive monitoring should be considered.
2. **Furosemide,** 40 mg, should be administered but dehydration should not be exacerbated if present. The concurrent hypokalemia or hypomagnesemia must be corrected. Thiazide diuretics should not be used (worsens hypercalcemia). If the preceding treatments are not effective, the physician should administer **calcitonin** 0.5 to 4 MRC U/kg intravenously over 24 h or intra-

muscularly divided every 6 h, along with **hydrocortisone,** 25 to 100 mg intravenously every 6 h.

Hypocalcemia ($Ca^{2+} < 8.5$ or Ionized Level < 2.0)

Clinical Features

The signs and symptoms of hypocalcemia are usually seen with ionized Ca^{2+} levels below 1.5. Clinically patients have paresthesias, increased deep tendon reflexes (DTR), cramps, weakness, confusion, and seizures. Patients may also demonstrate Chvostek's sign (twitch of the corner of mouth on tapping with finger over cranial nerve VII at zygoma) or Trousseau's sign (more reliable, carpal spasm when the blood pressure cuff is left inflated at a pressure above the systolic blood pressure for longer than 3 min). If the patient is alkalotic, ionized calcium (physiologically active) may be very low, even with normal total calcium levels. In refractory CHF, Ca^{2+} can be low. Severely alkalotic patients may have a normal total Ca^{2+} yet have hypocalcemia.

Diagnosis and Differential

Common causes include shock, sepsis, renal failure, pancreatitis, drugs (cimetidine mostly), hypoparathyroidism, phosphate overload, Vitamin D deficiency, fat embolism, strychnine poisoning, hypomagnesemia, and tetanus toxin. The ECG often shows a prolonged QT interval.

Emergency Department Care and Disposition

1. If the patient is asymptomatic oral **calcium gluconate** tablets, 1 to 4 g/d divided every 6 h, with or without **Vitamin D** (calcitrol, 0.2 μg two times daily) should be used. Milk is not a good substitute (low Ca^{2+}).
2. In more urgent situations with symptomatic patients, **calcium gluconate** or **calcium chloride,** 10 mL of a 10% solution can be given over 10 min with a slow intravenous line.

Hypomagnesemia

Clinical Findings

Mg^{2+}, K^+, and PO_4^- move together intra- and extracellularly. Hypomagnesemia can present as a CNS disorder—depression, vertigo, ataxia, seizures, increased DTR, tetany or as a cardiovascular disorder—dysrhythmias, prolonged QT and PR, worsening of digitalis effects. Also seen are anemia, hypotension, hypothermia, and dysphagia.

Diagnosis and Differential

The diagnosis should not be based on Mg^{2+} levels, since total depletion can occur before any significant laboratory changes. It must therefore be suspected along with CNS manifestations. In the United States, the most common cause is alcoholism, followed by poor nutrition, cirrhosis, pancreatitis, correction of diabetic ketoacidosis, or excessive GI losses. Difficulty treating hypokalemia can be a presentation of low Mg^{2+}.

Emergency Department Care and Disposition

First, volume deficit and any decreased potassium, calcium, or phosphate must be corrected. If the patient is an alcoholic in delirium tremens (DTs) or pending DTs, 2 g **magnesium sulfate** must be administered in the first hour, followed by 6 g (in the first 24 h). A check for DTRs should be made every 15 min. DTRs disappear when the serum magnesium level rises above 3.5 meq/L, at which time the magnesium infusion should be stopped.

Hypermagnesemia

Clinical Features

Signs and symptoms manifest progressively; DTRs disappear with a serum magnesium level above 3.5 meq/L, muscle weakness at a level above 4 meq/L, hypotension at a level above 5 meq/L, and respiratory paralysis at a level above 8 meq/L.

Diagnosis and Differential

Hypermagnesemia is a rare encounter in most emergency departments (EDs). Common causes are renal failure with concomitant ingestion of magnesium-containing preparations (antacids) and lithium ingestion. Serum levels are diagnostic. Increased potassium and phosphate should be suspected.

Emergency Department Care and Disposition

Rehydrate with NS and **furosemide,** 20 to 40 mg intravenously (in the absence of renal failure.) Acidosis should be corrected with ventilation and sodium bicarbonate, 50 to 100 meq, if needed. In symptomatic patients, 5 mL (10% solution) of CaCl intravenously antagonizes the magnesium effects.

Phosphate and Chloride Abnormalities

Hypophosphatemia rarely occurs, except in patients receiving total parental nutrition. Hyperphosphatemia occurs mainly with renal failure and can be treated with hydration, acetazolamide, or dialysis. Chloride abnormalities usually occur in association with other metabolic disorders, such as metabolic alkalosis (hypochloremia) or dehydration (hyperchloremia). Treatment for chloride disorders is the correction of the volume deficit with NS, the acid-base abnormality, or the potassium deficit.

ACID-BASE PROBLEMS

The lungs and kidneys primarily maintain the acid-base regulation. *Acidosis* is due to gain of acid or loss of alkali; causes may be metabolic (fall in serum HCO_3^-) or respiratory (rise in PCO_2). *Alkalosis* is due to loss of acid or addition of base and is either metabolic (rise in serum HCO_3^-) or respiratory (fall in PCO_2). The difference between acidosis and acidemia is very important: a patient can have a normal pH (no acidemia) but have an underlying acidosis compensated for by an alkalosis. Metabolic disorders prompt an immediate compensatory change in ventilation, either venting CO_2 or retaining it. The effect of the kidneys in response to metabolic disorders is to excrete hydrogen ions (with chloride) and retain HCO_3^-.

Several conditions should alert the clinician to possible acid-base disorders: history of renal, endocrine, or psychiatric disorders (drug ingestion) or signs of acute disease (tachypnea, cyanosis, Kussmaul's respiration, respiratory failure, shock, changes in mental status, vomiting, diarrhea, or other acute fluid losses).

General Approach

The compensatory mechanisms will return the pH toward, but not to, normal. The type of acid-base disturbance the patient has can be determined by several steps: drawing blood and then determining the presumptive type of acid-base disorder from the pH, the PCO_2, the CO_2 content (serum bicarbonate), and the anion gap. In a mixed disorder, the pH, PCO_2, and HCO_3^- may be normal, and the only clue to a metabolic acidosis is a widened anion gap. Presumptive types of acid-base disorders are diagnosed by comparing actual laboratory values to values calculated by formulas that predict the anticipated compensatory changes.

1. *Blood Draw.* After initial attention to the ABCs, a complete history (including review of systems, ROS), and physical examination, blood should be sent for ABG measurement; electro-

lytes, BUN, and creatinine levels; and serum osmolality and urine should be dipped for ketones and glucose. If a patient has a normal pH, normal PCO_2, normal CO_2, and AG, the patient does not have an acid-base problem.
Use as normals: $pH = 7.4$, $HCO_3^- = 24$ mm/L, $PCO_2 = 40$ mmHg.
2. *Presumptive Type.* Determine the type of acid-base disorder from the following: any listed increase or decrease uses the preceding normals as reference points.

Type	pH	PCO_2	HCO_3^-
Respiratory acidosis	Decreased	Increased	Increased
Respiratory alkalosis	Increased	Decreased	Decreased
Metabolic acidosis	Decreased	Decreased	Decreased
Metabolic alkalosis	Increased	Increased	Increased
Mixed disorder	Variable	Variable	Variable

The following steps should be a guide when confirming the presumptive type.

Respiratory Acidosis

Using historical information, respiratory acidosis can be further divided into acute respiratory acidosis (e.g., hypoventilation from narcotic overdose) and chronic respiratory acidosis (e.g., chronic obstructive pulmonary disease with CO_2 retention). Only in chronic conditions does the kidney have time to compensate for the respiratory changes (takes 48 to 72 h). Formulas to calculate the expected changes in pH (from 7.4) and HCO_3^- (from 24 mm/L) using the observed change in PCO_2 (from 40 mmHg) include the following:

Acute respiratory acidosis. Predicted decrease in $pH = (0.007) \times$ (observed change in PCO_2); predicted increase in $HCO_3^- = (0.1) \times$ (observed change in PCO_2).
Chronic respiratory acidosis. Predicted decrease in $pH = (0.003) \times$ (observed change in PCO_2); predicted increase in $HCO_3^- = (0.35) \times$ observed change in PCO_2).

If these conditions do not hold true, you do not have a primary respiratory disorder. (See "Metabolic Acidosis" later.)

Respiratory Alkalosis

Using historic information, respiratory alkalosis can be further divided into acute respiratory alkalosis (e.g., hyperventilation from anxiety) and chronic respiratory alkalosis (e.g., untreated hyper-thyroidism). Only in chronic conditions do the kidneys have time to compensate for the respiratory changes (takes 48 to 72 h). Formulas to calculate the expected changes in pH (from 7.4) and HCO_3^- (from 24 mm/L) using the observed change in PCO_2 (from 40 mmHg) include the following:

Acute respiratory alkalosis. Predicted increase in pH = (0.007) × (observed change in PCO_2); predicted decrease in HCO_3^- = (0.2) × (observed change in PCO_2). Usually the HCO_3^- is not less than 18 in acute conditions.

Chronic respiratory alkalosis. Predicted increase in pH = (0.0017) × (observed change in PCO_2); predicted decrease in HCO_3^- = (0.5) × (observed change in PCO_2). Usually the HCO_3^- is not less than 14 in chronic conditions.

If these conditions do not hold to be true, the patient does not have a primary respiratory disorder (See "Metabolic Alkalosis" later).

Pure Metabolic Acidosis

If the acid-base disorder is a simple metabolic acidosis, the clinician should be able to predict the decrease in PCO_2 (from 40 mmHg) using the observed change in HCO_3^-. (from 24 mm/L) with the following formula: Predicted decrease in PCO_2 = (1.0 to1.5) × observed decrease in HCO_3^-. If these conditions do not hold to be true, the patient has a mixed disorder.

Pure Metabolic Alkalosis

If the acid-base disorder is a simple metabolic acidosis, the clinician should be able to predict the decrease in PCO_2 (from 40 mmHg) using the observed change in HCO_3^- (from 24 mm/L) with the following formula: Predicted increase in PCO_2 = (0.25 to 1.0) × observed increase in HCO_3^-. If the clinician has determined that the patient has a mixed disorder, the treatments listed in both the respiratory and metabolic sections that follow should be con-sidered.

Respiratory Acidosis

Clinical Features

Respiratory acidosis may be life-threatening and a precursor to respiratory arrest. The clinical picture is often dominated by the underlying disorder. Typically, respiratory acidosis depresses men-tal function, which may progressively slow the respiratory rate. Patients may be confused, somnolent, and, eventually, uncon-scious. Although frequently hypoxic, in some disorders the fall in oxygen saturation may lag behind the elevation in PCO_2. Pulse oximetry may be misleading, making ABG essential for the diagnosis. The differential diagnosis includes: COPD, drug overdose, CNS disease, chest wall disease, pleural disease, and trauma.

Emergency Department Care and Disposition

1. Ventilation must be increased. In many cases, this requires intubation. The hallmark indication for intubation in respiratory acidosis is depressed mental status. Only in opiate intoxication is it acceptable to await treatment of the underlying disorder (rapid administration of naloxone) before reversal of the hypoventilation.
2. The underlying disorder must be treated. It must be remembered that high-flow oxygen therapy may lead to exacerbation of CO_2 narcosis in patients with COPD and CO_2 retention. These patients must be monitored closely when administering oxygen and intubated if necessary.

Respiratory Alkalosis

Clinical Features

Hyperventilation syndrome is a problematic diagnosis for the emergency physician, as a number of life-threatening disorders present with tachypnea and anxiety: asthma, pulmonary embolism, diabetic ketoacidosis, and others. Symptoms of respiratory alkalosis often are dominated by the primary disorder promoting the hyperventilation. Hyperventilation by virtue of the reduction of PCO_2, however, lowers both cerebral and peripheral blood flow, causing distinct symptoms. Patients complain of dizziness, painful flexion of the wrists, fingers, ankles, and toes (carpal-pedal spasm), and, frequently, a chest pain described as tightness.

The diagnosis of hyperventilation due to anxiety is a diagnosis of exclusion. ABGs can be used to rule out acidosis and hypoxia. (See Chap. 26, "Pulmonary Embolism," for discussion of calculating the alveolar-arterial oxygen gradient.) Causes of respiratory alkalosis to consider include hypoxia, fever, hyperthyroidism, sympathomimetic therapy, aspirin overdose, progesterone therapy, liver disease, and anxiety.

Emergency Department Care and Disposition

1. The underlying cause must be treated. Only when more serious causes of hyperventilation are ruled out should the treatment of anxiety be considered. Anxiolytics may be helpful, such as lorazepam 1 to 2 mg, intravenously or orally.

2. Rebreathing into a paper bag can cause hypoxia and should not be used.

Metabolic Acidosis

When considering metabolic acidosis, causes should be further divided into elevated and normal anion-gap acidosis. The term *anion gap* is misleading because in serum, there is no gap between total positive and negative ions; however, more positive ions are commonly measured than negative ions. The anion gap, therefore, is measured as follows:

$$\text{Anion gap} = Na^+ - (Cl^- + HCO_3^-)$$
$$= \text{approximately 10 to 12 meq/L}$$

Clinical Features

No matter what the etiology, acidosis can cause nausea and vomiting, abdominal pain, change in sensorium, and tachypnea, and sometimes a Kussmaul's respiratory pattern. It also leads to decreased muscle strength and force of cardiac contraction, arterial vasodilation, venous vasoconstriction, and pulmonary hypertension. Patients may present with nonspecific complaints or shock.

Diagnosis and Differential

Causes of metabolic acidosis can be divided into two main groups: (*a*) those associated with increased production of organic acids (increased anion-gap metabolic acidosis; see Table 4-5); and (*b*) those associated with a loss of bicarbonate or addition of chloride (normal anion-gap metabolic acidosis; see Table 4-6). A mnemonic to aid the recall of the causes of increased anion-gap metabolic acidosis is *A MUD PILES*—*a*lcohol, *m*ethanol, *u*remia, *d*iabetic ketoacidosis, *p*araldehyde, *i*ron and *i*soniazid, *l*actic acidosis, *e*thylene glycol, and *s*alicylates and *s*tarvation. A mnemonic that can aid the recall of normal anion-gap metabolic acidosis is *USED CARP*—*u*reterostomy, *s*mall bowel fistulas, *e*xtra chloride, *d*iarrhea, *c*arbonic anhydrase inhibitors, *a*drenal insufficiency, *r*enal tubular acidosis, and *p*ancreatic fistula.

Emergency Department Care and Disposition

After the ABCs have been assured, the following general treatment is recommended.

1. Supportive care should be given by improving perfusion, administering fluids as needed, and improving oxygenation and ventilation.

TABLE 4-5 Causes of High Anion-Gap Metabolic Acidosis

Lactic acidosis
  Type A—Decrease in tissue oxygenation
  Type B—No decrease in tissue oxygenation

Renal failure (acute or chronic)

Ketoacidosis
  Diabetes
  Alcoholism
  Prolonged starvation (mild acidosis)
  High-fat diet (mild acidosis)

Ingestion of toxic substances
  Elevated osmolar gap
    Methanol
    Ethylene glycol
  Normal osmolar gap
    Salicylate
    Paraldehyde
    Cyanide

2. The underlying problem should be corrected. If the patient has ingested a toxin, lavage, administration of activated charcoal, the appropriate antidote, and dialysis should be performed, as directed by the specific toxicology chapters in this handbook. If septic, cultures should be performed and antibiotics administered, as directed by the appropriate chapters in this handbook. If in shock, the patient should be administered fluids and vasopressors as directed by the appropriate chapters in section 2 of this book. If the patient is in DKA, he or she should be treated as directed in Chap. 125 with intravenous fluids and insulin.
3. When pH < 7.1 or the HCO_3^- < 8 to 10, treatment should be considered with sodium bicarbonate (controversial). The pH

TABLE 4-6 Causes of Normal Anion-Gap Metabolic Acidosis

With a tendency to hyperkalemia	With a tendency to hypokalemia
Subsiding DKA	Renal tubular acidosis type I
Early uremic acidosis	Renal tubular acidosis type II
Early obstructive uropathy	Acetazolamide therapy
Renal tubular acidosis type IV	Acute diarrhea (losses of HCO_3^-
Hypoaldosteronism	and K^+)
Potassium-sparing diuretics	Ureterosigmoidostomy

Abbreviations: DKA, diabetic ketoacidosis; HCO_3^-, bicarbonate; and K^+, potassium.

should be raised to approximately 7.25, using 1 meq/kg of HCO_3^- over 20 to 30 min. It is important to beware of sodium overload, particularly in neonates and patients in pulmonary edema. Reassessment for pH, PCO_2, and HCO_3^- should be made and the need for further therapy determined. It is important to remember that giving HCO_3^- in the face of inadequate ventilation exacerbates the acidosis from a build-up of CO_2. The key is to administer HCO_3^- as slowly as the situation permits.

Metabolic Alkalosis

The two most common causes of metabolic alkalosis are excessive diuresis (with loss of potassium, hydrogen ion, and chloride) and excessive loss of gastric secretions (with loss of hydrogen ion and chloride). Other causes of hypokalemia should also be considered.

Clinical Features

Symptoms of the underlying disorder (usually fluid loss) dominate the clinical presentation, but general symptoms of metabolic alkalosis include muscular irritability, tachydysrhythmias, and impaired oxygen delivery. The diagnosis of metabolic alkalosis is made from laboratory studies revealing a bicarbonate level above 26 meq/L and a pH above 7.45. In most cases, there is also an associated hypokalemia and hypochloremia. The differential diagnosis includes dehydration, loss of gastric acid, excessive diuresis, administration of mineralocorticoids, increased intake of citrate or lactate, hypercapnia, hypokalemia, and severe hypoproteinemia.

Emergency Department Care and Disposition

1. Fluids should be administered in the form of NS in cases of dehydration.
2. Potassium should be administered as KC, not faster than 20 meq/h, unless serum potassium is above 5.0 meq/L.

For further reading in *Emergency Medicine: A Comprehensive Study Guide,* 5th ed., see Chap. 21, "Acid-Base Disorders," by David D. Nicolaou and Gabor D. Kelen; Chap. 22, "Blood Gases: Pathophysiology and Interpretation," by Mark P. Hamlin and Peter J. Pronovost; and Chap. 23, "Fluid and Electrolyte Problems," by Michael Londner, Christine Carr, and Gabor D. Kelen.

5 | Therapeutic Approach to the Hypotensive Patient

John E. Gough

Over 1 million patients in shock present to emergency departments each year. Shock occurs when circulation is insufficient to meet the resting metabolic demands of the tissues. Such tissue hypoperfusion is associated with decreased venous oxygen content and metabolic acidosis (lactic acidosis). Shock is classified into four categories based on etiology: (1) hypovolemic, (2) cardiogenic, (3) distributive (e.g., neurogenic anaphylaxis), and (4) obstructive.

Clinical Features

Factors that influence the clinical presentation of a patient in shock include the etiology, duration, and severity of the shock state as well as the underlying medical status of the patient. Often the precipitating cause of shock may be readily apparent [e.g., acute myocardial infarction, trauma, gastrointestinal (GI) bleeding, or anaphylaxis]. It is not uncommon for the patient to present with nonspecific symptoms (e.g., generalized weakness, lethargy, or altered mental status). A targeted history of both the presenting symptoms and previously existing conditions (e.g., cardiovascular disease, GI bleeding, adrenal insufficiency, or diabetes) will aid in identifying the cause and guide the initial treatment of shock. Drug use (both prescribed and nonprescribed) is an essential element of the initial history. Medication use may be either the cause or a contributing factor to the evolution of shock. For example, diuretics can lead to volume depletion, and cardiovascular medications (e.g., beta blockers and digoxin) can depress the pumping action of the heart. The possibility of drug toxicity and anaphylactic reactions to medications should also be considered.

Assessment of vital signs is a routine part of the physical examination; however, no single vital sign or value is diagnostic in the evaluation of the presence or absence of shock. The patient's temperature may be elevated or subnormal. The presence of hyper- or hypothermia may be a result of endogenous factors (e.g., infec-

53

tions or hypometabolic states) or exogenous causes (e.g., environmental exposures). The heart rate is typically elevated; however, bradycardia may be present with many conditions, such as intraabdominal hemorrhage (probably secondary to vagal stimulation), cardiovascular medication use (e.g., beta blockers or digoxin), hypoglycemia, and preexisting cardiovascular disease.

The respiratory rate is frequently elevated early in shock. Increased minute ventilation, increased dead space, bronchospasm, and hypocapnia may all be seen. As shock progresses hypoventilation, respiratory failure, and respiratory distress syndrome may occur.

The systolic and diastolic blood pressures (BP) may initially be normal or elevated in response to compensatory mechanisms such as tachycardia and vasoconstriction. As the body's compensatory mechanisms fail, BP typically falls. Postural changes in BP, commonly seen with hypovolemic states, will precede overt hypotension. The pulse pressure, the difference between systolic and diastolic BP measurements, may be a more sensitive indicator. The pulse pressure usually rises early in shock and then decreases before a change in the systolic BP is seen.

In addition to the abovementioned vital sign abnormalities, other cardiovascular manifestations may include neck vein distention or flattening, and cardiac dysrhythmias. An S3 may be auscultated in high-output states. Decreased coronary perfusion pressures can lead to myocardial ischemia, decreased ventricular compliance, increased left ventricular diastolic pressures, and pulmonary edema.

Decreased cerebral perfusion leads to mental status changes such as weakness, restlessness, confusion, disorientation, delirium, syncope, and coma. Patients with long-standing hypertension may exhibit these changes without severe hypotension. Cutaneous manifestations may include pallor, pale or dusky skin, sweating, bruising, petechiae, cyanosis [may not be evident if severe anemia (hemoglobin level less than 5 g/dL) is present], altered temperature, and decreased capillary refill.

GI manifestations resulting from low flow states may include ileus, GI bleeding, pancreatitis, acalculous cholecystitis, and mesenteric ischemia. In an effort to conserve water and sodium, levels of aldosterone and antidiuretic hormone are increased. This results in a reduced glomerular filtration rate, redistribution of blood flow from the renal cortex to the renal medulla, and oliguria. In sepsis, a paradoxical polyuria may occur and be mistaken for adequate hydration.

Early in shock a common metabolic abnormality is a respiratory alkalosis. As the shock state continues and compensatory mechanisms begin to fail, anaerobic metabolism occurs, leading to the formation of lactic acid and resulting in a metabolic acidosis. Other metabolic abnormalities that may be seen are hyperglycemia, hypoglycemia, and hyperkalemia.

Diagnosis and Differential

The clinical presentation and presumed etiology of shock will dictate the diagnostic studies, monitoring modalities, and interventions utilized. The approach to each patient must be individualized; however, frequently performed laboratory studies include complete blood count; platelet count; electrolytes, blood urea nitrogen, and creatinine determinations; prothrombin and partial thromboplastin times; and urinalysis. Other tests commonly utilized are arterial blood gas, lactic acid, fibrinogen, fibrin split products, D-dimer, and cortisol determinations; hepatic function panel; cerebrospinal fluid studies, and cultures of potential sources of infection. A pregnancy test should be performed on all females of childbearing age. Other common diagnostic tests include radiographs (chest and abdominal), electrocardiograms, ultrasound or computed tomography scans (chest, head, abdomen, and pelvis), and echocardiograms.

Continuous monitoring of vital signs should be instituted in all patients. In addition to commonly monitored parameters such as pulse, blood pressure, respiratory rate, and temperature, other modalities, such as pulse oximetry, end-tidal CO_2, central venous pressure (CVP), central venous O_2 saturation, cardiac output, and calculation of systemic vascular resistance, may be indicated.

A search to determine the etiology of the shock must be undertaken. Lack of response to appropriate stabilization measures should cause the clinician to evaluate the patient for a more occult cause. First the physician must be certain that the basic steps of resuscitation have been carried out appropriately. Consider whether or not the patient has been adequately volume resuscitated. Early use of vasopressors may elevate the CVP and mask the presence of continued hypovolemia. Ensure that all equipment is connected and functioning appropriately. Carefully expose and examine the patient for occult wounds. Consider less commonly seen diagnoses, such as cardiac tamponade, tension pneumothorax, adrenal insufficiency, toxic or allergic reactions, and occult bleeding (e.g., rupture of ectopic pregnancy, or occult intraabdominal or pelvic bleeding) in a patient who is not responding as expected.

Please refer to the other chapters in this book regarding the evaluation of the specific forms of shock.

Emergency Department Care and Disposition

The goal of the interventions is to restore adequate tissue perfusion in concert with the identification and treatment of the underlying etiology.

1. Aggressive airway control, often involving endotracheal intubation, is indicated.
2. All patients should receive supplemental high-flow **oxygen**. The tachypnea that often accompanies shock adds to oxygen consumption and therefore may contribute to lactic acid production.
3. Early surgical consultation is indicated for internal bleeding. Most external hemorrhage can be controlled by direct compression. Rarely, clamping or tying off of vessels may be needed. Use of tourniquets is discouraged. All patients require adequate venous access. Cannulation of peripheral veins with large-bore catheters usually provides an adequate route for providing fluid resuscitation. For monitoring and treatment purposes (e.g., long-term vasopressors or pacemakers), however, central venous access may be necessary.
4. Volume replacement. The type, amount, and rate of fluid replacement remain areas of controversy. Most utilize **isotonic crystalloid** intravenous (IV) fluids (0.9% NaCl, Ringer's lactate) in the initial resuscitation phase. Use of colloids [5% albumin, purified protein fraction, fresh-frozen plasma (FFP), and synthetic colloid solutions (hydroxyethyl starch or dextran 70)] continue to be advocated by some. Due to the increased cost, lack of proven benefit, and potential for disease transmission (with FFP), the routine use of colloids is questionable. Standard therapy in the hemodynamically unstable patient typically has been 20 to 40 mL/kg given rapidly (over 10 to 20 min). Since only about 30 percent of infused isotonic crystalloids remain in the intravascular space, it is recommended to infuse approximately three times the estimated blood loss. However, the benefits of early and aggressive fluid replacement in the ED or prehospital setting remain unproven. Studies have suggested that rapid fluid administration may contribute to ongoing hemorrhage by both mechanical effects and dilution of clotting factors. While it is not appropriate to totally withhold fluids, some amount of "underresuscitiation" (i.e., maintaining mean arterial BP around 70 mmHg) may be beneficial until surgical control of the bleeding site can be accomplished. **Blood** remains the ideal resuscitative fluid. Ideally, fully cross-matched blood is preferred. If the clinical situation dictates more rapid intervention, type-specific, type O (Rh negative to be given to females of childbearing years), or autologous blood may be uti-

lized. The decision to use platelets or FFP should be based on clinical evidence of impaired hemostasis and frequent monitoring of coagulation parameters. Platelets are generally given if there is ongoing hemorrhage and the platelet count is 50,000 or less; FFP is indicated if the prothrombin time is prolonged more than 1.5. The pneumatic antishock garment is no longer recommended in the treatment of shock but may be used to splint and control bleeding of the lower extremities.

5. Vasopressors are utilized after appropriate volume resuscitation has occurred and there is persistent hypotension. American Heart Association recommendations based on blood pressure determinations are **dobutamine** 2.0 to 20.0 μg/(kg/min) for systolic BP over 100 mmHg, **dopamine** 2.5 to 20.0 μg/(kg/min) for systolic BP 70 to 100 mmHg, and **norepinephrine** 0.5 to 30.0 μg/min for systolic BP under 70 mmHg.

6. Acidosis should be treated with adequate ventilation and fluid resuscitation. Sodium bicarbonate (1 meq/kg) use is controversial. If it is used, it is given only in the setting of severe acidosis refractory to the abovementioned methods.

7. Early surgical or medical consultation for admission or transfer is indicated.

For further reading in *Emergency Medicine: A Comprehensive Study Guide*, 5th ed., see Chap. 26, "Approach to the Patient in Shock," Emanuel P. Rivers, Mohamed Y. Rady, and Robert Bilkovski; and Chap. 27, "Fluid and Blood Resuscitation," Steven C. Dronen and Eileen M. K. Bobek.

---

6 | Septic Shock

John E. Gough

Sepsis is a heterogenous clinical syndrome that can be caused by any class of microorganism. The incidence of sepsis has risen over the past three decades, affecting approximately 300,000 to 500,000 patients annually in the United States. About one-half of these patients will develop shock with a mortality rate ranging from 20 to 80 percent. The most frequent sites of infection are the lungs, abdomen, and urinary tract. Gram-positive and gram-negative bacteria account for the majority of sepsis. Predisposing factors for gram-negative bacterial sepsis include diabetes mellitus, lymphoproliferative diseases, cirrhosis, burns, invasive procedures, and chemotherapy. Risk factors for gram-positive sepsis include vascular catheters, burns, indwelling mechanical devices, and intravenous drug use. Nonbacterial sepsis is more commonly seen in immunocompromised individuals.

CLINICAL FEATURES

Hyperpyrexia is commonly seen with infectious diseases; however hypothermia is not uncommon with sepsis and septic shock (particularly with the extremes of age and immunocompromised patients). Other abnormalities concerning vital signs may include tachycardia, wide pulse pressure, tachypnea, and hypotension.

Mental status changes are commonly seen ranging from mild disorientation to coma. Ophthalmic manifestations include retinal hemorrhages, cotton wool spots, and conjunctival petechiae.

Early cardiovascular manifestations include vasodilatation resulting in warm extremities. Cardiac output is initially maintained through a compensatory tachycardia. Myocardial depression may occur early in sepsis. As sepsis progresses, hypotension may occur. Patients in septic shock may demonstrate a diminished response to volume replacement.

Respiratory symptoms include tachypnea and hypoxemia. Sepsis remains the most common condition associated with acute respiratory distress syndrome (ARDS), which may occur within minutes to hours from the onset of sepsis.

Renal manifestations include azotemia, oliguria, and active urinary sediment. Azotemia and oliguria are usually attributed to acute tubular necrosis (ATN). While the exact pathogenesis of ATN is unknown, predisposing factors include hypotension, dehydration, aminoglycoside administration, and pigmenturia.

Liver dysfunction is common, with the most frequent presentation being cholestatic jaundice. Increases in transaminases, alkaline phosphatase (up to 3 times that of normal levels), and bilirubin are often seen. Severe or prolonged hypotension may induce acute hepatic injury or ischemic bowel necrosis. Painless mucosal erosions may occur in the stomach and/or duodenum and predispose the patient to upper GI bleeds.

Cutaneous lesions may be the result of (*a*) direct invasion (cellulitis, erysipelas, or fasciitis), (*b*) a consequence of hypotension and/or disseminated intravascular coagulation (DIC; acrocyanosis or necrosis of peripheral tissues), and (c) secondary to infective endocarditis (microemboli or immune complex vasculitis).

Frequent hematologic changes include neutropenia, neutrophilia, thrombocytopenia, and DIC. A "left shift," resulting from demargination and release of less mature granulocytes from the marrow, is common. Neutropenia, which occurs rarely, is associated with increased mortality.

The hemoglobin and hematocrit are usually not affected unless the sepsis is prolonged or there is an associated GI bleed. Thrombocytopenia may be associated with DIC, although isolated thrombocytopenia may be present in over 30 percent of patients with sepsis and may be an early clue to bacteremia. More commonly associated with gram-negative sepsis, DIC may have either a "compensated" or "decompensated" form. The compensated form occurs when there is increased coagulation factor production in the liver, release of platelets from storage sites, and increased synthesis of inhibitors. Uncompensated DIC presents with clinical bleeding and/or thrombosis. Laboratory studies suggesting DIC include thrombocytopenia, prolonged prothrombin time (PT) and partial thromboplastin time (PTT), decreased fibrinogen level and antithrombin levels, and increased fibrin monomer, fibrin split values, and D-dimer values.

Hyperglycemia may be the result of increased catecholamines, cortisol, and glucagon. Increased insulin resistance, decreased insulin production, and impaired utilization of insulin may further contribute to hyperglycemia. Rarely, depletion of glucagon and inhibition of gluconeogenesis lead to hyperglycemia.

Early in sepsis, blood-gas determinations often reveal hypoxemia and a respiratory alkalosis. As perfusion worsens and glycolysis increases, a metabolic acidosis occurs. This acidosis is further exacerbated by lactic acid production.

DIAGNOSIS AND DIFFERENTIAL

Septic shock should be suspected in any patient with a temperature of $> 38°$ or $< 36°C$, systolic blood pressure of < 90 mmHg, and evidence of inadequate organ perfusion. Hypotension should not reverse with volume replacement. Other clinical features include mental obtundation, hyperventilation, hot or flushed skin, and a widened pulse pressure. History and physical examination, coupled with other diagnostic modalities, will often aid in identifying the source of the infection.

Many diagnostic tests are available to aid in the identification of the source of sepsis; however, septic shock remains a clinical diagnosis. Laboratory tests such as a complete blood cell count, platelet count, DIC panel (PT, PTT, fibrinogen, D-dimer, and antithrombin concentration), electrolyte levels, liver function tests, renal function tests, arterial blood gas (ABG) analysis, and urinalysis are often utilized. Bacterial cultures of blood and urine should be obtained on all septic patients. Additionally, cultures of the cerebrospinal fluid, sputum, and other secretions should be obtained as indicated. A gram stain and counter immunoelectrophoresis (CIE) can help quickly identify pathogens and guide initial therapy. Radiographs of suspected foci of infection (chest, abdomen, etc.) should be obtained. Ultrasonography or computed tomography scanning may help identify occult infections in the cranium, thorax, abdomen, and pelvis. As acute meningitis is the most common central nervous system infection associated with septic shock, a lumbar puncture should quickly be performed when indicated. If meningitis is a serious consideration, empiric antibiotic therapy should be instituted as soon as possible. Differential diagnosis should include other noninfectious types of shock such as hypovolemic, cardiogenic, neurogenic, and anaphylactic.

EMERGENCY DEPARTMENT CARE AND DISPOSITION

1. The *ABC*s of resuscitation should be addressed. Aggressive airway management with high-flow oxygen and endotracheal intubation may be necessary.
2. **Hemodynamic stabilization.** Rapid infusion of crystalloid IV fluid (LR or not significant) at 500 mL (20 mL/kg in children) every 5 to 10 min. Often 4 to 6 L (60 mL/kg in children) may be necessary. In addition to blood pressure, mental status, pulse, capillary refill, central venous pressure, pulmonary capillary wedge pressure, and urine output (> 30 mL/h in adult, > 1 mL/kg per h in children) should be monitored. If ongoing blood loss (e.g., GI bleed) is suspected, blood replacement may be necessary.
3. **Dopamine** 5 to 20 μg/kg per min titrated to response should be used.
4. If blood pressure remains < 70 mmHg despite preceding measures, **norepinephrine** 8 to 12 μg/min loading dose and 2 to 4 μg/min infusion to maintain mean arterial blood pressure of at least 60 mmHg should be started.
5. The **source of infection** must be removed (e.g., removal of indwelling catheters and I&D of abscesses).
6. **Empiric antibiotic therapy.** This measure is ideally begun after obtaining cultures but administration should not be delayed. Dosages should be maximum allowed and given intravenously.

(Initial/loading doses listed.) When source is unknown, therapy should be effective against both gram-positive and gram-negative organisms. For antibiotic therapy in children, see Chap. 70. In adults a third-generation **cephalosporin** (e.g., **ceftriaxone** 1 g IV, or **cefotaxime** 2 g IV, **ceftazidime** 2 g IV) or an antipseudomonal β-lactimase-susceptible penicillin (**imipenum** 750 mg IV) can be used. Also recommended is the addition of an aminoglycoside (**gentamicin** 2 mg/kg IV, **tobramycin** 2 mg/kg IV) to this regimen. In immunocompromised adults **ceftazidime** 2 g IV, or **imipenem** 750 mg IV, or **meropenum** 1 g IV alone is acceptable. If there is high probability of gram-positive etiology (e.g., illicit drug use) **oxacillin** 2 g IV or **vancomycin** 15 mg/kg IV should be added. If an anaerobic source is suspected (e.g., intra-abdominal, genital tract, odontologic, and necrotizing soft tissue infection) **metronidazole** 7.5 mg/kg IV or **clindamycin** 0.45 g IV should additionally be administered. If *Legionella* is a potential source, **erythromycin** 0.5 g IV can be added. **Vancomycin** 15 mg/kg IV can be added if indwelling vascular devices are present.

7. Acidosis is treated with oxygen, ventilation, IV fluid replacement. If severe, administration of sodium bicarbonate 1 meq/kg IV is acceptable or as directed by ABGs.

8. DIC should be treated with **fresh frozen plasma** 15 to 20 mL/kg initially to keep PT at 1.5 to 2 times normal and treated with **platelet infusion** to maintain serum concentration of 50 to 100 times 10^9 per liter.

9. If adrenal insufficiency is suspected, glucocorticoid (**solucortef** 100 mg IV) should be administered.

For further reading in *Emergency Medicine: A Comprehensive Study Guide,* 5th ed., see Chap. 28, "Septic Shock," by Jonathan Jui.

---

7 | Cardiogenic Shock
John E. Gough

Cardiogenic shock results from an impairment of the heart's pumping ability such that there is inadequate perfusion to meet the resting metabolic demands of the tissues. The etiology is most commonly related to a loss of effective myocardial contractility as seen with acute myocardial infarction (AMI), left ventricular (LV) aneurysm, cardiomyopathies, myocarditis, myocardial contusion, and drug or toxin effects. Mechanical impairments to systemic blood flow such as valvular dysfunctions, pulmonary embolism, wall rupture, tamponade, and aortic dissection may also play a role in the development of cardiogenic shock. Cardiogenic shock is the most frequent cause of in-hospital death associated with an AMI. The median time for the development of cardiogenic shock after AMI is approximately 7 h from the onset of symptoms. Risk factors for the development of cardiogenic shock following AMI include: advanced age, female gender, large MI, anterior wall MI, previous MI, history of congestive heart failure (CHF), multivessel disease, proximal occlusion of the left anterior descending artery, and diabetes mellitus. Early recognition and aggressive intervention is essential as the mortality rate is extremely high.

CLINICAL FEATURES

The hallmark of all shock states is hypoperfusion. Cardiogenic shock commonly, but not always, presents with hypotension (systolic blood pressure < 90 mmHg). Other blood pressure parameters that may be more sensitive are a 30 mmHg decrease in mean arterial blood pressure and a pulse pressure of less than 20 mmHg. Sinus tachycardia is frequently seen and treatment should be directed at the underlying cause. Other common findings include cool, clammy skin and oliguria. Decreased cerebral perfusion and hypoxemia may lead to mental status changes such as anxiety and confusion. Concomitant left ventricular failure will frequently present with tachypnea, rales, wheezing, and frothy sputum. Jugular venous distention without pulmonary edema in the setting of hypotension should raise the suspicion of RV infarction, tamponade, or pulmonary embolus. Cardiac auscultation should be performed to identify the presence of an S_3 or S_4. The presence of a murmur may represent either valvular dysfunction or septal defects.

DIAGNOSIS AND DIFFERENTIAL

As with most patients encountered in the emergency department, a careful, directed history and physical examination is useful in the initial evaluation of a patient with suspected AMI and cardiogenic shock. Other clinical entities that may mimic cardiogenic shock include aortic dissection, pulmonary embolus, pericardial tamponade, acute valvular insufficiency, hemorrhage, and sepsis.

Perhaps the most important test that should be quickly obtained is the 12-lead electrocardiogram (ECG). Acute ST changes and conduction delays may confirm the presence of an AMI. Right-sided precordial leads should be performed in suspected acute inferior and posterior MIs. A chest radiograph should also be obtained quickly looking for evidence of CHF, wide mediastinum, or abnormalities of the cardiac silhouette.

Other ancillary tests such as baseline laboratory studies including a complete blood count, coagulation parameters, chemistries, serum lactate, and arterial blood gases should be obtained when appropriate. Serum markers of myocardial injury (CK-MB, troponin I, and troponin II) will also be useful in establishing the diagnosis of an AMI.

A bedside two-dimensional transthoracic echocardiogram (TTE) is a modality that can help differentiate the causes of cardiogenic shock as well as evaluate other causes of decreased cardiac output. TTE can identify regional hypokinetic, akinetic, or dyskinetic abnormalities. Detection of early signs of distress such as lack of compensatory hyperkinesis can guide in the initiation of inotropic support as well as the consultation of invasive cardiologists. Other causes of decreased cardiac output that can be evaluated with TTE include pulmonary hypertension seen with pulmonary embolism (RV dilation, tricuspid insufficiency, paradoxical septal motion, and high estimated RV, and pulmonary artery pressures); cardiac tamponade (pericardial effusion, collapse of right atrium, and diastolic RV collapse); RV infarction (loss of RV contractility, RV dilatation, and normal estimated pulmonary pressures); valvular stenosis or insufficiency; septal and free wall ruptures; and dissection involving the aortic root.

Invasive hemodynamic monitoring with a pulmonary artery catheter can provide important information. It is most commonly performed in the intensive care unit as opposed to the ED setting.

EMERGENCY DEPARTMENT CARE AND DISPOSITION

The priorities in the care of the patient with cardiogenic shock are the same as with all unstable patients, that is, rapid evaluation and treatment of life threats with attention to the ABCs of resuscitation. In light of the high mortality rate despite interventions, decisions as to withholding aggressive care should be determined based on patient and family wishes.

1. **Initial stabilization.** If there is a high flow of O_2, endotracheal intubation, intravenous access, cardiac rhythm, and pulse oximetry monitoring should be considered.

2. Rhythm disturbances, hypoxemia, hypovolemia, and electrolyte abnormalities should be identified and treated.
3. **Aspirin** 160 to 325 mg. The patient should chew and swallow unless there is an allergy or contraindication.
4. Intravenous nitroglycerin or morphine sulfate, titrated to response, should be administered as needed for chest pain, as well as hemodynamic parameters monitored.
5. For mild to moderate hypotension, in absence of hypovolemia, **dobutamine** 2.5 to 20.0 μg/kg per min should be administered. For severe hypotension **dopamine** 2.5 to 20.0 μg/kg per min should be used, titrated to desired effect and utilized at the lowest dose possible.
6. Intravenous **nitroglycerin** 5 to 100 μg/min and **sodium nitroprusside** 0.5 to 10.0 μg/kg per min should be used to improve cardiac output through reduction of preload and afterload.
7. **Intra-aortic balloon pump.** To decrease afterload the measure should be temporized and diastolic pressure and coronary perfusion augmented.
8. **Thrombolytic therapy**, percutaneous transluminal angioplasty (PCTA), emergent CABG should be used as indicated or available.
9. Cardiology and cardiac surgery should be consulted early. Transfer should be arranged if indicated.

For further reading in *Emergency Medicine: A Comprehensive Study Guide,* 5th ed., see Chap. 29, "Cardiogenic Shock," by Raymond E. Jackson.

---

8 | Neurogenic Shock

John E. Gough

Neurogenic shock occurs after an injury to the spinal cord. Sympathetic outflow is disrupted resulting in unopposed vagal tone. The major clinical signs are hypotension and bradycardia. Acute spinal cord injury is most commonly seen with blunt trauma accounting for approximately 85 to 90 percent of cases. The most commonly affected area is the cervical region, followed by the thoracolumbar junction, the thoracic region, and the lumbar region. Neurogenic shock must be differentiated from "spinal" shock. *Spinal shock* is defined as temporary loss of spinal reflex activity occurring below a total or near-total spinal cord injury.

CLINICAL FEATURES

Patients are generally hypotensive with warm, dry skin. The loss of sympathetic tone may impair the ability to redirect blood flow from the periphery to the core circulation leading to excessive heat loss and hypothermia. Bradycardia is a characteristic finding of neurogenic shock; however, it is not universally present. These symptoms can be expected to last from one to three weeks.

The anatomic level of the injury to the spinal cord impacts the likelihood and severity of neurogenic shock. Injuries above the T1 level have the capability of disrupting the spinal cord tracts that control the entire sympathetic system. Injuries occurring in the levels from T1 to L3 may only partially interrupt the sympathetic outflow. The higher the level of injury the more likely it is for the patient to exhibit severe symptoms.

Neurogenic shock may be present with both complete and incomplete spinal cord lesions. The initial presentation represents the acute traumatic injury to the cord. However, a secondary cord injury may evolve over the first few days to weeks following the initial injury. The secondary cord injury is thought to be a result of ischemia to the spinal cord and may lead to a higher level of dysfunction than originally present or to an incomplete injury becoming a complete lesion.

DIAGNOSIS AND DIFFERENTIAL

The diagnosis of neurogenic shock should be one of exclusion. Neurogenic shock must be differentiated from other types of shock, particularly hypovolemic. When dealing with a trauma patient, one must always assume that any hypotension is a result of ongoing blood loss. A patient suffering from neurogenic shock may also have concomitant injuries which may contribute to hemodynamic instability. Clinical clues such as hypotension, bradycardia, neurologic dysfunction, and warm, dry skin may lead the clinician to suspect neurogenic shock; however, only after other injuries have been identified and treated can the diagnosis of neurogenic shock safely be made.

EMERGENCY DEPARTMENT CARE AND DISPOSITION

The initial evaluation and care of the patient with potential neurogenic shock is the same as for all trauma patients, that is, rapid identification and stabilization of life-threatening injuries.

1. Airway control should be insured with spinal immobilization and protection.

2. **Crystalloid** IV fluids should be infused to maintain a mean arterial blood pressure above 70 torr. To prevent excessive fluid administration, a pulmonary artery catheter may be placed to monitor hemodynamic response. If fluid resuscitation is inadequate to insure organ perfusion, inotropic agents such as **dopamine** 2.5 to 20.0 μg/kg per min and **dobutamine** 2.0 to 20.0 μg/kg per min may be added to improve cardiac output and perfusion pressure. The doses should be titrated to the appropriate clinical response.

3. If necessary, severe bradycardia may need to be treated with **atropine** 0.5 to 1.0 mg IV (every 5 min for a total dose of 3.0 mg) or with a pacemaker.

4. In the presence of neurologic deficits, **high-dose methylprednisolone** therapy should be instituted within 8 h of injury. A 30 mg/kg bolus should be administered over 15 min followed by a continuous infusion of 5.4 mg/kg per h for the next 23 h.

5. Trauma surgery, neurosurgery, and orthopedic consultation should be obtained and arrangement made for transfer if necessary.

For further reading in *Emergency Medicine: A Comprehensive Study Guide,* 5th ed., see Chap. 31, "Neurogenic Shock," by Brian Euerle and Thomas M. Scalea.

9	Anaphylaxis and Acute Allergic Reactions

Christian A. Tomaszewski

Allergic reactions can range from trivial-appearing urticaria to full-blown anaphylaxis with cardiovascular collapse and respiratory compromise. The most common etiologies include intravenous penicillin and hymenoptera stings. Although most acute allergic reactions are type I, where an antigen interacts with IgE on mast cells and basophils, other hypersensitivity reactions include type II antigen interacting with IgG and IgM antibodies (e.g., blood transfusion reaction, idiopathic thrombocytopenic purpura); type III, deposition of antigen-antibody complexes (e.g., serum sickness, poststreptococcal glomerulonephritis); and type IV, delayed hypersensitivity reaction from T lymphocytes (e.g., poison ivy, skin test for tuberculosis).

Clinical Features

Anaphylaxis can occur within seconds, but can be delayed an hour, after a sensitized individual is exposed to such things as (*a*) drugs (e.g., penicillin and trimethoprim-sulfamethoxazole), (*b*) foods (e.g., shellfish, nuts, eggs, and preservatives such as sulfites and tetrazine dyes), and (*c*) stings (especially hymenoptera). In addition, such things as dextran, codeine, and radiocontrast material can cause an anaphylactoid reaction, which is non-IgE-mediated and requires no sensitizing exposure. Both anaphylaxis and anaphylactoid reactions have the same final common pathway, through mast-cell degranulation. Finally, aspirin and other nonsteroidal anti-inflmmatory drugs can cause anaphylactic symptoms through modulation of the cycloxygenase-arachidonic acid pathway.

Anaphylactic reactions range from local organ involvement to serious multisystem effects. Dermatologic features include pruritis, urticaria, erythema multiforme, and angioedema. The latter can be seen as an isolated response to angiotensin-converting enzyme (ACE) inhibitors. By definition, anaphylaxis includes either respiratory compromise or cardiovascular collapse. Respiratory features may include tracheal swelling, stridor, wheezing, and respiratory arrest. Gastrointestinal (GI) features include nausea, cramps, vomiting, and diarrhea. Untreated, anaphylaxis leads to shock with tachycardia and hypotension. Cardiac patients are susceptible to myocardial ischemia as well as an exaggerated allergic response if on β blockers. If patients survive the initial insult, a second phase of mediator release can occur at 4 to 8 h in up to 20 percent of cases.

Diagnosis and Differential

Diagnosis will be based on symptoms seen in any particular patient. Usually history will confirm exposure to a potential allergen, such as a new drug, food, or insect sting. There is no specific test available in the emergency department to confirm the diagnosis.

Workup, however, may include a complete blood cell count, glucose, electrolyte levels, urinalysis, and arterial blood gas analysis, depending on presenting symptoms. The differential includes myocardial infarction, asthma, carcinoid, hereditary angioedema, and vasovagal reactions.

Emergency Department Care and Disposition

The airway is the primary concern in the treatment of any allergic reaction. Patients with respiratory symptoms or abnormal vital signs should be placed on pulse oximetry and cardiac monitor with intravenous access. The combination of oxygen and epinephrine can usually reverse any impending respiratory compromise.

1. High-flow oxygen should be administered by face-mask, if necessary, to maintain adequate oxygenation. Endotracheal intubation, if required, can be difficult because of angioedema or laryngeal spasm; therefore, preparation should be made for transtracheal jet insufflation or cricothyroidotomy.
2. Any patient with airway symptoms or hypotension should receive **epinephrine**. This can be given subcutaneously 0.3 to 0.5 mg (0.3 to 0.5 mL) of 1:1000 (pediatric dose 0.01 mL/kg). In the presence of shock or respiratory arrest, a bolus of 100 μg of intravenous epinephrine as a 1:100,000 dilution (0.1 mL of 1:1000 in 10 mL normal saline) can be given over 5 to 10 min.
3. Attention must be made to termination of further exposure. This may be as simple as stopping an intravenous line of drug or removing a stinger.
4. Most patients, especially if hypotensive, will require large volumes of **crystalloid fluids**. If after 1 to 2 L, patients are still hypotensive, then intravenous epinephrine (1:10,000) should be administered at 1 to 4 μg/min (pediatric dose, 0.1 to 1 μg/kg/min).
5. Every patient with allergic symptoms requires antihistamines. **Diphenhydramine** can be given 25 to 50 mg (pediatric dose 1 mg/kg), intravenously in serious cases. In addition, an H_2 blocker such as **ranitidine** 50 mg intravenously (pediatric dose 0.5 mg/kg) can be helpful.
6. After treatment with epinephrine, any persistent bronchospasm can be treated with nebulized β **agonists,** such as **albuterol** 0.5 mL of 5% in 3 mL saline.
7. **Steroids** are useful in controlling persistent or delayed allergic reactions. Severe cases can be treated with **methylprednisolone** 125 mg (pediatric dose 1 to 2 mg/kg) intravenously. Milder reactions can be treated with oral **prednisone**, 60 mg to start.
8. If patients are taking β blockers, **glucagon** (1 to 2 mg every 5

min) can be used for hypotension refractory to epinephrine and fluids.

In mild reactions, patients may be observed several hours prior to discharge. Severe cases, with any evidence of hypotension or respiratory compromise, deserve prolonged observation (> 6 h) with repeated doses of antihistamines and steroids as needed. Patients can be discharged on an antihistamine and prednisone for 4 days. Remember, all serious cases deserve preventive therapy upon discharge. This includes a self-administration epinephrine kit, as well as referral to an allergist for desensitization therapy. The recurrence rate for anaphylaxis from insect stings is 40 to 60 percent.

For further reading in *Emergency Medicine: A Comprehensive Study Guide,* 5th ed., see Chap. 30, "Anaphylaxis and Acute Allergic Reactions," by Shaheed I. Koury and Lee U. Herfel.

ANALGESIA, ANESTHESIA, AND SEDATION

10 | Acute Pain Management and Conscious Sedation

Frantz R. Melio

The underutilization of sedation and analgesia in the emergency department has been well documented. Reasons for this include misunderstanding of a patient's response to pain, lack of knowledge of the pharmacokinetics of the various agents used, fear of serious side effects, and issues related to convenience. Patients at risk for receiving suboptimal treatment include children, those who cannot communicate with care givers, the elderly, and the cognitively impaired. It is crucial not to confuse sedation and analgesia.

Clinical Features

Physiologic responses to pain and anxiety include increased heart rate, blood pressure, and respiratory rate. Behavioral changes include facial expressions, posturing, crying, and vocalization. Pain is best assessed using objective scales. Subjective impressions are often incorrect. Pain relief is a dynamic process, and reassessment is mandatory.

Emergency Department Care and Disposition

When treating anxious patients or patients in need of uncomfortable procedures, one should begin with nonpharmacologic interventions (e.g., relaxation, distraction, psychoprophylaxis, biofeedback, and guided imagery). Communication should be appropriate for the developmental age of the patient. A gentle and unhurried approach is best. Procedures should be explained in a clear and honest manner, with time given for questions and answers. With children, discussing the procedure just before it is performed should minimize anticipation of painful procedures. Environmental adjustments, such as dimmed lights, a quiet room, and audiovisual input, may be helpful. Parents should be included in interventions, since their help may be crucial in comforting their child. Certain children will require restraints. Parents should be relieved of the responsibility of restraining their child. Once the necessity for pharmacologic interventions has been determined, consideration should be given to the need for sedation or analgesia, the route of delivery, and the desired duration of effects.

Systemic Analgesia and Sedation

Conscious sedation (CS) is a medically controlled state of depressed consciousness that allows protective reflexes to be maintained. Patients undergoing CS should be able to maintain a patent airway and respond to stimulation or commands. Indications for systemic analgesia and/or CS include treatment of severe pain, attenuation of pain and anxiety associated with procedures, rapid tranquilization, and the need to perform a diagnostic procedure.

Preparation Whenever systemic analgesia or sedation is used, the patient should be continuously monitored (cardiac monitor and pulse oximetry) and under constant observation by a dedicated health care provider who is trained in airway management. Oxygen, suction, and appropriately sized airway equipment should be readily accessible. Precalculated doses of reversal agents should be available: **naloxone**, 0.1 mg/kg per dose given every 2 to 3 min until desired effect to reverse opiates, **flumazenil**, 0.01 to 0.02 mg/kg, with additional 0.005 mg doses, to a maximum 0.2 mg per dose and 1 mg total. The half-life of naloxone and flumazenil may be shorter than that of the drugs they reverse. Therefore, patients who require reversal should be observed for a prolonged period of time to avoid rebound cardiovascular or respiratory depression. Flumazenil should not be used in patients on chronic benzodiazepine or tricyclic antidepressant therapy due to the risk of seizure. A baseline blood pressure, heart rate, respiratory rate, and level of consciousness should be assessed and documented every 5 to 10 min. Generally, administering medications intravenously (IV) is the best method for obtaining rapid and safe analgesia or sedation. Other routes may be appropriate (especially in children), but provide less reliable and slower clinical effects, limit the ability to titrate, and result in frequent under- or overmedication. The use of these agents should be individualized to the patient and planned procedure. The physician must consider his or her skill and expertise with the intended medications and what resources are available. Informed consent, with a discussion of the risks and benefits of CS, should be obtained. These agents have a narrow therapeutic index. Using the smallest effective total dose, given in small IV increments and allowing adequate time for peak effect, is generally the safest method of administering these agents.

Analgesia for brief procedures Opiates are the drugs of choice for analgesia. Fentanyl is a synthetic narcotic, that is 100 times more potent than morphine. It has almost immediate onset of action and approximately 30 min duration when administered IV. Fentanyl and other narcotics are relatively contraindicated in patients with hemodynamic or respiratory compromise, as well as those with altered mental status. Fentanyl is less likely to cause respiratory depression, histamine release, and cardiovascular compromise than are other opiates. Administering fentanyl slowly over 3 to 5 min can minimize respiratory depression. Fentanyl is associated with chest wall rigidity at higher doses (5 to 15 μg/kg), which may require naloxone reversal or neuromuscular blockage and intubation. The dose of **fentanyl** is 2 to 3 μg/kg, with additional doses titrated by 0.5 μg/kg until the desired level of analgesia is reached. Fentanyl is also available in a self-administered lozenge, which has been found practical in the pediatric patient.

Nitrous oxide is an effective analgesic that produces a state of conscious sedation with euphoria and dissociation. It can be used alone or in conjunction with local anesthetics. **Nitrous oxide** is delivered as a 30 to 50% mixture with oxygen. It should be self-administered through a system that is fail-safe against delivery of a hypoxic mixture. Peak effects are reached within 1 to 2 min, and the patient is fully aroused within minutes of cessation of therapy. Nitrous oxide has minimal respiratory or cardiovascular effects. It is contraindicated in patients who have recently been sedated with another agent, and those with altered mental status, balloon tipped catheters, dyspnea, severe chronic obstructive pulmonary disease, pneumothorax, eye injury, or obstructed viscous.

Ketamine is a dissociative analgesic that also has sedative properties. Ketamine is usually given intramuscularly (IM) or IV to adults. Oral (PO), rectal (PR), IM, and IV administration has been described in children. The dose of **ketamine** is 4 mg/kg when given PO, PR, and IM. A supplemental 2 mg/kg dose may be given. The IV dose is 1 mg/kg, with additional 0.25 mg/kg doses titrated to the desired effect. **Atropine** (0.01 mg/kg) is often used as an adjunct to control hypersalivation. Although airway reflexes are usually protected and bronchodilation occurs, ketamine can cause laryngospasm. Ketamine has catecholamine-releasing properties. It should be avoided in the setting of head trauma, and in patients with poor sympathetic tone or prolonged stress. Adults and older children may have unpleasant hallucinations when awakening from ketamine-induced sedation. Placing recovering patients in a darkened, quiet room may minimize this emergence reaction. **Low-dose midazolam** (0.01 mg/kg IM or IV or 0.1 mg/kg PO) attenuates this experience, but it may lead to respiratory depression.

Analgesia for longer procedures Morphine is the gold standard for this use. Meperidine is a synthetic derivative of morphine that is one-tenth as potent and has a shorter duration. Meperidine causes more histamine release than does morphine, and its primary metabolite, normeperidine, is bioactive and toxic (causing central nervous system excitation and seizures). Meperidine can cause a fatal reaction when used in patients taking monoamine oxidase inhibitors and can accumulate in patients with renal insufficiency. The IV dose of **morphine** is 0.1 mg/kg, with additional doses of 0.05 mg/kg titrated to the desired effect. The dose of **meperidine** is 1 mg/kg, with additional 0.5 mg/kg doses given, if necessary. Most adults will require a total dose of 1.5 to 3.0 mg/kg of meperidine for a painful procedure. An adult 1 mg dose of **hydromorphone** is equivalent to a 5 mg dose of morphine. The Demerol, Phenergar, Thorazine (DPT) cocktail is unreliable, can cause respiratory depression, and has a duration of action of more than 7 h. More appropriate regimens should be used in its place.

Hydroxyzine is synergistic with opiates and has intrinsic analgesic properties. **Hydroxyzine**, 0.5 mg/kg, can be given PO or IM in conjunction with narcotics. Hydroxyzine will reduce the incidence of nausea and vomiting associated with opiate administration.

Phenothiazines do not enhance analgesia and produce nonreversible sedation. Their use in this setting should be limited to the treatment of nausea.

Ketorolac is a nonsteroidal anti-inflammatory drug (NSAID) that can be given PO, IM, or IV. The IM and IV doses are 0.5 to 1 mg/kg (maximum 60 mg, 30 mg in the elderly). Ketorolac does not cause respiratory depression. It can be used in combination with opiate analgesics. The most common side effects are related to gastrointestinal irritation, platelet inhibition, and renal damage. Ketorolac has not been shown to be more effective than less expensive oral NSAIDs. It should not be used for more than 5 days.

Sedation for brief procedures Benzodiazepines are sedative agents that provide skeletal muscle relaxation, anxiolysis, and amnesia. They have no direct analgesic properties. When used in combination with opioids, it is generally safer to administer the benzodiazepine first for sedation or relaxation, followed by carefully titrating the opioid for analgesia. The dose of opioid required is usually lowered in these cases, and patients are more prone to developing respiratory compromise. Hypotension, another side effect of benzodiazepines, can be avoided by administering these agents slowly. **Midazolam** is a short-acting (30 to 40 min) benzodiazepine that has been successfully used by PO, PR, nasal, subcutaneous, IM, and IV routes. It is a potent sedative with excellent amnestic properties. An effective adult dosage regimen is 0.25 to 1 mg every 3 to 5 min, until sedation or muscular relaxation occurs. Lower dosages may be more appropriate for the elderly or intoxicated patient. Pediatric doses are IV 0.05 to 0.1 mg/kg per dose every 3 to 5 min (maximum single dose 2 mg, maximum total dose 0.2 mg/kg), IM 0.1 to 0.3 mg/kg, PO 0.5 to 0.75 mg/kg (maximum dose 15 mg), nasal 0.3 to 0.5 mg/kg (maximum dose 5 mg), and PR 0.25 to 0.5 mg/kg (maximum dose 15 mg).

The actions and side effects of barbiturates are similar to those of benzodiazepines. Two important differences must be noted: (1) barbiturates can increase airway tone and, therefore, should not be given to patients with moderate to severe airway disease; and (2) these agents must be used cautiously, since patients may rapidly progress from light sedation to deep sedation to general anesthesia.

Methohexital and thiopental are ultra–short-acting barbiturates, with methohexital having a shorter duration of action. **Methohexital**, 0.5 to 2 mg/kg, or **thiopental**, 1 to 5 mg/kg, will produce sedation within 1 to 2 min. These drugs are administered slowly by titrated incremental IV doses. Methohexital may be given rectally to children in doses of 20 mg/kg. Thiopental frequently causes hypotension, particularly when given rapidly. This effect is accentuated in the presence of hypovolemia, or preexisting heart disease. These agents may also cause laryngospasm and paradoxical excitation.

Propofol is an ultra–short-acting anesthetic. When given by infusion, its onset and resolution are rapid (5 to 10 min). It has antiemetic but no amnestic properties. Propofol can lead to profound cardiovascular and respiratory depression especially in the elderly. It is a relatively new drug for the emergency department. Its use in children is controversial. **Propofol** can be given as a bolus of 2.0 to 2.5 μg/kg, but an infusion is preferred, given at a rate of 25 μg/kg/min and titrated to the desired effect; then a maintenance infusion of 3 to 6 mg/kg/h is continued until the conclusion of the procedure.

Sedation for longer procedures Diazepam is a longer-acting benzodiazepine with anxiolytic and amnestic properties. It has been largely superseded by midazolam.

Pentobarbital is a barbiturate that induces sleep and can be administered by various routes. Within 1 min, IV administration can lead to sleep that lasts for 15 to 60 min. Recommended dosage varies greatly. An initial 2.5 mg/kg (maximum, 100 mg) IV dose can be given, followed, as needed, every 5 min by an additional 1.25 mg/kg (maximum total 300 mg). Intramuscular dosage is 2 to 5 mg/kg, with a maximum dose of 100 to 200 mg. Pentobarbital can cause respiratory and cardiovascular depression, particularly when administered rapidly or in conjunction with a narcotic.

Chloral hydrate has been used successfully, particularly in children under 4 years old. It is unlikely to cause respiratory depression. **Chloral hydrate** can be administered PO or PR at a dosage of 75 mg/kg. Its main disadvantage is its 30- to 60-min onset of action and its prolonged duration (up to several hours).

Disposition Patients are eligible for discharge only when fully recovered. When discharged, the patient must be accompanied by an adult and should not drive. Instructions for care must be given to responsible accompanying adults, since many of these systemic agents impair recall.

Local and Regional Anesthesia

Local and regional anesthesia are essential for emergency department pain management. Agents can be administered topically, by infiltration, and IV. This discussion focuses on topical and infiltrative anesthesia, with a discussion of finger and toe blocks. For discussion of other nerve and regional blocks, please refer to *Emergency Medicine: A Comprehensive Study Guide,* 5th ed., Chap. 32. Newer, less invasive methods are becoming available.

Infiltrative anesthesia There are two classes of local anesthetics (LAs): amides and esters. **Lidocaine** is an amide anesthetic with excellent efficacy and a low toxicity profile. The onset of action is 2 to 5 min and the duration 1 to 2 h. Injection of lidocaine is painful due to its acidic pH. Pain can be minimized by buffering the lidocaine with bicarbonate (in a proportion of 1 $NaHCO_3$:9 lidocaine), warming the medication before injection, using small gauge needles (27 or 30 gauge) for injection, and injecting the anesthetic slowly. The addition of epinephrine to lidocaine provides for a longer duration of anesthesia, provides wound homeostasis, and slows systemic absorption (thus decreasing toxicity). The addition of epinephrine increases the pain of injection by lowering the pH of the solution. Epinephrine also decreases local perfusion. It therefore cannot be used in an end-arterial field (i.e., digits, penis, nose, or ears). The vasoconstrictive properties of epinephrine may also make wounds more prone to infection. **Bupivacaine** has a longer duration than lidocaine and is preferred for prolonged procedures. The onset of action is similar to that of lidocaine. Buffering of bupivacaine is accomplished with 1 $NaHCO_3$:29 bupivacaine. **Procaine** and **tetracaine** are ester anesthetics that can be used in patients with allergies to amide anesthetics.

The toxicity of LAs can be severe and lead to cardiovascular collapse, seizures, and death. Toxicity is related to total dose and mode of delivery. The absorption of these agents is site dependent. The maximum dose of lidocaine is 4.5 mg/kg without epinephrine, and 7 mg/kg with epinephrine. The maximum toxic doses of bupivacaine are 2 mg/kg without and 3 mg/kg with epinephrine. When used for intercostal nerve blocks, the maximum safe dose is 10 times less than the mentioned doses for lidocaine and bupivacaine. Please refer to Chap. 32 in *Emergency Medicine: A Comprehensive Study Guide,* 5th ed., for a full discussion on toxic doses and effects. Allergic reactions to LAs are rare and usually due to preservatives. The safest approach in a patient who claims to be allergic to an LA is to skin test with 0.1 mL of preservative-free anesthetic from the other class of LA. An alternative approach is to use diphenhydramine (0.5 to 1%) for anesthesia. This is also associated with significant toxicity, and its effectiveness is questionable.

Local anesthetic infiltration The most common use of LA is infiltration for wound repair or invasive painful procedures. When repairing wounds, LA is infiltrated into the wound margins or as a "field block" surrounding the wound. When infiltrating intact skin, raising a wheal may cause less pain on subsequent infiltration. LA can also be used in orthopedic procedures, such as fracture and joint reduction, by directly injecting the LA into the affected joint or fracture hematoma.

Digital blocks Finger and toe blocks are advantageous in that less anesthetic is needed, better anesthesia is obtained, and tissues are not distorted. The onset of anesthesia is delayed when compared to LA. Neurovascular status must be assessed and documented before the procedure. Lidocaine or bupivacaine are the most commonly used agents, depending on the time needed to perform the procedure. Epinephrine should not be used in these procedures. Complications include nerve injury and intravascular injection leading to systemic toxicity. Always aspirate before injecting to avoid inadvertent intravascular injection of LA.

The procedure for digital blocks involves sterile preparation of the skin, followed by the introduction of a 27 gauge or smaller needle into the skin (a skin wheal may be raised before deeper injection) and into one side of the extensor tendon of the affected finger just proximal to the web. After aspiration, approximately 1 mL of LA is injected into the tissue on the dorsal surface of the extensor tendon. The needle is advanced toward the palm until its tip is seen beneath volar skin at the base of the finger just distal to the web. After aspiration, 1 mL of LA is injected. Before removing the needle, redirect it across the opposite side of the finger and inject approximately 1 mL across the dorsal digital nerve. Five minutes later repeat the procedure on the opposite side of the finger (Fig. 10-1). An alternative method is to inject a 27 gauge needle into the web space between the affected and adjacent finger, directing the needle to the metacarpal joint of the affected finger. After aspiration, inject 1 to 2 mL into the area of the digital nerve. Before removal of the needle, advance the needle first dorsally and then volarly, and inject 1 mL of LA; repeat on the opposite side. Toes can be blocked in a similar fashion. Great toes can also be blocked using a modified collar block. A 27 gauge

FIG. 10-1   Positions for needle (see text).

needle is introduced on the dorsolateral aspect of the base of the toe until it blanches the plantar skin. As the needle is withdrawn, 1.5 mL of LA is injected. Before the needle is removed, it is passed under the skin on the dorsal aspect of the toe, and 1.5 mL of LA is injected as the needle is withdrawn. The needle is reintroduced through the anesthetized skin on the dorsomedial aspect of the toe and advanced until the plantar skin is blanched; as the needle is withdrawn, 1.5 mL of LA is injected.

Topical anesthetics Common preparations of topical anesthetics (TAs) include tetracaine adrenaline cocaine (TAC) lidocaine epinephrine tetracaine (LET), lidocaine prilocaine (EMLA), and various preparations of lidocaine. TAC and LET are commonly used in place of infiltrative anesthesia. The advantages of these TAs are that they eliminate the need for injection, do not distort wound edges, provide good homeostasis, and are applied painlessly. TAC is a controlled substance, is more expensive, is more toxic, and is no more efficacious than LET. Both LET and TAC should be left in place for at least 20 min for maximal effect. Neither agent should be used on mucous membranes or in end-artery fields. TAC and LET are available in liquid preparations that are used to moisten a cotton applicator, which is then held on the wound. LET also is available in a gel form, which has the advantage of greater ease of application. Topical lidocaine is marketed in a solution, jelly, or ointment. Viscous lidocaine can be used for the temporary relief of inflamed mucous membranes. Lidocaine jelly should be used with the insertion of Foley catheters, the insertion of nasogastric tubes, and other painful procedures. As with infiltrative use of lidocaine, care must be taken not to exceed maximal doses. EMLA is a cream that is used on intact skin. It is particularly useful in the pediatric population to relieve pain associated with IV catheters, venipunctures, lumbar punctures, and other painful procedures. The main drawback of EMLA is that adequate analgesia usually requires 45 min to 1 h of application time.

For further reading in *Emergency Medicine: A Comprehensive Study Guide,* 5th ed., see Chap 32, "Acute Pain Management, Analgesia, and Anxiolysis in the Adult Patient," by Erica Liebelt and Nadine Levick; Chap. 33, "Systemic Analgesia and Sedation for Painful Procedures," by David D. Nicolaou; and Chap. 130, "Acute Pain Management and Sedation in Children," by Erica Liebelt and Nadine Levick.

11 | Management of Patients with Chronic Pain

David M. Cline

Chronic pain is defined as a painful condition that lasts longer than 3 months. It can also be defined as pain that persists beyond the reasonable time for an injury to heal or a month beyond the usual course of an acute disease. Complete eradication of pain is not a reasonable endpoint in most cases. Rather, the goal of therapy is pain reduction and return to functional status.

Clinical Features

Signs and symptoms of chronic pain syndromes are summarized in Table 11-1. Most of these syndromes will be familiar to emergency physicians.

Complex regional pain type I, also known as reflex sympathetic dystrophy, and complex regional pain type II, also known as causalgia, may be seen in the emergency department (ED) 2 weeks or more after an acute injury. These disorders should be suspected when a patient has classic symptoms: allodynia (pain provoked with gentle touch of the skin) and a persistent burning or shooting pain. Associated signs early in the course of the disease include edema, warmth, and localized sweating. Complex regional pain is an important diagnosis to make, since early steroid treatment may prevent ongoing symptoms.

Diagnosis and Differential

The most important task of the emergency physician is to distinguish chronic pain from acute pain that heralds a life- or limb-threatening condition. A complete history and physical examination should either confirm the chronic condition or point to the need for further evaluation when unexpected signs or symptoms are elicited.

Rarely is a provisional diagnosis of a chronic pain condition made for the first time in the ED. The exception is a form of post-nerve-injury pain, complex regional pain. The sharp pain from acute injuries, including fractures, rarely continues beyond 2 weeks duration. Pain in an injured body part beyond this period should alert the clinician to the possibility of nerve injury, and proper treatment, discussed later, should be instituted.

TABLE 11-1 Signs and Symptoms of Chronic Pain Syndromes

Disorder	Pain symptoms	Signs
Myofascial headache	Constant dull pain, occasionally shooting pain	Trigger points on scalp, muscle tenderness and tension
Transformed migraine	Initially migraine-like, becomes constant, dull; nausea, vomiting	Muscle tenderness and tension, normal neurologic examination
Fibromyalgia	Diffuse muscular pain, stiffness, fatigue, sleep disturbance	Diffuse muscle tenderness, >11 trigger points
Myofascial chest pain	Constant dull pain, occasionally shooting pain	Trigger points in area of pain
Myofascial back pain syndrome	Constant dull pain, occasionally shooting pain, pain does not follow nerve distribution	Trigger points in area of pain, usually no muscle atrophy, poor ROM in involved muscle
Articular back pain	Constant or sharp pain exacerbated by movement	Local muscle spasm
Neurogenic back pain	Constant or intermittent, burning or aching, shooting or electric shocklike, may follow dermatome; leg pain > back pain	Possible muscle atrophy in area of pain, possible reflex changes
Complex regional pain type I (RSD)	Burning persistent pain, allodynia, associated with immobilization or disuse	Early: edema, warmth, local sweating Late: above alternates with cold, pale, cyanosis, eventually atrophic changes
Complex regional pain type II (causalgia)	Burning persistent pain, allodynia, associated with peripheral nerve injury	Early: edema, warmth, local sweating Late: above alternates with cold, pale, cyanosis, eventually atrophic changes
Postherpetic neuralgia	Allodynia, shooting, lancinating pain	Sensory changes in the involved dermatome
Phantom limb pain	Variable: aching, cramping, burning, squeezing or tearing sensation	None

Abbreviations: ROM, range of motion; RSD, reflex sympathetic dystrophy.

Definitive diagnostic testing of chronic pain conditions is difficult, requires expert opinion, and, often, expensive procedures such as magnetic resonance imaging (MRI), computed tomography (CT), and thermography. Therefore, referral to the primary source of care and eventual specialist referral are warranted to confirm the diagnosis.

Emergency Department Care and Disposition

Treatment with opiates frequently contribute to the psychopathological aspects of the disease. Many pain specialists feel that they should not be used except for cancer pain. There are two essential points that affect the use of opioids in the ED on which there is agreement: (*a*) opioids should only be used in chronic pain if they enhance function at home and at work, and (*b*) a single practitioner should be the sole prescriber of narcotics or be aware of their administration by others. Finally, a previous narcotic addiction is a relative contraindication to the use of opioids in chronic pain.

The management of chronic pain conditions is listed in Table 11-2. The need for long-standing treatment of chronic pain conditions may limit the safety of the nonsteroidal anti-inflammatory drugs (NSAIDs). The newer cyclooxygenase 2 inhibitor types of NSAIDs, such as rofecoxib 50 mg first dose, then 25 mg daily, may be an alternative for patients who cannot tolerate standard NSAIDs.

Antidepressants are the most frequently used drugs for the management of chronic pain. Often, effective pain control can be achieved at doses lower than typically required for relief of depression. When antidepressants are prescribed in the ED, a follow-up plan should be in place. Discussion with a pain specialist is often beneficial. The most common drug and dose is amitriptyline, 10 to 25 mg, 2 h prior to bedtime.

Referral to the appropriate specialist is one of the most productive means to aid in the care of chronic pain patients who present to the ED. Chronic pain clinics have been successful at changing the lives of patients by eliminating opioid use, decreasing pain levels by one-third, and increasing work hours twofold.

MANAGEMENT OF PATIENTS WITH DRUG-SEEKING BEHAVIOR

The spectrum of drug-seeking patients includes those who have chronic pain and have been advised to avoid taking narcotics, drug

TABLE 11-2 Management of Chronic Pain Syndromes

Disorder	Primary ED treatment	Secondary treatment*	Possible referral outcome
Cancer pain	NSAIDs, opiates	Long-acting opiates	Optimization of medical therapy
Myofascial headache	NSAIDs, cyclobenzaprine	Antidepressants, phenothiazines	Trigger-point injections, optimization of medical therapy
Transformed migraine	NSAIDs, cyclobenzaprine	Antidepressants	Optimization of medical therapy, narcotic withdrawal
Fibromyalgia	NSAIDs	Antidepressants, exercise program	Optimization of medical therapy, dedicated exercise program
Myofascial chest pain	NSAIDs	Antidepressants	Trigger-point injections, optimization of medical therapy
Myofascial back pain syndrome	NSAIDs, stay active	Antidepressants	Trigger-point injections, optimization of medical therapy
Articular back pain	NSAIDs		Surgery, physical therapy
Neurogenic back pain	Acute: tapered solumedrol or prednisone	NSAIDs, muscle relaxants	Epidural steroids, surgery, exercise program
Complex regional pain types I and II (RSD and causalgia)	Acute: prednisone 60 mg/d × 4 days and taper to include 3 weeks of therapy	Chronic: Antidepressants, anticonvulsants	Sympathetic nerve blocks, TENS, spinal analgesia
Postherpetic neuralgia	Acute: simple analgesics	Chronic: antidepressants, capsaicin	Regional nerve blockade
Phantom limb pain	Simple analgesics	Antidepressants, anticonvulsants	TENS, sympathectomy

*If started in the ED, consultation and/or follow-up with pain specialist or personal physician recommended.

Abbreviations: NSAIDs, nonsteroidal anti-inflammatory drugs; RSD, reflex sympathetic dystrophy; TENS, transcutaneous electrical nerve stimulation.

addicts who are trying to supplement their habit, and "hustlers" who are obtaining prescription drugs to sell on the street.

Clinical Features

Because of the spectrum of drug-seeking patients, the history given may be factual or fraudulent. Drug seekers may be demanding, intimidating, or flattering. In one ED study, the most common complaints of patients who were drug seeking were (in decreasing order): back pain, headache, extremity pain, and dental pain. Many fraudulent techniques are used including "lost" prescriptions, "impending" surgery, factitious hematuria with a complaint of kidney stones, self-mutilation, and factitious injury.

Diagnosis and Differential

The diagnosis of drug-seeking behavior may not be possible in the ED. The medical record can provide a wealth of information regarding patients, including documentation proving that patients are supplying false information. Drug-seeking behaviors can be divided into two groups: "predictive" and "less predictive" (Table 11-3). The behaviors listed under "predictive" are illegal in many states and form a solid basis to refuse narcotics to patients.

TABLE 11-3 Characteristics of Drug-Seeking Behavior

Behaviors predictive of drug-seeking behavior*

Sells prescription drugs
Forges/alters prescriptions
Factitious illness, requests narcotics
Uses aliases to receive narcotics
Admits to illicit drug addiction
Conceals multiple physicians prescribing narcotics
Conceals multiple ED visits receiving narcotics

Less predictive for drug-seeking behavior

Admits to multiple doctors prescribing narcotics
Admits to multiple prescriptions for narcotics
Abusive when refused
Multiple drug allergies
Uses excessive flattery
From out of town
Asks for drugs by name

*Behaviors in this category are unlawful in many
 states.

Emergency Department Care and Disposition

The treatment of drug-seeking behavior is to refuse the controlled substance, consider the need for alternative medication or treatment, and consider referral for drug counseling.

For further reading in *Emergency Medicine: A Comprehensive Study Guide,* 5th ed., see Chap. 34, "Management of Patients with Chronic Pain," by David M. Cline.

EMERGENCY WOUND MANAGEMENT

12 | Evaluating and Preparing Wounds

Michael J. Utecht

Traumatic wounds are routinely encountered in the emergency department. The history should include the mechanism, time, and location of injury; symptoms (e.g., pain, swelling, paresthesias, and loss of function); prior wound care; handedness and occupation; and tetanus status. Allergies (e.g., to analgesics, anesthetics, antibiotics, or latex), medications, chronic medical conditions (e.g., diabetes, chronic renal failure, and immunosuppression) and previous scar formation (keloid) should be documented. When caring for wounds, the ultimate goal is to restore the physical integrity and function of the injured tissue without infection.

Wound repair has been traditionally divided into three categories. *Primary closure* (healing by primary intention) is performed with sutures, staples, or adhesives at the time of initial evaluation. *Secondary closure* (healing by secondary intention) is where the wound is allowed to granulate and fill, with only cleaning and débridement as needed. *Tertiary closure* (delayed primary closure) is where the wound is initially cleaned, débrided, and observed for typically 4 or 5 days before closure.

When treating a wound, the emergency physician should consider the time and mechanism of injury as well as its location, since these factors all play roles in the wound's potential for infection. Either shear, compressive, or tensile forces cause acute traumatic wounds. Shear forces are produced by sharp objects with relatively low energy, resulting in a wound with a straight edge and little contamination that can be expected to heal with a good result. Wounds caused by compression or tension forces are produced when a blunt object impacts the skin. The higher energy applied by such forces produces stellate and flap-type lacerations, respectively, whose surrounding devitalized tissue results in a wound one hundred times more susceptible to infection than those caused by shear forces.

In addition to the mechanism of injury, exogenous and endogenous sources of bacteria must be considered in assessing a wound's potential for infection. Over most of the body surface, the density of bacteria is quite low (trunk, upper arms, and legs). Moist areas harbor millions of bacteria, as do exposed anatomic areas (head, face, hands, and feet). Since these organisms reside in the most superficial layers of the skin, topically applied antiseptic agents provide sterility or near-sterility in most skin areas of the body, minimizing infection potential. Lacerations contacting the oral cavity are heavily contaminated with facultative and anaerobic organisms. Wounds sustained from contaminated objects or occurring in contaminated environments have an increased risk of infection. The most common foreign body in wounds is soil. Clay-containing soils and soils with large amounts of organic material have a high potential for infection, whereas sand and black dirt from a highway surface have a low potential. Animal bite wounds are common and pose a higher risk of infection. Wounds contacted by human or animal fecal contaminants also run a high risk for infection despite therapeutic intervention.

The body responds to an injury by initiating a series of restorative stages to recover tissue continuity and strength. Hemostasis, inflammation, epithelialization, angiogenesis, and fibroplasia occur over the first several days to weeks following an injury. Wound contraction and scar remodeling occur over the next several months. Contraction significantly modifies the cosmetic appearance of treated wounds. An important principle of wound repair is to take this expected contraction into account and repair lacerations with everted edges. It is impossible to predict the ultimate appearance of wounds at the time of suture removal; therefore, it is important to educate patients on wound remodeling.

WOUND EXAMINATION

Wound examination is greatly facilitated by a cooperative patient, good positioning, and adequate lighting. Sterile technique should be used. It is important to practice universal precautions to protect the patient and physician from cross-infection.

When examining the wound, location, size, shape, margins (i.e., smooth or jagged), and depth should be noted. Any sensory, motor, tendon, or vascular compromise should be documented, as should injuries to specialized ducts. When the injury occurs to an extremity and bleeding complicates thorough inspection of the wound, a sphygmomanometer placed proximal to the injury and inflated to a pressure greater than the patient's systolic blood pressure will provide excellent hemostasis. Palpation of the bone adjacent to the wound may detect tenderness or instability consistent with an underlying bone injury, which can be confirmed by roentgenograms. Careful examination of the surrounding soft tissue may reveal a foreign body that was not visible on roentgenogram (e.g., plastic, wood, and other organic material). Pieces of metal, glass, gravel, teeth, and bone larger than 1 mm are readily visible on plain radiographs.

Although an emergency physician can treat most traumatic wounds, consultation should be considered in certain cases. Injuries requiring open reduction of fractures, amputation, neurorrhaphy, vascular anastomosis, flexor tendon repair, and repair of specialized ducts, lid margin, and tarsal plate of the eyelid should be referred to the appropriate specialist. Any injury that in the opinion of the examining emergency physician may have a poor cosmetic or functional outcome should be treated by or in consultation with the appropriate specialist.

WOUND PREPARATION

Proper wound preparation is a critical step in emergency department wound care for restoring the integrity and function of the injured tissue while minimizing the risk of infection and maximizing cosmetic results.

Anesthesia

In general, pain control should be provided prior to extensive wound preparation. Local anesthesia and systemic analgesia will enable better preparation, evaluation, and treatment with a relaxed patient (see Chap. 10). A careful neurovascular examination of the involved area should be performed prior to the administration of local anesthesia.

Hemostasis

Control of bleeding is necessary for proper wound evaluation and treatment. Direct pressure is usually effective. Ligation of minor vessels in the extremity may be necessary and can be achieved by applying an absorbable suture material after isolating and clamping the involved vessel. Chemical means of hemostasis include epinephrine, absorbable gelation sponge (Gelform), and oxidized cellulose (Oxcel). Epinephrine is typically pre-mixed with lidocaine, providing local vasoconstriction and prolonged anesthesia. Epinephrine should not be used in end organs, such as fingers, toes, and tip of nose, ears, or penis. Gelform has no intrinsic hemostatic properties and works by the pressure it exerts as it becomes a fluid-filled sponge. Oxcel reacts with blood to form an artificial clot. Bipolar electrocautery can achieve hemostasis for blood vessels smaller than 2 mm in diameter, but caution should be used to avoid tissue necrosis if applied improperly. Battery-powered hand-held units do not generate sufficient heat to produce coagulation in vessels larger than capillaries.

Foreign-Body and Hair Removal

Visual wound inspection down to the full depth and along the full course of the wound is the important method of detecting foreign bodies. See Chap. 17 for discussion of foreign-body removal. hair, which can act as a foreign body, should be removed by clipping 1 to 2 mm above the skin with scissors. Shaving may damage the hair follicles, allowing bacterial invasion, and can increase the infection rate tenfold. Ointments can be used to clear hair away from wound edges as an alternative to clipping. Hair should never be removed from the eybrows.

Irrigation

High-pressure irrigation decreases bacterial count and helps to remove foreign bodies, thereby decreasing the risk of infection. Effective high-pressure irrigation can be achieved by using a 19-gauge needle or catheter attached to a 35-mL or 65-mL syringe. Although the precise voloume of irrigant required is not known, 60 mL/cm of wound length is a useful guideline, with a 200 mL minimum. Wound soaking is not effective in cleansing contaminated wounds. Saline solution is the least expensive irrigant and has the lowest toxicity. There is no added benefit to the addition of povidone-iodine or hydrogen peroxide.

Débridement

Devitalized tissue may increase the risk of infection and delay healing. Débridement not only removes foreign matter and bacterial and devitalized tissue but also creates a sharp wound edge that is easier to repair. Excision, utilizing a standard surgical blade and scissors, is the most effective type of débridement. Tissue that has a narrow base or lacks capillary refill will require débridement. Wounds with an extensive amount of nonviable tissue may require a large amount of tissue removal and will need more delayed wound closure or grafting. In general, a surgical specialist should be consulted to manage such wounds.

Antibiotics

To reduce the incidence of wound infections, antibiotics have been used for years, although their benefit for most patients is not clear. If used for the treatment of traumatic wounds in the emergency department, antibiotic prophylaxis should be (1) started rapidly, ideally within 1 h and before significant tissue manipulation; (2) performed with agents that are effective against predicted pathogens; and (3) administered by routes that rapidly achieve desired blood levels. Generally, this will require an intravenous, broad-spectrum antibiotic. Oral administration may also work if done before manipulation. Reasonable coverage can be expected from penicillinase-resistant penicillin (e.g., dicloxacillin) or a first-generation cephalosporin (e.g., cephalexin). See Chap. 18 for discussion of dog, cat, and human bites. Full-thickness oral lacerations should be treated with penicillin. Wounds contaminated by fresh water and plantar puncture wounds through athletic shoes may require a fluoroquinolone to cover *Pseudomonas.* (Quinolones are not recommended for children.) Antibiotics should be continued for up to 5 days.

Tetanus Prophylaxis

Guidelines for tetanus prophylaxis in wound management have been developed by several public and professional organizations. See Chap. 89 and Table 89-1 for the Centers for Disease Control and Prevention guidelines. Since the incubation period is from 7 to 21 days, it is acceptable to give the absorbed tetanus toxoid days after injury. Immunization and immunoglobulin administration are safe during pregnancy.

For further reading in *Emergency Medicine: A Comprehensive Study Guide,* 5th ed., see Chap. 35, "Evaluation of Wounds," by Louis J. Kroot; and Chap. 36, "Wound Preparation," by Susan C. Stone and Wallace A. Carter.

---

13 | Methods for Wound Closure
       | *Michael J. Utecht*

Wounds can be closed primarily in the emergency department (ED) by the placement of sutures, surgical staples, skin-closure tapes, and adhesives. All wounds heal with some scarring; the goal is to use techniques that make the scar as small and invisible as possible. In closing a laceration it is important to match each layer of a wound edge to its counterpart. Care must be taken to avoid having one wound edge rolled inward. The rolled-in edge occludes the capillaries, promoting wound infection. The dermal side will not heal to the rolled epidermal side, causing wound dehiscence when the sutures are removed, resulting in an inferior scar appearance. The techniques described are an overview of basic wound closure, which should aid the practitioner in achieving acceptable results.

WOUND CLOSURE MATERIALS

Sutures

Sutures are generally divided into two general classes based on their rate of degradation. Sutures that degrade rapidly, losing all their tensile strength within 60 days are considered "absorbable" sutures. Sutures that maintain their tensile strength for longer than 60 days are "nonabsorbable" sutures. Most absorbable sutures lose half their tensile strength within 4 weeks, and some nonabsorbable sutures lose some strength during this 60-day interval.

Sutures are sized according to their diameter. In general ED use, 6-0 material is the smallest and is used for percutaneous closure on the face and other cosmetically important areas. Suture sizes 5-0 and 4-0 are progressively larger and used on the trunk and extremities. Very thick skin as is found on the scalp and sole, may require closure with 3-0 sutures.

All sutures compromise local tissue defenses increasing the potential for infection. The perisutural cuff may provide an avenue of contamination in addition to the trauma of inserting a needle that can incite an inflammatory response. Sutures that are tied too tightly impair blood flow and cause tissue necrosis of the wound edges. The quantity of suture and the chemical reactivity of the material may increase susceptibility to infection as well. Sutures made of natural fiber potentiate infection more than other nonabsorbable sutures and should be avoided in contaminated wounds. Synthetic monofilament poses a lower risk of infection than does comparable multifilament material and is the recommended suture material for most percutaneous skin closures.

Staples

Skin closure by metal staples is quick and economical, with the advantage of low tissue reactivity. The skin staple, however, does not provide the same coaptation for lacerations with irregular skin edges that sutures can achieve and should be reserved for lacerations where the healing scar is not readily apparent (e.g., scalp). When placing staples, the wound edges should be held together with tissue forceps. The device should be placed gently against the skin and the trigger squeezed slowly. A properly placed staple should have its topside off the skin surface (Fig. 13-1).

Skin-Closure Tapes

Skin-closure tapes are used as an alternative to sutures and staples and for additional support after suture and staple removal. Tapes work best on flat, dry, nonmobile surfaces where the wound edges fit together without tension. Taped wounds are more resistant to infection than sutured wounds. They can be used for skin flaps, where sutures may compromise perfusion, and for lacerations with thin, friable skin that will not hold sutures. Adherence of tapes is enhanced by the use of benzoin to the skin surface 2 to 3 cm beyond the wound edges. Individual tapes are applied with some space between them but not so much that the wound edges gap open between the individual tapes (Fig. 13-2). Tapes should stay in place about as long as an equivalent suture and will spontaneously detach as the underlying epithelium exfoliates.

Tissue Adhesives

Tissues adhesives close wounds by forming an adhesive layer on top of intact epithelium. Cyanoacrylate adhesives should never be applied within wounds due to their intense inflammatory reaction with subcutaneous tissue. Adhesives should not be applied to mucous membranes, infected areas, joints, areas with dense hair (e.g.,

FIG. 13-1   A cutaneous staple properly placed will evert the skin edges and not be in contact with the skin surface.

FIG. 13-2   Skin-closure tapes should be applied perpendicular to the wound edges and spaced so that the edges do not gape.

scalp), or on wounds exposed to body fluids. Adhesives are most useful when they are used on wounds that close spontaneously, have clean or sharp edges, and are located on clean, nonmobile areas. Wounds where the edges are separated more than 5 mm are unlikely to stay closed with tissue adhesives alone. In this case, subcutaneous sutures can be inserted to relieve this tension. Lacerations longer than 5 cm are prone to shear forces and are unlikely to remain closed with tissue adhesives alone. Once applied, Cyanoacrylate should not be covered with ointment, bandage, or dressing. Patients should be instructed not to pick at edges of the adhesive. After 24 h, the area can be gently washed with plain water but should not be scrubbed, soaked, or exposed to moisture for any length of time. The adhesive will spontaneously slough in 5 to 10 days. Should a wound open, the patient should immediately return for closure.

SUTURING TECHNIQUES

Percutaneous Suture

Percutaneous sutures that pass through both the epidermal and dermal layers are the most common sutures used in the ED. Dermal, or subcuticular, sutures reapproximate the divided edges of the dermis without penetrating the epidermis. Occasionally, these two sutures are used together in a layered closure. Sutures can be applied in a continuous fashion ("running" sutures) or as interrupted sutures.

Percutaneous sutures should be placed to achieve eversion of the wound edges. To accomplish this, the needle should enter the skin at a 90° angle. The needle point should also exit the opposite side at 90°. The depth of the suture should be wider than the width. Sutures placed in this manner will encompass a portion of tissue that will evert when the knot is tied (Fig. 13-3). An adequate number of interrupted sutures should be placed so that the wound edges are closed without gaping.

Sutures are secured by tying the free ends into a series of square knots, beginning with the surgeon's knot, where the initial double throw offers better knot security with less slipping of the suture material as the wound is pulled together. The knots should be constructed by carefully snuggling each throw tightly against the preceding one. Ideally, the knotted suture should reapproximate the divided wound edges without strangulating the tissue encircled by the suture loop. For monofilament and multifilament nylon sutures 2-0 to 4-0 size, two square knots (four throws) placed snugly against each other are adequate for knot security. Finer sutures, 5-0 and 6-0, should have three square knots (six throws).

Straight, shallow lacerations can be closed with percutaneous sutures only, sewing from one end toward the other and aligning edges with each individual suture bite. Deep, irregular wounds with uneven, unaligned, or gaping edges are more difficult to

FIG. 13-3   A single interrupted percutaneous suture with everted edges.

suture. Certain principles have been identified for these more difficult wounds:

1. Wounds where the edges cannot be brought together without excessive tension should have dermal sutures placed to partially close the gap.
2. Adipose tissue beneath the skin should not be sutured as obliteration of this potential dead space increases the incidence of infection.
3. When wounds edges of different thicknesses are to be reunited, the needle should be passed through one side of the wound and then drawn out before reentry through the other side to ensure that the needle is inserted at a comparable level.
4. Uneven edges can be aligned by first approximating the midportion of the wound with the initial suture. Subsequent sutures are placed in the middle of each half, until the wound edges are aligned and closed.

Simple interrupted sutures are the most versatile and are good for realigning irregular wound edges and stellate lacerations (Fig. 13-4). An advantage of interrupted sutures is that only the involved sutures need to be removed in the case of wound infection.

Continuous Sutures

Continuous ("running") sutures are best when repairing linear wounds. An advantage of the continuous suture is that it accommo-

FIG. 13-4   Stellate laceration closed with interrupted sutures.

dates to the developing edema of the wound edges during healing. However, a break in the suture may ruin the entire repair and may cause permanent marks if placed too tightly. Continuous suture closure of a laceration can be accomplished by two different patterns. In the first pattern, the needle pathway is at a 90° angle to the wound edges and results in a visible suture that crosses the wound edges at a 45° angle (Fig. 13-5A). In the other pattern, the needle pathway is at a 45° angle to the wound edges, so that the visible suture is at a 90° angle to the wound edges (Fig. 13-5B). In either case, the physician starts at the corner of the wound farthest away and sutures toward him/herself. A variation on the continuous running suture is to "lock" the running suture (Fig. 13-6). This technique aids in hemostasis and is employed on the scalp and vagina most frequently.

FIG. 13-5   **A.** Running suture crossing wound at 45°. **B.** Running suture crossing wound at 90°.

FIG. 13-6   Running locked suture.

Dermal Sutures

Dermal (subcuticular) sutures can be used alone or as adjuncts to percutaneous sutures in wounds subjected to strong skin tensions. When dermal closure alone is used, it is generally applied in a continuous manner with the ends brought out of the skin so that the suture can be removed. Both synthetic absorbable and nonabsorbable sutures are used. It is advisable to close the skin with surgical tapes or wound adhesive for more accurate approximation of the epidermis when using dermal sutures alone.

Interrupted dermal sutures are started by entering the skin near the base of the wound and exiting just beneath the dermal-epidermal junction; this assures that the knot will be buried in the depth of the wound (Fig. 13-7). Continuous dermal sutures are useful in wounds subject to strong skin tensions, patients prone to keloid formation, and those individuals who are unable to contact a health professional for suture removal. Absorbable sutures are ideal. Continuous dermal sutures are begun as an interrupted dermal suture (Fig. 13-8). The physician cuts the free end close to the knot, and the next stitch is passed horizontally from the end of the wound through the superficial dermis. After the dermis is exited, pulling the suture across at right angles to the wound identifies the position of the next bite. Accurate positioning is

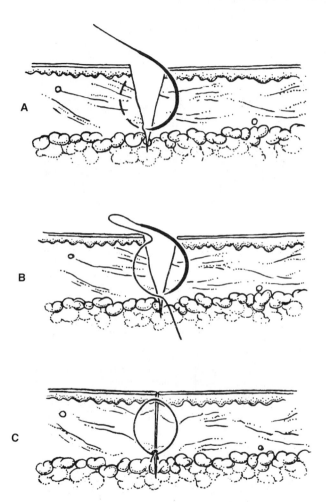

FIG. 13-7   Dermal suture. **A.** Entry is at base of wound on one side and exit at the dermal-epidermal junction. **B.** Entry on the opposite side is at the dermal-epidermal junction with exit at the base. **C.** The tied loop has the knot buried in the wound and not close to the skin surface.

FIG. 13-8 Continuous subcuticular suture. **A.** Linear laceration. **B.** Course of suture underneath skin. **C.** Placement of sutures.

assured by slight backtracking of each bite. At a point one bite from the end of the wound a loop of suture is used to construct the terminal square knots.

Mattress Sutures

Vertical mattress (Fig. 13-9) and horizontal mattress sutures (Fig. 13-10) are also employed in certain situations. The vertical mattress suture is useful in areas of lax skin (elbow and dorsum of hand) where the wound edges tend to fold into the wound. It can act

FIG. 13-9 Vertical mattress suture.

FIG. 13-10 Horizontal mattress suture.

FIG. 13-11 Purse-string suture.

as an "all-in-one" suture, avoiding the need for a layered closure. Horizontal mattress sutures are faster and better at eversion than vertical mattress. It is especially useful in areas of increased tension such as fascia, joints, and callus skin. In order to avoid tissue strangulation, care must be taken not to tie the individual sutures too tightly.

Purse-String Suture

Purse-string suture is very useful at reapproximating multiple flap tips and corner wounds (Fig. 13-11). It is used in these areas in order to preserve the blood supply and minimize tissue destruction at the tips of the skin edges.

Dog-Ear Maneuver

The dog-ear maneuver is a technique used to handle excess tissue at one end of a wound (Fig. 13-12). The wound is extended from the apex toward the long side in the form of a hockey stick. Then

FIG. 13-12 Dog-ear maneuver. **A.** Incision is carried off one end of the wound at 45° toward the side with excess tissue. **B.** The excess tissue is pulled over the incision and cut away. **C.** The sutured laceration now has a "hockey stick" angulation.

the triangular piece of excess skin is removed and the skin edges are sewn together.

For further reading in *Emergency Medicine: A Comprehensive Study Guide,* 5th ed., see Chap. 37, "Methods for Wound Closure," by Julia Martin and Rob Herfel.

---

14 | Lacerations to the Face and Scalp
David M. Cline

SCALP AND FOREHEAD

The scalp and forehead (which includes eyebrows) are parts of the same anatomic structure (Fig. 14-1). Eyebrows should never be clipped or shaved because their delicate contour and form are valuable landmarks for the meticulous reapproximation of the wound edges. After the wound has been cleansed and hemostasis achieved, the base of the wound should always be palpated for possible skull fracture. All depressed fractures should be evaluated by computed tomography scanning.

When the edges of a laceration of either the eyebrow or the scalp are devitalized, débridement is mandatory. When débriding these sites, the scalpel should cut an angle that is parallel to that of the hair follicles. In some cases, it may be necessary to control scalp hemorrhage by direct pressure or by clamping vessels at the wound edges. Wound closure should be initiated first with approximation of the galea aponeurotica with buried, interrupted absorbable 4-0 sutures. The divided edges of muscle and fascia must also be closed with buried, interrupted, absorbable 4-0 synthetic sutures to prevent further development of depressed scars. The skin can be closed by staples or by simple interrupted nylon sutures (sutures that are a different color than the patient's hair should be considered). Some authors recommend single-layer closure with 3-0 nylon sutures for scalp wounds on nonbalding patients.

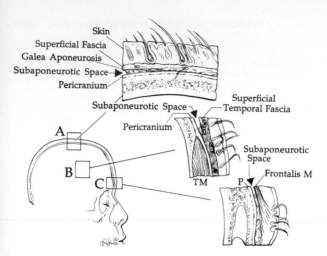

FIG. 14-1 The layers of the scalp and forehead.

FIG. 14-2 Key stitches in the forehead.

The skin edges of anatomic landmarks on the forehead should be approximated first with key stitches, using interrupted, nonabsorbable monofilament 5-0 synthetic sutures (Fig. 14-2). Accurate alignment of the eyebrow, transverse wrinkles of the forehead, and the hairline of the scalp is essential. It may be necessary to have younger patients raise their eyebrows to create wrinkles for accurate placement of the key stitches. A firm pressure dressing placed around the head can close any potential dead space, encourage hemostasis, and prevent hematoma formation. This pressure dressing should be left in place for 48 h.

EYELIDS

A complete exam of the eye's structure and function is essential. A search should be made for foreign bodies (see Chap. 145). The lid should be examined for involvement of the canthi, the lacrimal system, or penetration through the tarsal plate or lid margin. The following wounds should be referred to an ophthalmologist: (*a*) those involving the inner surface of the lid, (*b*) those involving the lid margins, (*c*) those involving the lacrimal duct, (*d*) those associated with ptosis, and (*e*) those that extend into the tarsal plate. Failure to recognize and properly repair the lacrimal system can result in chronic tearing.

Uncomplicated lid lacerations can be readily closed using nonabsorbable 6-0 suture. Tissue adhesive is contraindicated near to the eye.

NOSE

Lacerations of the nose may be limited to skin or involve the deeper structures (sparse nasal musculature, cartilaginous framework, and nasal mucous membrane). They are repaired by accurate reapproximation of each tissue layer. Inexperienced operators should refer such cases to an otolaryngologist or plastic surgeon. Local anesthesia of the nose can be difficult because of the tightly adhering skin. Topical anesthesia may be successful with lidocaine, epinephrine, and tetracaine.

When the laceration extends through all tissue layers, closure should begin with a marginal, nonabsorbable, monofilament 5-0 synthetic suture that aligns the skin surrounding the entrances of the nasal canals, to prevent malapposition and notching of the alar rim. Traction upon the long, untied ends of the marginal suture approximates the wounds and aligns the anterior and posterior margins of the divided tissue layers. The mucous membrane should then be repaired with interrupted, braided, absorbable 5-0 synthetic sutures, with their knots buried in the tissue. The area is reirrigated gently from the outside. The cartilage may rarely need to be approximated with a minimal number of 5-0 absorbable sutures. In sharply demarked linear lacerations, closure of the overlying skin is usually sufficient. The cut edges of the skin, with its adherent musculature, are closed with interrupted, nonabsorbable, monofilament 6-0 synthetic sutures. Removal of the external sutures may take place in 3 to 5 days.

Following any nasal injury, the septum should be inspected for hematoma formation using a nasal speculum. The presence of bluish swelling in the septum confirms the diagnosis of septal hematoma. Treatment of the hematoma is evacuation of the blood clot. Drainage of a small hematoma can be accomplished by aspiration of the blood clot through a #18 needle. A larger hematoma should be drained through a horizontal incision at the base. Bilateral hematomas should be drained in the operating room by a specialist. Reaccumulation of blood can be prevented by nasal packing. Antibiotic treatment is recommended to prevent infection that may cause necrosis of cartilage. Oral penicillin, cephalosporin, or macrolide is acceptable.

LIPS

The technique of closure will depend largely on the type of lip wound. Isolated intraoral lesions may not need to be sutured. Through-and-through lacerations that don't include the vermilion border can be closed in layers. A 5-0 absorbable suture should be used first for the mucosal surface, followed by reirrigation and closure of the orbicularis oris muscle with 5-0 absorbable suture. The skin should be closed with 6-0 nylon suture or tissue adhesive.

Repair of a complex lip laceration requires a three-layered closure (Fig. 14-3). Using skin hooks, traction is applied to align the anterior and posterior borders of the laceration. Closure of the wound should start at the vermilion-skin junction with a nonabsorbable, monofilament 6-0 synthetic suture. The orbicularis oris muscle is then repaired with interrupted, braided, absorbable 4-0 synthetic sutures. The vermilion-mucous membrane junction is approximated with a braided, absorbable 5-0 synthetic suture. The suture ligature's knot is buried in the subcutaneous tissue. The divided edges of the mucous membrane and vermilion are then closed using interrupted, braided, absorbable 5-0 synthetic sutures with a buried-knot construction. Skin edges of the laceration are usually jagged and irregular, but they can be fitted together as

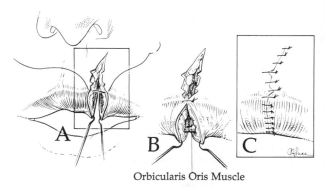

Orbicularis Oris Muscle

FIG. 14-3   Irregular-edged vertical laceration of the upper lip. **A.** Traction is applied to the lips and closure of the wound is begun first at the vermilion-skin junction. **B.** The orbicularis oris muscle is then repaired with interrupted, absorbable 4-0 synthetic sutures. **C.** The irregular edges of the skin are then approximated.

the pieces of a jigsaw puzzle using interrupted, nonabsorbable, monofilament 6-0 synthetic sutures with their knots formed on the surface of the skin.

CHEEKS AND FACE

In general, facial lacerations are closed with 6-0 nonabsorbable, simple interrupted sutures and are removed after 5 days. Tissue adhesive is an alternative. Attention to anatomic structures including the facial nerve and parotid gland is necessary (Fig. 14-4). If these structures are involved, operative repair is indicated.

EAR

Superficial lacerations of the ear can be closed with 6-0 nylon suture. Exposed cartilage should be covered. Debridement of the skin is not advisable, since there is very little excess skin. In most through-and-through lacerations of the ear, the skin can be approximated and the underlying cartilage will be supported adequately (Fig. 14-5). Following repair of simple lacerations, a small piece of nonadherent gauze may be applied over the laceration only and a pressure dressing applied. Gauze squares are placed behind the ear to apply pressure, and the head is wrapped circumferen-

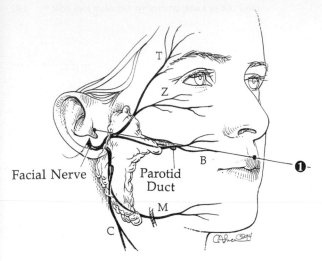

FIG. 14-4 Anatomic structures of the cheek. The course of the parotid duct is deep to a line drawn from the tragus of the ear to the midportion of the upper lip.

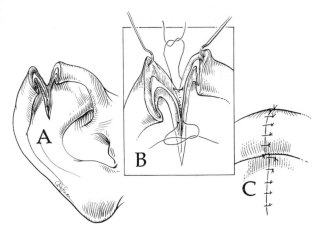

FIG. 14-5 **A.** Laceration through auricle. **B.** One or two interrupted, 6-0 coated nylon sutures will approximate divided edges of cartilage. **C.** Interrupted nonabsorbable 6-0 synthetic sutures approximate the skin edges.

tially with gauze. Sutures should be removed in 5 days. An otola-ryngologist or plastic surgeon should be consulted for more complex lacerations, ear avulsions, or auricular hematomas.

For further reading in *Emergency Medicine, A Comprehensive Study Guide,* 5th ed., see Chap. 38, "Lacerations to the Face and Scalp," by Wendy C. Coates.

---

15 | Fingertip and Nail Injuries

Stephanie B. Abbuhl

Fingertip injuries can be divided into four categories: (1) digital tip amputation with skin or pulp loss only, (2) digital tip amputation with exposed bone, (3) injury of the perionychium, and (4) fracture of the distal phalanx. Successful repair of fingertip injuries requires a knowledge of anatomy (Fig. 15-1) and an understanding of techniques of reconstruction.

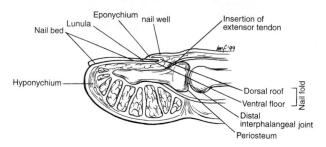

FIG. 15-1   Anatomy of the perionychium. [From Zook EG: The perionychium, in Green DP (ed): *Operative Hand Surgery,* 2d ed. New York, Churchill Livingstone, 1988, p 1332, with permission.]

DISTAL TIP AMPUTATION WITH SKIN OR PULP LOSS ONLY

Distal fingertip amputations that are 1 cm^2 or less in size without exposed bone can usually be treated conservatively with serial dressing changes alone. This is a desirable option because healing occurs by secondary intention and results in very little scarring. In children under 12, conservative management is preferred because spontaneous regeneration of the fingertip occurs, usually with excellent results. The patient should be instructed to soak the fingertip once a day in warm water with an antibacterial soap added. This is followed by tap water irrigation and application of a sterile nonadherent dressing. Follow-up should be arranged in 2 days for a wound check.

In cases were the amputated portion is greater than 1 cm^2 and the severed tip is available, an alternative treatment is to use the amputated portion as a full-thickness skin graft. A split or full-thickness skin graft harvested from a distant site is another means of wound closure. In these cases, consultation with a specialist is appropriate. Complications of skin grafts include decreased sensibility of the fingertip, scar tenderness both at donor and graft sites, poor cosmetic quality, and hyperpigmentation in patients with dark skin.

DIGITAL TIP AMPUTATION WITH EXPOSED BONE

If a significant loss of tissue to the fingertip causes exposure of the tuft of the distal phalanx, skin grafting will be unsuccessful, since bone does not provide adequate vascularity to support the donor tissue. Several treatment options exist, and the best choice is determined by the size and geometry of the injury, the angle of the tip amputation, and the presence of the amputated tip. Rongeuring of a small protruding portion of the phalanx may be performed to shorten the fingertip and allow healing by secondary intention. Another choice is microsurgical reimplantation when the amputated part is at the level of the lunula or proximal to it. In a child, reimplantation of an amputated single digit at this level should always be considered. Consultation with a specialist is indicated in all patients with specific occupational concerns and when the injured digit is the thumb or index finger.

INJURY OF THE PERIONYCHIUM

The perionychium, or nail, includes the entire complex of the nail plate, nail bed, nail matrix, and surrounding paronychium. A force that can break the durable nail plate can disrupt the nail matrix and bed and will often heal by scar formation, resulting in a split, absent, or nonadherent nail. For example, a hammer injury frequently results in multiple stellate lacerations of the nail bed and matrix. Meticulous repair of the nail matrix and bed will reduce the scar formation and should be done as soon as possible after the injury. There is an associated distal tuft fracture in approximately 50 percent of nail bed injuries, and therefore all patients require the standard three radiographic views of the involved digit.

Subungual hematomas characteristically cause severe throbbing pain, requiring decompression by simple trephination of the nail plate. Various tools have been used effectively for this purpose, including a heated paper clip, electric nail drill, electrocautery, 18-gauge needle, and scalpel. Upon discharge, patients are instructed to soak the affected finger in warm water containing antibacterial soap two to three times a day.

In the past, it has been said that hematomas that have separated over 50 percent of the nail plate from the nail bed or matrix require removal of the nail plate for complete inspection of the nail bed. However, recently two prospective studies have suggested that simple trephination alone produces good to excellent results in eighty-five percent of these patients regardless of the size of the hematoma, presence of nondisplaced fracture, or infection.

It can be difficult to decide when it is necessary to remove a nail plate and inspect the nail bed and matrix for laceration. Nail removal is recommended if there is a significant crush injury, associated nail avulsion, or surrounding nail fold disruption. Removal of the nail is also indicated when a displaced tuft fracture is found on x-ray. Nail plate removal can be accomplished by using appropriate anesthesia and establishing a cleavage plane between the nail plate and bed by opening and closing the blades of iris scissors. Using the same technique, a similar plane is also developed between the eponychium and the nail plate. Gentle distal traction on the nail plate will then separate the plate from the proximal nail sulcus. Lacerations of the nail bed are carefully repaired using 6-0 or 7-0 absorbable sutures. Crush injuries often result in stellate lacerations, which may require extensive repair with a magnifying loupe.

Occasionally lacerations of the nail bed are associated with partial avulsions of the nail matrix from the sulcus. When this happens, the germinal matrix may lie on top of the eponychium. Management entails replacement of the matrix in its anatomic position using a series of three horizontal mattress sutures (Fig. 15-2). Two incisions can be made perpendicular to the lateral curved margin of the eponychial fold to better visualize the injured matrix.

A

B

FIG. 15-2 Technique for repair of an avulsion of the germinal matrix using three horizontal mattress sutures. (From Chudnofsky CR, Sebastian S: Special wounds: Nail bed, plantar puncture, and cartilage. *Emerg Med Clin North Am* 10:808, 1992, with permission.)

After the nail bed and matrix are reapproximated, the nail plate should be thoroughly cleansed and then replaced in the proximal sulcus to serve as a stent and protective covering for the bed and matrix. The nail plate is trephinated to allow drainage of any blood. The nail plate is held in place with an interrupted, monofilament 5-0 nylon suture passed through the distal end of the nail plate to fingertip skin. The fingertip is dressed with nonadherent gauze, and a volar splint is placed to protect the injured part and restrict movement. The dressing can be removed 5 days later to check for formation of hematoma, which should be evacuated if present. The suture is removed in 3 weeks, although the nail plate will frequently adhere to the nail bed and matrix for 1 to 3 months, until dislodged by the new nail.

If the nail plate is destroyed or too damaged to be used as a splint, nonbiologic stents made of silastic or silicone may be used to elevate the eponychium and protect the nail bed. Similarly, a sterile piece of aluminum foil used to wrap suture materials may be used.

AVULSION OF THE NAIL BED AND MATRIX

When a nail plate is avulsed, fragments of the nail bed may remain attached to the nail plate. These fragments, along with all other retrievable fragments unattached to the nail plate, should be replaced as free grafts. The graft should be carefully approximated to the nail bed segments using 7-0 chromic sutures attached to a microsurgical spatula needle. A pressure dressing is applied to prevent accumulation of blood and serum beneath the graft. When the avulsed nail bed fragment is not available or in the case of a large defect, a full-thickness nail bed graft can be harvested from the patient's toe and sutured into the nail bed of the affected finger. Consultation with a specialist is appropriate in such cases.

FRACTURE OF THE DISTAL PHALANX

When a fracture of the distal phalanx has occurred and the nail is avulsed out of the proximal eponychial fold, this usually indicates a nail bed laceration, which should be repaired. There is usually excellent soft tissue support of a distal phalanx fracture because of the dorsal nail plate and the volar pulp and fibrous septa. When the soft tissue support is lost, fixation of the fracture with a Kirschner wire is required, usually by a specialist. Splinting of the fracture is necessary for 10 to 14 days.

When a child is struck on the fingertip, the injury that often results is an open fracture of the base of the distal phalanx with the nail plate lying superficial to the eponychium. Because the epiphyseal plate is weaker than the insertion of the extensor tendon, an epiphyseal separation, rather than a mallet finger, occurs. Management includes closed reduction by hyperextension and replacement of the nail plate under the proximal nail fold after thorough cleansing.

RING TOURNIQUET SYNDROME

Acute or chronic digital swelling can leave a ring tightly trapped at the base of the proximal phalanx, resulting in nerve damage, ischemia, and digital gangrene if not promptly removed. The finger should be assessed for lacerations, sensory function (two-point discrimination), and perfusion (color and capillary refill). Diminished sensation or perfusion requires rapid ring removal, usually by cutting the ring off with a ring cutter.

If removal can be attempted with slower techniques that preserve the ring, there are several options. The simplest technique is lubrication. A variety of lubricants can be applied to the digit and the ring removed with circular motion and traction.

Another option, the string technique, uses a length of string wound circumferentially around the finger; when the string is unwrapped, the ring is advanced. String, umbilical tape, or O-gauge silk sutures can be used, but synthetic monofilament sutures should be avoided because they tend to cut the skin. First one end of the string is passed under the ring, and then the finger is wrapped, starting next to the ring and winding clockwise, with each loop snug against the previous one, from proximal to distal (Fig. 15-3). Wrapping and compression is a painful process and usually requires regional anesthesia. To remove the ring, the proximal end

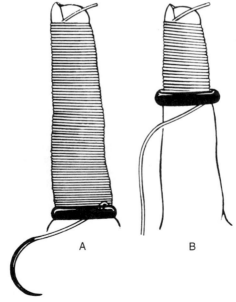

FIG. 15-3 String technique for ring removal. **A.** Completely wrapped. **B.** Unwrapping, with ring advancing off with the string.

of the string is slowly unwrapped in a counterclockwise manner, advancing the ring toward the distal end as the string unwinds.

For further reading in *Emergency Medicine: A Comprehensive Study Guide,* 5th ed., see Chap. 39, "Fingertip and Nail Injuries," by Robert S. Chang and Wallace A. Carter.

---

16   Lacerations of the Joints and Extremities

Martin J. Carey

Clinical and Diagnostic Features

Evaluation of wounds in general is discussed in Chap. 12. It is important to determine the position of the limb at the time of injury, which will help to uncover occult tendon injuries. The dominant limb should be documented.

Assessment for associated nerve, vessel, or tendon injury is mandatory. The limb should be inspected prior to the use of anesthetic. At this time, sensory neurologic function should be evaluated using light touch and two-point discrimination testing (with a distance of 5 mm between the points) for the fingers. Motor function may be better assessed after the wound is anesthetized (see Table 16-1). At this time, the wound can also be explored. The limb should be moved through its full range of motion, in order to exclude tendon injury. Each tendon function should be tested individually (see Table 16-2), but the tendon should still be visibly inspected to rule out a partial laceration.

The use of ancillary studies in the investigation of wounds is discussed in Chap. 12. See Chap. 17 for management of suspected foreign bodies.

Emergency Department Care and Disposition

See Chap. 12 for discussion of wound evaluation and preparation. Most lacerations of the extremities can be closed with simple

TABLE 16-1 Motor Function of Peripheral Nerves

Nerve	Motor function
Radial	Wrist extension Digit extension
Ulnar	Finger abduction Finger adduction Thumb adduction
Median	Thumb flexion Thumb opposition Thumb abduction
Superficial peroneal	Foot eversion
Deep peroneal	Foot inversion Ankle dorsiflexion
Tibial	Ankle plantar flexion

TABLE 16-2 Tendon Function of the Upper and Lower Extremities

Tendon	Motor function
Flexor digitorum profundus	DIP joint flexion
Flexor digitorum superficialis	PIP joint flexion
Flexor carpi ulnaris	Flexion at wrist with ulnar deviation
Flexor carpi radialis	Flexion at wrist with radial deviation
Extensor carpi ulnaris	Extension at wrist with ulnar deviation
Extensor carpi radialis	Extension at wrist with radial deviation
Extensor digitorum communis	Extension of digits 2–5
Flexor pollicis longus	Thumb flexion
Extensor pollicis longus	Thumb extension at DIP
Extensor pollicis brevis	Thumb extension at MCP
Abductor pollicis longus	Thumb abduction
Extensor hallicis longus	Great toe extension with ankle inversion
Tibialis anterior	Ankle dorsiflexion and inversion
Achilles tendon	Ankle plantar flexion and inversion

Abbreviations: DIP, distal interphalangeal; PIP, proximal interphalangeal; MCP, metacarpophalangeal.

interrupted sutures. Deeper wounds may require a two-layer closure, with absorbable 4-0 or 5-0 material to the deeper layer. This is particularly important in areas of high tension. Cyanoacrylite glue is usually not used in areas where there is any tension or movement. Lacerations involving the joint capsule or tendons should be splinted in a position of function.

Specific Areas

Wrist Patients with lacerations to the wrist should be asked about a possible suicide attempt. The function of all tendons must be assessed. Often, lacerations at the wrist are multiple and parallel. Fig. 16-1 demonstrates a technique to close these lacerations. The suture should be at a uniform depth throughout.

Hand Lacerations to the palm can be difficult to anesthetize, and a regional nerve block at the wrist may be required. Any lacerations to the flexor tendons or tendon sheaths, revealed during the obligatory careful inspection, should be referred to a hand surgeon. Repair can be delayed, and these patients should have the wound closed, the hand splinted in a position of function, and referral arranged within a few days. Every effort should be made when repairing palmar lacerations to correctly reapproximate the skin creases and to avoid injury to the underlying tendon sheaths and tendons.

The dorsum of the hand can be anesthetized using a radial nerve block. Repair is usually with interrupted nonabsorbable sutures. Any injury over the metacarpophalangeal (MCP) joints suggests a potential "clenched fist" injury (CFI). (See Chap. 18 for management.)

Extensor tendon laceration not over the MCP joint should be discussed with a hand surgeon. A hand surgeon should repair any extensor tendon injury to the thumb, but experienced emergency physicians can repair extensor tendon injuries to the fingers. Usually a "figure of eight" knot using a 4-0 nonabsorbable suture is used, with the knot tied to the side of the tendon (see Fig. 16-2). Lacerations to the extensor tendon over the distal interphalangeal joint results in a mallet finger deformity, while injuries to the extensor tendon over the proximal interphalangeal joint results in a boutonniere deformity. Both of these injuries are treated with splinting if closed, and operative repair if open.

Lower extremities Wounds on the lower extremities are usually under greater tension than are those on the upper limb. Conse-

FIG. 16-1   Horizontal mattress sutures for multiple parallel lacerations.

quently, a layered closure with 4-0 absorbable material to the fascia and interrupted 4-0 nonabsorbable sutures to the skin is preferred. Deep sutures should be avoided in diabetics and patients with stasis changes, because of the increased risk of infection.

Knee   Wounds over the knee, as for all wounds over joints, should be examined throughout the range of movement. If there is a possibility that the joint may be breached, 60 mL of sterile saline

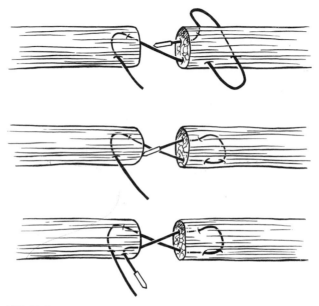

FIG. 16-2   Extensor tendon laceration repair with a figure-of-eight stitch.

can be injected into the joint at a point separate from the wound and the presence of leakage sought. The popliteal artery, the popliteal nerve, and the tibial nerve are all at risk around the knee: their integrity should always be ascertained. After closure, the knee should be splinted to prevent excessive tension on the wound edges.

Ankle and foot Lacerations to the ankle and foot can easily damage underlying tendons. The joints should be moved through their full range with direct inspection of the wound to ensure there is no partial injury to the tendon. Particularly at risk are the Achilles tendon, the tibialis anterior, and the extensor hallucis longus. If any of these tendons are injured, they should be formally repaired. The Thompson test can be utilized to assess the Achilles tendon. While kneeling on a chair, the patient's calf is gently squeezed at the midpoint. Absent plantar flexion of the foot indicates complete Achilles tendon laceration (a partial injury may still yield plantar flexion).

Lacerations of the sole of the foot must be carefully explored to ensure both the absence of tendon injury, but also the absence of foreign bodies. The patient lying prone, with the foot supported on a pillow, or overhanging the bed assists inspection. Regional anesthesia is often best for exploration and repair of lacerations in this area. Large needles are required in order to penetrate adequately the thick dermis of the sole. Absorbable material is usually avoided in the foot. Nonabsorbable 3-0 or 4-0 material is used. Injuries to the dorsum of the foot can be repaired with 4-0 or 5-0 nonabsorbable sutures. Lacerations between the toes can be difficult to repair. The presence of an assistant can be a great help, holding the toes apart. An interrupted mattress suture is often required, in order to ensure adequate skin apposition. Crutches and a walking boot may be required after repair of any laceration on the foot. Other potentially serious injuries to the foot may be caused by lawn mowers and by bicycle spokes. Extensive soft tissue injury can occur, together with underlying fractures and tendon lacerations. These severe injuries require the services of an orthopedic specialist. Finally, an unusual type of injury can be seen in infants, where a strand or strands of hair wrap around one of the toes. The hair must be completely cut to avoid compromising the neurovascular bundle to the toe. This is best accomplished by making an incision on the extensor surface of the toe down to the extensor ligament.

Disposition

Patients should be instructed to keep wounds clean and dry. Sutures should be removed in 7 to 10 days for upper limb lacerations, 10 to 14 days for the lower limb, and 14 days for lacerations over joints. Patients should receive routine wound care instructions. Elevation of the affected limb will reduce edema and aid healing.

For further reading in *Emergency Medicine: A Comprehensive Study Guide,* 5th ed., see Chap. 40, "Lacerations of the Extremities and Joints," by Madonna Fernández and Wendy C. Coates; and Chap. 41, "Foot Lacerations," by Earl J. Reisdorff.

17   Soft Tissue Foreign Bodies

Martin J. Carey

The potential presence of foreign bodies should be considered when evaluating fresh wounds or assessing complications in older wounds. Many times, the foreign body is not obvious to either the patient or the physician. A high index of suspicion and good history taking are essential.

Clinical Features

An increased risk of a foreign body is found in wounds caused by objects that splinter, shatter, or break. Important considerations include glass shards from a breaking bottle, wood splinters (pieces of which may be broken off on attempting to remove the splinter), needles that break off within the wound, or material (e.g., pieces of cloth or a shoe sole) driven into the wound at the time of injury.

Patients have a healed wound, but complain of pain in the wound on pressure or movement. A delayed nerve, tendon, or vessel injury at the site of an old wound requires investigation. A wound that fails to heal or an infection that seems resistant to therapy may indicate a retained foreign body. New onset arthritis in a joint near a wound may be an indication of a thorn-induced synovitis.

Patients' perceptions of a possible foreign body should be regarded seriously. Palpation of the wound may elicit pain, or a foreign body may be felt. Most foreign bodies are found during careful, deliberate exploration of the wound. Adequate lighting, hemostasis, and anesthesia, together with patient cooperation, maximize the chances of finding a foreign body. If necessary, the wound may need to be extended to ensure adequate exploration. Blind exploration with a hemostat is occasionally acceptable, especially if the wound is deep, and extending the wound is not desirable. Glass or metallic objects can be felt to "grate" against the hemostat. Should a foreign body be felt, it should be removed under direct vision.

Diagnosis and Differential

If exploration does not reveal a foreign body, when there is a high degree of suspicion of the presence of one, imaging studies should be performed. If a radiopaque object caused the wound, and no foreign body is seen on adequate radiographs, then the search can end. If the object is not radiopaque, computed tomography (CT) scanning should be considered. Ultrasound is less reliable, but is effective in guiding removal of the foreign body.

Plain Radiography

Plain radiography identifies up to 98 percent of radiopaque objects (glass, metal, gravel, mammalian and some fish bones, teeth, pencil lead, some plastics, and sand). "Soft tissue" radiographs should be obtained, using multiple projections. Radiography is unable to identify vegetative matter, many plastics, and some fish bones. Occasionally there may be indirect evidence of a nonradiopaque foreign body (e.g., a periosteal reaction or air around an object).

Computed Tomography

CT is able to identify a wider range of foreign bodies, as it is 100 times more sensitive at differentiating densities. However, it may not be able to identify some thorns, spines, or certain types of wood. Its disadvantage is the cost and the increased radiation dose.

Ultrasonography

There is a wide range of reported sensitivities and specificities with the use of ultrasound in the detection of foreign bodies such as wood, spines, and other vegetative matter. This variability is due to differences in the size and sonographic nature of the foreign material, the presence of confounding objects such as air or blood around the foreign body, and the skill and experience level of the operator. Once an object has been identified, either by touch, radiography, or ultrasound, ultrasound can be used in place of fluoroscopy to guide retrieval. A 7.5 MHz transducer can find objects up to 3 cm below the skin surface.

Emergency Department Care and Disposition

General Principles

Not all foreign bodies need to be removed; though it is important to identify their presence in the initial visit. Examples include asymptomatic bullets deep in muscle or small inert objects. Vegetative foreign bodies and heavily contaminated objects should always be removed. Multiple small particulate matter (e.g., road grit) should also be removed by careful scrubbing, or traumatic dermal tattooing will result.

Localization of the foreign body is sometimes enhanced through the use of two or three needles inserted around the wound, followed by radiographs taken in multiple planes. If objects cannot be located, or their inert nature does not require immediate removal, patients should be referred to plastic or orthopedic surgeons for foreign body removal.

Specific Foreign Bodies and Removal Procedures

Metallic needles Long, thin objects may be difficult to locate. If the needle is superficial and can be palpated, an incision can be made over one end, and the needle removed. If the needle is deeper, then the incision can be made at the midpoint of the needle and the needle grasped with a hemostat and pushed back out through the entrance wound. If the needle is perpendicular to the skin, the incision may need to be extended. Pressure on the wound edges may then displace the needle so that it can be grasped and removed.

Wood splinters and organic spines As these objects can disintegrate, wood splinters and organic spines should not be simply pulled out of a wound, unless they are very superficial and small. If the splinter is parallel to the skin surface, the splinter should be exposed along its length and removed under direct vision. Alternatively, an elliptical incision can be made to either side of the splinter, and the block of tissue with the embedded splinter removed.

Subungual splinters should be removed either with a splinter forceps or by excising a triangular area of nail over the splinter and then removing the splinter. Cactus spines should be removed with forceps or extracted using facial gel, rubber cement, or household glue. Deeply embedded spines should be removed by incision or excision.

Fishhooks A number of techniques have been described for the removal of fishhooks. In each case, the skin around the site of entry should be anesthetized prior to attempting removal. If very superficial, the hook may be pulled backward out of the skin while gentle downward pressure is placed on the shank of the hook. A piece of string looped around the hook and then firmly tugged, again while downward pressure is applied to the shank, is a variation on this (Fig. 17-1). Care must be taken that the hook does not fly off and injure bystanders. Other methods include sliding a needle along the shank of the hook, eventually finding and covering the barb. The needle and hook are then removed together (Fig. 17-2). Alternatively, the hook can be pushed out through the skin, the barb cut off with wire cutters, and the shank then withdrawn. A further method involves excising the skin over the hook, and then removing the hook through the wound. Care must be taken to avoid significant structures, but this approach has the advantage of allowing adequate cleaning of the site, and ensuring

FIG. 17-1   String-pull technique. String or suture material is tied to the curve of the hook. The hook is positioned as described in the simple retrograde technique, and a quick pull on the string will dislodge the hook.

the removal of any foreign matter, such as the bait, that may have been introduced into the wound.

Postremoval Treatment

After removal, the wound should be adequately cleaned and irrigated. This may require extension of the incision to ensure complete cleaning. If the potential for infection is low and the wound has been completely cleaned, it may be closed primarily. If there is a potential for infection, delayed primary closure is preferred. All patients should have adequate tetanus immunization. If a foreign body is deliberately left in place, the patient should be fully informed.

FIG. 17-2   Needle-cover technique. The area is anesthetized, and an 18-gauge needle is inserted into the entrance wound along the hook. The lumen of the needle is placed over the barb to cover it, and both the hook and needle are backed out of the wound.

Delayed Removal

Patients referred for delayed removal should be reassured of the safety of the practice. If the foreign body is near a tendon or joint, the limb should be splinted. Antibiotics are indicated if the wound is infected, but the utility of prophylactic antibiotics has not been studied.

For further reading in *Emergency Medicine: A Comprehensive Study Guide,* 5th ed., see Chap. 42, "Soft Tissue Foreign Bodies," by Richard L. Lammers.

---

18 | Puncture Wounds and Animal Bites

Michael E. Chansky

PUNCTURE WOUNDS

Puncture wounds may injure underlying structures, introduce a foreign body, and plant inoculum for infection. Infection occurs in up to 11 percent of puncture wounds, with *Staphylococcus aureus* predominating. *Pseudomonas aeruginosa* is the most frequent etiologic agent in postpuncture wound osteomyelitis, particularly when penetration occurs through the sole of an athletic shoe. Postpuncture wound infections and failure of an infection to respond to antibiotics suggests the presence of a retained foreign body. Organized evaluation and management is necessary to minimize complications.

Clinical Features and Diagnosis (See also Chap. 12.)

Wounds over 6 h old with large and deep penetration and obvious visible contamination, which occurred outdoors with penetration through footwear and involving the forefoot carry the highest risk of infectious complications. Patients with a history of diabetes mellitus (DM), peripheral vascular disease (PVD), or immunosuppression (IS) are at increased risk of infection.

On physical examination, the likelihood of injury to structures beneath the skin must be determined. Distal function of tendons, nerves, and vessels should be carefully assessed. The site should be inspected for location, condition of the surrounding skin, and the presence of foreign matter, debris, or devitalized tissue. Infection is suggested when there is evidence of pain, swelling, erythema, warmth, fluctuance, decreased range of motion, or evidence of drainage from the site.

A high index of suspicion must be maintained for a retained foreign body. Multiple view "soft tissue" plain-film radiographs should be obtained of all infected puncture wounds and of any wound suspicious for a retained foreign body. See Chap. 17 for recommendations on the diagnosis and management of retained foreign bodies.

Emergency Department Care and Disposition

Many aspects of the treatment of puncture wounds remain controversial.

1. Uncomplicated, clean punctures < 6 h after injury require only low-pressure **irrigation** and **tetanus prophylaxis** as indicated. Soaking has no proven benefit. Healthy patients do not appear to require prophylactic antibiotics.
2. Prophylactic antibiotics "may" benefit patients with PVD, DM, and IS. Plantar puncture wounds, especially those in high-risk patients, located in the forefoot, or those through athletic shoes should be treated with prophylactic antibiotics. Fluoroquinolones (such as **ciprofloxacin** 500 mg bid) are broad-spectrum antibiotics that rapidly achieve high blood levels following an oral dose and are acceptable alternatives to parenteral administration of both a cephalosporin and aminoglycoside. In general prophylactic antibiotics should be continued for 5 to 7 days.
3. Ciprofloxacin is not recommended for use in children for prophylaxis. **Cephalexin** 25 to 50 mg/kg per day divided qid up to 500 mg can be used with close follow-up.
4. Wounds infected at presentation need to be differentiated into cellulitis, abscess, deeper spreading soft tissue infections, and bone or cartilage involvement. **Plain radiographs** are indicated to detect the possibility of a radiopaque foreign body, soft tissue gas, or osteomyelitis.
5. Cellulitis is usually localized without significant drainage, developing within 1 to 4 days. There is no need for routine cultures, and antimicrobial coverage should be directed at gram-positive organisms, especially *S. aureus*. Effective agents include **diclox-**

acillin (500 mg PO tid), first-generation cephalosporins (e.g., **cephalexin**), or **ciprofloxacin.**

6. A local abscess may develop at the puncture site, especially if a foreign body remains. Treatment includes incision, drainage, and careful exploration for a retained foreign body. Serious, deep soft tissue infections require surgical exploration and debridement in the OR.

7. Any patient who relapses or fails to improve after initial therapy should be suspected of having osteomyelitis or septic arthritis. Radiographs, WBC, ESR, and orthopedic consultation should be obtained. Definitive management frequently necessitates operative intervention for debridement. Pending cultures, antibiotics are started that cover *Staphylococcus* and *Pseudomonas* species. A reasonable regimen would be parenteral **nafcillin,** 1 to 2 g IV q 4 h, and **ceftazidime,** 1 to 2 g IV q 8 h.

8. Conditions for admission include wound infection in patients with DM, PVD, or other immunocompromised states; wounds with progressive cellulitis and lymphangitic spread; osteomyelitis; septic arthritis; and deep foreign bodies necessitating operative removal.

9. Tetanus prophylaxis should be provided according to guidelines (see Chap. 89). Outpatients should avoid weight-bearing, elevate and soak the wound in warm water, and have follow-up within 48 h.

NEEDLE-STICK INJURIES

Needle-stick injuries carry the risk of bacterial infection in addition to the risk of infection with hepatitis and human immunodeficiency virus (HIV). Each hospital should have a predesigned protocol developed by infectious disease specialists for the expeditious evaluation, testing, and treatment of needle-stick injuries, because recommendations in this area are complex and changing.

HIGH-PRESSURE-INJECTION INJURIES

High-pressure-injection injuries may present as a puncture wound, usually to the hand or foot. This equipment is designed to force liquids (usually paint or oil) through a small nozzle under high pressure—sometimes up to several thousand pounds per square inch. These injuries are severe owing to intense inflammation incited by the injected liquid spreading along fascial planes. Patients have pain and minimal swelling. Despite an innocuous appearance, serious damage can develop. Pain control should be achieved with parenteral analgesics; digital blocks are contraindicated so as to avoid increases in tissue pressure with resultant further compromise in perfusion. An appropriate hand specialist should be consulted immediately and early surgical debridement implemented for an optimal outcome.

HUMAN BITES

Human bites produce a crushing or tearing of tissue, with potential for injury to underlying structures and inoculation of tissues with normal human oral flora. Human bites are most often reported on the hands and upper extremities. Infection is the major serious sequelae.

Clinical Features (See also Chap. 12.)

Of particular concern is the clenched fist injury (CFI), which occurs at the metacarpophalangeal (MCP) region as the fist strikes the mouth and teeth of another individual. These hand injuries are at increased risk for serious infection, and any questionable injury in the vicinity of the MCP joint should be considered a CFI until proved otherwise.

The physical examination should include assessment of the direct injury and a careful evaluation of the underlying structures, including tendons, vessels, nerves, deep spaces, joints, and bone. Local anesthesia is usually required to perform a careful wound exploration. In a CFI, the wound must be examined through a full range of motion at the MCP joint to detect extensor tendon involvement, which may have retracted proximally in the unclenched hand. The exam must also assess a potential joint-space violation. Radiographs are recommended, particularly of the hand, to delineate foreign bodies and fractures.

Human bites to the hand are frequently complicated by cellulitis, lymphangitis, abscess formation, tenosynovitis, septic arthritis, and osteomyelitis. The most frequent aerobic organism isolated is *Streptococcus viridans,* followed by *Staph. epidermidis, Corynebacterium* sp., *Staph. aureus, Eikenella* sp., and *Haemophilus* sp. Common anaerobic isolates include *Bacteroides* sp., *Fusobacterium* sp., and anaerobic cocci (e.g., *Peptostreptococcus* sp.). Human bites to locations other than the hand appear to have similar rates of infection as nonbite lacerations. Human bites in children and bites to the face have exhibited low rates of infection, often less than 5 percent.

Diagnosis

History and physical exam usually will reveal a straightforward diagnosis. There are times, however, when a patient may try to conceal or deny the true etiology of a human bite and a high degree of suspicion is warranted, particularly when the wound is on the hand. It is important to keep in mind that viral diseases can also be transmitted by human bites (e.g., herpes simplex, herpetic whitlow, and hepatitis B.) The potential risk of acquiring HIV through a human bite appears to be negligible due to low levels of HIV in saliva.

Emergency Department Care and Disposition

1. Copious wound **irrigation** with a normal saline solution and judicious limited debridement of devitalized tissue are critical to initial management.
2. Human bites to the hand should initially be left open. Other sites can undergo primary closure unless there is a high degree of suspicion for infection.
3. Prophylactic antibiotics should be considered in all human bites of the hands and other locations in high-risk patients (i.e., those with asplenia, diabetes mellitus, and HIV). Three to five days of treatment with an acceptable regimen covering mouth flora (such as **amoxicillin/clavulanate,** 500 mg PO tid, or a fluoroquinolone) should be initiated.
4. Uncomplicated fresh CFI wounds should be left open with an appropriate dressing. The hand should be immobilized and elevated for 24 h, and prophylactic antibiotics should be administered. The patient should be reevaluated in 1 to 2 days. If there is a laceration to either the extensor tendon or joint capsule, or radiographic findings, a hand specialist should be consulted for possible exploration in the operating room and admission for parenteral antibiotics.
5. Wounds that are infected at presentation require systemic antibiotics after cultures are obtained. Local cellulitis in healthy and reliable patients may be managed on an outpatient basis with immobilization, antibiotics, and close follow-up. Moderate-to-severe infections require admission for surgical consultation and parenteral antibiotics. Appropriate coverage includes **ampicillin/sulbactam,** 1.5 g q 6 h IV, or **cefoxitin,** 2.0 g q 8 h IV. Penicillin-allergic patients may be treated with clindamycin plus ciprofloxacin.
6. All patients should receive tetanus immunization according to guidelines.

DOG BITES

Dog bites account for 80 to 90 percent of reported animal bites, with school-age children sustaining the majority of reported bites. Infection occurs in approximately 5 percent of cases and is more common in patients over 50 years old, those with hand wounds or deep puncture wounds, and those who delay in seeking initial treatment over a 24-h period.

Clinical Features

A thorough history and exam as outlined in the section on human bites are required to assess the extent of the wound and the likelihood of infection. Radiographs are recommended if there is evidence of infection, suspicion of a foreign body, bony involvement, or large dog intracranial penetration bites to the heads of small children. Infections from dog-bite wounds are often polymicrobial and include both aerobic and anaerobic bacteria. *Staph. aureus, Pasteurella multocida,* β- and γ-hemolytic streptococci, *E. corrodens,* and *Actinomyces* and *Bacteroides* species are among the most frequent isolates. *Capnocytophaga canimorsus* is a fastidious, thin, gram-negative bacillus that has been associated with severe infection in immunocompromised patients (i.e., those with asplenia), causing sepsis, DIC, acute renal failure, and cardiopulmonary failure.

Emergency Department Care and Disposition

1. All dog-bite wounds require appropriate local wound care with copious **irrigation** and debridement of devitalized tissue.
2. Primary closure can be utilized in wounds to the scalp, face, torso, and extremities other than the feet and hands. Lacerations of the feet and hands should be left open initially. Large, extensive lacerations, especially in small children, are best explored and repaired in the operating room.
3. Puncture wounds, wounds to the hands and feet, and wounds in high-risk patients should receive 3 to 5 days of prophylactic antibiotics with **amoxicillin/clavulanate** 500 mg PO tid or clindamycin plus ciprofloxacin. In children, clindamycin plus trimethoprim-sulfamethoxazole should be used.
4. **Penicillin** (500 mg qid) is the drug of choice for *C. canimorsus* and should be used prophylactically in high-risk immunocompromised patients (i.e., those with asplenia, alcoholism, or chronic lung disease). Cephalosporins, tetracyclines, erythromycin, and clindamycin are reasonable alternatives.
5. Wounds obviously infected at presentation need to be cultured

and antibiotics initiated. Reliable, low-risk patients with only local cellulitis and no involvement of underlying structures can be managed as outpatients with close follow-up. Infection developing within 24 h after injury suggests *P. multocida,* and treatment with **penicillin,** ciprofloxacin, or trimethoprim-sulfamethoxazole is recommended. Wound infection developing beyond 24 h after the bite implicates *Staphylococcus* and *Streptococcus,* and these patients should receive **dicloxacillin** (12 to 25 mg/kg per day divided qid: 500 mg qid in adults) or first-generation cephalosporin (e.g., **cephalexin,** 25 to 50 mg/kg per day divided qid: 500 mg qid in adults).

6. Significant wound infections require admission and parenteral antibiotics. Examples include infected wounds with evidence of lymphangitis, lymphadenitis, tenosynovitis, septic arthritis, osteomyelitis, systemic signs, and injury to underlying structures, such as tendons, joints, or bones. Radiographs may reveal fractures, soft tissue air or dislodged teeth. Cultures should be obtained from deep structures, preferably during exploration in the operating room. Initial antibiotic therapy should begin with ampicillin/sulbactam or clindamycin plus ciprofloxacin. If the gram stain reveals gram-negative bacilli, a third- or fourth-generation cephalosporin or aminoglycoside should be added.

7. Tetanus prophylaxis should be provided according to standard guidelines.

CAT BITES

Cat bites account for 5 to 18 percent of reported animal bites, with the majority resulting in puncture wounds on the arm, forearm, and hand. Up to 80 percent of cat bites become infected, primarily due to the high percentage of puncture wounds and a higher likelihood of *P. multocida* in feline oral flora.

Clinical Features

P. multocida is the major pathogen, isolated in 53 to 80 percent of infected cat bite wounds. *Pasteurella* causes a rapidly developing intense inflammatory response with prominent symptoms of pain and swelling. It may cause serious bone and joint infections, and bacteremia. Many patients with septic arthritis due to *P. multocida* have altered host defenses due to glucocorticoids or alcoholism.

Emergency Department Care and Disposition

Treatment for cat-bite wounds is essentially the same as for dog-bite wounds.

1. All cat-bite wounds require appropriate local wound care with copious **irrigation** and debridement of devitalized tissue.
2. Primary wound closure is usually indicated, except in puncture wounds and lacerations smaller than 1 to 2 cm, as they cannot be adequately cleaned. Delayed primary closure can also be employed in cosmetically important areas.
3. Prophylactic antibiotics should be administered to high-risk patients including those with punctures of the hand; immunocompromised patients; and patients with arthritis or prosthetic joints. The case can be made that all cat bites should receive prophylactic antibiotics because of the high risk of infection. **Amoxicillin/clavulanate, cefuroxime, or doxycycline,** administered 3 to 5 days, are appropriate.
4. For cat bites that develop infection, evaluation and treatment is similar to dog-bite infections. Radiographs may reveal dislodged teeth in puncture wounds. Penicillin is the drug of choice for *Pasteurella multocida* infections.
5. **Tetanus prophylaxis** should be provided according to standard guidelines.

CAT-SCRATCH DISEASE

Clinical Features

Cat-scratch disease (CSD) occurs most often in young patients, with persistent regional lymphadenopathy in the area of the body draining the site of a recent cat scratch or bite. Often this is preceded by an erythematous papule or pustule at the inoculation site. Although most patients with cat-scratch disease are not seriously ill and spontaneous resolution is common, up to 2 percent can suffer from involvement in the CNS, liver, spleen, bone, and skin. The precise etiologic agent has been difficult to determine, but most investigations implicate *Bartonella henselae,* a small gram-negative rod.

Diagnosis

Diagnosis is made with (*a*) history of cat exposure, (*b*) typical lymphadenopathy, (*c*) no other cause of lymph gland swelling, and (*d*) a positive serologic test for *B. hensalae.* Serologic assay using the polymerase chain reaction is the most accurate method.

Emergency Department Care and Disposition

Most patients with CSD are not seriously ill, spontaneous resolution is common, and antibiotic therapy has not been studied in large controlled clinical trials. Most reviews do not recommend antibiotic therapy for uncomplicated cases. Antimicrobial susceptibility testing has shown favorable MIC values to rifampin, gentamicin, doxycycline, and the macrolides, which all penetrate human cells where the bacterium resides. Severely ill patients, those with systemic complications, and immunocompromised patients should be treated with either **rifampin** or **trimethoprim-sulfamethoxazole.**

For further reading in *Emergency Medicine: A Comprehensive Study Guide,* 5th ed., see Chap. 43, "Puncture Wounds and Bites," by Charles A. Eckerline, Jr., Jim Blake, and Ronald F. Koury.

---

19 | Postrepair Wound Care

Eugenia B. Smith

DRESSINGS

Wound dressings provide a moist environment, which facilitates epithelialization during the first 24 to 48 h. Face and scalp lacerations may be simply dressed with a layer of antibiotic ointment. Iodine-containing preparations should be avoided as they may impair wound healing. Wounds that are not on the face or scalp are generally dressed.

The basic wound dressing has four layers: (*a*) a nonadherent layer adjacent to the wound, (*b*) gauze sponges to absorb any exudate, (*c*) wrapping to hold the first two layers in place, and (*d*) tape or elastic bandage to secure the entire package.

Reasons for wound dressing include the following:

1. General cleanliness as the dressing absorbs exudate.
2. Protection from external contamination when the patient returns home or to work.
3. Camouflage, so that the patient or others do not have to see the wound.

4. Prevention of premature suture removal from spontaneous un-raveling or due to the patient's curiosity.
5. Prevention from excessive movement by providing a "soft" splint.
6. Satisfying the patient's expectation that the repaired wound will be dressed.

Dressing Changes

Generally, wound dressings should be changed as often as needed to maintain cleanliness and to remove drainage or exudate. A routine change in 24 h is recommended to inspect the wound for early signs of infection, check for bleeding, and remove exudate. The wound should be redressed, and often a simpler dressing may be applied.

PAIN CONTROL

Patients who receive appropriate analgesia while in the emergency department (ED) and postdischarge will be more comfortable and satisfied with their care. If narcotic analgesia is requested, it is generally not required after 48 h.

ANTIBIOTIC PROPHYLAXIS

The following types of wounds have shown evidence that supports the use of appropriate antibiotic prophylaxis upon discharge from the ED:

1. Intraoral lacerations: penicillin.
2. Complicated human bites: amoxicillin/clavulanate.
3. Complicated dog bites: amoxicillin/clavulanate.
4. Cat bites: amoxicillin/clavulanate.
5. Plantar puncture wounds, particularly through athletic shoes: ciprofloxacin (not for children).
6. See Chap. 18 for treatment alternatives and more information.

RECHECKS

Selective rechecks are appropriate for patients with complicated wounds at risk for infection, those with comorbid conditions such

TABLE 19-1 Timing for Removal of Cutaneous Sutures and Staples

Area	Number of days
Face	4–5
Scalp	7–10
Trunk	10
Arm (surface)	10
Arm (joint)	10–14
Hand	10–14
Leg (surface)	10
Leg (joint)	10–14
Foot	14

as immunosuppression, or those who do not seem to understand signs of infection.

CLOSURE REMOVAL

Facial sutures are removed at 4 to 5 days in order to avoid potential "railroad track" appearance, and wounds may require adhesive closure strips for an additional 3 to 4 days. Sutures and staples in other areas may be removed in 7 to 14 days (Table 19-1). Sutures and staples applied over highly mobile areas such as major joints may require an additional 3 to 4 days.

INSTRUCTIONS FOR PATIENTS

1. Washing: Scalp, face, and neck wounds may be washed after 8 to 24 h, wounds in other areas may be washed in 12 to 24 h. Immersion or soaking of the wound should be avoided.
2. Bleeding: A small amount of bloody discharge is expected, if more bleeding occurs the patient should return for a recheck.
3. Infection: The patient should return for a recheck if there is increased pain, redness, purulent drainage, fever, or red streaks.
4. Dehiscence: The patient should return if the wound opens.
5. Cosmesis: Scar appearance depends on wounding mechanism, type of wound, location, and comorbid diseases. Sunscreens may be required for several months. If necessary, wound revision should wait 6 to 9 months after initial injury.

CONCLUSION

Simple and specific instructions upon discharge are an important aspect of wound management and will enhance patient satisfaction.

For further reading in *Emergency Medicine: A Comprehensive Study Guide,* 5th ed., see Chap. 44, "Postrepair Wound Care," by Louis J. Kroot.

CARDIOVASCULAR DISEASES

| 20 | Approach to Chest Pain and Possible Myocardial Ischemia |

Thomas Rebbecchi

Patients with acute nontraumatic chest pain are among the most challenging patients cared for by emergency physicians. They may appear seriously ill or completely well and yet remain at significant risk for sudden death or an acute myocardial infarction.

Clinical Features

The typical pain of myocardial ischemia has been described as retrosternal or epigastric squeezing, tightening, crushing, or pressure-like discomfort. The pain may radiate to the left shoulder, jaw, arm, or hand. In many cases, particularly in the elderly, the predominant complaint is not of pain, but of a poorly described visceral sensation with associated dyspnea, diaphoresis, nausea, light-headedness, or profound weakness. The onset of symptoms may be sudden or gradual, and symptoms usually last minutes to hours. In general, symptoms that last less than 2 min, or are constant over days, are less likely to be ischemic in origin. Symptoms that are new to the patient, or are familiar, yet now occur with increasing frequency, severity, or at rest are called unstable and warrant urgent evaluation even if they are absent at the time of presentation. Cardiac risk factors should only be used to predict coronary artery disease (CAD) within a given population and not in an individual patient. It should also be mentioned that women may have more subtle signs of ischemia.

Physical Examination

Patients with acute myocardial ischemia may appear clinically well or be profoundly hemodynamically unstable. The degree of hemodynamic instability is dependent on the amount of myocardium at risk, associated dysrhythmias, and/or preexisting valvular or myocardial dysfunction. Worrisome signs may be clinically subtle, particularly the presence of sinus tachycardia, which may be due to pain and fear, or may be an early sign of physiologic compensation for left ventricular failure. Patients with acute ischemia often have a paucity of significant physical findings. Rales, a third or fourth heart sound, cardiac murmurs, or rub are all clinically relevant and important findings. The presence of chest wall tenderness has been demonstrated in patients with acute myocardial infarction, and so its presence should not be used to exclude the possibility of acute myocardial ischemia. Also, response to a particular treatment should not be taken as evidence of a certain disease.

Diagnosis and Differential

Electrocardiography

Of all the diagnostic tools clinically used in assessing chest pain, the electrocardiogram (ECG) is the most reliable when used and interpreted correctly. Patients with acute infarctions may have ECG findings that range from acute ST-segment elevations to completely normal. This means that the ECG is useful only when it has a positive, or diagnostic, finding. New ST-segment elevations, Q waves, bundle branch block, and T-wave inversions or normalizations are highly suggestive of ischemia and warrant aggressive management in the emergency department (ED). The presence of a normal or unchanged ECG does not rule out the diagnosis of acute myocardial ischemia.

Serum Markers

Serum markers, if positive, are highly specific for acute myocardial infarction and include myoglobin, creatinine phosphokinase (CK) and its MB isoenzyme, troponin I and T, and others. The documentation of normal serum markers in the bloodstream does not exclude the diagnosis of acute myocardial infarction. The use of these markers can aid the clinician in assessing risk for chest pain patients including disposition within the hospital.

Echocardiography

Emergency two-dimensional echocardiography may have value in the evaluation of chest pain when the ECG is nondiagnostic, for example, in patients with pacemakers, have a bundle branch block, or have a baseline abnormal ECG. The finding of regional wall-motion abnormalities in acutely symptomatic patients is highly suggestive of active ischemia. Two-dimensional echocardiography may also aid in the diagnosis of other conditions that may mimic ischemic disease, such as pericarditis, aortic dissection, or hypertrophic cardiomyopathy.

Provocative Tests

A number of tests are now being performed in some EDs that will unmask otherwise unrecognized, clinically significant ischemic disease. Patients with atypical chest pain and normal stress thallium or technetium scans have a very low incidence of both short- and long-term subsequent ischemic events.

Differential Diagnosis

The priority must always be to exclude life-threatening conditions, and ED physicians should organize their test ordering strategies to screen for those conditions first. (For a list of possible causes of nontraumatic chest pain, see Table 20-1.)

Specific Causes of Chest Pain

Angina Pectoris

The pain of chronic stable angina is episodic and lasts 5 to 15 min. It is precipitated by exertion and relieved with rest or sublingual nitroglycerin within 3 min. The pain is typically visceral in nature (aching, pressure, and squeezing) with radiation to the neck, jaw, arm, or hand. In individual patients the character of each attack varies little with recurrent episodes. Most patients can differentiate their usual angina from other causes of pain. Physicians evaluating patients with stable angina should carefully screen for changes in the pattern that would suggest a shift from stable to unstable angina or even suggest a different diagnosis.

Unstable Angina

Patients who complain of recent onset of angina, changing character of their angina, or angina at rest are thought to have an unstable pattern of their angina. They are at risk for an acute myocardial infarction or sudden cardiac death. (See Chap. 22 for management.)

Variant (prinzmetal) Angina

This form of angina is thought to be due to spasm of the epicardial vessels in patients with either normal coronary arteries (one-third of patients) or in patients with underlying atherosclerotic disease (two-thirds of patients). Pain typically occurs at rest and may be precipitated by the use of tobacco or cocaine. The ECG typically shows ST-segment elevations during an acute attack.

Acute Myocardial Infarction

Ischemic pain that lasts longer than 15 min, is not relieved by nitroglycerin, or is accompanied by diaphoresis, dyspnea, nausea,

TABLE 20-1 Etiology of Nontraumatic Chest Pain

Cardiac causes
  Coronary artery disease
  Stable angina
  Unstable angina
  Variant angina
  Acute myocardial infarction

Pericarditis

Valvular disease
  Aortic stenosis
  Subaortic stenosis
  Mitral valve prolapse

Vascular causes
  Aortic dissection
  Pulmonary embolus
  Pulmonary hypertension

Pulmonary causes
  Pleural irritation from infection, inflammation, infiltration
  Barotrauma from pneumothorax, pneumomediastinum
  Tracheobronchitis

Musculoskeletal causes
  Costochondritis
  Intercostal muscle strain
  Cervical thoracic spine problems

Gastrointestinal causes
  Esophageal reflux/spasm
  Mallory Weiss syndrome
  Biliary colic
  Dyspepsia
  Pancreatitis

Miscellaneous causes
  Herpes zoster
  Chest wall tumors

or vomiting, suggests the diagnosis of acute myocardial infarction. The clinician must understand the limitations of the screening tools used in the ED and should have a high level of suspicion for acute myocardial infarction in patients with risk factors and prolonged or persistent symptoms for whom there is no other clear diagnosis. (See Chap. 22.)

Aortic Dissection

This diagnosis should be suspected in patients who complain of sudden onset of severe, tearing pain in the retrosternal or midscapular area. High-risk patients are also those at risk for acute myocardial infarction, specifically the middle-aged hypertensive male. Patients may be hypertensive or hypotensive in shock. There may be a diastolic murmur of aortic regurgitation indicating a proximal dissection or distal pulse deficits, indicating a distal dissection. The dissection may occlude coronary ostia, resulting in myocardial infarction, or the carotids, resulting in cerebral ischemia and stroke. (See Chap. 28 for a complete discussion of aortic dissection.)

Pericarditis

Patients with pericarditis will typically complain of pain that is constant, retrosternal, and radiating to the back, neck, or jaw. Pain is classically worsened by lying supine and is relieved by sitting forward. The presence of a pericardial friction rub supports the diagnosis. ECG may show PR-segment depressions, diffuse ST-segment elevations, or T-wave inversions that are typically diffuse. (See Chap. 25 for a complete discussion of pericarditis.)

Acute Pericardial Tamponade

Patients with acute tamponade may complain of positional or pleuritic chest pain, dyspnea, and palpitations. Their exam will reveal tachycardia, hypotension, jugular venous distension, and distant heart sounds. If cardiovascular collapse is imminent, emergent pericardiocentesis is indicated.

Pulmonary Embolus

Patients typically complain of sudden onset of pleuritic chest pain associated with dyspnea, tachypnea, tachycardia, or hypoxemia. The absence of any of these findings does not preclude the diagnosis, and a high index of suspicion is essential. (See Chap. 26 for a complete discussion of pulmonary embolism.)

Musculoskeletal Causes

Chest pain due to irritation or inflammation of structures in the chest wall is commonly seen in the ED. Possible causes include costochondritis, intercostal strain due to severe coughing, and pectoralis muscle strain in the setting of recent physical exertion. Patients will complain of sharp pain that is worsened with movement of the chest wall, and coughing, and some pain that can be elicited by palpation of the chest wall. These findings in patients without any other symptoms and no history of significant cardiac disease support the diagnosis of musculoskeletal pain. This pain is generally responsive to nonsteroidal anti-inflammatory drugs (NSAIDs). It is important to emphasize that the presence of chest wall tenderness does not rule out the possibility of myocardial ischemia.

Gastrointestinal Causes

Esophageal reflux, dyspepsia syndromes, and esophageal motility disorders can produce chest pain that is difficult to distinguish from ischemic pain. Patients may complain of burning, gnawing pain associated with an acid taste radiating into the throat. Pain may be exacerbated by meals, worse when supine and associated with belching. Clinicians should determine whether the symptoms are due to a gastrointestinal (GI) disorder based on the clinical presentation and the absence of findings and/or risk factors suggesting an ischemic cause. Diagnostic decisions should not be made on the basis of a response to a therapeutic trial of antacids, GI cocktails, or nitroglycerin. (See Chaps. 36, 38, and 40 for more discussion of GI causes of chest pain.)

Emergency Department Care and Disposition

It should be assumed that every patient complaining of chest pain might be having an acute myocardial infarction. Patients with suspicious histories should have a large-bore intravenous line established, a cardiac monitor, and an ECG obtained as soon as possible. Vital signs and pulse oximetry should be continuously monitored.

1. Patient should be asked about cardiac risk factors, preexisting CAD, quality of chest pain, time of onset and duration of symptoms, and whether the pattern has been stable, unstable, continuous, or intermittent. Physicians should ask specifically for clues to noncardiac causes of chest pain: ability to elicit pain by movement or cough; relationship to meals; pain that is of sudden onset, referred to the back, or pleuritic in nature.
2. Patients should be examined noting evidence of heart failure or valvular insufficiency, pericardial rubs, or tenderness of the chest wall. Specifically, physicians should ask whether pain elicited on palpation of the chest wall exactly reproduces the patient's pain.
3. An ECG should be obtained on all patients for whom there is a reasonable suspicion of myocardial ischemia. A normal ECG, although minimizing the likelihood of an acute myocardial infarction, does not definitively rule out the possibility of MI.
4. If the etiology of chest pain remains unclear in some patients, clinicians should consider obtaining arterial blood gases, chest x-rays, and echocardiograms, as guided by clinical suspicion and findings.

5. Clinicians should not use patients' clinical response to GI cocktails, nitroglycerin, or NSAIDs to exclude the possibility of myocardial ischemia.
6. In patients with nondiagnostic ECGs for whom there is a clinical suspicion for ischemia, clinicians should consider provocative testing, echocardiography, or admission and observation. Physicians should not rely on serum enzyme testing to rule out the possibility of clinically significant disease.

For further reading in *Emergency Medicine: A Comprehensive Study Guide,* 5th ed., see Chap. 45, "Approach to Chest Pain and Possible Myocardial Ischemia," by Gary B. Green and Peter M. Hill.

---

21 | Syncope
Christian A. Tomaszewski

Syncope, which accounts for up to 3 percent of all emergency department (ED) visits, is a transient loss of consciousness accompanied by loss of postural tone. Although syncope typically is a benign vasovagal event, it may represent a life-threatening dysrhythmia particularly in the elderly. One-half of all patients will never have a definite etiology established for their syncopal episode.

Clinical Features

The most common cause of syncope is reflex-mediated, where a sympathetic response to stress is suddenly withdrawn leading to pronounced vagal tone with hypotension and/or bradycardia. The hallmark of vasovagal syncope is the prodrome of dizziness, nausea, diminished vision, pallor, and diaphoresis. In addition, the clinician should look for appropriate stimuli (i.e., blood drawing, injury, and fear) in combination with standing, before making the diagnosis of vasovagal syncope. An elderly patient may relate that they were wearing a tight collar, shaving, or turning their head immediately prior to fainting, thus suggesting carotid sinus hypersensitivity. In situational syncope, the autonomic reflexive response may result from a specific physical stimulus, such as micturation, defecation, or extreme coughing.

A sudden change in posture after prolonged recumbence, with the inability to mount an adequate increase in heart rate and/or peripheral vascular resistance results in orthostatic syncope. Often this is due to autonomic dysfunction, such as peripheral neuropathy, spinal cord injury, and Shy-Drager's syndrome. More serious causes of orthostatic syncope are disorders that cause volume depletion, such as vomiting, diarrhea, bleeding, diuresis, and sepsis.

Cardiac syncope is due to either a dysrhythmia or a structural cardiopulmonary lesion. Tachydysrhythmias, such as ventricular tachycardia, torsades de pointes, and supraventricular tachycardia, are common causes of syncope. But one is more likely to encounter incidental bradycardia on examination and electrocardiogram (ECG). Syncope from dysrhythmias is usually sudden, with a brief (< 3 s) prodrome, if any. Structural abnormalities of the heart are unmasked as syncope during exertion or vasodilatory drugs. In the elderly, this is most commonly due to aortic stenosis. In the young patient, it is most commonly hypertrophic cardiomyopathy. Approximately 10 percent of patients with pulmonary embolism will have pulmonary outflow obstruction that leads to syncope.

Cerebrovascular disorders are a rare cause of syncope. If brainstem ischemia is the cause, then usually patients report other posterior circulation deficits—diplopia, vertigo, and nausea—associated with the "drop attack." If patients relate that upper extremity exercise preceded the event, then they may be suffering from obstruction of the brachiocephalic or subclavian artery, i.e., subclavian steal syndrome. A transient rise in intracranial pressure with subarachnoid hemorrhage is probably the cause of syncope in patients with a severe "thunderclap" headache.

Because of poor autonomic responses and multiple medications, the elderly are particularly prone to syncope, usually due to cardiac causes. Antihypertensive agents, such as β blockers and calcium channel antagonists, blunt tachycardic reflexes to orthostatic or vasodilatory stress. In addition, they may cause cardiac blocks and life-threatening dysrhythmias. Diuretics also contribute to orthostatic hypotension from volume depletion. Syncope is a dual threat to elderly patients—it causes falls with orthopedic injuries and it portends sudden cardiac death in many cases.

Diagnosis and Differential

Although an etiology for the syncopal episode may be difficult to establish, the most important tools in the workup of syncope are a good history, physical examination, and ECG. The history should be directed to high-risk factors, including age, medications, and prodromal events. Sudden events without warning suggest dysrhythmias; exertion may imply a structural cardiopulmonary lesion. Associated symptoms are helpful for detecting a cardiac (i.e., palpitations and chest pain) or neurologic (i.e., vertigo and focal weakness) cause for syncope. Back or abdominal pain may suggest a leaking abdominal aortic aneurysm or ruptured ectopic pregnancy. Trauma without defensive injuries or single vehicle crashes may distract one from an initial syncopal event as the precipitating cause. Additionally, past medical history is useful in revealing cardiac or psychiatric (e.g., hyperventilation) causes for syncope.

Physical examination may reveal the ultimate cause of syncope. The cardiac exam may uncover a ventricular flow obstruction problem. A cardiac murmur may represent aortic stenosis or hypertrophic cardiomyopathy. An accentuated pulmonary gallop can be a clue to pulmonary embolism. A complete neurologic assessment and rectal examination may yield further secondary causes for syncope.

Although the yield is low, the ECG is useful in detecting ischemia and dysrhythmias. The ECG can also show a propensity to dysrhythmias such as prolonged QT interval leading to torsades de pointes, or shortening of the PR interval and a delta wave seen in Wolf-Parkinson-White syndrome. Prolonged monitoring may reveal a transient, but recurring, dysrhythmia.

Selected laboratory testing is the norm. A hematocrit or rectal exam for occult gastrointestinal bleeding may explain syncope associated with orthostatic hypotension. Women of childbearing age warrant a pregnancy test. Although not recommended routinely, electrolytes may reveal a depressed bicarbonate after a seizure and are indicated in patients with weakness or irritable myocardium.

There are a variety of bedside tests that may provide clues in selected cases, such as reproducing presyncopal symptoms with hyperventilation. A blood pressure check in both arms with more than a 20 mmHg difference suggests subclavian steal syndrome. Carotid sinus massage can be performed in selected patients without bruits if one suspects carotid sinus hypersensitivity. Orthostatic hypotension (autonomic instability from drugs or disease) is defined as a systolic blood pressure drop of at least 20 mmHg. The caveat of making this diagnosis is that symptoms should recur with standing.

Seizure is the most common disorder mistaken for syncope. The hallmarks of seizure, i.e., tongue biting and incontinence, can also be seen with convulsive syncope, which are brief clonic jerks due to cerebral anoxia. The most helpful differentiating factor is that true seizures are followed by a postictal phase with disorientation and slow return to normal consciousness.

Emergency Department Care and Disposition

By definition, syncope results in spontaneous recovery of consciousness. Therefore, the main goal of ED care is to identify those patients at risk for further medical problems. Patients can be divided into three classes after a careful history, physical examination, and ECG:

1. *If the diagnosis is established,* then patients can be appropriately managed directing attention to the underlying cause of their syncopal event. Patients with syncope in whom a life-threatening etiology is identified, including neurologic or cardiac causes, warrant admission. If the diagnosis is not established, then patients can be further stratified:

2. *High-risk patients* are those at risk for sudden cardiac death or ventricular dysrhythmia: i.e., abnormal ECG, age > 45 years, or history of ventricular dysrhythmia or congestive heart failure. With admission, the workup of these patients can be expedited to determine a possible structural or electrical cause of cardiac syncope.

3. *Low-risk patients* are those unlikely to have a cardiac etiology for their syncope. These patients are young (age < 45 years) and have a normal physical examination and ECG. Usually their syncope is due to vasovagal mechanisms and they do not require further workup for an isolated episode. They can be discharged safely home with instructions to return if there is a recurrence of presyncopal symptoms. Worrisome or recurrent cases may benefit from further outpatient workup including Holter monitoring. They should also be advised not to work at heights or drive their vehicle until a diagnosis is established.

For further reading in *Emergency Medicine: A Comprehensive Study Guide,* 5th ed., see Chap. 46, "Syncope," by Barbara K. Blok.

22 | Acute Coronary Syndromes: Myocardial Ischemia and Infarction and Their Management

Frantz R. Melio

MYOCARDIAL ISCHEMIA AND INFARCTION

Ischemic heart disease and its complications are the leading causes of death in the United States. Approximately 1.3 million nonfatal acute myocardial infarcts and 500,000 to 700,000 deaths occur yearly. Of these patients, 50 to 60 percent will die prior to hospital arrival. The majority of additional deaths will occur early during initial hospitalization. Currently, the greatest potential to decreasing mortality and morbidity is to minimize the time between injury and treatment.

Clinical Features

Myocardial ischemia results from the imbalance between myocardial oxygen supply and demand. Seven major risk factors for coronary artery disease (CAD) have been identified: age, male sex, family history, cigarette smoking, hypertension (HTN), hypercholesterolemia, and diabetes (DM). Cocaine is directly myotoxic, accelerates atherosclerosis and CAD, and causes, myocardial infarction (MI) in patients with no coronary artery disease. The progression from ischemia to infarction (cell death) is a continuum. After acute coronary occlusion, ischemia and infarction progress from the subendocardium to the epicardium over a 6 h period. Reperfusion within these 6 h has the potential to salvage myocardium and decrease morbidity and mortality.

Angina pectoris represents cardiac ischemia. Anginal pain is typically retrosternal and may radiate to the neck, jaw, shoulders, or the inside of the left or both arms. Anginal pain is often described as "discomfort." Patients may experience chest pressure, heaviness, fullness, and squeezing sharp or stabbing pain. Reproducible chest wall tenderness is not uncommon. Associated symptoms include dizziness, palpitations, diaphoresis, dyspnea, nausea, and vomiting. Stable angina is characterized by episodic chest pain, usually lasting 5 to 15 min. The pain is provoked by exertion, cold, or stress and relieved by rest or nitroglycerin (NTG). Stable angina is usually due to a fixed coronary lesion. Unstable angina represents a clinical state between stable angina and MI. Physiologically, unstable angina is due to plaque rupture and thrombosis. There are three forms of unstable angina: (a) new-onset angina (within 2 months); (b) increasing angina (increased threshold, frequency, or duration); (c) angina at rest (within one week). The natural history of unstable angina is 40 percent incidence of MI and 17 percent incidence of death within 3 months.

Variant (Prinzmetal) angina occurs primarily at rest (without provocation), but can be provoked by cocaine or tobacco use. Coronary artery spasm is thought to cause variant angina.

Myocardial infarction patients have severe anginal pain of 15 to 30 min duration. Elderly patients and those with diabetes may have silent ischemia (painless) or atypical presentations (nonretrosternal chest pain, atypical radiation, weakness, dizziness, or dyspnea). Patients with inferior MIs may have abdominal pain, nausea, or vomiting.

Ischemia alters normal cellular contractility and electrical activity. This leads to the major complications of cardiac ischemia or infarction, dysrhythmias, and impaired ventricular function. The major determinant of prognosis in MI is the amount of infarcted myocardium. Heart failure usually develops when 25 percent of left ventricular (LV) muscle is impaired. Cardiogenic shock occurs with 40 percent LV impairment. Right ventricular (RV) MI occurs with 20 to 40 percent of inferior MIs. RV MI may cause hypotension, which is worsened by NTG. Other complications of MI include mural thrombosis, systemic arterial embolism (strokes, etc.), congestive heart failure (CHF), rupture of the ventricular wall (cardiac rupture), ventricular septum, or papillary muscle (typically seen with inferior MI).

Dysrhythmic complications are frequent and can be fatal. The incidence of lethal dysrhythmias is greatest in the early phases of MI. Premature ventricular contractions are seen in virtually all MIs. Tachydysrhythmias are noted more frequently in anterior MI. Sinus bradycardia, first-degree atrioventricular blocks (AVB), and Mobitz I AVB are usually due to increased vagal tone seen in inferior MI. Mobitz II and complete AVB are usually due to structural damage to the conduction system seen in large anterior MI. Ventricular tachycardia and fibrillation occurring early in the setting of MI do not appear to have a large effect on prognosis. Delayed ventricular tachycardia and fibrillation are associated with significant mortality.

Pericarditis can occur during the first week post-MI. Dressler's syndrome occurs in the post-MI period and is characterized by chest pain, fever, pericarditis, and pleural effusions.

Diagnosis and Differential

The diagnosis of angina is based on history. Physical examination of patients with ischemia or infarction is often unremarkable. The clinician must determine if complications are present (dysrhythmias, heart failure, and shock). New systolic murmurs may represent papillary muscle rupture. Friction rubs may be heard in the presence of pericarditis.

The most important diagnostic test is the electrocardiogram (ECG). Only one-half of MI patients, however, will have diagnostic changes on the initial ECG. A normal or nonspecific ECG does not rule out ischemia or negate the need for hospitalization. The diagnostic yield of ECGs can be improved by recording additional leads (right-sided, 22 lead) and by obtaining serial or continuous recordings. Acute ischemia can be subendothelial (ST-segment depression) or transmural (ST-segment elevation). Ischemic T waves are deep, symmetrical, and inverted. Infarcted, electrically dead tissue eventually produces Q waves. In the setting of MI, ST-segment changes are seen early, T-wave changes are variable, and Q waves take hours to develop. In general, the more elevated the ST segments and the more ST segments that are elevated, the more extensive the injury. Infarcts can be localized by determining the ECG leads affected (Table 22-1). ECG evaluation for ischemia can be difficult with paced rhythms or bundle branch block. MI in the setting of left bundle branch block or paced rhythms is suggested by (a) ST elevation of >1 mm concordant with the QRS complex; (b) ST depression of >1 mm in leads V_1, V_2, or V_3; and (c) discordant ST elevation of .5 mm.

Injured cardiac muscle cells release cardiac enzymes. Serial measurement of these enzymes is used to diagnose MI, but the role of these markers is limited in the emergency department (ED).

TABLE 22-1 Localization of MI Based on ECG Findings

V_2–V_4—anterior

II, III, aVF, V_5, V_6—inferior

V_1–V_3—anteroseptal

I, aVL, V_4–V_6–lateral

V_1–V_6—anterolateral

V_{4R}–V_{6R}—right ventricular (often associated with inferior)

Posterior MI has large R $>$ .04 mm, R/S $>$ 1, and ST depression in V_1 and V_2

Abbreviations: MI, myocardial infarction; ECG, electrocardiogram.

Many of these enzymes are not specific to myocardial injury [creatine phosphokinase (CPK), lactic acid dehydrogenase (LDH), myoglobin (MB), troponin T]. The cardiac isoform of troponin I is not found in skeletal muscle. Patients who are early in the course of MI may not have elevated CK-MB, troponin I, or LDH. The sensitivity of CK-MB immunoassays is 50 percent on presentation to the ED and rises to 90 percent if the duration of pain is greater than 9 h. Troponin I has similar sensitivity and specificity to CK-MB. Troponin I is more sensitive for MI in the subset of patients with trauma, surgery, cocaine use, renal failure, or skeletal muscle disease. Myoglobin, troponin T, and CK-MB isoforms are released earlier than CK-MB. Patients with unstable angina will not show serial elevations in CK-MB. Elevations of troponin I and T are predictive of cardiovascular complications in patients with acute coronary syndromes (ACS).

Echocardiography (ECHO) is useful in diagnosing impaired wall motion and anatomic complications of MI (ruptured papillary muscle or ventricular wall and pericardial effusion). Nuclear scans may also be used to diagnose MI. These modalities have been shown to be sensitive, but not specific, in the ED diagnosis of MI.

Differential diagnosis of cardiac ischemia or infarction includes pericarditis, cardiomyopathies, cardiac valvular disease, pulmonary embolism, pneumonia, pneumothorax, asthma or chronic obstructive pulmonary disease, gastrointestinal disorders (especially esophageal disease), chest trauma, chest wall disorders, hyperventilation, aortic aneurysm and dissection, and mediastinal disorders.

Emergency Department Care and Disposition

Strict attention should be paid to the ABCs. All patients suspected of having cardiac pain should be placed on a cardiac monitor, receive an intravenous line, and supplemental oxygen. A rapid screening, including risk factors, indications, and contraindications for thrombolytics, should be performed. ECGs should be obtained within 5 min of the patient's presentation to the ED. Many of these steps can be accomplished in the prehospital arena.

Treatment of ACS should be individualized based on symptoms, history, physical exam, and ECG findings. Treatment of angina starts with a correction of modifiable risk behavior (smoking, diet, control of underlying diseases). Nitroglycerin, aspirin, β blockers, and calcium channel agonists are all useful in the treatment of cardiac ischemia. There are three facets to the treatment of MI patients: (*a*) establish early coronary patency; (*b*) maintain patency; and (*c*) protect myocardium from further damage. Patency is established by thrombolytic therapy, angioplasty, or coronary artery bypass surgery. Maintenance of patency is achieved by anti-coagulation and antiplatelet agents. Protection of the myocardium is accomplished by reducing the heart's oxygen demand and increasing the oxygen delivery. Dysrhythmias should be treated if the effect on heart rate exacerbates oxygen supply or demand imbalance, or if the dysrhythmia seems capable of deteriorating into cardiac arrest.

1. Aspirin has been shown to reduce cardiac deaths by 20 percent. **Aspirin,** 160 to 325 mg, should be given as soon as possible, chewed for more rapid onset. Aspirin and Indocin are used to treat Dressler's syndrome.

2. **Nitroglycerin** (NTG) reduces cardiac mortality by 20 to 30 percent. Oral and transdermal NTG are useful in preventing angina. Sublingual NTG (spray or tablet) is usually effective for the treatment of acute anginal pain within 3 min. A sublingual dose should be repeated 3 times at 2- to 5-min intervals. If there is no improvement with sublingual NTG, intravenous NTG should be started at 5 to 10 μg/min. The dose should be titrated to pain and hypotension by 5 to 10 μg/min increments every 3 to 5 min. Doses above 100 μg/min have been associated with paradoxically increased ischemia. They should be used carefully in the setting of hypotension, as they may further worsen perfusion to ischemic myocardium. NTG is not indicated in the setting of RV infarcts. A common side effect of NTG is headache.

3. **Thrombolytic agents** open occluded arteries, salvage ischemic myocardium, and reduce the morbidity and mortality of MI. Maximum benefit occurs when thrombolytics are given within 1 to 2 h of symptom onset, and they should be administered within 30 min of a patient's ED arrival. As thrombolytics have potentially fatal side effects, the appropriate selection of candidates for use is important. Indications for thrombolytic administration are noted in Table 22-2; contraindications are listed in Table 22-3. Because of this need for selection, only 20 to 25 percent of all MI patients receive thrombolytics.

The decision to administer thrombolytics should be individualized. For example, elderly patients ($>$ 75 years) have more complications but benefit the most from thrombolytics. There is evidence that treatment 6 to 12 h after onset of symptoms may decrease mortality. The risk for cerebrovascular accident (CVA), CHF, and cardiac rupture, however, is also increased. CVA (occurring in approximately 1 percent of patients) is more common in patients older than 66, weighing less than 70 kg, and hypertensive on presentation. Cardiology consultation

TABLE 22-2 Indications for Thrombolysis

Symptoms consistent with MI with onset <12 h

ECG criteria:
> 1 mm ST elevation in 2 or more contiguous limb leads
> 2 mm ST elevation in 2 or more contiguous chest leads
New left bundle branch block

No contraindications (see Table 22-3)

Absence of cardiogenic shock, unless mechanical reperfusion will be delayed > 60 min., then use tPA

Abbreviations: MI, myocardial infarction; ECG, electrocardiogram; tPa, tissue plasminogen activator.

TABLE 22-3 Contraindications for Thrombolysis

Absolute
  Active or recent (<10 days) internal bleeding
        Active bleeding
        History of CVA < 2–6 months or any hemorrhagic CVA
        Intracranial or intraspinous surgery or trauma < 2 months
        Intracranial or intraspinous neoplasm, aneurysm, AV malformation
        Trauma or surgery at a non-compressible site <10 days
        Suspected aortic dissection or pericarditis
        Allergy to specific thrombolytic

Relative
  Known bleeding diathesis
        Severe uncontrolled HTN (SBP > 200 mmHg and/or DBP > 120 mmHg)
        Active peptic ulcer disease
        Cardiopulmonary resuscitation >10 min
        Use of oral anticoagulants (PT > 15 sec, INR > 2)
        Hemorrhagic ophthalmic conditions
        Ischemic or embolic CVA > 6 mo
        Uncontrolled HTN (SBP >180 mmHg and/or DPB >110 mmHg)
        Puncture of noncompressible blood vessel <10 days
        Significant trauma or major surgery > 2 weeks but < 2 months
        Pregnancy

Abbreviations: CVA, cerebrovascular accident; AV, atrioventriclar; HTN, hypertension; SBP, systolic blood pressure; DBP, diastolic blood pressure; PT, prothrombin time; INR, international normalized ratio.

before initiating thrombolytics in cases of delayed presentation is appropriate. Before administering thrombolytics, informed consent should be obtained (with particular attention paid to an understanding of the risks). Indications and contraindications should be sought and noted (this includes examination for equal pulses, stool guaiac, and pericardial rubs). Blood tests should be drawn when intravenous lines are started. Arterial puncture should be avoided, as should venipuncture or central line placement in areas that are not readily compressible.

Streptokinase (SK) activates circulating plasminogen and is not fibrin-specific. It is derived from β-hemolytic streptococcus and is capable of generating an allergic reaction (minor 5 to 5.7 percent, anaphylaxis < 0.2 to 0.7 percent). Hypotension, usually responsive to fluids and slowing drug infusion, occurs in 13.3 to 15 percent of patients. Antibodies may develop 5 days after treatment and persist for 6 months. Repeated doses of SK are not recommended within this time period. Other contraindications to the use of SK include the presence of hypotension, and streptococcal infections within 12 months. The dose of SK is 1.5 million U given over 60 min. The half-life of SK is 23 min, and systemic fibrinolysis persists for 24 h. Heparin should be given within 4 h of starting SK. **Tissue plasminogen activator** (tPA) is a naturally occurring human protein and is not antigenic. tPA is fibrin-specific and has a half-life of 5 min. The dose of tPA is listed in Table 22-4. When compared with traditional dosing, front-loaded tPA has been shown to have superior 90-min patency rates and reocclusion rates without increased bleeding risk. **Reteplase** is a modification to tPA with a prolonged half-life of 18 min versus 3 min. The GUSTO study found similar mortality and stroke rates between the two agents. Reteplase may have a faster time to perfusion. The advantage of reteplase is that it is given in two

TABLE 22-4 Thrombolytic Dosages

Streptokinase—1.5 million U over 1 h.
Front-loaded tPA
    15 mg IV over 2 min, followed by 0.75 mg/kg (50 mg max) IV over 30 min, followed by 0.5 mg/kg (35 mg max) IV over 60 min.

Traditional tPA
    Total dose 1.25 mg/kg (max 100 mg) over 3 h—60% given over 1 h (6–10% of the total dose) over 1–2 min, the rest over the h, then the remaining 40% given over the next 2 h.
Reteplase—2 boluses, 10 mg each, 30 min apart.

10 mg boluses 30 min apart. The cost is similar to tPA. Intravenous heparin must be given simultaneously with tPA and reteplase. Compared with SK, reteplase and tPA are more expensive ($2000 vs. $300), have a greater 90-min (but not 24 h) patency rate, cause a higher incidence of intracranial bleeding (0.94 vs. 0.52 percent), and may (there were flaws in the GUSTO study) be associated with a decrease in mortality (based on a meta-analysis of GUSTO 1, ISIS 3, and GISS 2 studies).

The most significant complication of thrombolytics is hemorrhage, especially intracranial bleeding. External bleeding can usually be controlled by prolonged external pressure. Significant bleeding, especially internal, requires cessation of thrombolytics, heparin, and aspirin. Crystalloid and red blood cell infusion may be necessary. Cryoprecipitate (cryo) and fresh frozen plasma (FFP) will reverse fibrinolysis due to thrombolytics. Initially, 10 U of cryo are given, and fibrinogen levels are obtained. If the fibrinogen level is < 1 g/L, the dose of cryo should be repeated. If bleeding continues despite a fibrinogen level > 1 g/L, or if the fibrinogen level is < 1 g/L after 20 U of cryo, then 2 U of FFP should be administered. If this does not control hemorrhage, then platelets or antifibrinolytic agents (aminocaproic acid or tranexamic acid) are indicated. Intracranial hemorrhage requires all of the preceding steps to be initiated.

4. **Heparin** is used for its anticoagulative properties, which prevent the progression of coronary artery and mural thrombosis. Heparin may be used as a third-line agent (after aspirin and NTG) in unstable angina. Heparin bolus given early in the course of MI is an effective alternative to thrombolytics. In addition, heparin is a mandatory adjunct to thrombolytic therapy. The recommended intravenous dose is 5000 to 10,000 U bolus followed by a 1000 to 1500 U/h infusion. Weight-based nomograms may prove to be a more appropriate dosing schedule. Subcutaneous dosing can be used with streptokinase. The dose is 12,500 U twice a day. Heparin use is associated with an increased risk of bleeding. Anticoagulation due to heparin can be reversed with protamine. The dosage is 1 mg of protamine per 100 U of heparin (heparin given as a bolus or infused in the previous 4 h). Low molecular weight heparins (LMWH) have greater bioavailability, lower protein binding, longer half-life, and more reliable anticoagulative effect than their counterparts. They are administered in fixed subcutaneous doses. Initial studies comparing LMWH with heparin in ACS have demonstrated decreased ischemia and MI without increased bleeding complications.

5. Primary angioplasty (PTCA) refers to the practice of emergent coronary angiography followed by angioplasty (balloon, rotary, and laser), coronary artery stenting, or atherectomy in lieu of thrombolysis. PTCA is successful in reducing stenosis to < 40 percent in 94 percent of patients. In-hospital mortality is 7.2 percent in centers with significant expertise (1.8 percent in patients eligible for thrombolytics). Compared with tPA, PTCA has a lower incidence of reinfarction and recurrent ischemia, bleeding complications (including CVA), and death. PTCA is also associated with greater improvements in LV function. There are three subsets of patients for which PTCA is especially attractive: (*a*) patients with MI in cardiogenic shock; (*b*) patients with nondiagnostic ECG; (*c*) patients with contraindications to thrombolysis; and (*d*) patients with refractory symptoms. Angiography also has the advantage of identifying patients who require bypass surgery.

6. β blockers can reduce both the short- and long-term mortality in patients with MI. β_1-blocking (cardioselective) agents are preferred (metoprolol). Indications and contraindications to the use of β blockers are shown in Table 22-5. Used in the setting of MI, the greatest benefit is seen when treated within 8 h. The targeted optimal heart rate is 60 to 90 beats per min in the setting of MI. Dosage of **metoprolol** is 5 mg given intravenously over 1 min (smaller doses may be used in patients with relative contraindications). This bolus is repeated twice every 5 to 15 min, for a total of 15 mg. **Esmolol,** a short-acting β blocker, also can be used. An initial 500 $\mu g/kg$ bolus is infused over 1 min, and a 50 $\mu g/kg/min$ infusion is then titrated to a maximum dose of 200 $\mu g/kg/min$.

7. Glycoprotein IIB/IIIa antagonists are agents that bind to and inhibit platelet aggregation. Abciximab, eptifibatide, and tirofiban are currently available. These agents have been used as: (*a*) adjuncts to angioplasty; (*b*) medical stabilization of ACS; and (*c*) in combination with low-dose thrombolytics. Abciximab with heparin and aspirin, when used in conjunction with angioplasty, decreases mortality, MI, and urgent repeat intervention. An initial study supports the same benefit with eptifibatide. Tirofiban, abciximab, and eptifibatide have been shown to decrease short- and long-term mortality, recurrent ischemia, and MI in patients with medically treated unstable angina or non-Q-wave MI. Preclinical studies of abciximab with low-dose thrombolytics have demonstrated more rapid and stable vessel patency (theoretically with less intracranial hemorrhage). There is a 0.1 percent incidence of intracranial bleeding, but a 6 percent chance of significant catheter site bleeding

TABLE 22-5 Indications and Contraindications to β blockade

Indications
  Transmural MI (ST elevation and/or Q waves)
  Reflex tachycardia or tachydysrhythmias
  Hypertension
  Continued or recurrent pain
  In conjunction with thrombolytics
  Possible benefit: non-Q-wave MI and pain of > 6 h duration

Contraindications

Absolute
  Heart rate < 60
  SBP <100 mmHg
  Moderate-to-severe LV dysfunction
  Signs of peripheral hypoperfusion
  Severe COPD
  Second- or third-degree AVB

Relative
  Asthma
  Severe peripheral vascular disease
  Concurrent use of Ca channel blockers
  Difficult-to-control diabetes
  First-degree AVB

Abbreviations: MI, myocardial infarction; SBP, systolic blood pressure; LV, left ventricular; COPD, chronic obstructive pulmonary disease; AVB, atrioventricular block; Ca, calcium.

(which requires transfusion). Due to the significant cost and the preliminary nature of the studies, the use of these agents in the ED should be discussed with local cardiologists.

8. **Morphine sulfate** (2 to 10 mg intravenously, given in 2-mg increments) can be used to reduce anginal pain. Morphine has not been consistently shown to affect preload. Morphine may decrease cardiac output. Morphine should be used with caution in the presence of hypotension and in patients with inferior MI.

9. Calcium channel blockers have little benefit in the treatment of unstable angina and MI.

10. Meta-analysis of trials has demonstrated a 20 percent decrease in mortality (thought to be related to decreased incidence of dysrhythmia) when intravenous **magnesium** is given in acute-stage MI. Current recommendations support correction of documented hypomagnesemia and treatment of torsade-type tachycardia with prolonged QT. Magnesium use in high-risk patients may be beneficial. The recommended dose of magne-

sium is 1 to 2 g over 10 to 20 min, followed by a continuous infusion of 1 to 2 g/h.

11. Prophylactic lidocaine is not recommended and has been shown to have a trend toward increased mortality.

12. Angiotensin-converting enzyme inhibitors have been shown to decrease mortality when used in the setting of CHF and in the postinfarction period. Their use in the acute treatment of unstable angina is more controversial. When used within 24 h of MI, enalapril increases mortality and should not be used. ACE inhibitors should be started in patients with MI and ST elevation in two or more precordial leads, or in the setting of heart failure. Contraindications include hypotension, bilateral renal artery stenosis, renal failure, cough, or angioedema due to ACE inhibitors in the past.

13. Right ventricular infarcts are treated somewhat differently than LV infarcts. Patients with RV infarcts are dependent on elevated RV filling pressures to maintain cardiac output. Diuretics and NTG should be avoided. Volume infusion should be used to increase cardiac output. Dobutamine is indicated if an inotropic agent is needed. Nitroprusside to decrease afterload or intraaortic balloon counterpulsation may be of benefit in refractory cases.

14. Dysrhythmias should be treated as per ACLS protocols (see Chap. 2).

15. See Chap. 7 for the management of cardiogenic shock.

Nitroprusside, NTG, and diuretics must be used with extreme caution in the setting of hypotension. MI patients with continued hemodynamic instability and pain or those who have not reperfused after administration of thrombolytics are candidates for rescue angioplasty. Emergent coronary artery bypass surgery may also be indicated for these patients. Patients in refractory cardiogenic shock should undergo emergent angioplasty. Intraaortic balloon pump or other LV assisting devices may also be indicated for these patients. Cardiology consultation is recommended.

Admission

Patients with acute MI or unstable angina who have either ongoing chest pain, ECG changes, dysrhythmias, or hemodynamic compromise often require cardiac intensive care. Patients with unstable angina with resolved chest pain, normal or nonspecific ECG changes, and no complications should be admitted to a monitored bed. Chest-pain-free patients with normal or nonspecific ECGs can be admitted to a step-down unit. Chest-pain patients with low likelihood of MI can undergo serial ECG and cardiac enzyme testing in a chest-pain observation unit and MI can be ruled out within 24 h.

For further reading in *Emergency Medicine: A Comprehensive Study Guide,* 5th ed., see Chap. 47, "Acute Coronary Syndromes: Unstable Angina, Myocardial Ischemia, and Infarction," by Judd E. Hollander; and Chap. 48, "Intervention Strategies for Acute Coronary Syndrome," by Judd E. Hollander.

---

23 | Heart Failure and Pulmonary Edema
David M. Cline

Acute pulmonary edema is one of the most dramatic presentations of the many clinical effects of heart failure. The most common precipitating factors of heart failure are (*a*) cardiac tachydysrhythmias, such as atrial fibrillation; (*b*) acute myocardial infarction or ischemia; (*c*) discontinuation of medications, such as diuretics; (*d*) increased sodium load; (*e*) drugs that impair myocardial function; and (*f*) physical overexertion.

CLINICAL FEATURES

Patients with acute pulmonary edema usually have symptoms of left ventricular heart failure, severe respiratory distress, frothy pink or white sputum, moist pulmonary rales, and an S_3 or S_4. Patients frequently are tachycardic, have cardiac dysrhythmias such as atrial fibrillation or premature ventriculor contraction (PVCs) and are hypertensive. There may be a history of exertional dyspnea, paroxysmal nocturnal dyspnea, and orthopnea. Patients with right ventricular heart failure have dependent edema of the extremities and may have jugular venous distention, hepatic enlargement, and, less commonly, ascites.

DIAGNOSIS AND DIFFERENTIAL

The diagnosis of acute pulmonary edema is made with clinical findings and a chest x-ray; the severity of illness may demand that a portable anterior-posterior film be taken. Additional tests that should be ordered to help management include an electrocardiogram, electrolyte levels, BUN levels, creatinine level, complete blood cell count, arterial blood gas level, and possibly cardiac enzyme levels. The diagnosis of right-sided heart failure is made clinically, but if the cause is left-sided heart failure, the heart will be enlarged on chest x-ray. In the differential diagnosis, consider the common causes of acute respiratory distress: asthma, chronic obstructive pulmonary disease (COPD), pneumonia, allergenic reactions, and other causes of respiratory failure. The second consideration is the cause of interstitial edema: pulmonary edema associated with the preceding precipitating factors earlier and the causes of noncardiac pulmonary edema, such as drug-related alveolar capillary damage, or that seen with acute respiratory distress syndrome (ARDS).

EMERGENCY DEPARTMENT CARE AND DISPOSITION

The treatment of patients in acute pulmonary edema includes oxygen, preload reducers, diuretics, afterload reducers, and inotropic agents.

1. 100% **oxygen** by face mask must be administered to achieve an oxygen saturation of 95% by pulse oximetry. Immediate intubation should be considered for unconscious or visibly tiring patients.
2. If hypoxia persists despite oxygen therapy, **continuous positive airway pressure** (*CPAP*) should be applied via face mask.
3. **Nitroglycerin** 0.4 mg must be administered sublingually (may be repeated every 5 min), or as a topical paste, 1 to 2 in. If the patient does not respond, or the ECG shows ischemia, nitroglycerin 10 μg/min should be given as an IV drip, and titrated.
4. After nitrates, a potent intravenous diuretic must be administered, such as **furosemide** 40 to 80 mg IV, or bumetanide (bumex) 0.5 to 1 mg IV. Electrolytes should be monitored, especially serum potassium.
5. For patients with resistant hypertension, or those who are not responding well to nitroglycerin, **nitroprusside** may be used, starting at 2.5 μg/kg per min and titrated.
6. For hypotensive patients or patients in need of additional inotropic support, **dopamine** should be started at 5 to 10 μg/kg per min and titrated to a systolic BP of 90 to 100. Dobutamine

can be given in combination with dopamine or as a single agent, providing the patient is not in severe circulatory shock. **Dobutamine** should be started at 2.5 μg/kg per min and titrated to the desired response.

7. CPAP should be administered by face mask if the patient has not responded to the preceding therapy.

Acute mitral valve or aortic valve regurgitation should be considered as a cause of pulmonary edema, especially if the heart is of normal size. The patient may need emergency surgery. The initial electrocardiogram (ECG) may fail to demonstrate acute myocardial infarction, for patients who deteriorate or fail to improve, a repeat of the 12-lead ECG should be considered, as well as thrombolytic therapy if indicated.

Coexisting dysrhythmias (see Chap. 2) or electrolyte disturbances (see Chap. 4) should be treated, avoiding those therapies that impair the inotropic state of the heart. **Morphine** can be given (1 to 2 mg IV) and repeated as needed. Its use is controversial, however, and may cause respiratory depression and add little to oxygen, diuretics, and nitrates. Digoxin acts too slowly to be of benefit in acute situations. Rotating tourniquets do not reduce preload and should not be used. For anuric (dialysis) patients, sorbitol, and phlebotomy may have some benefit, but, dialysis is the treatment of choice in these patients who prove resistant to nitrates.

Patients with acute pulmonary edema should be admitted to the ICU and may require invasive hemodynamic monitoring. In the presence of new arrhythmias, uncontrolled hypertension, or suspected MI, the patient should be admitted for evaluation and optimization of drug therapy, usually to a telemetry bed.

Long-term treatment of congestive heart failure includes dietary salt reduction, chronic use of diuretics such as furosemide, 20 to 80 mg daily, afterload reducers such as captopril, 6.25 to 25 mg bid/tid, and digoxin 0.125 to 0.25 mg daily. Patients with an exacerbation of chronic CHF without chest pain or complicating factors who respond to diuretics may be discharged home if follow-up is arranged.

For further reading in *Emergency Medicine: A Comprehensive Study Guide,* 5th ed., see Chap. 49, "Heart Failure and Pulmonary Edema," by Charles B. Cairns.

24 | Valvular Emergencies and
Endocarditis

David M. Cline

VALVULAR HEART DISEASE

The majority of valvular heart disease is chronic in nature. Acute life-threatening valvular incompetence, however, may occur in association with myocardial infarction (mitral incompetence), endocarditis (mitral and aortic incompetence), or aortic dissection (aortic incompetence). Acute right-sided valvular heart disease is most frequently found in association with endocarditis in IV drug users. Chronic valvular disease may present with acute symptoms due to increased demands on cardiac output, such as exertion, tachycardia, anemia, pregnancy, or infection. When considering the treatment of tachycardia, remember that tachycardia may significantly reduce regurgitant flow and improve cardiac output in aortic regurgitation, whereas it compromises ventricular filling and cardiac output in aortic stenosis.

Clinical Features

Acute mitral incompetence presents with dyspnea, tachycardia, and pulmonary edema, with or without ischemic-type chest pain. Acute aortic incompetence may present with acute pulmonary edema; however, patients may also complain of fever and chills if endocarditis is the cause, or of (tearing) chest pain radiating between the shoulder blades if aortic dissection is the cause. Aortic regurgitation may also present with systemic emboli or persistent tachycardia.

The most common presenting symptom in chronic valvular heart disease is dyspnea, usually on exertion. Mitral stenosis may also present with atrial fibrillation, systemic emboli, or hemoptysis. Aortic stenosis may present with syncope on exertion, angina, or myocardial infarction. Mitral valve prolapse is most commonly asymptomatic, but may present with atypical chest pain, palpitations, fatigue, and dyspnea unrelated to exertion. A comparison table of murmurs and signs is listed in Table 24-1. Acute right-sided valvular heart disease presents with symptoms associated with endocarditis, including fever, chills, dyspnea, and sepsis.

TABLE 24-1 Comparison of Heart Murmurs, Sounds, and Signs

Valve disorder	Murmur	Heart sounds and signs
Mitral stenosis	Mid-diastolic rumble, crescendos into S_2	Loud snapping S_1, apical impulse is small and tapping due to underfilled left ventricle.
Mitral regurgitation	Acute: harsh apical systolic murmur that starts with S_1 and may end before S_2 Chronic: high pitched apical holosystolic murmur that radiates to the axilla	S_3 and S_4 may be heard.
Mitral valve prolapse	Click may be followed by a late systolic murmur that crescendos into S_2	Mid-systolic click; S_2 may be diminished by the late systolic murmur.
Aortic stenosis	Harsh systolic ejection murmur	Paradoxic splitting of S_2, S_3, and S_4 may be present; pulse of small amplitude; pulse has a slow rise and sustained peak.
Aortic regurgitation	High pitched blowing diastolic murmur immediately after S_2	S_3 may be present; wide pulse pressure.
IHSS	Harsh systolic crescendo-decrescendo best heart at the apex or left sternal border	No opening snap; apical impulse may be double; pulse has a brisk rise and double peak.

Diagnosis

In the emergency department, diagnosis is often suspected by auscultatory findings. The electrocardiogram (ECG) is not confirmatory. Chest x-ray may show the following: straightening of the border on the left side of the heart in mitral stenosis; pulmonary edema with less cardiac enlargement than expected in acute left-sided valvular incompetence; or, possibly, aortic dilation in cases of aortic dissection. A clinically suspected diagnosis should be confirmed by echocardiography or by consultation with a cardiologist. The urgency for an accurate diagnosis and appropriate referral depends on the severity of symptoms and the suspected diagnosis.

Acute mitral or aortic incompetence should always be suspected in patients presenting with acute pulmonary edema, especially when the heart is smaller than expected on chest radiography, or the patient does not respond to conventional therapy. When aortic dissection is suspected as the cause of acute aortic incompetence and the patient is sufficiently stable, computed tomography (CT) scanning of the chest is useful. Angiography may still be required after CT scanning.

Emergency Department Care

1. Pulmonary edema should be treated with oxygen and intubation for failing respiratory effort. Diuretics (i.e., **furosemide** 40 mg IV) should be used and combined with nitrates (*nitroglycerin* IV, started at 10 μg/min and titrated up) if tolerated. Patients with aortic stenosis will usually have normal-to-low BP and will not tolerate afterload reducers. In contrast, patients with mitral incompetence or aortic incompetence can benefit from IV nitroprusside or nitroglycerin even with normal blood pressures. In these patients, reducing afterload helps to reduce regurgitation and relieve pulmonary edema.

2. The hypertension associated with aortic dissection should be controlled with beta adrenergic blockade (e.g., **labetalol** 20 mg IV) or intravenous **nitroprusside** (started at 0.5 μg/kg/min and titrated up).

3. Patients with valvular heart disease and acute pulmonary edema should be considered for Swan-Ganz catheter insertion. Valvular disease, especially stenosis, may complicate the procedure.

4. Rapid atrial fibrillation, which may precipitate symptoms in patients with silent valvular disease, should have rate control with intravenous **diltiazem** (20 mg IV). Emergency cardioversion may be needed in severely compromised patients, but recurrence is common. The most common cause of arrhythmia in valvular heart disease—a dilated atrium—remains unchanged by cardioversion. The danger of embolization is greater in patients with atrial fibrillation.

5. In the event of embolization, anticoagulation should be undertaken with IV **heparin** (5000 U IV, followed by 1000 U/h), provided there is no history of bleeding. This is especially needed in the setting of atrial fibrillation.

6. Prophylaxis for infective endocarditis is recommended during procedures that are prone to bacteremia in patients at risk for developing endocarditis. Patients considered at risk include those with a prosthetic heart valve, a history of endocarditis, rheumatic heart disease, acquired and congenital valvular dis-

ease, idiopathic hypertrophic subaortic stenosis, or mitral valve prolapse with a murmur. Common procedures requiring prophylaxis are listed in Table 24-2.

Patients with acute onset of valvular incompetence will be acutely ill and will require admission. Patients with aortic stenosis who have syncope on exertion should be considered for admission. Consultation with a cardiologist may be required to determine the need for hospital admission. In patients that do not respond to medical management consider intra-aortic balloon counterpulsation; however, this is contraindicated in wide-open aortic regurgitation.

Emergency surgery should be considered in all cases of acute symptomatic valvular disease, especially mitral and aortic regurgitation. Because stenotic lesions are slowly progressive, emergency surgery is rarely needed for stenotic defects, but a patient with new onset of syncope in association with aortic stenosis should be considered for urgent repair.

PROSTHETIC VALVE DISEASE

Patients who receive prosthetic valves are instructed to carry a card in their wallet that describes their valve. Prosthetic valves tend to be slightly stenotic and a very small amount of regurgitation is common because of incomplete closure. Systemic embolism, originating from a thrombus on the prosthetic valve, is the most important complication of mechanical models. Endocarditis occurs frequently during the first 2 months postsurgery, and *Staphylococcus epidermidis* and *Staphylococcus aureus* dominate. Late cases of endocarditis are similar to the those affecting native valves.

Clinical Findings

Many patients have persistent dyspnea and reduced effort tolerance after successful valve replacement. Mechanical valves have loud metallic-sounding closing sounds. Patients with bioprostheses usually have normal S_1 and S_2, with no abnormal opening sounds.

Diagnosis

New or progressive symptoms referable to the heart suggest a prosthetic valve disorder. Therefore, new or progressive dyspnea of any form, new onset or worsening of congestive heart failure, decreased exercise tolerance, or a change in chest pain compatible with ischemia all suggest valvular dysfunction.

TABLE 24-2 Prophylaxis for Infective Endocarditis

Procedure	Standard regimen*	Alternate regimen
Dental procedure known to cause bleeding	Amoxicillin 2.0 g PO 1 h prior to the procedure, or Ampicillin 2.0 g IM or IV 30 min prior to procedure	Clindamycin 600 mg PO 1 h before procedure, or Cephalexin 2.0 g PO 1 h prior to the procedure, or Cefadroxil 2.0 g PO 1 h prior to the procedure, or Azithromycin 500 mg PO 1 h prior to the procedure, or Clarithromycin 500 mg PO 1 h prior to the procedure
Urethral catheterization if infection is present Urethral dilation	Ampicillin 2.0 g IV/IM plus gentamicin 1.5 mg/kg IV/IM (not to exceed 120 mg) 30 min before procedure followed by half the original dose of ampicillin 6 h later	Vancomycin 1.0 g IV over 1 h plus gentamicin 1.5 mg/kg IV/IM (not to exceed 120 mg), complete infusion within 30 min of starting procedure. For moderate risk patients, amoxicillin 2 g PO 1 h prior to procedure
Incision and drainage of infected tissue	Cefazolin 1.0 g IV/IM 30 min before procedure, or Cephalexin 2.0 g PO 1 h prior to the procedure, or Cefadroxil 2.0 g PO 1 h prior to the procedure	Vancomycin 1.0 g IV over 1 h plus gentamicin 1.5 mg/kg IV/IM (not to exceed 120 mg), complete infusion within 30 min of starting procedure

*Includes patients with prosthetic heart valves and others at high risk. Initial pediatric doses are as follows: amoxicillin, 50 mg/kg, ampicillin 50 mg/kg, cephalexin 50 mg/kg, cefadroxil 50 mg/kg, azithromycin 15 mg/kg, clarithromycin 15 mg/kg, clindamycin 20 mg/kg, gentamicin 2 mg/kg, and vancomycin 20 mg/kg. Pediatric doses should not exceed listed adult doses.

Emergency Department Management

Patients with a prosthetic valve suspected of having acute valvular dysfunction or endocarditis require admission to the hospital and evaluation of the valve for possible replacement.

INFECTIVE ENDOCARDITIS

Infective endocarditis can be divided into acute and subacute forms, depending on the virulence of the infecting organism. Endocarditis can be further divided into disease of the left and right side of the heart. Left-sided disease (aortic and/or mitral valves) is the most common. The most common organisms include *Streptococcus viridans* (declining in frequency), *Staphylococcus aureus* (increasing in frequency), *Enterococcus,* and fungal organisms. *Pseudomonas* and *Serratia* are important etiologic agents in IV drug users in certain areas of the country, especially Detroit and San Francisco, respectively.

Right-sided disease (tricuspid and/or pulmonic valves) is usually seen in IV drug abusers (60 percent) and is caused by *Staphylococcus aureus* (75 percent), *Streptococcus pneumonia* (20 percent), and gram-negative organisms (4 percent).

Clinical Features

Acute left-sided disease presents with a picture of sepsis, with or without cardiac failure. Typically patients appear ill with fever, chills, and tachycardia, and they may have significant congestive heart failure symptoms, such as dyspnea, frothy sputum, and chest pain. Patients may quickly deteriorate, with acute rupture of mitral or aortic valves. Murmurs are typically that of aortic or mitral regurgitation, however, the murmur is often absent or unable to be heard over lung sounds in acute cases. Neurologic symptoms secondary to aseptic meningoencephalitis and embolization of vegetations account for 29 percent of ED presentations. These complications most commonly are mental status changes, hemiplegia, aphasia, ataxia, or severe headache. Patients may complain of monocular blindness.

Patients with subacute left-sided disease have recurrent intermittent fever and constitutional symptoms, such as malaise, anorexia, or weight loss. The majority of patients with left-sided subacute disease have a murmur of aortic or mitral regurgitation or a change in their previous murmur at the time of their admission to the hospital. Many admitted patients, however, have murmurs not previously detected. Patients may have Roth spots, which are retinal hemorrhages with central clearing. Peripheral evidence of endocarditis includes Osler's nodes, which are tender nodules on the tips of the toes and fingers, and Janeway lesions, which are nontender plaques on the soles of the feet and palms of the hands.

Right-sided disease is usually acute and presents with fever and respiratory symptoms: cough, chest pain, hemoptysis, and dyspnea. Chest radiography often reveals pulmonary effusions and multiple pulmonary infiltrates of variable size and shape.

Diagnosis

The diagnosis of endocarditis is based on positive blood cultures and evidence of valvular injury or vegetations. Three separate cultures from different veins should be obtained. Aerobic, anaerobic, and fungal cultures should be obtained before antibiotics are started. Echocardiography is helpful but should not delay appropriate stabilizing treatments. Nonspecific laboratory findings that support this diagnosis include leukocytosis, elevated C-reactive proteins, normocytic anemia, hematuria (25 to 50 percent), and pyuria.

Emergency Department Care

The first priority in the care of patients with acute infective endocarditis is stabilization of respiratory and cardiac symptoms.

1. For patients with mental status changes and hypoxia or a compromised airway, control of the airway with oral intubation may be required. Cardiac decompensation is usually due to left-sided valvular incompetence or rupture.
2. Acute rupture of the mitral or aortic valve should be stabilized with afterload reducers, such as sodium nitroprusside, with insertion of a Swan-Ganz catheter for monitoring therapy as soon as possible. Preparation for emergency surgery should be made for patients suspected of acute valvular rupture. Aortic balloon counterpulsation may be helpful for mitral valve rupture, but is contraindicated for wide-open aortic valve rupture.
3. The second priority is drawing three blood cultures from different sites and then starting empiric antibiotic therapy.
4. For acute infective endocarditis, a penicillinase-resistant penicillin, such as **nafcillin** 1.5 g every 4 h, should be given with an aminoglycoside chosen on the basis of local patterns of susceptibility. In geographic areas where there is a high incidence of methicillin-resistant *Staphylococcus,* or with patients already taking oral antibiotics **vancomycin** 1 g IV should be used in addition to an aminoglycoside.
5. Patients with prosthetic valve endocarditis should be treated with antibiotics that cover *Staphylococcus epidermidis,* usually vancomycin 1 g IV, in addition to an aminoglycoside.

6. Although subacute cases are frequently caused by *Streptococcus viridans,* which is covered by penicillin G, patients with subacute presentations that require admission should be started on a newer cephalosporin, such as **ceftriaxone** 1 g IV, in addition to an aminoglycoside, until cultures and sensitivities are known.

In general, patients with suspected endocarditis should be admitted to the hospital.

For further reading in *Emergency Medicine: A Comprehensive Study Guide,* 5th ed., see Chap. 50, "Valvular Emergencies and Endocarditis," by David M. Cline.

25	The Cardiomyopathies, Myocarditis, and Pericardial Disease
	David Dubow

THE CARDIOMYOPATHIES

Cardiomyopathies are the third most common form of heart disease in the United States and are the second most common cause of sudden death in the adolescent population. It is a disease process that directly affects the cardiac structure and alters myocardial function. Four types are currently recognized: (*a*) dilated cardiomyopathy (DCM), (*b*) hypertrophied cardiomyopathy (HCM), (*c*) restrictive cardiomyopathy, (*d*) dysrhythmic right ventricular cardiomyopathy. Unclassified cardiomyopathy is an additional category that includes primary heart muscle disorders that do not fit into any of the four groups.

Dilated Cardiomyopathy

Dilation and compensatory hypertrophy of the myocardium result in depressed systolic function and pump failure leading to low cardiac output. Eighty percent of cases of DCM are idiopathic. Other etiologies include toxins (e.g., alcohol, cocaine, and antiretroviral drugs), infections (e.g., viral, bacterial, and fungal), collagen vascular disorders, hypersensitivity, peripartum, metabolic disorders (e.g., nutritional, endocrine, and electrolyte disturbances), neuromuscular diseases, and familial. Blacks and males have a 2.5-fold increased risk as compared to whites and females. The most common age at the time of diagnosis is 20 to 50 years.

Clinical Features

Systolic pump failure leads to signs and symptoms of congestive heart failure (CHF) including dyspnea on exertion, orthopnea, and paroxysmal nocturnal dyspnea. Chest pain due to limited coronary vascular reserve may also be present. Mural thrombi can form from diminished ventricular contractile force, and there may be signs of peripheral embolization (e.g., flank pain, hematuria, and extremity cyanosis). Holosystolic murmur may be heard along the lower left sternal border or at the apex. Other findings include a summation group, an enlarged and pulsatile liver, bibasilar rales, and dependent edema.

Diagnosis and Differential

Chest x-ray usually shows an enlarged cardiac silhouette, biventricular enlargement, and pulmonary vascular congestion. The electrocardiogram (ECG) shows left ventricular hypertrophy, left atrial enlargement, Q or QS waves, and poor R wave progression across the precordium. Atrial fibrillation and ventricular ectopy are frequently present. Echocardiography confirms the diagnosis and demonstrates ventricular enlargement, increased systolic and diastolic volumes, and a decreased ejection fraction. Differential diagnosis includes acute myocardial infarction, restrictive pericarditis, acute valvular disruption, sepsis, or any other condition that results in a low cardiac output state.

Emergency Department Care and Disposition

Patients with newy diagnosed, symptomatic DCM require admission to a monitored bed or intensive care unit. Initial management is symptom-directed.

1. Intravenous access, supplemental oxygen, and continuous monitoring should be established.
2. Intravenous diuretics (e.g, **furosemide** 40 mg intravenously) and **digoxin** (maximum dose 0.5 mg intravenously) can be administered. These drugs have a symptomatic benefit, but have not been shown to increase survival.
3. Angiotensin-converting enzyme (ACE) inhibitors (e.g., **enala-**

pril 1.25 mg intravenously every 6 h) and β blockers (e.g., **carvedilol** 3.125 mg orally) can be administered. These drugs have been shown to improve survival in DCM with CHF.

4. **Amiodarone** (loaded 150 mg intravenously over 10 min, then 1 mg/min for 6 h) for complex ventricular ectopy can be administered.

5. Anticoagulation should be considered to reduce mural thrombus formation.

Patients with known DCM who have mild-to-moderate exacerbations of their symptoms are most likely noncompliant with their medications or dietary restrictions. These patients can often be managed in the emergency department with intravenous diuretics, reinstitution of their medications, counseling, and prompt follow-up with their primary physician. It is important to search for other causes of exacerbations of DCM such as myocardial ischemia or infarction, anemia, infection, new-onset atrial fibrillation, bradydysrhythmias, valvular insufficiency, renal dysfunction, pulmonary embolism, or thyroid dysfunction.

Hypertrophic Cardiomyopathy

This illness is characterized by asymmetrically increased left ventricular and/or right ventricular muscle mass involving the intraventricular septum without ventricular dilatation. The result is abnormal compliance of the left ventricle leading to impaired diastolic relaxation and diastolic filling. Cardiac output is usually normal. Fifty percent of cases are hereditary.

Clinical Features

Symptom severity progresses with age. Dyspnea on exertion is the most common symptom, followed by angina-like chest pain, palpitations, and syncope. Patients may be aware of forceful ventricular contractions and call these palpitations. Physical exam may reveal a hyperdynamic apical impulse, a precordial lift, and a systolic ejection murmur best heard at the lower left sternal border or apex. The murmur may be increased with the Valsalva maneuver or standing after squatting. The murmur can be decreased by squatting, forceful hand-gripping, or passive leg elevation with the patient supine. (See Chap. 24 for contrasting murmurs.)

Diagnosis and Differential

The ECG demonstrates left ventricular hypertrophy in 30 percent of patients and left atrial enlargement in 25 to 50 percent. Large septal Q waves (greater than 0.3 mV) are present in 25 percent.

Another ECG finding is upright T waves in those leads with QS or QR complexes (T-wave inversion in those leads would suggest ischemia). Chest x-ray is usually normal. Echocardiography is the diagnostic study of choice.

Emergency Department Care and Disposition

Symptoms of HCM may mimic ischemic heart disease and treatment of those symptoms is covered in Chap. 22. Otherwise, general supportive care is indicated. β blockers are the mainstay of treatment for patients with HCM and chest pain. Patients should be discouraged from engaging in vigorous exercise. Those with suspected HCM who have syncope should be hospitalized.

Restrictive Cardiomyopathy

This is one of the least common cardiomyopathies. In this form of the disease the ventricular volume and wall thickness is normal, but there is decreased diastolic volume of both ventricles. Most causes are idiopathic, but systemic disorders have been implicated, such as amyloidosis, sarcoidosis, hemochromatosis, scleroderma, carcinoid, hypereosinophilic syndrome, and endomyocardial fibrosis.

Clinical Features

Symptoms of CHF predominate, including dyspnea, orthopnea, and pedal edema. Chest pain is uncommon. Physical exam may reveal an S_3 or S_4 cardiac gallop, pulmonary rales, jugular venous distension, Kussmaul's sign (inspiratory jugular venous distension), hepatomegaly, pedal edema, and ascites.

Diagnosis and Differential

The chest x-ray may show signs of CHF without cardiomegaly. Nonspecific ECG changes or, in the case of amyloidosis or sarcoidosis, conduction disturbances and low voltage QRS complexes may be seen.

Emergency Department Treatment and Disposition

Treatment is symptom-directed with the use of diuretics and ACE inhibitors. Corticosteroid therapy is indicated for sarcoidosis. Chelation is used for the treatment of hemochromatosis. Admission is determined by the severity of the symptoms and the availability of prompt subspecialty follow-up.

Dysrhythmogenic Right Ventricular Cardiomyopathy

This is the most rare form of cardiomyopathy, and the majority of patients present after an episode of near sudden death. All these patients require extensive workup and hospitalization.

MYOCARDITIS

Inflammation of the myocardium may be the result of a systemic disorder or an infectious agent. Viral etiologies include Coxsackie B, echovirus, influenza, parainfluenza, Epstein-Barr, and HIV. Bacterial causes include *Corynebacterium diptheria, Neisseria meningitides, Mycoplasma pneumoniae,* and β-hemolytic streptococci. Pericarditis frequently accompanies myocarditis.

Clinical Features

Systemic signs and symptoms predominate, including fever, tachycardia "out of proportion" to the fever, myalgias, headache, and rigors. Chest pain due to coexisting pericarditis is frequently present. A pericardial friction rub may be heard in patients with concomitant pericarditis. In severe cases, there may be symptoms of progressive heart failure (CHF, pulmonary rales, pedal edema, etc.).

Diagnosis and Differential

Nonspecific ECG changes, atrioventricular block, prolonged QRS duration, or ST-segment elevation (in the setting of associated pericarditis) are seen. Chest x-ray is normal. Cardiac enzymes may be elevated. Differential diagnosis includes cardiac ischemia or infarction, valvular disease, and sepsis.

Emergency Department Care and Disposition

Supportive care is the mainstay of treatment. If a bacterial cause is suspected, antibiotics are appropriate. Many patients have progressive CHF, therefore hospitalization in a monitored environment is usually indicated. (See Chap. 23 for management of CHF.)

ACUTE PERICARDITIS

Inflammation of the pericardium may be the result of viral infection (e.g., coxsackie virus, echovirus, and HIV), bacterial infection (e.g., *staphylococcus, S. pneumoniae,* β-hemolytic *streptococcus, Mycobacterium tuberculosis*), fungal infection (e.g., *Histoplasmosis capsulatum*), malignancy (leukemia, lymphoma, melanoma, and metastatic breast cancer), drugs (procainamide and hydralazine), radiation, connective tissue disease, uremia, myxedema, postmyocardial infarction (Dressler's syndrome), or may be idiopathic.

Clinical Features

The most common symptom is sudden or gradual onset of sharp or stabbing chest pain that radiates to the back, neck, left shoulder, arm, or trapezial ridge (especially distinguishing). The pain is typically aggravated by movement or inspiration and by lying supine. Sitting up and leaning forward reduces the pain. Associated symptoms include low-grade intermittent fever, dyspnea, and dysphagia. A transient, intermittent friction rub heard best at the lower left sternal border or apex is the most common physical finding.

Diagnosis and Differential

ECG changes come in stages. Initially there is ST-segment elevation in leads I, V_5, and V_6 with PR-segment depression in leads II, aV_F and V_4 through V_6. As the disease resolves the ST segment normalizes and the T-wave amplitude decreases and inverts. In the final stage, the ECG returns to normal. It is difficult to distinguish these ECG changes from those of early repolarization. A ST segment/T-wave amplitude ratio greater than 0.25 in leads I, V_5, or V_6 is indicative of acute pericarditis. Pericarditis without other underlying cardiac diseases does not typically produce dysrhythmias. Chest x-ray is usually normal, but should be done to rule out other disease. Echocardiography is the best diagnostic test. Other tests that should be completed include complete blood cell count with differential, blood urea nitrogen and creatinine levels (to rule out uremia), streptococcal serology, appropriate viral serology, other serology (e.g., antinuclear and anti-DNA antibodies), thyroid function studies, erythrocyte sedimentation rate, and creatinine kinase levels with isoenzymes (to assess for myocarditis).

Emergency Department Care and Disposition

Patients with idiopathic or presumed viral etiologies are treated as outpatients with nonsteroidal anti-inflammatory agents (e.g., ibuprofen 400 to 600 mg orally four times daily) for 1 to 3 weeks. Patients should be treated for a specific cause if one is identified. Any patient with myocarditis or hemodynamic compromise should be admitted into a monitored environment.

NONTRAUMATIC CARDIC TAMPONADE

Tamponade occurs when the pressure in the pericardial sac exceeds the normal filling pressure of the right ventricle resulting in restricted filling and decreased cardiac output. Causes include metastatic malignancy, uremia, hemorrhage (over-anticoagulation), idiopathic disorder, bacterial/tubercular disorder, or chronic pericarditis, and other (e.g., systemic lupus, postradiation, or myxedema).

Clinical Features

The most common complaints are dyspnea and decreased exercise tolerance. Other nonspecific symptoms include weight loss, pedal edema, and ascites. Physical findings include tachycardia, low systolic blood pressure, and a narrow pulse pressure. Pulsus paradoxus, neck vein distension, distant heart sounds, and right upper quadrant pain (due to hepatic congestion) may also be present. Pulmonary rales are usually absent.

Diagnosis and Differential

Low-voltage QRS complexes, and ST-segment elevation with PR-segment depression may be present on the ECG. Chest x-ray is usually normal. Echocardiography is the diagnostic test of choice.

Emergency Department Care and Disposition

Tamponade is a true emergency. Standard supportive measures as previously discussed should be instituted promptly. An intravenous fluid bolus of 500 to 1000 mL of normal saline may temporarily improve the hemodynamics. Pericardiocentesis is both therapeutic and diagnostic. These patients require admission to an intensive care unit or monitored setting.

CONSTRICTIVE PERICARDITIS

Constriction occurs when fibrous thickening and loss of elasticity of the pericardium results in interference of diastolic filling. Cardiac trauma, pericardiotomy (open-heart surgery), intrapericardial hemorrhage, fungal or bacterial pericarditis, and uremic pericarditis are the most common causes.

Clinical Features

Symptoms develop gradually and mimic those of restrictive cardiomyopathy, including CHF, exertional dyspnea, and decreased exercise tolerance. Chest pain, orthopnea, and paroxysmal nocturnal dyspnea are uncommon. On physical exam patients may have pedal edema, hepatomegaly, ascites, jugular venous distension, and Kussmaul's sign. A pericardial "knock" (an early diastolic sound) may be heard at the apex. There is usually no friction rub.

Diagnosis and Differential

The ECG is not usually helpful, but may show low-voltage QRS complexes and inverted T waves. Pericardial calcification is seen in up to 50 percent of patients on the lateral chest x-ray. Doppler echocardiography, cardiac computed tomography, and magnetic resonance imaging are diagnostic. Other diseases that should be considered include acute pericarditis or myocarditis, exacerbation of chronic ventricular dysfunction, or a systemic process resulting in decreased cardiac performance (e.g., sepsis).

Emergency Department Care and Disposition

General supportive care is the initial treatment. Symptomatic patients will require hospitalization and pericardiectomy.

For further reading in *Emergency Medicine: A Comprehensive Study Guide,* 5th ed., see Chap. 51, "The Cardiomyopathies, Myocarditis, and Pericardial Disease," by James T. Niemann.

---

26 | Pulmonary Embolism

David M. Cline

Pulmonary embolism (PE) is a common deadly disorder difficult to diagnose. Risk factors include congestive heart failure, acute myocardial infarction (MI), chronic obstructive pulmonary disease (COPD), pregnancy, prolonged immobilization, previous history of PE, history of deep-vein thrombosis (DVT), marked obesity, burns, malignancy, estrogen use and other hypercoagulable states, surgery in the last 3 months, or lower extremity trauma. Most patients will have at least one risk factor, but some may have an occult risk factor unknown at the time of presentation.

Clinical Features

The diagnosis of PE should be considered in any patient at risk who experiences acute dyspnea, chest pain, syncope, or shock. Common symptoms in decreasing order of frequency include dyspnea, pleuritic chest pain, anxiety, cough, hemoptysis, sweats, nonpleuritic chest pain, and syncope. Common signs in decreasing order of frequency include respirations > 16, rales, pulse > 100, temperature > 37.8°C (100.4°F), phlebitis or DVT, cardiac gallop, diaphoresis, edema, and cyanosis. Pleural friction rub and wheezes are infrequent signs of PE. The presence or absence of any symptom or sign does not confirm or exclude the diagnosis of pulmonary embolism. Massive PE (5 percent of cases) presents with hypotension and hypoxia.

Diagnosis and Differential

First the clinician must suspect the diagnosis of PE in patients at risk. Second, supplementary tests, including an arterial blood gas (ABG) analysis, 12-lead electrocardiogram (ECG), and chest x-ray will help to direct further testing and treatment. The diagnosis can be excluded or confirmed only with more sophisticated tests, such as a ventilation-perfusion lung scan ($\dot{V}/\dot{Q}$ scan) or pulmonary angiography. The ABG will demonstrate a PaO_2 less than 81 mmHg in 80 percent of patients with PE. As many as 5 percent of patients with PE will have a PaO_2 greater than 90 mmHg. The presence of an increased alveolar-arterial (A-a) gradient is more sensitive (85 percent) for PE and is calculated with the following formula:

$$\text{A-a gradient} = [150 - 1.2(PCO_2)] - PaO_2$$

The preceding value should be compared to the expected normal A-a gradient calculated with the following formula: [(patient age/ 4) − 4]. Patients with an increased A-a gradient should have further testing. The A-a gradient is less reliable in the elderly. A D-dimer level less than 500 U/mL has a negative predictive value of 90 percent for PE. However, the D-dimer assay has a high incidence of false positives. The classic $S_1Q_3T_3$ pattern on the ECG is highly suggestive of PE but is present in only 12 percent of patients. The most common ECG finding is nonspecific ST-T wave changes. A completely normal ECG is seen in less than 10 percent of cases. The chest x-ray may be normal, but an elevated dome of one diaphragm is seen in 50 percent of patients. The chest x-ray also should be used to correlate the abnormalities seen with radionuclide studies. Other supplemental tests include complete blood cell count to aid in the differential diagnosis, prothrombin time, and partial thromboplastin time in anticipation of possible anticoagulation.

Venography can be helpful, as radiographic evidence of DVT will be seen in 90 percent of patients with PE (clinical signs are seen in only 33 percent). Some centers achieve a 95 percent sensitivity for DVT with impedance plethysmography.

The $\dot{V}/\dot{Q}$ scan is a sensitive test for PE, and a completely normal study rules out the disorder. Pulmonary angiography is the gold standard for diagnosing PE and is a much more specific test than the $\dot{V}/\dot{Q}$ scan. Angiography exposes the patient to more potential complications, especially in elderly patients. Angiography may be needed to confirm the diagnosis if the $\dot{V}/\dot{Q}$ scan demonstrates equivocal results, such as medium or low probability for PE, in a patient at risk. Spiral computed tomography has compared favorably to $\dot{V}/\dot{Q}$ scanning, but its overall utility is still uncertain. Magnetic resonance imaging may also have future utility in confirming the diagnosis of PE.

Disorders in the differential diagnosis include respiratory disorders, such as asthma, COPD, pneumonia, spontaneous pneumothorax, and pleurisy. Cardiac disorders that may mimic PE include myocardial infarction and pericarditis. Musculoskeletal disorders that may mimic PE include muscle strain, rib fracture, costochondritis, and herpes zoster. Intraabdominal disorders that irritate the diaphragm or stimulate breathing may also present similar to PE. Finally, hyperventilation syndrome may mimic PE, however, this is a diagnosis of exclusion.

Emergency Department Care and Disposition

The treatment of PE consists of initial stabilization, anticoagulation with heparin, and thrombolytic therapy in extreme cases. Patients should be hooked up to a cardiac monitor, noninvasive blood pressure device, pulse-oximetry monitor, and an intravenous line.

1. Sufficient oxygen should be administered to maintain a pulse-oximetry reading of 95% O_2 saturation. Lower O_2 saturation levels may be acceptable in patients with chronic hypoxia. If an ABG is desired off O_2, the clinician should ensure that the patient is stable enough to endure the period of potential hypoxia.
2. Crystalloid intravenous fluids should be given initially for hypotension, and a central venous pressure or Swan-Ganz catheter should be considered if the patient does not respond to the

fluid bolus of 500 to 1000 mL of normal saline. If thrombolytic therapy is considered, central lines should be avoided.

3. For hypotension in the absence of hypovolemia, **dopamine** can be started at 2 to 5 μg/kg/min and titrated to maintain a systolic blood pressure of 90 mmHg.

4. **Heparin** should be started with an intravenous bolus of 10,000 to 20,000 U, followed by a continuous drip of 1000 U/h to be adjusted using the partial thromboplastin time, aiming for 1.5 to 2 times control. Contraindications to anticoagulation include active internal bleeding, uncontrolled severe hypertension, recent trauma, recent surgery, recent stroke, intracranial or intraspinal neoplasm. Heparin can be used safely in the nonbleeding pregnant patient but must be discontinued prior to delivery.

5. Low molecular heparin has been shown to be safe and effective in the treatment of DVT and PE. Examples include enoxaparin 1 mg/kg, subcutaneously as the initial dose.

6. For persistent hypotension despite medical management with the preceding measures, thrombolytic therapy should be considered. **Tissue plasminogen activator,** 50 to 100 mg intravenously over 2 to 6 h, has been recommended. **Streptokinase** can be given in a dose of 250,000 U intravenously over 30 min followed by a continuous intravenous infusion of 100,000 U/h for the next 12 to 24 h. Ideally, consultation with an intensivist should be done prior to starting thrombolytic therapy.

Patients who demonstrate any degree of clinical instability should be admitted to the intensive care unit. Stable patients may be admitted to a telemetry bed. Heparin does not prevent the embolization of existing clots. Further embolization and shock most commonly occur within 4 h of initial symptoms. Patients should be stable and beyond this initial high-risk period if admission to a nonmonitored bed is considered. For patients with contraindications to anticoagulation or thrombolytic therapy, a Greenfield filter can be inserted percutaneously.

For further reading in *Emergency Medicine: A Comprehensive Study Guide,* 5th ed., see Chap. 52, "Pulmonary Embolism," by Charles N. Schoenfeld.

27   Hypertensive Emergencies

Vincent Nacouzi

Successful management of hypertensive disease in the emergency department (ED) can be done using the following classification:

1. *Hypertensive emergency:* This entails an elevated blood pressure (BP) associated with acute central nervous system (CNS), cardiac, and/or renal dysfunction. Immediate recognition and treatment is required. Hypertensive crisis or malignant hypertension (HTN) falls under this category.

2. *Hypertensive urgency:* This requires a diastolic blood pressure (DBP) > 115 mmHg without any signs or symptoms of acute organ dysfunction. If allowed to persist, injury may occur. Decreasing the BP over 24 to 48 h and follow-up the next day is recommended.

3. *Acute hypertensive episode:* This includes a systolic blood pressure (SBP) > 180 and DBP > 110 mmHg without signs or symptoms. Usually no immediate treatment is required but the patient should have follow-up the next day.

4. *Transient HTN:* These patients usually become normotensive once the precipitating event is resolved. Examples include pregnancy, severe anxiety, alcohol withdrawal, and cocaine/drug use. The treatment varies according to the condition.

The clinician must insure that the BP cuff size is appropriate for the patient's size; a small cuff gives a falsely elevated BP reading.

Clinical Features

Essential historic items include a prior diagnosis of HTN; cessation of BP medications; cardiovascular, renal, or cerebrovascular disease; diabetes, chronic obstructive pulmonary disease (COPD), or asthma. Precipitating causes such as pregnancy, illicit drug use (cocaine and methamphetamines), monoamine oxidase inhibitor, or decongestants should be considered. Patients should be asked about CNS symptoms (headaches, visual changes, weakness, seizures, and confusion), cardiovascular symptoms (chest pain, palpitations, dyspnea, pedal edema, or tearing pain radiating to the back or abdomen), and renal symptoms (anuria, edema, hematuria, or flank pain). The patient should be examined for evidence of papilledema, retinal exudates, neurologic deficits, seizures, meningismus, or encephalopathy; the presence of any findings constitutes a hypertensive emergency. Also the patient should be assessed for carotid bruits, heart murmurs, gallops, symmetric pulses (coarctation Vs aortic dissection), abdominal masses, and pulmonary rales. In the pregnant (or postpartum) patient the clinician should look for hyperreflexia with peripheral edema indicating pre-eclampsia.

Diagnosis and Differential

An elevated blood urea nitrogen, creatinine, or potassium level in the presence of hematuria and proteinuria indicates renal injury. Worsening renal function in the presence of acute HTN, blood, or red blood cell casts in the urine is a hypertensive emergency. A toxicology profile helps identify illicit drug use. On the electrocardiogram (ECG) the clinician should look for acute ST changes suggesting ischemia, strain, or left ventricular hypertrophy. The chest x-ray helps to identify congestive heart failure (CHF), aortic dissection, or coarctation. A pregnancy test should be done on all hypertensive women of childbearing age.

Emergency Department Care and Disposition

In the presence of a hypertensive emergency intravenous access should be established and the patient placed on a cardiac monitor and kept well oxygenated. Following the ABCs, the treatment goal is to lower the mean arterial pressure = (SBP + 2 DBP)/3 by 20 to 25 percent over 30 min using the following regimens:

1. For *hypertensive encephalopathy,* **sodium nitroprusside** should be used. It should be started at 0.5 mg/kg/min and titrated to a maximum of 10 mg/kg/min. Rapid correction of the BP should be avoided to prevent cerebral ischemia secondary to hypoperfusion.

2. **Labetalol** is a second-line agent for hypertensive encephalopathy but a steady and consistent drop in the BP makes it useful. The clinician should avoid using it in patients with reactive airway disease, heart block, or cocaine intoxication. It is best to start with 20-mg increments intravenously with a maximum effect in 10 min, the maximum dose is 300 mg. A continuous infusion at 2 mg/min can also be used. The infusion should be stopped after the desired effect is achieved.

3. For *HTN associated with stroke,* increased BP is often a protective response to stroke. When the DBP is ≥ 135 mmHg, it should be reduced slowly by 20 percent using 5-mg increments of intravenous **labetalol**. With hemorrhagic strokes, oral **nimodipine** (60 mg PO every 4°) or **nicardipine** (2 mg intravenous bolus then 4 to 12 mg/h infusion) can reverse vasospasm for SAH.

4. For *HTN associated with pulmonary edema* intravenous **nitroglycerin** (5 to 20 μg/min) or nitroprusside (started at 0.3 μg/kg/min) should be used. Diuretics and morphine sulfate are used as well.

5. For *HTN associated with myocardial ischemia,* **nitroglycerin** (5 to 20 μg/min) is the first-line therapy. Diuretics and morphine can be added. Nitroprusside, hydralazine, and other antihypertensives that increase oxygen demand and tachycardia should be avoided.

6. For *HTN associated with aortic dissection,* treating the BP may limit the dissection. Either **labetalol** alone (given in 20-mg increments as described earlier) or a combination of **nitroprusside** (started at 0.3 μg/kg/min) and **esmolol** (500 μg/kg over 1 min, followed by an effusion of 50 to 150 μg/kg/min) can be used. Propranolol and metoprolol are alternatives.

7. For *HTN associated with renal failure,* **nitroprusside**, 5 to 20 μg/kg/min, is the preferred agent. Diuresis, clonidine (dose shown later), and emergency dialysis are other options.

8. For *asymptomatic hypertensive urgency,* the choice of the oral agent should be based on coexisting conditions if any. Diuretics should be used in patients with renal disease, CHF, and in the elderly, such as **hydrochlorothiazide (HCTZ)** 25 mg/d (the clinician should consider oral potassium supplement). For patients with angina or post myocardial infarction a β blocker should be considered, such as **metoprolol** 50 mg orally two times daily. Angiotensin-converting enzyme (ACE) inhibitors can be used in those with CHF or diabetes mellitus, such as **captopril** 25 mg two to three times daily. Alternative agents include **clonidine**, 0.2 mg oral loading dose, followed by 0.1 mg/h until the diastolic BP is below 115.

For a discussion of hypertension associated with pregnancy, see Chap. 59.

CHILDHOOD HYPERTENSIVE EMERGENCIES

Children often will have nonspecific complaints such as throbbing frontal headache or blurred vision. Physical findings associated with hypertension are similar to those found in adults.

The most common etiologies in this age group are renovascular lesions for which **diazoxide** intravenously (3 mg/kg) and/or intravenous **labetalol** (1 to 3 mg/kg/h) have been used extensively. Another alternative is **captopril** 1 mg/kg/24 h in 2 to 4 divided doses. Pheochromocytoma is the other common etiology presenting with nervousness, palpitations, sweating, blurry vision, and sometimes skin flushing. The treatment is surgical excision, managing the BP is with α-adrenergic blockage such as phentolamine. Pediatric hypertension that requires intervention in the ED will likely require admission.

For further reading in *Emergency Medicine: A Comprehensive Study Guide,* 5th ed., see Chap. 53, "Hypertension," by Melissa M. Wu and Arjun Chanmugam.

---

28 | Aortic Dissection and Aneurysms

Lance Brown

Aortic dissection and abdominal aortic aneurysms (AAAs) are important causes of morbidity and death that require rapid diagnosis and frequently require prompt operative repair to offer the patient any chance of survival. Diagnosing these conditions can be challenging and carries a high risk of misdiagnosis.

ABDOMINAL AORTIC ANEURYSMS

Clinical Features

Four clinical scenarios arise regarding abdominal aortic aneurysms (AAA): acute rupture, aortoenteric fistula, chronic contained rupture, and an incidental finding.

Acute rupturing AAA is a true emergency that if not identified and repaired rapidly will lead to death. The classic presentation is of an older (> 60 years) male smoker with atherosclerosis who experiences syncope without warning, regains consciousness, and complains of severe abdominal or back pain. Classically, such patients will have a tender pulsatile abdominal mass on physical examination. Hypotension may persist through presentation or may be transient, with a temporary normalization of vital signs. Femoral pulsations are typically normal. Patients usually present with some variation on this classic presentation. The patient may complain of unilateral flank pain, groin pain, hip pain, or pain localizing to one quadrant of the abdomen. There may be minimal complaint of pain. On examination, obesity may mask a pulsatile abdominal mass, or tenderness may be minimal or absent. Retroperitoneal hemorrhage may be appreciated as periumbilical ecchymosis, flank ecchymosis, or scrotal hematomas. If blood compresses the femoral nerve, a neuropathy of the lower extremity may be present.

Aortoenteric fistulas present as gastrointestinal bleeding. The classic presentation is of a patient who has previously undergone aortic grafting (e.g., AAA repair) and presents with massive life-threatening gastrointestinal bleeding. The patient may present with hematemesis, melenemesis, melena, or hematochezia. A continuum of severity exists, and the patient may present with a deceptively minor "sentinel" bleed or with massive bleeding and hemorrhagic shock.

Chronic contained rupture of AAA is an uncommon presentation. If an AAA ruptures into the retroperitoneum, there may be significant fibrosis and a limiting of blood loss. The patient typically appears quite well and can have had the pain for an extended period of time.

Incidentally finding an AAA can be lifesaving. These aneurysms are, by definition, asymptomatic and are usually identified when a radiologic study is performed for some other purpose [e.g., a computed tomography (CT) scan performed for trauma]. Those aneurysms greater than 5 cm in diameter are at a higher risk for rupture.

Diagnosis and Differential

In the setting of syncope, back pain, and shock with a tender pulsatile abdominal mass the diagnosis may be straightforward. The differential diagnosis depends on the variation in presentation. For example, the patient may present with syncope and shock but have minimal pain and the differential diagnosis is that of syncope: cardiac dysrhythmias, medication reaction, and so on. Other diagnoses that might be considered include renal colic (when flank pain dominates the clinical picture), musculoskeletal back pain, pancreatic disease, intraabdominal processes (diverticulitis, cholecystitis, appendicitis, mesenteric ischemia, etc.), scrotal or testicular disorders, and disorders that lead to gastrointestinal bleeding (esophageal varices, tumors, gastric ulcers, etc.).

If the diagnosis of rupturing AAA is clear on clinical grounds, the best course of action is to have the operating vascular surgeon immediately evaluate the patient in anticipation of taking the patient to the operating room. Diagnostic studies should not delay surgical repair. However, the diagnosis may not be entirely clear, and confirming studies may be required. In the unstable patient, bedside abdominal ultrasonography has a very high sensitivity for identifying AAA and can measure the diameter of the aneurysm. Aortic rupture cannot be reliably identified with ultrasound. Obesity and bowel gas may technically limit the study. In the stable patient, CT can identify the AAA and delineate the anatomic details of the aneurysm and any associated rupture. It is unclear what the role of plain radiography is in the diagnosis of rupturing AAA, since a calcified bulging aortic contour is present in only 65 percent of patients with symptomatic AAA.

Emergency Department Care and Disposition

The primary role of the emergency physician is in identifying AAA and determining which of the four clinical scenarios is present.

1. For suspected rupturing AAA or aortoenteric fistula, prompt surgical consultation in anticipation of emergency surgery is critical. No diagnostic testing should delay surgical repair.
2. Stabilize the patient utilizing large-bore intravenous access, judicious fluid administration for hypotension, treatment of hypertension (see Chap. 27), and typing and cross-matching of several units of packed red blood cells with transfusion as needed. Since patients may rapidly deteriorate clinically, those who undergo diagnostic testing should not be left unattended in the radiology department.
3. For chronic contained rupturing AAA, consultation with a vascular surgeon for urgent repair and intensive care unit admission should be sought.
4. For AAA identified as an incidental finding, the patient can potentially be discharged home, depending on the aneurysmal size and comorbid factors. Phone consultation with a vascular surgeon for admission or close office follow-up is usually adequate.

AORTIC DISSECTION

Clinical Features

Aortic dissection is typically a disease of the thoracic aorta commonly involving the ascending aorta or descending aorta in the region of the ligamentum arteriosum. Most patients are over the age of 50 years with a history of hypertension. Another group of patients are younger and have identifiable risk factors, such as Marfan's syndrome, other connective tissue disorders, congenital heart disease, and pregnancy. Patients who have undergone aortic catheterization or cardiac surgery may develop iatrogenically induced aortic dissection. More than 90 percent of patients will have the abrupt onset of severe tearing or ripping chest or upper back pain (between the scapulae). Accompanying nausea, vomiting, and diaphoresis are common.

The clinical presentation depends on the location of the dissection. Presentations include aortic valve insufficiency, coronary artery occlusion with myocardial infarction, carotid involvement with stroke symptoms, occlusion of vertebral blood supply with paraplegia, cardiac tamponade with shock and jugular venous distention, compression of the recurrent laryngeal nerve with hoarseness of the voice, and compression of the superior cervical sympathetic ganglion with Horner's syndrome. The dissection may progress down into the abdomen, causing abdominal or flank pain. As the dissection progresses, seemingly unrelated symptoms or confusing symptom complexes may present themselves. The dissection may develop a new opening into the true aortic lumen with a marked decrease in the severity of symptoms, leading to a false sense of reassurance.

The patient's physical examination findings will depend on the location and progression of the dissection. A diastolic murmur of aortic insufficiency may be heard. One-half of patients have decreased pulsation in the radial, femoral, or carotid arteries. Hypertension and tachycardia are common, but hypotension may also be present. Although one might expect a difference in extremity blood pressures, no specific threshold values have been defined. Forty percent of patients have neurologic sequelae, which can include strokes or paraplegia.

Diagnosis and Differential

The differential diagnosis to be considered depends on the location and progression of the dissection. Other causes of aortic insufficiency, myocardial infarction, esophageal rupture, other causes of strokes, spinal injury or tumor, vocal cord tumors, and other causes of cardiac tamponade, including pericardial disease, may need to be considered.

The diagnosis of aortic dissection depends on radiographic confirmation once the diagnosis is suspected. The chest x-ray shows an abnormal aortic contour 90 percent of the time. Widening of the mediastinum with deviation of the trachea, mainstem bronchi, or esophagus is also seen. The "calcium sign" may be present, with intimal calcium seen distant from the edge of the aortic contour. CT, angiography, and transesophageal echocardiograms are all quite sensitive and specific. The use of these studies is institutionally dependent, and they should be ordered in conjunction with the consulting vascular or thoracic surgeon.

Emergency Department Care and Disposition

All patients with aortic dissection or strongly suspected aortic dissection require emergent vascular or thoracic surgical consultation and prompt radiographic confirmation of the diagnosis, which is best directed by the operating surgeon. In general, patients with dissection of the ascending aorta require prompt surgical intervention. The operative care of dissection of only the descending aorta is controversial and should be evaluated on a case-by-case basis. Stabilization of the patient typically requires large-bore intravenous access, electrocardiogram, chest x-ray, and management of hypertension (see Chap. 27).

For further reading in *Emergency Medicine: A Comprehensive Study Guide*, 5th ed., see Chap. 54, "Aortic Dissection and Aneurysms," by Gary A. Johnson.

---

29 | Nontraumatic Peripheral Vascular Disorders

Lance Brown

SUPERFICIAL THROMBOPHLEBITIS

Superficial venous occlusion typically occurs in the lower extremity involving the saphenous vein and its varicosities and tributaries. Typical clinical features include localized pain, redness, induration, and tenderness along the course of the involved vein. Localized bruising and bleeding may also be seen. On occasion, it may be difficult to differentiate superficial thrombophlebitis from deep vein thrombosis, cellulitis, or lymphangitis on clinical exam. Although not typically required, a doppler ultrasound is the study of choice as flow in the involved vein reliably excludes the diagnosis of superficial thrombophlebitis, and deep venous thrombosis can also be evaluated. Treatment consists of warm compresses, analgesia, nonsteroidal anti-inflammatory medications, elevation of the extremity, support stockings or elastic support bandages, and daily activities as tolerated. The patient should have reliable follow-up and expect weeks of slowly improving symptoms.

DEEP VENOUS THROMBOSIS OF THE LOWER EXTREMITY

Deep venous thrombosis (DVT) is difficult to evaluate on clinical exam and can have life-threatening consequences, the most concerning of which is pulmonary embolism.

Clinical Features

The classic features of DVT include swelling of the lower extremity, tenderness, pain, redness, increased localized warmth, and possibly low-grade fever. Homan's sign (pain in the calf with forced dorsiflexion of the foot while the knee is held in extension) is diagnostically unreliable. Swelling and tenderness are the most common findings (each seen in over 75 percent of patients). The physical findings depend on the location and degree of venous obstruction. Significant proximal thrombosis may be present with minimal clinical findings.

Diagnosis and Differential

Examination findings are unreliable for the diagnosis of DVT. There are, however, historical risk factors that increase the likelihood of DVT. These include pelvic or lower extremity trauma, hypercoagulable condition (e.g., protein c disease), estrogen replacement, intravenous drug abuse, age greater than 40 years, malignancy, birth control pills, obesity, postpartum status, smoking, recent surgery, or immobilization (bed rest, casting, and prolonged sitting).

There are two tests that are readily available and useful in evaluating the patient with possible DVT: the D-dimer and ultrasound. The D-dimer is useful for its negative predictive value. The D-dimer is a blood laboratory test that can be elevated in DVT, pulmonary embolus, trauma, cancer, infections, surgery, and other conditions. However, a negative value (less than 250 mg/mL) can essentially rule out proximal DVT in the low-risk patient. The most commonly used test for DVT is ultrasound. Ultrasound is noninvasive, safe, quick, readily accessible, and accurate for proximal (proximal to the popliteal fossa) DVT. When a negative ultrasound is combined with a negative D-dimer, there is a negative predictive value for DVT of about 99 percent. Other tests include impedance plethysmography, venogram, nuclear medicine studies, and MRI. The use of these studies will be institutionally dependent.

Emergency Department Care and Disposition

The primary objective in treating DVT is prevention of pulmonary embolism. The mainstay of therapy is anticoagulation.

1. In the setting of ultrasound-documented proximal DVT with other complications, hospital admission is appropriate.
2. Either low-molecular-weight heparin (LMWH) or unfractionated **heparin** (with weight-based dosing of a bolus of 80 U/kg followed by an infusion of 18 U/kg per h) may be used. The available LMWHs include dalteparin, enoxaparin, or tinzaparin. An example treatment regimen would be **enoxaparin** 1 mg/kg of lean body weight subcutaneously twice daily. When using unfractionated heparin, the goal is a PTT of 1.8 to 2.8 times normal.
3. If anticoagulation is contraindicated, if a clot is extending proximally in spite of medical treatment, or if there is significant bleeding with the anticoagulants, consultation should be obtained for the placement of a Greenfield filter in the inferior vena cava.
4. In the setting of ultrasound-documented proximal DVT, discharge to home on LMWH can be considered. The patient should have few or no comorbid illnesses, be able to ambulate unassisted, have good social support at home, have a physician familiar with the use of LMWH who can follow up with the patient within 24 h, be able and willing to self-administer injections at home, and have no other reason for admission to the hospital. Warfarin therapy would then be initiated by the follow-up physician.
5. In the setting of unilateral leg swelling and an ultrasound negative for venous thrombosis proximal to the popliteal fossa (presumed calf DVT), discharge with a follow-up ultrasound in 5 to 7 days is recommended. Generally, no anticoagulation needs to be started except in very high risk groups including those with previous proximal DVT or pulmonary embolus, poor ambulation, a known hypercoagulable state, or extensive cardiovascular comorbidity. With a known or presumed calf DVT, the risk of pulmonary embolus within 7 days after an initial negative ultrasound is near zero, even without anticoagulation.

AXILLARY AND SUBCLAVIAN VEIN THROMBOSIS

Far fewer DVTs of the upper extremity occur than they do of the lower extremity. Clinical features include abrupt or gradual onset of swelling in the arm with dilated veins in the hand and forearm, a heavy feeling in the arm, and pain on physical activity relieved with rest. Risk factors are similar to those for DVT of the lower extremity (especially indwelling central lines, intravenous drug abuse, malignancy, hyper coagulable states). Predisposing anatomic variants (cervical web, hypertrophied scalene muscle, congenital web, etc.) are commonly found. Current therapy options include anticoagulation alone or preceded by catheter-directed thrombolysis. Diagnostic approach and treatment should be individualized, and consultation with a vascular surgeon is recommended in all cases.

ACUTE ARTERIAL OCCLUSION

Acute arterial occlusion is a limb-threatening emergency that requires prompt recognition and early vascular surgery consultation.

Clinical Features

The earliest symptom is extremity pain followed soon thereafter by skin ischemia with pallor and abnormal sensation (including paresthesias). Muscle weakness is expected. Anesthesia and paralysis develop, as the ischemic insult progresses. Pulselessness is expected, however, loss of palpable pulses may be a finding of chronic vascular disease. Late findings include skin and fat necrosis. An embolus from the heart is the most common cause of an acute arterial occlusion and a history of (or presentation of) atrial fibrillation or myocardial infarction should be sought.

Diagnosis and Differential

Maintaining a high degree of clinical suspicion is warranted, particularly in patients with atrial fibrillation and the acute onset of nontraumatic limb pain. Besides clot emboli from the heart, vegetations from heart valves, parts of prosthetic valves or vascular access devices, atheromatous plaques, or vasospasm should be considered in the differential. The most worrisome condition in the differential diagnosis is occlusion of arterial flow from the false lumen of a propagating thoracic aortic dissection. This is one instance whereby anticoagulation is strictly contraindicated.

Diagnostic studies can include intraoperative angiography and should be directed by the operating vascular surgeon.

Emergency Department Care and Disposition

Definitive therapy for acute arterial occlusion is surgical, and consultation with a vascular surgeon should be made upon suspicion of the diagnosis. Therapeutic options include surgical or catheter embolectomy and intraarterial thrombolysis.

For further reading in *Emergency Medicine: A Comprehensive Study Guide,* 5th ed., see Chap. 55, "Nontraumatic Peripheral Vascular Disorders," by Anil Chopra.

PULMONARY EMERGENCIES

---

30 | Respiratory Distress

Michael E. Chansky

Respiratory distress is a frequent sign or symptom in emergency patients. The etiologies are diverse and include the nonspecific findings of dyspnea, hypoxia, hypercapnia, and cyanosis. A pertinent history and exam are helpful in ordering the appropriate tests, making the proper diagnosis, and initiating appropriate therapy.

DYSPNEA

Dyspnea is a subjective feeling of difficult, labored, or uncomfortable breathing. It does not result from a single pathophysiologic mechanism, yet two-thirds of patients complaining of dyspnea have either a cardiac or pulmonary disorder.

Clinical Features

The patient presents with shortness of breath or breathlessness and must be rapidly evaluated for tachypnea, tachycardia, use of accessory respiratory muscles, and stridor. Alarming signs and symptoms include agitation or lethargy due to hypoxia, inability to speak, and paradoxical abdominal movements. In patients with any of these signs or symptoms, airway control and mechanical ventilation must be anticipated. Lesser degrees of dyspnea allow for a detailed medical history, which often identifies the primary responsible process (Table 30-1).

Diagnosis and Differential

In addition to accurate interpretation of the history and examination, ancillary tests aid in determining the severity and specific cause of dyspnea. Pulse oximetry is a rapid but insensitive screen

TABLE 30-1 Most Common Disorders Causing Dyspnea

Airway	*Vascular*
Foreign body	Pulmonary embolism
Angioedema	Sickle cell
Cardiac	*Neuromuscular*
LV failure	CVA
Arrhythmia	Guillain-Barre
Tamponade	Myasthenia gravis
Ischemia	Neuropathy
Lung parenchymal	Spinal cord trauma
Asthma	*Miscellaneous*
Pneumonia	Anemia
ARDS	Shock
Pleural and chest wall	CO poisoning
Pneumothorax	
Effusion	
Pregnancy	

for disorders of gas exchange. Arterial blood gas (ABG) analysis is more sensitive but cannot evaluate the work of breathing. A chest x-ray may indicate the category of primary disease (infiltrate, effusion, or pneumothorax) but may be normal. An electrocardiogram (ECG), hemoglobin levels, and spirometry may help identify the specific process, though challenging cases may require cardiac stress testing, echocardiography, formal pulmonary function testing, neuromuscular tests, electromyogram, or pulmonary biopsy.

Emergency Department Care and Disposition

There is no specific cause or treatment of dyspnea. Aggressive management of the underlying disorder is indicated after maintaining airway support and oxygenation. Supplemental **oxygen** should be provided with a goal of maintaining a P_{O_2} of over 60 mmHg. This can be lowered to 50 mmHg in patients with severe chronic obstructive pulmonary disease (COPD) and known hypoxia. All patients with unclear causes of dyspnea and hypoxia require **admission** to a monitored bed.

HYPOXIA

Hypoxia is defined as an insufficient delivery of oxygen to the tissue, and it results from any combination of five distinct mechanisms:

1. Hypoventilation-hypoxia and elevated P_{CO_2} (example: narcotic OD)

2. Right-to-left shunt-unoxygenated blood entering systemic arteries (example: atelectasis)
3. Ventilation/perfusion mismatch-regional alteration of ventilation or perfusion (example: PE or asthma)
4. Diffusion impairment-alveolar blood barrier abnormality (example: ARDS, sarcoid, and congestive heart failure (CHF)
5. Low-inspired oxygen (example: high altitude)

Hypoxemia is defined as an abnormally low arterial oxygen tension, arbitrarily $P_{O_2} < 60$ mmHg. Patients with hypoxemia may not be dyspneic, and patients with dyspnea may not have hypoxemia.

Clinical Features

Signs and symptoms of hypoxemia are nonspecific. Tachypnea and tachycardia may be present, and CNS manifestations include agitation, headache, somnolence, seizures, and coma. At $P_{O_2} < 20$ mmHg, there is a central depression of respiratory drive. Dyspnea may be present, but cyanosis is not a sensitive or specific indicator of hypoxemia.

Diagnosis and Differential

The diagnosis of arterial hypoxemia requires clinical suspicion and objective measurement. Formal diagnosis requires ABG analysis, although pulse oximetry is useful for screening gross alterations in P_{O_2}. Calculation of the arterial alveolar oxygen difference $(A\text{-}a)_{O_2}$, where A = forced inspiratory oxygen $(F_{I_{O_2}})$ $(760 - P_{H_2O}) - 1.2$ (P_{CO_2}) and a_{O_2} = ABG value can further quantitate the degree of hypoxemia. The history and examination should help delineate the exact etiology of hypoxia (see preceding examples). Disorders causing dyspnea can lead to hypoxia (see Table 30-1).

Emergency Department Care and Disposition

Regardless of the specific cause of hypoxemia, the initial approach remains the same: Aggressive management of the underlying disorder (if identified), with a goal of maintaining an arterial $O_2 > 60$ mmHg. All hypoxic patients require hospitalization and monitoring until control of the underlying process is achieved. An arterial line is indicated if multiple ABGs are anticipated.

HYPERCAPNIA

Hypercapnia is arbitrarily defined as a $Pa_{CO_2} > 45$ mmHg and is exclusively due to alveolar hypoventilation. It is almost never due to intrinsic lung disease or increased CO_2 production.

Clinical Features

The signs and symptoms of hypercapnia depend on the absolute value of P_{CO_2} and its rate of change. Acute elevations result in increased intracranial pressure, and patients may complain of headache, confusion, lethargy, seizures, and coma. Acute $P_{CO_2} >$ 100 mmHg can result in cardiovascular collapse, whereas chronic hypercapnia may be well tolerated.

Diagnosis and Differential

The diagnosis requires clinical suspicion and an ABG analysis. Pulse oximetry can be normal. The ABG analysis will reveal an acute respiratory acidosis with little metabolic compensation (low pH, high P_{CO_2}, low P_{O_2}, normal bicarbonate). The differential includes drug overdosage, hypoglycemia, severe asthma or COPD, neuromuscular disorders, severe obesity, and upper airway obstruction.

Emergency Department Care and Disposition

Aggressive specific therapy, while maintaining airway and ventilatory support, is indicated. A patient with a heroin overdose will respond more rapidly than a patient with Guillain-Barre syndrome. Disposition depends primarily on the underlying etiology and severity. Many patients will require hospitalization to a monitored bed.

CYANOSIS

Cyanosis causes a bluish skin color and mucous membranes that results from an increase in the absolute amount of reduced hemoglobin or abnormal hemoglobin in the blood. Cyanosis may be detected when the deoxyhemoglobin concentration is as low as 1.5 g/100 mL but generally requires 5 g/100 mL for bedside detection.

Clinical Features

The presence of cyanosis suggests tissue hypoxia or abnormal hemoglobin, such as methemoglobin. However, severe states of tissue hypoxia are possible without the presence of cyanosis. Central cyanosis is caused by unsaturated arterial blood or abnormal hemoglobin, and is typically seen on mucous membranes and skin (see Table 30-2). Skin thickness and pigmentation may make detection difficult. The tongue is considered a sensitive site for observing central cyanosis, while earlobes and nailbeds are less reliable. Peripheral cyanosis is secondary to decreased peripheral blood

TABLE 30-2 Common Causes of Cyanosis

Central cyanosis	Peripheral cyanosis
Hemoglobinopathies	Decreased cardiac output: shock
Methemoglobinemia: acquired,	Cold exposure
hereditary	Venous congestion
Sulfhemoglobinemia: acquired	Arterial thrombosis or embolus
Decreased arterial oxygen	
saturation	
Pulmonary etiologies: shunt,	
diffusion, V/Q mismatch	
Hypoventilation	
High altitude	
Anatomic shunts	
Cardiac: VSD, ASD, TOF	
Intrapulmonary	

flow and greater extraction of oxygen from arterial blood. Differentiation between these two states may be difficult.

Diagnosis and Differential

The presence of cyanosis must be taken in context with the entire clinical picture. Low flow states, hypoxemia, and methemoglobinemia must be considered. ABG analysis with co-oximetry is the gold standard test for assessment of the cyanotic patient. Pulse oximetry has limitations, as patient's with abnormal hemoglobins (methemoglobinemia, sulfhemoglobinemia, and carboxyhemoglobinemia) will often exhibit normal pulse oximetry, yet measured oxygen saturation by ABG analysis will be low. Carboxyhemoglobin produces "cherry red" cyanosis, hence it is not true cyanosis. Central cyanosis will exhibit diminished oxygen saturation associated with hypoxia. In peripheral cyanosis, the O_2 saturation should be normal. Abnormal hemoglobinemias will reveal a normal Pa_{O_2} (normal dissolved O_2 in the blood), normal calculated O_2 saturation, and abnormal measured O_2 saturation.

A complete blood cell count may reveal anemia or polycythemia. Anemic patients may not show clinical signs of cyanosis due to the absolute amount of reduced hemoglobin required. Polycythemia causes peripheral cyanosis by sludging. If the Pa_{O_2} and hemoglobin concentration are normal, cyanosis may be due to abnormal hemoglobin or skin pigmentation. Methemoglobinemia and sulfhemoglobinemia are usually acquired states secondary to chemicals or medications and should be suspected in the cyanotic patient with normal cardiopulmonary function. Benzocaine, nitrates, and nitrites are the most common agents implicated in drug-induced methemoglobinemia. In methemoglobinemia, venous blood will appear chocolate brown, and visible cyanosis is evident with as little as 1.5 g 100 mL of blood. Sulfhemoglobinemia commonly results from either phenacetin or acetanilid (Bromo Seltzer) and can produce cyanosis at a level of less than 0.5 g per 100 mL of blood. Industrial aniline compounds may produce met- or sulfhemoglobinemia. Since abnormal hemoglobin levels cannot bind oxygen, symptoms are secondary to hypoxia, and severity is related to the quantity of abnormal hemoglobin present.

Emergency Department Care and Disposition

Rapid identification and treatment of the underlying etiology of cyanosis is critical. Patients with central cyanosis not responsive to supplemental oxygen have either impaired circulation or abnormal hemoglobin. Patients with acquired methemoglobinemia require therapy for signs of hypoxia (i.e., angina, arrhythmias, seizures, hypotension, or coma). **Methylene blue** in a dose of 1 to 2 mg/kg of body weight given intravenously over 5 min as a 1% solution is the antidote, and should be administered after consultation with a toxicologist or physician familiar with its use. Peripheral cyanosis should respond to specific therapy for the underlying condition.

For further reading in *Emergency Medicine: A Comprehensive Study Guide,* 5th ed., see Chap. 58, "Respiratory Distress," by J. Stephan Stapczynski.

---

31 | Bronchitis and Pneumonia

David F. M. Brown

PNEUMONIA

Pneumonia is the sixth leading cause of death in the United States. Bacterial causes are the most common. Pneumococcus is responsible for up to 90 percent of all bacterial pneumonia, with *Escherichia coli, Pseudomonas aeruginosa, Klebsiella pneumoniae, Staphylococcus aureus, Haemophilus influenzae,* and group A streptococci accounting for most of the rest. *Legionella* species and anaerobes are less frequent causes of bacterial pneumonia, with the latter primarily the result of aspiration. Respiratory viruses, *Mycoplasma,* and *Chlamydia* account for the bulk of atypical pneumonia, which accounts for a third or more of all cases of pneumonia. Patients with chronic diseases, such as congestive heart failure, cancer, bronchiectasis, chronic obstructive pulmonary disease (COPD), diabetes, sickle-cell anemia, AIDS, and other immunodeficiencies, are at greater risk for pneumonia, as are smokers and postsplenectomy patients. Aspiration pneumonia occurs more frequently in alcoholics and patients with seizures, stroke, or other neuromuscular diseases. *Pneumocystis* pneumonia is a common complication of HIV infection and is discussed in Chap. 88.

Clinical Features

Patients with bacterial pneumonia generally present with some combination of fever, dyspnea, cough, pleuritic chest pain, and sputum production (Table 31-1). Pneumococcus classically presents abruptly with fever, rigors, and rusty brown sputum; *H. influenzae* is more common in smokers and those at the extremes of age. *S. aureus* frequently follows a viral respiratory illness, especially influenza and measles. Pneumonia due to *Legionella* is spread via airborne, aerosolized water droplets rather than by person-to-person contact. This form of pneumonia presents as do *Mycoplasma, Chlamydia,* and viral pneumonia, with fever, chills, malaise, dyspnea, and a nonproductive cough. *Legionella* also commonly causes gastrointestinal symptoms of anorexia, nausea, vomiting, and diarrhea. Mental status changes may also be present.

Physical findings of pneumonia vary with the offending organism and the type of pneumonia each causes, although most are associated with some degree of tachypnea and tachycardia. Lobar pneumonias, such as those caused by pneumococcus and *Klebsiella,* exhibit signs of consolidation, including bronchial breath sounds, egophony, increased tactile and vocal fremitus, and dullness to percussion. A pleural friction rub and cyanosis may be present. Bronchopneumonias, such as those caused by *H. influenzae,* reveal rales and rhonchi on examination without signs of consolidation. A parapneumonic pleural effusion may occur in either setting; empyemas are most common with *S.*

TABLE 31-1 Characteristics of Bacterial Pneumonia

Organism	Symptoms	Sputum	Chest X-ray	Therapy
Streptococcus pneumoniae	Sudden onset, fever, rigors, pleuritic chest pain, productive cough, dyspnea	Rust-colored; gram-positive; encapsulated diplococci	Lobar, occasionally patchy, occasional pleural effusion	Penicillin V 500 mg PO qid for 10 d or erythromycin 500 mg PO qid for 10 d or aqueous penicillin G 10–20/d IV q 4–6 h or ceftriaxone 1 g IV qd
Group A streptococci	Abrupt onset, fever, chills, productive cough, pleuritic chest pain	Purulent, bloody; gram-positive cocci in chains and pairs	Patchy, multilobar large pleural effusion	See above
Haemophilus influenzae	Gradual onset, fever, dyspnea, pleuritic chest pain; especially in elderly and COPD	Short, tiny, gram-negative encapsulated coccobacilli	Patchy, frequently basilar, occasional pleural effusion	Ceftriaxone 1 g IV qd or cefuroxime 0.75–1.5 g IV q 8 h or amoxacillin clavulanate 875 mg PO bid for 10 d
Klebsiella pneumoniae	Sudden onset, rigors, dyspnea, chest pain, bloody sputum; especially in alcoholics or nursing home patients	Brown "currant jelly"; thick, short, plump, gram-negative encapsulated paired coccobacilli	Upper lobes, bulging fissure sign, abscess formation	Cefazolin 0.5–1.0 g q 8 h IV or gentamicin 3–5 mg/kg/d divided q 8 h IV
Staphylococcus aureus	Gradual onset of productive cough, fever, dyspnea, especially just after viral illness	Purulent; gram-positive cocci in clusters	Patchy, multilobar; empyema, lung abscess	Oxacillin 8–12 g/d IV or vancomycin 500 mg IV q 6 h

Organism	Clinical features	Sputum	Radiographic	Treatment
Legionella pneumophila	Fever, chills, headache, malaise, dry cough, dyspnea, anorexia, diarrhea, nausea, vomiting	Few neutrophils and no predominant bacterial species	Multiple patchy nonsegmented infiltrates, progresses to consolidation, occasional cavitation and pleural effusion	Erythromycin 1 g IV q 6 h ± rifampin 600 mg PO qd
Pseudomonas aeruginosa	Recently hospitalized, debilitated, or immunocompromised patient with fever, dyspnea, cough	Gram-negative coccobacilli	Patchy with frequent abscess formation	Tobramycin 3 mg/kg divided q 8 h IV and either piperacillin 100 mg/kg divided q 6 h IV or ceftazidime 50 mg/kg divided q 8 h IV
Chlamydia pneumoniae	Gradual onset, fever, dry cough, wheezing, occasionally sinus symptoms	Few neutrophils, organisms not visible	Patchy subsegmental infiltrates	Erythromycin 500 mg PO qid for 10 d or azithromycin 500 mg on day 1, then 250 mg qd for 4 more days or clarithromycin 500 mg PO bid for 10 d
Mycoplasma pneumoniae	Upper and lower respiratory tract symptoms, nonproductive cough, bullous myringitis, headache, malaise, fever	Few neutrophils, organisms not visible	Interstitial infiltrates, (reticulonodular pattern), patchy densities, occasional consolidation	Same as for *Chlamydia pneumoniae* above
Anaerobic organisms	Gradual onset, putrid sputum, especially in alcoholics	Purulent; multiple neutrophils and mixed organisms	Consolidation of dependent portion of lung; abscess formation	Clindamycin 450–900 mg IV q 8 h or ticarcillin-clavulanate 3.1 g IV q 6 h

aureus, Klebsiella, and anaerobic infections. *Legionella,* which begins with findings of patchy bronchopneumonia and progresses to signs of frank consolidation, has other common signs, including a relative bradycardia and confusion. Interstitial pneumonias, such as those caused by viruses, *Mycoplasma,* and *Chlamydia,* may exhibit fine rales, rhonchi, or normal breath sounds. Bullous myringitis, when present in this setting, is pathognomonic for *Mycoplasma* infection.

Clinical features of aspiration pneumonitis depend on the volume and pH of the aspirate, the presence of particulate matter in the aspirate, and bacterial contamination. Although acid aspiration results in the rapid onset of symptoms of tachypnea, tachycardia, and cyanosis, and often progresses to frank pulmonary failure, most other cases of aspiration pneumonia progress more insidiously. Physical signs develop over hours and include rales, rhonchi, wheezing, and copious frothy or blood sputum. The right lower lobe is most commonly involved due to the anatomy of the tracheobronchial tree and to gravity.

Diagnosis and Differential

The differential diagnosis includes acute tracheobronchitis; pulmonary embolus or infarction; exacerbation of COPD; pulmonary vasculitides, including Goodpastures's disease and Wegener's granulomatosis; bronchiolitis obliterans; and endocarditis. The diagnosis of pneumonia is made on the presenting signs and symptoms, examination of the sputum, and chest radiograph (see Table 31-1). Other tests include a white blood cell count with differential count, pulse oximetric analysis, blood cultures, and pleural fluid examination. Arterial blood gas analysis may be performed in ill-appearing patients. If *Legionella* is being considered, serum chemistry studies and liver function tests should be performed, as hyponatremia, hypophosphatemia, and elevated liver enzyme levels are commonly found. Also, when appropriate, urine should be tested for *Legionella* antigen, and serologic testing for *Mycoplasma* can be performed, although these tests will have no impact on the emergency management of the patient. Results of bedside cold agglutinin tests may be positive in cases of *Mycoplasma* but are nonspecific.

Emergency Department Care and Disposition

The emergency department treatment and disposition of pneumonia depends primarily on the severity of the clinical presentation and radiographic findings. Sputum Gram's stain results are also useful.

1. Oxygen should be administered as needed, and antibiotic treatment should be initiated.

2. Therapies directed against specific organisms are listed in Table 31-1, although empiric antibiotic coverage is generally recommended unless the clinical features and sputum Gram's stain strongly suggest a specific cause.

3. For outpatient management in otherwise healthy patients under 60 years old, **erythromycin** 500 mg daily for 10 to 14 days is an excellent choice for empiric therapy. **Clarithromycin** 500 mg twice a day for 10 days and **azithromycin** 500 mg on day 1 followed by 250 mg daily for 4 additional days are more expensive alternatives with fewer side effects and better compliance. Newer fluoroquinolones, such as **levofloxacin** 500 mg daily for 10 to 14 days, are also highly effective but are expensive and restricted to patients over 18 years of age.

4. For outpatient management of patients over 60 years old or those with comorbid diseases, **levofloxacin** is a good choice as a single agent. Otherwise, **azithromycin** *or* **clarithromycin** in combination with either **cefuroxime** 500 mg orally (PO) daily for 10 days or **amoxicillin-clavulanate** 875 mg PO twice a day for 10 days are excellent dual drug regimens.

5. Close follow-up is necessary to monitor response to therapy.

6. Hospital admission should be reserved for patients at the extremes of life, pregnant women, and those with clinical signs of toxicity (i.e., tachycardia, tachypnea, hypoxemia, hypotension, and volume depletion) or serious comorbid conditions (e.g., renal failure, diabetes, or cardiac disease).

7. Patients requiring admission generally also receive empiric antibiotic therapy. Recommended treatments include **erythromycin** 500 mg intravenously (IV) every 6 h, **ceftriaxone** 1 to 2 g IV daily, or **levofloxacin** 500 mg IV daily.

8. Patients at high risk for gram-negative pneumonia or *Legionalla* (e.g., alcoholics, diabetics, and institutionalized or intubated patients) should be treated with either **levofloxacin** as monotherapy or with a combination of a microlide such as **erythromycin** 1 g IV every 6 h and either **ampicillin-sulbactam** 3 g IV every 6 h or **ceftriaxone** 1 to 2 g IV daily.

9. If *Pseudomonas* is suspected, double coverage with an antipseudomonal penicillin (e.g., ticarcillin) or cephalosporin (e.g., ceftazidime) and either an antipseudomonal aminoglycoside (e.g., tobramycin) or a fluoroquinolone (e.g., ciprofloxacin) is recommended.

10. Local antibiotic sensitives and resistance patterns, as well as local standards of care, should help determine final antibiotic selection.

11. Aspiration pneumonitides require a different therapeutic approach. Witnessed aspirations should be treated with immediate tracheal suctioning, and the pH of the aspirate should be ascertained. Bronchoscopy is indicated for the removal of large particles and for further clearing of the airways. Irrigation of the tracheobronchial tree with neutral or alkaline solutions is contraindicated, since it is of no proven benefit and may promote the spread of the aspirate deeper into the terminal airways. Patients requiring intubation should also be treated with positive end-expiratory pressure. Oxygen should be administered, but steroids and prophylactic antibiotics are of no value and should be withheld. For patients at risk of aspiration who present with signs and symptoms of infection, antibiotics are indicated. Appropriate choices include **clindamycin** 450 to 900 mg IV every 8 h and **ticarcillin-clavulanate** 3.1 mg IV every 6 h.

12. Failure of outpatient therapy generally requires hospital admission and broader-spectrum intravenous antibiotics. Patients with hypoxemia desite oxygen therapy or those with impending respiratory failure should be treated with endotracheal intubation and mechanical ventilation. This will improve oxygen delivery to the alveoli and facilitate pulmonary toilet.

BRONCHITIS

Acute bronchitis is an infection of the conducting airways of the lung. Most cases are caused by viruses. Diagnosis is made in the setting of an acute cough (usually productive), normal blood oxygenation, and no evidence of pneumonia, sinusitis, or chronic lung disease. A chest radiograph is not required in patients who appear nontoxic. Wheezing is frequently encountered and should be treated with bronchodilators. Otherwise, supportive treatment is the rule. Most cases are self-limited and do not require antibiotic therapy. Full recovery may take as long as 3 to 4 weeks.

For further reading in *Emergency Medicine: A Comprehensive Study Guide,* 5th ed., see Chap. 59, "Bronchitis and Pneumonia," by Donald A. Moffa, Jr., and Charles L. Emerman; Chap. 60, "Aspiration Pneumonia, Lung Abscess, and Pleural Empyema," by Eric Anderson and Maxime Alix Gilles.

32   Tuberculosis

              Amy J. Behrman

The incidence of tuberculosis (TB) rose sharply in the United States between 1984 and 1992, driven by factors including rising rates of incarceration, human immunodeficiency virus (HIV) infection, drug-resistant TB strains, and immigration from areas with endemic TB. Stronger TB control programs targeting high-risk groups have reversed this trend; since 1993, TB case rates have fallen steadily. However, TB remains an important public health problem. Patients with undiagnosed TB frequently present to emergency department (ED) for evaluation and care.

CLINICAL FEATURES

Primary TB

Primary TB infection is usually asymptomatic and noncontagious, presenting most frequently with only a new positive reaction to TB skin testing. Some patients may, however, present with active pneumonitis or extra pulmonary disease. Immunocompromised patients are much more likely to develop rapidly progressive primary infections.

Reactivation TB

The lifetime reactivation rate after primary TB infection is 5 to 10 percent. Rates are higher in the very young, the elderly, those with recent primary infection, those with major chronic diseases, and those with compromised immune systems. Most patients present subacutely with fever, cough, weight loss, fatigue, and night sweats.

Most patients with active TB have pulmonary involvement characterized by constitutional symptoms and (usually productive) cough. Hemoptysis, pleuritic chest pain, and dyspnea may develop. Rales and rhonchi may be found, but the pulmonary examination is usually nondiagnostic. Extra pulmonary TB develops in up to 15 percent of cases. Lymphadenitis, with painless enlargement and possible draining sinuses, is the most common example. Pleural effusion may occur when a peripheral parenchymal focus or local lymph node ruptures. Pericarditis, with typical symptoms, may develop by extension of infection from local lymph nodes or pleura. TB peritonitis usually presents insidiously after extension from local lymph nodes. TB meningitis may follow hematogenous spread, presenting with fever, headache, meningeal signs, and/or cranial nerve deficits. The course is often more acute in children. Miliary TB is a multisystem disease caused by massive hematogenous dissemination. It is most common in immunocompromised hosts and children. Symptoms and findings may include fever, cough, weight loss, adenopathy, hepatosplenomegaly, and cytopenias. Extra pulmonary TB may also involve bone, joints, skin, kidneys, and adrenals.

HIV and TB

Immunocompromised patients and HIV patients, in particular, are extremely susceptible to TB and far more likely to develop active infections with atypical presentations. TB must be considered in the evaluation of any HIV patient with pulmonary findings. Disseminated extra pulmonary TB is also far more common in HIV patients and should be considered in the evaluation of nonpulmonary complaints as well.

Drug-Resistant TB

Prior partially treated TB is the major risk factor for drug-resistant TB. It should be considered when TB is diagnosed, especially among those with suboptimal prior care such as immigrants from endemic areas, prisoners, homeless persons, and drug users. Multidrug-resistant TB (MDR TB) is more common in HIV patients than the general population and has a high fatality rate in this group.

DIAGNOSIS AND DIFFERENTIAL

Consider the diagnosis of TB in any patient with respiratory systemic complaints to facilitate early diagnosis, protect hospital staff, and make appropriate dispositions.

Radiology

Chest radiographs (CXRs) are the most useful diagnostic tools for active TB in the ED. Classic findings in active primary TB are parenchymal infiltrates with or without adenopathy. Lesions may calcify. Reactivation TB typically presents with lesions in the upper lobes or superior segments of the lower lobes. Cavitation, calcification, scarring, atelectasis, and effusions may be seen. Miliary TB may cause diffuse nodular infiltrates. TB can present with a wide range of CXR abnormalities. Patients coinfected with HIV and TB are particularly likely to present atypical or normal CXRs.

Microbiology

Acid-fast staining of sputum can detect mycobacteria in 60 percent of patients with pulmonary TB. This test can be performed in the ED or hospital lab. Atypical mycobacteria will yield false positives; many patients will have false negatives on a single sputum sample. Microscopy of nonsputum samples (e.g., pleural fluid and CSF) is less sensitive. Definitive cultures generally take weeks, but new genetic tests employing DNA probes or polymerase chain reaction technology can confirm the diagnosis in days or hours.

Skin Testing

Intradermal skin testing with purified protein derivative (PPD) identifies most patients with prior or active TB infection. Results are read 48 to 72 h after placement, limiting the usefulness of this test for ED patients. (See full textbook for PPD skin test interpretation criteria.) All PPD reactors should be evaluated for active disease and possible preventive therapy. Patients with HIV or other immunosuppressive conditions and patients with disseminated TB may be anergic.

EMERGENCY DEPARTMENT CARE AND DISPOSITION

1. *Treatment.* Successful treatment of active TB requires a combination of antimicrobials for extended time periods. Treatment is begun with at least 4 drugs until laboratory tests of cultures can rule out drug resistance. Initial therapy usually includes isoniazid (INH), rifampin, pyrazinamide, and either streptomycin or ethambutol for 2 months. At least 2 drugs (usually INH and rifampin) are continued for 4 more months. Medications can be tailored to culture and sensitivity results. Patients with immune compromise or MDR TB may require more drugs for longer periods. Daily and intermittent regimens are available. Some patients require directly observed therapy (DOT) to ensure compliance. Table 32-1 summarizes usual initial daily drug doses and side effects. (See *Emergency Medicine: A Comprehensive Study Guide,* 5th ed., for more information.) Persons with positive PPDs and no active TB disease should be evaluated for prophylactic treatment with INH to prevent reactivation TB.
2. *Outpatient Treatment.* Patients with active TB who are discharged from the ED must have documented immediate referral to a physician or Public Health Department for long-term treatment. Patients should be educated about home isolation, follow-up, and screening of household contacts.

TABLE 32-1 Dosages and Common Side Effects of Some Drugs Used in TB

Drug	Daily dose (max.)	Potential side effects
INH	Adult: 5 mg/kg (300 mg) Child: 10–20 mg/kg (300 mg) Route: PO	Hepatitis, neuritis, abdominal pain, acidosis, hypersensitivity drug interactions
Rifampin	Adult: 10 mg/kg (600 mg) Child: 10–20 mg/kg (600 mg) Route: PO	Hepatitis, thrombocytopenia, GI disturbance, fever, drug interactions
Pyrazinamide	Adult: 15–30 mg/kg (2 g) Child: same Route: PO	Hepatitis, rash, arthralgia, GI disturbance, hyperuricemia
Ethambutol	Adult: 15–25 mg/kg (2.5 g) Child: same Route: PO	Optic neuritis, headache, peripheral neuropathy, GI disturbance
Streptomycin	Adult: 15 mg/kg (1 g) Child: 20–30 mg/kg (1 g) Route: IM	8th cranial neuropathy, rash, renal failure, proteinuria
Ciprofloxacin	Adult: 750 mg bid Child: contraindicated Route: PO	Arthropathy, GI disturbance, CNS disturbance

3. *Admission.* Admission is indicated for clinical instability, diagnostic uncertainty (such as a febrile HIV patient with pulmonary infiltrates), unreliable outpatient follow-up or compliance, and active known MDR TB. Admission to respiratory or "droplet" isolation is mandatory.
4. *ED Infection Control.* ED staff should be trained to identify patients at risk for active TB as early as possible in their ED and prehosptial course. Patients with suspected TB should be masked or placed in respiratory isolation rooms. They should be transported wearing masks and admitted to respiratory isolation areas. Staff caring directly for patients with suspected TB should wear OSHA-approved respirators and masks. Engineering controls in the ED can minimize transmission from undiagnosed

cases. ED staff should receive regular PPD skin testing to detect new primary infections, rule out active disease, and consider INH prophylaxis.

For further reading in *Emergency Medicine: A Comprehensive Study Guide,* 5th ed., see Chap. 61, "Tuberculosis," by Janet M. Poponick and Joel Moll.

---

33 | Pneumothorax
Gary D. Wright

Pneumothorax is defined as an abnormal collection of air between the visceral and parietal pleura. Most commonly, the origin will be secondary to penetrating or blunt trauma, however, spontaneous pneumothorax is well recognized. This abnormal collection of air in the pleural space may result in malfunction of the thoracic pump mechanism, leading to hemodynamic and pulmonary compromise. Tension pneumothorax is caused by accumulation of air under pressure in the pleural space; this is a true medical emergency, which requires immediate intervention. Spontaneous pneumothorax can occur without any identified source of trauma. When this occurs in patients with no known lung disease, it is called *spontaneous pneumothorax*. In patients with underlying lung disease such as chronic obstructive pulmonary disease (COPD) and emphysema, it is defined as a secondary pneumothorax. Traumatic pneumothorax is very common and occurs secondary to blunt and penetrating trauma. Iatrogenic origin from barotrauma and invasive procedures is a common problem that must be considered when performing procedures. Pneumothorax is the most commonly described significant complication of subclavian vein catheterization. Postprocedure chest x-rays should be routinely obtained in these patients. Positive pressure ventilation can cause barotrauma to the alveoli and lead to pneumothorax. This condition should always be considered in the patient who deteriorates while on mechanical ventilation. Inappropriate placement of NG or feeding tubes has also been described as a source of pneumothorax. Careful evaluation of placement of these devices is critical to avoid complications.

CLINICAL FEATURES

Common symptoms of pneumothorax are chest pain and dyspnea. The pain is most commonly described on the side of the pneumothorax and is pleuritic in nature. Dyspnea, tachypnea, and tachycardia may be present depending upon the amount of air accumulated and the amount of physiologic impairment. The physical examination may show decreased breath sounds and hyperesonance on percussion over the affected side. Other physical findings include subcutaneous emphysema and, if tension is present, tracheal deviation, jugulovenous distention, hypotension, and cyanosis.

DIAGNOSIS AND DIFFERENTIAL

In stable patients, a chest x-ray confirms the diagnosis of pneumothorax. If tension pneumothorax is suspected, immediate treatment with needle thoracostomy is indicated. Expiratory lung films have not been shown to be any more effective at diagnosing pneumothorax than inspiratory films and do not allow for as adequate evaluation to the lung parenchyma. Chest computed tomography (CT) is very sensitive at diagnosing pneumothorax. Differential diagnosis of suspected pneumothorax includes the wide differential associated with chest pain. Most notably one should consider costochondritis, esophageal origin, myocardial infarction or ischemia, pericarditis, pleurisy, pneumonia, and pulmonary embolus.

EMERGENCY DEPARTMENT CARE AND DISPOSITION

The initial treatment of pneumothorax involves the determination of stability of the patient. Considerations for treatment must be individualized based on the origin and degree of stability.

1. If tension pneumothorax is suspected, immediate needle thoracostomy, followed by tube thoracostomy is indicated. X-rays should not be obtained before treatment.
2. If the patient is relatively asymptomatic with a small spontaneous pneumothorax, inpatient or outpatient observation without intervention may be appropriate. Pleural space air is gradually

reabsorbed; supplemental oxygen increases the rate of reabsorption.

3. Tube thoracostomy is indicated in patients with collapse of the lung, severe underlying pulmonary disease, significant dyspnea, unsuccessful aspiration, or where access to the patient may be difficult, such as helicopter transport. Consideration of the source of the injury should be used to guide selection of the tube size. In patients with a history of penetrating trauma from gunshots and stabs, a large bore tube should be considered, enabling adequate flow of suspected hemothorax.

If the pneumothorax is increasing in size, or if general anesthesia is going to be performed, tube thoracostomy should be performed. Simple catheter aspiration may be performed in the uncomplicated spontaneous pneumothorax. Immediate postprocedure x-ray should be obtained to confirm success of aspiration. Patients with full expansion of the lung on a 6 h postprocedure x-ray may be discharged. Appropriate discharge instructions are crucial. Rapid reexpansion of the collapsed lung has been shown to be associated with pulmonary edema. Close monitoring of these patients is prudent.

For further reading in *Emergency Medicine: A Comprehensive Study Guide,* see Chap. 62, "Spontaneous and Iatrogenic Pneumothorax," by William Franklin Young, Jr., and Roger Loyd Humphries.

---

34 | Hemoptysis

David F. M. Brown

Hemoptysis is the expectoration of blood from the bronchopulmonary tree. Massive hemoptysis is defined as greater than 600 mL per 24 h or greater than 100 mL/d for 3 to 7 d and requires prompt intervention to prevent asphyxiation from impaired gas exchange.

Minor hemoptysis is the production of smaller quantities of blood, often mixed with mucus.

CLINICAL FEATURES

Hemoptysis may be the presenting symptom for a variety of conditions. A history of underlying lung disease should be sought, as well as any history of tobacco use. The acute onset of fever, cough, and bloody sputum suggests pneumonia or bronchitis, whereas a more indolent productive cough indicates bronchitis or bronchiectasis. Dyspnea and pleuritic chest pain are hallmarks of pulmonary embolism. Fever, night sweats, and weight loss may reflect tuberculosis (TB) or bronchogenic carcinoma. Chronic dyspnea and minor hemoptysis may represent mitral stenosis or alveolar hemorrhage syndromes, with or without renal disease. The physical examination is aimed at assessing the severity of hemoptysis and the underlying disease process but is unreliable in localizing the site of bleeding. Common signs include fever and tachypnea. Hypotension is uncommon except in massive hemoptysis. The cardiac examination may reveal a diastolic rumble of mitral stenosis or a pronounced P2 suggesting pulmonary embolus. Pulmonary examination may reveal rales, wheezes, or focal consolidation. More commonly, however, the heart and lung examinations are normal. The oral and nasal cavities should be carefully inspected to rule out an extra pulmonary source of bleeding.

DIAGNOSIS AND DIFFERENTIAL

A careful history and physical, as described earlier, will generally suggest a diagnosis. Pulse oximetry and a chest x-ray are the most important tests. PA and lateral projections should be performed except in the unstable patient. Depending on the clinical presentation, other supplemental tests may include hemoglobin/hematocrit levels, platelet count, coagulation studies, arterial blood gas (ABG) analysis, urinalysis, and electrocardiogram (ECG). Less urgently, a PPD can be placed and sputum can be sent for gram stain, AFB smear, and appropriate cultures. The differential diagnosis includes infection (bronchitis, bronchiectasis, bacterial pneumonia, TB, fungal pneumonia, and lung abscess), neoplasms (bronchogenic carcinoma, and bronchial adenoma), cardiogenisis (mitral stenosis and LV failure), trauma and foreign body aspiration, pulmonary embolism, primary pulmonary hypertension, pulmonary vasculitis, and bleeding diathesis. No definitive diagnosis is made in up to 25 percent of cases.

EMERGENCY DEPARTMENT CARE AND DISPOSITION

The treatment of hemoptysis in the ED depends on its severity and persistence. Initial management should focus on controlling the ABCs. Cardiac and pulse oximetry monitors along with noninvasive blood pressure (BP) machines should be utilized, and large-bore intravenous lines should be placed.

1. Supplemental oxygen should be administered to keep O_2 saturation above 95%.
2. IV crystalloid should be administered initially for hypotension.
3. Blood should be typed and cross-matched; packed red blood cells should be transfused as needed.
4. Fresh frozen plasma (2 U) should be given to patients with coagulopathies; platelets should be administered to those with thrombocytopenia.
5. Patients with ongoing massive hemoptysis should be placed in the decubitus position with the bleeding lung down to minimize spilling of blood into the contralateral lung.
6. Cough suppression with **codeine** (15 to 30 mg) or other opioids is indicated.
7. For persistent hemoptysis and worsening respiratory status, endotracheal intubation should be performed with a large (8.0 mm) tube. This will allow for better suctioning and permits the passage of a flexible bronchoscope.
8. Indications for admission—frequently to the ICU—include massive hemoptysis *or* minor hemoptysis whose underlying cause carries a high risk of proximate massive bleeding. Some underlying conditions may warrant admission regardless. All admissions should include consultation with a pulmonologist or a thoracic surgeon for help with decisions regarding bronchoscopy, computed tomography (CT) scanning, or angiography for bronchial artery embolization. If the appropriate specialists are unavailable, the patient should be transferred after stabilization.
9. Patients who are discharged should be treated for several days with cough suppressants (i.e., **codeine** 15 to 30 mg q 4–6 h), inhaled β-agonist bronchodilators and, if an infectious etiology is suspected, appropriate antibiotics. Close follow-up is warranted.

For further reading in *Emergency Medicine: A Comprehensive Study Guide,* 5th ed., see Chap. 63, "Hemoptysis," by William Franklin Young, Jr., and Michael W. Stava.

35 | Asthma and Chronic Obstructive Pulmonary Disease

Frantz R. Melio

Asthma is a common chronic affliction with wide clinical variability. Although most patients have mild disease, asthma can be rapidly fatal. Patients with chronic obstructive pulmonary disease (COPD) often present in distress, expending tremendous effort to combat hypoxia. Uncomplicated medical or surgical disease will become more serious or life-threatening as the impact of COPD is unmasked.

Clinical Features

Asthma is reversible airway obstruction associated with hyperresponsiveness of the tracheobronchial tree. Features include bronchospasm, which can be reversed within minutes, and, with prolonged attacks, mucous plugging and inflammatory changes, which do not resolve for days to weeks. Patients with attacks lasting more than several days, steroid-dependent patients, and those with prior attacks requiring intubation are at higher risk for respiratory failure with hypoxia and hypercapnia.

The most common cause of COPD is cigarette smoking. Other causes include environmental toxins, genetic aberrations, and sustained bronchospastic airflow obstruction. There are two dominant clinical forms of COPD: (1) pulmonary emphysema, characterized by abnormal, permanent enlargement and destruction of the air spaces distal to the terminal bronchioles; and (2) chronic bronchitis, a condition of excess mucus secretion in the bronchial tree with a chronic productive cough occurring on most days for at least 3 months in the year for at least 2 consecutive years. Elements of both forms are often present, although one predominates. Airway resistance, especially to expiration, is a fundamental feature of either condition. Airflow obstruction is generally progressive, may be accompanied by airway hyperactivity, and may be partially reversible. Hypoxemia and hypercapnia result from ventilation-perfusion mismatches and alveolar hypoventilation. Pulmonary arterial hypertension develops, leading to right ventricular hypertrophy and cor pulmonale. Clinically, compensated patients present with exertional dyspnea, chronic productive cough (frequently with minor hemoptysis), and expiratory wheezing. Coarse crackles are heard in patients with primarily bronchitic disease. An expanded thorax, impeded diaphragmatic motion, and diminished breath sounds are noted in those with emphysema.

Acute exacerbations of asthma and COPD are usually due to increased bronchospasm, smoking, and exposure to other noxious stimuli (e.g., pollutants, cold, stress, antigens, and exercise), adverse response to medications (e.g., antihistamines, decongestants, β-blockers, NSAIDs, sulfating agents, food additives and preservatives, hypnotics, and tranquilizers), allergic reactions, and noncompliance with prescribed therapies. Respiratory infection, pneumothorax, myocardial infarction, dysrhythmias, pulmonary edema, chest trauma, metabolic disorders, and abdominal processes are triggers and complications of asthma and COPD.

Patients with exacerbations of asthma or COPD present complaining of dyspnea, chest tightness, wheezing, and cough. Physical examination reveals wheezing with prolonged expiration. Wheezing does not correlate with the degree of airflow obstruction. A "quiet chest" indicates severe airflow restriction. Patients and physicians often underestimate the severity of attacks. Patients with severe attacks may demonstrate sitting-up-and-forward posturing, pursed-lip exhalation, accessory muscle use, paradoxical respirations, and diaphoresis. Pulsus paradoxicus of 20 mmHg or more may be noted. Hypoxia is characterized by tachypnea, cyanosis, agitation, apprehension, tachycardia, and hypertension. Signs of hypercapnia include confusion, tremor, plethora, stupor, hypopnea, and apnea.

Diagnosis and Differential

ED diagnosis of asthma or COPD usually is made clinically. The clinician should attempt to determine the severity of the attack and the presence of complications. Objective measurements of airflow obstruction, such as sequential peak expiratory flow rate, have been shown to be more accurate than clinical judgment in determining the severity of the attack and the response to therapy. Laboratory examinations should be used selectively. Chest x-ray is used to diagnose complications such as pneumonia and pneumothorax. Arterial blood gas (ABG) measurements should not be obtained routinely but are more useful in evaluation of acute exacerbations of COPD. ABG values serve primarily to evaluate hypercapnia in moderate to severe attacks. Hypoxia can usually be evaluated by pulse oximetry. ABG results should be interpreted in light of the total clinical picture. Compensated hypercapnia and hypoxia are common in COPD patients; therefore, comparison with previous ABG values is helpful. Normal Pco_2 in the setting of an acute asthmatic attack is an ominous finding if the patient is doing poorly. An arterial pH below that consistent with renal compensation implies either acute hypercarbia or metabolic acidosis. Electrocardiograms are useful to identify dysrhythmias or ischemic injury. Measurements of methylxanthine levels should be obtained.

The differential diagnosis of decompensated asthma and COPD includes many of the disorders listed above as complications. In addition, interstitial lung diseases, pulmonary embolism, pulmonary neoplasia, aspirated foreign bodies, pleural effusions, and exposure to asphyxiants should be considered.

Emergency Department Care and Disposition

Although patients with COPD often have more underlying illnesses than do asthmatics, the therapy for acute bronchospasm and that for inflammation are similar. Treatment should precede history taking in acutely dyspneic patients, since patients may decompensate rapidly. These patients should be placed on a cardiac monitor and a noninvasive blood pressure device and have continuous pulse oximetry. An intravenous line should be started in patients with moderate and severe attacks. The primary goal of therapy is to correct tissue oxygenation.

1. Empiric supplemental **oxygen** should be administered. The need for supplemental oxygen in the setting of COPD must be balanced against progressive hypercarbia and suppression of hypoxic ventilatory drive. Arterial saturation should be corrected to above 90%.
2. Beta-adrenergic agonists produce prompt effects and are the drugs of choice to treat bronchospasm. Aerosolized or parenteral forms should be used in critical settings. Aerosol therapy minimizes systemic toxicity and is preferred. **Albuterol** sulfate 1.25 to 5 mg and metaproterenol 10 to 15 mg are the most β_2-specific agents. Isoetharine 2.5 to 5 mg or bitolterol mesylate 0.5 to 1.5 mg can also be delivered by nebulizer. Delivering doses in rapid succession or continuously maximizes results. Frequency of dosing depends on clinical response and signs of drug toxicity. Metered dose inhalers (MDIs) with spacer devices may be reasonable to use in less ill patients. Subcutaneous **terbutaline** sulfate (0.25 to 0.5 mL) or **epinephrine** 1:1000 (0.1 to 0.3 mL) may also be administered. Salmeterol, a long-acting β agonist indicated for maintenance therapy, should not be used for the treatment of acute exacerbations. Epinephrine should be avoided in the first trimester of pregnancy and possi-

bly in patients with underlying cardiovascular disease. β-adrenergic agonists may inhibit uterine contractions when used near term.

3. Steroids should be given immediately to patients with severe attacks as well as patients who are currently taking, or have recently taken, these drugs. Although their use is well established in asthma and severe COPD, there is a lack of supporting evidence for the use of steroids in the treatment of chronic/compensated or mild to moderate exacerbations of COPD. The optimal daily dose is the equivalent of 60 to 180 mg/d of **prednisone**, with an initial dose being the equivalent of 40 to 80 mg **prednisone**. The choice of steroid is not critical. If the patient is unable to take oral medication, intravenous (IV) **methylprednisolone** 60 to 125 mg may be used. Additional doses may be given every 4 to 6 h. Hydrocortisone should be avoided, however, because of excess mineralocorticoid effect. Inhaled steroids are extremely useful in the treatment of chronic asthma and COPD but should not be used for the treatment of acute symptoms. A 3- to 10-d course of oral steroids (**prednisone** 40 to 60 mg/d) is beneficial for discharged patients who have previously been on steroids, are high-risk patients, or were placed on steroids during their emergency department care.

4. Anticholinergics are useful adjuvants when given with other therapies. Ipratropium bromide has recently replaced nebulized atropine sulfate and glycopyrrolate as the agent of choice. Nebulized **ipratropium** (500 mg = 2.5 mL) may be administered either alone or mixed with albuterol. Ipratropium is available as a nebulized solution or as a metered-dose inhaler. A combined ipratropium and albuterol MDI is available. The effects of ipratropium peak in 1 to 2 h and last 3 to 4 h. Dosages may be repeated every 1 to 4 h. When used with β-agonist agents, effects may be additive. The use of nebulized anticholinergics has been reported to cause attacks of narrow-angle glaucoma due to topical ophthalmic absorption.

5. The role of methylxanthines in the treatment of acute asthma and COPD has been seriously challenged. See *Emergency Medicine: A Comprehensive Study Guide,* 5th ed., Chaps. 64 and 65, for administration guidelines.

6. Broad-spectrum antibiotics (trimethoprim-sulfamethoxazole DS, doxycycline, macrolides, cephalosporins, and newer fluoroquinolones) are indicated for treatment of bacterial respiratory infections. Preventive polyvalent pneumococcal and trivalent influenza vaccination may be administered to stable COPD patients.

7. While some authors have reported that 1 to 2 g of IV magnesium sulfate reduces bronchospasm, no consistent clinical benefit has been demonstrated.

Sedatives, hypnotics, and other medications that depress respiratory drive are generally contraindicated. β blockers may exacerbate bronchospasm. Antihistamines and decongestants should also be avoided, since they diminish the ability to clear respiratory secretions. Mucolytics may provoke further bronchospasm. The benefit of iodides and glyceryl guaiacolate in asthma and of doxapram in COPD is unproven. Mast cell and leukotriene modifiers have no role in the treatment of acute exacerbations of asthma or COPD. Many asthmatics respond poorly to ultrasonic nebulization and intermittent positive-pressure breathing.

Criteria for admission of patients with asthma are presented in Table 35-1. Patients with acute exacerbations of COPD are more likely to require admission. Indications for admission are presented in Table 35-2.

Several studies have demonstrated that an 80%:20% mixture of helium and oxygen (heliox) can lower airway resistance and aid in drug delivery in patients with very severe asthma exacerbation. Care must be taken with use of this therapy in oxygen-dependent patients. Ketamine has been successfully used in cases of refractory asthma. The bronchodilatory properties of ketamine make it a good choice, especially in combination with low-dose benzodiazepam for sedation of mechanically ventilated patients with bronchospasm.

TABLE 35-1 Criteria for Hospital Admission in Acute Asthma

Emergency visit within the preceding 3 days

Failure of subjective improvement following treatment

Failure of posttreatment FEV_1 to increase by > 500 mL, or absolute value < 1.6 L

Failure of posttreatment PEFR to increase more than 15% above initial value, or absolute value < 200 L/min, or PEFR $< 50\%$ predicted

Change in mental status (lethargy, agitation, exhaustion, and confusion)

Failure of hypercarbia to resolve after treatment

Presence of pneumothorax

Note: Presence of any of these conditions warrants admission to the hospital.
Abbreviations: FEV_1, forced expiratory volume; PEFR, peak expiratory flow rate.

TABLE 35-2 Criteria for Hospital Admissions in Acute Exacerbation of COPD

One or more of the following: inability to walk between rooms, to sleep or eat due to dyspnea, or to manage at home without additional resources, which are not available

Prolonged or progressive symptoms prior to ED visit

Altered mental status

Worsening hypoxia, hypercarbia, or acidosis (pH < 7.30)

High-risk comorbid conditions or complications

Unresponsive new or worsening cor pulmonale

Planned invasive procedure that may worsen pulmonary function

Respiratory muscle fatigue

In selected cooperative patients, noninvasive, positive-pressure ventilation (IPAP, CPAP, or BiPAP) may avert artificial ventilation. Assisted mechanical ventilation is indicated for inability to maintain O_2 saturation above 90% or severe hypercarbia associated with stupor, altered mental status, exhaustion, narcosis, or acidosis. Oral intubation is preferred, since larger endotracheal tubes can be used. Larger tubes facilitate suctioning, fiberoptic bronchoscopy, and ventilator weaning. Initially, high inspired oxygen concentrations may be used. A volume-cycled ventilator should always be used. Excessive tidal volumes (over 15 mL/kg ideal body weight) and air trapping (due to bronchospasm) can cause barotrauma and hypotension. Utilizing high flow rates at a reduced respiratory frequency (12 to 14 breaths/min) allows for adequate expiration. The goal of this approach, referred to as controlled mechanical hypoventilation, is to maintain adequate oxygenation with little regard for hypercarbia. Therapy should be guided by pulse oximetry and ABG results. Sedation and continued therapy for bronchospasm should continue after the patient has been placed on artificial ventilation. Close follow-up care must be arranged for discharged patients to ensure resolution of the exacerbation and to review the management plan. Despite appropriate therapy these patients have high relapse rates. Education of asthma and COPD patients prior to discharge (i.e., review of medications, inhaler techniques, use of peak flow measurements, avoidance of noxious stimuli, and need to follow-up) should be an integral part of emergency department care. (See *Emergency Medicine: A Comprehensive Study Guide,* 5th ed., Chap. 64, for discussion.)

For further reading in *Emergency Medicine: A Comprehensive Study Guide*, 5th ed., see Chap. 64, "Acute Asthma in Adults," by Rita K. Cydulka and Sorabh Khandelwal; and Chap. 65, "Chronic Obstructive Pulmonary Disease," by Rita K. Cydulka and Sorabh Khandelwal.

GASTROINTESTINAL EMERGENCIES

36	Acute Abdominal Pain
	Peggy E. Goodman

Acute abdominal pain, or nontraumatic abdominal pain in postpubescent patients lasting less than 1 week, is one of the most common and most challenging complaints to evaluate in the emergency department. It may be due to numerous etiologies, including gastrointestinal, genitourinary, cardiovascular, pulmonary, and other sources.

There are three categories of pain: poorly localized, visceral pain due to stimulation of autonomic nerve fibers; parietal pain caused by local irritation of peritoneal nerve fibers; and referred pain, which occurs at a location distant from the affected organ. Pain is then classified according to intraabdominal or extraabdominal sources. Intraabdominal sources of pain include peritonitis due to disease or injury of the abdominal or pelvic viscera; obstruction of the intestine, ureter, or biliary tree; gynecologic disorders; and vascular disorders, such as bowel infarction and aortic dissection, leakage, or rupture. Other sources of pain perceived as abdominal can be extraabdominal, metabolic, or neurogenic. Extraabdominal sources of pain include abdominal wall, thoracic, and pelvic pain. Abdominal wall pain is usually traumatic in origin. Intrathoracic disease, including pneumonia, pulmonary embolism, pneumothorax, esophageal disease, and acute myocardial ischemia, may be accompanied by vague abdominal distress, nausea, vomiting, and diaphoresis. Pelvic sources of pain, such as salpingitis, tubo-ovarian abscess, ovarian cyst torsion or rupture, abortion, and ectopic pregnancy also need to be considered in the differential diagnosis. Metabolic disorders, including diabetic ketoacidosis, sickle cell crisis, porphyria, spider and scorpion bites, heavy metal intoxication, and autoimmune disease, as well as neurogenic disorders, such as preeruptive herpes zoster and spinal disk disease, may be interpreted as abdominal pain.

Diagnosis and Differential

When evaluating a patient with abdominal pain, it is important to consider immediate life threats that might require emergency intervention. Important aspects of the patient's history include time of onset of pain; character, severity, and location of pain and its referral; aggravating and alleviating factors; and any changes in these symptoms. Cardiorespiratory symptoms, such as chest pain, dyspnea, and cough; genitourinary symptoms, such as urgency, dysuria, and vaginal discharge; and any history of trauma should be elicited. In older patients it is also important to obtain a history of myocardial infarction, other ischemic states, dysrhythmias, coagulopathies, and vasculopathies. Past medical and surgical history should be elicited, and a list of medications, particularly steroids, antibiotics, or nonsteroidal anti-inflammatory drugs (NSAIDs), should be noted. A thorough gynecologic history is indicated in female patients.

The physical examination should include the patient's general appearance. Patients with visceral pain tend to move about, whereas patients with peritonitis tend to lie still. The skin should be evaluated for pallor or jaundice. The vital signs should be inspected for signs of hypovolemia due to blood loss or dehydration. Due to medications or the physiology of aging, tachycardia may not always occur in the face of hypovolemia. A core temperature should be obtained; however, absence of fever does not rule out infection, particularly in the elderly. The abdomen should be inspected for contour, scars, peristalsis, masses, distention, and pulsation. Palpation is the most important aspect of the physical examination. The abdomen and genitals should be assessed for tenderness, guarding, masses, organomegaly, and hernias. However, retroperitoneal disorders may exhibit no "classic" abnormalities on examination. A pelvic examination is recommended in all postpubertal females. During the rectal examination, the lower pelvis should be assessed for tenderness and masses.

Elderly patients with abdominal pain present significant challenges in diagnosis and management. It can be difficult to obtain an accurate history from the patient or from care givers, and there may be delays in presentation. Elderly patients often fail to manifest the same signs and symptoms as younger patients, with decreased pain perception, and decreased febrile or muscular response to infection or inflammation. Hypotension from volume contraction, hemorrhage, or sepsis can be missed if a normally hypertensive patient appears normotensive. Comorbid diagnoses, such as cardiovascular, pulmonary, or renal disease, are more common. Older patients are generally at higher initial operative risk, so that observation is more likely if the diagnosis is unclear.

As a result, emergent surgical intervention for deterioration, such as sepsis, perforation, or rupture, has much higher complication and mortality rates than in younger patients. Conditions more common in the elderly include biliary tract disease, sigmoid volvulus, diverticulitis, acute mesenteric ischemia, and abdominal aortic aneurysm. Mesenteric ischemia should be considered in any patient over age 50 with abdominal pain out of proportion to physical findings; arteriography is the diagnostic test of choice.

Laboratory evaluation is supplementary to a careful history and physical examination. Complete blood count values can be normal in the presence of disease; however, an elevated white blood cell count should alert the clinician, and a source should be sought more diligently. Serial hematocrits may be of value in patients with acute blood loss, although it may take several hours for a change to be evident. Urinalysis may reveal hematuria in cases of renal colic or pyuria in urinary tract infection or other intraabdominal inflammation near the urinary tract. A pregnancy test should be obtained in women of childbearing age and is useful in the assessment for ectopic pregnancy. Serum amylase elevation and electrolyte abnormalities are neither specific nor sensitive diagnostic tools. An electrocardiogram should be considered, particularly in patients over 40 years old or with upper abdominal or nonspecific symptoms.

Imaging studies most useful as adjuncts to diagnosis include radiographs, ultrasound, and computed tomography (CT). Radiographs provide nonspecific assessment for calculi and calcifications, and air and fluid patterns. Their routine use is generally low yield, with low sensitivity and specificity, misleading findings, and lack of impact on management. Ultrasonography is a valuable diagnostic technique for the diagnosis of cholelithiasis, choledocholithiasis, cholecystitis, biliary duct dilatation, pancreatic masses, hydroureter, intrauterine or ectopic pregnancies, ovarian and tubal pathology, free intraperitoneal fluid, suspected appendicitis, and abdominal aortic aneurysm. They are also useful in some cases when CT is contraindicated due to dye allergy or renal insufficiency. Disadvantages include technical difficulties, including variations in the performance and interpretation of the study. CT is rapidly becoming the preferred imaging method for pancreatitis, biliary obstruction, aneurysm, appendicitis, and urolithiasis. There have been continuing improvements in scan speed and picture resolution, and reductions in the amount of radiopaque contrast material needed. Limitations include availability of equipment and rapid interpretation of studies. Barium contrast and radioisotope studies are rarely available or useful in the emergent setting and may limit the ability to perform other, more definitive tests.

Emergency Department Care and Disposition

Resuscitative and stabilizing measures should be instituted as appropriate. Unstable patients should be diagnosed clinically, with immediate intervention and surgical consultation.

1. During the initial evaluation the patient should have nothing by mouth. Consider intravenous hydration with normal saline or **lactated Ringer's** solution.

2. Upon completion of a thorough history and physical examination, the judicious use of analgesics is appropriate but still controversial. Judicious use of **opiates** may decrease guarding and improve localization of abdominal pain, and, if necessary, the effects can be reversed by naloxone. NSAIDs may be of use in patients with renal colic, but their use in other conditions is controversial. NSAIDs may cause further gastrointestinal irritation and may mask diagnostic signs and symptoms by their anti-inflammatory effects. **Antiemetics**, such as intravenous prochlorperazine 5 to 10 mg, also increase the patient's comfort and facilitate assessment of the patient's signs and symptoms without increasing gastrointestinal motility. Appropriate antibiotic therapy should be initiated, depending on the suspected source of infection.

3. Surgical or obstetric-gynecologic **consultation** should be obtained for patients with suspected acute abdominal or pelvic pathology requiring immediate intervention, including, but not limited to, abdominal aortic aneurysm, intraabdominal hemorrhage, perforated viscus, intestinal obstruction or infarction, and ectopic pregnancy.

Despite of the abovementioned measures, approximately 40 percent of patients presenting to the emergency department for acute abdominal pain will receive no definite diagnosis. Indications for admission (or continued observation with serial examinations) include toxic appearance, unclear diagnosis in elderly or immunocompromised patients, inability to reasonably exclude serious etiologies, intractable pain or vomiting, altered mental status, inability to follow discharge or follow-up instructions. Many patients with nonspecific abdominal pain may be discharged safely with appropriate instructions to return immediately for increased pain, vomiting, fever, or failure of symptoms to resolve.

For further reading in *Emergency Medicine: A Comprehensive Study Guide,* 5th ed., see Chap. 68, "Acute Abdominal Pain," by E. John Gallagher; and Chap. 69, "Abdominal Pain in the Elderly," by Robert McNamara.

37 | Gastrointestinal Bleeding

Peggy E. Goodman

Gastrointestinal (GI) bleeding is a potentially life-threatening problem. Upper GI bleeds, which are more common among males and elderly patients, occur proximal to the ligament of Treitz. Causes include peptic ulcer disease, erosive gastritis, esophagitis, esophageal and gastric varices, Mallory-Weiss syndrome, and aortoenteric fistula. Lower GI bleeding occurs distal to the ligament of Treitz. The most common cause of apparent lower GI bleeding is upper GI bleeding, but true lower GI bleeding is usually caused by diverticulosis or angiodysplasia. Malignancies, polyps, gastroenteritis, inflammatory bowel disease, and hemorrhoids are other etiologies of bleeding, but rarely cause massive hemorrhage.

Clinical Features

GI bleeding can present with signs of hypovolemia or shock, such as hypotension, tachycardia, decreased pulse pressure, angina, syncope, weakness, and confusion. "Coffee-ground" emesis or hematemesis suggest a proximal lesion and hematochezia or melena suggest a distal lesion. Weight loss or changes in bowel habits are classic symptoms of malignancy, and vomiting followed by hematemesis is suggestive of a Mallory-Weiss tear. Use of glucocorticoids, nonsteroidal anti-inflammatory agents, and alcohol suggest esophagitis, gastritis, and duodenitis. History of other medication use, such as anticoagulants, should also be elicited.

Diagnosis and Differential

The patient should be evaluated for hypovolemia from other sources, and the skin should also be examined for signs of liver disease or coagulopathy, such as ecchymoses, petechiae, and purpura. Ear, nose, and throat and pulmonary examinations should be performed to rule out factitious bleeding. The abdomen should be carefully examined for tenderness, masses, ascites, and organomegaly. A rectal examination should be performed to evaluate for the presence of masses and to obtain a specimen for stool guaiac. Certain substances, such as iron or bismuth, can simulate melena; however, stool guaiac will be negative. Essential laboratory studies include cross-matching of blood products and a hematocrit, although the initial hematocrit often will not reflect the actual amount of blood loss. Coagulation studies, electrolyte levels, and liver function tests should also be obtained. Upper GI hemorrhage may result in elevated blood urea nitrogen due to absorption of hemoglobin. An electrocardiogram should be obtained to determine if there is silent ischemia secondary to decreased oxygen delivery. Routine abdominal radiographs are of limited value. Use of barium limits the ability to perform endoscopy or angiography, so it should be avoided. Angiography can be used to determine sites of bleeding and to perform embolization or infusion of vasoconstrictive agents if bleeding is brisk (> 0.5 mL/min). Technetium-labeled red blood cell scans can be used to localize bleeding sites at lower rates of bleeding. Endoscopy can be both diagnostic and therapeutic and is the recommended intervention if qualified personnel are readily available.

Emergency Department Care and Disposition

Primary Treatment

Resuscitation is the most important step in management. GI hemorrhage compromises the airway from regurgitation and aspiration of blood, and decreased oxygen delivery. Ischemia and circulatory collapse can occur due to hypovolemia, decreased oxygen delivery, and cardiac stress.

1. High-flow oxygen should be administered and airway patency assured, with consideration of endotracheal intubation.
2. Large-bore intravenous access should be obtained, with infusion of **crystalloid**.
3. If the patient is elderly, continues bleeding, or does not respond to 2 L of crystalloid infusion, **packed red blood cells** should be considered, with replacement of coagulation factors as necessary.
4. A urinary catheter should be placed to evaluate adequacy of resuscitation and tissue perfusion.
5. A nasogastric (NG) tube should be placed in all patients with significant GI bleeding to help determine the etiology. A nonbloody NG aspirate can result from intermittent bleeding, pyloric spasm, or mucosal edema. If bright red blood or blood clots are found, gentle lavage with room temperature water should be performed via a large-bore NG tube. Vasoconstrictive agents and iced solutions have no proven benefit

and overvigorous suction should be avoided to avoid mucosal trauma.

Secondary

Endoscopy is the most accurate method of diagnosing the source of a GI bleed and also provides numerous therapeutic benefits. Esophageal varices can be endoscopically treated by injection sclerotherapy or by band ligation. Other sources of GI bleeding can also have hemostasis achieved endoscopically. For lower GI bleeding, protoscopy and colonoscopy may also be used therapeutically to achieve hemostasis. Drug therapy with infusion of **somatostatin** or **octreotide** (25 to 50 μg intravenous bolus, then 25 to 50 μg/h) are effective in decreasing bleeding. Both agents work more effectively in conjunction with sclerotherapy. These agents have largely replaced vasopressin because they do not have the side effects of hypertension, arrhythmias, ischemia, and gangrene. Other drugs such as betablockers or antibiotics are useful; however, first-line drugs in cases of hemorrhage and H_2 antagonists have not been proved to be of benefit. Balloon tamponade can be used as a temporizing measure if medical therapy fails and endoscopy is not available, but it carries risks of mucosal ulceration, esophageal or gastric rupture, asphyxiation, tracheal compression, and aspiration pneumonia. Endotracheal intubation to ensure airway patency is generally recommended when balloon tamponade is performed.

Surgical consultation and intervention may be needed on an emergent basis for patients who do not respond to medical therapy or to endoscopic intervention. Patients with GI hemorrhage should be admitted to the hospital with elderly endoscopic and surgical consultation. GI bleeds have a higher morbidity if a patient has an initial hematocrit less than 30 percent, initial systolic blood pressure lower than 100 mm, bright red blood in the lavage fluid or hematemesis, history of liver disease, hemodynamic instability, repeated bleeding, coexistent acute or chronic illness, and is over 60 years old. Studies have attempted to identify a low-risk population that can safely be treated on an outpatient basis, but thus far, endoscopy has been required to identify these patients prior to discharge.

For further reading in *Emergency Medicine: A Comprehensive Study Guide,* 5th ed., see Chap. 70, "Gastrointestinal Bleeding," by David T. Overton.

38 Esophageal Emergencies
Cary C. McDonald

DYSPHAGIA

The vast majority of patients with dysphagia, defined as difficulty swallowing, will have an identifiable, organic process causing their symptoms.

Clinical Features

Transfer, or oropharyngeal, dysphagia is difficulty in initiating swallowing. Transport, or esophageal, dysphagia occurs after swallowing is initiated and is reported as a sensation of food "getting stuck." Functional or motility disorders usually cause dysphagia that is intermittent and variable. Mechanical or obstructive disease is usually progressive. Physical examination of patients with dysphagia, which is often normal, should focus on the head, neck, and neurologic examination. Signs of a previous cerebrovascular accident, muscle disease, or Parkinson's disease can be present. Cachexia and cervical or supraclavicular adenopathy can be observed in patients with esophageal cancer.

Diagnosis and Differential

Initial evaluation can include anteroposterior and lateral neck and chest radiographs. Direct laryngoscopy can be used to identify structural lesions. Oropharyngeal dysphagia is best evaluated with videoesophagography. Traditional barium swallow can be used for evaluating transport dysphagia. Manometry and esophagoscopy can also be helpful.

Structural or obstructive causes of dysphagia include neoplasm, esophageal web or stricture, Schatzki's ring, and diverticulum. Neuromuscular disorders causing dysphagia include achalasia, scleroderma, cerebrovascular accident, dermatomyositis, and polymyositis.

Emergency Department Care and Disposition

Consultation with a gastroenterologist should be made regarding choice of the best diagnostic procedure and determining the disposition based upon the patient's clinical condition and provisional diagnosis.

CHEST PAIN OF ESOPHAGEAL ORIGIN

Differentiating esophageal pain from cardiac chest pain can be difficult. The incidence of esophageal disease as the cause of chest pain in patients with normal coronary arteries has been reported as ranging from 20 to 60 percent. The more common causes include gastroesophageal reflux disease (GERD) and esophagitis.

Clinical Features

Heartburn, or pyrosis, is the most common symptom and sometimes sole manifestation of GERD and is due to local lower esophageal mucosal inflammation. The pain frequently occurs after meals and can radiate to the back, neck, or arms. Like cardiac pain, GERD pain may be squeezing or pressure-like, and include a history of onset with exertion and offset with rest. Other associated symptoms include nausea, vomiting, diaphoresis, odynophagia, dysphagia, acid regurgitation, and hypersalivation. Complications of GERD over time include esophagitis, esophageal stricture, ulceration, and Barrett's esophagitis.

Esophagitis is an inflammatory response or infection of the esophageal mucosa and can cause long periods of chest pain as well as odynophagia. In addition to GERD, multiple medications have been implicated as an inflammatory cause, including nonsteroidal anti-inflammatory drugs (NSAIDs), potassium chloride, and antibiotics. Infectious esophagitis is seen in the immunocompromised population. The most common pathogens include *Candida* species, herpes simplex, and cytomegalovirus.

Diagnosis and Differential

Pain arising from the esophagus is the most alarming esophageal symptom, since it most often mimics chest pain due to cardiac ischemia or mediastinitis. At a minimum, an electrocardiogram (ECG) and chest radiographs should be obtained in all patients with ambiguous presentations. Both cardiac and esophageal patients can have ECG ST abnormalities.

Emergency Department Care and Disposition

Any patient with cardiac risk factors and pain of unclear origin should be strongly considered for cardiologic consultation and admission. Outpatient treatment for GERD includes

1. **H$_2$ blockers** and **proton-pump inhibitors** are mainstays of therapy. Dosage is titrated for each patient. A prokinetic drug may also decrease symptoms.

2. Eliminate risk factors for the disease: NSAIDs, ethanol, caffeine, nicotine, chocolate, and fatty foods. The patient should avoid eating 3 h before bedtime and should sleep with the head of the bed elevated (30°).
3. Advanced esophagitis and other upper gastrointestinal (GI) complications are diagnosed by endoscopy.

ESOPHAGEAL PERFORATION

Clinical Features

Esophageal injury is iatrogenic in up to 75 percent of esophageal perforations. The most commonly related intraluminal procedures include endoscopy, stricture dilation, Sengstaken-Blakemore tube insertion, and palliative laser cancer treatment. Postemetic perforation (Boerhaave's syndrome) is attributed to 10 to 15 percent of perforations. Less common causes of esophageal perforation include foreign-body or caustic ingestion, penetrating or blunt trauma, and malignancy.

Symptoms include acute, severe, unrelenting, and diffuse pain in the chest, neck, and abdomen radiating to the back and shoulders. Dysphagia, dyspnea, hematemesis, and cyanosis can be present as well. If esophageal contents leak into the mediastinum, a fulminant, necrotizing mediastinitis with polymicrobic infection can ensue that can rapidly lead to shock and death. Perforation into the pleural and peritoneal spaces can have a similar course.

Diagnosis and Differential

Physical examination varies with the severity of the rupture and the elapsed time until presentation. Abdominal rigidity with fever and hypotension often occur early. Tachycardia and tachypnea are common. Subcutaneous emphysema is common in cervical esophageal perforations. Mediastinal emphysema is less commonly detected by physical or radiologic examination. Hamman's crunch can sometimes be auscultated. Pleural effusion develops in 50 percent of patients with intrathoracic perforation. The differential diagnosis includes myocardial infarction, pulmonary embolus, aortic catastrophe, peptic ulcer disease, and acute abdominal causes.

Chest radiography and water-soluble contrast esophagoscopy most often make the diagnosis. Endoscopy, computerized tomography, and thoracentesis can be useful if esophagoscopy (10 to 25 percent false-negative rate) is unrevealing in the face of high clinical suspicion.

Emergency Department Care and Disposition

Rapid, aggressive management is integral to minimizing the associated morbidity and mortality rates. The resuscitation of shock, the administration of broad-spectrum antibiotics, and emergent surgical consultation should be implemented as soon as the diagnosis is seriously entertained.

ESOPHAGEAL BLEEDING

The general approach to esophageal bleeding is similar to the approach for bleeding from other upper GI sources.

Clinical Features

Presentation is usually acute onset of upper GI bleeding, but some patients report hematochezia, melena, isolated abdominal pain, or syncope as the initial complaint.

Diagnosis and Differential

Esophageal varices develop in patients with chronic liver disease in response to portal hypertension. Patients who develop varices as a result of ethanol dependence have a higher risk of bleeding. Mallory-Weiss syndrome is arterial bleeding from longitudinal lacerations of the distal esophagus–proximal stomach, usually at the gastroesophageal junction. Less than half of patients with Mallory-Weiss tears, which are responsible for 5 to 15 percent of upper GI bleeding, report vomiting prior to hematemesis. Esophageal cancer often results in heme-positive stools but is an uncommon cause of significant GI bleeding. The differential diagnosis includes sources of bleeding distal to the esophagus.

Emergency Department Care and Disposition

Gastric lavage through a nasogastric or larger-bore gastric tube is generally accepted, and airway management should be considered. Initiate a prompt mobilization of resources, including blood products, gastroenterology consult, and an appropriate inpatient level of care. Early endoscopy can be both diagnostic and therapeutic via electrocoagulation, sclerotherapy, or laser photocoagulation. Pharmacologic treatment with vasopressin-nitroglycerin combination, somatostatin, or octreotide can be used as well. Balloon tamponade is considered a last-resort therapy when pharmacologic management has failed and endoscopy is neither feasible secondary to massive bleeding or has been ineffective. Angiographic embolization or surgical intervention remain options as well.

About 60 percent of variceal bleeding will resolve with supportive care alone. The rate of spontaneous cessation is higher for nonvariceal sources of GI bleeding. The spectrum of bleeding in Mallory-Weiss syndrome is broad, but a low incidence of surgical intervention or adverse outcome is seen.

For further reading in *Emergency Medicine: A Comprehensive Study Guide*, 5th ed., see Chap. 71, "Esophageal Emergencies," by Moss H. Mendelson.

---

39 | Swallowed Foreign Bodies

Peggy E. Goodman

Foreign-body ingestion occurs in all age groups. Most cases occur in children, who swallow coins, toys, and other small objects. Many of the remaining cases occur in edentulous adults, psychiatric patients, or prisoners. Adults generally ingest meat or bones, and psychiatric and prison inmates ingest atypical foreign bodies, such as toothbrushes, spoons, and razor blades. Objects lodge in areas of physiologic narrowing, where they can cause airway obstruction, stricture, or perforation, with infection, abscess, and fistula. Once an object has passed through the pylorus, it will generally pass without difficulty.

Clinical Features

Objects lodged in the esophagus can produce anxiety, retrosternal discomfort, retching, vomiting, dysphagia, coughing, choking, or aspiration, and the patient may be unable to swallow secretions. The adult patient can usually provide an accurate history regarding the type of foreign body and the time of its impaction. In the pediatric patient it may be necessary to rely on such clues as refusal to eat, vomiting, gagging, choking, stridor, neck or throat pain, dysphagia, and increased salivation.

Diagnosis and Differential

Physical examination includes evaluation of the entire upper airway, including the neck and subcutaneous tissues. Direct or indirect laryngoscopy should be performed; in the absence of a foreign body, findings consistent with foreign-body ingestion, particularly in the pediatric age group, consist of red throat, palatal abrasion, temperature elevation, and peritoneal signs. Radiopaque objects can be visualized on standard x-rays of the neck, chest, or abdomen, or visualized by laryngoscopy or endoscopy.

Emergency Department Care and Disposition

General Care

Aspiration of the foreign body or built-up secretions should be prevented. If necessary, a tube should be placed proximal to the foreign body to remove unswallowed fluids or secretions. Serial abdominal examinations should be performed to detect early signs of developing peritonitis secondary to perforation. The progression of the foreign body through the gastrointestinal (GI) tract can be monitored with the use of serial x-ray films or handheld metal detectors.

Food Impaction

If the patient is able to manage secretions, conservative treatment is appropriate. If the food does not pass within 12 h or the patient is unable to swallow fluids, intervention is necessary. Lower esophageal sphincter relaxation, to facilitate bolus passage, can be attempted by the administration of intravenous **glucagon** 1 mg, sublingual **nitroglycerin** 0.3 to 0.4 mg, or sublingual nifedipine 10 mg, monitoring carefully for hypotension. Endoscopy is the preferred method of bolus removal; therefore, esophagogram, which impairs visualization, should be avoided if possible. Use of proteolytic enzymes (e.g., papain) should be avoided due to risks of esophageal perforation. The majority of patients with an impacted food bolus have an esophageal lesion that will require further evaluation to avoid recurrence.

Coin Ingestion

Approximately one-third of children with a coin lodged in their esophagus will be asymptomatic. Radiographs should be performed on all children suspected of swallowing coins to determine the presence and location of the object. Coins in the esophagus lie in the frontal plane, while coins in the trachea lie in the sagittal plane. Coins usually pass spontaneously but can be removed endoscopically if lodged in the esophagus.

Button Battery Ingestion

Button battery ingestion is a true emergency because of the rapid caustic action. Esophageal burns have occurred within 4 h, with perforation within 6 h. Lithium cells entail a high incidence of adverse outcomes, and mercuric oxide cells fragment more frequently than do other cells, although heavy-metal poisoning does not appear to be a significant complication. Blood and mercury levels should be monitored if a mercury-containing cell has opened while in the GI tract. If the button battery is suspected in the esophagus, the location should be documented by radiograph, followed by emergent endoscopy. Button batteries that have passed the esophagus in an asymptomatic patient may be treated conservatively, unless the battery has not passed the pylorus after 48 h of observation. Most batteries pass through the body within 48 to 72 h. Symptomatic patients should have early surgical consultation due to risks of mucosal damage and perforation. Battery identification assistance is available from the National Button Battery Ingestion Hotline, 202-625-3333.

Ingestion of Sharp Objects

Management is controversial. Objects longer than 5 cm and wider than 2 cm rarely pass the stomach, and objects with extremely pointed edges, such as open safety pins or razor blades, may cause intestinal perforation, most commonly at the ileocecal valve. For children who have swallowed sharp objects, an initial radiograph and examination should be performed. Asymptomatic children can be managed conservatively with serial radiographs.

Cocaine Ingestion

Cocaine packet ingestion is used for drug concealment. Multiple small packets of cocaine may be contained within a condom. Conservative treatment and full-bowel irrigation have been used.

Foreign-Body Retrieval

Endoscopy is the procedure of choice for foreign-body retrieval, except for cocaine, due to risks of packet rupture. It should be performed for objects lodged in the esophagus, heavy objects, sharp objects, coins and batteries that do not pass through the pylorus within 48 h, and open batteries, and in all other symptomatic patients. Fewer than 1 percent of ingested foreign bodies require surgical treatment. Surgical intervention is the safest method of cocaine packet recovery and may be necessary in cases of GI obstruction or perforation, or when endoscopic retrieval is not successful.

For further reading in *Emergency Medicine: A Comprehensive Study Guide,* 5th ed., see Chap. 72, "Swallowed Foreign Bodies," by Wade R. Gaasch and Robert A. Barish.

---

40 | Peptic Ulcer Disease and Gastritis
| *Christian A. Tomaszewski*

Peptic ulcer disease (PUD) is a chronic affliction marked by recurrent gastroduodenal ulcerations affecting up to 10 percent of the population at any time. The two independent risk factors for PUD are nonsteroidal anti-inflammatory drug (NSAID) use and *Helicobacter pylori* infection. Associated disorders are gastritis (i.e., inflammation of the gastric mucosa) and dyspepsia (i.e., upper abdominal discomfort).

Clinical Features

PUD classically presents with burning epigastric pain, 1 to 3 h after meals, often awakening the patient at night. Pain is typically relieved by food, milk, or antacids, but then recurs hours later. Elderly patients may have less pain associated with their ulcers and instead have nausea, vomiting, anorexia, weight loss, and bleeding.

A history of frequent vomiting, weight loss, early satiety, or nausea should suggest gastric outlet obstruction. Hemodynamic instability, hematemesis, or melena all confirm hemorrhagic complications. Although not commonly bleeding, a perforation will usually present with severe pain or peritoneal signs. Sudden mid-back pain may signify pancreatitis from posterior perforation.

Diagnosis and Differential

Typically the diagnosis of PUD is based on history and examination. Patients may have very mild epigastric tenderness. A succussion splash in the presence of excessive vomiting suggests gastric outlet obstruction. Directed laboratory work, such as complete blood cell count, lipase levels and liver function tests, may confirm associated illness. Rectal exam and nasogastric aspiration may aid in diagnosing bleeding complications. In the presence of bleeding, one should consider clotting studies. Radiological studies that might be useful include an upright chest (or left lateral decubitus) to detect free air, and an ultrasound or helical CT of the abdomen to rule out cholelithiasis or aortic aneurysm.

The definitive diagnosis of PUD can only be made with an upper gastrointestinal (GI) series using barium or by direct endoscopic visualization. Such tests are usually reserved for patients with severe pain or bleeding. Because of the prevalence of infection as an etiology of PUD, most clinicians advocate testing for *H. pylori*. The easiest test in the emergency department is a rapid serological detection of IgG antibodies with sensitivity and specificity approaching 90 percent. Although the test may be useful in patients with severe or refractory symptoms, it is not a test of cure because antibodies can remain present for years.

Many disorders mimic PUD in pattern and location of pain. Pancreatitis is usually associated with worse pain and more commonly radiates to the back. Similarly, the pulsatile epigastric mass representative of an abdominal aortic aneurysm may present with back pain. With gastroesophageal reflux the patient may relate positional pain originating substernally. Clues to biliary colic include a history of fatty food intolerance (rather than relief of pain with food), typically in a middle-age obese female. In addition to cholecystitis, right upper quadrant pain may signify hepatitis. The most serious diagnosis confused with PUD is myocardial ischemia or infarction, which should be considered in any patient over 40 years or with cardiac risk factors. Other GI disorders that mimic PUD include gastroesophageal reflux disease, with burning into the chest, and gastric cancer, with chronic pain and weight loss.

Emergency Department Care and Disposition

The treatment of PUD is primarily done on an outpatient basis unless complications exist. Traditional treatment has been simply to promote healing through decreasing or neutralizing hydrochloric acid in the gut with antacids or H_2-receptor antagonists. However, actual cure of this disease requires eradication of *H. pylori* infection. Finally, any NSAID use must be discontinued to prevent further recurrence.

1. Pain can be relieved with **liquid antacids** (e.g., magnesium/ aluminum hydroxide gel), 15 mL 1 and 3 h after each meal, and at bedtime.
2. Peptic ulcer disease is most conveniently treated with H_2-receptor antagonists: **cimetidine** (may cause drug interactions), 300 mg intravenously or 800 mg orally every bedtime; **ranitidine,** 50 mg intravenously or 300 mg orally every bedtime; **famotidine,** 20 mg intravenously or 20 to 40 mg orally every bedtime; and **nizatidine,** 300 mg orally every bedtime.
3. **Sucralfate,** 1 g four times daily, heals ulcers but may interfere with absorption of other medications.
4. In cases of resistant ulcers, one can use proton pump inhibitors such as **omeprazole** (may cause drug interactions), 20 mg daily, or **lansoprazole,** 15 mg daily.
5. **NSAID avoidance** must be encouraged. The safety of the newer cyclooxygenase-2 inhibitor type drugs is now being evaluated in PUD patients nationally.
6. Patients with positive serological testing require eradication of *H. pylori* with one of several combination therapies for 14 days; e.g., (*a*) bismuth subsalicylate 2 tablets four times daily with meals and bedtime + metronidazole 500 mg with meals + tetracycline 500 mg four times daily with meals and bedtime ± omeprazole 20 mg every day; (*b*) Helidac four times daily; or (*c*) Prevpac two times daily.

Patients who demonstrate any complication of PUD should be stabilized and admitted to the hospital. For hemorrhage, this includes intravenous fluids (Ringer's lactate or normal saline) with PRBCs and FFP as dictated clinically. Gastric lavage with room temperature water will help the clinician assess the extent of bleeding and prepare the patient for diagnostic and therapeutic endoscopy (see Chap. 37, "Gastrointestinal Bleeding"). Perforation requires nasogastric suction, broad-spectrum antibiotics, and surgical consultation. Gastric outlet obstruction requires correction of fluid and electrolyte abnormalities, with referral for possible surgical correction.

Stable patients with benign examination can be discharged on antacids or H_2-receptor antagonists. They should be referred for definitive diagnosis if symptoms persist. In addition, worrisome patients with anorexia, dysphagia, anemia, or weight loss or who are elderly will require early endoscopy to rule out cancer. All patients require counseling against the use of aspirin, NSAIDs, tobacco, and alcohol. In addition, they should be told to return for worsening and confounding symptoms (e.g., vomiting, bleeding, syncope, chest pain, or fever) or lack of improvement in 24 to 48 h.

For further reading in *Emergency Medicine: A Comprehensive Study Guide,* 5th ed., see Chap. 73, "Peptic Ulcer Disease and Gastritis," by Matthew C. Gratton.

---

41 | Appendicitis

Peggy E. Goodman

Appendicitis is a relatively common disorder that affects approximately 6 percent of the population. In many cases, some or all of the "classic" signs and symptoms are absent, leading to difficulty in diagnosis. Morbidity and mortality rates are related to the time from onset of symptoms to definitive diagnosis. Complications from misdiagnosis of appendicitis include intraabdominal abscess, wound infection, adhesion formation, bowel obstruction, and infertility.

Clinical Features

Abdominal pain is the most reliable symptom in appendicitis. The visceral innervation of the inflamed appendix results in dull pain originating in the periumbilical or epigastric region with localization to the right lower quadrant as peritoneal irritation occurs. Other symptoms classically associated with appendicitis include anorexia, nausea, and vomiting, which occur after the onset of abdominal pain. Although 60 percent of patients will have some combination of these symptoms, they are by themselves neither specific nor sensitive for appendicitis. The symptoms generally increase over approximately a 24-h period and may also be accompanied by dysuria, tenesmus, or other symptoms related to irritation of the abdominal or pelvic viscera. McBurney's point is the classic location of maximal tenderness, just below the middle of a line connecting the umbilicus and the anterior superior iliac spine. Palpation of the left lower quadrant with pain referred to the right lower quadrant is referred to as Rovsing's sign. The psoas sign is elicited by placing the patient in the left lateral decubitus position and extending the right leg at the hip. The obturator sign is elicited by passively flexing the right hip and knee and internally rotating the hip. If either the psoas muscle or obturator muscle is irritated by an inflamed appendix, these maneuvers will be painful. Patients with a pelvic appendix may be most tender on rectal examination, and patients with a retrocecal appendix may have more prominent right flank pain than abdominal pain. Fever is a relatively late finding in appendicitis and rarely exceeds 39°C (102.2°F) unless rupture or other complications occur.

Diagnosis and Differential

The diagnosis of acute appendicitis is primarily clinical. Factors that increase the likelihood of appendicitis, listed in decreasing order of importance, are right lower quadrant pain, rigidity, migration of pain to the right lower quadrant, pain before vomiting, positive psoas sign, rebound tenderness, and guarding. Additional studies, such as complete blood count, urinalysis, pregnancy test, and imaging studies, may be performed if the diagnosis is unclear. Elevation of the white blood cell count is sensitive but has very low specificity and is of limited value. Urinalysis is useful to rule out other diagnoses, such as urolithiasis or urinary tract infection, but pyuria and hematuria can occur if an inflamed appendix overlies the ureter. A pregnancy test should be obtained as part of the evaluation of abdominal pain in any fertile female. The role of imaging studies in the diagnosis of appendicitis is controversial. Plain radiographs of the abdomen are often abnormal but are not specific; even if a fecalith or an ileus is noted, correlation to the patient's acute presentation is unclear. Ultrasonography has a high sensitivity but is limited in evaluating a ruptured appendix or an abnormally located (e.g., retrocecal) appendix. Computed tomography is more sensitive than ultrasound, with comparable specificity, and may provide an alternative diagnosis. Patients with atypical presentations may be observed with serial abdominal examinations in order to avoid premature surgical intervention or discharge of the patient with an uncertain diagnosis.

Certain patient populations have higher rates of misdiagnosis of appendicitis, with increased morbidity and mortality rates. Patients under the age of 6 years have a high misdiagnosis rate due to poor communication skills and the association of many nonspecific symptoms, such as lethargy, upper respiratory symptoms, and urinary symptoms. Elderly patients may have decreased perception of symptoms due to the physiology of aging, medications, and comorbid conditions. The most significant predictors of acute appendicitis in the elderly are tenderness, rigidity, pain at diagnosis, fever, and previous abdominal surgery.

Pregnant patients are at risk for misdiagnosis, since nausea and vomiting may be incorrectly attributed to the pregnancy, and appendiceal displacement by the gravid uterus may result in tenderness and pain located in the right upper quadrant. Appendicitis is the most common extrauterine surgical emergency in pregnancy, and fetal mortality rates are high if perforation and peritonitis occur. Patients with AIDS are susceptible to complications from appendicitis because of delays in diagnosis due to their immunocompromise. Computed tomography is recommended to help make the diagnosis.

Emergency Department Care and Disposition

Prior to surgery, patients should have nothing by mouth and should have intravenous (IV) access, analgesia, and institution of antibiotic therapy.

1. Narcotic analgesics, such as **morphine** 0.1 mg/kg, are preferred, since they can be reversed by naloxone if needed.
2. Antibiotics are most effective when given prior to surgery, and several antibiotic regimens have been recommended. Choices include **metronidazole** 15 mg/kg IV (up to 1 g) plus **ampicillin** 50 mg/kg IV (up to 2 g) plus **gentamicin** 1 mg/kg IV, or single-agent coverage with a second- or third-generation cephalosporin, such as **cefoxitin** 20 to 40 mg/kg IV (up to 2 g).

If no precise diagnosis exists after workup and surgical consultation, patients should not be given any specific diagnostic label. These patients may be discharged if they have appropriate medical follow-up and specific discharge instructions. They should be seen within 24 h by their primary care physician or another primary care provider to evaluate the course of their illness, should avoid strong analgesics, and should return if they develop increased pain, fever, nausea, or other signs or symptoms of illness that is worsening or is not resolving.

For further reading in *Emergency Medicine: A Comprehensive Study Guide,* 5th ed., see Chap. 74, "Appendicitis," by Denis J. FitzGerald and Arthur M. Pancioli.

42 | Intestinal Obstruction

N. Heramba Prasad

Intestinal obstruction can either be caused by mechanical factors or by the loss of normal peristalsis. The latter, known as adynamic or paralytic ileus, is more common but is usually self-limiting. Mechanical bowel obstruction is caused by various intrinsic or extrinsic factors. Commonly, mechanical small bowel obstruction (SBO) occurs from adhesions resulting from previous surgical procedures or inflammatory diseases. Incarcerated inguinal hernia is the second most common cause of SBO. Occasionally, hernias at other sites such as the umbilicus, femoral canal, or obturator foramen may cause incarceration and obstruction. Intraluminal causes such as polyps, lymphomas, and adenocarcinomas are some rare causes of SBO.

Inflammatory bowel diseases such as regional enteritis, granulomatous colitis, ulcerative colitis, and diverticulitis may also affect the intestines at various levels. Congenital causes, such as atresia and stenosis, and foreign bodies such as bezoars, worms, gallstones, and hematomas should be considered in appropriate circumstances. Fecal impaction and carcinomas are common problems causing large bowel obstruction (LBO) in the elderly. Finally, intussusception in children and volvulus in the elderly should be kept in mind. Adynamic ileus is usually due to electrolyte abnormalities, peristaltic defects, infections, or retroperitoneal injuries. The site of obstruction should be determined clinically and with x-rays, as the treatment of SBO and LBO varies.

Clinical Features

Crampy, intermittent abdominal pain is the main feature of intestinal obstruction. Vomiting, bilious in early stages and feculent in late stages, is usually present. Inability to have a bowel movement or to pass flatus is often a presenting complaint. Physical signs vary, ranging from abdominal distention, localized or general tenderness, to obvious signs of peritonitis. Localization of pain may provide clues as to the site of obstruction. Although most small intestinal disorders tend to cause periumbilical pain initially, colonic diseases localize in the hypogastric region. Active, high-pitched bowel sounds are usually heard in mechanical SBO. Organomegaly, if present, may suggest the cause for the obstruction. Presence of abdominal surgical scars, hernias, and other mass lesions should be noted. Systemic symptoms and signs will depend upon the extent of dehydration and the presence of bowel necrosis or infection. Patients may be septic and acutely dehydrated. Rectal examination may reveal fecal impaction, rectal carcinoma, or occult blood. Empty rectal ampulla may be strongly suggestive of intestinal obstruction. Presence of preexisting stool in the rectum does not rule out obstruction. Pelvic examination may reveal any gynecologic infectious or neoplastic processes.

Diagnosis and Differential

Intestinal obstruction should be suspected in any patient with abdominal pain, distention, and vomiting and especially in those with previous abdominal surgery or groin hernias. Flat and upright abdominal radiographs and an upright chest x-ray should be obtained. In severely ill patients who cannot be upright, a left lateral decubitus film will be helpful. Distended intestines in the flat plate and stepladder pattern of air-fluid levels in the upright or decubitus film will confirm the diagnosis. X-rays are helpful in localizing the site of obstruction to large or small bowel. Films should be closely examined for the presence of free air from perforation, pneumonitis, pleural effusion, presence of gallstones, and mass lesions such as enlarged viscera or phlegmon from inflammatory processes.

Laboratory tests should include a complete blood cell count; electrolyte, blood urea nitrogen (BUN) creatinine, serum amylase, and lipase levels, and a urinalysis. Liver function tests and typing and cross-matching for blood products may be required. Extreme dehydration from vomiting and fluid sequestration in the bowel may cause hematocrit and BUN to be elevated. Leukocytosis with left shift may suggest abscesses, gangrene, or peritonitis. High white blood cell counts may suggest mesenteric vascular occlusion. High urine specific gravity, ketonuria, and metabolic acidosis may indicate the severity of the obstruction. Sigmoidoscopy and barium enema may be necessary to determine site and etiology of obstruction. Some have advocated contrast enhanced computed tomography to differentiate between partial and complete obstruction. This may not be clinically indicated.

Emergency Department Care and Disposition

Once the diagnosis of mechanical obstruction is established, surgical intervention is usually necessary.

1. **Surgical consultation** should be obtained without delay. In the emergency department, the bowel should be decompressed with a nasogastric tube. Use of long intestinal tubes, generally, has no role in the treatment of SBO.

2. **Intravenous crystalloid** replacement should be initiated. The patient's response to fluid therapy should be monitored closely with the blood pressure, pulse, and urine output. Impending shock should be recognized, and the patient should be vigorously resuscitated.
3. Most patients will need broad-spectrum antibiotic coverage (such as **cefoxitin** 2 g intravenously). When the diagnosis is uncertain, or if adynamic ileus is suspected, conservative measures, such as nasogastric decompression, intravenous fluids, and observation without surgical intervention, may be appropriate.

Pseudoobstruction commonly occurs in the low-colonic region. Depression of intestinal motility from medications such as anticholinergic agents or tricyclic antidepressants will cause large amounts of gas to be retained in the large intestine. Colonoscopy will be diagnostic as well as therapeutic. Surgery is not indicated.

For further reading in *Emergency Medicine: A Comprehensive Study Guide,* 5th ed., see Chap. 75, "Intestinal Obstruction," by Salvator J. Vicario and Timothy G. Price.

---

43 | Hernia in Adults and Children

Gary Wright

A hernia is an external or internal protrusion of a body part from its normal cavity. Typically, hernia is most commonly used to describe a protrusion of bowel externally through the abdominal wall. The most common types of abdominal hernias are inguinal, femoral, umbilical, and anterior abdominal wall. Predisposing factors include family history, lack of developmental maturity, undescended testes, genitourinary abnormalities, conditions of increased abdominal pressure (e.g., ascites or pregnancy), and surgical incision sites.

Clinical Features

Most hernias are detected on routine physical examination or inadvertently by the patient. When the contents of a hernia can be easily returned to the original cavity by manipulation, it is defined as reducible; when it cannot, it is irreducible or incarcerated. Strangulation refers to vascular compromise of the incarcerated contents. Incarcerated hernias may have acute inflammation and edema, leading to bowel obstruction and/or strangulation. When not relieved, strangulation may produce gangrene. Perforation may occur as a complication of strangulation.

Symptoms other than an obvious protruding mass from the abdominal wall include localized pain, nausea, and vomiting. Children may exhibit irritability. Careful evaluation for obstruction is recommended.

Diagnosis and Differential

Physical examination is the predominate means of diagnosis. Laboratory testing has no reliable indicators; however, leukocytosis and acidosis may be indicative of ischemic bowel. An upright chest x-ray should be obtained to detect free air if perforation is suspected. Flat and upright abdominal films may be helpful in evaluation for obstruction. Additional hernias may be diagnosed by the use of computed tomography or abdominal ultrasound.

The differential diagnosis of groin masses includes hernia, testicular torsion, tumor, lymph node, and hydrocele. Lymph nodes are generally multiple, firm, and movable. Hydroceles will transilluminate. Incarcerated hernias do not transilluminate and may be tender. In children, retracted or undescended testes may be mistaken for inguinal hernias.

Emergency Department Care and Disposition

If there is a history consistent with recent incarceration, attempt to reduce the hernia. If there is a question of the duration of the incarceration, no attempt to reduce should be made. The goal is to not introduce dead bowel into the abdomen.

To reduce a hernia,

1. Place the patient in Trendelenburg position.
2. Give sedation.
3. Place a warm compress on the area.
4. Gently compress the hernia, avoiding prolonged use of excessive force.

Since inguinal hernias have a high risk of incarceration in the first year of life, infants with inguinal hernias reduced in the emergency department should generally have repair within 24 h. Umbilical hernias in children are common. Unless there is evidence of obstruction or incarceration, immediate treatment is not recommended. These patients should be followed longitudinally by their primary care provider. Referral for surgical evaluation is recommended in children over 4 years or with hernias greater than 2 cm in diameter. In adults with reducible hernias, refer for outpatient surgical evaluation and repair. Discharge instructions should include avoidance of heavy lifting and return to the emergency department if the hernia was unable to be reduced promptly. Signs of obstruction should also be discussed.

Emergent surgical intervention is the treatment of choice for incarcerated hernias that are tender and unable to be reduced or are strangulated. Patients should be monitored closely, given nothing by mouth, and have intravenous fluid replacement. In these cases, insertion of a nasogastric tube is indicated. Broad-spectrum antibiotics are indicated if there is evidence of perforation. Vigorous fluid resuscitation may be necessary in case of shock.

For further reading in *Emergency Medicine: A Comprehensive Study Guide,* 5th ed., see Chap. 76, "Hernia in Adults and Children," by Frank W. Lavoie.

---

44 | Ileitis, Colitis, and Diverticulitis

Cary C. McDonald

CROHN'S DISEASE

Crohn's disease, also described as regional enteritis, terminal ileitis, and granulomatous ileocolitis, is an idiopathic gastrointestinal (GI) tract disease. Segmental involvement of any part of the GI tract from the mouth to the anus by a nonspecific granulomatous process characterizes the disease.

Clinical Features

Abdominal pain, anorexia, diarrhea, and weight loss are present in up to 80 percent of cases, although the clinical course is variable and unpredictable. Patients commonly experience an insidious onset of recurring fever, abdominal pain, and diarrhea over several years without a definitive diagnosis. Many patients develop perianal fissures or fistulas, abscesses, or rectal prolapse. Fistulas occur between the ileum and sigmoid colon, the cecum, another ileal segment, or the skin. Abscesses are characterized as intraperitoneal, retroperitoneal, interloop, or intramesenteric. Obstruction, hemorrhage, and toxic megacolon also occur. Half of all cases of toxic megacolon, frequently associated with massive GI bleeding, occur in patients with Crohn's disease.

Up to 30 percent of patients develop extraintestinal manifestations, including arthritis, uveitis, or liver disease. Common hepatobiliary complications include gallstones, pericholangitis, and chronic active hepatitis. Some patients develop thromboembolic disease as a result of a hypercoagulable state and have a 25 percent mortality rate. Malabsorption, malnutrition, and chronic anemia develop in long-standing disease, and the incidence of GI tract malignant neoplasm is triple that of the general population.

Diagnosis and Differential

The definitive diagnosis of Crohn's disease is usually established months or years after the onset of symptoms. Common misdiagnoses are appendicitis and pelvic inflammatory disease. A careful and detailed history for previous bowel symptoms that preceded acute presentation may provide clues for correct diagnosis. The absence of true guarding or rebound is noted. Peritonitis and leukocytosis may be masked in patients taking glucocorticoids.

The differential diagnosis of Crohn's disease includes lymphoma, ileocecal amebiasis, tuberculosis, Kaposi's sarcoma, *Campylobacter* enteritis, and *Yersinia* ileocolitis. Most of these conditions are uncommon, and the latter two can be differentiated by stool cultures.

Emergency Department Care and Disposition

Initial evaluation should determine the severity of the attack and identify significant complications such as hemorrhage, obstruction, or abscess. The aim of therapy includes relief of symptoms, suppression of the inflammatory disease, avoidance or management of complications, and maintenance of hydration and nutrition. Laboratory evaluation should include a complete blood count, chemistries, and blood bank testing when indicated. Plain abdominal x-rays will identify obstruction and toxic megacolon, which may appear as a long, continuous segment of airfilled colon greater than 6 cm in diameter. Computerized tomography or ultrasound of the abdomen best identifies abscesses and fistulas. A definitive diagnosis is confirmed by an upper GI series, an air-contrast barium enema, and colonoscopy. Available pharmacologic agents are as follows:

1. **Sulfasalazine** 3 to 4 g/d is effective for mild to moderate active Crohn's disease but has multiple toxic side effects, including GI and hypersensitivity reactions. See Chap. 77, *Emergency Medicine: A Comprehensive Study Guide,* 5th ed., for alternatives.
2. Glucocorticoids (**prednisone**) 40 to 60 mg/d are reserved for severe small intestine disease and ileocolitis.
3. Immunosupressive drugs, **6-mercaptopurine** 1 to 1.5 mg/kg/d or **azathioprine** 2 mg/kg/d, are used as steroid-sparing agents, in healing fistulas, and in patients with serious surgical contraindications.
4. **Metronidazole** 10 to 20 mg/kg/d or **ciprofloxacin** 500 to 750 mg twice daily is useful in patients with perianal complications and fistulous disease.
5. Diarrhea can be controlled by **loperamide** 4 to 16 mg/d, **diphenoxylate** 5 to 20 mg/d, or **cholestyramine** 4 g one to six times daily.

Patients who should be admitted include those who demonstrate signs of fulminant colitis, peritonitis, obstruction, significant hemorrhage, severe dehydration, or electrolyte imbalance, or patients with less severe cases that fail outpatient management. Surgical intervention is indicated in patients with intestinal obstruction or hemorrhage, perforation, abscess or fistula formation, toxic megacolon, or perianal disease, and in some patients who fail medical therapy. The recurrence rate after surgery is nearly 100 percent. When patients can be discharged from the hospital, alterations in therapy should be discussed with a gastroenterologist, and close followup must be ensured. Patients are advised to contact their physician or return to the emergency department if they develop increasing abdominal pain, fever, or malaise.

ULCERATIVE COLITIS

Ulcerative colitis is an idiopathic chronic inflammatory and ulcerative disease of the colon and rectum characterized clinically most often by bloody diarrhea.

Clinical Features

Ulcerative colitis is commonly characterized by intermittent attacks of acute disease with complete remission between bouts. Patients with mild disease (60 percent of cases) may present with constipation and rectal bleeding, fewer than four bowel movements per day, no systemic symptoms, and few extraintestinal manifestations. Severe disease (15 percent of cases) is associated with more than six bowel movements per day, weight loss, fever, tachycardia, anemia, and more frequent extraintestinal manifestations, including peripheral arthritis, ankylosing spondylitis, episcleritis, uveitis, pyoderma gangrenosum, and erythema nodosum. Ninety percent of deaths from ulcerative colitis occur in patients with severe disease.

The most common complications are hemorrhagic blood loss and toxic megacolon. Abscess and fistula formation, which is much more common in patients with Crohn's disease, occurs in 20 percent of patients with ulcerative colitis. Obstruction secondary to stricture formation and acute perforation are other complications. There is a ten- to thirtyfold risk of developing colon carcinoma. Other complications are similar to those of Crohn's disease.

Diagnosis and Differential

The diagnosis of ulcerative colitis may be considered with a history of abdominal cramps, diarrhea, and mucoid stools. Laboratory findings are nonspecific and may include leukocytosis, anemia, thrombocytosis, decreased serum albumin levels, abnormal liver function test results, and negative results on stool studies for ova, parasites, and enteric pathogens. Rectal biopsy can exclude amebiasis and metaplasia. Barium enema can confirm the diagnosis and defines the extent of colonic involvement, but colonoscopy is the most sensitive method. These procedures should not be performed in moderately or severely ill patients. Rigid or fiberoptic proctosigmoidoscopic examination is abnormal in 95 percent of patients with ulcerative colitis and may be used in severely ill patients. The differential diagnosis includes infectious, ischemic, irradiation, pseudomembranous, and Crohn's colitis. When the disease is limited to the rectum, consider sexually acquired diseases, such as rectal syphilis, gonococcal proctitis, lymphogranuloma venerum, and inflammation caused by herpes simplex virus, *Entamoeba histolytica*, *Shigella*, and *Campylobacter*.

Emergency Department Care and Disposition

Patients with severe disease should be admitted for intravenous fluid replacement and electrolyte abnormality correction as well as the following treatment:

1. Patients who have not previously been treated with steroids respond best to **ACTH** 120 U/d.
2. Patients on steroids should receive **hydrocortisone** 300 mg/d, **methylprednisolone** 48 mg/d, or **prednisone** 60 mg/d.
3. Cyclosporine 4 mg/kg/d has been advocated for cases of fulminant colitis that have failed treatment with intravenous steroids.

Complete bowel rest and parenteral nutrition remain controversial in patients with fulminant disease. Patients with significant GI hemorrhage, toxic megacolon, and bowel perforation should be admitted with consultation to both a gastroenterologist and a surgeon.

The majority of patients with mild and moderate disease can be treated as outpatients. Therapy listed below should be discussed with a gastroenterologist, and close followup must be ensured.

1. **Prednisone** 40 to 60 mg/d is usually sufficient and can be adjusted depending on the severity of the disease. Once clinical remission is achieved, steroids should be slowly tapered and discontinued, since there is no evidence that maintenance dosages of steroids reduce the incidence of relapses.
2. **Sulfasalazine** 1.5 to 2 g/d is inferior to steroids in treating acute attacks and is most useful in maintenance therapy by reducing the recurrence rate. Alternatives to sulfasalazine can be found in Chap. 77, *Emergency Medicine: A Comprehensive Study Guide,* 5th ed.
3. Topical steroid preparations, such as beclomethasone, hydrocortisone, tixocortol, or budesonide, can be used acutely and to maintain remission.
4. Supportive measures include replenishment of iron stores, dietary elimination of lactose, and addition of bulking agents, such as psyllium (Metamucil). Antidiarrheal agents can precipitate toxic megacolon and should be avoided.

PSEUDOMEMBRANOUS COLITIS

Pseudomembranous colitis is an inflammatory bowel disorder in which membrane-like yellowish plaques of exudate overlay and replace necrotic intestinal mucosa. The incidence is increasing, and three syndromes have been described: neonatal pseudomembranous enterocolitis, postoperative pseudomembranous enterocolitis, and antibiotic-associated pseudomembranous colitis.

Clinical Features

Clinical manifestations can vary from frequent, watery, mucoid stools to a toxic picture, including profuse diarrhea, crampy abdominal pain, fever, leukocytosis, and dehydration. Examination of the stool may reveal fecal leukocytes. Toxic megacolon or colonic perforation occurs rarely.

Diagnosis and Differential

Any antibiotic, but most commonly broad-spectrum antibiotics, such as clindamycin, cephalosporins, and ampicillin, alter the gut flora to allow toxin-producing *Clostridium difficile* to flourish within the colon. The disease typically begins 7 to 10 days after the institution of antibiotics, but the range is between a few days up to 8 weeks. The diagnosis is confirmed by the demonstration of *C. difficile* in the stool and by the detection of toxin in stool filtrates. Colonoscopy is not routinely needed to confirm the diagnosis.

Emergency Department Care and Disposition

The treatment of pseudomembranous colitis includes discontinuing antibiotic therapy and initiating intravenous fluid replacement and electrolyte abnormality correction. This is effective without additional treatment in 25 percent of patients.

1. Oral **metronidazole** 500 mg three times daily or oral **vancomycin** 125 to 250 mg four times daily is the treatment of choice in patients with mild to moderate disease who do not respond to supportive measures. Vancomycin should be reserved for cases where the patient has not responded to or is intolerant of metronidazole and in pregnancy.
2. Patients with severe diarrhea, those with a systemic response (e.g., fever, leukocytosis, or severe abdominal pain), and those whose symptoms persist despite appropriate outpatient management must be hospitalized and should receive vancomycin 125 to 250 mg four times daily for 10 d. The symptoms usually resolve within a few days.
3. Antidiarrheal agents may prolong or worsen symptoms and should be avoided.

Relapses occur in 10 to 20 percent of patients. Steroids and surgical intervention are rarely needed. Patients are advised to contact their physician or return to the emergency department if they develop increasing abdominal pain, fever, or malaise.

DIVERTICULITIS

Diverticulitis is an acute inflammatory process caused by bacterial proliferation within an existing colonic diverticulum. Clinical diverticulitis occurs in 10 to 25 percent of patients with diverticulosis. One-third of the U.S. population will have acquired the disease by age 50 and two-thirds by age 85. Only 2 to 4 percent of patients with diverticulitis are under the age of 40, but the younger age group tends to have a more virulent form of the disease, with frequent complications requiring earlier surgical intervention.

Clinical Features

The most common symptom is a steady, deep discomfort in the left lower quadrant of the abdomen. Other symptoms include tenesmus and changes in bowel habits, such as diarrhea or increasing constipation. The involved diverticulum can irritate the urinary tract and cause frequency, dysuria, or pyuria. If a fistula develops between the colon and the bladder, the patient may present with recurrent urinary tract infections or pneumaturia. Paralytic ileus with abdominal distention, nausea, and vomiting may develop secondary to intraabdominal irritation and peritonitis. Small bowel obstruction and perforation can also occur. Right lower quadrant pain, which may be indistinguishable from acute appendicitis, can occur with ascending colonic diverticular involvement and in patients with a redundant right-sided sigmoid colon.

Physical examination frequently demonstrates a low-grade fever, but the temperature may be higher in patients with generalized peritonitis and in those with an abscess. The abdominal examination reveals localized tenderness, often with voluntary guarding and rebound tenderness. A fullness or mass may be appreciated over the affected area of colon. Twenty-five percent of patients demonstrate occult blood. A pelvic examination should be performed in female patients to exclude a gynecologic source of symptoms.

Diagnosis and Differential

The differential diagnosis includes appendicitis, peptic ulcer disease, pelvic inflammatory disease, endometriosis, ischemic colitis, aortic aneurysm, renal calculus, irritable bowel syndrome, lactate intolerance, colon carcinoma, intestinal lymphoma, Kaposi's sarcoma, sarcoidosis, collagen vascular disease, irradiation colitis or proctosigmoiditis, fecal impaction, foreign-body granuloma, and any bacterial, parasitic, or viral infectious cause.

Laboratory studies should include routine screening blood tests, urinalysis, and an abdominal radiographic series. Leukocytosis is present in only 36 percent of patients with diverticulitis. The abdominal series may be normal or may demonstrate an associated ileus; partial small bowel obstruction; colonic obstruction; free air, indicating bowel perforation; or extraluminal collections of air, suggesting a walled-off abscess. Computerized tomography of the abdomen is the diagnostic procedure of choice and may demonstrate presence of diverticulae, inflammation of pericolic fat, bowel wall thickening, or peridiverticular abscess. Abdominal ultrasonography lacks specificity and is operator dependent. Barium contrast studies can easily demonstrate diverticulae but are insensitive in detecting the presence of diverticulitis. Controversy exists regarding the use of sigmoidoscopy or contrast radiographic studies during the acute inflammatory state because of the possible risk of precipitating colonic perforation.

Emergency Department Care and Disposition

Initial resuscitation of patients should include appropriate fluid and electrolyte replacement and focus on determining the severity of the illness. Admission is indicated in patients who demonstrate signs of toxicity, such as fever, tachycardia, leukocytosis, and severe abdominal pain.

1. Inpatient treatment includes intravenous antibiotics, usually an aminoglycoside, such as **gentamicin** or **tobramycin** 1.5 mg/kg, and either **metronidazole** 500 mg or **clindamycin** 300 to 600 mg, for aerobic and anaerobic organism coverage. Ticarcillin-clavulanic acid or imipenem has been used as an alternative agent.
2. The patient is placed on bowel rest, nothing by mouth is given, and intravenous fluids are administered. Nasogastric suction may be indicated in patients with bowel obstruction or adynamic ileus, and surgical consultation should be obtained.
3. Outpatient management is acceptable for patients with localized pain without signs and symptoms of local peritonitis or systemic infection. Treatment consists of bowel rest and broad-spectrum oral antibiotic therapy. Common agents effective against aerobic organisms include **ampicillin** (500 mg every 6 h), **trimetho-prim-sulfamethoxazole** 2 tablets every 12 h, **ciprofloxacin** 500 mg every 12 h, or **cephalexin** 500 mg every 6 h. One of these medications is taken in combination with an agent effective against anaerobic organisms, such as **metronidazole** 500 mg every 8 h or **clindamycin** 300 mg every 6 h. Patients should limit activity and maintain a liquid diet for 48 h. If symptoms improve, low-residue foods are added to the diet. Patients are advised to contact their physician or return to the emergency

department if they develop increasing abdominal pain, fever, or malaise.

For further reading in *Emergency Medicine: A Comprehensive Study Guide*, 5th ed., see Chap. 77, "Ileitis, Colitis, and Diverticulitis," by Howard A. Werman, Hagop S. Mekhjian, and Douglas A. Rund.

---

45 | Anorectal Disorders

N. Heramba Prasad

Anorectal disorders may be due to local disease processes or underlying serious systemic disorders. Whenever a patient has rectal bleeding or pain, the following disorders discussed should be considered. Anorectal manifestations of sexually transmitted diseases are discussed in Chap. 86. Pilonidal cysts are discssed in Chap. 93.

ANATOMY

The endodermal intestine joins with the ectodermal anal canal at the dentate line, at approximately 1 to 2 cm from the anal verge. The rectal ampulla narrows proximal to the dentate line, causing the mucosa to form pleated columns of Morgagni. At the dentate line, the columns form small anal crypts. These crypts may sometimes contain small anal glands that extend through the internal sphincter. The submucosa of the rectum contains blood vessels that thicken at the dentate line, forming the internal hemorrhoidal plexus. The inner circular muscle layer of the rectum forms the internal sphincter. Voluntary muscles of the pelvic floor, levator ani, and puborectalis form the external sphincter (Fig. 45-1).

Examination

After a detailed history of the complaints, a digital examination of the rectum, followed by anoscopy or rectosigmoidoscopy, must be performed. Patients should be placed in one of three positions:

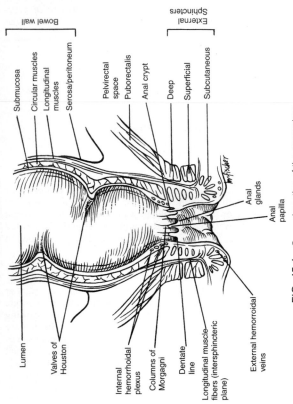

FIG. 45-1 Coronal section of the anorectum.

1. The left lateral or Sim's position, with the left leg extended and the right leg flexed at the knee and hip, is probably the most common position used in the emergency department (ED).
2. The supine or lithotomy position should be used for debilitated patients.
3. Knee-chest position in patients who are cooperative provides for a thorough examination.

HEMORRHOIDS

The internal hemorrhoidal veins are part of the portal system whereas the external hemorrhoidal veins drain into the systemic circulation through the iliac and pudendal veins. Engorgement, prolapse, or thrombosis of these veins is termed *hemorrhoids*. Internal hemorrhoids are not readily palpable and are best visualized through an anoscope. They are constant in location and are found at 2, 5, and 9 o'clock positions when patients are prone. Constipation and straining at stool, pregnancy, and increased portal venous pressure are some of the common causes of hemorrhoids. Tumors of the rectum and sigmoid colon should be considered in patients over 40 years of age.

Clinical Features

Painless, self-limited, bright-red rectal bleeding is the usual symptom in uncomplicated hemorrhoids. Pain is usually associated with thrombosed hemorrhoids. Large hemorrhoids may result in prolapse that may spontaneously reduce or require periodic manual reduction by patients. They may become incarcerated and gangrenous, requiring surgical intervention. Prolapse may cause mucous discharge and pruritus. Strangulation, severe bleeding, and thrombosis are common complications.

Emergency Department Care and Disposition

Unless complication is present, management is usually nonsurgical.

1. Hot sitz baths for at least 15 min 3 times per day and after each bowel movement will ameliorate pain and swelling. Following the sitz baths, the anus should be gently but thoroughly dried. Use of topical steroids, antibiotics, and analgesics are usually of no value and, in fact, may cause harm.
2. Bulk laxatives, such as psyllium seed compounds or stool softeners, should be used after the acute phase has subsided. Laxatives causing liquid stool are best avoided as they may result in cryptitis and sepsis.

3. Surgical treatment for hemorrhoids is indicated for severe, intractable pain, continued bleeding, incarceration, or strangulation.

4. Thrombosed external hemorrhoids may need surgical decompression and excision of the clots. If they have been present for less than 48 h and the pain is tolerable, sitz baths and bulk laxatives may be tried initially. Acute and recently thrombosed painful hemorrhoids should be treated with excision of the clots. After analgesia with appropriate conscious sedation and local infiltration, an elliptical skin incision is made over the hemorrhoids and the thrombosed vein is removed along with the elliptical skin (Fig. 45-2). Packing and a pressure dressing will usually control the bleeding. The pressure dressing may be removed after about 6 h, when the patient takes the first sitz bath.

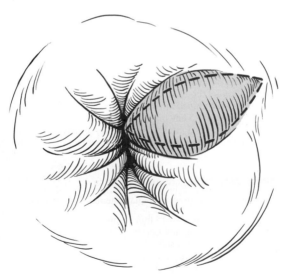

FIG. 45-2   Elliptical excision of thrombosed external hemorrhoid. (*From Goldberg SM et al: Essentials of Anorectal Surgery. Philadelphia, Lippincott, 1980. With permission.*)

CRYPTITIS

Sphincter spasm and repeated trauma from large hard stools cause breakdown of the mucosa over the crypts. This may lead to inflamed anal glands and abscess formation, fissures, and fistulae.

Clinical Features

Anal pain, especially with bowel movements, and itching, with or without bleeding, are the usual symptoms of cryptitis. Diagnosis is confirmed by palpation of tender, swollen crypts with associated hypertrophied papillae. The anoscope provides a definitive diagnosis. The crypts commonly involved are in the posterior midline of the anal ring.

Emergency Department Care and Disposition

Bulk laxatives, additional roughage, hot sitz baths, and warm rectal irrigations will enhance healing. Surgical treatment may be needed in refractory cases.

FISSURE IN ANO

Anal fissures are the most common cause of painful rectal bleeding. Swelling of the surrounding tissues produces hypertrophied papillae proximally and sentinel pile distally. Most anal fissures occur in the midline posteriorly. A fissure not in the midline should alert physicians to other potentially life-threatening causes, such as Crohn's disease, ulcerative colitis, carcinomas, lymphomas, syphilis, and tuberculosis.

Clinical Features

Sharp cutting pain occurs with defecation and subsides between bowel movements, which distinguishes fissures from other anorectal disorders. Bleeding is bright and in small quantities. Rectal examination is very painful and often not possible without application of topical anesthetic agents. In many instances, sentinel pile and the distal end of the fissure can be seen after gently retracting the buttocks, and further rectal examination may be deferred.

Emergency Department Care and Disposition

Treatment is aimed at relieving sphincter spasm and pain and at preventing stricture formation. Hot sitz baths and the addition of bran (fiber) to the diet are helpful. Use of topical anesthetics, while temporarily helpful, may cause a hypersensitivity reaction. Topical steroids are not recommended, as they may retard wound healing. Surgical excision of the fissure may be required if the area does not heal after adequate treatment.

ANORECTAL ABSCESSES

Abscesses start from the anal crypts and spread to involve the perianal, intersphincteric, ischiorectal, or the deep perianal space. Perianal abscess is the most common form seen at the anal verge. When not associated with any other perirectal infection or systemic symptoms, perianal abscess is the only one that can be safely incised in the ED.

Clinical Features

Pain can be dull, aching, or throbbing and becomes worse before defecation, but persists between bowel movements. Fever and leukocytosis may be present.

Emergency Department Care and Disposition

Most abscesses should be drained in the operating room. Simple perianal abscesses may be drained in the ED, if surgical consultation is not readily available. After adequate local analgesia with conscious sedation, a cruciate incision is made over the abscess, and the dog-ears excised. Packing is usually not required. Sitz baths should be started the next day.

FISTULA IN ANO

Fistulae commonly result from perianal or ischiorectal abscess. Crohn's disease, ulcerative colitis, tuberculosis, gonococcal proctitis, and carcinomas should be considered in the etiology. Persistent bloody, malodorous discharge occurs as long as the fistula remains open. Blockage of the tract causes recurrent bouts of abscess formation.

Emergency Department Care and Disposition

Surgical excision is the definitive treatment. Sitz baths and local cleansing will temporize the condition until surgery.

RECTAL PROLAPSE

Prolapse (procidentia) may involve either just the mucosa or all the layers of the rectum. In addition, intussusception of the rectum may present as a prolapse.

Clinical Features

Most patients will complain of a protruding mass, mucous discharge, associated bleeding, and pruritus.

Emergency Department Care and Disposition

In children, under proper analgesia and sedation, the prolapse can be gently reduced. Every effort should be made to prevent children from being constipated. Surgical correction is usually necessary in all other age groups.

RECTAL FOREIGN BODIES

Emergency Department Care and Disposition

Most rectal foreign bodies are low lying and can be removed in the ED. If the size and shape are such that perforation is suspected, a follow-up proctoscopy or x-ray may be required. Adequate sphincter relaxation is essential for removal of foreign bodies. Local infiltration anesthesia injected through a 30-gauge needle into the internal sphincter muscle circumferentially will provide good relaxation. The examiner's finger in the rectum will help guide the needle into the sphincter. Large bulbar objects may create a vacuum-like effect proximally, making removal by simple traction impossible. In these cases, the vacuum can be overcome by passing a catheter around the foreign body into the ampulla and injecting air. Occasionally, passing a Foley catheter proximal to the foreign body, inflating the balloon, and applying gentle traction may help maneuver the foreign body into a more desirable position for ease of removal.

PRURITUS ANI

Clinical Features and Emergency Department Care and Disposition

Although primary or idiopathic pruritus does occur, other causes should be ruled out. These include fissures, fistulae, hemorrhoids, and prolapse and such dietary factors as caffeine, milk, chocolate, tomatoes, citrus fruits, pinworms, *Candida trichophyton,* and local irritants. Treatment will depend upon the underlying condition.

For further reading in *Emergency Medicine: A Comprehensive Study Guide,* 5th ed., see Chap. 78, "Anorectal Disorders," by James K. Bouzoukis.

46 | Vomiting, Diarrhea, and Constipation

Christian A. Tomaszewski

Although vomiting, diarrhea, and constipation are typically due to gastrointestinal disorders, the clinician must be mindful of systemic causes as well. The initial duty is to define what the patient means by such complaints. One can then decide whether the complaints represent a benign condition requiring symptomatic relief or a harbinger of an emergent condition requiring surgical intervention.

VOMITING AND DIARRHEA

Clinical Features

Vomiting

History is essential in determining the cause of vomiting. Vomiting with blood could represent gastritis, peptic ulcer disease, or carcinoma. However, aggressive nonbloody vomiting followed by hematemesis is more consistent with a Mallory-Weiss tear. The presence of bile rules out gastric outlet obstruction, such as from pyloric stenosis or strictures. An associated symptom such as fever would direct one to an infectious or inflammatory cause. Radiation of the pain to the chest suggests myocardial infarction or pneumonia. Radiation to the back can be seen with aortic aneurysm or dissection, pancreatitis, pyelonephritis, or renal colic. Headache with vomiting suggests increased intracranial pressure, such as with subarachnoid hemorrhage or head injury. Vomiting in a pregnant patient is consistent with hyperemesis gravidarum in the first trimester; but in the third trimester it could represent preeclampsia if accompanied by hypertension. Associated medical conditions are also useful in discerning the cause of vomiting: insulin use suggests ketoacidosis, peripheral vascular disease suggests mesenteric ischemia, previous surgery suggests intestinal obstruction, and medication use (e.g., lithium or digoxin) suggests toxicity.

The physical examination in a vomiting patient includes a careful assessment of the gastrointestinal, pelvic, and genitourinary systems. In addition, assessment of hydration status is important. Other clues to specific causes for vomiting may come from the dermal examination (e.g., hyperpigmentation with Addison's disease) or pulmonary examination (e.g., clues of pneumonia).

Diarrhea

By definition, diarrhea represents a daily stool output of more than 200 g but generally refers to any increase in frequency or liquidity. Other important historical factors include duration of illness and presence of blood. Acute diarrhea of less than 2 to 3 weeks' duration is more likely to represent a serious cause, such as infection, ischemia, intoxication, or inflammation. Associated factors, such as fever, pain, or type of food ingested, may help in the diagnosis of infectious gastroenteritis. Neurologic symptoms can be seen in certain diarrheal illnesses, such as seizure with shigellosis or theophylline toxicity, or paresthesias with ciguatoxin.

Details about the host can also better define the diagnosis. Malabsorption from pancreatic insufficiency or HIV-related bowel disorders need not be considered in a healthy host. History of foods ingested, such as meat, dairy products, seafood, or unpasteurized products, may isolate the vector and narrow the differential diagnosis for infectious diarrhea considerably (e.g., oysters suggest *Vibrio;* rice suggests *Bacillus cereus;* eggs suggest *Salmonella;* and meat suggests *Campylobacter, Staphylococcus, Yersinia, Escherichia coli,* or *Clostridium).* Certain medications, particularly antibiotics, colchicine, lithium, and laxatives, can all contribute to diarrhea. Travel may predispose the patient to *E. coli* or *Giardia.* Social history, such as sexual preference, drug use, and occupation, may suggest such diagnoses as HIV-related illness or organophosphate poisoning.

The physical examination usually concentrates initially on assessment of fluid status. Abdominal examination can narrow the differential diagnosis as well as reveal the need for surgical intervention. Even appendicitis can present with diarrhea in up to 20 percent of cases. Rectal examination can rule out impaction or presence of blood, the latter suggesting inflammation, infection, or mesenteric ischemia.

Diagnosis and Differential

A mnemonic to prompt the physician's recall of disease groupings causing vomiting and diarrhea is GASTROENTERITIS: *g*astrointestinal diseases, *a*ppendicitis or aorta, *s*pecific disease (e.g., glaucoma), *t*rauma, medications (*R*x), *o*bstetric-gynecologic disorders, *e*ndocrine disorders, *n*eurologic disease, *t*oxicology, *e*nvironmental disorders, *r*enal disease, *i*nfection, *t*umors, *i*schemia, and *s*upratentorial.

Vomiting

All women of childbearing age warrant a pregnancy test. In vomiting associated with abdominal pain, liver function tests, urinalysis, and lipase or amylase determinations may be useful. Electrolyte determinations and renal function tests are usually of benefit only in patients with severe dehydration or prolonged vomiting. In addition, they may confirm addisonian crisis with hyperkalemia and hyponatremia. The electrocardiogram and chest radiograph can be reserved for patients with suspected ischemia or pulmonary infection. An acute abdominal series can be used to confirm the presence of obstruction.

Diarrhea

The most specific tests in diarrheal illness all involve examination of the stool in the laboratory. Wright's stain for fecal leukocytes has an 82 percent sensitivity and 83 percent specificity for the presence of invasive bacterial pathogens. Because of its poor sensitivity and the safety of antibiotics, even in noninvasive diarrhea, this test has lost its popularity. Instead, fecal blood testing may provide similar information at lower cost. A more expensive proposition, stool culture, also has poor sensitivity. Therefore, it is reserved for those patients with immunocompromise or persistent diarrhea, or toxic patients with severe dehydration. In addition, it may be useful for patients involved in public health sensitive occupations. In patients with chronic persistent diarrhea, an examination for ova and parasites may be useful to rule out *Giardia* or *Cryptosporidium*. Although not extremely sensitive, *Clostridium difficile* toxin assay may be useful in ill patients with antibiotic-associated diarrhea. Because of the low sensitivity and delay in results, laboratory testing in routine diarrheal cases is not indicated.

General laboratory testing in patients with diarrhea is usually unnecessary. However, in extremely dehydrated or toxic patients, electrolyte determinations and renal function tests may be useful. In an infant with bloody diarrhea, the presence of renal failure and anemia suggest hemolytic uremic syndrome, usually due to *E. coli* O157:H7. If toxicity is suspected, tests for levels for theophylline, lithium, or heavy metals will aid in the diagnosis. Radiographs are reserved for ruling out obstruction or pneumonia, particularly *Legionella*. In addition, angiography may be indicated in acute mesenteric ischemia.

Emergency Department Care and Disposition

The treatment of vomiting and diarrhea consists of correcting fluid and electrolyte problems. In addition, one must initiate specific therapy for any life-threatening cause identified in the initial workup of vomiting and diarrhea.

1. Replacement of fluids can be intravenous (IV; bolus 500 mL in adults, 10 to 20 mL/kg in children) with normal saline solution in seriously ill patients. Mildly dehydrated patients may tolerate an oral rehydrating solution containing sodium (at least 45 meq/L in children) as well as glucose to enhance fluid absorption. The World Health Organization advocates a mixture of 1 cup orange juice, 4 tsp sugar, 1 tsp baking powder, and $\frac{3}{4}$ tsp salt in 1 L boiled water. The goal is 50 to 100 mL/kg over the first 4 h.

2. Nutritional supplementation should be started as soon as nausea and vomiting subside. Patients can quickly advance from clear liquids to solids, such as rice and bread. Patients may benefit from avoiding caffeine and sorbitol-containing products.

3. Antibiotics are recommended for adult patients with severe or prolonged diarrhea. In addition, they are indicated for travelers from tropical or Third World countries. Although single-dose fluoroquinolones show some effectiveness, these antibiotics are usually given for 3 to 5 days: **ciprofloxacin** 500 mg orally (PO) bid, **norfloxacin** 400 mg PO bid, or **ofloxacin** 300 mg PO bid. Although inferior, **trimethoprim-sulfamethoxazole** (TMP-SMX), TMP 10 mg/kg/d:SMX 50 mg/kg/d (maximum dose TMP 160 mg:SMX 800 mg) is indicated for children or nursing patients, if antibiotics are truly necessary. It should be noted that antibiotics are of questionable value in infectious diarrhea from *E. coli* O157:H7.

4. **Metronidazole** 15 mg/kg PO divided tid for 5 days (maximum 1000 mg/d) is indicated for *C. difficile*, *Giardia*, or *Entamoeba* (treat for 10 days) infection. Antibiotics are especially indicated in patients or workers in the food industry or institutional settings such as day care centers and nursing homes.

5. Antidiarrheal agents, especially in combination with antibiotics, have been shown to shorten the course of diarrhea. **Loperamide** is given 4 mg PO initially and then 2 mg PO after each diarrheal stool to a maximum of 16 mg/d (for children over 2 years, 0.8 mg/kg/d is given, with one-third of the dose given initially and one-third of the dose after the next two diarrheal stools).

6. Antiemetic agents are useful in actively vomiting patients with dehydration. Traditionally, **promethazine** 25 mg (12.5 mg in children over 2 years) intramuscularly (IM), IV, or rectally (PR) every 6 h is prescribed. **Prochlorperazine** 10 mg IV or IM or 25 mg PR or PO is particularly useful if vomiting is accompanied by headache. Finally, **metoclopramide** 10 to 20 mg (1 mg/kg)

is very useful for nausea and can be given in pregnancy (category B).

Patients with a life-threatening cause of vomiting or diarrhea require admission. In addition, toxic or severely dehydrated patients, particularly infants and the elderly, or those still intolerant of oral fluids after hydration warrant admission. Patients with an unclear diagnosis but favorable examination findings after hydration can be discharged safely home with antiemetics. Work excuses are indicated for patients in the food, day care, and health industries.

CONSTIPATION

Clinical Features

Constipation is the most common digestive complaint in the United States. The usual definition of this disorder is the presence of hard stools that are difficult to pass. Acute onset implies obstruction until proven otherwise. Chronic constipation is less ominous and can be managed on an outpatient basis. Associated symptoms, such as vomiting and inability to pass flatus, confirm obstruction. Associated illnesses can help disclose the underlying diagnosis: cold intolerance (hypothyroidism), diverticulitis (inflammatory stricture), or nephrolithiasis (hyperparathyroidism).

Physical examination should focus on detection of hernias or abdominal masses. Rectal examination will detect masses, such as fecal impaction, anal fissures, or fecal blood. The latter, accompanied by weight loss or decreasing stool caliber, may confirm colon carcinoma. The presence of ascites in postmenopausal women raises suspicion of ovarian or uterine carcinoma.

Diagnosis and Differential

Chronic constipation requires few laboratory tests. Directed testing in acute constipation, based on suspicion, can include a complete blood count (to rule out anemia), a thyroid panel (to rule out hypothyroidism), and electrolyte determinations (to rule out hypokalemia or hypercalcemia). Flat and erect abdominal films may be useful in confirming obstruction or assessing stool burden. Barium enema is diagnostic for such disorders as intussusception, Hirschsprung's disease, and volvulus. Ultrasound studies, particularly in pediatric cases, can discern the cause of obstruction, including pyloric stenosis and intussusception.

The differential diagnosis for constipation is extensive; however, chronic constipation is a functional disorder that can be worked up on an outpatient basis. Nevertheless, complications of chronic constipation, such as fecal impaction and intestinal pseudo-obstruction, will require either manual or colonoscopic intervention.

Emergency Department Care and Disposition

Treatment of constipation is directed at symptomatic relief as well as correction of patients' habits. Occasionally, specific treatment is required for complications of constipation or for underlying disorders that can lead to organic constipation.

1. The most important prescription for functional constipation is a dietary and exercise regimen that includes fluids (1.5 L/d), fiber (10 g/d), and exercise. Fiber in the form of bran (1 cup/d) or psyllium (Metamucil 1 tsp tid) increases stool volume and gut motility.
2. **Medications** can provide temporary relief for this chronic problem. Stimulants can be either given PO, as with anthraquinones (e.g., Peri-Colace 1 to 2 tablets PO at bedtime) or PR, as with bisacodyl (Dulcolax 10 mg PR tid in adults or children). In the absence of renal failure, magnesium (e.g., milk of magnesia 15 to 30 mL daily to bid or magnesium citrate 200 mL once) is useful. In children mineral oil (15 to 30 mL/year of age daily or bid PO for up to 3 d) has been advocated.
3. **Enemas** of soapsuds (1500 mL PR) or phosphate (e.g., Fleets I unit PR, 1 oz/10 kg in children) are generally reserved for severe cases or after fecal disimpaction.
4. Fecal impaction should be removed manually using local anesthetic lubricant. In female patients, transvaginal pressure with the other hand may be helpful. An enema or suppositories to complete evacuation can follow.

All patients with apparent functional constipation can be managed as outpatients. One caveat is that fecal impaction must be checked for in both adults and children and manually relieved prior to emergency department discharge. Early follow-up is indicated in patients with recent severe constipation or systemic symptoms, such as weight loss, anemia, or change in stool caliber. Patients with organic constipation from obstruction require hospitalization and surgical evaluation. Intestinal pseudoobstruction and sigmoid volvulus can sometimes be corrected colonoscopically.

For further reading in *Emergency Medicine: A Comprehensive Study Guide*, 5th ed., see Chap. 79, "Vomiting, Diarrhea, and Constipation," by Annie Tewel Sadosty and Brian J. Browne.

47 | Jaundice, Hepatic Disorders, and Hepatic Failure

Gregory S. Hall

JAUNDICE

Jaundice, a yellowish discoloration of the skin, sclerae, and mucous membranes, results from hyperbilirubinemia (breakdown of hemoglobin) and thus the deposition of bile pigments. It has many etiologies (see Table 47-1). Hyperbilirubinemia can be divided into two types. The unconjugated form results from increased bilirubin production or a liver defect in its uptake or conjugation. The conjugated form occurs in the setting of intra- or extrahepatic cholestasis, resulting in decreased excretion of conjugated bilirubin. The total serum bilirubin should be elevated in a jaundiced patient. Clinically, jaundice usually becomes noticeable at a serum bilirubin level of 2.0 to 2.5 mg/dL and is often first seen in the sclera. An indirect fraction of serum bilirubin of 85 percent or higher is consistent with the unconjugated type, whereas a direct fraction of 30 percent or above indicates the conjugated form. Conjugated bilirubin is water soluble and is detectable in the urine even with low serum levels.

Clinical Features

Jaundice is a symptom with a myriad of possible underlying causes. Sudden onset of jaundice in a previously healthy young person, together with a prodrome of fever, malaise, myalgias, and a tender enlarged liver, points to hepatitis (probably viral) as a likely cause. Heavy ethanol use suggests alcoholic hepatitis. In the setting of alcoholic liver disease and cirrhosis, jaundice usually develops gradually (discussed later). A history of drug or toxin ingestion should always be obtained from the jaundiced patient. A family history of jaundice or a history of recurrent mild jaundice that spontaneously resolves usually accompanies inherited causes of jaundice such as Gilbert syndrome. Cholecystitis in itself may not cause jaundice unless there is acute biliary obstruction present such as with a retained common bile duct gallstone. Painless jaundice in an older patient classically suggests pancreatic or hepatobiliary malignancy. Patients with a known prior malignancy and a hard, nodular liver accompanied by jaundice are likely to be found to have liver metastases. Bilitary tract scarring or strictures must always be suspected as a cause of jaundice in patients with a

TABLE 47-1 Causes of Jaundice

Unconjugated	Conjugated
Hemolytic anemia	Intrahepatic
Hemoglobinopathy	Infectious
	Viral hepatitis
Transfusion reaction	Leptospirosis
	Infectious mononucleosis
Gilbert disease	Toxins (drugs/chemicals)
Crigler-Najjar syndrome	Familial
	Rotor syndrome
Premature neonates	Dubin-Johnson syndrome
Congestive heart failure	Alcoholic liver disease
	Other
Sepsis	Sarcoidosis
	Lymphoma
	Liver metastasis
	Cirrhosis
	Pregnancy
	Amyloidosis
	Extraheptic
	Gallstones
	Pancreatic tumors/cysts
	Cholangiosarcoma
	Bile duct stricture
	Sclerosing cholangitis

prior history of biliary tract surgery, pancreatitis, cholangitis, or inflammatory bowel disease. Hepatomegaly with jaundice, accompanied by pedal edema, jugular venous distention, and a gallop rhythm suggest chronic heart failure.

Diagnosis and Differential

Initial laboratory tests that should be obtained in the workup of a jaundiced patient include serum bilirubin level (both total and direct fraction—indirect fraction can be deduced by simple subtraction), serum aminotransferases and alkaline phosphatase levels, urinalysis to check for bilirubin and urobilinogen, and a complete blood cell count (CBC). Additional laboratory tests may be indicated based on the clinical setting [serum amylase and lipase levels, prothrombin time (PT), electrolytes and glucose levels, blood urea nitrogen (BUN) and creatinine levels, viral hepatitis panels, drug levels, and pregnancy test]. With normal liver enzyme levels, the jaundice is more likely to be caused by sepsis or systemic infection, inborn errors of metabolism, or pregnancy, rather than by primary hepatic disease. With abnormally elevated liver enzymes, the pattern of abnormalities may suggest the etiology. Aminotransferase elevation, if predominant, suggests hepatocellular diseases such as viral or toxic hepatitis or cirrhosis, whereas markedly elevated alkaline phosphatase levels (2 to 3 times that of normal levels) and GGT points to intra- or extrahepatic obstruction (gallstones, stricture, malignancy). A Coombs test and hemoglobin electrophoresis may be useful if anemia is present, along with normal liver aminotransferase levels (hemolysis and hemoglobinopathy). If clinical features and initial laboratory results reveal conjugated hyperbilirubinemia, ultrasound studies of the biliary tract, liver, and pancreas should be performed to rule out gallstones, dilated extrahepatic biliary ducts, or mass/tumor in the liver, pancreas, and portal region. A computed tomography scan may also be considered but is often more costly and is not as sensitive as ultrasound for detection of gallstones in the gallbladder.

Emergency Department Care and Disposition

Jaundice by itself is not an adequate justification for hospital admission. In some situations discharge from the emergency department pending further outpatient workup may be appropriate, if a patient is hemodynamically stable with new onset jaundice and has no evidence of liver failure or acute biliary obstruction, and if appropriate laboratory studies have been ordered, timely follow-up is available, and the patient is reliable and has adequate social support. If extrahepatic biliary obstruction is suspected, surgical consultation should be obtained in the emergency department. For other possible admission indicators, see the remaining sections of this chapter as well as Chap. 48.

HEPATITIS

Hepatitis is defined by liver inflammation with hepatocellular necrosis. In the United States, it is commonly associated with viral infection or ethanol use (as well as other toxins—see chapters on toxicology). Risk factors for viral hepatitis include male homosexuality, hemodialysis, intravenous drug abuse, raw seafood ingestion, blood product transfusion, tattoos or body piercing, needle punctures, foreign travel, or close contact with an infected source patient. Both viral and toxin-induced hepatitis may lead to fulminant hepatic failure, chronic liver disease, cirrhosis, and end-stage liver disease (ESLD). In the United States, the majority (50 percent) of cases of ESLD results from alcohol abuse. The remainder of this section will focus on viral hepatitis, while the next section will deal with alcoholic hepatitis and cirrhosis.

Clinical Features

Viral hepatitis may range in severity from asymptomatic infection to fulminant hepatic failure to chronic cirrhosis. Symptomatic patients usually report sudden or insidious onset of prodrome of anorexia, nausea, emesis, fatigue, malaise, and altered taste. Low-grade fever, accompanied by pharyngitis, coryza, and headache, may confuse the picture and lead to an initial misdiagnosis of upper respiratory infection or flulike illness. A few days of generalized pruritis and dark urine may precede the onset of gastrointestinal (GI) symptoms and jaundice. Malaise usually persists while the other prodromal symptoms resolve. Right upper quadrant pain with an enlarged tender liver and splenomegaly may be found. Many patients do *not* become clinically jaundiced, and most will recover gradually over the ensuing 3 to 4 months. Rarely, fulminant hepatic failure develops with a clinical picture of encephalopathy, coagulopathy, and rapidly worsening jaundice. Chronic persistent infection (usually with hepatitis B or C) can lead to the development of cirrhosis with gradual jaundice, ascites, peripheral edema, and liver failure over a period of 10 to 20 years.

A number of different viral agents have been implicated in the etiology of hepatitis. Hepatitis A (HAV) is transmitted predominantly by the fecal oral route and is commonly seen in Americans. Children and adolescents are more commonly affected, but often subclinically, whereas most adults are symptomatic with a longer, more severe course. Symptom onset is often more abrupt than with other viruses. Epidemic outbreaks have been seen in children at day care centers, institutionalized patients, and in patients exposed to a common source case via contaminated food or water. Fulminant liver failure—though rare—may occur, but chronic infection is not seen.

Hepatitis B (HBV) is acquired primarily via a percutaneous exposure to infected blood or body fluids. Most cases are subclinical without jaundice. Often symptom onset is insidious and in 5 to 10 percent of cases is preceded by a serum sickness-like syndrome with polyarthritis, proteinuria, and angioneurotic edema. Symptomatic patients usually have a more severe and protracted course than those with HAV. Chronic HBV infection occurs in 6 to 10 percent of patients who may go on to develop cirrhosis, ESLD, and hepatocellular carcinoma. An effective vaccine against HBV has resulted in a decline in the prevalence of HBV in the U.S. population.

Hepatitis C (HCV) is the most common of all blood infections in the United States and may be contracted via parenteral, sexual, and perinatal contact. Most patients remain asymptomatic or have milder symptoms than those with HBV or HAV. Unfortunately, chronic HCV infection occurs in 85 percent of patients, the majority of whom remain subclinically infected. Up to 70 percent of chronic HCV cases progress to the development of chronic liver disease (cirrhosis and ESLD) and are at increased risk for hepatocellular carcinoma.

Hepatitis D (HDV) can only coinfect in the setting of acute or chronic HBV infection. Acute HDV superinfection of an HBV carrier, often in the setting of intravenous drug abuse, frequently leads to fulminant liver failure with a high mortality rate. Hepatitis E is a small RNA virus (HEV) and has been seen in sporadic water-borne outbreaks in Asia, India, Africa, Mexico, and the former Soviet Union. Imported cases of HEV have been reported in the United States. The clinical course is similar to HAV, but results in a higher incidence of acute hepatic failure and death, particularly in pregnancy. Acute illness with associated liver function test abnormalities may also occur with infections by other viruses such as cytomegalovirus (CMV), herpes simplex, Cocksackie, and Epstein-Barr (EBV). However, clinically evident hepatitis and jaundice are unusual in otherwise healthy individuals affected by one of these viruses. Non-A, non-B hepatitis is caused by other hepatotropic viruses that have yet to be characterized (formerly HCV was the predominant virus in this group) and are transmitted via blood exposure causing infection and course similar to HCV.

Establishment of a diagnosis of viral hepatitis depends primarily on liver function abnormalities coupled with the clinical picture. Serum transaminase levels (GGT, AST, ALT) should be checked—elevations are suggestive of hepatitis. Values in the hundreds of units per liter are consistent with viral inflammation but elevations into the thousands suggest hepatocellular necrosis, extensive liver injury, and more fulminant disease. In acute and chronic viral hepatitis, the ratio of AST:ALT is usually < 1 (whereas a ratio > 2 is more suggestive of alcoholic hepatitis). Serum alkaline phosphatase level should also be determined—if elevated more than threefold above normal, cholestasis should be suspected. (A concurrently elevated GGT supports this.) Total serum bilirubin level along with its direct fraction (indirect fraction can be deduced by simple subtraction) may also be useful since a conjugated (direct) fraction of 30 percent or higher is consistent with viral hepatitis. The magnitude of transaminase elevation is, however, not a reliable marker of disease severity, but a persistent total bilirubin level > 20 mg/dL or a PT prolonged by more than a few seconds indicates a poor prognosis (hence PT time should be checked). Serum electrolyte, BUN, and creatinine levels should be checked if there is clinical suspicion of volume depletion or electrolyte abnormalities. Abnormal mental status should prompt an immediate determination of serum glucose level, which may be low due to poor oral intake or hepatic failure. (Other causes of abnormal mental status such as hypoxia, sepsis, intoxication, structural intracranial process, or encephalopathy must also be considered.) A CBC may be useful, as an early transient neutropenia followed by a relative lymphocytosis with atypical forms is often seen with viral hepatitis. Anemia, if present, may be more suggestive of alcoholic hepatitis, decompensated cirrhosis, GI bleeding, or a hemolytic process. Serologic studies to determine the specific viral agent responsible may be ordered in the emergency department to facilitate the final diagnosis, but these results are rarely immediately available and thus play no significant role in emergency department management. Important differential diagnoses include alcohol- or toxin-induced hepatitis, infectious mononucleosis, cholecystitis, ascending cholangitis, sarcoidosis, lymphoma, liver metastases, and pancreatic or biliary tumors.

Emergency Department Care and Disposition

Supportive care is the mainstay of therapy for acute viral hepatitis.

1. Most patients can be successfully managed as outpatients with emphasis on rest, adequate oral intake, strict personal hygiene, and avoidance of hepatotoxins (ethanol and drugs). Patients should be instructed to return for worsening symptoms, particularly vomiting, fever, jaundice, or abdominal pain. Follow-up arrangements should be made.
2. Patients with any of the following should be admitted to the hospital: encephalopathy, PT prolonged by more than a few seconds, intractable vomiting, hypoglycemia, bilirubin > 20 mg/dL, age > 45 years, immunosuppression, or suspected toxin-induced hepatitis.
3. Volume depletion and electrolyte imbalances should be corrected with intravenous crystalloid. Hypoglycemia should be initially treated with 1 amp of 50% dextrose in water intravenously followed by the addition of dextrose to intravenous fluids and careful monitoring.
4. Fulminant hepatic failure should warrant admission to the intensive care unit with aggressive support of circulation and respiration, monitoring and treatment of increased intracranial pressure if present, correction of hypoglycemia and coagulopathy,

administration of oral lactulose or neomycin, and a protein-restricted diet. (See following section on treatment of cirrhosis.) Consultation with a hepatologist and liver transplant service are indicated.

5. Glucocorticoid therapy has no value in acute viral hepatitis, even with fulminant hepatic failure, and should be avoided.

ALCOHOLIC LIVER DISEASE AND CIRRHOSIS

Three clinical syndromes best describe liver injury secondary to alcohol: hepatic steatosis (fatty liver), alcoholic hepatitis, and alcoholic cirrhosis. An enlarged, non- or mildly tender liver from steatosis is usually seen in a relatively asymptomatic alcoholic patient. Alcohol-induced hepatitis may present as a very mild or severe acute illness in a chronic alcohol user, whereas cirrhosis from alcohol abuse or other causes represents a chronic process with intermittent exacerbations or associated complications, which usually prompt most emergency department visits.

Clinical Features

Alcoholic hepatitis is typically found in the chronic alcoholic who has gradual onset of anorexia, nausea, fever, dark urine, jaundice, weight loss, abdominal pain, and generalized weakness. Physical exam reveals a tender, enlarged liver, low-grade fever, and icteric mucous membranes, sclera, or skin. Patients suffering from cirrhosis generally report a gradual deterioration in their health with anorexia, muscle loss (often masked by edema or ascites), fatigue, nausea, emesis, diarrhea, and increasing abdominal girth (ascites). Low-grade intermittent or continuous fever may also be present, while hypothermia may be seen at end-stage disease. Abdominal palpation may reveal a small firm liver and possibly splenomegaly. Jaundice, pedal edema, ascites, and spider angiomata are also common. Hepatic encephalopathy, characterized by a fluctuating level of consciousness and confusion and, possibly, hyperreflexia, spasticity, and generalize seizures may also be present. Asterixis ("liver flap") is characteristic, but not specific for encephalopathy due to liver failure. Patients with cirrhosis often come to the emergency department because of worsening ascites or edema, complications such as GI or variceal bleeding (see Chap. 37, "Gastrointestinal Bleeding"), encephalopathy, spontaneous bacterial peritonitis (abdominal pain), and various concurrent infections (urinary tract infection, pneumonia, etc.)

Diagnosis and Differential

Alcoholic hepatitis and cirrhosis may be diagnosed by their clinical features and laboratory findings. Laboratory studies that should be checked include levels of serum transaminases (GGT, ALT, AST), serum alkaline phosphatase, total bilirubin (and its fractions), serum albumin, serum glucose and electrolytes, BUN, and creatinine, CBC, and PT. In the setting of alcoholic hepatitis, serum transaminase levels are usually elevated to a range of 2 to 10 times that of normal with AST: ALT ratio of > 1.5 to 2.0 (AST production is stimulated by ethanol). With cirrhosis, transaminase levels are often only mildly elevated. Alkaline phosphatase and bilirubin levels are usually only mildly elevated with both alcoholic hepatitis and cirrhosis. Anemia, leukopenia, and thrombocytopenia are commonly seen in chronic ethanol abusers. If concurrent pancreatitis is suspected, serum lipase and amylase levels should be checked. Fever with or without leukocytosis in a chronic alcoholic warrants a chest x-ray to rule out pneumonia; cultures of blood, urine, and ascitic fluid; and a thorough search for other sources of sepsis (meningitis, cholecystitis, cellulitis, perirectal abscess, etc.) Elevated serum ammonia level unfortunately does not correlate well with acute deterioration of liver function due to cirrhosis and, while it may be checked as a marker of encephalopathy, it cannot be used as an index of its severity or response to treatment.

Spontaneous bacterial peritonitis (SBP), the most common complication of cirrhotic ascites, should be suspected in any cirrhotic patient with fever, abdominal pain or tenderness, worsening ascites, subacute functional decline, or encephalopathy. Other subtle clues to SBP include deteriorating renal function, hypothermia, and diarrhea. SBP may be confirmed through sampling of ascitic fluid by paracentesis, ideally under ultrasound guidance to minimize the risk of bowel puncture. (See Chap. 82, *Emergency Medicine: A Comprehensive Study Guide,* 5th ed., for details on this procedure.) Ascitic fluid should be tested for total protein and glucose levels, lactic (acid) dehydrogenase (LDH), Gram stain, and white blood cell count (WBC) with differential. A total WBC count > 1000 per cubic millimeter or neutrophil (PMN) count > 250 per cubic millimeter is diagnostic for SBP. (A total WBC count > 10,000 per cubic millimeter, total protein > 1 g/dL, glucose < 50 mg/dL, or elevated LDH point to the possibility of generalized peritonitis due to a local focus of infection—e.g., cholecystitis or appendicitis.) Culture results from ascitic fluid are often negative, but placing 10 mL of ascitic fluid in a blood culture bottle may have an improved yield. Gram-negative Enterobacteriaceae (*E. coli, Klebsiella*, etc.) account for 63 percent of SBP, followed by the pneumococcus (15 percent) and the enterococcus (6 to 10 percent). Hepatorenal syndrome, a refractory form of acute renal failure that occurs in cirrhotic patients, may develop in the setting of sepsis, acute dehydration, overzealous diuresis, or high-volume paracentesis. The differential diagnosis includes other forms of hepatitis (drugs, toxins, etc.), as well as other causes of upper abdominal pain (cholecystitis, biliary colic, gastritis or peptic ulcer disease, pancreatitis, etc.) Cirrhosis is often caused by ethanol or chronic viral hepatitis—uncommon causes include drugs or toxins, hemochromatosis, Wilson's disease, and primary (idiopathic) biliary cirrhosis.

Emergency Department Care and Disposition

Alcoholic Hepatitis

1. Hospital admission is required for all but the mildest of cases of alcoholic hepatitis.
2. Fluid therapy with dextrose-containing intravenous fluids should be given with the goal of maintaining adequate intravascular volume while avoiding fluid overload in the edematous or ascitic patient. In some cases, central venous pressure monitoring may be needed to help guide fluid therapy. **Thiamine** (100 mg) should always be given with initial intravenous fluids and dextrose. Vitamin supplements should also be given to any malnourished alcoholic. Correction of electrolyte abnormalities should be initiated (many alcoholic patients will require supplemental magnesium and potassium.)
3. Careful attention to any additional drug therapies must be maintained so as to avoid the use of any hepatotoxic agents and to account for possible alterations in normal drug metabolism.
4. Identified bacterial coinfections should be promptly treated with appropriate parenteral antibiotics and broad spectrum coverage should be initiated in any alcoholic with suspected sepsis, pending culture results (see Chap. 6).

Cirrhosis and Liver Failure

1. Abstinence from alcohol and other hepatotoxins (drugs, etc.) is essential for outpatient management. Adjunctive measures may include salt and water restriction, cautious diuretic use (spironolactone), protein-restricted diet, and therapeutic paracentesis for relief of abdominal distention.
2. Emergency management often includes changing diuretic dosage, correction of fluid or electrolyte abnormalities, and blood transfusion for symptomatic anemia.
3. New onset or worsening encephalopathy warrants hospital admission. Management includes supplemental oxygen, support of perfusion, respiration as needed and supplemental dextrose in intravenous fluids. Precipitating factors such as a coexisting infection, GI bleeding, or renal failure must be carefully investigated and aggressively treated. **Lactulose** (30 mL) may be given

orally by NG tube or by enema, up to 3 times a day until 1 to 2 soft stools per day are produced. Alternatively, neomycin may be given to help clear the gut of bacteria and nitrogenous products.

4. **Cefotaxime** 2 g intravenously followed by 1 to 2 g intravenously every 6 h is the current antibiotic regimen of choice for spontaneous bacterial peritonitis (alternatives include ticarcillin-clavulanate, piperacillin-tazobactam, ampicillin-sulbactam, or the quinolones).

5. Acute liver failure from any cause (with prolonged PT, hypoglycemia, coagulopathy, encephalopathy, marked jaundice, etc.) should warrant admission to the intensive care unit, aggressive treatment, and consultation with a hepatologist and transplant team if available.

6. Any cirrhotic patient whose clinical stability is in doubt should always be considered for admission. All patients with clearly decompensated cirrhosis, fever, hypothermia, or complications such as concurrent infection, SBP, GI bleeding, encephalopathy, and acute or worsening renal function should be admitted.

7. Discharged patients should have timely follow-up arranged with their primary care provider and should be given careful instructions to return for any worsening of their baseline status or for such symptoms such as abdominal pain, fever, melena, hematemesis, vomiting, worsening diarrhea, or mental status changes.

For further reading in *Emergency Medicine: A Comprehensive Study Guide,* 5th ed., see Chap. 80, "Jaundice," by Richard O. Shields, Jr., and Chap. 82, "Hepatic Disorders and Hepatic Failure," by Rawden W. Evans.

---

48 | Cholecystitis and Biliary Colic
Gregory S. Hall

Biliary tract emergencies most often result from obstruction of the gallbladder or biliary duct by gallstones. The four most common biliary tract emergencies caused by gallstones include biliary colic, cholecystitis, gallstone pancreatitis, and ascending cholangitis. The first two, biliary colic and cholecystitis, are more frequently encountered in patients at emergency departments. Gallstones, though common in the general population, remain asymptomatic in some patients. Classically, the patient with symptomatic gallstone disease is an obese, fertile female between 20 and 40 years of age. Biliary disease, however, can affect all age groups, especially those with diabetes and the elderly. Common risk factors associated with gallstones and cholecystitis include increased age, female sex and parity, obesity, familial tendency, oral contraceptives, clofibrate, Asian descent, chronic liver disease, sickle cell anemia, and hereditary spherocytosis.

Clinical Features

Patients with acute biliary colic may have a wide range of symptoms and, unfortunately, the location, radiation, and duration of their abdominal pain is not always a reliable guide to the presence of gallbladder disease. Biliary colic may present with either epigastric or right upper quadrant pain, which may range from mild to severe, and, while classically described as intermittent or colicky, may instead be constant. It is often accompanied by nausea and vomiting. Pain may be referred to the right shoulder or left upper back. It may begin after eating but bears no association to meals in at least one-third of patients. Acute episodes of biliary colic typically last for 2 to 6 h, followed by a gradual or sudden resolution of symptoms. Often patients experience some mild residual abdominal soreness or aching for another 24 h. Recurrent episodes are usually infrequent, generally at intervals of greater than 1 week. Biliary colic seems to follow a circadian pattern with highest incidence of symptoms between 9 P.M. and 4 A.M. At presentation, physical exam commonly reveals right upper quadrant or epigastric tenderness without findings of peritonitis. Volume depletion due to emesis may be evident. Symptoms and findings are easy to confuse with dyspepsia, peptic ulcer disease, gastritis, and esophageal reflux.

Acute cholecystitis presents with pain similar to biliary colic that persists for longer than the typical 6 h of colic. Fever, chills, nausea, emesis, and anorexia are common. Past history of similar attacks or known gallstones may be reported. As the gallbladder becomes progressively inflamed, the initial poorly localized upper abdominal pain often becomes sharp and localized to the right upper quadrant. The patient may have moderate-to-severe distress and may appear toxic. Other findings may include abdominal distention, hypoactive bowel sounds, and Murphy's sign—increased pain or inspiratory arrest during deep subcostal palpation of the right upper quadrant during deep inspiration. Generalized abdominal rigidity, though rare, suggests perforation and diffuse peritonitis if present. Volume depletion is common, but jaundice is unusual. Acalculous cholecystitis occurs in 5 to 10 percent of patients with cholecystitis, has a more rapid, aggressive clinical course, and occurs more frequently in patients with diabetes, the elderly, trauma or burn victims, following prolonged labor or major surgery, or with systemic vasculitides.

Depending on the population studied, biliary calculi are involved in 30 to 70 percent of cases of acute pancreatitis. Of all patients with gallstones, 15 to 20 percent will develop pancreatitis due to obstruction of the ampulla of Vater by a stone. Clinical presentation will be similar to other forms of pancreatitis, including epigastric or diffuse abdominal pain radiating to the back, nausea, emesis, and fever. Acute cholecystitis may be concurrently present. Ascending cholangitis, a life-threatening condition with high mortality, results from complete biliary obstruction (often a common duct stone, less commonly a tumor) with bacterial superinfection and septicemia. Patients often present in extremis with jaundice, fever, mental confusion, and shock. Charcot's triad of fever, jaundice, and right upper quadrant pain is suggestive, but all 3 features may be present in only 25 percent of patients.

Diagnosis and Differential

Suspicion of gallbladder or biliary tract disease must be maintained in any patient at risk with upper abdominal pain. Patients with uncomplicated biliary colic usually have normal laboratory findings. Laboratory studies that may aid in diagnosis include a white blood cell count (WBC)—leukocytosis with left shift suggests acute cholecystis, pancreatitis, or cholangitis, but a normal WBC does not exclude them. With either biliary colic or cholecystitis, serum bilirubin and alkaline phosphatase levels may be normal or mildly elevated. Serum amylase and/or lipase levels should be checked to exclude pancreatitis. Urinalysis with sediment exam should be performed to rule out urinary tract infection, and all women of child-bearing potential should have a serum or urine pregnancy test to rule out obstetrical causes of abdominal pain. Levels of serum electrolytes, glucose, blood urea nitrogen, and creatinine should be obtained to exclude diabetic ketoacidosis and may aid evaluation of the patient's volume status. Pain x-ray films of the abdomen may reveal other causes of upper abdominal pain (e.g., bowel obstruction), but gallstones will be radiopaque in only 10 to 20 percent. Chest x-rays may aid in excluding right lower lobe pneumonia or pleural effusion. A 12-lead electrocardiogram should be obtained in older patients to rule out myocardial infarction or ischemia.

Ultrasound scan of the hepatobiliary tract is presently the initial diagnostic study of choice for patients suspected of biliary colic or obstruction. It can detect stones as small as 2 mm as well as signs of cholecystitis—thickened gallbladder wall, gallbladder distention, and pericholecystic fluid. A positive sonographic Murphy's sign, if elicited during the scan, is highly suggestive of cholecystitis.

Computed tomography (CT) scanning of the abdomen is most useful when other intraabdominal processes are suspected in the differential diagnosis. Gallstones, wall thickening, and pericholecystic fluid may all be found, but unfortunately CT has only 50 percent sensitivity for cholecystitis. Radionuclide cholescintigraphy (HIDA or DISIDA scans) offers a sensitivity of 97 percent and a specificity of 90 percent for cholecystitis. A reasonable emergency department approach to suspected cholecystitis would be to first obtain an ultrasound scan, followed by a radionuclide scan only if ultrasound fails to establish the diagnosis.

The differential diagnosis of patients with upper abdominal pain must include gastritis, peptic ulcer, hepatitis or hepatic abscess, pancreatitis, Fitz-Hugh-Curtis syndrome, pelvic inflammatory disease with or without abscess, pyelonephritis, pleurisy-pneumonia, acute myocardial infarction and diabetic ketoacidosis.

Emergency Department Care and Disposition

Emergency department management of any patient with abdominal pain should always begin with the ABCs of resuscitation and supportive care. Uncomplicated biliary colic will resolve spontaneously, while cholecystitis, pancreatitis, and cholangitis require hospital admission.

1. Isotonic crystalloid intravenous fluids should be given to correct volume deficits and electrolyte imbalances. Septic shock, if present, should be aggressively resuscitated with crystalloids and intravenous vasopressors if necessary to support perfusion.
2. Symptomatic treatment for emesis is best achieved with antiemetics (**promethazine** 12.5 to 25 mg intravenously) or antispasmodics (glycopyrrolate 0.1 mg intravenously). Gastric decompression with nasogastric tube suctioning should be instituted if vomiting is intractable.

3. For analgesia, **meperidine**, 0.5 to 1.0 mg/kg intravenously or intramuscularly, is preferred over other opiates because it causes less spasm of the sphincter of Oddi. **Ketorolac tromethamine,** 15 to 30 mg intravenously or 30 to 60 mg intramuscularly, may help relieve the pain of gallbladder distention in patients without cholecystitis.

4. Early antibiotic therapy should be initiated in any patient suspected of cholecystitis. Single-agent therapy with a parenteral third-generation cephalosporin (**cefotaxime** 1 to 2 g intravenously every 8 h, **ceftazidime** 1 to 2 g intravenously every 8 h, **ceftizoxime** 1 to 2 g intravenously every 8 to 12 h, or **ceftriaxone** 1 to 2 g intravenously every 24 h in single or every 12 h in divided doses) may be adequate for patients without sepsis. Those with sepsis or obvious peritonitis are best managed with triple coverage using **ampicillin** (0.5 to 1.0 g intravenously every 6 h), **gentamicin** (3 mg/kg/d intravenously divided every 8 h) and **clindamycin** (1200 to 2700 mg/d intravenously divided into 2, 3, or 4 equal doses), or the equivalent substitutes (e.g., metronidazole for clindamycin, third-generation cephalosporins or piperacillin/tazobactam for ampicillin, etc.)

5. Patients diagnosed with acute cholecystitis, gallstone pancreatitis, or ascending cholangitis require immediate surgical consultation with hospital admission. Signs of systemic toxicity or sepsis warrant admission to the intensive care unit pending surgical treatment.

6. Patients accurately diagnosed with uncomplicated biliary colic whose symptoms abate with supportive therapy within 4 to 6 h of onset can be discharged home if they are able to maintain oral hydration. Oral narcotic-acetoaminophen analgesics may be prescribed for the next 24 to 48 h for the common residual abdominal aching. Timely outpatient follow-up should be arranged with a surgical consultant or the patient's primary care physician. The patient should be carefully instructed to return to the emergency department if fever develops, abdominal pain worsens, intractable vomiting returns, or another significant attack occurs prior to follow-up.

For further reading in *Emergency Medicine: A Comprehensive Study Guide,* 5th ed., see Chap. 81, "Cholecystitis and Biliary Colic," by Tom P. Aufderheide, William J. Brady, and Judith E. Tintinalli.

49 | Acute Pancreatitis
Michael E. Chansky

Acute pancreatitis (AP) is a common cause of abdominal pain, and the diagnosis is primarily made based on clinical presentation. The severity of the disease may range from mild glandular edema to frank necrosis and hemorrhage and is most often related to alcohol abuse, cholelithiasis, and trauma (Table 49-1).

Clinical Features

Symptoms are dependent on the degree of glandular destruction. The typical presentation includes midepigastric constant boring pain radiating to the back, which is associated with nausea, vomiting, abdominal distention, and hyperamylasemia or high serum lipase. Refractory hypotensive shock, blood loss, hypocalcemia, prerenal azotemia, and respiratory failure may accompany the most severe forms. The patient is usually in moderate distress with tachycardia and epigastric tenderness.

Diagnosis and Differential

The diagnosis must be suspected by the history, examination, and presence of abnormal laboratory tests, which most often reveal nonspecific elevations of serum amylase and lipase. Amylase is primarily found in the pancreas and salivary glands, but lower levels exist in fallopian tubes, ovaries, testes, lung, and small bowel. Unfortunately elevated amylase may have an extra pancreatic source, and AP may present with a normal amylase. Most studies suggest a sensitivity of 80 to 90 percent and, at a level of 3 times the upper limit of normal, a specificity of 75 percent. Lipase has a longer half-life than amylase (7 versus 2 h), is more accurate in the diagnosis of AP, and can be utilized without a serum amylase study in patients with undifferentiated abdominal pain. As with most inflammatory conditions, leukocytosis is usually present, but rarely exceeds 20,000 per milliliter in uncomplicated AP. An elevated blood urea nitrogen level is common secondary to third spacing, and an elevated alkaline phosphatase level suggests biliary disease. Persistent hypocalcemia (< 7 mg per 100 mL), hypoxia, and metabolic acidosis are associated with poor prognosis.

Plain radiographs play little role in the diagnosis of AP, although calcification, when present, suggests preexisting pancreatic disease. Their role is to exclude other diseases in the differential. Patients

TABLE 49-1 Common Etiologic or Contributing Factors in
Acute Pancreatitis

Ethanol ingestion

Biliary tract disease

Trauma, penetrating or blunt

Penetrating peptic ulcer

Following endoscopic procedures

Obstruction secondary to neoplasms, diverticula, and polyps

Metabolic disturbances
  Hyperlipemia (Frederickson types I, IV, V)
  Hypercalcemia
  Diabetes mellitus, diabetic ketoacidosis
  Uremia

Viral Infections
  Viral hepatitis
  Infectious mononucleosis
  Coxsackie group B
  HIV

Pregnancy—any trimester, postpartum

Collagen vascular disease

Liver disease

Generalized infections

Drugs
  Oral contraceptives
  Azathioprine
  Glucocorticoids
  Tetracyclines
  Isonazid
  Indomethacin
  Thiazides
  Salicylates
  Calcium
  Warfarin

with AP may have a partial ileus or gaseous distention of the colon
with a distally collapsed colon. The hypoxic patient may show
signs of adult respiratory distress syndrome (ARDS) or a left
pleural effusion. Ultrasound may identify diagnostic gallstones or
biliary tree dilation, but lacks diagnostic value in other etiologies
of AP. A computed tomography scan may reveal edema indicative
of AP but lacks sensitivity in mild or early disease.

The differential diagnosis of AP includes left lower lobe pneumonia, rupture of a pseudocyst, gallbladder disease (cholecystitis or choledocholithiasis), peritonitis (appendicitis, diverticulitis, or perforated viscus), peptic ulcer disease (gastritis or gastric outlet obstruction), small bowel obstruction, renal colic, dissecting aortic aneurysm, diabetic ketoacidosis, and gastroenteritis. AP may be a difficult diagnosis to establish, and repeated observation and surgical consultation is often necessary.

Emergency Department Care and Disposition

Treatment of AP revolves around fluid resuscitation, prevention of vomiting, pain control, and pancreatic rest (nothing per oral, NPO).

1. **Crystalloid intravenous fluids** are the mainstay of treatment, along with bolus normal saline to maintain blood pressure and adequate urine output. A central venous pressure or Swan-Ganz catheter should be considered if the patient is hypoxic with ARDS on chest film or has hypotension unresponsive to aggressive fluid resuscitation and pressor support.
2. **Oxygen** should be administered to maintain a pulse-oximetry reading of 95% oxygen saturation. Respiratory failure is rare but a well-described complication of AP.
3. A **nasogastric tube** (NG) to low suction should be considered if the patient is distended or actively vomiting. The NG tube theoretically reduces pancreatic stimulation and prevents vomiting, although no controlled trial has shown its value.
4. Parenteral analgesia and antiemetics are often necessary for patient comfort. Intravenous or intramuscular narcotics should be used on a short term basis. H_2 blockers are frequently utilized but have no proven benefit.
5. Patients with acute biliary obstruction may require urgent decompression via endoscopic sphincterotomy of the ampulla of Vater.
6. Prophylaxis for alcohol withdrawal in the appropriate setting is indicated.
7. Patients with severe systemic disease will require intubation, intensive monitoring, Foley catheterization, and transfusion of blood and blood products as needed. Peritoneal lavage should be considered for ill patients who fail to respond to initial supportive measures.

Patients with mild AP may be managed as outpatients with close follow-up provided they can tolerate clear liquids and oral analgesics. Most patients will require hospital floor admission to a medical or surgical service. Patients who demonstrate poor prognostic signs (dropping hemoglobin, poor urine output, persistent hypotension, hypoxia, acidosis, and hypocalcemia) despite aggressive early treatment should be admitted to the intensive care unit with surgical consultation.

For further reading in *Emergency Medicine: A Comprehensive Study Guide,* 5th ed., see Chap. 83, "Acute and Chronic Pancreatitis," by Robert J. Vissers and Riyad B. Abu-Laban.

---

50 | Complications of General and Urologic Surgical Procedures

N. Heramba Prasad

Outpatient surgical procedures are becoming increasingly common. Emergency physicians, therefore, will see more and more postoperative complications. Fever, respiratory complications, genitourinary complaints, wound infections, vascular problems, and complications of drug therapy are some common postoperative disorders seen in the emergency department (ED). Most of these are discussed elsewhere in this book; certain specific problems will be mentioned here. The causes of postoperative fever are listed as the five Ws: *W*ind (respiratory), *W*ater urinary tract infection (UTI), *W*ound, *W*alking deep venous thrombosis (DVT), and *W*onder drugs (pseudomembranous colitis, PMC).

Clinical Features

Fever in the first 24 h is usually due to atelectasis, necrotizing fasciitis, or clostridial infections. In the 24 to 72 h period, pneumonia, atelectasis, intravenous-catheter-related thrombophlebitis, and infections are the major causes. UTIs are seen 3 to 5 days postoperatively. DVT typically occurs 5 days after the procedure, and wound infections generally manifest 7 to 10 days after surgery. Antibiotic-induced PMC is seen 6 weeks after surgery.

Respiratory Complications

Postoperative pain and inadequate clearance of secretions contribute to the development of atelectasis. Fever, tachypnea, tachycardia, and mild hypoxia are usually seen. Pneumonia may develop 24 to 96 h later. Hypoxia widened A-a gradient and respiratory distress should point to the diagnosis of pulmonary embolism (see Chap. 26 for diagnosis and management).

Genitourinary Complications

UTIs are more common after instrumentation of the urinary tract. Urinary retention occurs in 4 percent of all surgical patients and in 60 percent of patients after urethral surgery. It is more common in elderly males, especially after excessive fluid administration and after spinal anesthesia. Lower abdominal pain, urgency, and inability to void should alert the clinician to suspect urinary retention. Oliguria or anuria commonly results from volume depletion. Intrinsic factors such as acute tubular necrosis (ATN), drug nephrotoxicity, and postrenal obstructive uropathy also may lead to acute renal failure.

Wound Complications

Hematomas result from inadequate hemostasis. Careful evaluation to rule out infections must be undertaken. Seromas are collections of clear fluid under the wound. Extremes of age, diabetes, poor nutrition, necrotic tissue, poor perfusion, foreign bodies, and wound hematomas contribute to the development of wound infections. Necrotizing fasciitis is characterized by extremely painful, erythematous, swollen, and warm areas without sharp margins. This staphylococcal infection spreads rapidly. Patients will exhibit marked systemic toxicity, and crepitance and bullae may be present. Wound dehiscence can occur due to diabetes, poor nutrition, chronic steroid use, and inadequate or improper closure of the wound. Dehiscence of an abdominal wound may result in evisceration of abdominal organs.

Vascular Complications

Superficial thrombophlebitis usually occurs in the upper extremities after intravenous catheter insertion or in the lower extremities because of stasis and varicosity of veins. DVT commonly occurs in the lower extremities. Swelling and pain of the calf are commonly encountered. (See Chap. 29 for diagnosis and management.)

Drug Therapy Complications

Many drugs are known to cause fever and antibiotic-induced diarrhea. PMC, a dreaded complication, is caused by *Clostridium difficile* toxin. Bloody, watery diarrhea, fever, and crampy abdominal pain are the usual complaints.

Diagnosis and Differential

Patients with suspected respiratory complications should have chest x-rays. They may reveal platelike or discoid atelectases, pneumonia, or pneumothorax. Pneumothorax occurs early after certain surgical procedures or catheter insertion, and a chest x-ray will help confirm the diagnosis.

Patients with oliguria or anuria should be evaluated for signs of hypovolemia or urinary retention. Diagnosis of PMC is established by demonstrating *C. difficile* cytotoxin in the stool. In 27 percent of the cases, however, the assay can be negative.

Emergency Department Care and Disposition

Always discuss patients and proposed treatments with the surgeon who initially cared for the patients. Although debilitated patients may need hospitalization, many patients with atelectasis can be treated as outpatients. Postoperative pneumonia is polymicrobial, and an antipseudomonas antibiotic with an aminoglycoside is usually recommended. Most patients with UTI can be managed as outpatients with oral antibiotic therapy (see Chap. 53).

Insertion of a Foley catheter and prompt drainage will alleviate urinary retention. There is no need for clamping the catheter periodically. Prophylactic antibiotics are reserved for patients who have had urinary tract instrumentation, those with prolonged retention, and those at risk for infection.

Wound hematomas may require removal of some sutures and evacuation. Surgical consultation before treatment is appropriate. Seromas can be treated with needle aspiration and wound cultures. Admission may not always be necessary.

Most wound infections can be treated with oral antibiotics (usually the surgeon's choice), unless patients manifest systemic symptoms and signs. Perineal infections usually require hospital admission and parenteral antibiotics. As surgical débridement and parenteral antibiotics are indicated for necrotizing fasciitis, physicians should start **clindamycin** 900 mg and **penicillin G,** 6 million units intravenously.

Most patients with superficial thrombophlebitis can be treated with local heat and elevation of the affected area, if there is no evidence of cellulitis or lymphangitis. Patients with suppurative thrombophlebitis, characterized by erythema, lymphangitis, fever, and severe pain, should be hospitalized and treated with excision of the affected vein.

Fluid resuscitation, oral vancomycin, and metronidazole, orally or intravenously, are currently available treatment modalities for drug-induced PMC (see Chap. 46, "Vomiting, Diarrhea, and Constipation").

SPECIFIC CONSIDERATIONS

Complications of Breast Surgery

Wound infections, hematomas, pneumothorax, necrosis of the skin flaps, and lymphedema of the arms after mastectomy are common problems seen after breast surgery. Lymphedema of the arm occurs in 5 to 10 percent of patients. Elevation and minor activity restriction will help reduce swelling.

Complications of Gastrointestinal Surgery

Intestinal obstruction. Neuronal dysfunction following any surgery where the peritoneum is entered causes paralytic ileus. Following gastrointestinal (GI) surgery, small bowel tone returns to normal within 24 h, gastric function within 2 days, and colonic function within 3 days.

Prolonged ileus should alert clinicians to peritonitis, abscesses, hemoperitoneum, pneumonia, sepsis, and electrolyte imbalance. Clinical features include nausea, vomiting, obstipation, constipation, abdominal distention, and pain.

Abdominal x-rays; complete blood cell count; electrolyte, blood urea nitrogen, and creatinine levels; and urinalysis should be obtained. Treatment of adynamic ileus consists of nasogastric suction, bowel rest, and hydration. Mechanical obstruction is usually due to adhesions and may require surgical intervention.

Intraabdominal abscesses are caused by preoperative contamination or postoperative anastomotic leaks. Diagnosis can be confirmed by computed tomography (CT) scan or ultrasonography. Surgical exploration, evacuation, and parenteral antibiotics will be required.

Pancreatitis occurs especially after direct manipulation of the pancreatic duct. Patients typically have nausea, vomiting, abdominal pain, and leukocytosis. Lumbar pain, left pleural effusion, Turner's sign (discoloration of the flank), and Cullen's sign (periumbilical ecchymosis) may be present. Serum amylase and lipase levels are usually elevated. (See Chap. 49 for management.)

Cholecystitis and biliary colic have been reported as postoperative complications. Elderly patients are more prone to develop acalculous cholecystitis.

Fistulas, either internal or external, may result from direct bowel injury and require surgical consultation and hospitalization. *Anastomotic leaks* are especially devastating after esophageal or colon surgery. Esophageal leaks occur 10 days after the procedure. Dramatic presentation with shock, pneumothorax, and pleural effusion is usually seen.

Dumping syndrome is noticed in gastric bypass procedures. It is due to the sudden influx of hyperosmolar chyle into the small intestine resulting in fluid sequestration and hypovolemia. Patients experience nausea, vomiting, epigastric discomfort, palpitations, dizziness, and sometimes syncope.

Alkaline reflux gastritis is caused by the reflux of bile into the stomach. Endoscopic evaluation will establish the diagnosis. Postvagotomy diarrhea and afferent loop syndrome are seen in some patients.

Complications of percutaneous endoscopic gastrostomy (PEG) tubes include infections, hemorrhage, peritonitis, aspiration, wound dehiscence, sepsis, and obstruction of the tube.

Complications arising from stomas are due to technical errors or from underlying diseases such as Crohn's disease and cancer. Ischemia, necrosis, bleeding, hernia, and prolapse are sometimes seen.

Colonoscopy may cause hemorrhage, perforation, retroperitoneal abscesses, pneumoscrotum, pneumothorax, volvulus, and infection.

Rectal surgery complications include urinary retention, constipation, prolapse, bleeding, and infections.

Finally, tetanus has been known to occur following surgical wounds.

Complications of Urologic Surgery

Epididymitis, scrotal swelling, and hemorrhage are sometimes seen following vasectomies. Hematuria, urinary retention, strictures, and infections may occur following prostate surgery. After extracorporeal shockwave lithotripsy, pain and hematuria persist for some time. Suspected perineal hematomas from subcapsular renal hemorrhage can be confirmed by CT or ultrasonography. Ureteric reobstruction from stone fragments can be diagnosed by intravenous pylogram. UTIs occur infrequently.

For further reading in *Emergency Medicine: A Comprehensive Study Guide,* 5th ed., see Chap. 84, "Complications of General Surgical Procedures," by Edmond A. Hooker; and Chap. 94, "Complications of Urologic Procedures," by Elaine B. Josephson and Anthony Gomez.

SECTION 8

RENAL AND GENITOURINARY DISORDERS

51 | Acute Renal Failure

Marc D. Squillante

Renal dysfunction and acute renal failure (ARF) present with a wide variety of manifestations, depending on the underlying etiology. Although the initial symptoms may be those of the primary cause, ultimately patients will develop deterioration of renal function. Risk factors include cardiac disease, hypovolemia from any cause, vascular or thrombotic disorders, glomerular diseases, diseases affecting the renal tubules, use of nephrotoxic drugs, and a variety of anatomic problems of the genitourinary tract.

Clinical Features

Deterioration in renal function leads to excessive accumulation of nitrogenous waste products in the serum. ARF can be classified as *oliguric* (< 400 mL urine per 24 h) and *nonoliguric* (> 400 mL per 24 h). Patients usually have signs and symptoms of their underlying causative disorder, but eventually develop stigmata of renal failure. Volume overload, hypertension, pulmonary edema, mental status changes or neurologic symptoms, nausea and vomiting, bone and joint problems, anemia, and increased susceptibility to infection (a leading cause of death) can occur, as patients develop more chronic uremia.

Diagnosis and Differential

History and physical examination usually provide clues to etiology. Signs and symptoms of the underlying causative disorder (Table 51-1) should be vigorously sought. Physical exam should assess vital signs, volume status, establish urinary tract patency and output, and search for signs of chemical intoxication, drug usage, muscle damage, or associated systemic diseases. Diagnostic studies

TABLE 51-1 Common Causes of Acute Renal Failure (ARF)

Prerenal	Renal	Postrenal
Decreased cardiac output	Vascular/ischemia	Penile lesions
Myocardial ischemia/infarction	Renal vasculature thrombosis, TTP, DIC,	Phimosis
Valvular heart disease	NSAIDs, severe hypertension, hemolytic-uremic	Meatal stenosis
Cardiomyopathy	syndrome	Urethral stricture
Pericardial tamponade		
High-output failure	Glomerular	Prostatic enlargement—BPH, cancer
	Primary glomerular diseases (acute	
Hypovolemia	glomerulonephritis), or systemic disease with	Upper urinary tract/ureteral diseases (usually
Blood loss/hemorrhagic shock	glomerular involvement (SLE, vasculitis, HSP,	requires bilateral involvement/obstruction)
Vomiting/diarrhea	endocarditis)	Calculi, tumors, blood clots
Diuretics		Papillary necrosis
Postobstructive diuresis	Tubulointerstitial	Vesicoureteral reflux
Fluid sequestration	Ischemic ATN, rhabdomyolysis, toxin induced	Stricture
Cirrhosis	tubular damage (aminoglycosides, radio	AAA
Pancreatitis	contrast, solvents, heavy metals, ethylene	Retroperitoneal fibrosis
Burns	glycol, myoglobin/hemoglobin), acute interstitial	
General anesthesia	nephritis, infiltrative and autoimmune diseases,	
Septic shock	infectious agents	

Abbreviations: DIC, disseminated intramuscular coagulation; NSAIDs, nonsteroidal anti-inflammatory agents; ATN, acute tubular necrosis; TTP, thrombotic thrombocytopenic purpura; SLE, systemic lupus erythematosus; HSP, Henoch-Schönlein purpura; BPH, benign prostatic hypertrophy; AAA, abdominal aortic aneurysm.

include urinalysis; blood urea nitrogen (BUN) and creatinine levels, serum electrolyte levels, urinary sodium and creatinine levels, and urinary osmolality. Analysis of these tests allows most patients to be placed in either the prerenal, renal, or postrenal group. Fractional excretion of sodium and renal failure index can be calculated to help in this categorization (Table 51-2). Normal urinary sediment may be seen in prerenal and postrenal failure, hemolytic-uremic syndrome, and thrombotic thrombocytopenic purpura. The presence of albumin may indicate glomerulonephritis or malignant hypertension. Granular casts are seen in acute tubular necrosis (ATN), glomerulonephritis, and interstitial nephritis. Albumin and red blood cell casts are found in both glomerulonephritis and malignant hypertension. White blood cell casts are seen in interstitial nephritis and pyelonephritis. Crystals can be present with renal calculi and certain drugs (sulfas, ethylene glycol, and radio contrast agents). Ultrasonography is the radiologic procedure of choice in most patients with acute renal failure when hydronephrosis is suspected.

Prerenal failure is produced by conditions that decrease renal perfusion (Table 51-1). Prerenal failure is a common precursor to

TABLE 51-2 Laboratory Studies Aiding in the Differential Diagnosis of Acute Renal Failure

Test employed	Prerenal	Renal[a]	Postrenal[b]
Urine sodium (meq/L)	< 20	> 40	> 40
FE_{Na} (%)[c]	< 1	> 1	> 1
Renal failure index (RFI)[d]	< 1	> 1	> 1
Urine osmolality (mosm/L)	> 500	< 350	< 350
Urine/serum creatinine ratio	> 40:1	< 20:1	< 20:1
Serum urea nitrogen/creatinine ratio	> 20:1	= 10:1	> 10:1

[a] FE_{Na} may be < 1 in intrinsic renal failure patients with glomerulonephritis, hepatorenal syndrome, radio contrast acute tubular necrosis, myoglobinuric and hemoglobinuric acute renal failure, renal allograft rejection, and with certain drugs (captopril and nonsteroid antiinflammatory agents).

[b] Can see indices similar to prerenal early in course of obstruction. With continued obstruction, tubular function is impaired and indices mimic those of renal causes.

[c] Fractional excretion of sodium (%) = $\dfrac{\text{Urine sodium/serum sodium}}{\text{Urine creatinine/serum creatinine}} \times 100$

[d] RFI = $\dfrac{\text{Serum sodium}}{\text{Urine creatinine/serum creatinine}} \times 100$

ischemic and nephrotoxic causes of intrinsic renal failure, as well as an independent cause of ARF. Prerenal failure is the most common cause of ARF (in 40 to 80 percent of cases). *Intrinsic renal failure* have vascular and ischemic etiologies; glomerular and tubulointerstitial diseases are causative as well. ATN due to severe and prolonged prerenal etiologies causes most cases of intrinsic renal failure. Nephrotoxins are the second most common cause of ATN. *Postrenal azotemia* occurs primarily in elderly men with high-grade prostatic obstruction. Lesions of the external genitalia (i.e., strictures) are also common causes.

Emergency Department Care and Disposition

Initial care of patients with ARF focuses on treating the underlying cause and correcting fluid and electrolyte derangement. Efforts should be made to prevent further renal damage and provide supportive care until renal function has recovered. (See Chap. 4 for treatment of electrolyte and acid base disorders.)

Prerenal Failure

Effective intravascular volume should be restored with isotonic fluids (normal saline and lactated Ringer's) at a rapid rate in appropriate patients. If cardiac failure is causing prerenal azotemia, intravascular volume should be reduced (i.e., with diuretics) to improve cardiac output and renal perfusion.

Postrenal Failure

Appropriate urinary drainage should be established. The exact procedure will vary depending on the level of obstruction. A Foley catheter should be placed to relieve obstruction caused by prostatic hypertrophy. Percutaneous nephrostomy may be required for ureteral occlusion until definitive surgery to correct the obstruction can take place when the patient's status is stabilized. For the acutely anuric patient, obstruction is the major consideration. If no urine is obtained on initial bladder catheterization, emergency urologic consultation should be considered. With chronic urinary retention, postobstructive diuresis may occur due to osmotic diuresis or tubular dysfunction. Patients may become suddenly hypovolemic and hypotensive. Urine output must be closely monitored, with appropriate fluid replacement.

Renal Failure

ATN from ischemia or nephrotoxic agents is the most common cause of intrinsic ARF. History, physical exam, and baseline laboratory tests should provide clues to the diagnosis. Nephrotoxic agents (drugs and intravenous contrast) should be avoided. Diuretics (i.e., **furosemide** 20 to 80 mg intravenously) occasionally can augment diuresis and convert oliguric into nonoliguric renal failure. Patients with nonoliguric ARF have improved mortality and renal function recovery. (Volume must be restored in these patients before using diuretics.) Low-dose **dopamine** (1 to 5 μg/kg/min) may improve renal blood flow and urine output, but does not lower mortality rates or improve recovery. It is probably best used in ARF patients with congestive heart failure. Mannitol may be protective against myoglobinuric ARF in early rhabdomyolysis.

Adequate circulating volume must be restored first. Renally excreted drugs (digoxin, magnesium, sedatives, and narcotics) should be used with caution since therapeutic doses may accumulate to excess and cause serious side effects. Fluid restriction (500 mL plus daily urine output) may be required.

Dialysis

If treatment of the underlying cause fails to improve renal function, hemodialysis or peritoneal dialysis should be considered. Decisions about dialysis are usually made by the nephrology consultant. Dialysis is often initiated when the BUN level is > 100 mg/dL or the serum creatinine level is > 10 mg/dL. Patients with complications of ARF such as cardiac instability (due to metabolic acidosis and hyperkalemia), intractable volume overload, hyperkalemia, and uremia (i.e., encephalopathy, pericarditis, and bleeding diathesis) not easily corrected by other measures should be considered for emergency dialysis.

Disposition

Patients with new-onset ARF usually require hospital admission, often to an intensive care unit. Transferring patients to another institution should be considered if nephrology consultation and dialysis facilities are not available.

For further reading in *Emergency Medicine: A Comprehensive Study Guide,* 5th ed., see Chap. 88, "Acute Renal Failure," by Richard Sinert.

52 | Emergencies in Dialysis Patients

David M. Cline

Dialysis patients sustain multiple complications of their disease process and treatment. (See the appropriate chapters for discussion on the management of hypertension, heart failure, bleeding disorders, and electrolyte disorders.)

UREMIC PERICARDITIS

The classic symptom is chest pain, which is partially relieved by sitting up and leaning forward. A pericardial friction rub may not be heard or may be heard intermittently. Low-grade fever and atrial arrhythmias (paroxysmal atrial tachycardia, atrial flutter–atrial fibrillation) are common as well. Echocardiography often demonstrates a pericardial effusion. The pericardial fluid may impede venous return, leading to congestive heart failure and hypotension. Treatment of simple pericarditis in uremic patients is intensive dialysis. Symptomatic tamponade is relieved by pericardiocentesis.

CARDIAC ARRHYTHMIAS AND CARDIAC ARREST

The most common cause of cardiac arrest in uremic patients is hyperkalemia. The treatment should include administration of calcium gluconate (10 mL of 10% solution), followed by infusion of 50 mL of 50% glucose, along with 20 U of regular insulin, and infusion of 50 to 100 meq of intravenous sodium bicarbonate. Hemo- or peritoneal dialysis, using a lower concentration of $K+$ in the dialysate, is the most effective way to reduce the potassium level and should be employed as soon as possible.

HYPOTENSION

A sudden drop in blood pressure is a common complication during dialysis and, if not promptly treated, can lead to cardiac arrest. Subjective symptoms such as muscle cramps, nausea, yawning, and mental confusion may precede the actual hypotension in most patients, but not in all. Treatment consists of the rapid infusion of isotonic saline. Patients usually respond to 500 mL or less. In rare instances, the use of vasopressors may be required. Other causes of hypotension, including pericardial disease, sepsis, gastrointestinal (GI) bleeding, or cardiac dysfunction, should be ruled out.

NEUROLOGIC COMPLICATIONS

Uremic encephalopathy presents with cognitive defects, memory loss, slurred speech, and asterixis. The progressive neurologic symptoms of uremia are the most common indications for initiating dialysis. Dialysis disequilibrium demonstrated by symptoms of increased intracranial pressure, including nausea, vomiting, headache, and mental confusion, can develop soon after or within a few hours of a dialysis treatment. It is common after first dialysis, but also can occur on a rare occasion, even in patients treated with chronic dialysis. Therapy is mannitol 0.5 gm/kg intravenously. Subdural hematoma is more common in hemodialysis patients and should be differentiated from the above disorders with a computed tomography scan.

GASTROINTESTINAL DISORDERS

Upper GI bleeding may result from uremic gastritis, peptic ulcer disease, or excess anticoagulation. Management does not differ from that in nonuremic patients. Caution should be exercised, however, in using large doses of magnesium-containing antacids. Since magnesium is normally excreted by the kidney, abnormal levels could accumulate in the plasma of the uremic patient, leading to mental obtundation and respiratory depression.

PROBLEMS PECULIAR TO PERITONEAL DIALYSIS

Infection of the peritoneal membrane is the most frequent and critical complication in patients receiving chronic peritoneal dialysis. The symptoms may be subtle and include abdominal discomfort, pain during inflow, and fever. Physical examination may reveal abdominal tenderness, particularly around the catheter site, and decreased bowel sounds. Laboratory evaluation should include complete blood cell count and analysis of peritoneal fluid for cell count, Gram-stain, protein, culture, and sensitivity. A bag of drained dialysate should be used for culture and analysis. A variety of microorganisms (bacterial, fungal, and parasitic) have been found after culturing the fluid from the peritoneal cavity of dialysis patients. The mainstay of therapy is the infusion of an appropriate antimicrobial agent into the peritoneal cavity. Depending upon the results of gram-stain, usually **cephalothin** 500 mg/L is added to the dialysate. Alternatively **vancomycin** (1 g) is given and, possibly, **gentamicin** (100 mg) is added. To avoid fibrin formation 1000 U of heparin are added to the infusion. If a patient experiences recurrent bouts of peritonitis, tunnel infection, or intraabdominal abscess, the catheter should be changed. Appropriate surgical drainage of intraabdominal abscess is also warranted to prevent relapse.

PROBLEMS RELATED TO VASCULAR ACCESS

The most frequent complications associated with the external shunts are clotting and infection. When the shunt is acutely clotted, the vascular surgeon must be notified immediately. Declotting procedures using a Fogarty balloon catheter are normally accomplished by the surgeon in the operating suite. In some instances, however, instillation of urokinase, 5000 to 10,000 U, into the arterial and venous parts of the clotted shunt may dissolve the clot and prevent the need for further intervention.

Infection of the cannula site is a significant problem in the hemodialysis patient. Coagulase-positive staphylococci and *S. epidermidis* are frequently cuultured from the exit site. Physical examination may reveal local inflammation, tenderness over the cannula tips, and purulent drainage at the exit sites. Vancomycin is the drug of choice, 1 g intravenously.

For further reading in *Emergency Medicine: A Comprehensive Study Guide,* 5th ed., see Chap. 89, "Emergencies in Renal Failure and Dialysis Patients," by Richard Sinert.

---

53 | Urinary Tract Infections and Hematuria

Stephen H. Thomas

Urinary tract infection (UTI) is defined as significant bacteriuria in the presence of symptoms. It is a frequently occurring condition accounting for a significant number of emergency department (ED) visits, with acuity ranging from commonplace cystitis to life-threatening gram-negative urosepsis.

Atraumatic hematuria, commonly associated with UTI, can also be seen in a wide variety of other conditions, such as nephrolithiasis or neoplasm. In most cases, the primary goal in management of hematuria is to address the underlying condition.

Clinical Features

The diagnosis of UTI should be considered in patients presenting with dysuria, urinary frequency, lower abdominal pain, and suprapubic tenderness. Fever, chills, malaise, flank pain, and costovertebral angle tenderness (upper tract signs) may occur with lower tract infections but are more likely to be associated with pyelonephritis. Although pyelonephritis may sometimes be difficult to distinguish clinically from lower urinary tract infection, a history of several days of dysuria and frequency followed by upper tract signs is suggestive.

Diagnosis of presence of hematuria is straightforward. In macroscopic hematuria, the patient notes alteration of urine appearance ranging from discoloration to passage of frank blood and clots. Microscopic hematuria is present when urinary red blood cells are identified by analytic (e.g., dipstick or microscope) methods.

Diagnosis and Differential

The first step in establishing the diagnosis of UTI or hematuria is collection of an adequate urine specimen for analysis and culture. A properly performed midstream urine collection enables reliable urinalysis while avoiding discomfort and potential complications (e.g., iatrogenic UTI) of urethral catheterization. In patients who are unable to provide a midstream sample, urethral catheterization is indicated. Inspection and smell of the urine sample provide little useful information except when gross blood or clots are present.

Laboratory analysis of the specimen will provide information on pyuria, bacteriuria, hematuria, and nitrate and leukocyte esterase tests. A urine culture should be obtained in the following settings: pyelonephritis, patients requiring hospitalization, patients with chronic indwelling urinary catheters, and all children and adult males. Significant pyuria corresponds to two to five leukocytes per high-power field (HPF) in a centrifuged specimen. In males, in whom urethritis and prostatitis are the most common causes of pyuria, one to two leukocytes per HPF may be significant. False-negative test results can occur with large urine volumes, self-medication, or obstructed kidneys. Significant hematuria is present when there are more than five red blood cells per HPF. False-positive results may occur with vaginal contamination during menses.

The presence of any bacteria on Gram's stain of uncentrifuged urine is significant, as is the presence of more than 15 bacteria per HPF in a centrifuged sample. False-positive results may occur with vaginal or fecal contamination. False-negative results are common in patients with *Chlamydia* or low-colony-count UTI.

Hematuria may be seen in (hemorrhagic) cystitis. The nitrate test is a specific but insensitive indicator of UTI. Similarly, the leukocyte esterase test suffers from relatively low sensitivity. Thus, the information provided by these tests can be helpful, but their function as screening tools is limited.

The differential diagnosis for UTI includes mechanical or chemical urethritis, urolithiasis, vulvovaginitis, cervicitis, and salpingitis. The differential diagnosis for (atraumatic) hematuria includes (but is not limited to) nephrolithiasis, glomerulonephritis, prostatic hypertrophy, neoplasm, Henoch-Schönlein purpura, and shistosomiasis. Gross hematuria is most often associated with lower tract disease, whereas microscopic hematuria is most commonly seen with upper tract pathology. Hematuria indicated by urine dipstick testing when laboratory microscopy fails to detect red blood cells may be seen in the setting of myoglobinuria (rhabdomyolysis syndrome).

Emergency Department Care and Disposition

Urinary Tract Infection

Primary decisions to be considered in treatment of patients with UTI are whether patients have pyelonephritis and whether patients with pyelonephritis require hospitalization. The majority of patients with UTI have lower tract disease and are treated as outpatients. Indications for culture have been discussed. In patients with hematuria, the issues are the identification and treatment of the specific cause of the hematuria. As is the case with UTI, the majority of patients with atraumatic hematuria can be managed on an outpatient basis. Considerations for ED management and disposition of UTI are primarily related to institution of appropriate antibiotic therapy and determination of which patients warrant hospitalization.

1. The most common etiologic agents of UTI are *Escherichia coli* (over 80 percent of cases) and other gram-negative organisms. To cover these, initial oral antibiotic therapy should usually consist of 10 d of one of the following: **cotrimoxazole** 1 double-strength tablet bid; **nitrofurantoin** 100 mg qid; **amoxicillin-clavulanate** 875/125 mg bid, or a **quinolone** such as ciprofloxacin 250 to 500 mg bid.
2. Shorter (3-d) courses of therapy may be appropriate for certain patient populations with uncomplicated lower tract UTI.
3. Patients with new sexual partners, sexual partners with urethritis, signs or symptoms of cervicitis, or pyuria without bacteriuria should be treated with **doxycycline** 100 mg bid for 10 d and cultured for gonococcus.

4. Bacteriuria and symptoms should dissipate within 24 to 48 h. A short course of a urinary tract anesthetic (**phenazopyridine** 200 mg tid) should be considered when patients have significant dysuria.
5. The decision to admit patients with pyelonephritis is based on age, host factors, and response to initial ED interventions. Unremitting fever and loss of vasomotor tone are indications for admission, as are intractable nausea and vomiting. Intravenous antibiotic choices for these patients are **trimethoprim-sulfamethoxazole** (TMP-SMX) 160/800 mg TMP-SMX every 12 h, **ceftriaxone** 1 g every 12 h, or **gentamicin** 2 mg/kg load and then 1 mg/kg every 8 h. Patients with factors associated with poor outcome should also be admitted: old age and general debility, renal calculi or obstruction, recent hospitalization or instrumentation, diabetes mellitus, evidence of chronic nephropathy, sickle cell disease, underlying carcinoma, or intercurrent cancer chemotherapy. These patients must be admitted and covered with broad-spectrum antibiotics (including antipseudomonal agents). All admitted patients must have adequate hydration instituted in the ED.
6. Any pregnant patient with bacteriuria, even if asymptomatic, should be treated.
7. Patients not responding to appropriate antibiotics should first be confirmed to have UTI with a urine culture, and organism-specific therapy should be instituted. Patients with a UTI who have failed standard therapy may respond to a change in antibiotics or may have hitherto undetected structural or immunologic compromise.

Hematuria

Considerations for ED management and disposition of hematuria are primarily related to the differential diagnosis, since treatment is directed at the underlying cause.

1. In younger patients, hematuria is most often due to nephrolithiasis or UTI and much less commonly due to neoplasm (e.g., Wilms' tumor) or glomerulonephritis.
2. Red, clotted blood in the urine indicates a source below the kidneys.
3. Hematuria varying with menstruation may indicate endometriosis.
4. Hematuria occurring in the presence of back or flank pain may be associated with expanding abdominal aortic aneurysm.
5. In patients over the age of 40 any hematuria, even with a clear diagnosis of UTI or stone, warrants close follow-up and

retesting of urine because of the chance of coexisting urinary tract cancer.

6. The most common cause of hematuria worldwide is schistosomiasis; this entity should be considered in patients with appropriate travel history.

7. Hematuria in a pregnant woman may be a harbinger of preeclampsia, pyelonephritis, or obstructing nephrolithiasis; there should be a low threshold for consultation and admission in this population.

8. Hemodynamically stable patients with minimal or no symptoms who are able to tolerate oral fluids and have no significant comorbid conditions (e.g., renal failure or anemia) may be discharged for outpatient follow-up, which should consist of (at least) repeat urinalysis within a week.

For further reading in *Emergency Medicine: A Comprehensive Study Guide*, 5th ed., see Chap. 90, "Urinary Tract Infections," by David S. Howes and William F. Young; and Chap. 93, "Hematuria and Hematospermia," by David S. Howes and Mark P. Bogner.

---

54 | Male Genital Problems

Stephen H. Thomas

Few problems encountered in the emergency department (ED) match the anxiety of a male with acute genital pain. In addition to the psychological impact, symptoms are severe because of extensive sensory innervation.

TESTES AND EPIDIDYMIS

Testes

Testicular torsion must be the primary consideration in any male (of all age groups) complaining of testicular pain. Pain usually occurs suddenly, is severe, and is felt in the lower abdominal quadrant, the inguinal canal, or the testis. The pain may be constant or intermittent but is not positional, since torsion is primarily an ischemic event. When the diagnosis is obvious, urologic consultation is indicated for exploration, since imaging tests can be too time-consuming. In indeterminate cases, color-flow duplex ultrasound and, less commonly, radionuclide imaging may be helpful. The ED physician can attempt manual detorsion. Most testes torse in a lateral to medial direction, so detorsion is performed in a medial to lateral direction, similar to the opening of a book. The endpoint for successful detorsion is pain relief; urologic referral is still indicated.

Torsion of the appendages is more common than testicular torsion but is not dangerous, since the appendix testis and appendix epididymis have no known function. If the patient is seen early, diagnosis can be supported by the following: pain is most intense near the head of the epididymis or testis; there is an isolated tender nodule; or the pathognomonic blue dot appearance of a cyanotic appendage is illuminated through thin prepubertal scrotal skin. If normal intratesticular blood flow can be demonstrated with color Doppler, immediate surgery is not necessary, since most appendages calcify or degenerate over 10 to 14 days and cause no harm. If the diagnosis cannot be assured, urologic exploration is needed to rule out testicular torsion.

Epididymitis

Epididymitis is characterized by gradual onset of pain due to inflammatory causes. Bacterial infection is the most common, with infecting agents dependent on the patient's age. In patients younger than 40 years old, epididymitis is primarily due to sexually transmitted diseases (STDs). Common urinary pathogens predominate in older men. Epididymitis causes lower abdominal, inguinal canal, scrotal, or testicular pain alone or in combination. Due to the inflammatory nature of the pain, patients with epididymitis may note transient pain relief when elevating the scrotal contents while recumbent. Initially, tenderness is well localized to the epididymis, but progression of inflammation results in the physical examination finding of a single, large testicular mass (epididymoorchitis) difficult to differentiate from testicular torsion or carcinoma. At this stage the patient may appear toxic and require admission for intravenous antibiotics (e.g., **ceftriaxone** 1 to 2 g every 12 h or **trimethoprim-sulfamethoxazole** 5 mg/kg trimethoprim component every 6 h), scrotal elevation and ice application, NSAIDs, opioids for analgesia, and stool softeners. Outpatient treatment is an option in patients who do not appear toxic; urologic follow-up within a week is indicated. Oral antibiotic regimens should include 10 d of therapy with one of the following: **doxycycline** 100 mg bid or **ofloxacin** 300 mg bid for patients under age

40; for patients age 40 and older, **trimethoprim-sulfamethoxazole** one double-strength tablet bid or a quinolone, such as **ciprofloxacin** 500 mg bid.

Orchitis in isolation is rare; it usually occurs with viral or syphilitic disease and is treated with disease-specific therapy, symptomatic support, and urologic follow-up. Testicular malignancy should be suspected in patients presenting with asymptomatic testicular mass, firmness, or induration. Ten percent of tumors present with pain due to hemorrhage within the tumor. Urgent urologic follow-up is indicated.

SCROTUM

Scrotal abscesses may be localized to the scrotal wall or may arise from extensions of infections of intrascrotal contents (i.e., testis, epididymis, and bulbous urethra). A simple hair follicle scrotal wall abscess can be managed by incision and drainage; no antibiotics are required in immunocompetent patients. When a scrotal wall abscess is suspected of coming from an intrascrotal infection, ultrasound and retrograde urethrography may demonstrate pathology in the testis and/or epididymis, and the urethra, respectively. Definitive care of any complex abscess calls for a urology consultation.

Fournier's gangrene is a polymicrobial infection of the perineal subcutaneous tissues. Diabetic males are at highest risk. Prompt diagnosis is essential to prevent extensive tissue loss. Early surgical consultation is recommended for at-risk patients who present with scrotal, rectal, or genital pain. Aggressive fluid resuscitation with normal saline solution, broad-spectrum (i.e., gram-positive, gram-negative, and anaerobic) antibiotic coverage, surgical débridement, and hyperbaric oxygen are treatment mainstays.

PENIS

Balanoposthitis is inflammation of the glans (balanitis) and foreskin (posthitis). Upon foreskin retraction, the glans and prepuce appear purulent, excoriated, malodorous, and tender. Treatment consists of cleansing with mild soap, ensuring adequate dryness, application of antifungal creams (**nystatin** qid or **clotrimazole** bid), and urologic referral for follow-up and possible circumcision. An oral cephalosporin (e.g., **cephalexin** 500 mg qid) should be prescribed in cases of secondary bacterial infection.

Phimosis is the inability to retract the foreskin proximally. Hemostatic dilation of the preputial ostium relieves the urinary retention until definitive dorsal slit or circumcision can be performed.

Paraphimosis is the inability to reduce the proximal edematous foreskin distally over the glans. Paraphimosis is a true urologic emergency because resulting glans edema and venous engorgement can progress to arterial compromise and gangrene. If surrounding tissue edema can be successfully compressed, as by wrapping the glans with 2 x 2–inch elastic bandages for 5 min, the foreskin may be reduced. Making several puncture wounds with a small (22- to 25-gauge) needle may help with expression of glans edema fluid. Local anesthetic block of the penis is helpful if patients cannot tolerate the discomfort associated with edema compression and removal. If arterial compromise is suspected or has occurred, local infiltration of the constricting band with 1% plain lidocaine followed by superficial vertical incision of the band will decompress the glans and allow foreskin reduction.

Entrapment injuries occur when various objects are wrapped around the penis. Such objects should be removed, and urethral integrity (retrograde urethrogram) and distal penile arterial blood supply (Doppler studies) should be confirmed when indicated.

Penile fracture occurs when there is an acute tear of the penile tunical albuginea. The penis is acutely swollen, discolored, and tender in a patient with history of trauma during intercourse accompanied by a snapping sound. Urologic consultation is indicated.

Peyronie's disease presents with patients noting sudden or gradual onset of dorsal penile curvature with erections. Examination reveals a thickened plaque on the dorsal penile shaft. Assurance and urologic follow-up are indicated.

Priapism is a painful pathologic erection, which may be associated with urinary retention. Infection and impotence are other complications. Regardless of etiology, the initial therapy for priapism is **terbutaline** 0.25 to 0.5 mg subcutaneously in the deltoid area. Corporal aspiration and irrigation with either normal saline solution or an α-adrenergic antagonist is the next step and may need to be performed by the emergency physician when urologic consultation is not available. Even when emergency physicians provide stabilizing care, urologic consultation is indicated in all cases.

URETHRA

Urethral stricture is becoming more common due to the rising incidence of STDs. If a patient's bladder cannot be cannulated with a 14 F or 16 F Foley or Coudé catheter, the differential diagnosis includes urethral stricture, voluntary external sphincter spasm, bladder neck contracture, or benign prostatic hypertrophy. Retrograde urethrography can be performed to delineate the location and extent of urethral stricture. Endoscopy is necessary to confirm bladder neck contracture or define the extent of an obstructing prostate gland. Suspected voluntary external sphincter spasm can be overcome by holding the patient's penis upright and encouraging him to relax his perineum and breathe slowly during the procedure. After no more than three gentle attempts to pass a 12 F Coudé catheter into a urethra prepared with anesthetic lubricant, urologic consultation should be obtained. In an emergency situation, suprapubic cystotomy can be performed. The infraumbilical and suprapubic area is prepped with povidone-iodine solution. A 25- to 27-gauge spinal needle is used to locate the bladder (ED ultrasound study can be useful at this point), followed by placement of the cystotomy using the Seldinger technique. Urologic follow-up should occur within 48 h.

Urethral foreign bodies are associated with bloody urine and slow, painful urination. X-ray of the bladder and urethral areas may disclose a foreign body. Removal of the foreign body may be achieved with a gentle milking action; retrograde urethrography or endoscopy is required in such cases to confirm an intact urethra. Often, urologic consultation for endoscopy or open cystotomy is required for foreign-body removal.

Urinary Retention

Urinary retention syndromes can range from overt retention to insidious overflow incontinence. A detailed history, including over-the-counter cold and diet aids, may reveal the cause of urinary retention. Men do not void as completely when sitting down, and infrequent ejaculation may lead to a secondary prostatic congestion and symptoms of outlet obstruction. An intact sensory examination, anal sphincter examination, and bulbocavernosus reflex test differentiate chronic outlet obstruction from the sensory or motor neurogenic bladder and spinal-cord compression.

Physical examination should include search for meatal stenosis, palpation of urethral length for masses or fistulae consistent with urethral stricture disease or abscess formation, lower abdominal examination for palpation of suprapubic mass, and rectal examination to evaluate anal sphincter tone and prostate size and consistency. Most patients with bladder outlet obstruction are in distress, and passage of a urethral catheter alleviates their pain and their urinary retention. Copious intraurethral lubrication including a topical anesthetic should be used, and a 16 F Coudé catheter is recommended if straight catheters fail. Be certain to pass the catheter to its fullest extent, obtaining free urine flow, before inflating the balloon. The catheter should be left indwelling and connected to a leg drainage bag. Belladonna and opium suppositories (one every 4 to 6 h) can be prescribed to alleviate the constant urge to void secondary to bladder spasm, which frequently accompanies an indwelling catheter. In patients whose bladder catheter will be left in longer than 5 to 7 d, prophylactic antibiotics (e.g., **trimethoprim** 100 mg/d) should be instituted. Otherwise, antibiotics are indicated only if urinalysis is consistent with urinary tract infection. If urinary retention has been chronic, postobstructive diuresis may occur even in the presence of normal blood urea nitrogen and creatinine levels. In such patients, close monitoring of urinary output is indicated, and they should be observed for 4 to 6 h after catheterization.

In all cases of urinary retention, urologic follow-up is indicated for a complete genitourinary evaluation.

For further reading in *Emergency Medicine: A Comprehensive Study Guide*, 5th ed., see Chap. 91, "Male Genital Problems," by Robert E. Schneider.

55 | Renal Colic
Elicia Sinor Kennedy

Urologic stones can form anywhere in the urinary tract, although primary bladder stones are rare. The most common clinical presentation occurs when the stones migrate down the ureter causing some degree of obstruction and pain. This painful condition is called renal colic.

Clinical Features

Both adults and children present with kidney stones. In adults, the condition is three times more common in males than females and kidney stones usually occur in the third to fifth decade of life. Children constitute 7 percent of cases seen with the distribution being equal between the sexes. Patients usually present with an acute onset of severe pain which may be associated with nausea, vomiting and diaphoresis. The pain is sharp and episodic in nature due to the intermittent obstruction and is relieved after the stone passes. The pain typically originates in either flank, radiating around the abdomen toward the groin; however, as the stone passes distally it may become anterior abdominal or suprapubic in nature. Vesicular stones may present with intermittent dysuria and terminal hematuria. Patients are frequently anxious, pacing or writhing, and are unable to hold still or converse. Children may present in a similar fashion but up to 30 percent have only painless hematuria. Physical findings can include tachycardia and elevated blood pressure, which are secondary to pain. The patients are usually afebrile unless a urinary tract infection is concurrent. Examination may reveal costovertebral tenderness or abdominal tenderness over the site of the impacted stone.

Diagnosis and Differential

Upon clinical suspicion of a kidney stone, an initial dipstick urine test and complete urinalysis expedites the differential diagnosis and rules out infection. Microscopic hematuria is present 90 percent of cases, although there is no correlation between the quantity of blood present and the degree of obstruction. A kidneys, ureters, bladder x-ray (KUB) can be helpful in excluding other pathologic conditions and in visualizing stones since 90 percent are radiopaque. Historically the gold standard for diagnosis of renal stone and colic was the intravenous pyelogram (IVP). With the advent of newer-generation computed tomography (CT) scanners, the use of noncontrast helical CT scanning has dramatically increased and in some institutions it has become the diagnostic procedure of choice. Its accuracy is equal, if not superior, to that of the IVP. Images are obtained from the top of the kidney to the bottom of the bladder. Positive findings include ureteral caliber changes, suspicious calcifications, stranding of perinephric fat, and dilation of the collecting system. Advantages of the CT are the speed with which it can be obtained and the avoidance of exposure to contrast agents. Disadvantages are that it does not evaluate renal function and depends on the availability of newer-generation CT scanners and the skill of the radiologist in using this modality. The IVP gives both functional and anatomical information. Prior to obtaining an IVP, the patient should be questioned regarding allergy to contrast media and appropriate materials for managing allergic reactions should be readily available. A pregnancy test should be obtained for any patient at risk. Pregnant patients and children are preferentially evaluated with ultrasound to decrease radiation exposure. Blood urea nitrogen and creatinine levels should be determined prior to the IVP for any patient at risk of contrast agent nephrotoxicity. This is most likely in patients with preexisting renal insufficiency, diabetes mellitus, dehydration, hypovolemia, hypotension, advanced age (> 70 years), multiple myeloma, hypertension, hyperuricemia, a history of contrast media within 72 h, and those with cardiovascular disease on a diuretic. Maintaining adequate urinary output with administration of intravenous (IV) fluids also decreases the risk of renal injury. Positive findings include distention of the renal pelvis, calyceal distortion, dye extravasation, hydronephrosis, ureteral column dye cutoff and a delay in appearance of a nephrogram. Postvoid films are useful in diagnosing distal stones. False-negative IVP results can occur in the radiolucent, partially obstructing stone. Ultrasound, an anatomic rather than functional test, is useful in patients that are not candidates for IVP. It detects hydronephrosis and larger stones but is not sensitive for midureteral stones or small stones (less than 5 mm). Differential diagnosis of renal stones includes pyelonephritis, renal infarction, papillary necrosis, biliary colic, and acute muscle strain. The most critical alternative diagnosis to consider is rupturing or dissecting aortic abdominal aneurysm, which can have a similar presentation. Other diagnoses to consider are ruptured ectopic pregnancy or appendicitis, since they can be life threatening if missed. Patients receiving outpatient extracorporeal shock wave lithotripsy for urolithiasis may present to the ED with renal colic as the resulting "sludge" is passed in the urine.

Emergency Department Care and Disposition

In most cases the diagnosis of urologic stones and renal colic is clinical. Management consists of excluding infection and other diagnoses, supportive care, analgesia and appropriate referral. Patients should be monitored if possible, and an IV line established for hydration and pain medication administration.

1. Crystalloid IV fluids should be given to maintain adequate urinary output in the event an IVP is ordered.
2. Adequate analgesia may require large doses of titrated narcotics, such as morphine or its equivalent. Narcotics may be accompanied by nonsteroidal anti-inflammatory drugs (NSAIDs) but should not be their replacement, since the onset of pain relief with NSAIDs is much slower. NSAIDs should be used with caution in patients with suspected compromise of overall renal function (e.g., elderly, hypovolemic, or diabetic patients or those with renal insufficiency) in order to avoid worsening or precipitating decline in renal function.
3. An IVP or noncontrast helical CT scan should be performed to confirm the diagnosis and ensure the presence of two anatomically normal kidneys. In patients who are not candidates for IVP or CT, ultrasound is an appropriate diagnostic adjunct. If diagnosis is very clinically evident or the diagnosis already established, a KUB is sufficient. It is controversial whether all patients require ED imaging. For healthy young patients in whom the diagnosis

is very straightforward, it may be appropriate to delay workup to be performed on an outpatient basis. For older patients with a more complicated differential diagnosis, the diagnosis should be confirmed by some imaging modality.
4. While the patient is in the ED, all urine should be collected and strained for pathologic analysis of collected stones. In cases of complicating urinary tract infection, antibiotics should be started.

Discharge is appropriate for patients with small unilateral stones (less than 6 mm), no infection, and pain controlled by oral analgesics. Patients may be given a urinary strainer, prescriptions for oral narcotics and urologic follow-up within 5 days. If the stone is passed in the ED, no treatment is necessary other than elective urologic follow-up. Patients should be instructed to return if they develop fever, vomiting or uncontrolled pain. Urologic consultation on an emergent basis is prudent in the patient that appears to have classic urolithiasis and does not appear to be responding to appropriate pain medication. Admission is indicated for patients with infection and concurrent obstruction, a solitary kidney with obstruction, uncontrolled pain or emesis, and large or proximal stones. Hospitalization should be discussed with a urologist for patients with renal insufficiency, severe underlying disease, an IVP indicating extravasation or complete obstruction, a suspected vesicular stone, or multiple visits to the ED.

For further reading in *Emergency Medicine: A Comprehensive Study Guide,* 5th ed., see Chap. 92, "Urologic Stone Disease," by Joel Moll and W. F. Peacock IV.

---

56 | Complications of Urologic Devices
David M. Cline

COMPLICATIONS OF URINARY CATHETERS

Infection is the most common complication of urinary catheters, and management is discussed in Chap. 53. Minor traumatic complications of urinary catheters may require no therapy, while major complications (such as bladder perforation) require consultation with a urologist.

Nondraining Catheter

Obstruction is suggested if the catheter does not easily flush or if there is no return of the irrigant. Obstruction of the catheter by blood clots often creates a situation in which the catheter is easily flushed, but little or no irrigant is returned. If this occurs, the catheter can be replaced with a triple-lumen catheter so that the bladder can be easily irrigated. If, after clearing the bladder of all clots, evidence of continued bleeding is present, urologic consultation is recommended for possible cystoscopy. Some physicians advocate the use of single-lumen catheters to lavage the bladder, as its larger lumen may aid in the evacuation of larger clots.

Nondeflating Retention Balloon

If the obstruction is distal, the result of a crush or defective valve, the catheter can be cut proximal to the defect. If this does not deflate the balloon, a lubricated guidewire can be introduced into the cut inflation channel in an attempt to clear the obstruction. The balloon can be ruptured within the bladder. Utilizing overinflation with sterile water often requires 10 to 20 times the normal balloon volume. Urologic consultation may be required if simple measures are not successful.

COMPLICATIONS OF URETERAL STENTS

Dysuria, urinary urgency, frequency, and abdominal and flank discomfort are common complaints in patients with ureteral stents. The baseline discomfort in a functioning, well-positioned stent can range anywhere from minimal to debilitating. However, an abrupt change in the character, location, or intensity of the pain requires further evaluation for stent malposition and malfunction.

Ureteral stents may remain in place for weeks to months and often function with no complication during the entire period. However, stents can often become encrusted with mineral deposits and may obstruct. Complete obstruction of urine flow is possible, although this tends to occur more often in patients with stents in place for long-term use. These patients may require urologic consultation and in some cases may require stent replacement.

Urinary Tract Infection Versus Stent Migration and Malfunction

Changing abdominal or flank pain, or bladder discomfort, may be indicative of stent migration. X-ray examination is indicated with comparison to a previous film to evaluate stent position, and urologic consultation with further studies to evaluate stent position may eventually be necessary.

When a urinary tract infection occurs in the presence of a stent, stent removal is not mandatory, because most infections can be managed with outpatient antibiotics. If pyelonephritis or systemic infection is evident, however, then further evaluation and emergent intervention are indicated. Plain x-ray examination to check for stent migration, and urologic consultation for evaluation of stent migration and malfunction, are indicated, as well as initiation of antibiotic therapy.

For further reading in *Emergency Medicine: A Comprehensive Study Guide,* 5th ed., see Chap. 95, "Complications of Urologic Devices," by C. Richard Ross and Edward Lee.

GYNECOLOGY AND OBSTETRICS

57 | Vaginal Bleeding and Pelvic Pain in the Nonpregnant Patient

Rebecca S. Rich

PREPUBERTAL CHILDREN

In prepubertal girls, vaginitis is the most common cause of pelvic pain and bleeding. Vaginal bleeding can be secondary to maternal estrogen withdrawal in neonates. Trauma to the genital area must alert physicians to the possibility of sexual assault. Vaginal foreign bodies may present with intermittent bloody, foul-smelling discharge. Other conditions to consider are congenital vaginal abnormalities, precocious puberty and menarche, urethral prolapse. and dermatologic lesions. See Chap. 62.

VAGINAL BLEEDING IN ADOLESCENTS AND ADULTS

Once pregnancy is excluded, consider structural and traumatic causes of bleeding. A thorough pelvic examination may show the source. Bleeding can arise from the uterus or cervix and may be due to cervicitis, endometrial or cervical polyps, cervical or endometrial (especially in older women) cancer, submucosal fibroids, local trauma to the genitalia, or a retained foreign body. In postmenopausal women, the two most common causes are exogenous estrogens and atrophic vaginitis or endometritis (each 30 percent of cases), as well as endometrial cancer (15 percent of cases), polyps, and endometrial hyperplasia. Most of these patients can be referred for definitive gynecologic care.

Anovulatory dysfunctional uterine bleeding (irregular shedding of a thickened endometrium) is a likely cause if the findings on pelvic examination are normal. Anovulation is especially common in perimenarcheal girls and perimenopausal women, although in the latter malignancy is the most worrisome concern. Patients with anovulatory cycles present with prolonged menses or intermenstrual bleeding. Usually the bleeding is not heavy, but the most severe cases occur in adolescents shortly after menarche.

Consider coagulopathy as a cause of vaginal bleeding, especially in young women. Primary coagulation disorders account for 19 percent of menorrhagia in teens, including von Willebrand's disease, myeloproliferative disorders, and immunothrombocytopenia. Skin signs such as petechiae may be absent.

Emergency Department Care and Disposition

Most patients with vaginal bleeding require no immediate interventions. Hemodynamically unstable patients require standard resuscitation, and prompt dilation and curettage (D and C) is usually indicated. Hemodynamically stable patients thought to have anovulatory dysfunctional uterine bleeding can be managed medically with hormonal manipulation.

1. For patients with severe bleeding, intravenous (IV) conjugated **estrogen** 25 mg may be given. More commonly, oral (PO) therapy is given: conjugated estrogen 2.5 mg qid. Add **medroxyprogesterone** 10 mg/d when the bleeding subsides; continue both for 7 to 10 d.
2. Alternatively, a **PO contraceptive** is given: ethinyl estradiol 35 μg and norethindrone 1 mg, 4 tablets per day for 7 d. A slow taper may be given: ethinyl estradiol 35 μg and norethindrone 1 mg 4 tablets for 2 d, 3 tablets for 2 d, 2 tablets for 2 d, and then 2 tablets for 3 d.

Alternatively, medroxyprogesterone 10 mg/d PO for 10 d can stabilize an immature endometrium. Bleeding occurs 3 to 10 days after stopping progesterone but may be heavy. Older patients in whom there is concern about underlying malignancy should not be started on hormones in the emergency department (ED) but should be referred to a gynecologist for cervical biopsy. Nonsteroidal anti-inflammatory drugs (NSAIDs) are useful adjuncts to decrease bleeding.

PELVIC PAIN

Although most female patients with pelvic pain have gynecologic problems, consider nongynecologic conditions, such as inflammatory bowel disease, gastroenteritis, diverticulitis, urinary-tract infection or obstruction, and, particularly, appendicitis. Pelvic inflammatory disease, a serious and common cause of pelvic pain, is covered in detail in Chap. 63.

Ovarian Cysts

The most common noninfectious cause of pelvic pain is rupture of an ovarian cyst or solid ovarian, tubal, or uterine mass. With the exception of persistent corpus luteum cysts, ovarian cysts occur in women in normal menstrual cycles. Ovarian enlargement is initially asymptomatic or causes poorly defined visceral pain due to poor afferent innervation. When leakage or rupture occurs, acute pain results from irritation of the parietal peritoneum from the cyst or mass contents. In the case of a dermoid tumor, chemical peritonitis can occur.

Follicular cysts are very common and generally regress spontaneously in 1 to 3 months. These cysts may rupture and cause sharp pain that resolves over several days. There may be associated peritoneal signs due to irritation from cystic fluid or blood. Corpus luteum cysts are less common and also usually resolve at the end of the menstrual cycle if pregnancy does not occur. However, persistent corpus luteum cysts can cause unilateral pelvic pain with associated menstrual cycle abnormalities. Cyst rupture can cause sharp pain, peritoneal irritation, and bleeding.

Pregnancy must be excluded, since rupture of a corpus luteum cyst can mimic ectopic pregnancy. Ultrasound is the most useful test for detection of adnexal pathology and free fluid. Patients with unruptured cysts should be referred for gynecologic follow-up. If a cyst has ruptured and the patient is hemodynamically stable, she may be discharged with analgesics and follow-up. Rupture of a hemorrhagic corpus luteum cyst may cause hemoperitoneum, which requires surgical intervention.

Ovarian Torsion

Ovarian and adnexal torsion is rare. It often occurs in an enlarged or abnormal ovary. Over half of these patients will have tumors, usually benign dermoids. The ovary twists on its pedicle, with compromise of its blood supply and necrosis. Torsion of tubal masses and pedunculated fibroids can present similarly. Patients have sudden onset of severe pelvic pain. Many patients have nausea and vomiting, suggesting appendicitis. There may be a history of previous similar episodes. On pelvic examination, patients have unilateral adnexal tenderness, pain, and usually a mass. Ultrasound may be helpful, but often the diagnosis is not made until the time of surgery. Laparoscopic ovarian or adnexal detorsion or removal is the treatment of choice.

Mittelschmerz

Mittelschmerz (middle pain) is midcycle pain at ovulation, occurring around days 14 to 16 of the menstrual cycle. The pain is typically unilateral, is mild to moderate, and often lasts a day or less. There may be light spotting. The diagnosis is clinical, and more serious causes of adnexal pain should be ruled out. The pelvic examination may reveal adnexal tenderness without mass. Mittelschmerz is self-limited and is treated symptomatically using analgesics.

Endometriosis

In this disease, normal endometrium occurs in ectopic locations. All pelvic structures, including the gutters, cul-de-sac, ligaments, and pelvic peritoneum may be affected.

After primary dysmenorrhea, this is the most common cause of midcycle pain. Symptoms include pelvic pain, usually at menses; dyspareunia; and dysmenorrhea. Endometriosis can also cause infertility. Pelvic examination may entail pain and tenderness, but this symptom is not specific. Rupture of an ovarian endometrioma may present with acute, severe pain with peritoneal signs.

The diagnosis may be suspected in the ED but cannot be established noninvasively. The extent of disease often correlates poorly with symptoms. To confirm the diagnosis, visualization via laparoscopy or laparotomy is necessary. The most appropriate ED management is analgesia and referral.

Leiomyomas

Commonly called fibroids, leiomyomas are benign muscle tumors. They are the most common pelvic tumor, occurring in one in four white and one in two African American women. They are often multiple. Up to 30 percent of women with fibroids have associated pelvic pain and bleeding. Acute pain is rare, but severe pain may be associated with torsion of a pedunculated fibroid. In pregnant women, fibroids may degenerate (infarct) due to rapid growth with outstripping of the blood supply, causing acute severe pain. The diagnosis is usually suggested on pelvic examination by an enlarged uterus or palpable masses. Ultrasound is confirmatory. With degeneration, an acute abdomen may occur, but most patients can be managed with analgesia and referral.

Dysmenorrhea

Primary dysmenorrhea is most common in young girls just after menarche. Pain is crampy and may be associated with nausea, backache, and headache. NSAIDs are very helpful. An oral contraceptive can be useful as second-line therapy. Acquired secondary dysmenorrhea occurs later in life in association with other gynecologic problems, such as infection, fibroids, endometriosis, and adhesions.

For further reading in *Emergency Medicine: A Comprehensive Study Guide*, 5th ed., see Chap. 98, "Vaginal Bleeding and Pelvic Pain in the Nonpregnant Patient," by Laurie Morrison and Julie Spence.

---

58 | Ectopic Pregnancy
Sally S. Fuller

Ectopic pregnancy (EP) occurs in 2 percent of all pregnancies and is the leading cause of maternal death in the first trimester. Twenty percent of EPs are ruptured at the time of presentation. Important risk factors include a history of pelvic inflammatory disease; surgical procedures on the fallopian tubes, including tubal ligation; previous EP; abortions; peritubular adhesions from endometriosis or appendicitis; diethylstilbestrol exposure; intrauterine device use; and treatment with infertility drugs. This diagnosis must be considered in every woman of childbearing age presenting with abdominal pain.

Clinical Features

The classic triad of abdominal pain, vaginal bleeding, and a positive pregnancy test result used to describe EP may be present, but many cases occur with more subtle findings. Presenting signs and symptoms may be different in ruptured versus nonruptured EP. Only 90 percent of women with EP complain of abdominal pain; 80 percent have vaginal bleeding; and only 70 percent give a history of amenorrhea. The pain described may be extreme or relatively minor. The pain may be localized to the pelvis or diffuse. The presence of hemoperitoneum causing diaphragmatic irritation may cause pain to be referred to the shoulder or upper abdomen. Vaginal bleeding is usually light; heavy bleeding is more commonly seen with threatened abortion or other complications of pregnancy. Presenting vital signs may be entirely normal or may indicate advanced hemorrhagic shock. See Table 58-1 for the normal physiologic changes of pregnancy. Relative bradycardia may be present even in cases with rupture and intraperitoneal hemorrhage. Physical examination findings are highly variable. The abdominal examination may show signs of localizing or diffuse tenderness with or without peritoneal signs. The pelvic examination findings may be normal but more often reveal cervical motion tenderness, adnexal tenderness with or without a mass, and possibly an enlarged uterus. Fetal heart tones are only rarely audible.

TABLE 58-1 Physiologic Changes in Pregnancy

Cardiac output	Elevated 30–50%
Blood volume	Elevated 45%
Mean hemoglobin level	10.2–11.6 g/dL
Heart rate	Increased 15–20 beats/min
Blood pressure	Decreased 5–10 mmHg systolic; decreased 10–15 mmHg diastolic
Normal arterial blood gas levels	pH 7.4–7.45; P_{O_2} 95–105 mmHg; P_{CO_2} 28–32 mmHg
GFR	Elevated 50%
Normal serum creatinine level	0.5–0.75 mg/dL
ESR	Markedly elevated in normal pregnancy
Coagulation	Thromboembolism is the number 1 cause of maternal mortality; risk of thromboembolism is increased 1.8 times normal in postpartum period
WBC count	10,000–15,000/μL
Insulin requirements in IDDM	Dramatically increased in early pregnancy

Abbreviations: ESR, erythrocyte sedimentation rate; GFR, glomerular filtration rate; IDDM, insulin-dependent diabetes mellitus; WBC, white blood cell.

Diagnosis and Differential

Urine pregnancy testing [for urinary beta human chorionic gonadotropin (β-HCG)] should be performed immediately. Dilute urine may result in a false negative result; serum testing will provide a definitive result in such situations. (A negative serum pregnancy test result definitively rules out EP.) Pelvic ultrasound is the test of choice for identifying EP. If an intrauterine pregnancy is identified, the chance of a coexisting EP is extremely small in most patients. However, if a patient has been on fertility drugs, has had in vitro fertilization, or has multiple risk factors for EP, further evaluation for EP is warranted. Sonographic findings of an empty uterus with an adnexal mass (other than a simple cyst) with or without free fluid in the abdomen is highly suggestive of EP. Sonographic findings of an empty uterus without free fluid or an adnexal mass in a woman with a positive pregnancy test result is considered indeterminate. In such situations, the findings must be evaluated in context with the patient's quantitative β-HCG level. A high β-HCG level (greater than 6000) with an empty uterus is suggestive of EP. If the β-HCG is low (less than 1500), then the pregnancy may indeed be intrauterine or ectopic but too small to be visualized on ultrasound. In this situation, repeat quantitative β-HCG testing in 2 days must be performed. A normal intrauterine pregnancy should show at least a 66 percent increase in the β-HCG level in that period of time; EP would show a much slower rate of increase. Levels between 1500 and 6000 may warrant dilation and curretage (D and C) or laparoscopy to diagnose EP following evaluation by an obstetric-gynecologic consultant. Individual hospitals may vary in the expertise of the sonographers available, and levels other than 1500 and 6000 may be reasonable guidelines in certain institutions. Differential diagnosis in the patient presenting with abdominal pain, vaginal bleeding, and early pregnancy includes threatened, incomplete, or missed abortion; recent elective abortion; or endometritis.

Emergency Department Care and Disposition

Treatment of patients with suspected EP is dependent on the patient's vital signs, physical signs, and symptoms. Close communication with the obstetric-gynecologic consultant is essential.

1. For unstable patients, start **two large bore intravenous lines** for rapid infusion of crystalloid and/or packed red blood cells to maintain blood pressure.
2. Perform a bedside urine **pregnancy test**.
3. Notify an obstetric-gynecologic **consultant** immediately for the

unstable patient, even before laboratory and diagnostic tests are complete.

4. Draw blood for a complete blood count, blood typing and Rh factor determination (or cross matching for unstable patients), quantitative β-HCG determination (if indicated), and serum electrolyte determinations.

5. If the patient is stable, proceed with the diagnostic workup. In reliable patients with indeterminate ultrasound results and a low β-HCG level, discharge with ectopic precautions and arranged follow-up in 2 days for repeat β-HCG determination and obstetric-gynecologic reevaluation is appropriate.

6. Definitive treatment, as determined by the obstetric-gynecologic consultant, may involve laparoscopy, D and C, or medical management with methotrexate.

For further reading in *Emergency Medicine: A Comprehensive Study Guide*, 5th ed., see Chap. 100, "Ectopic Pregnancy," by Richard S. Krause and David M. Janicke.

---

59 | Emergencies during Pregnancy and the Postpartum Period

Sally S. Fuller

The major emergencies associated with pregnancy and the postpartum period include hemorrhagic complications, infectious complications, and complications related to hypertension, preeclampsia, and the HELLP (hemolysis, elevated liver enzymes, and low platelets) syndrome. The assessment, management, and disposition of these diseases vary according to gestational age. Nausea and vomiting of pregnancy is also commonly encountered in the emergency department (ED). See Table 58-1 for the normal physiologic changes during pregnancy.

VAGINAL BLEEDING IN THE FIRST HALF OF PREGNANCY

Vaginal bleeding during the first half of pregnancy is very common and occurs in up to 40 percent of pregnancies. The differential diagnosis includes spontaneous abortion, ectopic pregnancy (see Chap. 58), and bleeding due to vaginal or cervical infections such as gonorrhea, *Chlamydia*, and bacterial vaginosis (see Chap. 62). Spontaneous abortion occurs in up to 30 percent of pregnancies, most during the first 8 weeks. Risk factors include advanced maternal age, previous abortions, syphilis, HIV, anatomic abnormalities of the genital tract, and exposure to tobacco, drugs, or other toxic agents.

Clinical Features

The clinical features associated with abortion include vaginal bleeding and abdominal pain, both of which may vary in severity. Passage of tissue may occur along with the bleeding. History taking should attempt to quantify the amount of bleeding (in pads used per hour) and screen for concurrent diseases. The physician should pay careful attention to presenting and repeated vital sign determinations for indications of hemodynamic instability (see Table 58-1). On physical examination, the physician should examine carefully for fetal heart sounds, the site of bleeding, signs of infection (cervical cultures or DNA probes should be sent), dilated cervix, passage of fetal tissue, or for signs of ectopic pregnancy (see Chap. 58). If fetal tissue is present, it must be preserved and sent for pathologic examination.

Diagnosis and Differential

Blood should be drawn for a complete blood count (CBC), blood typing and Rh factor determination (or typing and cross matching in unstable patients), and quantitative serum β-HCG analysis. Urinalysis should be performed to screen for urinary tract infection (which is associated with a higher incidence of abortion). Ultrasound is frequently necessary to differentiate spontaneous abortion or threatened abortion from ectopic pregnancy, to determine fetal viability, and to check for retained products of conception (incomplete abortion). A patient with β-HCG level greater than 2000 mIU/mL should have a visible gestational sac on ultrasound if the pregnancy is a normal intrauterine pregnancy. Absence of a visible gestational sac with a β-HCG level greater than 2000 is suggestive of spontaneous abortion or ectopic pregnancy.

Emergency Department Care and Disposition

Management in the ED consists of intravenous (IV) **fluid resuscitation** in patients with unstable vital signs, and obstetric-gynecologic **consultation** for patients with heavy bleeding, unstable vital signs, fever, or visible products of conception. Every Rh-negative woman with vaginal bleeding should receive **Rh$_O$ (D) immune globulin** (RhoGam) 300 μg. Heavy bleeding can be managed by giving oxytocin 20 U in 1 L of normal saline solution infused at 150 to 200 mL/h. Stable patients with threatened abortion may be discharged if follow-up is ensured, with instructions to return in case of heavy bleeding, fever, or passage of tissue. Limited activity and pelvic rest (avoidance of intercourse and use of tampons) are frequently advised. Patients with incomplete or inevitable abortions should be admitted for dilation and curretage. A patient with completed abortion, as determined by ultrasound and/or complete passage of products of conception, may be discharged with close follow-up and instructions to return for heavy bleeding. See *Emergency Medicine: A Comprehensive Study Guide,* 5th ed., Chap. 101, for a discussion of molar pregnancy.

NAUSEA AND VOMITING OF PREGNANCY

Nausea and vomiting are very frequent occurrences in pregnancy. Intractable nausea and vomiting with greater than 5 percent weight loss and hypokalemia or ketonemia (i.e., hyperemesis gravidarum) may result in low birth weight infants. The clinical features include nausea, vomiting, and volume depletion without significant abdominal pain. (Presence of pain should alert the physician to rule out other diagnoses, such as cholecystitis, pancreatitis, gastroenteritis, hepatitis, ulcer disease, pyelonephritis, ectopic pregnancy, and fatty liver of pregnancy.) Diagnostic workup should include a CBC; electrolyte, blood urea nitrogen, and creatinine determinations; and urinalysis (with special attention to urinary ketones). ED treatment consists of rehydration with IV fluid of **5% dextrose in normal saline solution** or 5% dextrose in lactated Ringer's solution, and antiemetic medication (**promethazine** 12.5 to 50 mg IV) may be given. The patient should be reevaluated after IV hydration to see whether urinary ketones have cleared and to determine whether oral fluids can be tolerated. If so, she may be discharged with promethazine 25 mg suppositories every 4 to 6 h as needed. Close follow-up should be arranged, since the problem frequently recurs. Patients who fail to tolerate oral fluids, who have persistent electrolyte abnormalities, or who have 10 percent weight loss should be admitted.

HYPERTENSION, PREECLAMPSIA, AND RELATED DISORDERS

Hypertension with pregnancy is associated with a number of dangerous complications, such as preeclampsia, eclampsia, HEELP syndrome, abruptio placenta, preterm birth, and low birth weight infants.

Clinical Features and Diagnosis

Differentiation between transient hypertension of pregnancy (a benign condition) and more serious conditions can be difficult; frequently the distinction cannot be made until the postpartum period. For this reason, all hypertensive women should be evaluated thoroughly and obstetric-gynecologic consultation obtained. Hypertension in pregnancy is defined as a blood pressure greater than 140/90, a 20 mmHg rise in systolic blood pressure, or a 10 mmHg rise in diastolic blood pressure above the prepregnancy level.

Preeclampsia complicates 7 percent of pregnancies (most commonly primigravidas) and occurs between the twentieth week of gestation and 1 to 2 weeks postpartum. The clinical presentation can be variable, but the classic case is characterized by hypertension, proteinuria, and edema; presenting complaints may include headache, visual disturbances, or abdominal pain. Eclampsia is preeclampsia complicated by seizures.

The HELLP syndrome is a variant of preeclampsia seen primarily in multigravidas. The presenting complaint is usually abdominal pain, and the blood pressure may not be elevated initially; thus, it is important to differentiate between the HELLP syndrome and other gastrointestinal causes or urinary tract infection. Laboratory tests are key to making the diagnosis of HELLP syndrome: blood tests may show schistocytes on peripheral smear, platelet count less than 150,000/mL, elevated aspartate aminotransferase (AST) and alanine aminotransferase (ALT) levels, and abnormal coagulation profile.

Emergency Department Care and Disposition

ED management of these syndromes consists of seizure prevention or control and blood pressure control.

1. **$MgSO_4$,** loading dose 4 to 6 g in 100 mL of fluid over 20 min, followed by maintenance infusion of 2 g/h in 100 mL of fluid, is effective for seizure control. Magnesium levels and reflexes should be monitored to avoid excessive neuromuscular depression.

2. **Hydralazine** 2.5 mg initially, followed by 5 to10 mg every 10 min IV or intramuscular (IM), or **labetalol** 20 mg IV initial bolus, with repeat boluses of 40 to 80 mg if needed to a maximum of 300 mg may be used for blood pressure control.

Emergent consultation by an obstetrician is necessary. Delivery of the fetus is necessary for definitive care.

VAGINAL BLEEDING IN THE SECOND HALF OF PREGNANCY

Vaginal bleeding during the second half of pregnancy is potentially life threatening to the mother and fetus. Common causes include abruptio placentae, placenta previa, cervicovaginal lesions, and PROM. Pelvic speculum and digital examination should not be performed until ultrasound has definitively ruled out placenta previa as the cause for bleeding.

Abruptio placentae is the premature separation of the placenta. Risk factors include hypertension, advanced maternal age, multiparity, smoking, cocaine use, previous abruption, and abdominal trauma. Clinical features include vaginal bleeding, abdominal pain, back pain, uterine tenderness, and uterine irritability. The amount of pain and bleeding are highly variable, and are not reliable indicators of the severity of the abruption. Complications include fetal distress or death, maternal death due to hemorrhage, hypotension, disseminated intravascular coagulation (DIC), fetomaternal transfusion, and amniotic fluid embolism. Whenever the diagnosis is suspected, emergent obstetrical consultation should be sought. Ultrasound is useful in determining the extent of abruption and fetal viability but should not delay consultation. Blood tests should be obtained, including CBC, typing and cross matching, coagulation and DIC profile, and renal function studies. ED management includes **crystalloid IV fluids** and/or packed red blood cells for hemodynamically unstable patients. Frequent fetal and maternal monitoring should be performed. Emergency delivery may be indicated to save the life of the fetus and/or mother. Tocolytics are not indicated. **RhoGam** 300 μg should be given to Rh negative mothers.

Placenta previa is the implantation of the placenta over the cervical os. Risk factors include multiparity and prior cesarean section. Classic clinical features are painless bright red vaginal bleeding. Maternal and/or fetal death are potential complications. Vaginal speculum or digital examination should not be performed, since they may precipitate catastrophic hemorrhage. Diagnosis is made by ultrasound. The obstetrician should be consulted emergently. CBC and type and cross match should be obtained. Hemodynamically unstable patients should receive **crystalloid IV fluids** and/or packed red blood cells if needed. **RhoGam** 300 μg should be given to Rh negative patients.

Preterm Labor

Preterm labor is defined as labor prior to 37 weeks gestation. It occurs in 10% of deliveries and is the leading cause of neonatal death. Risk factors include PROM, abruptio placentae, drug abuse, multiple gestation, polyhydramnios, cervical incompetence, uterine abnormalities, prior preterm labor, and infection. Clinical features include regular uterine contractions with cervical changes of effacement. The diagnosis is made by observation over an extended period of time, with external fetal monitoring and serial cervical sterile speculum examinations. Digital examinations should be avoided. ED management of preterm labor begins with maternal hydration. The ED physician should consult the obstetrician emergently for admission and for decision regarding tocolytics. Women in preterm labor between 24 and 36 weeks' gestation may be candidates for tocolysis. However, risks must be discussed; all currently available regimens have serious side effects. If tocolytic protocols are initiated, the mother should receive glucocorticoids (**betamethasone** 12 mg IM every 24 h or **dexamethasone** 6 mg IM every 6 h for 4 doses) to hasten fetal lung maturity. Since the risk for group B streptococcus is higher in preterm infants, mothers should receive 5 million U **penicillin G** if they are not allergic to it.

PREMATURE RUPTURE OF MEMBRANES

PROM is rupture of membranes prior to the onset of labor. Labor will occur within 24 h in 90 percent of term patients and 50 percent of preterm patients. The clinical presentation of PROM is usually a copious rush of fluid or continuous leakage of fluid from the vagina. Sterile speculum examination may be undertaken to confirm the diagnosis, but digital cervical examination should be avoided to minimize the risk of infection. The diagnosis of PROM may be confirmed by identifying a pool of fluid in the posterior fornix of the vagina with pH greater than 6.5 (dark blue on nitrazine paper) and ferning pattern on smear. Ultrasound may confirm abnormally low amniotic fluid. False positive results with the nitrazine test may be observed with semen, blood, or certain infectious discharges. Tests for *Chlamydia*, gonorrhea, bacterial vaginosis, and group B streptococcus should be performed. Patients with suspected PROM should be admitted. Tocolytics are generally not used.

EMERGENCIES DURING THE POSTPARTUM PERIOD

Hemorrhage and infection are the most common postpartum complications in the ED. Postpartum preeclampsia or eclampsia, amniotic fluid embolism, and postpartum cardiomyopathy are rare but life threatening complications that may be seen.

Hemorrhage

The differential diagnosis of postpartum hemorrhage includes uterine atony (most common), uterine rupture following cesarean section, laceration of the lower genital tract, retained placental tissue, uterine inversion, and coagulopathy. Careful physical examination should be performed to look for signs of trauma, the enlarged and "doughy" uterus of uterine atony (the normal postpartum uterus feels firm and should not extend above the umbilicus), or a vaginal mass suggestive of an inverted uterus. Uterine bleeding in spite of good uterine tone and normal size may be an indication of retained products of conception; ultrasound should be performed to confirm the diagnosis. ED management consists of hemodynamic stabilization with **crystalloid IV fluids** and/or packed red blood cells if needed. Uterine atony is treated with **oxytocin** 20 to 30 U in 1 L of IV fluids given 200 mL/h. Minor lacerations of the cervix or vagina can be repaired using local anesthesia. Extensive lacerations, retained products of conception, uterine inversion, or uterine rupture require emergency evaluation and operative treatment by the obstetrician.

Infection

Postpartum endometritis occurs in 3 percent of vaginal deliveries and 15 to 30 percent of cesarean deliveries. Most infections are polymicrobial. Clinical features included fever, malaise, lower abdominal pain, and foul-smelling lochia. The severity of the disease may vary from minor illness to sepsis with necrotizing fasciitis.

Risk factors for more severe disease include obesity, diabetes, and hypertension. Diagnosis is made by physical examination revealing uterine fundus tenderness, cervical motion tenderness, and, often, purulent discharge. Laboratory tests including a CBC, urinalysis, and cervical cultures should be performed. Blood cultures should be obtained on septic appearing patients. Most patients require hospitalization for broad spectrum antibiotic treatment, such as **cefotaxime** 1 to 2 g IV every 6 to 8 h or combination therapy with **ampicillin** 1 g IV every 6 h and **gentamicin** 1.5 mg/kg IV every 8 h.

Mastitis is cellulitis of the periglandular breast tissue occurring most commonly in lactating women. Clinical features include pain, induration, redness, and warmth of the affected breast, with axillary adenopathy, fever, chills, and malaise. Outpatient treatment with dicloxacillin 500 mg qid or cephalexin 500 mg qid is usually effective. The patient should be instructed to continue nursing on the affected breast. Breast milk cultures are not indicated. Occasionally, abscess formation may occur and require incision and drainage.

Amniotic Fluid Embolism

Amniotic fluid embolism is a sudden, catastrophic illness of unknown cause with mortality rates of 60 to 80 percent. Clinical features include sudden cardiovascular collapse with seizure-like activity and profound hypoxemia. In patients who survive the first hour, DIC is frequently seen. Care is supportive: cardiovascular resuscitation, intubation and oxygenation, and treatment for DIC. Delivery, if not already complete, should be immediate.

For further reading in *Emergency Medicine: A Comprehensive Study Guide*, 5th ed., see Chap. 101, "Emergencies during Pregnancy and the Postpartum Period," by Gloria J. Kuhn.

---

60 | Comorbid Diseases in Pregnancy

Sally S. Fuller

See Table 58-1 for the normal physiologic changes during pregnancy.

DIABETES

Diabetes complicates 2 to 3 percent of pregnancies. Of these patients, 90 percent are gestational diabetics. Diabetics are at increased risk for hypertensive diseases, preterm labor, spontaneous abortion, pyelonephritis, fetal demise, hypoglycemia, and diabetic ketoacidosis (DKA). Some gestational diabetics can control their diabetes through diet; the rest, including the chronic diabetics, require insulin during pregnancy. Oral hypoglycemic agents are contraindicated. For patients with preexisting diabetes, the amount of insulin required increases throughout the pregnancy from about 0.7 U/(kg/d) initially to 1.0 U/(kg/d) at term. Typically, two-thirds of the insulin is given in the morning (two-thirds NPH and one-third regular) and one-third is given in the evening (one-half NPH and one-half regular). DKA in pregnancy tends to occur more rapidly and at lower glucose levels than in nonpregnant patients. Beta-adrenergic tocolytics tend to increase the risk for DKA. Patients should be treated with continuous insulin intravenous (IV) infusion. General management guidelines are the same as in the nonpregnant patient. Hypoglycemia presents with the same signs and symptoms as in nonpregnant patients. For mildly hypoglycemic awake patients, oral treatment with milk and crackers every 15 min is recommended to avoid overcorrection and hyperglycemia associated with concentrated glucose solutions. Obtunded patients are treated with 50 mL of 50% dextrose solution IV or glucagon 1 to 2 mg intramuscularly.

HYPERTHYROIDISM AND THYROID STORM

Hyperthyroidism in pregnancy can increase the risk of preeclampsia and neonatal morbidity and can cause hyperemesis gravidarum. Propylthiouracil (PTU) is the treatment of choice, and the patient should be monitored closely for signs of toxicity (purpuric rash and agranulocytosis). Thyroid storm has a high mortality rate and presents with fever, volume depletion, and sometimes cardiac failure. PTU, along with sodium iodide and propanol (unless cardiac failure is present), are useful to control the symptoms. Radioactive iodine therapy is not used in pregnancy.

DYSRHYTHMIAS

Dysrhythmias are encountered rarely in pregnancy. Lidocaine, digoxin, and procainamide have been found to be safe in pregnancy in the usual dosages. Beta blockers may be used acutely for control of tachydysrhythmias but should not be used long term. Verapamil has been shown safe for treatment of supraventricular tachycardia. If anticoagulation is needed in pregnancy for atrial fibrillation, heparin is the drug of choice. Cardioversion has not been shown to be harmful to the fetus.

THROMBOEMBOLISM

Deep venous thrombosis (DVT) is five times more common in the pregnant and postpartum population, and is most prevalent in postpartum and postcesarean patients. Advanced maternal age, increasing parity, and multiple gestation are other risk factors uniquely associated with pregnancy. Other risk factors and clinical features for DVT and pulmonary embolism (PE) are similar in the pregnant and nonpregnant populations. Diagnostic modalities useful in pregnancy for diagnosis of DVT include impedance plethysmography and technetium-99m radionuclide venography. Iodine-125 fibrinogen scanning should not be used. Diagnosis of PE in pregnancy is unchanged from that in the nonpregnant population. Hydration and frequent voiding should be encouraged during ventilation-perfusion scanning to minimize the radiation exposure to the fetus, since the isotope is excreted in the urine. Treatment of DVT and PE is with heparin; warfarin is contraindicated in pregnancy. See Chaps. 26 and 29 for more information on diagnosis and management of these conditions.

ASTHMA

Clinical features, diagnosis, and management of asthma are similar in pregnant and nonpregnant patients. The possibility of PE should be considered when new onset of asthmatic symptoms occurs in pregnancy. In monitoring asthmatics, peak expiratory flow rates are unchanged in pregnancy. Interpretation of arterial blood gas values, however, should take into account that normal pregnancy P_{CO_2} values are 27 to 32 mmHg. The finding of a P_{CO_2} of 39 in a pregnant asthmatic represents significant CO_2 retention. During treatment, patients should be maintained in a near sitting position, with pelvis tilted toward the left to maximize placental circulation. Clinical decision making regarding intubation or admission is similar in pregnant and nonpregnant patients. Standard agents for rapid-sequence intubation can be used.

URINARY TRACT INFECTIONS

Urinary tract infection is the most common bacterial infection during pregnancy. Asymptomatic bacteriuria should be cultured and treated if the culture result is positive. Simple cystitis may be treated with 7 to 10 days of **nitrofurantoin** 100 mg twice a day, **amoxicillin** 500 mg twice a day, or **cephalexin** 500 mg four times a day. Trimethoprim is contraindicated in pregnancy, and sulfa drugs should be avoided in patients near term. A urine culture should be obtained prior to treatment. Patients with pyelonephritis should be admitted for IV antibiotics because of increased incidence of preterm labor with pyelonephritis. Urine cultures and blood cultures should be obtained; IV antibiotics and IV hydration should be started as soon as possible. Drugs of choice for IV therapy include **cefazolin** 1 g every 8 h, or **ampicillin** 1 g every 6 h plus **gentamicin** 1.5 mg/kg every 8 h. Quinolone antibiotics are contraindicated. Antibiotic suppression should be continued for the rest of the pregnancy following a case of pyelonephritis.

SICKLE CELL DISEASE

Women with sickle cell disease are at higher risk for miscarriage, preterm labor, and vasoocclusive crises. Clinical features, evaluation, and treatment for acute pain crises are similar in pregnant and nonpregnant patients. Women with pregnancies of potentially viable gestational age should be admitted for monitoring during crises. Nonsteroidal antiinflammatory medications should be avoided after 32 weeks gestation. Hydroxyurea, frequently used for maintenance therapy, should be discontinued during pregnancy because of teratogenicity. Aplastic crises are rare but may be associated with parvovirus infection and hydrops fetalis.

MIGRAINE

Treatment mainstays during pregnancy are acetaminophen, codeine, and meperidine. Ergot alkaloids should not be used, and there is currently insufficient information available regarding the use of sumatriptan.

SEIZURE DISORDERS

Management of pregnant patients with seizure disorders is similar to that for the nonpregnant patient. Valproic acid should be avoided whenever possible because of a 1 to 3 percent incidence of fetal neural tube defects. Serum therapeutic levels of anticonvulsants are unchanged; however, the dosage to maintain the level may need to be increased. Status epilepticus with prolonged maternal hypoxia and acidosis has a high mortality rate for the mother and infant and should be treated aggressively with early intubation and ventilation. The patient should be placed on oxygen and positioned in the left lateral position to maximize placental oxygenation.

HIV INFECTION

All pregnant HIV-infected women beyond 14 weeks gestation should be on zidovudine therapy to reduce the risk of transmission to the fetus. Patients with CD4 counts less than 200 should be on prophylaxis for *Pneumocystis carinii*. Treatment for opportunistic infections is unchanged in pregnant women. Early and aggressive treatment of hypoxia with intubation and ventilation may improve fetal outcome.

SUBSTANCE ABUSE

Cocaine use is associated with increased incidence of fetal death in utero, placental abruption, preterm labor, premature rupture of membranes, spontaneous abortion, intrauterine growth restriction, and fetal cerebral infarcts. Treatment of acute cocaine toxicity is unchanged in pregnancy.

Opiate withdrawal in pregnant women is treated with methadone or clonidine. **Clonidine** dosage is 0.1 to 0.2 mg sublingually every hour up to 0.8 mg until signs of withdrawal resolve, followed by maintenance doses of 0.8 to 1.2 mg/d in divided doses for 7 days. The clonidine is then tapered over 3 days. Patients on methadone should not have the methadone withdrawn because of increased risk of fetal death in utero.

Alcohol use of more than two drinks per day may increase rates of spontaneous abortion, low birth weight, premature labor, and perinatal mortality. Acute alcohol withdrawal may be treated with short-acting barbiturates; benzodiazepines should be avoided in early pregnancy due to possible teratogenic effects. Disulfiram should be avoided altogether.

DOMESTIC VIOLENCE

Approximately 15 percent of pregnant women are victims of domestic violence during their pregnancy. They are at risk for placental abruption, uterine rupture, preterm labor, and fetal fractures. Physicians must maintain a high index of suspicion for domestic abuse and refer to the appropriate law enforcement and social service agencies.

DRUG USE IN PREGNANCY

Table 60-1 provides general recommendations regarding drug use in pregnancy. For any drug not listed in the table, the manufacturer's recommendations should be checked prior to administration.

DIAGNOSTIC IMAGING IN PREGNANCY

The threshold for teratogenesis from ionizing radiation is 10 rad, with 8 to 15 weeks gestation being the most vulnerable period. No single test exceeds this threshold; however, the effects of multiple tests are cumulative and may exceed the threshold. Ultrasonog-

TABLE 60-1 Drug Use in Pregnancy

Drug	Category*	Comment
Antibiotics		
Cephalosporins	B	May use
Penicillins	B	May use
Erythromycin	B	Estolate salt contraindicated due to hepatotoxicity; otherwise may use
Azithromycin	B	May use
Nitrofurantoin	B	May use
Clindamycin	B	May use
Metronidazole	B	Should be avoided during first trimester
Isoniazid	C	May use when necessary
Ethambutol	B	May use
Antivirals		
Acyclovir	C	May use in life-threatening maternal illness
Antihypertensive agents		
Alpha-methyldopa	B	May use
Beta blockers	B, C	May use when necessary
Calcium channel blockers	C	May use when necessary
Prazosin	C	May use when necessary
Hydralazine	C	Widely used
Anticonvulsants		
All	C, D	Congenital malformations reported with all anticonvulsants, but benefits may outweigh risks; use of folic acid (1 mg/d) may help prevent teratogenesis; valproic acid has especially high risk of neural tube defects
Corticosteroids	C	May be used in pregnancy for serious maternal conditions; gestational diabetes may develop

Anticoagulants		
Heparin	C	Drug of choice for pregnant women requiring anticoagulation
Analgesics		
Acetaminophen	A	May use
Propoxyphene	C	Caution advised when used close to term; neonatal withdrawal may occur
Opiates	C	Caution advised when used close to term; neonatal withdrawal may occur; avoid aspirin combinations
Nonsteroidal anti-inflammatory drugs	B, C, D	May be used for short duration (48–72 h) and not at all after 32 weeks; ibuprofen widely used
Antiemetics		
Meclizine	B	May use
Dimenhydrinate	B	May use
Diphenhydramine	B	Avoid first trimester
Trimethobenzamide	C	Used widely
Phenothiazines	C	Used widely
Over-the-counter cold medications		
Pseudoephedrine	C	Topical sprays preferable
Phenylpropanolamine	C	Topical nasal sprays preferable
Vaccines		
Live vaccines (measles-mumps-rubella)	X	Contraindicated
Inactivated viral vaccines (rabies, hepatitis B, influenza)	C	May be given
Pneumococcal vaccine	C	May be given
Tetanus and diphtheria	C	May be given

*Categories A, safe, human studies; B, presumed safe, animal studies; C, uncertain safety, animal studies show an adverse effect; D, unsafe, use may be justifiable in certain circumstances; X, contraindicated.

raphy and magnetic resonance imaging have not shown any teratogenic effects.

For further reading in *Emergency Medicine: A Comprehensive
Study Guide*, 5th ed., see Chap. 102, "Comorbid Diseases in
Pregnancy," by Jessica L. Bienstock and Harold E. Fox.

---

61 | Emergency Delivery
David M. Cline

PREPARATION FOR EMERGENCY DELIVERY

Any pregnant woman arriving in the emergency department who
is beyond 20 weeks gestation and appears to be actively contracting
should be rapidly evaluated with a bimanual pelvic examination
to assess cervical dilatation. Maternal vital signs and fetal heart rate
should also be checked. The gravida with active vaginal bleeding,
however, should be evaluated with ultrasound to rule out placenta
previa before the pelvic examination is attempted. If significant
pain and a "rock-hard" uterus is found in association with marked
bleeding, placental abruption should be ruled out. Also, if there is
suspicion of ruptured membranes, the patient should be evaluated
with a sterile speculum and with Nitrazine paper and ferning tests
to confirm a diagnosis of ruptured membranes unless delivery
appears imminent. The speculum examination will show the size
of cervix to estimate dilatation.

If the cervix is 6 cm or more dilated in a woman experiencing
active contractions, further transport, even short distances, may be
hazardous. Preparations should be made for emergency delivery.
An intravenous line should be established, if there is time before
delivery, in case the administration of medications, fluids, or blood
products is needed immediately postpartum. Minimal blood testing
should include hemoglobin or hematocrit measurement (or a complete blood cell count), hepatitis-B surface antigen (HBsAG), and
blood typing (if unknown). Also, a clotted tube of blood should be
made available for emergency cross-matching, if necessary. If possible, urine should be tested for protein and glucose.

Emergency Delivery Procedure

As the baby's head descends, imminent delivery can be anticipated by the bulging of the perineum and the appearance of the fetal scalp at the introitus. At this point, no attempt should be made to delay delivery, but a controlled delivery is important in preventing both fetal and maternal injury.

1. If the dorsal lithotomy position is chosen, the mother should be tilted slightly to one side to lessen vena caval compression and should be brought to the edge of the bed or stretcher, or the buttocks raised on pillows, to allow room for delivery of the baby's head and shoulders. The mother's legs should be widely separated and supported with her knees flexed.

2. With each contraction, the vaginal outlet bulges to accommodate a greater portion of the fetal head; this process may be aided by gentle digital stretching of the perineum. Episiotomy may be performed at this time if necessary to allow delivery without spontaneous lacerations. A local anesthetic should be injected just prior to episiotomy with 5 to 10 mL of 1% lidocaine in a syringe with a small-gauge needle. A midline perineal incision should be made, taking care not to extend into the rectum.

3. As the head emerges, the palm of one hand should be placed over the head to assist with the normal extension of the head and at the same time prevent the head from suddenly popping out of the vagina. At this point the mother is asked not to push in order to minimize the trauma associated with uncontrolled expulsive efforts. The best method to inhibit the overwhelmingly strong desire to bear down when the fetal head is distending the perineum is reassurance and asking the mother to pant or breathe through her nose.

4. With expulsive efforts under control, and one hand on the infant's crowning head, the second hand, draped with a sterile cloth, can be used to gently lift the infant's chin posterior to the maternal anus. This facilitates further extension and a slow, controlled emergence of the baby's head (modified Ritgen's maneuver). As the head is delivered, usually with the face down, it tends to return to one or the other lateral positions.

5. The baby's neck region should be palpated immediately after delivery of the head to check for a nuchal cord, which may be found about 25 percent of the time. If the cord is relatively loose, it can be slipped out of the way over the baby's head. If the cord is tight, two clamps should be placed close together on the most accessible portion of the cord (usually anteriorly) and the cord cut in betwen. The cord can then be unwound if there are multiple loops.

6. Before the delivery of the shoulders and thorax is continued, the baby's face should be wiped off and the mouth and nose aspirated with a soft rubber bulb syringe to clear the airway. This is especially important to prevent meconium aspiration if there has been meconium staining of the amniotic fluid. If no bulb syringe is available, the mouth should be scooped out with the finger as well as possible. Squeezing the nose between the fingers and stroking the upper neck from the larynx toward the mandible may also be helpful.

7. Attention should then be turned toward delivery of the shoulders. This can be facilitated by placing a hand on either side of the baby's head; a gentle downward traction will ease the anterior shoulder under the pubic symphysis. Care should be taken not to use undue force, as this may result in brachial plexus injury. If there is resistance, an assistant should be asked to use suprapubic pressure (not fundal pressure) to avoid impaction of the shoulder behind the symphysis.

8. When the anterior shoulder is visible, gentle upward traction will deliver the posterior shoulder. The posterior shoulder should not pop out uncontrolled, as this may result in a laceration of the anal sphincter into the rectum (third-degree perineal laceration).

9. The baby will be very slippery, especially if there is thick vernix (white, cheesy desquamated skin). The posterior hand should slide down onto the posterior shoulder as it is delivered and then behind the back of the neck to support the baby's head. The anterior hand should then be brought along the baby's back as the body delivers spontaneously. Placing the index finger between the lower legs, and the third finger and thumb around each leg, ensures a safe grip.

10. If the baby is breathing spontaneously and is close to term, there is no need to rush cutting the cord. The baby can be dried off, wrapped in a warm blanket, and placed on the mother's abdomen to help minimize heat loss.

11. The cord should be doubly clamped before cutting with sterile scissors. If sterile scissors are unavailable, it is better to leave the cord uncut until sterile instruments can be found. (See Chap. 3 for details of neonatal resuscitation.)

Management of Shoulder Dystocia

The first step in dealing with shoulder dystocia is to position the mother for maximum room and maneuverability. The maternal perineum should be at the end of the examining table, and the maternal legs should not be in stirrups but sharply flexed toward the abdomen in the McRoberts maneuver. A generous episiotomy should be cut with adequate local anesthesia. At this time suprapubic, not fundal, pressure should be applied by an assistant. Shoulder dystocia is likely to be further aggravated by fundal pressure, but suprapubic pressure can help dislodge the anterior shoulder impacted behind the pubic symphysis. If these measures fail, manual rotation of one or both shoulders toward the anterior surface of the fetal chest should be attempted to try to produce a smaller shoulder-to-shoulder diameter and displace the anterior shoulder from behind the pubic symphysis. A variation of this, the Woods corkscrew maneuver, consists of progressively rotating the posterior shoulder 180° in a corkscrew fashion, resulting in the release of the impacted anterior shoulder. Of course, any maneuvering in the birth canal may be difficult with a large, macrosomic infant filling it. At the same time, suprapubic pressure may be applied, but at a 45° lateral angle in the direction of the attempted rotation of the anterior shoulder.

Management Immediately Postpartum

The placenta should be allowed to separate spontaneously, unless there is considerable active bleeding. Pulling on the cord risks cord rupture or the possible catastrophe of inversion of the uterus. The usual signs of placenta separation are a gush of blood and lengthening of the cord. As the placenta is expelled, the membranes may be teased out by rotating the placenta and twisting the membranes. After the placenta is out, the uterus should be massaged to help it to contract and remain firm. **Oxytocin,** 10 U, may be given slowly intravenously (or mixed in the intravenous bag) or intramuscularly if no intravenous line is available to help maintain uterine contraction. Uterine atony often results after precipitous labor (total labor less than 3 h). Excessive bleeding calls for vigorous uterine massage, increased amount of intravenous crystalloid solutions, and additional oxytocin or methylergonovine (Methergine) 0.2 mg intravenously. Bleeding sites for lacerations should also be identified and controlled with clamps or direct pressure. Episiotomy or laceration repair should await the availability of an experienced practitioner or obstetrician.

For further reading in *Emergency Medicine: A Comprehensive Study,* 5th ed., see Chap. 103, "Emergency Delivery," by Michael J. VanRooyen and Julia B. VanRooyen.

62 | Vulvovaginitis

Rebecca S. Rich

Vulvovaginitis is a common problem whose causes include infections, irritants and allergies, foreign bodies, and atrophy. The normal vaginal flora helps maintain an acidic pH between 3.5 and 4.1, which decreases pathogen growth.

For coverage of genital herpes, see Chap. 86.

BACTERIAL VAGINOSIS

Bacterial vaginosis (BV) is the most common cause of vaginal discharge and odor in women, although many women who meet the clinical criteria described below are asymptomatic. BV occurs when vaginal lactobacilli are replaced by anaerobes, *Gardnerella vaginalis*, and *Mycoplasma hominis*.

There is an association between BV and preterm labor or premature rupture of the membranes, and postsurgical infection.

Clinical Features

When symptomatic, women with BV have vaginal discharge and may have itching. Examination findings range from mild vaginal redness to a frothy gray-white discharge.

Diagnosis and Differential

The diagnostic criteria of the Centers for Disease Control and Prevention include three of the following: (*a*) discharge, (*b*) pH greater than 4.5, (*c*) fishy odor when 10% KOH is added to the discharge (positive amine test result), (*d*) clue cells, which are epithelial cells with clusters of bacilli stuck to the surface, seen on saline wet preparation. Often, however, the diagnosis of BV is suspected from a compatible presentation along with absence of *Candida* and *Trichomonas*.

Emergency Department Care and Disposition

Metronidazole 500 mg orally (PO) bid for 7 d is standard treatment of BV. **Clindamycin** 300 mg PO bid for 7 d is an alternative. Treatment is not recommended for male partners or asymptomatic women. Routine treatment of pregnant women with BV is not recommended. Pregnant women at high risk of preterm labor should be treated. During the first trimester, use metronidazole 0.75%, one applicator intravaginally bid for 5 d, or clindamycin.

CANDIDAL VAGINITIS

Candida albicans is a normal vaginal commensal in up to 20 percent of women, and candidiasis is not considered a sexually transmitted disease, although it can be transmitted sexually. Conditions that promote candidal vaginitis include systemic antibiotics, diabetes, pregnancy, birth control pills, and the postmenopausal state.

Clinical Features

Symptoms of candidal vaginitis include vaginal discharge, itching, dysuria, and dyspareunia. Signs include vulvar and vaginal edema, erythema, and a thick "cottage cheese" discharge.

Diagnosis and Differential

Examine vaginal secretions microscopically in a few drops of saline solution or make a KOH preparation. Ten percent KOH dissolves vaginal epithelial cells, leaving yeast buds and pseudohyphae intact and easier to see. The sensitivity of the KOH technique is 80 percent.

Emergency Department Care and Disposition

The imidazoles (**clotrimazole** 1% cream or **miconazole** 2% cream) are the drugs of choice, applied topically for 3 to 7 d. **Fluconazole** 150 mg PO is an alternative. Treatment of sexual partners is not necessary unless candidal balanitis is present.

TRICHOMONAL VAGINITIS

Trichomoniasis, caused by a protozoan *Trichomonas vaginalis*, is almost always a sexually transmitted disease. However, up to 25 percent of women harboring the organism are asymptomatic.

Clinical Features

Most patients have vaginal discharge. Other symptoms include perineal irritation, dysuria, spotting, and pelvic pain. Discharge may be frothy and malodorous. Vaginal erythema and irritation are common.

Diagnosis and Differential

Saline wet preparation shows motile, pear-shaped, flagellated trichomonads that are slightly larger than leukocytes. The sensitivity of this test is 40 to 80 percent.

Emergency Department Care and Disposition

A single 2-g oral dose of **metronidazole** is the drug of choice. For treatment failures, metronidazole 500 mg bid for 7 d is recommended. Concomitant alcohol use may induce a disulfiram-like reaction. Most infected men are asymptomatic; male partners need treatment to avoid retransmission of disease. Metronidazole can be used in pregnancy, with a single dose recommended, but it is not approved until the second trimester. Topical clotrimazole is less effective but safe. If symptoms persist and are severe, metronidazole can be given after the first trimester. During lactation, the single 2-g oral dose is recommended, with no breast feeding for 24 h.

CONTACT VULVOVAGINITIS

Common causes of contact vulvovaginitis include douches, soaps, bubble baths, deodorants, perfumes, feminine hygiene products, topical antibiotics, and tight undergarments. Patients complain of perineal burning, itching, swelling, and often dysuria. The examination shows a red and swollen vulvovaginal area. In severe cases, there may be vesicles and ulceration. Vaginal pH changes may promote overgrowth of *Candida,* obscuring the primary problem.

Try to identify the precipitating agent and rule out infectious causes. Most cases resolve spontaneously when the precipitant is withdrawn. For more severe reactions, cool sitz baths, compresses with Burow's solution, and topical corticosteroids may help. Oral antihistamines are drying but may be helpful if a true allergy is identified.

VAGINAL FOREIGN BODIES

In younger girls, common items are toilet paper, toys, and small household objects. Later, a forgotten or unretrievable tampon or diaphragm is often the culprit. Patients present with a foul-smelling or bloody discharge. Removal of the object is usually curative without other therapy.

ATROPHIC VAGINITIS

Lack of estrogen after menopause leads to vaginal mucosal atrophy. The epithelium becomes pale, thin, and less resistant to minor trauma or infection. Bleeding can occur. The vaginal pH also increases, and subsequent changes in the vaginal flora can predispose to bacterial infection with purulent discharge. Treatment is a topical vaginal **estrogen** $\frac{1}{2}$ to 1 application for 1 to 2 weeks. A sulfa cream should be used for secondary infection. Estrogen creams should not be prescribed in the emergency department for women with prior reproductive tract cancer or postmenopausal bleeding. Since carcinoma is a major concern, such patients should be referred to a gynecologist.

For further reading in *Emergency Medicine: A Comprehensive Study Guide*, 5th ed., see Chap. 104, "Vulvovaginitis," by Gloria J. Kuhn.

---

63 | Pelvic Inflammatory Disease

Rebecca S. Rich

Pelvic inflammatory disease (PID) is the most common serious infection in reproductive-age women in the United States. The disease ranges from mild to severe, including salpingitis, endometritis, tuboovarian abscess, perihepatitis, and pelvic peritonitis. *Neisseria gonorrheae* and *Chlamydia trachomatis* (see Chap. 86) cause most cases, but PID is polymicrobial in 30 to 40 percent of cases. Bacteria ascend from the lower genital tract to the normally sterile endometrium and adnexae. The vast majority of cases are sexually transmitted. Risk factors for PID include prior sexually transmitted diseases (STDs), multiple partners, adolescence, substance abuse, intrauterine device (IUD), and frequent douching. Patients with prior tubal ligation can get PID, but the disease may be milder. Pregnancy does reduce the risk, but PID can occur in the first trimester and lead to fetal loss. Long-term sequelae of PID include ectopic pregnancy, tubal infertility, and chronic pelvic pain.

Clinical Features

Symptoms include abdominal and pelvic pain, fever, vaginal discharge, vaginal bleeding, and dyspareunia. Anorexia, nausea, and vomiting are common, mimicking appendicitis or gastroenteritis. Urinary irritative symptoms may occur, suggesting urinary tract infection. Onset of symptoms often occurs after menses.

Diagnosis and Differential

Diagnostic criteria are listed in Table 63-1. Disproportionate unilateral adnexal tenderness and/or adnexal mass or fullness may indicate tuboovarian abscess. Abdominal guarding and rebound tenderness will develop with peritonitis. Associated right upper quadrant tenderness suggests Fitz-Hugh-Curtis syndrome, a localized form of peritonitis, perihepatitis, due to infection around the liver. Laboratory studies should include a pregnancy test and cultures for gonorrhea and *Chlamydia* at a minimum, with other tests depending on the clinical presentation. Send an RPR for syphilis in any patient with PID, since STDs frequently coexist. The differential diagnosis includes appendicitis, gastroenteritis,

TABLE 63-1 Diagnostic Criteria for Pelvic Inflammatory Disease

All major criteria below must be present:
  Lower abdominal pain
  Tenderness on lower abdominal examination
  Cervical motion tenderness
  Adnexal tenderness

In addition, one or more of the following criteria will enhance the specificity of the diagnosis:
  Temperature >100.4°F (38°C)
  Abnormal cervical or vaginal discharge
  Laboratory evidence of *Chlamydia trachomatis* or *Neisseria gonorrhoeae*
  Elevated erythrocyte sedimentation rate or C-reactive protein
  White blood cell count >10,000/mL

The following definitive criteria are warranted in selective cases:
  Positive transvaginal ultrasound, or other imaging technique, showing thickened, fluid-filled tubes with or without tuboovarian abscess or free pelvic fluid, *or*
  Positive endometrial biopsy, *or*
  Positive laparoscopy

Source: Adapted from *MMWR* 47:79, 1998.

TABLE 63-2 Outpatient Antibiotic Management of Pelvic Inflammatory Disease

Ceftriaxone 250 mg IM, *or*

Cefoxitin 2 g IM plus probenecid 1 mg PO, *or*

Other parenteral third-generation cephalosporin

  plus

Doxycycline 100 mg PO bid × 14 d, *or*

Ofloxacin 400 mg PO bid × 14 d plus metronidazole 500 mg PO bid × 14 d

Source: Adapted from *MMWR* 47:79, 1998.

urinary tract infection, ureteral colic, pregnancy complications, and ovarian cyst or torsion. Although no ancillary tests are required to make the diagnosis of PID, pelvic ultrasound may be helpful to exclude tuboovarian abscesses, pregnancy complications, or appendicitis.

Emergency Department Care and Disposition

The Centers for Disease Control and Prevention publish treatment guidelines for PID (see Tables 63-2 and 63-3). Consider inpatient parenteral treatment for the following: inability to rule out surgical emergencies, such as appendicitis; uncertain diagnosis;

TABLE 63-3 Inpatient Antibiotic Management of Pelvic Inflammatory Disease

Cefotetan 2 g IV q 12 h, *or*

Cefoxitin 2 g IV q 6 h

  plus

Doxycycline 100 mg IV/PO q 12 h

  or

Clindamycin 900 mg IV q 8 h

  plus

Gentamycin loading dose IV/IM (2 mg/kg) and then maintenance 1.5 mg/kg q 8 h

Source: Adapted from *MMWR* 47:79, 1998.

immunosuppressed patient; suspected or demonstrated pelvic abscess; IUD in place; adolescent patient; patient with significant fertility issues; severe illness with systemic toxicity or peritoneal signs; nausea and vomiting precluding oral treatment; unreliable patient; or failure to respond to outpatient oral therapy. The majority of tuboovarian abscesses (60 to 80 patient) will resolve with antibiotic administration alone, but these patients should be admitted and surgical intervention discussed with a gynecologist. Instruct discharged patients to be rechecked within 72 h. Treat male partners to prevent reinfection. Counsel patients to avoid sexual contact until patient and partner have completed treatment and counseling about condom use.

For further reading in *Emergency Medicine: A Comprehensive Study Guide,* 5th ed., see Chap. 105, "Pelvic Inflammatory Disease," by Amy J. Behrman and Suzanne Moore Shepherd.

64	Complications of Gynecologic Procedures
	David M. Cline

The most common reasons for emergency department visits during the postoperative period following gynecologic procedures are pain, fever, and vaginal bleeding. A focused but thorough evaluation should be performed including cervical cultures and bimanual examination. (Complications common to gynecologic and general surgery are covered in Chap. 50.)

COMMON COMPLICATIONS OF ENDOSCOPIC PROCEDURES

Laparoscopy

The major complications associated with the use of the laparoscope are the following: (*a*) thermal injuries to the bowel; (*b*) bleeding at the site of tubal interruption or sharp dissection; and (c) rarely, ureteral or bladder injury, large-bowel injury, and pelvic hematoma or abscess. Of these complications, the most serious and dreaded is that of thermal injury to the bowel. These patients generally appear 3 to 7 days postoperatively, depending upon the degree of necrosis, with signs and symptoms of peritonitis, including bilateral lower abdominal pain, fever, elevated white blood cell (WBC) count, and direct and rebound tenderness. X-rays show an ileus or free air under the diaphragm. Although gas has been used to insufflate the abdomen, it should be absorbed totally within 3 postoperative days. Patients who have increasing pain after laparoscopy, either early or late, have a bowel injury until proved otherwise. If thermal injury is a serious consideration and cannot be distinguished from other causes of peritonitis, it is best to err on the side of early laparotomy.

Hysteroscopy

Complications of hysteroscopy include the following: (a) reaction to the distending media, (b) uterine perforation, (c) cervical laceration, (d) anesthesia reaction, (e) intraabdominal organ injury, (f) infection, and (g) postoperative bleeding. Postoperative bleeding will be the most likely cause of a hospital revisit. After hemodynamic stabilization of the patient, the gynecologist can insert a pediatric Foley or balloon catheter to tamponade the bleeding. Infection as a result of the hysteroscopic procedure is uncommon. Treatment should be commensurate with presentation and symptoms. Uterine perforations are mentioned only because they are relatively common complications associated with the procedure but seldom require more than observation.

MISCELLANEOUS COMPLICATIONS OF MAJOR GYNECOLOGIC PROCEDURES

Cuff Cellulitis

Cuff cellulitis refers to infections of the contiguous retroperitoneal space immediately above the vaginal apex and including the surrounding soft tissue. It is a common complication following both abdominal and vaginal hysterectomy. It usually produces a fever between postoperative days 3 to 5. These patients complain of fever and lower quadrant pain. Pelvic tenderness and induration are prominent during the bimanual examination. A vaginal cuff abscess may be palpable. The treatment of choice is readmission, drainage, and intravenous antibiotics as determined by the gynecologist.

Postconization Bleeding

The most common complication associated with major gynecologic procedures is bleeding. If delayed hemorrhage occurs, it usually occurs 7 days postoperatively. Bleeding following this procedure can be rapid and excessive. Visualization of the cervix is the key to controlling such bleeding. Application of **Monsel's solution** is a reasonable first step if it is easily available. Usually suturing of the bleeding arteriole is necessary. Quite often, the patient must be taken to the operating room for repair secondary to poor visualization.

Induced Abortion

Retained products of conception and a resulting endometritis are the most common complications. Patients usually complain of excessive bleeding, fever, and abdominal pain 3 to 5 days posttermination; but may not return with complaints for up to 2 weeks. Pelvic examination will reveal a subinvoluted tender uterus with foul-smelling blood vaginally. An elevated WBC count is common. Treatment must include evacuation of intrauterine contents and intravenous antibiotic therapy. Triple antibiotic therapy (ampicillin, gentamycin, and clindamycin) is the standard; however, there is increasing evidence that **ampicillin with sulbactam** 3 g IV is equally effective. If the patient has pain, bleeding, or both—but unaccompanied by fever—missed ectopic pregnancy must be ruled out.

Vesicovaginal Fistulas

Vesicovaginal fistulas may occur after total vaginal hysterectomy. Patients return 10 to 14 days after surgery with watery vaginal discharge. Gynecologic consultation is necessary.

For further reading in *Emergency Medicine: A Comprehensive Study Guide,* 5th ed., see Chap. 108, "Complications of Gynecologic Procedures," by Michael A. Silverman and Karen J. Morrill Hardart.

SECTION 10
PEDIATRICS

65 | Fever

Juan A. March

Fever is the single most common complaint of children presenting to the emergency department and accounts for about 30 percent of all pediatric outpatient visits. The physician evaluating the febrile child must differentiate the mildly ill from the seriously ill child. Many factors, such as clinical assessment, physical findings, age of the patient, and height of the fever, can influence evaluation and management decisions.

Clinical Features

It is important to recognize that fever represents a symptom of some underlying disease, and one must determine the actual disease process. Body temperature normally varies from morning to evening with the body's circadian rhythm. Current practice guidelines suggest that a temperature of 38°C (104°F) is a sufficient fever to warrant an evaluation. In general, higher temperatures are associated with a higher incidence of bacteremia. A retrospective study of hyperpyrexia reported that the incidence of meningitis was twice as high in children with fever above 41.1°C (105.9°F) as it is compared to children with fever between 40.5° and 41.0°C (104.9° and 105.8°F). Fever alone, however, is not a reliable indicator of the presence or absence of meningitis.

Diagnosis and Differential

Infants up to 3 months. The age of the patient influences the extent of the workup. Early studies suggested that infants under the age of 3 months are at high risk for serious life-threatening infection. Clinical assessment of the severity of illness in a young, febrile infant is problematic. Young infants lack social skills, such as the social smile, and lack the ability to interact with the examiner.

The history and physical examination may provide clues to the diagnosis. A history of lethargy, irritability, or poor feeding suggests a serious infection. The physical examination may reveal a focus of infection such as an inflamed eardrum. Inconsolable crying

343

or increased irritability during examination is frequently seen in infants with meningitis. Cough or tachypnea with a respiratory rate over 40 might suggest a lower respiratory infection and the need for a chest x-ray.

The absence of any diagnostic abnormalities on history or physical examination suggests the need for extensive laboratory tests to detect occult infection. These tests would include a complete blood cell count (CBC) and differential, blood culture, lumbar puncture, chest x-ray, urinalysis and culture, and a stool culture if there is a history of diarrhea. Urinary tract infections may not produce symptoms other than fever, so a urinalysis obtained via catheter and culture should be included routinely in the evaluation. Antibiotic therapy and hospitalization should be instituted as suggested by the results of these studies.

The recognition of occult serious infection in the well-appearing young, febrile infant is problematic. No single variable can correctly identify these infants. Combinations of variables in nontoxic-appearing infants are more helpful in the differentiation process including: white blood cell count (WBC) between 5000 and 15,000/mm^3, band count less than 1500/mm^3, no evidence of soft-tissue infection, normal urinalysis and stool with less than 5 WBC/hpf in infants with diarrhea. In low-risk patients, absence of these variables is usually (but not always) associated with the absence of serious illness (0.2 percent).

Some clinicians have recommended that these young febrile infants should receive antibiotic coverage with ceftriaxone (50 mg/kg), pending culture results (cefotaxime 50 mg/kg should be used if less than 1 week old). However, this management algorithm is no longer the standard of care. The need for hospitalization in the up to 3 months age group presents another area of disagreement. Some physicians hospitalize all febrile infants under 3 months old, whereas others hospitalize only those under 1 month of age. Because the differentiation between a sick and well infant is so difficult, all such febrile infants need extensive septic workups. The decision to use prophylactic antibiotics is not a substitute for a complete septic workup. The decision not to hospitalize must be made after careful assessment and after ensuring the reliability of follow-up.

Infants 3 to 24 months. Clinical judgment appears to be more reliable in the assessment of the older infant. Characteristics to note are willingness to make eye contact, playfulness, response to noxious stimuli, alertness, and consolability. The history and physical examination will frequently reveal the source of the infection. Pneumonia is commonly of viral etiology, however, it is appropriate to institute antibiotic therapy, see Chap. 71. Nuchal rigidity or Kernig's or Brudzinski's signs may not be apparent in the child under 2 years old. A bulging fontanelle, vomiting, irritability that increases when the infant is held, inconsolability, or a seizure may be the only signs suggestive of meningitis. Up to 20 percent of children with petechiae will have bacteremia or meningitis, most frequently with *Neisseria meningitidis* or *H. influenzae.* The organism most commonly causing bacteremia in this age group is *S. pneumoniae.* It is apparent that bacteremia patients do better if they receive antibiotics early. Blood cultures appear to be useful for following patients who may not be returning for periodic evaluations. Controlled trials investigating efficacy have demonstrated a reduction in the incidence of meningitis in bacteremic children treated with ceftriaxone (50 mg/kg) given twice, 24 h apart, as compared to those treated with oral or no antibiotics. However, only 0.019 percent of children aged 3 to 36 months with occult bacteremia develop meningitis and widespread prophylactic antibiotics are not recommended. Parenteral ceftriaxone should never be initiated without appropriate antecedent or coincident diagnostic studies.

Older Febrile Children. Children over 3 years of age are easier to evaluate because they can specify their complaints. The risk of bacteremia appears lower in this age group. Pneumonia in this age group may be caused by *Mycoplasma pneumoniae.* Rales may not be present early in the course, and bedside cold agglutinins may assist with the diagnosis of *M. pneumoniae.* See Chap. 71 for treatment recommendations.

Emergency Department Care and Disposition

Although fever may provoke febrile seizures, fever is not known to produce any harmful effects in children. However fever does cause the patient discomfort and as such should be treated. One can facilitate heat loss in a child using any combination of measures.

1. *Increasing heat loss.* Unwrapping a bundled child increases heat loss through radiation.
2. Drug dosage for **ibuprofen** is 5 to 10 mg/kg per dose at 6 h intervals (maximum dose 600 mg), and dosage for **acetaminophen** is 10 to 15 mg/kg per dose at 4 h intervals. Alternating these two drugs, every 3 h, in an effort to avoid the recrudescence of fever is common practice. Aspirin should not be used in children with chickenpox or with influenza-like illnesses due to its link with Reye's syndrome.

All patients with positive blood cultures should be recalled for repeat evaluation. If clinically well and afebrile, they should be instructed to complete the current course of therapy. However, any patient who remains febrile or does poorly, even if on oral antibiotics, should receive a complete septic evaluation (CBC, blood culture, lumbar puncture, chest film, and urine culture), be hospitalized, and receive parenteral antibiotics.

For further reading in *Emergency Medicine: A Comprehensive Study Guide,* 5th ed., see Chap. 110, "Fever," by Carol D. Berkowitz.

---

66 | Common Neonatal Problems

David M. Cline

NORMAL VEGETATIVE FUNCTIONS

Most bottle-fed infants will want 6 to 9 feedings per 24 h by the first week of life, whereas breast-fed infants may require feeding every 2 to 4 h. Intake is satisfactory if infants are no longer losing weight by 5 to 7 days and are gaining weight by 12 to 14 days of age. Stool frequency may vary from 1 to 7 times per day, with frequent loose stools in breast-fed infants. Breast-fed infants, however, may occasionally go 5 to 7 days without a bowel movement. Stool color is of no significance unless blood is present.

CRYING, IRRITABILITY, LETHARGY

Infants who have an episode of acute inconsolable crying should be observed closely for an underlying cause (Table 66-1).

Intestinal Colic

The most common cause of crying is intestinal colic. This usually occurs in normal, healthy, thriving babies in the second or third week of life and persists until 3 months of age. Episodes commonly occur in the late afternoon or evening. The infants typically scream, draw up their knees as if in pain, and may pass flatus.

TABLE 66-1 Conditions Associated with Uncontrollable Crying, Irritability, or Lethargy in Neonates

Intestinal colic

Traumatic conditions
  Battered child syndrome (fractures, burns, etc.)
  Falls (skull or extremity fractures)
  Open diaper pin
  Strangulation of digit or penis
  Corneal abrasion or foreign body

Infections
  Meningitis
  Generalized sepsis
  Otitis media
  Urinary tract infection
  Gastroenteritis

Surgical
  Incarcerated hernia (umbilical or inguinal)
  Testicular torsion
  Anal fissure

Improper feeding practices

Diagnosis is made when the typical episodic history is found and there is no evidence of physical illness. A careful history, physical examination, and appropriate laboratory investigations will enable the emergency physician to diagnose colic and exclude other serious conditions listed in Table 66-1.

Emergency Department Care and Disposition

1. Changes in care-taking styles can be suggested, such as increased carrying and rocking, decreased interfeed intervals, and use of pacifier.
2. Changes in the environment (e.g., background music or rides in the car and stroller can be suggested.
3. A trial of feeding change can be suggested in refractory cases, such as visible peristalsis, persistent regurgitation, or severe symptoms after ingesting cow's milk protein. For breast-fed infants, removing cow's milk from the diet of the mother may help. For milk-protein formula-fed infants, switching to soy-based formula may be required.

ABUSE AND TRAUMA

An inconsistent or implausible history may lead the physician to suspect a diagnosis of child abuse, while physical examination may reveal unexplained injuries (bruises at varying ages, skull fractures, extremity fractures, cigarette burns, etc.). If a diagnosis of abuse is suspected, the child should be admitted to the hospital for protection and further investigations. An examination of the eye is essential since the presence of retinal hemorrhage, especially in the absence of external signs of trauma, suggests whiplash injury due to severe shaking. Examination of the eye is also useful in ruling out an eyelash in the eye or a corneal abrasion as reasons for the infant's symptoms.

GASTROINTESTINAL TRACT SYMPTOMS

Surgical Lesions

The most common signs of surgical lesions in the gastrointestinal (GI) tract are irritability and crying, followed by poor feeding, vomiting, constipation, and abdominal distention. Physical examination may reveal a red, edematous, tender lump at the site of the hernia or testicular torsion. Anal fissures may also occur at this age and may be difficult to diagnose.

Feeding Difficulties

Most visits for feeding difficulties are due to parental perception that the infant's food intake is inadequate. If weight gain is satisfactory and the infant is satisfied after feedings, intake is adequate. Rarely, anatomic abnormalities can cause difficulty in feeding and swallowing. A careful history usually pinpoints these difficulties as occurring from birth. These infants appear malnourished and dehydrated. In contrast, previously normal infants with a recent decrease in intake have an acute disease, usually an infection. Improper feeding practices may result in an irritable infant with periods of inconsolable crying. This usually results from overfeeding, with inadequate burping during feeds.

Regurgitation

Regurgitation of small amounts is common in the neonate and is due to reduced lower-esophageal sphincter pressure and relatively increased intragastric pressure. Parents may confuse regurgitation with vomiting. Vomiting results from forceful contraction of the diaphragm and abdominal muscles, whereas regurgitation is independent of any effort and probably represents the ultimate degree of GI reflux. If the neonate is thriving, parents can be reassured that regurgitation is of no clinical significance and will decrease as the infant grows. Infants who are not thriving or having respiratory symptoms should be investigated for anatomic causes of regurgitation or chronic aspiration.

Vomiting

Acute vomiting may be part of the symptom complex of some diseases (see Table 66-1), especially increased intracranial pressure and infections (sepsis, urinary tract infections, and gastroenteritis). Projectile vomiting is usually seen in infants with pyloric stenosis and assumes its characteristic pattern after the second and third week of life. This condition usually occurs in first-born males and is characterized by projectile vomiting at the end of feeding or shortly thereafter. The vomitus does not contain bile or blood. Examination of these infants should be done with the infant relaxed and the stomach empty. Prominent gastric waves may be seen going from left to right as well as a firm olive mass felt by palpating up and down under the liver edge. Malnutrition and dehydration may be evident. Hospitalization is necessary for rehydration and surgical referral.

In any infant who is vomiting, signs of dehydration and candidiasis of the mouth should be sought. Signs and symptoms of hepatobiliary disease (e.g., jaundice), urinary tract disease, and central nervous system disease should be sought. Vomiting may also be due to inborn errors of metabolism and may present with nonspecific signs, as well as metabolic abnormalities such as hypoglycemia and metabolic acidosis. Infants who are vomiting should be admitted for evaluation and therapy.

Diarrhea

Diarrhea is associated with the excessive loss of fluid and electrolytes in stools. When an infant is feeling well and gaining weight appropriately, the only treatment necessary is to reassure parents that all is well. Infectious diarrhea is usually associated with fever and viral etiology, with rota- and enteroviruses being most common. Bacterial and parasitic causes (*Giardia, Entamoeba histolytica*) are rare in neonates. Causes of bloody diarrhea in the neonate include necrotizing enterocolitis, bacterial enteritis, antibiotic-associated diarrhea, milk allergy, and, rarely, intussusception. Infants who are moderately or severely dehydrated should be admitted to the hospital for treatment.

Necrotizing enterocolitis usually presents with other signs of sepsis (jaundice, lethargy, fever, poor feeding, abdominal distention, and discoloration). Abdominal radiography may demonstrate pneumatosis intestinalis. True milk allergy presents with abdominal distention, explosive bloody diarrhea, and, in severe cases, shock.

Abdominal Distention

Abdominal distention is normal in the neonate and is usually due to lax abdominal musculature and relatively large intraabdominal organs. In the majority of cases, if the infant is comfortable and feeding well and the abdomen is soft, there is no need for concern.

Constipation

Infrequent bowel movements in neonates do not necessarily mean that the infant is constipated. The breast-fed infant may on occasion go without a bowel movement for 5 to 7 days and then pass a normal stool. If the infant has never passed stools, however, the possibility of intestinal stenosis or atresia, Hirschsprung's disease, and meconium ileus or plug should be considered. Constipation occurring after birth but within the first month of life suggests Hirschsprung's disease, hypothyroidism, or anal stenosis.

CARDIORESPIRATORY SYMPTOMS

Cardiorespiratory symptoms in neonates are nonspecific and may be due to primary organ failure (cardiovascular or respiratory) and secondary to a variety of systemic diseases, such as sepsis and metabolic acidosis, abdominal pathology, and severe meningitis. Regardless of etiology, the first concern is the assessment and stabilization of airway, breathing, and circulation; and the second is establishing the diagnosis. (Causes of rapid breathing are listed in Table 66-2; pneumonia is discussed in Chap. 71; bronchiolitis is discussed in Chap. 72.) Normal respiratory rate ranges from 30 to 60 breaths per minute in infants.

Congenital Diseases

Occasionally, H-type tracheoesophageal fistulas may present in the first month of life or later with recurrent pneumonia, respiratory distress after feedings, and problems handling mucus. Rapid breathing due to cardiac disease is usually not associated with significant retractions and use of accessory muscles. As a general rule, the well-developed neonate who has unexplained cyanosis and tachypnea should be suspected of having congenital cardiac disease (see Chap. 67).

Cough and Nasal Congestion

Cough may be a prominent feature of most of the primary respiratory conditions listed in Table 66-2. Treatment of the underlying condition is the therapy of choice. Cough suppressants should be

---

TABLE 66-2 Causes of Rapid Breathing in the Neonate

Pneumonia
  Bacterial
  Viral
  Chlamydia
  Aspiration

Bronchiolitis

Illness to other organ systems
  Septicemia
  CNS (e.g., meningitis)
  Abdomen (e.g., distention, gastroenteritis)
  Metabolic acidosis

Congenital diseases
  Respiratory disease
    Delayed presentation of diaphragmatic hernia
    Tracheoesophageal fistula
    Lobar emphysema
    Tracheal stenosis, webs

Heart disease
  Cardiac failure
  Cyanotic disease (e.g., transposition of great arteries)

Neuromuscular disease
  Infantile botulism
  Muscle weakness

Abbreviation: CNS, central nervous system.

used with extreme caution in neonates. Nasal congestion is best treated with instillation of saline drops when necessary.

Noisy Breathing and Stridor

Noisy breathing is a common complaint in the neonate and is usually benign. Stridor is usually due to congenital anomalies (webs, cysts, atresia, stenosis, clefts, and hemangiomas) extending anywhere from the nose to the trachea and bronchi. Infants who were intubated in the neonatal period are prone to develop subglottic stenosis. Infection (croup, epiglottitis, and abscess) as a cause of stridor in the neonate is rare.

Apnea and Periodic Breathing

Periodic breathing, which may occur in normal neonates, should be differentiated from apnea. Apnea is defined as a cessation of respiration for 10 to 20 s with or without bradycardia and cyanosis.

Apnea may be precipitated by any of the disease conditions listed in Table 66-2 and usully indicates respiratory muscle fatigue and impending respiratory arrest.

Cyanosis and Blue Spells

If breathing is rapid but not labored, the most likely cause is cyanotic congenital heart disease with right-to-left shunting. If breathing is labored (grunting or indrawing), pulmonary disease (pneumonia or bronchiolitis) is likely. Infants with cyanosis should be admitted for monitoring and further investigation.

JAUNDICE

The most common causes of jaundice seen in the ED are physiologic (seen at 2 to 3 days of age), secondary to sepsis, breast-milk jaundice, and, occasionally, hemolysis due to autoimmune congenital causes. A proper history and physical examination will provide clues to the cause of jaundice. The well-looking child who is gaining weight and feeding well is unlikely to be septic. Laboratory evaluation should include complete blood cell count for anemia, smear for hemolysis, direct and total bilirubin level, reticulocyte count, and Coomb's test. In addition, hospital admission, applicable cultures, and antibiotics are appropriate for neonates who are unwell and have any of the signs and symptoms listed in Table 66-3. In all cases, arrangements should be made for monitoring of bilirubin and hemoglobin levels. Although most well infants can be monitored out of hospital, infants who are anemic or those with bilirubin levels approaching transfusion levels (approximately 20 mg/dL) should be admitted.

TABLE 66-3 Signs and Symptoms of Neonatal Sepsis

Temperature	Fever, hypothermia
CNS dysfunction	Lethargy, irritability, seizures
Respiratory distress	Apnea, tachypnea, grunting
Feeding disturbance	Vomiting, poor feeding, gastric distention, diarrhea
Jaundice	
Rashes	

Abbreviation: CNS, central nervous system.

DIAPER RASH AND ORAL THRUSH

Candida diaper dermatitis is an erythematous plaque with a scalloped border, sharply demarcated edge, and studded by satellite lesions. An oral course of treatment is usually warranted to prevent colonization of the gut. Oral lesions are white, flaky plaques covering the tongue, lips, gingiva, and mucous membranes. The underlying pathology of ill infants should be treated with oral antifungal therapy **nystatin** suspension, 100,000 U/mL, 1 to 2 drops each side of the mouth every 4 to 6 h after feedings for 7 to 14 days.

FEVER AND SEPSIS

Fever (see Table 66-3) is most commonly due to infections. Most infections occurring in the first 5 days of life are acquired by vertical transmission from the mother. Bacterial infections are usually caused by group B stretococci (30 percent), *Escherichia coli* (30 to 40 percent), other gram-negative enteric organisms (15 to 20 percent), and gram-positive cocci (10 percent). Infections in the neonate will manifest as a variety of symptoms and signs, such as feeding difficulties, fever, jaundice, or respiratory distress. A septic neonate may have normal or subnormal temperatures rather than fever. Urinary tract infections in neonates are often associated with nonspecific signs, such as irritability, diarrhea, or poor feeding, and diagnosis is established by urine culture rather than by urinalysis. All neonates with possible sepsis should be hospitalized and given broad-spectrum antibiotic therapy pending results of appropriate cultures (urine, blood, cerebrospinal fluid, etc.). (See Chap. 70.)

SUDDEN INFANT DEATH SYNDROME

Although sudden infant death syndrome should be considered, catastrophic deterioration is more likely due to infectious causes (septicemia or meningitis), trauma (intracranial bleeding or child abuse), and inborn errors of metabolism (medium-chain acyl dehydrogenase deficiency). When the cause of death is not known, physicians should obtain appropriate samples (blood, urine, skin biopsy, etc.) and obtain permission for an autopsy.

For further reading in *Emergency Medicine: A Comprehensive Study Guide,* 5th ed., see Chap. 112, "Common Neonatal Problems," by M. Yousuf Hasan and Niranjan Kissoon.

67 | Pediatric Heart Disease
C. James Corrall

There are six common clinical presentations of pediatric heart disease: cyanosis, congestive heart failure (CHF), pathologic murmur in an asymptomatic patient, abnormal pulses, hypertension, and syncope. Table 67-1 lists the most common lesions in each category. Congenital heart disease may also present with shock. Pediatric heart disease is frequently misdiagnosed as a viral upper respiratory tract illness or feeding intolerance. In fact, feeding intolerance may be the first symptom of congenital heart disease. This chapter will focus on conditions producing cardiovascular symptoms seen in the emergency department (ED). These conditions require immediate recognition, therapeutic intervention, and prompt referral to a pediatric cardiologist. Treatment of dysrhythmias is discussed in Chap. 3. Pediatric hypertension is discussed in Chap. 27. Syncope is discussed in Chap. 79. Evaluation of an asymptomatic murmur is an elective diagnostic workup that can be done on an outpatient basis.

CYANOSIS AND SHOCK

Determining the cause of cyanosis and respiratory distress in the critically ill neonate is difficult. The clinician should consider congenital heart disease, respiratory disorders, central nervous system disease, and sepsis. The hyperoxic test helps to differentiate respiratory disease from cyanotic congenital heart disease (although imperfectly). The infant should be placed on 100% oxygen. Persistence of hypoxemia suggests the presence of a shunt from congenital heart disease.

Clinical Features

Cyanosis associated with a heart murmur strongly suggests congenital heart disease, but the absence of a murmur does not exclude a structural heart lesion. Early signs of inadequate cardiac output in the neonate may be suggested by slow feeding or tachypnea, diaphoresis, or staccato cough with feeding.

Shock with or without cyanosis, especially during the first 2 weeks of life, should alert the clinician to the possibility of congenital heart disease associated with closure of a patient ductus arteriosus. Neonates with shunt-dependent lesions will experience profound symptoms with closure of the ductus. Shock in the neonate

TABLE 67-1 Clinical Presentation of Pediatic Heart Disease

Cyanosis	TGA, TOF, TA, Tat, TAVR
Congestive heart failure	See Table 67-3
Murmur/symptomatic patient	Shunts: VSD, PDA, ASD Obstructions Valvular incompetence

Abnormal pulses
  Bounding
  Decreased with prolonged amplitude
	
	PDA, AI, AVM
	Coarctation, HPLV

Hypertension	Coarctation

Syncope
  Cyanotic
  Acyanotic
	
	TOF
	Critical AS

Abbreviations: AI, aortic insufficiency; AS, aortic stenosis; ASD, atrial septal defect; AVM, arteriovenous malformation; HPLV, hypoplastic left ventricle; PDA, patent ductus arteriosus; TA, truncus arteriosus; Tat, tricuspid atresia; TAVR, total anomalous venous return; TGA, transposition of the great arteries; TOF, tetralogy of Fallot; VSD, ventricular septal defect.

is recognized by inspection of the patient's skin for pallor, cyanosis, and skin mottling and assessment of the mental status appropriate for age. Mental status changes may be fluctuating signs of apathy, irritability, or failure to respond to pain or parents. Tachycardia and tachypnea are commonly present. Tachypnea associated with congenital heart disease is typically effortless, without accessory muscle use commonly seen with respiratory disease. The workup for congenital heart disease begins with chest x-ray and electrocardiogram (ECG). Echocardiography is generally required to define the diagnosis.

Diagnosis and Differential

The differential diagnosis for cyanosis or shock due to congenital heart disease includes typically cyanotic lesions: transposition of the great vessels, tetralogy of Fallot, and other forms of right ventricular outflow tract obstruction or abnormalities of right heart formation. Typically acyanotic lesions that can present with shock include severe coarctation of the aorta, critical aortic stenosis, and hypoplastic left ventricle. It should be noted that cyanosis may accompany shock of any cause.

Transposition of the great vessels represents the most common cyanotic defect presenting with symptoms during the first week of life. This entity is easily missed due to the absence of cardiomegaly or murmur. Symptoms (prior to shock) include dusky lips, increased respiratory rate, and/or feeding difficulty.

Tetralogy of Fallot produces the following features: a holosystolic murmur of ventricular septal defect (VSD), a diamond-shaped murmur of pulmonary stenosis, and cyanosis. The toddler may relieve symptoms by squatting. Chest x-ray may reveal a boot-shaped heart with decreased pulmonary vascular markings. The ECG may reveal right ventricular hypertrophy and right axis deviation.

Hypercyanotic episodes, or "tet spells," may bring children with tetralogy of Fallot to the ED with dramatic presentations. Symptoms include paroxysmal dyspnea, labored respiration, increased cyanosis, and possibly syncope. If the condition is accompanied by polycythemia, the patient may suffer seizures, cerebrovascular accidents, or death. These episodes frequently follow exertion due to feeding, crying, or straining at stool and last from minutes to hours.

Left ventricular outflow obstruction syndromes may present with shock, with or without cyanosis. Several congenital lesions fall into this category, but in all these disorders, systemic blood flow is dependent upon a large contribution of shunted blood from a patent ductus arteriosus. When the ductus closes, these infants present with decreased or absent perfusion, hypotension, and severe acidosis.

Emergency Department Care and Disposition

1. Cyanosis and respiratory distress are first managed with high-flow oxygen, cardiac and **oxygen** monitoring, and a stable intravenous (IV) line.
2. Noncardiac causes of symptoms should be considered and treated appropriately, including a fluid challenge of 20 mL/kg of **normal saline** solution as indicated.
3. Immediate consultation should be obtained with a pediatric cardiologist and, if the patient is in shock, a pediatric intensivist.
4. Management of hypercyanotic spells consists of positioning the patient in knee-chest position and administration of **morphine** sulphate subcutaneously or intramuscularly 0.2 mg/kg. Resistant cases can be further treated with **propranolol** 0.05 to 0.1 mg/kg, especially when the patient has tachycardia.
5. For severe shock in infants suspected of having shunt-dependent lesions, **prostaglandin E$_1$** can be given in an attempt to

reopen the ductus. Start 0.05 to 0.1 mg/kg/min initially; this may be increased to 0.2 mg/kg/min if there is no improvement. Side effects include fever, skin flushing, diarrhea, and periodic apnea. Intubation and ventilation are often required.

By definition, these children are critically ill and require admission, usually to the pediatric intensive care unit.

CONGESTIVE HEART FAILURE

Clinical Features

The distinction between pneumonia and CHF in infants requires a high index of clinical suspicion and is a difficult one to make. Pneumonia can cause a previously stable cardiac condition to decompensate; thus, both problems can present simultaneously. The common symptoms and signs of an infant presenting in CHF are outlined in Table 67-2. Note that the tachypnea associated with congestive heart failure in infants is typically "effortless," in the absence of airway obstruction, as seen with respiratory disease.

Diagnosis and Differential

Cardiomegaly evident on chest x-ray is universally present except in constrictive pericarditis. A cardiothoracic index greater than 0.6 is abnormal. The primary radiographic signs of cardiomegaly on the lateral chest x-ray are an abnormal cardiothoracic index and lack of retrosternal air space due to the direct abutment of the heart against the sternum.

TABLE 67-2 Recognition of Congestive Heart Failure in Infants

Signs	Right-sided failure	Left-sided failure	Both
Cardinal	Hepatomegaly	Tachypnea Dyspnea and sweating on feeding Rales	Cardiomegaly Failure to thrive Tachycardia
Unusual	Jugular venous distention Peripheral edema Anasarca		

Once CHF is recognized, age-related categories simplify further differential diagnosis (Table 67-3). In contrast to the gradual onset of failure with a VSD, coarctation of the aorta can present with abrupt onset of congestive heart failure precipitated by a delayed closure of the ductus arteriosus during the second week of life. Onset of CHF after 3 months of age usually signifies acquired heart disease. The exception is when pneumonia, endocarditis, or other complications cause a congenital lesion to decompensate.

Myocarditis is often preceded by a viral respiratory illness and needs to be differentiated from pneumonia. As with pneumonia, the infant usually presents in distress with fever, tachypnea, and tachycardia. ECG may reveal diffuse ST changes, dysrhythmias, or ectopy, signaling increased risk of sudden death. Chest x-ray shows cloudy lung fields either from inflammation or pulmonary edema. Cardiomegaly with poor distal pulses and prolonged capillary refill, however, distinguish it from common pneumonia. Once cardiomegaly is discovered, hospital admission and an echocardiogram are indicated.

Usually pericarditis presents as cardiomegaly discovered on a chest x-ray. Clinical signs such as chest pain, muffled heart sounds, and a rub may be present. An echocardiogram is performed urgently to distinguish a pericardial effusion from dilated or hyper-

TABLE 67-3 Differential Diagnosis of Congestive Heart Failure Based on Age of Presentation

Age	Spectrum	
1 min 1 h	Noncardiac origin: anemia, acidosis, hypoxia, hypoglycemia, hypocalcemia, sepsis	Acquired
1 day 1 week 2 weeks 1 month	PDA in premature infants HPLV Coarctation Ventricular septal defect	Congenital
3 months 1 year 10 years	Supraventricular tachycardia Myocarditis Cardiomyopathy Severe anemia Rhematic fever	Acquired

Note: For meanings of acronyms, refer to Table 67-1.

trophic cardiomyopathy as well as to determine the need for peri-cardiocentesis.

If an infant presents in pure right-sided CHF, the primary problem is most likely to be pulmonary, such as cor pulmonale. In early stages, lid edema is often the first noticeable sign. This may progress to hepatomegaly and anasarca.

Emergency Department Care and Disposition

1. The infant who presents with mild tachypnea, hepatomegaly, and cardiomegaly should be seated upright in a comfortable position, oxygen should be given, and the child should be kept in a neutral thermal environment to avoid metabolic stresses imposed by either hypothermia or hyperthermia.
2. If the work of breathing is increased or CHF is apparent on chest x-ray, 1 to 2 mg/kg of **furosemide** parenterally is indicated.
3. Hypoxemia can usually be corrected by fluid restriction, diuresis, and an increased Fio_2, although continuous positive airway pressure is sometimes necessary.
4. Stabilization and improvement of left ventricular function can often first be accomplished with inotropic agents. **Digoxin** is used in milder forms of CHF. The appropriate first digitalizing dose to be given in the ED is 0.02 mg/kg.
5. At some point, CHF progresses to cardiogenic shock, in which distal pulses are absent and end-organ perfusion is threatened. In such situations, continuous infusions of inotropic agents, such as **dopamine** or **dobutamine,** are indicated instead of digoxin. The initial starting range is 2 to 10 mg/kg/min.
6. Aggressive management is often necessary for secondary derangements, including respiratory insufficiency, acute renal failure, lactic acidosis, disseminated intravascular coagulation, hypoglycemia, and hypocalcemia.
7. For definitive diagnosis and treatment of congenital lesions presenting in CHF, cardiac catheterization followed by surgical intervention is often necessary. See the previous section for recommendations regarding administration of prostaglandin E_1 as a temporizing measure prior to surgery.

For further reading in *Emergency Medicine: A Comprehensive Study Guide*, 5th ed., see Chap. 115, "Pediatric Heart Disease," by C. James Corrall.

68 | Otitis Media and Pharyngitis

Marilyn P. Hicks

OTITIS MEDIA

Otitis media (AOM), an infection of the middle ear, commonly affects infants and young children because of relative immaturity of the upper respiratory tract, especially the eustachian tube. *Streptococcus pneumoniae* is the most prevalent and most virulent cause, accounting for approximately 40 percent of infections. *Haemophilus influenzae* NT (nontypeable) and *Moraxella catarrhalis* account for another 40 percent and have a high rate of spontaneous resolution.

Clinical Features

The peak age is 3 to 24 months. Symptoms include fever, poor feeding, irritability, vomiting, ear pulling, and earache. Signs include dull, bulging, immobile tympanic membrane (TM), loss of visualization of bony landmarks within the middle ear, air-fluid levels or bubbles within the middle ear, and bullae on the TM.

Diagnosis and Differential

Diagnosis is based on presenting symptoms and changes of the TM and middle ear. A red TM alone does not indicate the presence of an ear infection. Fever, prolonged crying, and viral infections can cause hyperemia of the TM. Pneumatic otoscopy can be a helpful diagnostic tool; however, a retracted drum for whatever reason will demonstrate decreased mobility.

Emergency Department Care and Disposition

Treatment begins with antibiotics listed in Table 68-1. Amoxicillin remains the first drug of choice despite the increasing incidence of penicillin-resistant *Strep. pneumoniae* and the predominance of β-lactamase-producing *H. influenzae* NT and *M. catarrhalis*. An average of 20 percent of pneumococci have some degree of penicillin resistance; some geographic areas have rates as high as 40 percent. Approximately 50 percent of *H. influenzae* NT and > 90 percent of *M. catarrhalis* are β-lactamase-producing strains. Penicillin-resistant *Strep. pneumoniae* also exhibits resistance to erythromycin, trimethoprim-sulfamethoxazole, clindamycin, cefixime, ceftibuten, cefaclor, and loracarbef. Macrolides (clar-

TABLE 68-1 Drug Treatment for Otitis Media

1st line antibiotics	Amoxicillin	45–60 mg/kg/d tid × 10 d
	Trimethoprim-sulfamethoxazole	8–10 mg trimethoprim/kg/d × 10 d
	Erythromycin/sulfisoxazole	50 mg erythromycin/kg/d × 10 d
2d line antibiotics	Amoxicillin-	80–100 mg/kg/d × 10 d
	Amoxicillin-clavulanate	45 mg/kg/d × 10 d
	Cefpodoxime	10 mg/kg/d (max 400) × 10 d
	Cefuroxime axetil	20 mg/kg/d × 10 d
	Azithromycin	10 mg/kg × 1, 5 mg/kg × 4 d
	Ceftriaxone	50 mg/kg/d × 1–3 doses
Analgesics	Auralgan otic	3–4 ggts q4h
	Acetaminophen/codeine	0.5–1.0 mg codeine/kg/dose q4–6h
	Ibuprofen	10 mg/kg/dose q8h

ithromycin and azithromycin) have rapidly developed significant resistance to *Strep. pneumoniae* (35 to 55 percent).

Pharmacokinetic studies suggest higher doses of amoxicillin (80 to 100 mg/kg/d divided two times a day) are more active against moderately and highly resistant strains of *Strep. pneumoniae.* Risk factors for drug-resistant *Strep. pneumoniae* (DRSP) include age < 2 years, group day care, frequent AOM, frequent and/or recent antibiotics, and immunoincompetence. High-dose amoxicillin (80 to 100 mg/kg/d) should be considered for children at risk. Other antibiotics appropriate for DRSP include amoxicillin-clavulanate, cefpodoxime, and ceftriaxone. Cefuroxime axetil exhibits moderate activity against intermediate resistant *Strep. pneumoniae.*

Infants less than 30 days of age with AOM are at risk for infection with group B *Streptococcus, Staphylococcus aureus,* and gram-negative bacilli and should undergo evaluation and treatment for presumed sepsis.

Recurrent AOM is characterized as three or more episodes within 6 months or 4 or more within 12 months. Persistent AOM occurs when the signs and symptoms of AOM do not improve with appropriate antibiotic therapy. High-dose amoxicillin therapy or other antibiotics suitable for DRSP coverage should be considered for both recurrent and persistent AOM. When using ceftriaxone for the presumed treatment of DRSP, one intramuscular 50 mg/kg dose may not suffice; children should be followed on a 24-h basis until symptoms resolve. As many as three injections may be necessary.

In uncomplicated AOM, symptoms resolve within 48 to 72 h; however, the middle ear effusion may persist as long as 8 to 12 weeks. Routine follow-up is not necessary unless the symptoms persist or worsen.

OTITIS MEDIA WITH EFFUSION

Otitis media with effusion (OME) is fluid within the middle ear without the associated signs and symptoms of an acute infection. Chronic OME (duration > 3 months) can result in significant hearing loss and language delay.

Clinical Features

OME is characterized by a middle ear effusion, distortion of bony landmarks and decreased mobility of the TM. Absent are symptoms of acute infection such as fever, irritability, and otalgia.

Diagnosis and Differential

The diagnosis is based upon the appearance of the TM in the absence of systemic symptoms. Audiometry is of limited value for diagnosis, but is crucial to the evaluation of a hearing deficit.

Emergency Department Care and Disposition

Treatment of OME includes the following:

1. Careful observation for resolution (standard treatment of choice).
2. No indication for antihistamines, decongestants, or steroids.
3. Ear, nose, and throat (ENT) referral and hearing evaluation for chronic OME.
   a. Antibiotics achieve resolution in only 14 percent of cases.
   b. Bilateral myringotomy tubes.

OTITIS EXTERNA

Otitis externa (OE) is an inflammatory process involving the auricle, external auditory canal (EAC), and surface of the TM. It is commonly caused by gram-negative enteric organisms, *Staphylococcus, Pseudomonas,* or fungi.

Clinical Features

Peak seasons for OE are spring and summer, and the peak age is 9 to 19 years. Symptoms include earache, itching, and fever. Signs include erythema, edema of EAC, white exudate on EAC and

TM, pain with motion of tragus or auricle, and periauricular or cervical adenopathy.

Diagnosis and Differential

Diagnosis for OE is based on clinical signs and symptoms. A foreign body within the external canal should be excluded by carefully removing any debris that may be present.

Emergency Department Care and Disposition

The clinician should place a wick in the canal if significant edema obstructs the EAC. Cortisporin Otic solution, Otic Domeboro, or propylene glycol solution can be used. Oral antibiotics are indicated if otitis media or auricular cellulitis is present. Analgesics, including narcotics, may be necessary initially. Follow-up should be advised if improvement does not occur within 48 h; otherwise reevaluation at the end of treatment is sufficient.

Cultures of the EAC may identify unusual or resistant organisms. Patients with diabetes or other forms of immunoincompetence can develop malignant otitis externa. Malignant OE is characterized by systemic symptoms and auricular cellulitis. This condition can result in serious complications and requires hospitalization with intravenous antibiotics.

PHARYNGITIS

Etiologies include multiple viruses and bacteria, but only group A β-hemolytic Streptococcus (GABHS), Epstein-Barr virus, and *Neisseria gonorrhea* require accurate diagnosis. The identification and treatment of GABHS pharyngitis is important in order to prevent the suppurative complications and the sequelae of acute rheumatic fever.

Clinical Features

Peak seasons for GABHS are late winter or early spring, and the peak age is 4 to 11 years. Symptoms (sudden onset) include sore throat, fever, headache, abdominal pain, enlarged anterior cervical nodes, palatal petechiae, and tonsillar hypertrophy. With GABHS there is absence of cough, coryza, laryngitis, stridor, conjunctivitis, and diarrhea. A scarlatina-form rash associated with pharyngitis almost always is GABHS and is commonly referred to as scarlet fever. Diagnosis based on clinical findings alone results in only 50 to 70 percent accuracy at best.

Epstein-Barr virus (EBV) is a herpes virus and often presents much like streptococcal pharyngitis. Common symptoms are fever, sore throat, and malaise. Cervical adenopathy may be prominent and often is posterior as well as anterior. Hepatosplenomegaly may be present. EBV should be suspected in the child with pharyngitis nonresponsive to antibiotics, in the presence of a negative throat culture.

Gonococcal (GC) pharyngitis in children and nonsexually active adolescents should alert one to the possibility of child abuse. GC pharyngitis tends to have a more benign clinical presentation than GABHS pharyngitis.

Diagnosis and Differential

Definitive diagnosis of GABHS is made with the throat culture; however, this may not always be practical in the ED, because of the time involved and potential problems with follow-up. Rapid antigen-detection tests, if properly performed, achieve sensitivity and specificity close to that of the throat culture. A negative rapid strep test does not exclude GABHS and should be verified with a throat culture. Other etiologies of pharyngitis to recognize are Epstein-Barr virus (infectious mononucleosis) and *N. gonorrhea.*

TABLE 68-2 Treatment of GAS and GC Pharyngitis

GAS pharyngitis	Penicillin V	1 g bid × 10 d > 27 kg 500 mg bid × 10 d < 27 kg
	Amoxicillin	60 mg/kg/day tid × 10 d 750 mg qd × 10 d ≥ 5 y of age
	Benzathine PCN	1.2 million U IM > 27 kg; 600,000 U IM < 27 kg
	Erythromycin	E. estolate 20–40 mg/kg/d tid × 10 d E. ethylsuccinate 40–50 mg/kg/day tid × 10 d
	Cephalexin	25–50 mg/kg/d bid × 10 d (500 bid adolescent)
	Cefadroxil	30 mg/kg/day bid × 10 d
	Azithromycin	12 mg/kg qd × 5 d
Gonococcal pharyngitis	Ceftriaxone	125 mg IM < 45 kg; 250 mg IM > 45 kg
	Spectinomycin (PCN allergy) AND	40 mg/kg/IM × 7 d
	Erythromycin or doxycycline	40 mg/kg/d (< 8 y old) 100 mg bid (> 8 y old) × 7 d

With EBV, the white blood cell count will typically show a lymphocytosis with a preponderance of atypical lymphocytes. Diagnosis is confirmed with a positive heterophil antibody (mono spot). Diagnosis of GC pharyngitis is made by culture on Thayer-Martin medium. Vaginal, cervical, and rectal cultures should also be obtained if GC pharyngitis is suspected.

Emergency Department Care and Disposition

See Table 68-2 for antibiotic choices for GABHS and GC pharyngitis. Antipyretics and sometimes analgesics will be necessary during the first 48 to 72 h of treatment. Appropriate follow-up should be encouraged for treatment failure and symptomatic contacts. Follow-up for suspected GC pharyngitis should include child sexual abuse and social service investigations.

EBV is usually self-limited and requires only supportive treatment of antipyretics, fluids, and bed rest. Occasionally EBV is complicated by airway obstruction and can be effectively treated with **prednisone,** 2.5 mg/kg/d tapered over 5 days, or **dexamethasone,** 1 mg/kg to a maximum of 10 mg, then 0.5 mg/kg every 6 h.

For further reading in *Emergency Medicine: A Comprehensive Study Guide,* 5th ed., see Chap. 116, "Otitis and Pharyngitis in Children," by Kimberly S. Quayle, Susan Fuchs, and David M. Jaffe.

---

69 | Skin and Soft Tissue Infections

C. James Corrall

This chapter discusses several common skin and soft-tissue infections of childhood. Impetigo is discussed in Chap. 82.

CONJUNCTIVITIS

Conjunctivitis is an inflammation of the membranes lining the surface of the eye. It may be secondary to infection, allergy, or mechanical or chemical irritation. Conjunctivitis is the most common ocular infection of childhood and is usually a sporadic illness, but may occur with epidemic periodicity with viral pathogens in summer months. *Neisseria gonorrhea* poses the greatest threat to the integrity of the eye in the neonate. Later in childhood, the respiratory tract pathogens predominate, particularly untypable *Haemophilus* species.

Clinical Features

Older children with conjunctivitis may complain of photophobia, ocular pain, or the sensation of a foreign body in the eye, which is associated with crusting of the eyelids or conjunctival injection. A thorough examination of the structure and function of both eyes should be performed, including visual acuity and extraocular muscle function. Erythema and increased secretions characterize conjunctivitis, with intense redness and purulence being more common with infectious rather than allergic causes. Allergic conjunctivitis is typically recurrent, seasonal, and accompanied by pruritus and sneezing. Fever and other systemic manifestations do not occur with isolated conjunctivitis. The duration of symptoms with infectious causes is often 2 to 4 days.

Diagnosis and Differential

The diagnosis of infectious conjunctivitis depends on the clinical examination. A Gram stain should be performed in infants less than 1 month old or in confusing cases. It will show more than 5 white blood cells (WBCs) per field and, in many cases, bacteria. The finding of gram-negative intracellular diplococci identifies *N. gonorrhea*. Conjunctival scrapings or cultures may be performed to diagnose *Chlamydia trachomatis* or other viral or bacterial pathogens. Fluorescein staining helps to identify the dendrites of herpes simplex. Conjunctivitis may be a manifestation of a systemic disorder, such as measles or Kawasaki's disease.

Differential diagnosis of the red eye includes conjunctivitis, orbital and periorbital infection, retained foreign body, corneal abrasion, uveitis, and glaucoma.

Emergency Department Care and Disposition

Treatment is directed at the most common causes of conjunctivitis based on patients' ages and examination findings as well as slit-lamp exam, fluorescein staining pattern, and Gram staining if indicated.

1. Infants less than 1 month of age with exceptionally purulent conjunctivitis or gram-positive stain for *N. gonorrhoea* should

receive a single dose of **ceftriaxone,** 125 mg intramuscularly, hospital admission, or close follow-up the next day. Public health reporting and investigation are mandatory.

2. For infants under 3 months of age, treatment with **erythromycin** (50 mg/kg/d divided four times a day for 14 days) is instituted to treat *C. trachomatis* and to prevent later development of the associated vertically transmitted pneumonia syndrome.

3. Older children require only topical antibiotic instillation into the conjunctival sac such as sulfacetamide.

4. For herpes simplex infections, urgent consultation with an ophthalmologist is required. Topical and oral antiviral therapy is indicated. Examples include trifluridine drops 9 times daily and acyclovir.

5. Antihistamines—The administration of **diphenhydramine** (5 mg/kg/d divided every 4 to 6 h orally) or **hydroxyzine** (2 mg/kg/d divided every 6 h PO) may be useful for allergic conjunctivitis along with eradication of exposure to offending agents.

6. Cool moist compresses will lessen the edema and crusting.

All children with conjunctivitis should have reevaluation within 48 h of treatment if there is no improvement, and no child should be treated for longer than 5 days with topical therapy without improvement. Failure to improve indicates further investigation and ophthalmologic consultation.

SINUSITIS

Sinusitis is an inflammation of the paranasal sinuses that may be secondary to infection and allergy and may be acute, subacute, or chronic in time course. The major pathogens in childhood are *Streptococcus pneumoniae* and *Haemophilus influenzae.* Other agents have been identified but their role is unclear.

Clinical Features

Two major types of sinusitis may be differentiated on clinical grounds, acute severe sinusitis and mild subacute sinusitis. Acute severe sinusitis is associated with elevated temperature, headaches, and localized swelling and tenderness or erythema in the facial area corresponding to the sinuses. Such localized findings are most often seen in older adolescents and adults. Mild subacute sinusitis is manifest in childhood as a protracted upper respiratory infection (URI) with a predominance of purulent nasal discharge and the absence of swelling. Rather than improve in 3 to 7 days, these children have persistent symptoms in excess of 2 weeks. Fever is infrequent. This latter type of sinusitis may be confused with congestion of brief duration found with some URIs.

Diagnosis and Differential

The diagnosis is made on clinical grounds without laboratory or radiographic studies. Transillumination of the maxillary or frontal sinuses is seldom helpful. Standard radiographs should be obtained for patients with uncertain clinical diagnosis and in cases of severe sinusitis. The most diagnostic finding is an air-fluid level or complete opacification of the sinus. Computed tomography (CT) is a more accurate and expensive tool for cases that fail to respond to standard therapy. Few other conditions masquerade as sinusitis, and the differential is limited, particularly in children.

Emergency Department Care and Disposition

The first step in management of sinusitis is to differentiate bacterial sinusitis from nasal congestion of a URI. The former may mandate antibiotic therapy for resolution, and the latter responds spontaneously.

1. For acute severe disease, intravenous therapy is recommended: **cefuroxime** (100 mg/kg/d divided every 8 h) or **ceftriaxone** (75 mg/kg/d) or **ampicillin-sulbactam** (200 mg/kg/d of ampicillin divided every 8 h). Persistent disease demands ear, nose, and throat referral for surgical drainage.
2. Mild subacute disease can be treated with **amoxicillin** (40 mg/kg/d orally divided three times a day). Persistent subacute disease can be treated with **cefprozil** (30 mg/kg/d orally divided three times a day) or **erythromycin-sulfisoxazole** (40 mg/kg/d of erythromycin orally divided four times a day).

Untreated or inadequately treated infection may spread from the sinuses to surrounding structures and can be life-threatening. Complications include epidural, subdural, or brain abscess, meningitis, and cavernous sinus thrombosis. More commonly periorbital and orbital cellulitis develops. These complications necessitate immediate surgical consultation for drainage procedures and culture to direct antibiotic therapy.

CELLULITIS

Cellulitis is an infection of the skin and subcutaneous tissues that extends below the dermis, differentiating it from impetigo. It is a frequent infection in warm weather. Under normal circumstances, *Staphylococcus aureus, Streptococcus pyogenes,* and *H. influenzae* are the most commonly isolated organisms. Since the advent of effective conjugated vaccines against *H. influenzae,* such infections are rare in childhood but are now more common in adolescents.

Clinical Features

Cellulitis manifests a local inflammatory response at the site of infection with erythema, warmth, and tenderness. Fever is unusual, except in severe cases including those caused by *H. influenzae.*

Diagnosis and Differential

The diagnosis of cellulitis is made by inspection. Cellulitis must be differentiated from other causes of erythema and edema including trauma, allergic reaction, and cold-induced lesions. Laboratory studies, including WBC concentration, blood culture, and rarely, aspirate culture, are obtained in specific circumstances, to include immunocompromise, fever, severe local infection, facial involvement, and failure to respond to standard therapy.

Emergency Department Care and Disposition

Treatment is determined by severity of illness, facial involvement, and immunocompetence.

1. For toxic patients with fever and leukocytosis, or for facial involvement, intravenous therapy should be used: **ampicillin-sulbactam** (200 mg/kg/d of ampicillin divided every 8 h) or **cefuroxime** (100 mg/kg/d divided every 8 h) or **ceftriaxone** (75 mg/kg/d).
2. For nontoxic patients, **dicloxacillin** (50 to 100 mg/kg/d divided four times a day) or **cephalexin** (50 to 100 mg/kg/d divided four times a day) should be used.
3. For immunocompromised patients intravenous therapy should be used: **oxacillin** (150 mg/kg/d divided every 6 h) or **cefazolin** (100 mg/kg/d divided every 6 h) plus **gentamicin** (5 to 7.5 mg/kg/d divided every 8 h).

Patients must be followed carefully and should have improvement in erythema and induration within 72 h of institution of therapy. Patients who fail to respond to reasonable outpatient antibiotic therapy must be further evaluated and considered for admission and intravenous antibiotic therapy. Other underlying conditions, such as diabetes or immune compromise, must be sought.

PERIORBITAL/ORBITAL CELLULITIS

Periorbital cellulitis is an inflammatory process of the tissues anterior to the orbital septum or within the orbit (orbital cellulitis). *Staph. aureus* and *Strep. pneumoniae* are the principal etiologic agents. Orbital infections are most often due to *Staph. aureus,* particularly when puncture wounds are involved. Children under 3 years old are more likely to be bacteremic, thus experiencing the highest incidence of periorbital cellulitis. Orbital cellulitis can occur at any age but is usually seen in children less than 6 years old.

Clinical Features

Orbital and periorbital cellulitis causes the periorbital area to appear red and swollen. Periorbital edema is usually more pronounced with preseptal infections. Proptosis or limitation of extraocular muscle function indicates orbital involvement. The eye is usually painful to touch but is nonpruritic.

Diagnosis and Differential

Periorbital and orbital cellulitis are distinguished from noninfectious disorders on the basis of clinical findings and the WBC concentration. As with cellulitis at other locations, allergic and traumatic causes for edema must be considered. Tumors and metabolic disease may cause swelling and discoloration, particularly thyrotoxicosis in adolescents and neuroblastoma in the young child. Leukocytosis occurs frequently with cellulitis and more often with bacteremic preseptal infections. Blood cultures in patients with leukocytosis are often positive. CT is performed when orbital involvement is suspected and may easily demonstrate an inflammatory mass or tumor.

Emergency Department Care and Disposition

Admission and treatment with intravenous antibiotics is indicated to prevent complications of meningitis and subperiosteal abscess. Antibiotic choices are the same as those listed earlier under cellulitis with facial involvement.

Children initially treated with intravenous antibiotics should have rapid defervescence and improvement in clinical status within

48 to 72 h of therapy. Continued worsening or the development of proptosis or ophthalmoplegia should prompt CT of the orbit and consideration of an etiology other than infectious causes or a severe complication of infection such as retroorbital abscess or orbital cellulitis. Changing antibiotic therapy should be made only on the basis of culture and consultation. Surgical drainage may be necessary with abscess formation.

For further reading in *Emergency Medicine: A Comprehensive Study Guide*, 5th ed., see Chap. 117, "Skin and Soft Tissue Infections," by Richard Malley.

---

70 | Bacteremia, Sepsis, and Meningitis in Children

Marilyn P. Hicks

BACTEREMIA

Children from 3 months to 36 months of age are at increased risk of occult bacteremia (OB), which occurs in approximately 2.8 percent of patients with rectal temperatures of 39°C (102.2°F) or higher. Infants under 3 months of age are at significant risk of OB and serious bacterial infections (SBIs) due to immunologic immaturity and gastrointestinal colonization of invasive organisms to which they have minimal resistance. *Streptococcus pneumoniae* accounts for more than 90 percent of OB, with *Neisseria meningitidis*, group A streptococcus, and *Salmonella* responsible for the remainder.

Clinical Features

The hallmark symptom of OB is fever, and the incidence rises incrementally with rectal temperatures above 39°C (102.2°F). The child appears relatively well, exhibiting fever alone or in combination with signs of minor infection, such as upper respiratory infection, vomiting, or diarrhea. Because children with OB do not appear toxic, clinical signs are not reliable indicators of this condition.

Diagnosis and Differential

Definitive diagnosis of OB is made by blood culture. A white blood cell count greater than15,000/μL or an absolute neutrophil count greater than 10,000/μL is known to correlate with an increased incidence of bacteremia. Elevated erythrocyte sedimentation rate and C-reactive protein levels also correlate with an increased rate of OB but are not practical for use in the emergency department (ED) setting. Infants at high risk for SBIs include the following: (*a*) infants 0 to 90 days of age, (*b*) immunoincompetent children, (*c*) children not immunized for *Haemophilus influenzae* (HIB), (*d*) children with risk factors for drug resistant pneumococcus (e.g., day-care attendance, frequent otitis media, and/or antibiotics), and (*e*) children with unreliable caretakers.

Emergency Department Care and Disposition

1. All infants under 30 days of age who are febrile should undergo a septic workup, be given intravenous (IV) antibiotics (Table 70-1), and be admitted.
2. Infants 30 to 90 days of age may not require full septic evaluation if they have no risk factors, have reliable caretakers, and follow-up can be arranged within 12 h. Acceptable options are (*a*) a

TABLE 70-1 Antibiotic Therapy for Sepsis and Meningitis

Age	Antibiotic	Dose
<1 month	Ampicillin and gentamicin* or ampicillin and cefotaxime	200–400 mg/kg/d divided q 4–6 h 7.5 mg/kg/d divided q 8 h 200–400 mg/kg/d divided q 4–6 h 200 mg/kg/d divided q 6–8 h
1–2 months	Ampicillin and gentamicin or ceftriaxone or cefotaxime	200–400 mg/kg/d divided q 4–6 h 7.5 mg/kg/d divided q 8 h 100 mg/kg/d divided q 12–24 h 200 mg/kg/d divided q 6–8 h
>2 months	Ceftriaxone or cefotaxime	100 mg/kg/d divided q 12–24 h 200 mg/kg/d divided q 6–8 h

*During the first week of life, reduce gentamicin dose to 5 mg/kg divided q 12 h.

complete blood count (CBC), blood culture, catheter urinalysis, culture and sensitivities (C&S), no antibiotics, and follow-up within 12 h; (*b*) complete septic workup, no antibiotics, and follow-up within 12 h; (*c*) complete septic workup, ceftriaxone 50 mg/kg intramuscularly (IM), and follow-up within 12 h; or (*d*) complete septic workup, admission to the hospital, and IV antibiotics.

3. Children between 6 and 36 months of age have the highest incidence of OB but the lowest rate of SBIs. Evaluation in this age group is also dependent upon the extent of the fever, the presence of risk factors, and the ability to ensure adequate and timely follow-up. Options for evaluation in this age group are (*a*) no tests, no antibiotics, and follow-up in 12 to 24 h; (*b*) catheterized urinalysis C&S in males 6 months or less and females 2 years or less and follow-up in 12 to 24 h; (*c*) CBC, catheter urinalysis with C&S, blood culture if the white blood cell count is less than $5000/\mu L$ or greater than $15,000/\mu L$ (absolute neutrophil count greater than 10,000), with or without ceftriaxone 50 mg/kg IM, and follow-up in 12 to 24 h; and (*d*) complete septic workup, with or without ceftriaxone 50 mg/kg IM, and follow-up in 12 to 24 h.

4. If the clinical condition of the child deteriorates at any time during the evaluation or follow-up process, a full septic workup should be done (if not already performed) and IV antibiotics begun in conjunction with hospital admission.

SEPSIS

Sepsis is bacteremia with clinical evidence of systemic infection and can rapidly progress to multiorgan failure and death. Risk factors include prematurity, immunoincompetence, recent invasive procedures, and indwelling foreign objects, such as catheters. Sepsis in children tends to have age-related causes, often with common organisms (Table 70-2).

Clinical Features

Clinical signs may be vague and subtle in the young infant, including lethargy, poor feeding, irritability, or hypotonia. Fever is common; however, very young infants may be hypothermic. Tachypnea and tachycardia are usually present as a result of fever but may also be secondary to hypoxia and metabolic acidosis. Sepsis can rapidly progress to shock, manifested as prolonged capillary refill, decreased peripheral pulses, altered mental status, and decreased

TABLE 70-2 Common Organisms Causing Sepsis and Meningitis in Children

Age	Organisms
0–1 months	Group B streptococcus *Escherichia coli*
3 months–5 years	*Haemophilus influenzae* *Neisseria meningitidis* *Streptococcus pneumoniae*
>5 years	*N. meningitidis* β-Hemolytic streptococcus

urinary output. Hypotension is usually a very late sign of septic shock in children and, in conjunction with respiratory failure and bradycardia, indicates a grave prognosis.

Diagnosis and Differential

Diagnosis is based upon clinical findings and confirmed by positive blood culture results. All infants who are toxic appearing should be considered septic. The workup of a child with presumed sepsis should include a CBC, blood culture, catheterized urinalysis with C&S, chest x-ray, lumbar puncture, and stool studies in the presence of diarrhea. The critically ill child should also have coagulation studies, including fibrin split product and fibrinogen level determinations, as well as arterial blood gas analysis.

Emergency Department Care and Disposition

1. Administration of high-flow **oxygen,** cardiac monitoring, and securing IV access are first steps. Endotracheal intubation should be performed in the presence of respiratory failure.
2. Shock is treated with 20 mL/kg boluses of **normal saline** solution with serial assessments of perfusion.
3. If fluid resuscitation fails, **dopamine** 5 to 10 μg/kg/min or epinephrine 0.1 μg/kg/min may be necessary.
4. Hypoglycemia is corrected with 0.5 g/kg boluses of 25% **dextrose**.
5. Antibiotic therapy should begin as soon as IV access is achieved and should not be delayed due to difficulty with procedures such as lumbar puncture. Empiric antibiotic coverage is chosen based on the age of the patient (Table 70-1).

Consider the presence of drug-resistant organisms or immuno-incompetence and infection with unusual or opportunistic organisms.

MENINGITIS

Meningitis is usually a complication of a primary bacteremia and has a peak incidence in children between birth and 2 years of age. Prematurity and immunoincompetence put children at higher risk. Organisms responsible for meningitis are essentially the same as those that cause sepsis (see Table 70-2).

Clinical Features

Meningitis may present with the subtle signs that accompany less serious infections, such as otitis or sinusitis. Typical of these are irritability, inconsolability, hypotonia, and lethargy. In young infants suspicion should be especially high due to the often nonspecific presentation of the illness. Older children may complain of headache, photophobia, nausea, and vomiting, and exhibit the classic signs of meningismus and neck pain. Occasionally, meningitis presents as a rapidly progressive, fulminant disease characterized by shock, seizures, or coma.

Diagnosis and Differential

Diagnosis is made by lumbar puncture and analysis of the cerebrospinal fluid (CSF). The CSF should be examined for white blood cells, glucose, and protein and undergo Gram's-staining and culture. If white blood cells are present and previous antibiotic therapy has occurred, the CSF should be screened for bacterial antigens. In the presence of immunoincompetence, also consider infections with opportunistic or unusual viral organisms. Contraindications to lumbar puncture are cardiorespiratory compromise, increased intracranial pressure, and coagulopathy. Cranial computed tomography should be performed prior to lumbar puncture in the presence of focal neurologic signs or increased intracranial pressure.

Emergency Department Care and Disposition

Treatment should always begin with the ABCs and restoration of oxygenation and perfusion (see specific treatment recommendations under "Sepsis," above). Empiric antibiotic therapy is based on the patient's age (see Table 70-1). Antibiotic administration should not be deferred or delayed when meningitis is strongly suspected. **Dexamethasone** 0.6 mg/kg/d every 6 h for 4 d should be considered in children over 3 months of age who have *H. influenzae* or pneumococcal meningitis. If given, dexamethasone should be administered at the time or shortly after the first antibiotic dose to be most effective.

For further reading in *Emergency Medicine: A Comprehensive Study Guide,* 5th ed., see Chap. 118, "Bacteremia, Sepsis, and Meningitis in Children," by Peter T. Mellis.

---

71 | Pneumonia

Marilyn P. Hicks

In children, pneumonia is an age-related disease with a much higher frequency of serious illness in infants and young children (Table 71-1). Risk factors include the presence of chronic or debilitating disease, attendance at day care, and young age of the patient, especially prematurity.

Clinical Features

The clinical presentation is also age-based. Symptoms in the infant may be nonspecific, characterized by fever, poor feeding, vomiting, irritability, or lethargy. Auscultation of the chest in the infant or young child does not often yield localized rales due to the small chest size; however, one may hear decreased breath sounds, wheezing, or rhonchi. Cough, retractions, grunting, and hypoxia are more reliable signs of pulmonary pathology. Tachypnea is a very sensitive indicator of respiratory disease in infants and young children (Table 71-2). Older children may complain of chest pain or dyspnea, and auscultatory findings are more reliable. Occasionally fever and abdominal pain and distention may be the presenting symptoms, with respiratory signs absent or minimal. Impending respiratory failure is heralded by hypoxia, cyanosis, altered mental status, or shock.

TABLE 71-1 Common Organisms Causing Pediatric Pneumonia

Age Group	Organisms*
Newborn	Group B streptococci Gram-negative bacilli *Listeria monocytogenes* Herpes simplex Cytomegalovirus Rubella
0.5–4 months	Viruses *Chlamydia trachomatis* *Streptococcus pneumoniae* *Haemophilus influenzae*
4 months–4 years	*Staphylococcus aureus* Viruses *Streptococcus pneumoniae* *Haemophilus influenzae*
5–17 years	*Staphylococcus aureus* *Mycoplasma pneumoniae* Viruses *Streptococcus pneumoniae*

*Listed from top to bottom by greatest to lowest frequency of occurrence.

Diagnosis and Differential

Radiographic findings in viral pneumonia are interstitial infiltrates, atelectasis, peribronchial infiltrates, and cuffing. Bacterial pneumonia typically present as lobar or segmental consolidation. Pneumatocele, empyema, or pneumothorax suggests *Staphylococcus aureus* infection. *Mycoplasma* pneumoniae may appear as streaky interstitial infiltrates or lobar consolidation; the presence of upper respiratory symptoms and benign clinical course help differentiate *Mycoplasma* from bacterial causes. The white blood cell count is usually elevated with a shift to the left in bacterial pneumonia.

TABLE 71-2 Standards for Tachypnea in Infants and Children

Age, months	Upper limit of normal respiratory rate, breaths/min
<2	55
2–12	45
>12	35

Blood culture results are positive in 10 to 30 percent of bacterial pneumonia and should be obtained for all toxic-appearing children. All patients with pneumonia require pulse oximetric analysis, and hypoxic children require admission. Other indications for admission include vomiting, dehydration, and signs of impending respiratory failure or sepsis. All infants under 3 months of age should be considered for hospital admission.

Emergency Department Care and Disposition

1. During the newborn period, **ampicillin** 200 to 400 mg/kg/d every 6 h and **gentamicin** 5 mg/kg/d every 12 h during the first week of life and 7.5 mg/kg/d every 8 h after the first week of life may be used. Third-generation cephalosporins, **cefuroxime** or **cefotaxime** 150 mg/kg/d every 8 h may be a better choice due to the ototoxicity associated with gentamicin. Ceftriaxone should be avoided during the immediate newborn period due to its interference with bilirubin metabolism.
2. In hospitalized patients under 3 months of age, third-generation cephalosporins are the drugs of choice: **cefuroxime** and **cefotaxime** at 150 mg/kg/d every 8 h or **ceftriaxone** 75 to 100 mg/kg/d every 12 to 24 h. If staphylococcal pneumonia is considered, **nafcillin** 150 mg/kg/d should be added to the regimen. If the patient is at risk for penicillin-resistant pneumococcus, **vancomycin** 40 mg/kg/d should be given. **Erythromycin** 50 mg/kg/d IV every 6 h is the drug of choice for *Mycoplasma* and *Chlamydia*.
3. Outpatient treatment of uncomplicated pneumonia in children more than 3 months and less than 4 years of age is **amoxicillin clavulanate** 45 mg/kg/d or **azithromycin** single 10-mg/kg dose followed by 5 mg/kg/d for 4 d is an acceptable alternative. Azithromycin or **erythromycin** 50 mg/kg/d are the drugs of choice in children over 4 years of age and in penicillin-allergic children.
4. If bronchospasm is a prominent symptom, aerosolized **albuterol** therapy may be tried.
5. Oxygen should be administered to maintain the SaO_2 at greater than 94%.
6. Children with severe respiratory distress or impending respiratory failure should be admitted to the pediatric intensive care unit.
7. Attention should be paid to adequate hydration and fever control.

TABLE 71-3 Indications for Admission

Age < 3 months

Toxic appearance

Respiratory distress

Oxygen requirement

Dehydration

Vomiting

Failed outpatient therapy

Immunocompromise

Noncompliant or unreliable caretaker

8. Children who are discharged should have follow-up within 24 to 48 h, and specific instructions concerning complications should be given to the care giver.

Hospital admission (see Table 71-3) and administration of IV antibiotics should be considered.

For further reading in *Emergency Medicine: A Comprehensive Study Guide*, 5th ed., see Chap. 119, "Viral and Bacterial Pneumonia in Children," by Kathleen M. Brown and Thomas E. Terndrup.

72 | Asthma and Bronchiolitis

Marilyn P. Hicks

ASTHMA

Asthma affects approximately 10 percent of the pediatric population and is the most common chronic disease of childhood. The rate of incidence, as well as the death rate, has increased significantly in past years. Factors that put children at risk for death are listed in Table 72-1. Several factors contribute to exacerbation of asthma, the most common being infection. Allergens, exercise, and irritants, especially cigarette smoke, also often trigger asthma.

Clinical Features

Wheezing is the most common symptom of asthma; however, if there is severe bronchoconstriction one may only hear decreased breath sounds. Also, persistent nonproductive cough or exercise-induced cough may be the result of bronchospasm. Occasionally rales or rhonchi may be present in conjunction with wheezing. Tachypnea and tachycardia almost always accompany wheezing. Retractions, nasal flaring, and accessory muscle breathing usually reflect the severity of the attack. Cyanosis, altered mental status, and somnolence often indicate respiratory failure. Bradycardia and shock herald impending cardiac arrest.

Diagnosis and Differential

The chest x-ray usually reveals hyperinflation and flattening of the diaphragm and is not useful in the treatment of uncomplicated, chronic asthma. Children experiencing a first episode of wheezing may need a chest x-ray if the cause is unclear. Other indications for x-ray include unilateral wheezing or rales, productive cough, or fever. Measurement of peak flow is useful in older children; peak expiratory flow rate less than 50 percent of the predicted value indicates severe obstruction. All children should have initial pulse oximetry on room air and if oxygen saturation is less than 93 percent, continuous monitoring should occur. Arterial blood gases are indicated if the oxygen saturation is less than 88 percent or remains less than 90 percent despite therapy, or if at any time the child exhibits

TABLE 72-1 Risk Factors Associated with Asthma Death

Intubation for asthma
Two or more hospitalizations, three or more ED visits in past year
Hospitalization or ED visit in past month
Syncope or hypoxic seizure with asthma
Recent steroid use or dependence
Increased use of β_2 agonists
Poor access to health care and/or psychosocial problems

signs of fatigue or impending respiratory failure. Hypercarbia, not hypoxia, is often the initial sign of respiratory failure. A P_{CO_2} of 40 or greater is usually an early indication of impending respiratory failure.

The most common cause of wheezing in infants and young children is bronchiolitis, especially during fall and winter, when respiratory syncytial virus is prevalent. Infants with bronchopulmonary dysplasia often exhibit wheezing as a manifestation of chronic lung disease or secondary infections. These children also may develop wheezing as a symptom of congestive heart failure, as will children with sickle cell disease or congenital heart disease. Recurrent aspiration resulting from gastroesophageal reflux may cause wheezing in young infants. Structural abnormalities, such as vascular rings, bronchial stenosis, or mediastinal cysts, can cause wheezing. Often early cystic fibrosis will present with wheezing and may mimic asthma. Pneumonia in young children may also be accompanied by wheezing. Aspiration of a foreign body may manifest as unilateral wheezing and should be considered in association with sudden onset of respiratory distress preceded by choking.

Emergency Department Care and Disposition

Nebulized β_2-agonist therapy, specifically albuterol, is the mainstay of acute asthma therapy, along with the administration of supplemental oxygen and early use of corticosteroids.

1. **Oxygen** should be administered when oxygen saturation is below 94%.
2. **Albuterol** can be administered as episodic treatments at 0.15 mg/kg every 20 min or as continuous nebulization up to 0.5 mg/kg/h, depending on the severity of the patient.
3. Steroids used early can prevent progression of an attack, decrease incidence of emergency department (ED) visits and hospitalization, and reduce rates of morbidity. Indications for use are for children with mild asthma who do not respond to 3 albuterol nebulizations at 20-min intervals, with moderately severe asthma who do not respond to the first nebulization, with severe asthma, with frequent attacks in the recent past (1 week to 1 month), who are steroid dependent, or with a history of respiratory failure or intubation. Steroids may be given as **prednisone** or **prednisolone** 1 to 2 mg/kg/d and, if given for 5 d or less, need not be tapered. Steroids are contraindicated in varicella-susceptible patients who have had known exposure or might have potential exposure to varicella.
4. **Ipratropium** should be considered for patients with severe distress or those who do not respond readily to albuterol alone. It

can be administered at a dose of 250 μg in 2 mL saline solution or mixed with the first three doses of albuterol.

5. **Terbutaline,** also a β_2-agonist, may be given as an aerosol, as well as subcutaneously (SC) and intravenously (IV). The nebulized dose is 1 mg of a 0.1% solution in 2 mL of saline solution for children under 1 year of age and 2 mg for children over 1 year of age every 15 to 20 min (maximum dose 3 mg). Terbutaline may also be given SC 0.01 mL/kg every 15 to 20 min (maximum dose 0.25 mL).

6. SC injection of **epinephrine** is rarely used anymore but is an acceptable alternative when nebulized therapy is delayed or unavailable or as initial therapy for the child with severe hypoventilation or apnea. It is given at doses of 0.01 mL/kg SC every 15 to 20 min (maximum dose 0.3 mL).

7. **Magnesium sulfate** 50 to 75 mg/kg (maximum dose 2 g) IV over 20 min may benefit a subset of children with severe exacerbation.

8. Helium-oxygen (Heliox) may benefit children with severe exacerbation by decreasing airway resistance and work of breathing. Heliox is available as a 60/40 or 70/30 oxygen mixture and therefore cannot be used in children with O_2 requirements greater than 40%.

Children who have not returned to baseline after five to six β_2-agonist treatments require admission. Children in status asthmaticus may become dehydrated due to decreased oral intake and increased insensible water loss. IV fluids should be administered as maintenance therapy. Treatment of children with respiratory failure includes continuous β_2-agonist nebulization, intravenous β_2-agonist therapy, or mechanical ventilation. If mechanical ventilation is required, low inflating pressures and long expiratory times may reduce the risk of barotrauma. Ketamine (1 to 2 mg/kg/IV) is a useful induction agent for intubation due to its bronchodilating effects. Morphine, meperidine, and atracurium should be avoided because of increased bronchospasm from histamine release.

Children who are discharged should have a home nebulizer or a metered-dose inhaler (MDI) and spacer if they are 5 years old or older (2 puffs every 4 to 6 h). A small volume spacer with a face mask, may be used with an MDI for infants and younger children. If oral steroids are prescribed, they should be continued for no longer than 5 d at a dose of 1 to 2 mg/kg/d. Timely follow-up within 24 to 48 h should be arranged prior to discharge. Parents and children should be given clear instructions as to signs of worsening problems and to return to the ED if needed.

BRONCHIOLITIS

Bronchiolitis occurs typically during fall to early spring, affects infants less than 2 years old, and is primarily characterized by tachypnea and wheezing. Respiratory syncytial virus accounts for the majority of infections; however, other respiratory viruses have been isolated. Young infants (under 2 months of age) and those with history of prematurity, bronchopulmonary dysplasia, congenital heart disease, or immunosuppression are at particular risk.

Clinical Features

Although wheezing is the prominent clinical manifestation, symptoms of upper respiratory infection will precede the respiratory distress. Most infants will exhibit fever, and apnea can occur among those 6 months of age or less. Other signs of respiratory distress, such as tachypnea, retractions, nasal flaring, and grunting, may be present. Rales may be present as well, either alone or in conjunction with wheezing. Decreased breath sounds or absence of breath sounds signifies severe bronchoconstriction. Cyanosis and altered mental status are ominous signs of respiratory failure.

Diagnosis and Differential

All children should have a chest x-ray with the first episode of wheezing. The chest x-ray in bronchiolitis shows hyperinflation and peribronchial cuffing. Occasionally small areas of atelectasis may mimic pneumonic infiltrates. True consolidation is indicative of a primary pneumonia or bronchiolitis with superinfection.

Identification of respiratory syncytial virus can be made from nasal washings using fluorescent monoclonal antibody testing. This is particularly useful in identifying children at risk for severe disease and hospitalized children who require respiratory isolation. All children with respiratory distress should have initial pulse oximetry on room air, and if the Sao_2 is less than 93%, pulse oximetry should be continuous. Arterial blood gas analysis is indicated for children exhibiting signs of respiratory failure or shock and those whose Sao_2 remains low despite adequate β_2-agonist therapy. White blood cell count and blood culture are not useful unless a superimposed bacterial infection is suspected.

Emergency Department Care and Disposition

1. Children with bronchiolitis may respond to inhaled β agonists and should receive a trial of nebulized **albuterol** 0.15 mg/dose. If improvement occurs, treatments may be repeated as needed.
2. Nebulized **epinephrine** (1:1000) 0.5 mL in 2.5 mL normal saline

solution may be beneficial if albuterol fails. It can be administered every 2 h.

3. **Helium-oxygen** (Heliox) should be considered for children with severe symptoms but should not be used in patients with an oxygen requirement greater than 40%.

4. Dehydration may complicate bronchiolitis because increased work of breathing prevents adequate oral intake, as well as increasing insensible water loss. IV fluids should be administered to children requiring admission, and close attention should be given to the state of hydration of children discharged.

5. Corticosteroids are not indicated in bronchiolitis unless there is a history of underlying reactive airway disease, in which case a dose of 1 to 2 mg/kg should be administered.

6. Apnea and respiratory failure mandate endotracheal intubation and mechanical ventilation.

Indications for hospitalization include (1) apnea, (2) respiratory distress, (3) hypoxia, and (4) vomiting and/or dehydration. Infants who are not hypoxic, are well hydrated, and have minimal or no respiratory distress may be discharged from the ED. Infants who continue to be tachypneic in the absence of wheezing should be observed and considered for admission. Clear instructions should be given to the care giver regarding signs of worsening respiratory distress and dehydration. All infants should have follow-up within 24 to 36 h.

For further reading in *Emergency Medicine: A Comprehensive Study Guide*, 5th ed., see Chap. 120, "Pediatric Asthma and Bronchiolitis," by Maybelle Kou and Thom A. Mayer.

---

73 | Seizures and Status Epilepticus in Children

Michael C. Plewa

Both the causes and the manifestations of seizure activity are numerous, ranging from benign to life-threatening. Although the majority of seizures are idiopathic in nature (e.g., epilepsy), several risk factors include encephalitis, disorders of amino acid metabolism, structural abnormalities (e.g., hydrocephalus, microcephaly, or arteriovenous malformations), congenital infections, or neurocutaneous syndromes (e.g., tuberous sclerosis, neurofibromatosis, or Sturge-Weber syndrome). Precipitants of seizures can include fever, sepsis, hypoglycemia, hypocalcemia, hypoxemia, hyper- or hyponatremia, hypotension, toxin or medication exposure, and head injury.

Clinical Features

Symptoms of seizure may include any of the following: loss of or alteration in consciousness, including behavioral changes and auditory or olfactory hallucinations; involuntary motor activity, including tonic or clonic contractions, spasms, or choreoathetoid movements; and incontinence. Signs could include alteration in consciousness or motor activity; autonomic dysfunction, such as mydriasis, diaphoresis, hypertension, tachypnea or apnea, tachycardia, and salivation; and postictal somnolence.

Diagnosis and Differential

The diagnosis of seizure disorder is based primarily on history and physical examination, with laboratory studies (other than a bedside assay for glucose) obtained in a problem-focused manner. In patients with breakthrough seizures or status epilepticus, serum drug level determinations are useful for some antiepileptic agents (Table 73-1), while others, such as gabapentin, lamotrigine, topiramate, tiagabine, vigabatrin, and carbamazepine, may not be immediately available or useful in guiding therapy. Serum chemistry studies (i.e., electrolytes, magnesium, calcium, creatinine, and

TABLE 73-1 Therapeutic Antiepileptic Drug Levels, $\mu g/mL$

Drug	Total	Free
Phenytoin	10–22	1.0–2.2
Phenobarbital	15–20	NA
Carbamazepine	6–12	1.8–2.2
Primidone	5–12	NA
Valproic acid	50–130	10–25
Ethosuximide	50–100	NA

Abbreviation: NA, not applicable.

blood urea nitrogen levels) are usually not indicated except in neonatal seizures, infantile spasms, febrile seizures that are complex in nature (with duration over 15 min, focal involvement, or several recurrences in 24 h), status epilepticus, or suspected metabolic or gastrointestinal disorders. Serum ammonia, TORCH (*t*oxoplasmosis, *r*ubella, *c*ytomegalovirus, *h*erpes), titers, and urine and serum amino acid screening may be useful in neonatal seizures. Blood gas analysis is indicated in neonatal seizures and status epilepticus. Cardiac monitoring is useful to assess the PR and QT intervals and the possibility of cardiac dysrhythmia as the precipitant of seizure. Magnetic resonance imaging is the preferred neuroimaging procedure for most cases of new-onset seizures, whereas cerebral ultrasound is useful in neonates and immediate noncontrast computed tomography is indicated in cases of head trauma, nonfebrile status epilepticus, and focal seizures or focal neurologic signs. Lumbar puncture should be performed in patients with neonatal seizure, infantile spasms, complex febrile seizures under 18 months of age, meningeal signs, or persistent alteration in consciousness. Emergent electroencephalographic (EEG) monitoring is indicated for neonatal seizures, nonconvulsive status epilepticus, and refractory status epilepticus, especially when a paralytic agent is used.

It is important to differentiate true seizure activity from one of several nonepileptic paroxysmal disorders, such as neonatal jitteriness, hyperexplexia (startle disease), near-miss sudden death syndrome, breath-holding spells (of cyanotic or pallid types), hyperventilation, syncope, migraine, hysterical pseudoseizures, narcolepsy, cataplexy, night terrors, vertigo, Tourette's syndrome, chorea, or paroxysmal choreoathetosis, which are characterized by normal EEGs and are unresponsive to antiepileptic drugs.

Emergency Department Care and Disposition

1. Airway maintenance (supplemental oxygen, suctioning, airway opening, or intubation when necessary)
2. Seizure termination
3. Correction of reversible causes
4. Initiation of appropriate diagnostic studies
5. Arrangement of follow-up or admission, as appropriate

Termination of seizure activity is important to prevent irreversible pathologic changes and risk of persistent seizure disorder, especially in the setting of status epilepticus, defined as one seizure greater than 20 min in duration or a series of seizures greater than 30 min without interictal awakening. For this reason, seizures lasting greater than 10 min are treated as status epilepticus. Intravenous (IV) access is essential in cases of neonatal seizures, status epilepticus, and recurrent seizures.

First Seizure

Patients with an uncomplicated simple seizure should undergo evaluation and treatment of any underlying cause and may not require antiepileptic drugs. Patients with prolonged or repetitive witnessed seizures, especially with concomitant neurologic deficit, are started on antiepileptic drugs. Although any antiepileptic agent may be used, the decision is based on side effect profile, experience, and ease of administration. **Carbamazepine** 10 to 40 mg/kg/d in 2 to 4 daily doses, **phenytoin** 4 to 8 mg/kg/d in 2 to 3 daily doses, or **phenobarbital** 3 to 8 mg/kg/d in 1 to 2 daily doses is commonly used for partial seizures, and **valproate** 20 to 60 mg/kg/d in 2 to 4 daily doses is commonly used for generalized seizures. **Felbamate** 45 mg/kg/d in 3 daily doses or **gabapentin** 20 to 30 mg/kg/d in 3 daily doses is used for complex partial seizures. **Ethosuximide** 20 to 30 mg/kg/d in 2 to 3 daily doses, **iamotrigine** 5 to 15 mg/kg/d in 1 to 2 daily doses, or **valproate** is used for absence seizures (after confirmatory EEG). IV loading can be achieved with the IV form of valproate depacon 10 to 30 mg/kg over 15 min, or **fosphenytoin** 15 to 20 mg phenytoin equivalents (PE)/kg at 3 PE/kg/min, a phenytoin prodrug without infusion-related complications. Discharged patients should have close follow-up arranged.

Febrile Seizure

Identification and treatment of the cause of fever is the primary goal of therapy for febrile seizures. Fever can be controlled by acetaminophen or ibuprofen and tepid water baths. Antiepileptic drug therapy with oral phenobarbital or valproate should be considered in patients at high risk of recurrence, such as those with an underlying neurologic deficit (e.g., cerebral palsy), complex (prolonged or focal) febrile seizure, repeated seizures in the same febrile illness, onset under 6 months of age, or more than three febrile seizures in 6 months. A single dose of oral or rectal diazepam 0.2 to 0.5 mg/kg given at the onset of febrile illness may also be effective in these patients. Admit children with suspected sepsis or meningitis as well as those with recurrent seizures. Discuss antiepileptic drug administration or EEG monitoring and arrange close follow-up with the primary care physician for discharged patients.

Neonatal Seizures

The cause of neonatal seizures should be investigated and treated aggressively in an intensive care setting. Persistent or uncertain cause of seizures should be treated with empiric IV **pyridoxine** 100 mg/d; hypoglycemia with **25% glucose** solution 2 mL/kg IV or **10% glucose** 3 mL/kg in neonates; hypocalcemia with **calcium gluconate** 4 mL/kg or 200 mg/kg of 5% solution IV and **magnesium sulfate** 0.2 mL/kg of 2% solution IV or 0.2 mL/kg of 50% solution intramuscularly (IM); and biotinidase deficiency with **biotin** 10 mg/d. The first line agent is IV **phenobarbital** 20 mg/kg at 1 mg/kg/min followed by 3 to 4 mg/kg/d. Second line agents include IV **fosphenytoin** 20 mg PE/kg at 3 mg PE/kg/min and then 4 to 8 mg PE/kg/d, **midazolam** 0.2 mg/kg over 2 min, or **lorazepam** 0.1 mg/kg IV over 2 min. Refractory seizures are treated with continuous IV infusion of **midazolam** 0.04 to 0.5 mg/kg/h or **pentobarbital** 0.5 to 3.0 mg/kg/h.

Infantile Spasms

Prompt recognition of infantile spasms is essential to optimal outcome. Therapy with adrenocorticotropic hormone (ACTH; or with clonazepam or valproate) is often started in the inpatient setting after specialty consultation. Glucose transporter defect syndrome is treated with a ketogenic diet.

Head Trauma and Seizure

Immediate seizures following head trauma may require short-term treatment with fosphenytoin, especially following severe head injury. Early and late posttraumatic seizures may require long-term antiepileptic therapy if recurrent.

Breakthrough Seizures in the Known Epileptic

Patients with a single breakthrough seizure should have antiepileptic drug levels measured (Table 73-1), since low levels (secondary to noncompliance or altered metabolism) or, occasionally, toxic levels may be the cause. Those with recurrent or frequent tonic, tonic-clonic or clonic seizures and low antiepileptic drug levels should receive rapid loading of antiepileptic drug IV (phenobarbital, fosphenytoin, or Depacon) or rectally (liquid valproate, phenobarbital, phenytoin, primidone, or carbamazepine). Lamotrigine should not be loaded because of risk of rash. A second antiepileptic agent should be considered if levels are in the high therapeutic range, such as phenobarbital, phenytoin, or valproate for focal or partial seizures and lamotrigine, ethosuximide, valproate, clonazepam, or acetazolamide for absence seizures. Admission should be considered for patients with serious medical illness, toxic drug levels, or frequent or recurrent seizures despite therapeutic drug levels. Close outpatient follow-up should be arranged for discharged patients.

Status Epilepticus

Airway maintenance is of primary importance in status epilepticus because all therapeutic agents can result in respiratory depression. With IV access, **lorazepam** 0.1 mg/kg to a total of 8 mg, **diazepam** 0.2 to 0.5 mg/kg to a total of 2.6 mg/kg, or **midazolam** 0.2 mg/kg is the primary agent of choice. Without IV access, alternatives include rectal, nasal, or IM midazolam 0.1 to 0.2 mg/kg; rectal diazepam 0.5 mg/kg; rectal valproic acid 60 mg/kg; or intraosseous (IO) infusion of lorazepam, diazepam, or midazolam (in similar dosages as IV). **Phenobarbital** 20 to 30 mg/kg IV or IO repeated 10 mg/kg every 20 min to levels of 60 μg/mL should be started immediately after the primary agent, followed by **fosphenytoin** 20 mg PE/kg IV or IO if phenobarbital is ineffective. Hypoglycemia should be treated with **25% glucose** 2 mL/kg IV or IO. If seizures persist after fosphenytoin, consider continuous midazolam IV infusion 0.04 to 0.05 mg/kg/h or general anesthesia (along with continuous EEG monitoring) with pentobarbital 2 mg/kg bolus followed by 1 to 2 mg/kg/h IV infusion or inhalational agents. Continuous midazolam infusion or oral clonazepam 0.2 to 0.6 mg/kg/d by nasogastric tube can be used for noncontinuous status epilepticus.

Consider treatable causes, such as hypoglycemia, hyponatremia, toxin exposure (e.g., iron, lead, carbon monoxide, salicylates, stimulants, etc.) or infections (e.g., meningoencephalitis or brain abscess). Specific toxicologic therapy (e.g., activated charcoal, hyperbaric oxygen, or chelation therapy) should be used when appropriate for suspected toxin exposure.

For further reading in *Emergency Medicine: A Comprehensive Study Guide*, 5th ed., see Chap. 121, "Seizures and Status Epilepticus in Children," by Michael A. Nigro.

74 | Vomiting and Diarrhea

Debra G. Perina

Gastroenteritis is a major public health problem, accounting for up to one-fifth of all acute-care outpatient visits to hospitals. Most children who come to the emergency department because of vomiting have a self-limited viral disorder. Likewise, most cases of diarrhea result from self-limited enteric infections. Despite this, loss of water and electrolytes can lead to clinical dehydration in 10 percent of cases and may be life-threatening in 1 percent.

Clinical Features

Evaluation of the child's hydration state is most important, regardless of whether the presenting complaint is vomiting or diarrhea. Clinical assessment of the child's hydration status is discussed in further detail in Chap. 80, "Fluid and Electrolyte Therapy." Viral, bacterial, or other infectious organisms may cause gastroenteritis, and spread occurs by the fecal-oral route. Pathogenic agents may be isolated from up to 50 percent of children with diarrhea. Acute diarrhea is the most prominent symptom in infants and children. Viral etiologies are the most common cause of both. Viral pathogens cause disease by tissue invasion and alteration of intestinal absorption of water and electrolytes. Bacterial pathogens cause diarrhea by the production of enterotoxins and cytotoxins and invasion of the mucosal absorptive surface. Dysentery occurs when bacteria invade the mucosa of the terminal ileum and colon, producing diarrhea with blood, mucus, or pus. Table 74-1 lists common causative agents, clinical features, and treatment for diarrhea in children.

Diagnosis and Differential

The most important aspect of diagnosis is a thorough history and physical examination. Selective laboratory testing may be useful if enteric pathogens are suspected. Dehydration caused by diarrhea is usually isotonic, and serum electrolyte determinations are not necessary unless signs of severe dehydration are present. However, be alert for the development of hypoglycemia in the setting of protracted vomiting and/or diarrhea in infants and toddlers. Blood glucose determinations are useful in this setting. Stool cultures should be reserved for cases where the child is febrile, has numerous episodes of diarrhea, and has blood in the stool. The fecal leukocyte test, sometimes used as a screening tool, has poor sensi-

TABLE 74-1 Common Agents, Clinical Features, and Treatment
of Diarrhea

Agent	Clinical features	Treatment
Viral		
Rotavirus	Watery diarrhea, winter, most common agent	Rehydration
Enteric adenovirus	Watery diarrhea, concurrent respiratory symptoms	Rehydration
Norwalk	Watery diarrhea, epidemic, fever, headache, myalgias	Rehydration
Bacterial		
Campylobacter jejuni	Fever, abdominal pain, watery or bloody diarrhea, may mimic appendicitis, animal reservoir	Rehydration Erythromycin
Shigella	Fever, abdominal pain, headache, mucoid diarrhea	TMP-SMX or ampicillin
Salmonella	Fever, bloody diarrhea, animal reservoir; antibiotics prolong the carrier state	TMP-SMX if complicated
Escherichia coli		
Enterotoxigenic	Watery diarrhea	TMP-SMX
Enterohemorrhagic	Dysentery, associated with HUS	Rehydration; check CBC, BUN, creatinine
Vibrio cholerae	Rice-water diarrhea	TMP-SMX
Yersinia enterocolitica	Fever, vomiting, diarrhea, abdominal pain; may mimic appendicitis	Rehydration
Clostridium difficile	Recent antibiotic use	Metronidazole
Staphylococcus aureus	Food poisoning	Rehydration
Parasitic		
Giardia lamblia	Diarrhea, flatulence; exposure to day care centers, mountain streams	Rehydration Metronidazole
Entamoeba histolytica	Bloody, mucoid stools; hepatic abscess	Metronidazole

Doses: ampicillin 50 (mg/kg)/d divided qid; erythromycin 40 (mg/kg)/d divided qid; metronidazole 30 (mg/kg)/d divided bid; TMP-SMX based on 8–12 (mg/kg)/d of the TMP component divided bid.
Abbreviations: bid, twice a day; BUN, blood urea nitrogen; CBC, complete blood count; qid, four times a day; HUS, hemolytic-uremic syndrome; TMP-SMX, trimethoprin-sulfamethoxazole.

tivity. A positive result should be interpreted in relation to the patient's entire clinical picture. Vomiting and diarrhea may also be a nonspecific presentation for other disease processes, such as otitis media, urinary tract infection, sepsis, malrotation, increased intracranial pressure, metabolic acidosis, and drug or toxin ingestion. Particular attention should be paid to infants under 1 year of age, since they are at risk for rapid dehydration and hypoglycemia. Bilious vomiting in an infant under 2 years of age is worrisome and considered a sign of intestinal obstruction until proven otherwise. Special attention should be given to those children who have chronically debilitating illnesses, high-risk social situations, or malnutrition, since they are at particular risk for rapid decompensation.

Emergency Department Care and Disposition

If vomiting is the prominent symptom,

1. Since most cases are self-limited, oral rehydration is generally all that is necessary. Vomiting is not a contraindication to oral rehydration with glucose-electrolyte solutions. The key is to give small amounts of the solution frequently.
2. If oral rehydration is not possible or not tolerated by the patient, intravenous (IV) rehydration with normal saline solution may be necessary.
3. Antiemetics are controversial and generally not recommended. If they are used, the physician should be aware of potential adverse side effects associated with these drugs, such as dystonic reactions.

If diarrhea is the prominent symptom,

1. Children with mild diarrhea who are not dehydrated may continue routine feedings.
2. Children with moderate to severe dehydration should first receive adequate rehydration before resuming routine feedings. Food should be reinstated after the rehydration phase is completed and never delayed more that 24 h. There is no need to dilute formula, since over 80 percent of children with acute diarrhea can tolerate full-strength milk safely.
3. Dietary recommendations include a diet high in complex carbohydrates, lean meats, vegetables, fruits, and yogurt. Fatty foods

and foods high in simple sugars should be avoided. The BRAT diet is discouraged, since it does not provide adequate energy sources.

4. Antimotility drugs are not helpful and should not be used to treat acute diarrhea in children.
5. Antibiotics are considered if the diarrhea has persisted longer than 10 to 14 days or the patient has a significant fever, systemic symptoms, or blood or pus in the stool.

All infants and children who appear toxic or have high-risk social situations, significant dehydration, altered mental status, inability to drink, bloody diarrhea, or laboratory evidence of hemolytic anemia, thrombocytopenia, azotemia, or elevated creatinine levels should be admitted. Children who respond to oral or IV hydration can be discharged. Instructions should be given to return to the emergency department or seek care with the primary physician if the child becomes unable to tolerate oral hydration, develops bilious vomiting, becomes less alert, or exhibits signs of dehydration, such as no longer wetting diapers.

For further reading in *Emergency Medicine: A Comprehensive Study Guide*, 5th ed., see Chap. 122, "Vomiting and Diarrhea in Children," by Christopher M. Holmes and Ronald D. Holmes.

---

75 | Pediatric Abdominal Emergencies
Debra G. Perina

Abdominal pain in children is a diagnostic challenge to the emergency department (ED) physician. To provide effective treatment, the physician must be able to recognize clinical manifestations of common diseases, develop a differential diagnosis, and know how to approach a child. The child's age will influence the presenting signs and symptoms significantly. Abdominal disease processes can be classified in several ways: with or without fever, abdominal or extraabdominal, obstructive or nonobstructive, or a local or systemic process. Obtaining a thorough history from both parent and child if possible is very helpful in determining the diagnosis. The history should include fever, quality and location of pain, chronology of events, feedings, bowel habits, weight changes, and blood in stool. Physical examination should include completely disrobing the patient and inspection and nontouch maneuvers followed by palpation. Never omit the rectal examination and guaiac test. Remember to evaluate extraabdominal areas, such as the chest, pharynx, and neck. A palpated abdominal mass is worrisome at any age, since it may be the first presentation of a tumor or life-threatening pathology, such as neuroblastoma, Wilms' tumor, rhabdomyosarcoma, pyloric stenosis, intussusception, or ectopic pregnancy.

Clinical Features

Presenting signs and symptoms vary with the child's age. The key gastrointestional signs and symptoms are pain, vomiting, diarrhea, constipation, bleeding, jaundice, and masses. These symptoms can be the result of a benign process or indicate a life-threatening illness. The origin of abdominal pain may be extraabdominal, such as with pneumonia or pharyngitis. Pain in children less than 2 years usually manifests as fussiness, irritability, or lethargy. Pain may be peritonitic and exacerbated by motion or obstructive, spasmotic, and associated with restlessness. Pain of gastrointestinal (GI) origin is usually referred to the periumbilical area in children 2 to 6 years old. Associated symptoms or the presence of illness in other family members may be useful in arriving at a diagnosis.

Vomiting and diarrhea are common in children. These symptoms may be the result of a benign process or indicate the presence of a life-threatening process (see Chap. 74). Bilious vomiting is always indicative of a serious process. Constipation may be functional or pathologic. The shape and girth of the abdomen, presence of bowel sounds or masses, and abnormalities in the anal area should be noted. GI bleeding can be from upper or lower sources. Upper sources are vascular malformation, swallowed maternal blood, bleeding diathesis, foreign body, peptic ulcer disease, and Mallory-Weiss tear. Lower GI bleeding can be from fissures, intussusception, hemolytic uremic syndrome, swallowed maternal blood, vascular malformations, polyps, inflammatory bowel disease, or diverticulum. The cause of minimal to moderate amounts of blood in the stool is frequently never identified. Jaundice outside of infancy is usually an ominous sign.

Diagnosis and Differential

The likely etiologies of abdominal pain change with age. Table 75-1 lists common causes of abdominal pain seen in various age groups and identifies those that are potentially life-threatening. It is clinically useful to split the most serious causes of GI emergencies in the first year of life from older children. Common emergencies in the first year of life include malrotation of the gut, incarcerated hernia, intestinal obstruction, pyloric stenosis, and intussusception. Malrotation of the gut, although rare, can present with a volvulus, which can be life-threatening. Presenting symptoms are usually bilious vomiting, abdominal distention, and streaks of blood in the stool. The vast majority of cases present within the first month of life. Distended loops of bowel overriding the liver on abdominal radiographs are suggestive of this diagnosis.

The symptoms of incarcerated hernia include irritability, poor feeding, vomiting, and an inguinal or scrotal mass. The mass will not be detected unless the infant is totally undressed. The incidence of incarcerated hernia is highest in the first year of life. It is possible to manually reduce the hernia on examination in most cases (see Chap. 43). Intestinal obstruction may be caused by atresia, stenosis, meconium ileus, malrotation, intussusception, volvulus, incarcerated hernia, imperforate anus, and Hirschsprung's disease. Presentation includes irritability, vomiting, and abdominal distention, followed by absence of bowel sounds. Pyloric stenosis usually presents with nonbilious projectile vomiting occurring just after feeding. It is most commonly seen in the second or third week of life. It is familial and male predominant, with first-born males being particularly affected. Palpation of the pyloric mass, or "olive," in the left upper quadrant is diagnostic. Ultrasound may also aid in the diagnosis if clinically suspected and a mass is not palpated. Intussusception occurs when one portion of the gut telescopes into another. GI bleeding and edema give rise to bloody mucus-containing stools, producing the classic "current jelly" stool. The greatest incidence is between 3 months and 6 years of age. The classic presentation is sudden epigastric pain with pain-free intervals during which the examination can reveal the classic sausage-shaped mass in the right side of the abdomen. This mass is present in up to two-thirds of patients. A barium enema or insufflation can be both diagnostic and therapeutic, since the intussusception is reduced while doing the procedure in 80 percent of cases.

Common GI emergencies in children 2 years of age and older include appendicitis, bleeding, Meckel's diverticulum, colonic polyps, and foreign bodies. Appendicitis may present with the classic symptoms of pain, fever, and anorexia; however, presentation may

TABLE 75-1 Etiology of Abdominal Pain

Under 2 years	6-11 years
Appendicitis*	Appendicitis*
Colic (first 4 months)	Diabetic ketoacidosis
Congenital abnormalities*	Functional
Gastroenteritis	Gastroenteritis
Incarcerated hernia*	Henoch-Schönlein purpura
Intussusception*	Incarcerated hernia*
Malabsorption	Inflammatory bowel disease
Malrotation	Obstruction
Metabolic acidosis*	Peptic ulcer disease*
Obstruction	Pneumonia*
Sickle cell pain crisis	Renal stones
Toxins*	Sickle cell syndrome
Urinary tract infection	Streptococcal pharyngitis
Volvulus*	Torsion of ovary or testicle
	Toxins*
	Trauma*
	Urinary tract infection

2-5 years	Over 11 years
Appendicitis*	Appendicitis*
Diabetic ketoacidosis*	Cholecystitis
Gastroenteritis	Diabetic ketoacidosis*
Hemolytic uremic syndrome*	Dysmenorrhea
Henoch-Schonlein purpura	Ectopic pregnancy*
Incarcerated hernia*	Functional
Intussusception*	Gastroenteritis
Malabsorption	Incarcerated hernia*
Metabolic acidosis*	Inflammatory bowel disease
Obstruction	Obstruction
Pneumonia*	Pancreatitis
Sickle cell pain crisis	Peptic ulcer disease*
Toxins*	Pneumonia*
Trauma*	Pregnancy
Urinary tract infection	Renal stones
Volvulus*	Sickle cell syndrome
	Torsion of ovary or testicle
	Toxins*
	Trauma*
	Urinary tract infection

*Life-threatening causes of abdominal pain.

be extremely varied, making the diagnosis quite challenging. Guarding and rebound may or may not be found on examination, the temperature may be normal, the white blood cell count may be normal, the child may be asking for food and may not be anorexic, and associated gastroenteritis is fairly common. Appendicitis is seen in children younger than 1 year, and the perforation rate is higher in this age group due to the difficulty of making the diagnosis and frequent confusion with gastroenteritis. GI bleeding can be caused by several sources. Upper GI bleeding usually results from peptic ulcer disease, gastritis, or varices. Lower GI bleeding can be due to infectious colitis, inflammatory bowel disease, coagulopathies, hemolytic-uremic syndrome, and Henoch-Schönlein purpura. A small amount of blood in the diaper is most likely related to anal fissure or ingested foodstuffs. Portal hypertension, although rare, is one of the common causes of major upper GI bleeding and is associated with congenital liver disease and biliary atresia. Colonic polyps can be single, multiple, or classic familial polyposis. They can give rise to painless bright red lower GI bleeding. A single polyp is most common and frequently is palpated by the mother or noticed as a mass protruding from the anus. Foreign bodies in the GI tract are frequently seen in young children (see Chap. 39). Laxatives are contraindicated. Any foreign body caught in the esophagus must be removed by esophagoscopy. Pancreatitis is increasing in incidence in childhood. The most common cause is abdominal trauma followed by postviral process, drugs and toxin exposure, and idiopathic.

Emergency Department Care and Disposition

1. If the child is critically ill, resuscitation efforts should begin immediately, and the examination can be done concurrently.
2. Remove all clothing prior to examination. The examination should always include a rectal examination and testing of stool for occult blood.
3. The most important laboratory studies are complete blood count with differential, urinalysis, and guaiac test for occult blood. Other tests should be guided by how ill-appearing the child is. Determinations of electrolyte and amylase levels and pregnancy testing may be indicated.
4. Chest and abdominal radiographs can be useful to diagnose pneumonia, obstruction, or ileus. Abdominal ultrasound is useful in assessment of pyloric stenosis, ectopic pregnancy, or appendicitis. Abdominal computed tomography scan may be diagnostic with abdominal masses and appendicitis.

5. In some cases dehydration and electrolyte abnormalities may require correction with oral or intravenous rehydration.

For further reading in *Emergency Medicine: A Comprehensive Study Guide*, 5th ed., see Chap. 123, "Pediatric Abdominal Emergencies," by Robert W. Schafermeyer.

| 76 | The Child with Diabetes and Diabetic Ketoacidosis |

Leslie McKinney

Type 1, or insulin-dependent, diabetes mellitus (IDDM) is a common disease of childhood clinically detected by the presence of hyperglycemia in association with glucosuria. The diagnosis is typically characterized by polyuria, polydipsia, and polyphagia; however, other common complaints include failure to gain weight, weight loss, enuresis, anorexia, changes in vision and school performance. The diagnosis of the disease and management of diabetic ketoacidosis (DKA) are important skills for the emergency physician.

DIABETIC KETOACIDOSIS

Clinical Features

DKA is a common complication of IDDM and is responsible for the majority of deaths in diabetics less than 24 years old. DKA should be considered clinically in patients with hyperventilation, fruity breath odor of ketosis, dehydration, lethargy, vomiting, abdominal pain, fever, and polyuria.

Diagnosis and Differential

DKA is defined by hyperglycemia (blood glucose greater than 250mg/dL), ketonemia, and metabolic acidosis (pH less than 7.2 and plasma bicarbonate level less than 15 meg/L) associated with glucosuria and ketonuria. Most such patients are dehydrated and ill in appearance. Laboratory tests required to manage and diagnose

DKA include serum electrolyte determinations, urinalysis, blood pH, and serum ketone determination. Sepsis should be considered when the cause of DKA is not apparent and a complete blood count, a chest x-ray, and appropriate cultures should be obtained. Other causative factors include trauma, vomiting, noncompliance, and overall stress.

Emergency Department Care and Disposition

The treatment of DKA consists of volume replacement, insulin therapy, correction of electrolyte abnormalities, and a search for a causative factor. Patients should be placed on a cardiac monitor, noninvasive blood pressure device, and pulse oximetry, and intravenous lines should be established. Initially, hourly monitoring of electrolytes and pH is necessary.

1. In general, to calculate the total fluid deficit, compare the patient's presenting weight to a recent weight. If that is not available, assume a 10 percent (100-mL/kg) deficit. Volume replacement using a **normal saline** (NS) infusion of 10 to 20 mL/kg over 1 to 2 h should be given initially to most patients. If evidence of shock is present, administer a 20-mL/kg bolus of NS. After initial stabilization is complete, the remaining fluid deficit should be replaced over 24 to 48 h using 0.45% NS unless serum osmolality remains above 320 mosm/L; then continue NS until the osmolality approaches normal. Monitor glucose levels closely and begin 5% dextrose in 0.45% NS when blood glucose levels are between 300 and 250 mg/dL.

2. A regular **insulin** infusion of 0.1 U/kg/h should be initiated as soon as a glucose level above 250 mg/dL is obtained. There is debate regarding an initial insulin bolus of 0.1 U/kg, and most authorities begin with a continuous infusion. If the acidosis has not improved after 2 h of insulin therapy, increase the insulin infusion to 0.15 to 0.2 U/kg/h. Continue both the insulin infusion and 5% dextrose in 0.45% NS until the acidosis is corrected.

3. Restoration of **sodium** levels is accomplished by administration of NS and 0.45% NS fluid. Patients typically reveal sodium deficits of approximately 6 meq/kg. Also, the hyperglycemia and hyperlipoidemia associated with DKA cause a falsely low serum sodium level. Monitor serum sodium levels closely, since a decline of the sodium level is sometimes indicative of developing cerebral edema.

4. Management of **potassium** abnormalities is critical to the care of DKA patients. Because of the shift of potassium to the extracellular space secondary to the acidosis of DKA, one may see falsely elevated serum K^+ levels despite total body depletion. If the pH is 7.10 or less and the K^+ level is normal or low, begin

replacement therapy immediately by adding 40 meq K^+ to each liter of maintenance fluid. Consider doses as high as 60 meq/L if the potassium level is less than 3.0 meq/L. If the K^+ level is elevated (greater than 6.0 meq/L), consider holding K^+ therapy until urine output is present and K^+ is correcting. Use half KCL and half KPO_4. Monitor calcium levels, since excess phosphate can cause hypocalcemia.

5. Bicarbonate therapy remains controversial and should be used only in life-threatening situations, such as cardiac dysrhythmias or dysfunction.

6. A potentially fatal complication of DKA in children is development of cerebral edema. This typically occurs 6 to 10 h after initiating therapy and presents as mental status changes progressing to coma. Although the etiology of this complication is unknown, it is felt that several factors may contribute, including overly aggressive fluid therapy, rapid correction of blood glucose levels, bicarbonate therapy, and failure of the serum sodium level to increase with therapy. Treatment should include **mannitol** 1 to 2 g/kg, intracranial pressure monitoring, possible intubation with hyperventilation, and fluid restriction.

7. Most of these patients will require admission to a pediatric intensive care unit for intensive monitoring and ongoing therapy. Consultation with the patient's primary care physician should be made early in the course of therapy.

For further reading in *Emergency Medicine: A Comprehensive Study Guide,* 5th ed., see Chap. 124, "The Diabetic Child and Diabetic Ketoacidosis," by Maribel Rodriguez and Thom A. Mayer.

---

77 | Hypoglycemia in Children

Juan A. March

Hypoglycemia is a relatively common condition in pediatrics, particularly in acutely sick infants and children. The diagnosis and treatment of hypoglycemia in the emergency department should be prompt because persistent or recurrent hypoglycemia may have permanent catastrophic effects on the brain, particularly in infants. Hypoglycemia is defined as a serum or plasma glucose concentration less than 45 mg/dL.

Clinical Features

Hypoglycemia occurs as a primary or secondary feature of a large number of clinical conditions. Such conditions include, but are not limited to, infection, congenital heart disease, maternal toxemia of pregnancy, idiopathic ketotic hypoglycemia, hypopituitarism, and glycogen storage disease. In addition, ingested substances such as insulin, ethanol, oral hypoglycemics, salicylates, beta blockers, and quinidine can cause hypoglycemia. The symptoms vary and may be overshadowed by the dramatic appearance of the primary disease, such as meningococcemia. It is prudent, therefore, to assess for and treat hypoglycemia immediately.

Patients become symptomatic from hypoglycemia because of compensatory heightened adrenergic activity and the cerebral metabolic perturbances directly attributable to glucose deprivation. Older children usually have the same signs as adults. Manifestations tend to be subtler and nonspecific in infants and include poor feeding, lethargy, apnea, emesis, altered personality, hypotonia, and hypothermia. Infants and children with unexplained respiratory or cardiac arrest should be tested immediately for hypoglycemia. Older children present with the classic clinical signs of hypoglycemia with adrenergic excess, such as anxiety, tachycardia, perspiration, nausea, tremors, pallor, chest pains, weakness, abdominal pain, hunger, and irritability. Neuroglycopenic effects, such as confusion, ataxia, headache, depressed consciousness, blurred vision, lightheadedness, focal neurologic deficits, seizures, strabismus, staring, and paresthesia may also be apparent.

Diagnosis and Differential

In those patients suspected or at risk of being hypoglycemic, bedside glucose measurement can be diagnostic within 2 min. Take care to ensure that the testing strip is completely covered with blood and that isopropyl alcohol does not contaminate the specimen. When bedside glucose is unavailable, it is better to treat empirically than to delay appropriate treatment.

Emergency Department Care and Disposition

There are three important aspects of emergency patient care: (1) rapid diagnosis of hypoglycemia, (2) acquisition of germane blood and urine specimens, and (3) prompt restoration and maintenance of euglycemia. Clearly, it is imperative to replete the serum with glucose, but it is shortsighted to neglect the first two objectives.

1. After specimen collection, a bolus of **10% dextrose** in water ($D_{10}W$) 3 mL/kg is given intravenously (IV) or intraosseously. In older children $D_{25}W$ may be used, but $D_{25}W$, and especially $D_{50}W$, are very hyperosmolar and may cause phlebitis and tissue necrosis in smaller veins. Furthermore, hyperosmolar loading in premature neonates is associated with an increased risk of intracranial germinal matrix hemorrhage and subsequent periventricular leukomalacia.
2. Follow the bolus with a continuous infusion of 10% dextrose–50% normal saline solution in an age- and weight-appropriate fashion. However, when standard therapy fails, hydrocortisone is useful for those who cannot achieve euglycemia despite adequate dextrose administration. This is especially true of patients with hypopituitarism and adrenal insufficiency.
3. When IV access is unavailable, **glucagon** 0.025 to 0.05 mg/kg intramuscularly can be considered. Glucagon only works in patients with intact glycogen stores, and its use is controversial in the pediatric population. Thus, an intraosseous should be considered when IV access is not possible.

For further reading in *Emergency Medicine: A Comprehensive Study Guide*, 5th ed., see Chap. 125, "Hypoglycemia," by Randolph J. Cordle.

---

78 | Altered Mental Status in Children
Debra G. Perina

Altered mental status (AMS) in children is failure to respond to the external environment after appropriate stimulation in a manner consistent with the child's developmental level. In treating children with AMS, aggressive resuscitation, stabilization, diagnosis, and treatment must occur simultaneously to prevent morbidity and death.

Clinical Features

The spectrum of AMS ranges from confusion to lethargy, stupor, and coma indicative of either depression of the cerebral cortex or localized abnormalities of the reticular activating system. Pathologic conditions can be divided into supratentorial lesions, subtentorial lesions, and metabolic dysfunction. Supratentorial lesions present with focal motor abnormalities, rostral-to-caudal progression of dysfunction, and slow nystagmus toward the lesion with cold calorics. Motor abnormalities generally precede AMS. Subtentorial lesions produce rapid loss of consciousness, cranial nerve abnormalities, abnormal breathing patterns, and asymmetric or fixed pupils. Metabolic dysfunction produces decreased level of consciousness before exhibiting motor signs, which are symmetrical when present. Pupillary reflexes are intact except with profound anoxia, opiates, barbiturates, and anticholinergics.

Diagnosis and Differential

A thorough history and physical are paramount to determining the diagnosis. Key questions must include prodromal events and associated signs and symptoms, such as fever, headache, weakness, vomiting, diarrhea, gait disturbances, head tilt, rash, palpitations, abdominal pain, hematuria, and weight loss. Inquiries should also be made regarding past medical history, family history, and immunization status. The examination should look for signs of occult infection, trauma, toxicity, or metabolic disease. A useful tool for organizing diagnostic possibilities is the mnemonic AEIOU TIPS (Table 78-1).

Diagnostic adjuncts should be guided by the clinical situation but can include analysis of blood, gastric fluid, urine, stool, cerebrospinal fluid (CSF), electrocardiography, or selected radiographic studies. Rapid bedside glucose determination is a universally accepted standard. If meningitis or encephalitis is suspected, lumbar puncture and CSF analysis should be done as rapidly as possible after initial resuscitation and stabilization. A 12-lead electrocardiogram should be obtained in cases where there are pathologic auscultatory findings or rhythm disturbances.

Emergency Department Care and Disposition

At least two individuals are needed in caring for a child with AMS. One can be obtaining a medical history while the other performs resuscitation, followed by a more thorough physical examination.

TABLE 78-1 AEIOU TIPS:

A	**Alcohol.** Changes in mental status can occur with serum levels <100 mg/dL. Concurrent hypoglycemia is common. **Acid-base and metabolic.** Hypotonic and hypertonic dehydration. Hepatic dysfunction, inborn errors of metabolism, diabetic ketoacidosis, primary lung disease, and neurologic dysfunction causing hypercapnia. **Dysrhythmia (arrhythmia)/cardiogenic.** Stokes-Adams, supraventricular tachycardia, aortic stenosis, heart block.
E	**Encephalopathy.** Hypertensive encephalopathy can occur with diastolic pressures of 100–110 mmHg. Reye's syndrome. **Endocrinopathy.** AMS is rare as a presentation in this category. Addison's disease can present with AMS or psychosis. Thyrotoxicosis can present with ventricular dysrhythmias. Pheochromocytoma can present with hypertensive encephalopathy. **Electrolytes.** Hyponatremia becomes symptomatic around 120 meq/L. Hypernatremia and disorders of calcium, magnesium, and phosphorus can produce AMS.
I	**Insulin.** AMS from hyperglycemia is rare in children, but diabetic ketoacidosis is the most common cause. Hypoglycemia can be the result of many disorders. Irritability, confusion, seizures, and coma can occur with blood glucose levels <40 mg/dL. **Intussusception.** AMS may be the initial presenting symptom.
O	**Opiates.** Common household exposures are to Lomotil, Imodium, diphenoxylate, and dextromethorphan. Clonidine, an α agonist, can also produce similar symptoms.
U	**Uremia.** Encephalopathy occurs in over one-third of patients with chronic renal failure. Hemolytic uremic syndrome can also produce AMS in addition to abdominal pain. Thrombocytopenic purpura and hemolytic anemia can also cause AMS.
T	**Trauma.** Children with blunt trauma are more likely to develop cerebral edema than adults. Remember to look for signs of child abuse, particularly shaken baby syndrome with retinal hemorrhages. **Tumor.** Primary, metastatic, or meningeal leukemic infiltration. **Thermal.** Hypo- or hyperthermia.
I	**Infection.** One of the most common causes of AMS in children. Meningitis should be high on the differential list. **Intracerebral vascular disorders.** Subarachnoid, intracerebral, or intraventricular hemorrhages can be seen with trauma, ruptured aneurysm, or arteriovenous malformations. Venous thrombosis can follow severe dehydration or pyogenic infection of the mastoid, orbit, middle ear, or sinuses.
P	**Psychogenic.** Rare in the pediatric age group, characterized by decreased responsiveness with normal neurologic examination including oculovestibular reflexes. **Poisoning.** Drugs or toxins can be ingested by accident, through neglect or abuse, or in a suicide gesture.
S	**Seizure.** Generalized motor seizures are often associated with prolonged unresponsiveness in children. Seizure in a young febrile patient suggests intracranial infection.

1. Airway, breathing, and circulation must be ensured.
2. Continuous pulse oximetry and supplemental **oxygen** as needed to correct hypoxia should be provided, including bag-valve mask and intubation when appropriate.
3. Fluid resuscitation with 20-mL/kg fluid boluses of **isotonic crystalloid** is gven for hypotension. Fluid boluses may be repeated up to 60 mL/kg, after which the need for pressor agents, such as dopamine, should be considered.
4. Perform bedside glucose testing and administer **glucose** if indicated (see Chap. 77).
5. Control core body temperature to minimize metabolic demands.
6. If seizures are present, control with **benzodiazepines** (see Chap. 73).
7. Restore acid-base balance. **Bicarbonate** is used sparingly and only if pH is less than 7.0.

Most patients with AMS require admission and extended observation. Only those with transient, rapidly reversible causes of AMS can be treated and discharged from the emergency department after a period of observation.

For further reading in *Emergency Medicine: A Comprehensive Study Guide,* 5th ed., see Chap. 126, "Altered Mental Status in Children," by Nancy A. Pook, Natalie M. Cullen, and Jonathan I. Singer.

---

79 | Syncope and Sudden Death in Children and Adolescents

Debra G. Perina

Syncope is very common in adolescence. At least 15 percent of children experience syncope by the age 18. This condition is transient and usually self-limited, but it may be a symptom of serious cardiac disease.

The rate of sudden unexpected death in children is 2.3 percent of all pediatric deaths. Sudden cardiac death makes up about one-third of these cases. Except for trauma, sudden cardiac death is the most common cause of sports-related deaths, particularly with basketball, football, and track. Other causes of sudden cardiac death in children are myocarditis, cardiomyopathy, congenital heart disease, and conduction disturbances. Hypertrophic cardiomyopathy is the most common cause of sudden cardiac death in adolescents without known cardiac disease

TABLE 79-1 Causes of Syncope in Children and Adolescents

Neurally mediated: most common cause of syncope in children
  Orthostatic: light-headedness with standing
  Situational: urination, defecation, coughing, and swallowing may precipitate
  Familial dysautonomia

Cardiac dysrhythmias: events that usually start and end abruptly
  Prolonged Q-T syndrome
  Wolff-Parkinson-White syndrome
  Sick sinus syndrome: associated with prior heart surgery
  Supraventricular tachycardia
  Atrioventricular block: most common in children with congenital heart disease
  Pacemaker malfunction

Structural cardiac disease
  Hypertrophic cardiomopathy: exertional syncope most common presentation, but infants can present with congestive heart failure and cyanosis; echocardiography necessary to confirm
  Dilated cardiomyopathy: may be idiopathic, postmyocarditis, or with congenital heart disease
  Congenital heart disease
  Valvular diseases: aortic stenosis usually congenital defect, Ebstein's malformation, or mitral valve prolapse (which is not associated with increased risk of sudden death)
  Dysrhythmogenic right ventricular dysplasia
  Pulmonary hypertension: dyspnea on exertion, exercise intolerance, shortness of breath
  Coronary artery abnormalities: aberrant left main artery causing external compression during physical exercise

Endocrine abnormalities: hyperthyroid, hyperglycemia, adrenal insufficiency

Medications and drugs: antihypertensives, tricyclic antidepressants, cocaine, diuretics, antidysrhythmics

Gastrointestinal disorders: reflux

TABLE 79-2 Risk Factors for Serious Causes of Syncope

Exertion preceding the event
History of cardiac disease in patient
Recurrent episodes
Recumbent episode
Family history of sudden death, cardiac disease, deafness
Chest pain, palpitations
Prolonged loss of consciousness
Medications that affect cardiac conduction

Clinical Features

Syncope is sudden onset of falling accompanied by a brief episode of loss of consciousness. Involuntary motor movements may occur with all types of syncopal episodes but are most common with seizures. Two-thirds of children experience light-headedness or dizziness prior to the episode. There are many causes of syncope in children. Table 79-1 lists the most common causes of syncope by category.

Neurally mediated syncope is the most common cause in children and includes vasovagal, neurocardiogenic, reflex syncope, and simple fainting. Risk factors associated with serious causes of syncope are presented in Table 79-2. Events easily mistaken for syncope are presented in Table 79-3 along with common associated symptoms.

TABLE 79-3 Events Mistaken for Syncope

Basilar migraine: headache, loss of consciousness, neurologic symptoms
Seizure: loss of consciousness, simultaneous motor movements, prolonged recovery
Vertigo: no loss of consciousness, spinning or rotating sensation
Hysteria: no loss of consciousness, indifference to the event
Hypoglycemia: confusion, gradual onset associated with diaphoresis
Breath-holding spell: crying prior to the event, age 6–18 months old
Hyperventilation: severe hypocapnia can cause syncope

Diagnosis and Differential

No specific historical or clinical features reliably distinguish between vasovagal syncope and other causes. However, a thorough history and physical examination can help to arouse suspicion of serious causes. Particular attention should be given to the cardiac examination. The most important step in evaluation of children with syncope is a detailed history, including medications, drugs, intake, and food. Syncope during exercise suggests a more serious cause. Many of the diseases that cause syncope also cause sudden death in children. Approximately 25 percent of children who suffer sudden death have a history of syncope. If witnesses note that the patient appeared dead or cardiopulmonary resuscitation was performed, a search for serious pathologic conditions must be undertaken. The physical examination should include a complete cardiovascular, neurologic, and pulmonary examination. Any abnormalities noted in the cardiovascular examination require an in-depth cardiac workup.

Emergency Department Care and Disposition

1. Laboratory assessment is guided by the history, physical examination, and clinical suspicion. Routine laboratory studies are not needed if vasovagal syncope in suspected. Those with worrisome associated symptoms should have a chemistry panel and hematocrit. A pregnancy test should also be done in females of childbearing age. Serum drug screening or alcohol level determination may also be useful if ingestion is suspected.
2. A chest radiograph and an electrocardiogram (ECG) may also be helpful if there is suspicion of pulmonary or cardiac causes.
3. An echocardiogram should be obtained in patients with known or suspected cardiac disease.
4. If vasovagal syncope is diagnosed, only reassurance is needed.
5. If no clear cause is found, the child may be discharged to be further evaluated and followed by the primary care physician unless there are cardiac risk factors or exercise induced symptoms.
6. Children with documented dysrhythmias should be admitted. Patients with a normal ECG but a history suggesting a dysrhythmic event are candidates for outpatient monitoring and cardiac workup.

For further reading in *Emergency Medicine: A Comprehensive Study Guide*, 5th ed., see Chap. 127, "Syncope and Sudden Death," by William E. Hauda II and Thom A. Mayer.

80 | Fluid and Electrolyte Therapy
Juan A. March

Important differences exist between young children and adults in fluid and electrolyte metabolism and homeostasis. The physiologic consequences of fluid and electrolyte disturbances are more pronounced in children due to their higher metabolic rate than they are in adults. The turnover of fluid and solute per kilogram of body weight is 3 times that of adults. Also a high percentage of their body weight is from water. Due to the volubility of children to fluid and electrolyte loss in combination with the high incidence of gastroenteritis in the pediatric population, it is no wonder that fluid and electrolyte abnormalities are among the most common problem facing emergency physicians.

Clinical Features

Deficits and Dehydration

The most common mechanism for fluid deficits or dehydration in children is excessive fluid loss. It is imperative to recognize the child with a fluid deficit and treat accordingly in order to prevent cardiovascular collapse. When fluid is lost over a long period, a large deficit may be well tolerated and have a subtle clinical presentation. The rapid and massive loss of fluid associated with cholera or rotavirus can be fatal since there is insufficient time for the intracellular fluid (ICF) to shift into the vascular tree. Due to the relatively large percent of total body water contained in the extracellular space, infants are especially at risk. The most accurate way of assessing the degree of dehydration is by weight.

Unfortunately an accurate preillness weight is often not available, and the degree of dehydration must be estimated clinically. The history should include intake (quantity and type of fluid), output (site, type, and amount), and other medical problems (preexisting and acute). Vital signs including weight, temperature, heart rate, respiratory rate, blood pressure, and capillary refill time should be taken. Physical examination should be performed with emphasis on the general appearance of the child, anterior fontanelle, skin elasticity, and mucous membranes.

Dehydration is divided into three groups according to the degree of the fluid deficit: mild (< 5 percent dehydration), moderate (5 to 10 percent dehydration), and severe (> 10 percent dehydration). Diagnosis of mild dehydration is usually made from the history, as physical signs are minimal or absent. Pulse rate may be slightly increased, but blood pressure is normal.

The clinical signs of moderate dehydration are much more obvious. The skin may be dry with tenting and loss of turgor. Mucous membranes are tacky or dry. The anterior fontanelle and eyeballs will be sunken. The child will usually have an altered sensorium with lethargy, restlessness, or irritability, and prolonged capillary refill time (> 2 s). Patients are in the early stage of compensatory shock (evidence of marked intravascular volume depletion with a normal blood pressure).

In severe dehydration there is uncompensated shock and evidence of circulatory collapse. The skin is cold, clammy, and mottled. Capillary refill time is significantly delayed (> 3 to 5 s). Peripheral pulses may be absent, and evidence of poor central nervous system (CNS) perfusion, with varying degrees of altered sensorium, may be present.

Differential Diagnosis

Types of Dehydration

The types of dehydration refer to the osmolar load of the plasma relative to the degree of fluid loss. Since the main solute in plasma is sodium, serum osmolality is mainly a reflection of sodium concentration. The types of dehydration are isonatremic (isotonic), hyponatremic (hypotonic), and hypernatremic (hypertonic). Each type of dehydration is associated with special problems. Defining the type of dehydration will direct management.

The vast majority of pediatric patients with isonatremic dehydration will typically have diarrhea, vomiting, or poor oral intake, with a proportionate loss of water and electrolytes, and serum sodium levels within a normal range of 130 to 145 meq/L.

In hyponatremic dehydration, the serum sodium level is less than 130 meq/L and the sodium deficit is greater than the water deficit. This typically occurs when sodium-poor fluids (e.g., tap water) are given to replace gastrointestinal (GI) losses. In hypernatremic dehydration, the serum sodium level is greater than 150 meq/L. Hypernatremia occurs when free water replacement is inadequate (incorrectly diluted formulas), or if sodium intake is abnormally high (boiled skim milk or use of baking soda).

Emergency Department Care and Disposition

In mild-to-moderate dehydration it has been demonstrated that oral rehydration is as effective as intravenous therapy. The use of prepackaged oral electrolyte solutions has made an enormous impact in developing nations. Time constraints may limit the use of oral rehydration in emergency departments in the United States. Replacement of the fluid deficit occurs in three phases: (*a*) correction of shock; (*b*) restoration of extracellular fluid (ECF) volume; and (*c*) replacement of ICF stores or maintenance fluid.

Correction of Shock

Children may be in a compensated shock state and still maintain normal blood pressure. Hypotension is a very late and ominous sign. Accurate weight should be obtained on all pediatric patients.

1. Vascular access should be started and blood obtained for immediate analysis of electrolyte; glucose; blood urea nitrogen; or creatinine levels, and pH concentration. A bedside glucose measurement should be done. If peripheral access cannot be obtained, percutaneous cannulation of the femoral or external jugular vein is an alternative. For children less than 6 years old, an intraosseous infusion needle may be placed for initial volume expansion (see Chap. 3).
2. All patients in shock should receive supplemental **oxygen.**
3. For correction of shock from all types of dehydration, the initial fluid bolus is the same—20 mL/kg of isotonic crystalloid (0.9% **normal saline** (NS) or **lactated Ringer's solution**) over 5 to 20 min. Glucose-containing solutions should be avoided as they are poor volume expanders and, in addition, bolus amounts can lead to cerebral edema, hyperglycemia, and resulting osmotic diuresis.
4. If hypoglycemia is present, 0.5 to 1.0 g/kg of **glucose** using $D_{25}W$ or $D_{10}W$ should be administered.

Although crystalloids provide good volume expansion, if the child has underlying cardiac, pulmonary, or renal disease, 10 mL/kg boluses of colloids should be considered. After the fluid bolus is completed, the patient should be reassessed. If perfusion remains compromised, the fluid bolus should be repeated. In general, few patients require more than 40 to 60 mL/kg of isotonic crystalloid during the first hour of therapy.

The next phase of therapy is restoration of ECF volume. The aim of this phase is correction of the fluid deficit with restoration of the fluid compartments over 24 to 48 h. Fluid therapy for this phase depends on the degree and type of dehydration present.

Isonatremic Dehydration

For the patient with isotonic dehydration, the initial fluid boluses given are subtracted from the calculated fluid deficit. The remaining deficit is replaced over 24 h: one-half is given over the first 8 h, and the other half over the subsequent 16 h. After adequate urine output is established, 40 meq/L of potassium chloride should be added. To calculate the fluid deficit, the patient's preillness weight should be multiplied by the percent deficit. For example, the deficit for a 12-kg child with 10 percent dehydration would be calculated as follows: 12 kg × 0.1 = a deficit of 1.2 kg or 1200 cm.

Hyponatremic Dehydration

In hypotonic dehydration, the water deficit is calculated and replaced as earlier. The sodium deficit, however, is different. Initial fluid boluses are given as normal saline or lactated Ringer's solution, which are relatively hypertonic solutions. D_5NS can be given to slowly raise the serum sodium level to 125 meq/L. The remainder of the fluid deficit as well as the maintenance fluid is given as $D_50.45NS$. After adequate urine output is established 40 meq/L of potassium chloride can be added.

If the initial serum sodium level is less than 120 meq/L or the patient has persistent seizures, 3% saline may be considered to correct the sodium deficit acutely at a rate of 1 to 2 mL/kg/h to a maximum of 6 mL/kg. Frequent serum sodium levels are essential.

Hypernatremic Dehydration

In hypertonic dehydration, the serum sodium level must be lowered slowly. Rapid rehydration leads to rapid expansion of intracellular volume, especially in the CNS, and this may cause abrupt cellular swelling and cerebral edema. The goal is to decrease the serum sodium level by approximately 10 to 15 meq/L/d. Replacement of the fluid deficit is accomplished evenly over 48 or 72 h if the initial sodium is greater than 175 meq/L. D_5 0.45 normal saline is generally used. For initial serum sodium levels greater than 210 meq/L, dialysis may be required. The patient may not appear dehydrated and may not require initial fluid boluses. If in doubt, however, a bolus of normal saline should be administered. The remaining fluid deficit is added to the maintenance fluid requirement for the next 48 h.

Maintenance

The goal of maintenance fluid and electrolyte therapy is to provide the body with water, sodium, potassium, chloride, and bicarbonate in order to maintain a state of normal homeostasis. Normal maintenance requirements provide water and electrolytes to replace those that are lost through urine, stool, and insensible routes. There is a 1:1 relationship between calories expended and body water required. In other words, the body needs 1 mL of water for every kilocalorie (kcal) expended (Table 80-1).

A rapid means of calculating maintenance fluid rates is as follows: 4 mL/h for every kilogram up to 10, plus 2 mL/h for every kilogram between 10 and 20, plus 1 mL/h for every kilogram over 20. Daily maintenance requirements of sodium and potassium are

TABLE 80-1 Bodily Water Requirements

Weight, kg	Water requirement/24 h
≤10	100 mL/kg
11–20	1000 mL + 50 mL/kg for each kg >10
≥20	1500 mL + 20 mL/kg for each kg >20

2 to 3 meq/kg per 24 h. Five grams of glucose per 100 kcal expended provides approximately 20% of the total daily caloric expenditure and will prevent ketosis. Newborn infants may require 10 g of glucose per 100 kcal expended. Standard intravenous solutions that meet these requirements are 5% dextrose in 0.2 or 0.25 normal saline ($D_5$0.2NS or $D_5$0.25NS) with 20 meq/L of potassium chloride added. Many conditions can alter a child's metabolic rate. Maintenance fluid and electrolyte requirements may need to be adjusted accordingly.

Admission

Patients with intractable vomiting or profuse diarrhea are obvious candidates for admission. In addition, admission should be considered in neonates and young infants who are at relatively greater risk of cardiovascular compromise if the underlying gastroenteritis is likely to continue. If discharged, expedient follow up is critical.

For further reading in *Emergency Medicine: A Comprehensive Study Guide,* 5th ed., see Chap. 128, "Fluid and Electrolyte Therapy," by William Ahrens.

---

81 Upper Respiratory Emergencies

Juan A. March

GENERAL APPROACH

Diseases that cause upper respiratory tract (URT) obstruction account for a significant percentage of pediatric emergency department visits. Some diseases of the URT are common and quite benign, while others are much less common and life-threatening.

Clinical Features

Cyanosis may be absent despite the presence of hypoxia. Cyanosis depends on the hemoglobin level and the peripheral circulation. Young infants may demonstrate mild peripheral cyanosis with a normal Po_2 due to high hemoglobin levels and sluggish peripheral circulation. When cyanosis is found, it should be taken as an ominous sign.

Tachypnea, chest retractions, and nasal flaring are the triad of labored respirations. Signs of labored respiration appear early in the course and worsen, thus serving as a prognostic as well as a diagnostic sign. Tachypnea is not specific for respiratory tract disease and is seen in cardiac disorders, as well as diseases that cause metabolic acidosis. Chest retractions and nasal flaring are more specific for respiratory tract disorders than is tachypnea, and both appear early in the course of the disease. Coughing is uncommon in the young infant and, if there is a persistent cough, pertussis, *Chlamydia* pneumonia, or cystic fibrosis should be considered. Sneezing is more common and often insignificant.

Grunting is a valuable diagnostic sign as it localizes disease to the lower respiratory tract and correlates with disease severity. Stridor on inspiration is indicative of obstruction at or above the larynx. It appears early and correlates with severity. Biphasic stridor places the obstruction in the trachea, whereas expiratory stridor usually means obstruction below the carina.

Diagnosis and Differential

When confronted with stridorous children, physicians should ascertain the ages of the patients and the duration of symptoms. Children less than 6 months old with a long duration of symptoms characteristically have a congenital cause of stridor. Laryngomalacia accounts for 60 percent of all neonatal laryngeal problems and is due to a developmentally weak larynx. Another cause of stridor in children under 6 months of age includes vocal cord paralysis, which may result from difficulty in passing the endotracheal tube between the vocal cords. Patients over 6 months old with a short duration of symptoms characteristically have an acquired cause of stridor, such as viral croup, epiglottitis, foreign body (FB) aspiration, peritonsilar abscess, or retropharyngeal abscess.

EPIGLOTTITIS

Clinical Features

Epiglottitis is a life-threatening disease that can occur at any age. Since the introduction of the *Haemophilus influenzae* vaccine, the median age of presentation is 7, and most cases are due to gram-positive organisms including *Streptococcus pyogenes, Staphylococcus aureus, and Streptococcus pneumonia* with less then 25 percent accounted for by *H.influenzae.* Classically, there is an abrupt onset of high fever, sore throat, stridor, dysphagia, and drooling developing over 1 to 2 days. Physical examination reveals a toxic-appearing child with an ashen gray color, apprehensiveness, and anxiety, but with minimal movements in the characteristic sniffing position. Absence of a spontaneous cough differentiates epiglottitis from viral croup. The presentation in older children and adults is much more subtle. The only complaint may be a severe sore throat, with or without stridor. Epiglottitis should be considered whenever the symptoms of sore throat, dysphagia, and drooling are out of proportion to visible pharyngeal pathology.

Diagnosis and Differential

Each institution should have a written protocol for "suspected epiglottitis management" including immediate recognition and triage to a resuscitation area, continuous monitoring by an individual skilled in difficult airway management, rapid consultation with appropriate colleagues, and consideration of patient transfer and radiological studies.

Physicians must stay with the children at all times and not send the patients to the x-ray department unattended. If total airway obstruction or apnea occurs, children with epiglottitis can be effectively bagged.

Lateral neck x-rays must be taken with the neck extended and should be taken during inspiration. The epiglottis is normally tall and thin, but in epiglottitis it is very swollen and appears squat and flat, like a thumbprint.

Emergency Department Care and Disposition

1. Direct visualization of the epiglottis is safe and accurate when performed by clinicians skilled in difficult airway management. It is unacceptable to carefully observe patients with epiglottitis for signs of deterioration. What will surely be observed is sudden and total obstruction. The objective of airway management is to prevent this from occurring.

2. Supportive therapy should include humidified oxygen and nebulized racemic epinephrine. Clinicians most skilled in difficult airway management should intubate patients as soon as possible. Sedation, paralytics, and vagolytics are used as indicated.
3. Choices for intravenous antibiotics include **cefuroxime** 50 mg/kg every 8 h intravenously, **cefotaxime** 50 mg/kg every 8 h, or **ceftriaxone** 50 mg/kg every 24 h. Due to the increasing incidence of cephalosporin resistance, the addition of vancomycin may also be considered. Steroids are not necessary, but are frequently used. Blood cultures are positive in 80 to 90 percent of patients.

VIRAL CROUP (LARYNGOTRACHEOBRONCHITIS)

Clinical Features and Diagnosis

Viral croup is usually a benign, self-limited disease due to marked edema and inflammation. The age range for viral croup is 6 months to 3 years, and it occurs mainly in the late fall and early winter. The etiology is usually parainfluenza virus. The typical history is 2 to 3 days of an upper respiratory infection(URI) with a gradually worsening cough, especially at night. By day 4, a barking cough with biphasic stridor and dyspnea are present, in addition to varying degrees of anxiety. Physical examination reveals marked stridor, retractions, tachypnea, hoarseness, and possibly, mild cyanosis on room air. A typical case of croup can be differentiated from epiglottitis on clinical grounds, therefore x-rays are not necessary in every patient.

Emergency Department Care and Disposition

The patient should be monitored with pulse oximetry and treated with cool mist, oxygen, and hydration, either intravenously or orally. Antibiotics are not needed.

1. Steroids have been shown to be beneficial in croup. **Prednisone,** 1 to 2 mg/kg/d, or **dexamethasone,** 0.25 to 0.5 mg/kg per dose every 6 h for 3 days can be administered.
2. Racemic **epinephrine** can be used to treat severe cases. Unfortunately, due to rebound stridor, it is recommended that patients treated with racemic epinephrine should be monitored for at least 3 h prior to determining the disposition.
3. Spasmodic croup, almost always occurring at night and usually without a preceding URI or fever, is thought to be due to allergy and is very sensitive to mist.

Bacterial tracheitis, a more severe form of croup, has been increasing in the past few years. Also referred to as *membranous laryngotracheobronchitis,* it is usually caused by *S. aureus.* Patients with bacterial tracheitis have more respiratory distress than patients with epiglotitis and may present similar to it even though the x-ray shows the typical findings of croup. These patients usually need intubation as well as antibiotics.

FOREIGN BODY ASPIRATION

Clinical Features and Diagnosis

FB aspirations cause over 3000 deaths each year, and 90 percent occur in children under 4 years of age. In children under 6 months of age the cause is usually secondary to a "helpful sibling feeding the patient." The most common FBs are peanuts, raisins, grapes, hot dogs, and sunflower seeds, but almost any object may be aspirated.

Patients may have a variety of signs, depending on the location of the FB and the degree of obstruction. Symptoms may include wheezing, crackles, tachypnea, persistent pneumonia, stridor, coughing, or apnea. A significant portion of patients present without cough, wheeze, or stridor. As many as one-third of the aspirations are not witnessed or remembered by the parent. Physicians must highly suspect FBs. Most airway FBs are radiolucent. An FB will cause air to be trapped, which leads to hyperinflation of the obstructed lung and a shift of the mediastinum during expiration away from the obstructed side. Mediastinal shift also may be seen on bilateral decubitus x-rays of the chest. A single negative x-ray does not rule out the presence of an FB.

Emergency Department Care and Disposition

Treatment of an airway FB is usually laryngoscopy or rigid bronchoscopy in the operating room under anesthesia. In cases of sudden cardiopulmonary collapse, emergent laryngoscopy is indicated to obtain a patent airway. Patients with an airway FB will require respiratory care for 24 to 72 h after FB removal. Antibiotics, steroids, oxygen, mist, and chest physiotherapy may all be necessary.

PERITONSILAR ABSCESS

Clinical Features

Peritonsillar abscess in children most commonly presents in adolescents with an antecedent sore throat. Most commonly, patients appear acutely ill with fevers, chills, dysphagia, trismus, drooling, and a muffled or "hot potato" voice. When present, trismus is thought to be due to secondary inflammation of the neighboring ptergoid muscles. These children may also have ipsilateral ear pain and torticollis. Typically the uvula is displaced away from the affected side. The involved tonsil is anteriorly and medially displaced.

Diagnosis and Differential

Careful visualization of the oral cavity is a must to reliably rule out this infection. When uvular deviation, marked soft palate displacement, severe trismus, airway compromise, or localized areas of fluctuance are noted, the diagnosis of peritonsillar abscess can be made with confidence and no imaging study is required. In younger children, computed tomography (CT) or ultrasound imaging may be required to help differentiate these processes. In nontoxic-appearing adolescents with findings more consistent with a peritonsillar cellulitis, a trial of antibiotics may be the best choice for initial treatment if a good follow-up is assured.

Emergency Department Care and Disposition

The definitive treatment of peritonsillar abscess has changed significantly over the last decade. Today, the majority of cases are treated as outpatients with needle aspiration, antibiotics, and pain control. Antibiotic choices include **ampicillin/sulbactam** 40 mg/kg/d divided every 8 h or a third-generation cephalosporin (see doses in epiglottitis section). Clearly, definitive follow-up is a must. Very young and uncooperative children may be better served with formal incision and drainage in the operating room to prevent injury to the jugular vein and carotid artery.

RETROPHARYNGEAL ABSCESS

Clinical Features and Diagnosis

Although rare, retropharyngeal abscess is the second most commonly seen infection of the deep neck space, usually occurring in children aged 6 months to 3 years. It begins with an URI or trauma, which localizes to the retropharyngeal lymph nodes over several days. Dysphagia and refusal to feed occur before significant respiratory distress. Patients usually appear toxic, presenting with fever, drooling, dysphagia, and inspiratory stridor. They assume an almost opisthotonic posture. Classical teaching is that a lateral neck x-ray performed during inspiration will show a widened retropharyngeal mass, but definitive diagnosis with a CT scan may be required. Physical examination of the pharynx may show a retropharyngeal mass. Palpation of the mass is dangerous, as it may lead to rupture of the abscess.

Emergency Department Care and Disposition

The airway should be stabilized followed by antibiotic therapy. Antibiotic choice is controversial since most retropharyngeal abscesses contain mixed flora including *S. aureus, S. pyogenes, Strep. viridians, Klebsiella, Peptostreptococcus, Fusobacterium* and *Bacteroides.* Single-agent treatment with **ampicillin/sublactum** 40 mg/kg/d divided every 8 h may be best. Others believe that high-dose penicillin G is most appropriate. Early consultation with an ear, nose, and throat specialist for operative incision and drainage is important to prevent extension of the abscess into the mediastinum.

For further reading in *Emergency Medicine: A Comprehensive Study Guide,* 5th ed., see Chap. 129, "Upper Respiratory Emergencies," by Randolph J. Cordle and Nicholas C. Relich.

---

82 | Pediatric Exanthems

Rebecca S. Rich

BACTERIAL INFECTIONS

Bullous Impetigo

Bullous impetigo is a staphylococcal skin infection of infants and young children. Typical skin lesions are superficial, thin-walled bullae that occur mostly on the extremities. The bullae contain clear to yellow fluid but rupture easily, leaving a denuded base, which dries to a shiny coating. Diagnosis is based on the characteristic appearance of the lesions, but, if there is doubt, aspirated bullous fluid may be cultured for staphylococci. Treatment is with oral (PO) antistaphylococcal agents, such as **cephalexin** 50 mg/kg/d PO divided qid or **dicloxacillin** 50 mg/kg/d PO divided qid, along with local wound care and topical agents, such as bacitracin.

Impetigo Contagiosum

Impetigo is a superficial skin infection typically caused by group A β-hemolytic streptococci or, less often, *Staphylococcus aureus*. It usually occurs in small children, often at areas of insect bites or minor trauma. The lesions start as red macules and papules, which then form vesicles and pustules. As these rupture, the fluid forms a golden crust. There may be local lymphadenopathy, but fever and systemic signs are rare. The face, neck, and extremities are most commonly affected. Diagnosis is based on the appearance of the rash. Effective antibiotics include cephalosporins (see "Bullous Impetigo," above), erythromycin or newer macrolides, or antistaphylococcal penicillins combined with wound cleansing and use of topical bacitracin or mucopiricin.

Erysipelas

Erysipelas is cellulitis and lymphangitis of the skin due to group A β-hemolytic streptococci, usually associated with fever and systemic toxicity. The rash starts as a red plaque, which gradually enlarges with local redness, heat, and swelling. A key feature is the raised, sharply demarcated, indurated border. The face is the most common site, with the portal of entry often a skin wound or pimple. Diagnosis is clinical. If there is clear evidence by Gram's stain that the infection is streptococcal, then intravenous (IV) **penicillin G** 100,000 U/kg/d divided every 6 h is adequate. Otherwise, initial therapy should be broader: **ceftriaxone** 75 mg/kg/d IV, **cefuroxime** 100 mg/kg/d IV divided every 8 h, or another antistaphylococcal antibiotic.

Mycoplasma Infections

Mycoplasma pneumonia is a common cause of pneumonia, bronchitis, and upper respiratory infections in children and young adults. This infection should always be considered in patients with rash and pneumonia. Common symptoms are fever, cough, sore throat, headache, and rash. The rash is typically red, maculopapular, and, often, truncal. An even more frequent rash associated with mycoplasma is erythema multiforme and, sometimes, Stevens-Johnson syndrome. Effective antibiotics for mycoplasma include **erythromycin** 40 mg/kg/d PO divided qid. The newer macrolides clarithromycin or azithromycin are often more convenient and better tolerated.

Scarlet Fever

Scarlet fever is a streptococcal pharyngitis infection with a distinctive toxin-mediated rash. The etiologic agent is group A β-hemolytic streptococci, although recently group C streptococcus has been implicated. School-age children are most commonly affected. Symptoms include fever, sore throat, headache, vomiting, and abdominal pain, followed by rash in 1 to 2 days. The pharynx and tonsils are typically red with white exudate. The pharynx is bright red with a white coating (strawberry tongue). The rash starts on the neck, groin, and axillae. It is red and punctate, and blanches with pressure. The rash is often accentuated at the flexural creases (Pastia's lines). When palpated, the rash has a characteristic rough, sandpaper feel. Desquamation occurs with healing. Scarlet fever is diagnosed by the rash's appearance in the setting of fever and pharyngitis. Throat swabs yield streptococci. Treatment is as for streptococcal pharyngitis, with **penicillin VK** 50 mg/kg/d PO divided qid being the drug of choice (**erythromycin** 40 mg/kg/d PO divided qid for penicillin-sensitive patients).

Staphylococcal Scalded-Skin Syndrome

Staphylococcal scalded-skin syndrome (SSSS) is a febrile illness of neonates and infants characterized by generalized confluent skin exfoliation. The disease is caused by a toxin produced by *Staphylococcus aureus* arising, not in the affected skin, but at a separate site, such as the nose, the pharynx, a wound, or an abscess and inducing separation at the granular layer of the epidermis. The illness begins with fever and irritability, followed by diffuse erythroderma, which typically spares the palms, soles, and mucosa. Soon large thin-walled bullae appear, rupturing easily and leaving large areas of moist denuded skin. The skin separates readily in response to gentle stroking (Nikolsky's sign). Once again, the diagnosis is clinical. SSSS may be confused, however, with toxic epidermal necrolysis (TEN), a more serious skin disease also characterized by bullae and exfoliation. Skin biopsy shows that in SSSS the cleavage is in the granular layer, whereas in TEN the separation occurs more deeply, leading to greater morbidity. Therapy includes parenteral antistaphylococcal antibiotics (see "Bullous Impetigo," above) and eradication of any underlying focus of infection, local wound care, prevention of hypothermia, and fluid support. The skin usually heals without scarring unless superinfection occurs. Hospital admission is usually required.

VIRUSES

Enteroviruses

Enteroviruses are common causes of exantha in young children. They include coxsackieviruses and echoviruses and typically occur in summer and early fall.

Clinical Features

Clinical syndromes caused by these viruses include myo- and pericarditis, aseptic meningitis, orchitis, hepatitis, bronchitis, and pneumonia, as well as nonspecific febrile illness with vomiting and myalgias. Skin manifestations are also varied, ranging from macular, morbilliform, vesicular, petechial, purpuric, and scarlatiniform. In fact, it may be difficult to differentiate enterovirus infections with rash from more serious conditions, such as sepsis, with organisms such as meningococcus.

Diagnosis and Differential

Since there are no specific clinically available tests for enterovirus, diagnosis is by exclusion. Once other, more serious illnesses are ruled out, therapy for enterovirus illnesses is supportive. Although many enteroviral infections are clinically indistinguishable, hand-foot-and-mouth disease, due to coxsackie A 16, is very commonly seen and has distinctive features. Patients become febrile and then develop painful oral lesions and skin rash. The oral lesions are small vesicles that quickly ulcerate. Children are often irritable and will not eat or drink due to pain. The skin lesions start as red papules, which become grayish vesicles, occurring on the palms, soles, and buttocks. The oral and skin lesions heal without scarring in 7 to 10 days. Herpetic gingivostomatitis in toddlers may have similar oral lesions, although there is no skin rash.

Emergency Department Care and Disposition

Since the oral lesions often preclude eating, intravenous (IV) hydration is occasionally necessary. Cool foods, such as ice cream and custards, can be helpful, as can combinations of liquid antacids, liquid diphenhydramine, and careful use of viscous lidocaine ("magic mouthwash").

Erythema Infectiosum

Erythema infectiosum (EI) is an acute febrile illness with a unique rash caused by parvovirus B19. Outbreaks occur primarily in the spring, most often affecting children aged 5 to 15. EI starts abruptly with a bright red rash on the cheeks (slapped-cheek appearance).

There is circumoral pallor and sparing of eyelids and chin. The facial rash fades after 4 to 5 days. About 1 to 2 days after the facial rash appears, a nonpruritic erythematous macular or maculopapular rash occurs on the trunk and limbs. This stage may last 1 week. The rash fades with central clearing, giving a distinctive lacy or reticulated appearance. The palms and soles are rarely affected. The rash may recur intermittently over the next few weeks, sometimes after sun exposure. Associated constitutional, respiratory, and gastrointestinal symptoms are common. Arthralgias and arthritis tend to occur only in adults. There is no specific therapy for EI.

Measles

Measles used to be a common childhood illness before nationwide immunizations. It is much less common now, but there have been recent local epidemics. It is a highly contagious myxovirus infection, occurring in the winter and spring. The incubation period is 10 days, followed by a 3-day prodrome of upper respiratory symptoms and then malaise, fever, coryza, conjunctivitis, photophobia, and cough. Patients look quite ill. The rash develops at day 14 after exposure, spreading from head to feet. It is initially red, blanching, and maculopapular, but it rapidly coalesces, especially on the face. As the rash fades, it looks coppery brown and may desquamate with healing. The rash generally lasts about a week. Koplik's spots, an associated pathognomonic exanthem, occur just before the onset of rash. They are tiny white spots (grains of sand), usually found on the buccal mucosa opposite the lower molars. Measles is a self-limited disease; treatment is supportive.

Infectious Mononucleosis

Infectious mononucleosis (IM), caused by Epstein-Barr virus, affects primarily children, teens, and young adults. Symptoms include fever, malaise, and sore throat. On examination, the pharynx is inflamed, often with exudate, and may look just like streptococcal pharyngitis. Lymphadenopathy affects both anterior and posterior cervical chains and may be generalized. There is a 5 to 10 percent incidence of maculopapular rash in IM. Nearly all patients who are treated with ampicillin or a congener, however, develop rash. The diagnosis is suggested by increased atypical lymphocytes on blood smear and confirmed by a positive heterophil antibody (Monospot) test result; the Monospot test is more reliable in patients over age 5 than in younger children. Treatment of IM is supportive. The main emergency complications of IM are splenic rupture and airway obstruction. Patients with IM should avoid contact sports for 4 to 6 weeks. A short course of corticosteroids, such as **predni-sone** 1 to 2 mg/kg PO qd, is helpful in patients with enlarged tonsils and potential airway obstruction.

Rubella

Rubella (German measles) was more common before immuniza-tions but still occurs, usually in the spring. Incidence among teens is increasing. Rubella starts with a mild prodrome of fever and upper respiratory symptoms. The pink maculopapular rash begins on the face and spreads down and out, then coalescing. The rash is often fleeting and subtle. Lymphadenopathy, especially in the posterior cervical and auricular chains, is characteristic. Rubella is a mild disease and often hard to diagnose; it is important to recognize, however, due to serious congenital fetal malformations when contracted in pregnancy.

Varicella

Varicella (chicken pox), caused by varicella zoster virus, is a pru-ritic, generalized vesicular exanthem occurring most often in the winter. It is very contagious in the prodromal and vesicular stages. Most patients are less than 10 years old, but chicken pox occurs at all ages and is usually more severe in adults. There is a prodrome of fever and upper respiratory symptoms. The rash starts on the trunk or head as faint red macules. Within 24 h the lesions vesicu-late (i.e., take on the appearance of a dewdrop on a rose petal) and, over the next 1 to 2 weeks, dry and crust over. Successive fresh crops appear in the initial days, leading to the characteristic finding of lesions in all stages of development. Low-grade fever occurs, but systemic toxicity is not severe. Diagnosis is clinical, based on the rash and contact with chicken pox. Uncomplicated varicella requires no specific therapy. Aspirin should be avoided, since it may predispose to Reye's syndrome. PO antihistamines, such as **hydroxyzine** 2 mg/kg/d PO divided qid or **diphenhydramine** 5 mg/kg/d PO divided qid, can help the intense itching. Routine use of acyclovir is not recommended for most children, but immu-nocompromised patients should receive it. Superinfection of le-sions is the most common complication in normal hosts. Varicella zoster immune globulin should be considered in nonimmune im-munocompromised patients exposed to varicella.

Roseola Infantum

This common childhood febrile illness is caused by human herpes-virus 6. Most patients are between 6 months and 3 years old. The illness starts with high fever that persists for 3 to 5 days. Children may be quite irritable. The rash usually occurs as the child's fever is resolving and consists of blanching macular or maculopapular rose or pink, discrete lesions that are most prominent on the neck, trunk, and buttocks. Mucous membranes are not involved. The rash lasts 1 to 2 days and then rapidly fades. Although roseola is ultimately benign, febrile seizures may occur, and, until the rash occurs, it may be hard to differentiate from more serious febrile illness.

Erythema Nodosum

Currently, this inflammatory exanthem is most commonly associated with medications, especially oral contraceptives. Other common etiologies include sarcoidosis, inflammatory bowel disease, leukemia, and vasculitis. Infectious causes such as tuberculosis, fungal diseases, and streptococcal infections are less common now than in the past. Erythema nodosum is clinically distinctive, with bilateral tender nodules developing symmetrically, particularly over the shins and extensor prominences. The nodules are 1 to 5 cm in size but may merge. The overlying skin is red, smooth, and shiny. The eruption lasts several weeks. Constitutional symptoms often occur at the onset, including fever, arthralgias, myalgias, and fatigue. The diagnosis is made clinically. There is no known therapy, but analgesics are often indicated. Since underlying causes are often present, the physician should look for them during the emergency department workup and refer patients promptly.

Kawasaki Disease

Kawasaki disease (KD), or mucocutaneous lymph node syndrome, is a generalized vasculitis of unknown cause, particularly involving the coronary arteries. The peak age of onset is 1 to 2 years. Table 82-1 lists clinical criteria for the diagnosis. The fever is high and prolonged, lasting 1 to 2 weeks in untreated children. The conjunctivitis is nonexudative. The polymorphous rash usually consists of red, raised plaques, often affecting the perineum. The erythrocyte sedimentation rate is often dramatically elevated. The acute febrile phase lasts 7 to 14 days. During the next, subacute phase, lasting 2 to 4 weeks, there is desquamation of the hands and feet. Thrombocytosis also occurs during this phase, when the child is at greatest risk for coronary thrombosis.

Coronary artery aneurysmal dilatation occurs in 20 percent of untreated patients, peaking 4 weeks after onset of illness. Sudden death occurs in 1 to 2 percent of untreated patients.

TABLE 82.1 Diagnostic Criteria for Kawasaki Disease

Fever of at least 5-d duration (100%)

Presence of at least 4 of the following 5 conditions:
  1. Bilateral conjunctivitis (85%)
  2. Changes of the lips and oral mucosa (90%)
     Dry, red, fissured lips
     Strawberry tongue
     Oropharyngeal edema
  3. Changes of the extremities (75%)
     Erythema of palms and soles
     Edema of hands and feet
     Periungual desquamation
  4. Polymorphous rash (80%)
  5. Cervical lymphadenopathy (70%)

Illness not explained by other known disease process

Patients meeting diagnostic criteria are usually admitted. Intravenous immunoglobulin 2 g/kg over 10 h within the first 10 days of illness reduces the incidence of aneurysm. Aspirin 80 to 100 mg/kg/d divided 4 times a day is also used for its antiplatelet effect.

Pityriasis Rosea

Pityriasis rosea (PR) occurs mostly in patients from age 10 to 35 in the spring and fall. The disease is not contagious. PR often starts with a herald patch, one red lesion with a raised border, usually on the trunk. About 1 to 2 weeks later, there is a widespread eruption of pink maculopapular oval patches, often affecting the trunk. The lesions have a dry, scaly collarette border. The classical PR rash is the shape of a Christmas tree over the patient's back. There may be mucosal involvement. The illness may last 3 to 8 weeks, with successive new crops of skin lesions. PR is largely a clinical diagnosis, but it may resemble fungal diseases (a KOH preparation of skin scrapings may help differentiate) or viral exantha. Since the classic PR look-alike is secondary syphilis, an RPR must be obtained. There is no specific therapy. Since the rash can be very itchy, antihistamines or oatmeal baths may be helpful.

For further reading in *Emergency Medicine: A Comprehensive Study Guide*, 5th ed., see Chap. 131, "Pediatric Exanthems," by Michael S. Weinstock and Michael S. Catapano.

83 | Musculoskeletal Disorders in Children

Rebecca S. Rich

CHILDHOOD PATTERNS OF INJURY

The growth plate (physis) is the weakest point in children's long bones and the frequent site of fractures. The ligaments and periosteum are stronger than the physis, tolerating mechanical forces at the expense of physeal injury. The blood supply to the physis arises from the epiphysis, so separation of the physis from the epiphysis may be disastrous for future growth. The Salter-Harris classification is widely used to describe fractures involving the growth plate (see Fig. 83-1).

Type I Physeal Fracture

In type I physeal fracture (6 percent of all physeal injuries), the epiphysis separates from the metaphysis. The reproductive cells of the physis stay with the epiphysis. There are no bony fragments. Bone growth is undisturbed. Diagnosis of this injury is suspected clinically in children with point tenderness over a growth plate. On x-ray, the only abnormality may be an associated joint effusion. There may be epiphyseal displacement from the metaphysis. In the absence of epiphyseal displacement, the diagnosis is clinical, supported by the joint effusion. Treatment consists of splint immobilization, ice, elevation, and referral.

Type II Physeal Fracture

Type II physeal fracture is the most common (75 percent) physeal fracture. The fracture goes through the physis and out through the metaphysis. The periosteum remains intact over the metaphyseal fragment, but is torn on the opposite side. Growth is preserved since the physis remains with the epiphysis. Treatment is closed reduction with analgesia and sedation followed by cast immobilization.

Type III Physeal Fracture

The hallmark of type III physeal fracture is an intraarticular fracture of the epiphysis with the cleavage plane continuing along the physis. This injury usually involves the proximal or distal tibia and accounts for 8 percent of all physeal injuries. The prognosis for

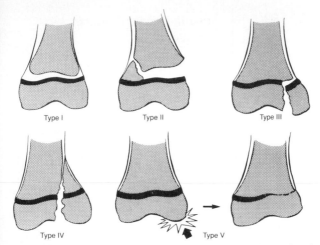

FIG. 83-1 Salter-Harris classification of physeal injuries. (Reproduced with permission from Tolo VT, Wood B: *Pediatric Orthopedics in Primary Care.* Baltimore, Williams & Wilkins, 1994.)

bone growth depends on the circulation to the epiphyseal bone fragment and is usually favorable. Reduction of the unstable fragment with anatomic alignment of the articular surface is critical. Open reduction is often required.

Type IV Physeal Fracture

The fracture line of type IV physeal fractures begins at the articular surface and extends through the epiphysis, physis, and metaphysis. This most often involves the distal humerus, accounting for 8 percent of all physeal injuries. Open reduction is required to reduce the risk of premature bone growth arrest.

Type V Physeal Fracture

Type V physeal fracture is a rare (1 percent) pattern usually involving the knee or ankle. The physis is essentially crushed by severe compressive forces. There is no epiphyseal displacement. The diagnosis is often difficult. An initial diagnosis of sprain or type I injury may prove incorrect when later growth arrest occurs. X-rays may look normal or demonstrate focal narrowing of the epiphyseal plate. There is usually an associated joint effusion. Treatment consists of cast immobilization, non-weight-bearing, and close orthopedic follow-up in anticipation of focal bone growth arrest.

Torus Fractures

Children's long bones are more compliant than those of adults and tend to bow and bend under forces where an adult's might fracture. Torus (also called *cortical* or *buckle*) fractures involve a bulging or buckling of the bony cortex, usually of the metaphysis. Patients have point tenderness over the fracture site and soft tissue swelling. Radiographs may be subtle but show cortical disruption. Torus fractures are not typically angulated, rotated, or displaced, so reduction is rarely necessary. Splinting or casting in a position of function for 3 to 4 weeks with orthopedic follow up is recommended.

Greenstick Fractures

In greenstick fractures, the cortex and periosteum are disrupted on one side of the bone but intact on the other. Treatment is closed reduction and immobilization.

Plastic Deformities

Plastic deformities are seen in the forearm and lower leg in combination with a completed fracture in the companion bone. The diaphyseal cortex is deformed, but the periosteum is intact.

FRACTURES ASSOCIATED WITH CHILD ABUSE

Certain injury patterns are consistently seen in abused children, particularly multiple fractures in various stages of healing. Twisting injuries create spiral fractures in long bones, highly specific for abuse in nonambulatory children. In ambulatory children, spiral fractures may occur accidentally, the classic example being the spiral fracture of the lower third of the tibia (toddler's fracture), but can also be seen with abuse. The injury pattern most closely associated with abuse is the chip fracture of the metaphysis. The tight attachment of the periosteum to the metaphysis will cause avulsion of little chips of the bone with pulling. There is exuberant callus formation and periosteal new bone formation. With direct trauma, subperiosteal hemorrhage characteristically lifts the periosteum off the bone, where it appears as an opacified line. Fragmentation of the clavicle and acromion and separation of the costochondral junctions of the ribs are very suggestive of abuse. Bony injuries from shaking are similar to twisting, but also include spinal compression fractures and other vertebral injuries. Distraction injuries to the long bones cause hemorrhagic separation of the distal metaphysis, creating a lucency proximal to the physis (bucket handle fracture). Squeezing injuries create rib fractures that are highly suggestive of abuse.

SELECTED PEDIATRIC ORTHOPEDIC PROBLEMS

Clavicle Fracture

A clavicle fracture is the most common fracture in children. Fractures may occur in newborns during difficult deliveries. Babies may have nonuse of the arm. If the fracture was not initially appreciated, parents may notice a bony callus at 2 to 3 weeks of age. In older infants and children, the usual mechanism is a fall onto the outstretched arm or shoulder. Care of patients with clavicle fractures is directed toward pain control. Even if anatomic alignment is not achieved in the emergency department (ED), displaced fractures usually heal well, although patients may have a residual bump at the fracture site.

Emergency Department Care and Disposition

"Figure of eight" shoulder abduction restraints have been the traditional treatment, but many patients have more pain with this device. Many orthopedists find a **sling-and-swathe** or **shoulder immobilizer** to be equally effective and less painful. Both devices should be worn day and night for 2 weeks, then during the day for another few weeks.

Supracondylar Fractures

The most common elbow fracture in childhood is the supracondylar fracture of the distal humerus. The mechanism occurs when children fall on their outstretched arms. The close proximity of the brachial artery to the fracture predisposes the artery to injury. Subsequent arterial spasm or compression by casts may further compromise distal circulation. A forearm compartment syndrome, Volkmann's ischemic contracture, may occur. Symptoms include pain in the proximal forearm upon passive finger extension, stocking-glove anesthesia of the hand, and hard forearm swelling. Pulses may remain palpable at the wrist despite serious vascular impairment. Injuries to the ulnar, median, and radial nerves are common too, occurring in 5 to 10 percent of all supracondylar fractures. Children complain of pain on passive elbow flexion and maintain the forearm pronated. X-rays show the injury, but the findings may be subtle. A posterior fat pad sign is indicative of intraarticular effusion and thus fracture. Normally, the anterior humeral line, a line drawn along the anterior distal humeral shaft, should bisect the posterior two-thirds of the capitellum on the lateral view. In subtle supracondylar fractures, the line often lies more anteriorly.

Emergency Department Care and Disposition

Splinting of the elbow in extension is recommended. In cases of neurovascular compromise, immediate fracture reduction is indicated. If an ischemic forearm compartment is suspected after reduction, surgical decompression or arterial exploration may be indicated. Admission is recommended for patients with displaced fractures or significant soft tissue swelling. **Open reduction** is often required. Outpatient treatment is acceptable for nondisplaced fractures with minimal swelling. Such children need orthopedic reassessment within 24 h.

Lateral and medial condylar fractures and intercondylar and transcondylar fractures carry risks of neurovascular compromise, especially to the ulnar nerve. These patients have soft tissue swelling and tenderness, maintaining the arm in flexion. Most patients require open reduction.

Radial Head Subluxation ("Nursemaid's Elbow")

Radial head subluxation is a very common injury seen most often in children between ages 1 to 4. The typical history is that children are lifted up by an adult pulling on the hand or wrist. Sometimes there is a history of trauma, and sometimes there is no event at all but children who refuse to use the arm. The arm is held close to the body, flexed at the elbow with the forearm pronated. Gentle exam reveals no tenderness to direct palpation, but any attempts to supinate the forearm or move the elbow cause pain. If the history and exam is classical, radiographs are not needed, but if the history is atypical or there is a point tenderness or signs of trauma, x-rays should be taken.

Emergency Department Care and Disposition

To reduce the injury, one hand should be held over the child's radial head and the other hand should hold the child's hand. Then, simultaneously, the physician should press down on the radial head with the thumb while fully flexing the elbow and supinating the forearm. There may be a "click" with reduction. (The child will scream and resist.) Usually the child will resume normal activity within 15 min if reduction is achieved. If the child is not better after a second reduction attempt, alternate diagnoses and radiographs should be considered. No specific therapy is needed after successful reduction. Parents should be reminded to avoid linear traction on the arm, as there is an increased risk of recurrence.

Slipped Capital Femoral Epiphysis

Slipped capital femoral epiphysis (SCFE) is more common in boys, with peak incidence between ages 12 to 15, and, in girls, between ages 10 to 13. With a chronic SCFE, children complain of dull pain in the groin, anteromedial thigh, and knee, which becomes worse with activity. With walking, the leg is externally rotated and the gait is antalgic. Hip flexion is restricted and accompanied by external rotation of the thigh. Acute SCFE is due to trauma or may occur in patients with preexisting chronic SCFE. Patients are in great pain, with marked external rotation of the thigh and leg shortening. The hip should not be forced through the full range of motion, as this may displace the epiphysis further.

The differential includes septic arthritis, toxic synovitis, Legg-Calvé-Perthes' disease, and other hip fractures. Children with SCFE are not febrile or toxic and have normal white blood cell counts (WBCs) and erythrocyte sedimentation rates (ESRs). On x-ray, medial slips of the femoral epiphysis will be seen on antero-posterior (AP) views while frog-leg views detect posterior slips. In the AP view, a line along the superior femoral neck should transect the lateral quarter of the femoral epiphysis, but not if the epiphysis is slipped.

Emergency Department Care and Disposition

The management of SCFE is operative. The main long-term complication is avascular necrosis of the femoral head.

Transient Tenosynovitis of the Hip

Transient tenosynovitis is the most common cause of hip pain in children less than age 10. The peak age is 3 to 6 years, with boys affected more than girls. The cause is unknown. Symptoms may be acute or gradual. Patients have pain in the hip, thigh, and knee and antalgic gait. Pain limits the hip's range of motion. There may be a low-grade fever, and patients do not appear toxic. The WBC and ESR are usually normal. Radiographs of the hip are normal or show a mild-to-moderate effusion. The main concern is differentiation from septic arthritis, particularly if patients are febrile, with elevation of the WBC or ESR and effusion. Diagnostic arthrocentesis is required, either with fluoroscopic or ultrasound guidance or in the operating room. The fluid in transient tenosynovitis is a sterile clear transudate.

Emergency Department Care and Disposition

Once septic arthritis and hip fracture have been ruled out, patients can be treated with crutches to avoid weight-bearing, anti-inflammatory agents such as **ibuprofen** 10 mg/kg, and close follow-up.

Acute Suppurative Arthritis

Septic arthritis occurs in all ages, but especially in children under 3. The hip is most often affected, followed by the knee and elbow. The diagnosis is critical because, left untreated, purulent joint infection leads to total joint destruction. Bacteria access the joint hematogenously, by direct extension from adjacent osteomyelitis, or from inoculation as in arthrocentesis or femoral venipuncture. The organisms vary with the children ages; *Haemophilus influenzae* has diminished due to widespread vaccination. Although systemic symptoms can be subtle in newborns, older children will appear ill, with high fever and irritability. The affected joint is very painful and shows warmth, swelling, and severe tenderness to palpation and movement. Children with hip or knee infection will limp or not walk at all. Children maintain an infected hip in flexion, abduction, and external rotation. X-rays show joint effusion, but this is nonspecific. The differential includes osteomyelitis, transient tenosynovitis, cellulitis, septic bursitis, acute pauciarticular juvenile rheumatoid arthritis (JRA), acute rheumatic fever, hemarthrosis, and SCFE. Distinguishing septic arthritis from osteomyelitis may be quite difficult. Osteomyelitis is more tender over the metaphysis, whereas septic arthritis is more tender over the joint line. Joint motion is much more limited in septic arthritis. Prompt arthrocentesis is the key to diagnosis, either at the bedside, or in the case of the hip, in the operating room or under ultrasound. Synovial fluid shows WBCs and organisms.

Emergency Department Care and Disposition

Prompt joint drainage is critical, either in the operating room in the case of the hip, or arthroscopically or via arthrocentesis in more superficial joints. Suggested antibiotics are listed in Table 83-1. The prognosis depends on the length of time between symptoms and treatment, which joint is involved (worse for the hip), presence of associated osteomyelitis (worse), and the patient's age (worse for youngest children).

AVASCULAR NECROSIS SYNDROMES

Legg-Calvé-Perthes' Disease

Legg-Calvé-Perthes' disease is essentially avascular necrosis of the femoral head with subchondral stress fracture. Collapse and

TABLE 83-1 Initial Antibiotic Therapy of Acute Suppurative Arthritis in Children

Age	Suspected organism	Antibiotics
Newborn (0–2 months)	*Staphylococcus aureus* Group B *Streptococcus*	Methicillin or nafcillin* Ampicillin or penicillin and gentamicin
	Gram-negative *bacilli*	Cefotaxime/ceftriaxone
	Neisseria gonorrhoeae	Cefotaxime/ceftriaxone
	Unknown	Methicillin or nafcillin* and cefotaxime/ceftriaxone
Infant (2–36 months)	*Haemophilus influenzae*	Cefuroxime or cefotaxime/ceftriaxone
	Strep. species	Penicillin G
	Staph. aureus	Methicillin or nafcillin*
	Gram-negative *bacilli*	Cefotaxime/ceftriaxone
	Unknown	Methicillin or nafcillin* and cefotaxime/ceftriaxone
Child (> 36 months)	*Staph. aureus*	Methicillin or nafcillin*
	Strep. species	Penicillin G, other β-lactams, clindamycin
	Gram-negative bacilli	Cefotaxime/ceftriaxone
	N. gonorrhoeae	Ceftriaxone or penicillin G
	Unknown	Methicillin or nafcillin* and cefotaxime/ceftriaxone

*Vancomycin if methicillinase-resistant *Staph. aureus* is suspected.

flattening of the femoral head ensues, with a potential for subluxation. The result is a painful hip with limited range of motion, muscle spasm, and soft tissue contractures. Onset of symptoms is between ages 4 to 9. The disease is bilateral in 10 percent of patients. Children have a limp and chronic dull pain in the groin, thigh, and knee, which becomes worse with activity. Systemic symptoms are absent. Hip motion is restricted; there may be a flexion-abduction contracture and thigh muscle atrophy. Initial radiographs (in the first 1 to 3 months) show widening of the cartilage space in the affected hip and diminished ossific nucleus of the femoral head. The second sign is subchondral stress fracture of the femoral head. The third finding is increased femoral head opacification. Finally, deformity of the femoral head occurs, with subluxation and protrusion of the femoral head from the acetabulum. Bone scan and magnetic resonance imaging are very helpful in making this diagnosis, showing bone abnormalities well before plain films. The differential diagnosis includes toxic tenosynovitis, tuberculous arthritis, tumors, and bone dyscrasias.

Emergency Department Care and Disposition

In the ED, the most important thing is to consider this chronic but potentially crippling condition. Nearly all children are hospitalized initially for traction.

Osgood-Schlatter's Disease

Osgood-Schlatter disease is a common syndrome that affects pre-teen boys more than girls. Repetitive stress on the tibial tuberosity by the quadriceps muscle initiates inflammation of the tibial tuberosity, without avascular necrosis. Children have pain and tenderness over the anterior knee, which becomes worse with knee bending and better with rest. The patellar tendon is thick and tender, with the tibial tuberosity enlarged and indurated. X-rays show soft tissue swelling over the tuberosity and patellar tendon thickening without knee effusion. Normally, the ossification site at the tubercle at this age will be irregular, but the prominence of the tubercle is characteristic of Osgood-Schlatter disease.

Emergency Department Care and Disposition

The disorder is self-limited. Acute symptoms improve after restriction of physical activities involving knee bending for 3 months. Crutches may be necessary, though a knee immobilizer or cylinder cast are only rarely needed. Exercises to stretch taut and hypertrophied quadriceps muscles are also helpful.

SELECTED PEDIATRIC RHEUMATOLOGIC PROBLEMS

Henoch-Schönlein Purpura

Henoch-Schönlein purpura (HSP) is a self-limited generalized leukocytoclastic vasculitis mediated by immune complexes. Palpable purpura, the classic vasculitic rash, appears on the trunk, buttocks, and legs. HSP also involves the glomeruli with resulting hematuria and proteinuria. Involvement of the bowel wall causes colicky abdominal pain and may lead to melena, hematochezia, or intussusception. A polymigratory periarticulitis occurs in most children. HSP is largely a clinical diagnosis; useful lab tests include urinalysis, complete blood cell count, tests of renal function, and, sometimes, tests for collagen vascular disease.

Emergency Department Care and Disposition

Hospital admission is indicated when the diagnosis is in doubt, dehydration occurs, or when gastrointestinal or renal complications require close observation. Arthritis, when present as an isolated symptom, can be treated with salicylates. Chronic renal damage, sometimes requiring dialysis, occurs in 7 to 9 percent of children with HSP.

Acute Rheumatic Fever

Acute rheumatic fever (ARF) is an acute inflammatory multisystem illness affecting primarily school-age children. It is not common in the United States, but there have been recent epidemics. ARF is preceded by infection with certain strains of group A β-hemolytic streptococcus, which stimulates antibody production to host tissues. Children develop ARF 2 to 6 weeks after symptomatic or asymptomatic streptococcal pharyngitis. Arthritis, which occurs in most initial attacks, is migratory and polyarticular, primarily affecting the large joints. Carditis occurs in one-third of patients and can affect valves, muscle, and pericardium. Sydenham's chorea occurs in 10 percent of patients and may occur months after the initial infection. The rash, erythema marginatum, is fleeting, faint, and serpiginous, usually accompanying carditis. Subcutaneous nodules, found on the extensor surfaces of extremities, are quite rare. Carditis confers greatest mortality and morbidity. Laboratory tests are used to confirm prior strep infection (throat culture and strep serology) or to assess carditis (electrocardiogram, chest x-ray, and echocardiogram). The differential includes JRA, septic arthritis, Kawasaki disease, leukemia, and other cardiomyopathies and vasculitides. In the ED, carditis is the main management issue. Most patients are admitted.

Emergency Department Care and Disposition

Significant carditis is managed with **prednisone** 1 to 2 mg/kg/d initially. Arthritis is treated with high-dose aspirin (75 to 100 mg/kg/d) to start. All children with ARF are treated with **penicillin** (or **erythromycin** if allergic): **benzathine PCN** 1.2 million U intramuscularly, **procaine PCN G** 600,000 U intramuscularly daily for 10 days, or oral **PCN VK** 25,000 to 50,000 U/kg/d divided four times a day for 10 days. Long-term prophylaxis is indicated for patients with ARF, and life-long prophylaxis is recommended for patients with carditis.

Poststreptococcal Reactive Arthritis

Because of increased group A β-hemolytic strep infections, post-streptococcal reactive arthritis (PSRA) is also increasing. PSRA is a sterile inflammatory nonmigratory mono- or oligoarthritis occurring with infection at a distant site with β-hemolytic strep and also *staphylococcus* and *salmonella*. Unlike ARF, PSRA is not associated with carditis, and in general is a milder illness. PSRA is responsive to nonsteroidal anti-inflammatory drugs (NSAIDs). The issue of penicillin prophylaxis, a mainstay of therapy in ARF, is unsettled and controversial in PSRA.

Juvenile Rheumatoid Arthritis

The group of diseases comprising JRA share chronic noninfectious synovitis and arthritis, with systemic manifestations. Pauciarticular disease is the most common form, usually involving a single large joint such as the knee. Permanent joint damage occurs infrequently. Polyarticular disease occurs in one-third of cases. Both large and small joints are affected, and there may be progressive joint damage. Systemic JRA occurs in 20 percent of patients. This form is associated with high fevers and chills. Extraarticular manifestations are common, including a red macular coalescent rash, hepatosplenomegaly, and serositis. The arthritis in this form may progress to permanent joint damage. In the ED, lab tests focus mostly on excluding other diagnoses. Arthrocentesis may be necessary to exclude septic arthritis, particularly in pauciarticular disease. X-rays initially show joint effusions but are nonspecific. The diagnosis of JRA will likely not be made in the ED.

Emergency Department Care and Disposition

Initial therapy for patients with an established diagnosis include aspirin or an NSAID. Glucocorticoids are occasionally used, for example, for unresponsive uveitis or decompensated peri- or myocarditis.

For further reading in *Emergency Medicine: A Comprehensive Study Guide*, 5th ed., see Chap. 132, "Musculoskeletal Disorders in Children," by Richard A. Christoph.

84 | Sickle Cell Anemia in Children

Cheryl Jackson

Sickle cell emergencies in children include vasoocclusive crises, hematologic crises, and infections. Children with sickle cell disease (SCD) can present great diagnostic and therapeutic challenges for emergency department (ED) physicians. All children with SCD presenting with fever, pain, respiratory distress, or a change in neurologic function require a rapid and thorough ED evaluation.

VASOOCLUSIVE CRISES

Vasoocclusive sickle episodes are due to intravascular sickling, which leads to tissue ischemia and infarction. Bones, soft tissue, viscera, and the brain may all be affected. Pain may be the only symptom; however, children may also have symptoms related to the affected organ system.

Pain Crises

Clinical Features

The classic sickle cell pain crisis is characterized by episodes of acute pain, sometimes triggered by stress, extremes of cold, dehydration, hypoxia, or infection. Most episodes occur without obvious cause. Typically there are no physical findings except pain and perhaps local tenderness, swelling, and warmth. It is rare for clinical symptoms of the disease to appear before 5 to 6 months of age. While young children tend to have pain in the limbs, older children may complain of pain in a variety of locations, including the abdomen and lumbosacral area.

Diagnosis and Differential

Infections can cause vasoocclusive pain crises; therefore, determining the presence of an infectious process is critical. Painful crises can be associated with low-grade fever and leukocytosis, but temperatures greater than 38.3°C (101°F) are more likely to be due to an infectious cause than to tissue ischemia. Vasoocclusive pain crises usually present in a stereotypical fashion. Atypical pain or new sites of pain warrant further investigation for infection or complications of sickle cell disease. Osteomyelitis or septic arthritis should be considered in the differential diagnosis (see Chap. 83).

Abdominal pain crises are common and are characterized by abrupt onset, lack of localization, and recurrent nature. It is important to determine whether the abdominal pain in SCD patients has substantially changed in character, quality, duration, severity, and associated symptoms. If such changes are present, infection or other related diagnoses, such as cholecystis, appendicitis, pancreatitis, hepatitis, perforated viscous, pelvic inflammatory disease, or other gynecologic pathology, should be considered and explored. Ultrasound examination and or computed tomography of the abdomen or pelvis may be useful in determining the diagnosis. If the diagnosis cannot be readily clarified and the cause of the abdominal pain is not clear, then prompt surgical consultation should be initiated.

Emergency Department Care and Disposition

Treatment objectives for painful crises are to thoroughly evaluate for underlying problems or pathologic conditions and to treat the pain. Pain management must be individualized, and an understanding of what treatment regimen has worked in the past is useful.

1. Aggressive hydration with either oral fluids as tolerated, or intravenous (IV) 5% dextrose (D_5) 0.25 normal saline solution (NS) or D_5 0.45 NS at $1\frac{1}{2}$ maintenance rate is also indicated.
2. Mild to moderate pain can often be managed with oral hydration and analgesics, such as narcotic-acetaminophen combinations and nonsteroidal anti-inflammatory drugs (NSAIDs).
3. Parenteral, long-acting narcotics, **morphine** 0.1 to 0.15 mg/kg IV or **hydromorphone** 0.015 mg/kg IV, are the next step.

Children should be admitted to the hospital if their pain is worsening, their oral fluid intake is inadequate, or they have not achieved adequate pain relief approximately 4 h after initiating IV analgesic medications and hydration. Children who have presented repeatedly for the same pain crisis should also be considered for admission. Any child discharged from the ED after being treated for a pain crisis should be reevaluated within 24 h by his or her pediatrician or hematologist.

Acute Chest Syndrome

Acute chest syndrome is believed to be attributable to a combination of pneumonia, pulmonary infarction, and pulmonary emboli from necrotic bone marrow. It is a major cause of death in all patients with SCD, especially those over the age of 10 years.

Clinical Features

Acute chest syndrome should be considered in all patients with SCD who present with complaints of chest pain, especially when it is associated with tachypnea, dyspnea, cough, and other symptoms of respiratory distress. Significant hypoxia and rapid deterioration to respiratory failure can occur.

Diagnosis and Differential

Chest x-rays should be obtained but may be normal during the first 72 h. There are no specific laboratory abnormalities typical of acute chest syndrome; however, a complete blood count (CBC), reticulocyte count, and blood culture should be obtained. Obtain sputum Gram's stain and culture when possible. Noninvasive pulse oximetry should be instituted, and arterial blood gas analysis is indicated in the presence of significant oxygen desaturation or respiratory distress. While ventilation and perfusion scans may be useful if the diagnosis of pulmonary embolus is being entertained, pulmonary angiography should be avoided, since contrast material can cause more pulmonary sickling.

Emergency Department Care and Disposition

All children in whom the diagnosis of acute chest syndrome is being considered, should be monitored closely for changes in work of breathing and oxygenation. Deterioration can be rapid.

1. Supplemental oxygen should be provided if respiratory distress is present or if oxygen saturation is persistently less than or equal to 94 percent.
2. Adequate analgesia for chest pain should be provided (see above), as well as IV hydration with $D_5 \frac{1}{2}$ NS at 1 to $1\frac{1}{2}$ **maintenance**.
3. Treat potential underlying bacterial pneumonia with empiric antibiotic therapy such as **ceftriaxone** 75 mg/kg/d or **cefotaxime** 50 to 75 mg/kg/d divided every 8 h.
4. Simple **red blood cell transfusion** (10 to 15 mL red blood cells per kilogram) or exchange transfusion should be considered in children with severe anemia (hemoglobin level less than 5 g/dL) or rapidly worsening hypoxia. Transfusion decisions should be made early and in consultation with a pediatric hematologist.

All children with suspected acute chest syndrome should be admitted to the hospital for further care.

Acute Central Nervous System Events

Clinical Features

Acute central nervous system (CNS) crisis should be considered in any patient with SCD who presents with sudden-onset headache or neurologic changes, including hemiparesis, seizures, speech defects, sensory hearing loss, visual disturbances, transient ischemic attacks, dizziness, vertigo, cranial nerve palsies, paresthesias, or inexplicable coma.

Diagnosis and Differential

When CNS vasoocclusion is suspected, a computed tomography (CT) scan or magnetic resonance imaging (MRI) of the brain should be obtained. A lumbar puncture is sometimes necessary to rule out subarachnoid hemorrhage. There are no specific hematologic changes associated with CNS vasoocclusion; however, a CBC and reticulocyte count should be obtained, and blood typing and screening should be ordered in case an exchange transfusion is necessary.

Emergency Department Care and Disposition

Suspected CNS vasoocclusion necessitates immediate stabilization and careful monitoring. Once intracranial hemorrhage or infarction is confirmed, $1\frac{1}{2}$- to 2-volume exchange transfusion should be begun as soon as possible in consultation with a pediatric hematologist. A pediatric neurosurgeon should be consulted once intracranial bleeding has been confirmed. All children with diagnosed or suspected CNS vasoocclusion should be admitted to the pediatric intensive care unit for close monitoring and further care.

Priapism

Priapism, a painful sustained erection in the absence of sexual stimulation, occurs when sickled cells accumulate in the corpora cavernosa. It can affect all males with SCD regardless of age, and severe prolonged attacks can cause impotence.

Patients with priapism should receive IV hydration with D_5 0.45 NS at $1\frac{1}{2}$ to 2 times maintenance, appropriate analgesia, and bladder catheterization if the patient is unable to void spontaneously. Treatment options include oral α-adrenergic agonists (e.g., terbutaline or pseudoephedrine), intrapenile injection of vasodilators (e.g., hydralazine), and/or needle aspiration of the corpora cavernosa. Management and admission decisions should be made promptly in consultation with a urologist and a pediatric hematologist.

HEMATOLOGIC CRISES

Acute Sequestration Crises

Clinical Features and Diagnosis

Sequestration crises are the second most common cause of death in children with SCD under the age of 5 years. The spleen of young children with sickle cell disease can massively enlarge, trapping a considerable portion of the circulating blood volume. This condition can quickly progress to hypotension, shock, and death. Such crises are often preceded by a viral infection.

Classically children present with sudden-onset left upper quadrant pain, pallor, and lethargy; a markedly enlarged, tender, and firm spleen on abdominal examination; and signs of cardiovascular collapse, including hypotension and tachycardia. A CBC reveals a profound anemia (hemoglobin drops to less than 6 g/dL or 3 g/dL lower than the patient's baseline level). Minor episodes can occur with insidious onset of abdominal pain, slowly progressive splenomegaly, and a more minor fall in the hemoglobin level (generally the hemoglobin level remains above 6 g/dL).

Splenic sequestration crises may be characterized by thrombocytopenia and higher than normal reticulocyte counts. Less commonly, sequestration can occur in the liver. Clinical features include an enlarged and tender liver with associated hyperbilirubinemia, severe anemia, and elevated reticulocyte count. Cardiovascular collapse is rare in this condition.

Emergency Department Care and Disposition

Early recognition and prompt initiation of treatment are the keys to successful management. The goal of treatment is to quickly expand the intravascular volume with the rapid infusion of large amounts of **NS** or **albumin** (start with 20 mL/kg). **Transfusion** with packed red blood cells or whole blood if available is often required and should be instituted immediately. Even children with minor episodes should be admitted to the hospital.

Aplastic Episodes

Potentially life-threatening, aplastic episodes are precipitated primarily by viral infections but can also be caused by bacterial infections, folic acid deficiency, or bone-marrow-suppressive or -toxic drugs.

Patients usually present with gradual onset of pallor, dyspnea, fatigue, and jaundice. CBC reveals an unusually low hematocrit (10 percent or lower) with decreased or absent reticulocytosis. White blood cell and platelet counts remain stable. Pain is not a hallmark of this crisis unless there is an associated vasoocclusive crisis. Obtain cultures if the source of infection is not apparent.

If anemia is severe, admit for red blood cell **transfusion** in order to avoid secondary cardiopulmonary complications.

Hemolytic Crises

Bacterial and viral infections in children with SCD can also precipitate an increasing degree of active hemolysis.

Onset is usually sudden. A CBC reveals a hemoglobin level decreased from baseline, with markedly increased reticulocytosis. Increased jaundice and pallor are noticed on physical examination, in addition to other signs and symptoms of the precipitating infection.

Specific therapy is rarely required. Hematologic values return to normal as the infectious process resolves. Care should be directed toward treating the underlying infection. Close follow-up to monitor hemoglobin level and reticulocyte count should be arranged at discharge.

Infections

Clinical Features

Children with SCD are functionally asplenic and have deficient antibody production and impaired phagocytosis. Therefore, bacterial infections, especially with encapsulated organisms, pose a serious and potentially fatal threat to young children with SCD.

Since sepsis can be rapid, overwhelming, and fatal, particularly in children less than 5 years of age, all children with SCD and fever should be quickly and carefully examined and managed aggressively.

The management and disposition of children with these variants of sickle cell disease should be made in conjunction with a pediatric hematologist.

Diagnosis and Differential

A CBC, reticulocyte count, and blood cultures should be obtained for all children with SCD and fever or history of fever. Other cultures (urine, throat, and sputum) should be obtained as indicated by the physical examination. The pulse oximetry reading should be checked and a chest x-ray obtained if the patient is hypoxic or there are signs of respiratory distress. A lumbar puncture is indicated if clinical signs and symptoms of meningitis are present. Knowledge regarding the child's immunization status (particularly whether he or she has been immunized against *Haemophilus influenzae* B and/or pneumococcus) and compliance with their home penicillin prophylaxis is helpful.

Emergency Department Care and Disposition

Children who are ill appearing on presentation should be treated parenterally with an antibiotic with activity against *Streptococcus pneumoniae* and *H. influenzae* (e.g., **ceftriaxone** 50 mg/kg IV or intramuscular) before evaluation is complete and test results are available. Consider vancomycin if patient is at high risk for penicillin-resistant pneumococcal infection. Manage septic shock aggressively with IV fluids, vasoactive medications, and possible transfusion. Admit to the hospital. Consider pediatric intensive care unit admission.

For further reading in *Emergency Medicine: A Comprehensive Study Guide,* 5th ed., see Chap. 133, "Sickle Cell Disease," by Peter J. Paganussi, Thom A. Mayer, and Maybelle Kou.

---

85 | Pediatric Urinary Tract Infections

Rebecca S. Rich

Bacteria enter the urinary tract after colonizing the perineum. In infants, urinary tract infection (UTI) can also occur with bacteremia. *Escherichia coli* predominates, but *Proteus, Enterobacter,* and *Klebsiella* are also important. *Enterococcus, Staphylococcus,* and group B *Streptococcus* are common gram-positive bacteria seen most often in neonates. In teenage girls, coagulase-negative *Staphylococcus* is a common pathogen. Adenovirus can cause cystitis, often in boys, presenting just as a bacterial infection would. UTIs occur in 4 to 7 percent of febrile infants. Under 3 months of age, the rate of bacteriuria is 1 percent. In febrile infants, bacteriuria occurs in 7 to 17 percent. At this age, sepsis accompanies UTI in 10 to 35 percent of cases. In infancy, boys have more UTIs, but after age 3 months and into adulthood, girls are at much higher risk. Symptomatic UTIs occur in 3 to 5 percent of school-age girls.

Clinical Features

Infants and young children usually present with nonspecific symptoms, such as fever, vomiting, diarrhea, and irritability. Older children may have dysuria, urinary frequency, enuresis, or abdominal pain. In older children there may be flank or suprapubic pain on examination. Differentiation of upper versus lower UTI can be difficult clinically, although fever, vomiting, and back pain suggest pyelonephritis. Vulvovaginitis is a common cause of dysuria and should be specifically sought on physical examination. Sexually transmitted diseases also share many symptoms with UTIs.

Diagnosis and Differential

Urine culture is the gold standard, but the results are not available in the acute setting. Since bag urine cultures are unacceptably contaminated, bladder catheterization or suprapubic tap is recommended. Older children can usually get an adequate clean specimen with good cleansing and coaching.

Unfortunately, neither urinalysis nor urine test strips are as accurate as urine culture. Although pyuria is suggestive of UTI, it is nonspecific and is absent in half of infants with culture-proven UTI. Pyuria, hematuria, and proteinuria are all very common in UTIs but occur often in the absence of infection. The sensitivity of positive test strip results for nitrate or leukocyte esterase for UTI is less than 50 percent. The combined presence of pyuria (0.5 white blood cells per high-power field) plus bacteria on urinalysis improves the sensitivity to 65 percent.

TABLE 85-1 Common Antimicrobial Drugs Used in Pediatric Urinary Tract Infections

Drug	Dosage and interval
Parenteral therapy	
Ampicillin	100 mg/kg/d 12h (<1 week old)
	q6–8h (>1 week old)
Ceftriaxone*	75 mg/kg/d q12–24h
Cefotaxime	150 mg/kg/d q6–8 h
Gentamicin	5 mg/kg/d q12h (<1 week old)
	7.5 mg/kg/d q8h (>1 week old)
Oral therapy	
Amoxicillin†	20–40 mg/kg/d q8h
Amoxicillin/ clavulanate	50 mg/kg/d q8h
TMP-SMX	6–12 mg/kg/d TMP, 30–60 mg/kg/d SMX q12h
Cephalexin	25–50 mg/kg/d q6h
Cefixime	8 mg/kg/d q12h

*Should not be used in neonates because of potential biliary sludge pseudolithiasis. If cocci are present in urinary sediment, ampicillin should be added until culture and sensitivities are available.
†*Escherichia coli* resistance should be considered.
Abbreviations: q, every; TMP-SMX, trimethoprim-sulfamethoxazole.
Source: Adapted from *Pediatr Emerg Med Rep* 2:107,1997.

Emergency Department Care and Disposition

Early treatment of UTIs in infants and children decreases the risks of kidney damage. Inpatient management with parenteral therapy is preferred for infants under 3 months with a febrile UTI; children who appear toxic or dehydrated, or are vomiting; and those with urinary stents or other foreign bodies, renal insufficiency, or immunocompromise. Children older than 3 months with febrile UTIs who appear nontoxic and are not significantly dehydrated or vomiting can receive initial parenteral treatment followed by a course of oral antibiotics with close outpatient follow-up. See Table 85-1 for specific drug recommendations and dosages.

Duration of therapy should be at least 10 days for pyelonephritis. Five days is probably adequate for uncomplicated bladder infections in children with normal anatomy. Follow-up is important, since some children will require evaluation for structural urinary tract abnormalities.

For further reading in *Emergency Medicine: A Comprehensive Study Guide*, 5th ed., see Chap. 136, "Pediatric Urinary Tract Infections," by Michael F. Altieri, Mary Camarca, and Thom A. Mayer.

INFECTIOUS DISEASES/IMMUNOLOGY

86 | Sexually Transmitted Diseases

Rebecca S. Rich

This chapter covers the major sexually transmitted diseases (STDs) in the United States with the exception of HIV, discussed in Chap. 88. Vaginitis and pelvic inflammatory disease (PID) are covered separately in Chaps. 62 and 63, respectively.

GENERAL RECOMMENDATIONS

When treating STDs in the emergency department (ED), keep in mind that STDs frequently occur concurrently, that compliance and follow-up are often limited, and that infertility may result from lack of treatment. For these reasons,

1. Treat even when an STD is only suspected, with emphasis on single-dose therapy if possible.
2. Perform serologic testing for syphilis on patients with other STDs.
3. Perform pregnancy tests on all female patients with STDs.
4. Counsel patients about STD prevention.
5. Counsel or refer patients for HIV testing.
6. Advise patients that partners must be treated to prevent reinfection. If partners are present during the ED visit, treat them at that time.

CHLAMYDIAL INFECTIONS

Chlamydia trachomatis is an obligate intracellular bacterium that causes urethritis, epididymitis, and proctitis in men and urethritis, cervicitis, PID, and infertility in women. In both sexes, asymptomatic infection is common. Patients with gonorrhea (GC) have a high incidence of concomitant *Chlamydia*. The incubation period is 1 to 3 weeks, with symptoms ranging from mild urinary burning to peritonitis. Diagnostic techniques include direct immunofluorescence, ELISA assays, DNA probes, and culture. Newer assays on urine are becoming available. As shown in Table 86-1, doxycycline or azithromycin are the treatments of choice.

GONOCOCCAL INFECTIONS

Neisseria gonorrhoeae causes urethritis, epididymitis, and prostatitis in men and urethritis, cervicitis, PID, and infertility in women. Rectal infection and proctitis can occur in both sexes. The incubation period ranges from 3 to 14 days. As with *Chlamydia*, asymptomatic infection is common. Disseminated GC is a systemic infection that occurs in 2 percent of patients with GC, most often women, and is the most common cause of infectious arthritis in young adults. Although there is overlap, disseminated GC tends to be biphasic. An initial febrile bacteremic stage includes skin lesions (tender pustules on a red base, usually on the extremities), tenosynovitis, and myalgias. Over the next week, these symptoms subside, followed by mono- or oligoarticular arthritis with purulent joint fluid. For uncomplicated GC, urethral or cervical cultures are the standard diagnostic tests. A Gram's stain of urethral discharge showing intracellular gram-negative diplococci is very useful in men, but cervical smears are unreliable in women. Diagnosis of disseminated GC is often clinical, since results of culture of blood, skin lesions, and joint fluid are positive in only 20 to 50 pecent of patients. Culturing the patient's cervix, rectum, and pharynx may improve the yield. A positive GC culture result from a partner is also very helpful. Several single dose therapies are available (see Table 86-1). Patients should be treated for *Chlamydia* as well. Disseminated GC is treated initially with parenteral ceftriaxone (1 g/d).

TRICHOMONAS INFECTIONS

Trichomonas vaginalis is a flagellated protozoan that causes vaginitis with discharge. Abdominal pain may also be present. In men, infection is often asymptomatic, but urethritis may be present. Diagnosis is based on finding the motile, flagellated organism on a saline wet preparation of vaginal discharge or urine. Metronidazole (2 g orally in a single dose) is the standard treatment for the patient and partner.

GENITAL WARTS

Human papilloma virus causes genital warts and may be related to cervical cancer. The warts appear after an incubation period

TABLE 86-1 Antimicrobial Therapy for Sexually Transmitted Diseases

Disease	Recommended treatment	Alternative
Chlamydial infection	Azithromycin 1 g PO single dose *or* Doxycycline 100 mg PO bid for 7 d	Ofloxacin 300 mg PO bid for 7 d *or* Erythromycin 500 mg PO qid for 7 d
Gonococcal infections	Ceftriaxone 125 mg IM single dose *or* Cefixime 400 mg PO single dose *or* Ciprofloxacin 500 mg PO single dose *or* Ofloxacin 400 mg PO single dose	
Gonococcal, disseminated	Ceftriaxone 1 g IV daily for 7–10 d, or for 2–3 d, followed by cefixime 400 mg PO bid or ciprofloxacin 500 mg PO bid to complete 7–10 d total therapy	Ceftizoxime or cefotaxime, 1 g IV q 8 h for 2–3 d or until improved, followed by cefixime 400 mg PO bid or ciprofloxacin 500 mg PO bid to complete 7–10 d total therapy
Trichomoniasis	Metronidazole 2 g PO single dose	Metronidazole 500 mg PO bid for 7 d
Syphilis, first-degree, second-degree, early latent	Benzathine penicillin G 2.4 million U IM single dose	Doxycycline 100 mg PO bid for 14 d
Syphilis, late latent or unknown	Benzathine penicillin G 2.4 million U IM 3 doses 1 week apart	Doxycycline 100 mg PO bid for 28 d
Herpes simplex infections	Acyclovir 400 mg PO tid for 7–10 d *or* Valacyclovir 1 g PO bid for 7–10 d	Famciclovir 250 mg PO tid for 7–10 d
Chancroid	Azithromycin 1 g PO single dose *or* Ceftriaxone 250 mg IM single dose	Ciprofloxacin 500 mg PO bid for 3 d Erythromycin base 500 mg PO qid for 7 d
Lymphogranuloma venereum	Doxycycline 100 mg PO bid for 21 d	Erythromycin 500 mg PO qid for 21 d

Abbreviations: bid, twice a day; IM, intramuscular; IV, intravenous; PO, oral; q, every; qid, four times a day; tid, three times a day.

Source: Adapted from Centers for Disease Control and Prevention: *MMWR* 47:RR-1, 1998.

of several months, and although they are not painful, they tend to coalesce and may cause discomfort due to their size and location. Diagnosis is clinical. Treatment is not usually undertaken acutely in the ED but includes cryotherapy with liquid nitrogen or podophyllin. Recurrence is frequent.

SYPHILIS

Treponema pallidum, the spirochete that causes syphilis, enters the body through mucous membranes and nonintact skin. Syphilis has been on the rise lately, thought to be related to the crack cocaine epidemic. Syphilis occurs in three stages. The primary stage is characterized by the chancre, a single painless ulcer with indurated borders found on the penis, vulva, or other areas of sexual contact (see Table 86-2). The incubation period is about 21 days, with the lesions disappearing after 3 to 6 weeks. There are no constitutional symptoms. The secondary stage occurs several weeks after the chancre disappears. Rash and lymphadenopathy are the most common symptoms. The rash starts on the trunk, spreading to the palms and soles, and is polymorphous, most often dull red and papular. The rash is not pruritic. Other constitutional symptoms are common, including fever, malaise, headache, and sore throat. Mucous membrane involvement includes oral lesions, and condylomata lata, cauliflower-resembling wartlike growths, may occur in the anogenital region. This stage also resolves spontaneously. Late stage syphilis, which is much less common, occurs years after the initial infection and affects the cardiovascular and neurologic systems. Specific manifestations include neuropathy (tabes dorsalis), meningitis, dementia, and aortitis with aortic insufficiency and thoracic aneurysm formation. Syphilis may be diagnosed in the early stages with dark-field microscopic identification of the treponemes from the primary chancre or secondary condylomata or oral lesions. Serologic tests include nontreponemal (VDRL and RPR) and treponemal (FTA-ABS). Nontreponemal test results are positive about 14 days after the appearance of the chancre. There is a false positive rate of about 1 to 2 percent of the population. Treponemal tests are more sensitive and specific but harder to perform. Syphilis in all stages remains sensitive to penicillin, which is the drug of choice. Treatment regimens are outlined in Table 86-1.

HERPES SIMPLEX INFECTIONS

Herpes simplex virus (HSV) type 2, and less often type 1, cause genital herpes, spreading through mucosal surfaces or nonintact

TABLE 86-2 Clinical Features of Genital Ulcers

Disease	Nature of genital ulcer	Incubation period (range)	Painful	Inguinal adenopathy
Syphilis	Indurated, clean base; heals spontaneously	2 weeks or longer	No	Firm, rubbery nodes; not tender
Herpes simplex infection	Multiple, small, grouped vesicles coalesce and form shallow ulcers; vulvovaginitis	2–7 d	Yes	Tender bilateral adenopathy
Chancroid	Irregular, purulent; undermined edges; not indurated; multiple ulcers	2–12 d	Yes	Present in 50%; usually unilocular; if fluctuant, very painful; may form crater
Lymphogranuloma venereum	Usually not observed; small and shallow; rapid spontaneous healing	5–21 d	No	More common in males; nodes in matted clusters; unilateral or bilateral, multiloculated

Source: Adapted from Scientific American Medicine: Sexually Transmitted Diseases, New York, Scientific American Medicine, 1997.

skin. In primary infections, painful pustules, vesicles, and ulcers occur about 1 week after contact with an infected person (see Table 86-2). Inguinal adenopathy is usually present. Patients with HSV infection may be asymptomatic and spread the virus to their partners. Systemic symptoms are common in first infections, including fever and myalgias. Dysuria is common, and urinary retention may occur. The untreated illness lasts 2 to 3 weeks, healing without scarring. The virus remains latent in the body, however, and recurrences occur in most patients but are usually briefer and milder without systemic symptoms. The diagnosis is usually clinical, based on the characteristic appearance. Viral cultures for HSV are more reliable than the Tzanck smear for intranuclear inclusions. Acyclovir is the treatment of choice for primary infections (see Table 86-1). The drug is less effective for recurrences but may be helpful if started at the onset of an attack.

CHANCROID

Caused by *Haemophilus ducreyi*, chancroid is more common in the tropics but is on the rise in the United States. After an incubation period of 3 to 10 days, a tender papule appears on the external genitalia and then enlarges to a painful purulent ulcer with irregular edges (see Table 86-2). Multiple ulcers may be present. Painful inguinal adenopathy, usually unilateral, follows in half of untreated patients, and these nodes may form a mass (bubo) that drains. Systemic symptoms are minimal. Diagnosis is usually clinical, with care to exclude syphilis. Sometimes the organism may be cultured from the ulcer or bubo. The drugs of choice are erythromycin, ceftriaxone, or azithromycin (see Table 86-1). Buboes should not be excised but may be aspirated for decompression to relieve pain.

LYMPHOGRANULOMA VENEREUM

Several serotypes of *C. trachomatis* cause lymphogranuloma venerum (LGV), which is endemic in other parts of the world but uncommon in the United States. The primary lesion usually occurs 5 to 21 days after exposure and is a painless small papule or vesicle that may go unnoticed and heals spontaneously in a few days (see Table 86-2). After anal intercourse, primary LGV may present as painful mucopurulent or bloody proctitis. Several weeks to months after the primary lesion, painful inguinal adenopathy occurs. The nodes mat together and often suppurate and form fistulae. Late sequelae include scarring; urethral, vaginal, and anal strictures; and occasionally lymphatic obstruction. Diagnosis is through serologic testing and culture of LGV from a lesion. Doxycycline is the drug of choice (see Table 86-1).

For further reading in *Emergency Medicine: A Comprehensive Study Guide*, 5th ed., see Chap. 137, "Sexually Transmitted Diseases," by Dexter L. Morris.

---

87 | Toxic Shock

Leslie C. McKinney

TOXIC SHOCK SYNDROME

Toxic shock syndrome (TSS) is a severe, life-threatening syndrome associated with colonization or infection with *Staphylococcus aureus*. Associated primarily with tampon use in the past, the overall incidence and number of cases associated with tampons has decreased dramatically over the past 20 years. Streptococcal toxic shock syndrome (STSS), or "flesh-eating bacteria," is now more prevalent than TSS. STSS presents in a similar fashion, is associated with a soft-tissue infection, and has a rapidly progressive course and a high mortality rate.

Clinical Features

TSS is characterized by high fever, hypotension, diffuse erythroderma, mucous membrane hyperemia, arthralgias, headache, and constitutional systems, which rapidly progress to multisystem dysfunction. When associated with menstruation, women typically present between the third and fifth day of menses. Diagnostic criteria are listed in Table 87-1.

Diagnosis and Differential

Other syndromes to consider when evaluating patients with the abovementioned findings include STSS, Kawasaki disease, staphylococcal scalded skin syndrome, Rocky Mountain spotted fever,

TABLE 87-1 Diagnostic Criteria for Toxic Shock Syndrome

An illness with the following clinical manifestations:
  Fever: temperature $\geq 38.9°C$ ($\geq 102.0°F$)
  Rash: diffuse macular erythroderma
  Desquamation: 1–2 weeks after onset of illness
  Hypotension

Multisystem involvement (three or more of the following):
  Gastrointestinal: vomiting or diarrhea at onset of illness
  Muscular: severe myalgia or CPK elevation twice normal
  Mucous membrane: vaginal, oropharyngeal, or conjunctival
  hyperemia
  Renal: blood urea nitrogen or creatinine at least twice the upper limit
  of normal for laboratory or urinary sediment with pyuria (≥ 5
  leukocytes per high-power field) in the absence of urinary tract
  infection
  Hepatic: total bilirubin, alanine aminotransferase enzyme, or
  aspartate aminotransferase enzyme levels at least twice the upper
  limit of normal for laboratory
  Hematologic: platelets $< 100,000/mL$
  Central nervous system: disorientation or alterations in
  consciousness

---

and septic shock. When considering TSS, evaluation should include arterial blood gas analysis; a complete blood count (CBC) with differential count; electrolyte determinations, including Mg^{++} and Ca^{++}; a coagulation panel; urinalysis; and a chest x-ray. Cultures of all potentially infectious sites should be obtained, and if a tampon is present it should be removed.

Emergency Department Care and Disposition

The treatment of TSS consists of initial management of circulatory shock, use of antistaphylococcal β-lactamase–stable antimicrobial agents, and the search for a focus of infection. All patients should be placed on a cardiac monitor, a noninvasive blood pressure device, pulse oximetry, oxygen, two intravenous (IV) lines, and Foley catheter.

1. Crystalloid IV fluids should be given initially for hypotension and consideration of a central venous pressure catheter or Swan-Ganz catheter may be necessary if there is no response to an initial fluid bolus of 1 to 2 L **normal saline** solution. Large volumes of fluid may be required over the first 24 h.
2. A **dopamine** infusion may be started at 3 μg/kg/min if there is no response to a fluid challenge, in order to maintain a systolic blood pressure of 90 mmHg.

3. Fresh-frozen plasma, packed red blood cells, or platelets may be given to correct any coagulation abnormalities.
4. Culture all potentially infected sites, including the blood, prior to starting antibiotic therapy.
5. Institute antistaphylococcal microbial therapy. Recommend either antistaphylococcal penicillin, such as **nafcillin** or **oxacillin** 1 to 2 g IV every 4 h, or a cephalosporin with β-lactamase stability, such as **cefazolin**, 2 g every 6 h. In penicillin-allergic patients, clindamycin, vancomycin, or, potentially, cephalosporins may be used.
6. Other considerations include the use of methylprednisolone and IV immunoglobulin in difficult cases.
7. Patients are typically admitted to the intensive care unit.

STREPTOCOCCAL TOXIC SHOCK SYNDROME

Initially defined in 1993, STSS has increased in incidence over the past 10 years to between 2000 and 3000 cases annually. STSS is very similar to TSS but is associated with a soft tissue infection that is culture positive for *Streptococcus pyogenes*.

Clinical Features

STSS typically presents with abrupt onset of pain and some signs of soft tissue infection, most commonly affecting the extremities, although truncal signs are possible. Patients are usually febrile, hypotensive, and confused and develop multisystem organ dysfunction. Necrotizing fasciitis may develop rapidly and carries a poor prognosis. Diagnostic criteria are listed in Table 87-2.

TABLE 87-2 Diagnostic Criteria for Streptococcal Toxic Shock Syndrome

An illness with the following clinical manifestations:
  Hypotension
  Multiorgan involvement characterized by two or more of the following:
    Renal impairment: creatinine level twice normal
    Coagulopathy
    Liver involvement: enzyme or bilirubin level twice normal
    Acute respiratory distress syndrome
    Generalized erythematous macular rash that may desquamate
    Soft tissue necrosis, including necrotizing fasciitis or myositis, or gangrene

Diagnosis and Differential

Consider TSS as well as other infections caused by group A streptococcus, *Clostridium perfringens,* and other bacteria; Kawasaki disease; Rocky Mountain spotted fever; and septic shock. When considering STSS, the physician should look for soft tissue infection and culture the suspected site. Laboratory evaluation includes a CBC with differential count; arterial blood gas analysis; liver function tests; serum electrolyte, Mg^{++}, and Ca^{++} determinations; a coagulation profile; blood cultures; chest x-ray; and urinalysis.

Emergency Department Care and Disposition

1. Refer to the treatment plan for TSS presented earlier and treat similarly, using aggressive fluid therapy and vasopressors as needed.
2. Begin antistreptococcal microbial therapy with IV **penicillin G** 24 million U/d in divided doses and IV **clindamycin** 900 mg every 8 h. Substitute erythromycin in penicillin-allergic patients.
3. Immediate surgical consultation is required, since débridement of wounds is mandatory.
4. IV immunoglobulin may be considered.
5. Patients require admission to the intensive care unit.

For further reading in *Emergency Medicine: A Comprehensive Study Guide,* 5th ed., see Chap. 138, "Toxic Shock Syndrome and Streptococcal Toxic Shock Syndrome," by Shawna J. Perry and Ann L. Harwood-Nuss.

---

88 | HIV Infection and AIDS
| *Arthur H. Tascone*

The spectrum of disease that results from human immunodeficiency virus (HIV) infection is commonly encountered in the practice of emergency medicine. Presentation may vary from primary infection to an asymptomatic phase to AIDS with life-threatening complications. Commonly associated risk factors include intravenous (IV) drug use, homosexuality, heterosexuality, bisexuality, receipt of blood transfusion before 1985, and maternal-neonatal transmissions.

Clinical Features

The spectrum of symptoms resulting from HIV infection and AIDS varies greatly. Virtually any organ system can be involved, and patients often present with symptoms from multiorgan disease to neurologic, pulmonary, gastrointestinal, cutaneous, and ophthalmologic systems. In addition, systemic illness is often found.

Neurologic disease occurs in 75 to 90 percent of AIDS patients. Dementia, meningitis, altered mental status, seizures, and focal neurologic deficits are commonly encountered. The most prominent pulmonary symptoms include cough, hemoptysis, dyspnea, chest pain, and fever. Gastrointestinal complications result in symptoms of dysphagia, odynophagia, abdominal pain, rectal bleeding, and proctitis. The most important dermatologic complications include rashes of disseminated herpes zoster, disseminated herpes simplex, and herpes zoster ophthalmicus. Ocular involvement from cytomegalovirus (CMV) infection results in retinitis and symptoms of visual change, ocular pain, and photophobia. Systemic illness results in symptoms of fever, weight loss, cachexia, and weakness. Given the profound impact of this complex medical condition, as well as its associated social stigma, patients may be depressed and suicidal.

Diagnosis and Differential

AIDS can be diagnosed if one or more of the opportunistic infections or malignancies listed in Table 88-1 is detected in the HIV patient. Due to the complexity of AIDS, many specific opportunistic infections and malignancies are difficult to diagnose in the emergency department setting. Emphasis should be placed on recognizing the specific organ systems involved and the severity of that involvement. Opportunistic infections and malignancies are more likely to occur in individuals with a CD4 lymphocyte count less than 200 cells/μL. If no CD4 count is available, finding a total lymphocyte count less than 1000 cell/uL on a standard complete blood count (CBC) has been shown to be strongly predictive of a CD4 count less than 200 cell/μL.

The most common causes of central nervous system (CNS) disease in the AIDS population include *Toxoplasma gondii, Cryptococcus neoformans,* and AIDS dementia. AIDS dementia is a

TABLE 88-1 AIDS-Defining Conditions

Esophageal candidiasis
Cryptococcosis
Cytomegalovirus retinitis
Herpes simplex virus
Kaposi's sarcoma
Brain lymphoma
Mycobacterium avium complex
Pnemocystis carinii pneumonia
Progressive multifocal leukoencephalopathy
Brain toxoplasmosis
HIV encephalopathy
HIV wasting syndrome
Disseminated histoplasmosis
Isosporiasis
Disseminated *Mycobacterium tuberculosis* disease
Recurrent *Salmonella* septicemia
CD4 count <200 cell/μL
Pulmonary tuberculosis
Recurrent bacterial pneumonia
Invasive cervical cancer

disorder marked by progressive memory and cognitive impairment. Computed tomography (CT) scan of the brain often reveals atrophy with ventricular enlargement. The clinician should exclude other diseases, such as drug ingestion, CNS infection, and toxins.

Toxoplasmosis is the most common cause of focal encephalitis in the AIDS population. CT scan with contrast and magnetic resonance imaging (MRI) of the brain may reveal ring-enhancing lesions. Lymphoma, fungal infection, and tuberculosis (TB) can also cause ring-enhancing lesions. Cryptococcal CNS infection occurs in up to 10 percent of AIDS patients. It can present with a focal CNS infection or with diffuse meningitis.

The evaluation of neurologic disease in the AIDS patient starts with a thorough physical examinaton. Standard testing should include CT scan and MRI if possible. Contrast CT should be considered if focal deficits are evident on examination. A lumbar puncture should be performed if no contraindications exist. Cerebrospinal (CSF) studies should include opening and closing pressures, cell count, glucose determination, protein determination, Gram's stain, India ink stain, bacterial culture, viral culture, fungal culture, toxoplasma and cryptococcal antigen determinations, and coccidiomycosis titer.

Pulmonary disease is common in the AIDS population. Besides community-acquired pathogens, opportunistic infections include *Pneumocystis carinii* pneumonia (PCP), *Mycobacterium tuberculosis* (MTB), CMV, *C. neoformans,* and *Histoplasma capsulatum.* Pulmonary neoplasms also occur. Table 88-2 lists the common

TABLE 88-2 Chest Radiographic Abnormalities: Differential Diagnosis in the AIDS Patient

Finding	Causes
Diffuse interstitial infiltration	PCP CMV MTB MAI Histoplasmosis Coccidioidomycosis Lymphoid interstitial pneumonitis
Focal consolidation	Bacterial pneumonia *M. pneumoniae* PCP MTB MAI
Nodular lesions	Kaposi's sarcoma MTB MAI Fungal lesions Toxoplasmosis
Cavitary lesions	PCP MTB Bacterial infection Fungal infection
Adenopathy	Kaposi's sarcoma Lymphoma MTB Cryptococcosis

Abbreviations: CMV, cytomegalovirus; MAI, *Mycobacterium avium intracellulare;* MTB, *Mycobacterium tuberculosis;* PCP, *Pneumocystis carinii* pneumonia.

chest radiograph findings along with their respective differential diagnoses.

PCP is the most common opportunistic pulmonary infection among AIDS patients. Typically, patients report a nonproductive cough and dyspnea. Chest radiographs often reveal diffuse interstitial infiltrates but may be falsely negative in 5 to 10 percent of cases. Hypoxemia and an increased alveolar-arterial gradient (greater than 35) on arterial blood gas (ABG) analysis support this diagnosis. Sputum analysis should be ordered, but in some patients bronchoscopy is necessary.

The incidence of MTB is increasing in the AIDS population. Cases of multidrug-resistant TB have been reported and pose a health threat to health care workers. Chest radiograph findings are varied but usually do not reveal an upper lobe distribution. All patients suspected of having TB should be placed on respiratory isolation during their evaluations. Sputum analysis for acid-fast bacilli should be undertaken. Cultures and bronchoscopy may be needed. A negative purified protein derivative (PPD) of tuberculin skin test result is not diagnostic in the immunocompromised patient.

Systemic illness, with its associated symptoms of fever, weight loss, cachexia, weakness, and malaise, account for a majority of emergency department presentations. Common causes of systemic illness and symptoms include *Mycobacterium avium intracellulare* (MAI) complex, CMV, non-Hodgkin's lymphoma, endocarditis, and AIDS-related fever. Appropriate laboratory investigation should include CBC, electrolyte determinations, review of CD4 counts, blood cultures (aerobic, anaerobic, and fundal), urinalysis, liver function tests, chest radiography, Venereal Disease Research Laboratories (VDRL) test, cryptococcal antigen determination, and *Toxoplasma* and *Coccidioides* serologic tests. A lumbar puncture should be considered if no source of infection is detected.

Gastrointestinal complications of AIDS are common. Emergency department evaluation should focus on severity of symptoms. Dysphagia and odynophagia are common with candidal, herpes simplex, and CMV oropharyngeal and esophageal disease. Debilitating symptoms warrant a gastroenterology consultation and endoscopy. Diarrhea is a common complication among AIDS patients. Emergency department evaluation includes testing of a stool sample for leukocytes, ova and parasites, acid-fast bacilli, and occult blood, and bacterial culture. The differential diagnosis includes *Shigella, Salmonella, Escherichia coli, Campylobacter, Giardia, Cryptosporidium, Isospora belli,* CMV, MAI, and antibiotic therapy.

Emergency Department Care and Disposition

The initial evaluation of HIV-infected and AIDS patients begins with a heightened awareness of the need for universal precautions. All blood and body fluid exposures should be considered infective. Respiratory isolation should be instituted for patients with suspected TB.

1. All unstable patients should have airway management as indicated, oxygen, pulse oximetry, cardiac monitoring, and IV access. Shock, with its myriad causes, should be managed in standard fashion (see Chaps. 5 and 6).
2. Seizures, altered mental status, gastrointestinal bleeding, and coma should be managed with standard protocols.
3. Suspected bacterial sepsis and focal bacterial infections should be treated with standard antibiotics. Unstable, ill-appearing AIDS patients with bacterial infections should be admitted. Specific opportunistic infections should be treated with medications as listed in Table 88-3. Ill-appearing febrile patients with a CD4 cell count less than 200 cell/μL should be admitted.
4. AIDS patients with pneumonia, hypoxemia worse than baseline, or suspected TB or PCP should be admitted. Antibiotics should be instituted early if a bacterial pathogen is suspected based on testing.
5. Admission should be considered for AIDS patients with new or changing neurologic disease. Treatment will be based on the specific cause detected on thorough testing. Neurologic consultation should occur early in such evaluations.
6. Diarrhea, leading to volume depletion, should be corrected with IV fluids. Specific treatment should be based on laboratory testing. Ill-appearing patients with fever, bloody stools, positive fecal leukocyte test results, or positive stool culture should have an appropriate antibiotic instituted. Chronic diarrhea in non-ill-appearing patients can have specific treatment based on culture and ova and parasite studies. Inability to correct orthostasis, intractable diarrhea, or inability of patients to care for themselves should prompt admission. Patients with dysphagia and odynophagia unresponsive to therapy or associated with inability to eat or drink should be hospitalized.
7. Patients with suspected CMV retinitis or herpes zoster ophthalmicus should have early consultation and admission. CMV is a common cause of blindness, and herpes zoster ophthalmicus causes ocular damage and glaucoma.
8. Patients with disseminated herpes zoster or disseminated herpes simplex require IV antiviral therapy.
9. AIDS patients with inability to care for themselves, poor social

TABLE 88-3 Treatment Recommendations for Common HIV-Related Infections

Organ system	Infection	Therapy
Systemic	*Mycobacterium avium*	Clarithromycin 500 mg PO bid plus ethambutol 15 mg/kg/d PO plus rifabutin 300 mg/kg/d PO
	CMV	Gancyclovir 5 mg/kg IV bid or foscarnet 60 mg/kg IV q8h
Pulmonary	PCP	TMP-SMX 15–20 TMP/kg/d and 75–100 mg SMX/kg/d PO or IV for 3 weeks or pentamidine 4 mg/kg/d IV or IM for 3 weeks; consider PO steroids for Pao_2 <70 mmHg or A-a gradient >35
	MTB	Rifabutin 10 mg/kg/d PO plus pyrazinamide 15–30 mg/kg/d PO plus streptomycin 15 mg/kg/d IM
CNS	Toxoplasmosis	Pyrimethamine 50–100 mg/d PO plus sulfadiazine 4–8 mg/kg/d plus folinic acid 10 mg/d PO
	Cryptococcosis	Amphotericin B 0.7 mg/kg/d IV with or without flucystosine; maintenance therapy required
Ophthalmologic	CMV	Ganciclovir 5 mg/kg bid for 2 weeks; maintenance therapy required daily
Gastrointestinal	Candidiasis (thrush)	Clotrimazole 10 mg 5 times daily troches or nystatin 500 kU 5 times daily gargle
	Esophagitis	Fluconazole 100 mg/d PO
	Salmonellosis	Ciprofloxacin 500 mg bid PO for 2–4 weeks; maintenance therapy required
	Cryptosporidiosis	No known effective cure
Cutaneous	Herpes simplex	Acyclovir 1000 mg/d PO or acyclovir 5–10 mg/kg/d IV
	Herpes zoster	Acyclovir 4000 mg/d PO; IV therapy required for ocular involvement or dissemination
	Candida, Tricophyton	Cotrimazole, miconazole, or ketoconazole, topical therapy bid to tid for 3 weeks

Abbreviations: bid, two times per day; tid, three times per day; TMP-SMX, trimethoprim-sulfamethoxazole.

support at home, poor access to follow-up, and advanced weakness and cachexia are candidates for admission. Patients with worsening depression and suicidal ideation need immediate attention and referral.

For further reading in *Emergency Medicine: A Comprehensive Study Guide,* 5th ed., see Chap. 139, "HIV Infection and AIDS," by Richard E. Rothman and Gabor D. Kelen.

---

89 | Tetanus and Rabies
C. James Corrall

TETANUS

Tetanus is an acute, frequently fatal spasmodic disease that results from a wound infected with the organism *Clostridium tetani.* The clinical manifestations of tetanus are all secondary to an exotoxin elaborated within the wound site with resultant generalized muscular rigidity and muscular contractions.

Clinical Features

In the United States the majority of cases occur in patients over 50 years old who are inadequately immunized. Tetanus occurs most frequently following an acute unreported injury, most commonly a puncture wound, but it can also develop after minor trauma, surgical procedures, abortions, or in neonates because of inadequate umbilical cord care. The majority of cases in the United States occur in rural southern states, predominately in California, Texas, and Florida.

The incubation period of tetanus can range from less than 24 h to over 30 days. Clinically, tetanus can be categorized into four forms based upon the site of inoculation and the incubation period: local, generalized, cephalic, and neonatal.

Local tetanus is manifested by persistent rigidity of muscles in close proximity to the injury site and usually resolves without sequelae. Generalized tetanus is the most common form of the disease and most frequently presents with pain and stiffness in the jaw and trunk muscles. Later, the rigidity leads to the development of trismus and the characteristic facial expression, *risus sardonicus* (devil's smile). Reflex spasms and tonic contractions of all muscle groups are responsible for the other symptoms of the disease, which include dysphagia, opisthotonos, flexing of the arms, fist clenching, and extension of the lower extremities. Patients are conscious and alert throughout these spasms unless laryngospasm and tetanic contraction of respiratory muscles causes respiratory compromise.

Autonomic nervous system dysfunction resulting in a hypersympathetic state occurs in the second week of the illness and is manifested as tachycardia, labile hypertension, profuse sweating, and hyperpyrexia. Such autonomic dysfunction contributes to morbidity and mortality and is difficult to manage.

Cephalic tetanus follows injuries to the head and neck area and occasionally results in dysfunction of cranial nerves, most often the seventh nerve. This form of tetanus has a particularly poor prognosis.

Neonatal tetanus carries an extremely high mortality rate and is uniformly associated with inadequate maternal immunization and poor umbilical cord care.

Diagnosis and Differential

Tetanus is diagnosed solely on the basis of the clinical examination. A history of active immunization with a booster within the previous 10 years eliminates tetanus as a diagnostic possibility. There are no confirmatory laboratory or microbiological tests. The differential diagnosis includes strychnine poisoning, dystonic reactions to the phenothiazines, hypocalcemic tetany, rabies, and temporomandibular joint disease.

Emergency Department Care and Disposition

Patients with tetanus should be managed in an intensive care unit due to the potential for respiratory compromise. Environmental stimuli must be minimized in order to prevent precipitation of reflex convulsive spasms. Identification and debridement of the inciting wound, if present, is necessary to minimize further toxin production.

1. **Tetanus immune globulin** (TIG), 500 U intramuscularly in a single injection should be given.

2. Antibiotics are of questionable value in the treatment of tetanus. If warranted, parenteral **metronidazole** (500 mg intravenously every 6 h) is the antibiotic of choice.

3. The benzodiazepines and, in particular, **diazepam** (5 mg intravenously every 3 h to effect) have been extensively used and result in sedation as well as amnesia, but **lorazepam** (2 mg intravenously to effect), because of its long duration of action, may be superior and the drug of choice. Midazolam is an alternative.

4. Neuromuscular blockade may be required to control ventilation and muscular spasm and to prevent fractures and rhabdomyolysis. In such cases, **vecuronium** (6 to 8 mg/h intravenously) is the agent of choice because of its minimal cardiovascular side effects. Sedation during neuromuscular blockade is mandatory.

5. The combined alpha- and beta-adrenergic blocking agent, **labetalol** (0.25 to 1 mg/min continuous intravenous infusion), has been used to treat the manifestation of sympathetic hyperactivity, but may precipitate myocardial depression. **Magnesium sulfate** (1 to 4 g/h intravenously) has been advocated as a treatment for this condition as well. **Morphine sulfate** (0.5 to 1 mg/kg/h) is also useful and provides sympathetic control without compromising cardiac output. **Clonidine** (300 μg every 8 h nasogastrically), an alpha-receptor agonist, may also be helpful in the management of cardiovascular instability.

6. Patients that recover from clinical tetanus *must* undergo active immunization because of lack of conference of immunity. Adsorbed tetanus toxoid should be administered intramuscularly at the time of injury and at 6 weeks and 6 months postinjury. Tetanus-diphtheria (Td) should be administered to patients > 7 years of age, and diphtheria-acellular pertussis-tetanus (DPT) administered to patients < 7 years of age. A summary of the guidelines for active immunization is presented in Table 89-1.

RABIES

Rabies is most commonly fatal and is transmitted by inoculation with infectious saliva or by salivary contact with a break in the skin or mucous membranes.

In the United States, dog and cat bites are the most common reason for implementation of postexposure prophylaxis, but the most important source of active rabies is wildlife transmission. Animal bites contracted outside the United States in an undeveloped country should be considered at high risk for rabies transmission.

TABLE 89-1 Summary Guide to Tetanus Prophylaxis in Wound Management

History of adsorbed tetanus toxoid (doses)	Clean, minor wounds		All other wounds*	
	T-d† 0.5 mL IM	TIG, 250 U IM	T-d† 0.5 mL IM	TIG, 250 U IM
Unknown or less than three	Yes‡	No	Yes	Yes
Three or more§	No‖	No	Yes#	No

*For example, wounds >6 h old, contaminated with soil, saliva, feces, or dirt; puncture or crush wounds; avulsions; wounds from missiles, burns, or frostbite.

†DPT for children <7 years of age (T-d if pertussis vaccine is contraindicated); T-d for persons >7 years of age.

‡The primary immunization series should be completed. Three doses total are required, with the second dose given at least 4 weeks after the first and the third dose 6 months later.

§If only three doses of fluid toxoid have been received, then a fourth dose of *absorbed* toxoid should be given.

‖Yes, if routine immunization schedule has lapsed in a child <7 years of age or if >10 years since last dose.

#Yes, if routine immunization schedule has lapsed in a child <7 years of age or if >5 years since last dose. Boosters more frequent than every 5 years may predispose to side effects.

Abbreviations: DPT, diphtheria-pertussis-tetanus; IM, intramuscular; T-d, tetanus-diphtheria; TIG, tetanus immune globulin.

Source: Adapted from the American College of Emergency Physicians, Scientific Review Committee: Tetanus immunization recommendations for persons seven years of age and older. *Ann Emerg Med* 15:1111, 1986; Tetanus immunization recommendations for persons less than seven years old. *Ann Emerg Med* 16:1181, 1987, with permission.

Rabid wildlife species include skunks, bats, raccoons, cows, dogs, foxes, and cats. Rodents (squirrels, chipmunks, rats, mice, etc.) and lagomorphs (rabbits, hares, and gophers) have never been implicated as carriers. Bites by these animals are *not* at risk for transmission. Most rabid animals are agitated and labile, may indiscriminately attack anything that moves, and may wander aimlessly. Feeble bark, drooling, stupor, and convulsions mark more advanced disease preceding death of the animal.

As human rabies has decreased in the United States, the proportion of rabies patients without animal-bite exposure has increased. In 60 percent of the cases in the 1980s, a source of infection was not identified. Incubation periods average 35 to 64 days; periods as short as 12 days or as long as 700 days have been reported.

Clinical Features

The initial symptoms of human rabies are nonspecific and last 1 to 4 days: fever, malaise, headache, anorexia, nausea, sore throat, cough, and pain, or paresthesia at the bite site (80 percent). Subsequently, central nervous system (CNS) involvement becomes apparent with restlessness and agitation, altered mental status, painful bulbar and peripheral muscular spasms, opisthotonos, and bulbar or focal motor paresis. Alternatively, in 20 percent, an ascending, symmetric, flaccid, and areflexic paralysis, comparable to the Landry-Guillain-Barré's syndrome, may be seen. Hypersensitivity to sensory stimuli and hydrophobia may occur at this stage, the latter resulting from the sight, sound, swallowing, or even mention of water. Progressively, lucid and confused intervals may become interspersed, cholinergic nervous abnormalities may manifest (hyperpyrexia, mydriasis, and increased lacrimation and salivation), and brainstem dysfunction (dysphagia, optic neuritis, and facial palsies) with hyperreflexia may occur. Extensor plantar responses may be positive and may mimic toxidromes and botulism. Common complications include adult respiratory distress syndrome, diabetes insipidus, SIADH, hypovolemia, electrolyte abnormalities, pneumonia, and cardiogenic shock with hypotension and dysrhythmia from rabies myocarditis. Coma, convulsions, and apnea are the final manifestation of rabid death.

Diagnosis and Differential

The diagnosis of rabies in the emergency department (ED) is clinical. A final diagnosis is made by postmortem analysis of brain tissue. Cerebrospinal fluid (CSF) and serum antibody titers should be sent to the lab. Elevated CSF protein and a mononuclear pleocytosis are also seen.

The differential diagnosis includes viral or other infectious encephalitis, polio, tetanus, viral process, meningitis, brain abscess, septic cavernous sinus thrombosis, cholinergic poisoning, and the Landry-Guillain-Barré syndrome. The diagnosis is especially difficult without history of exposure but should be considered for patients with a picture of progressive and unexplained encephalitis.

Emergency Department Care and Disposition

The treatment of rabies exposure consists of assessment of risk of rabies, public health and animal control notification, and, if warranted, the administration of specific immunobiological products to protect against rabies. These measures are usually performed in the ED together but may at times require time between modalities, although never at the risk of patient infection. The administration of rabies postexposure prophylaxis is a medical urgency, not a medical emergency and should not be taken casually. Pregnant patients should receive the same treatment as nonpregnant individuals.

1. Local wound care—Debridement of devitalized tissue, if any, is important in reducing the viral inoculum. Wounds of special concern should not be sutured as this promotes rabies virus replication.
2. Prophylactic antibiotics—These may be indicated for other reasons, but have no effect on the replication of rabies virus.
3. Tetanus prophylaxis—Tetanus should always be considered and primary or reimmunization prophylaxis should be administered.
4. **Human Rabies Immune Globulin** (HRIG)—This is administered only once at the outset of therapy. The dose is 20 IU/kg, with half the dose (based upon tissue volume constraints) infiltrated locally at the exposure site and the remainder administered intramuscularly.
5. **Human Diploid Cell Vaccine** (HDCV)—For active immunization, it is available in two formulations of the same vaccine. In the author's experience this is the preferred vaccine, due to less adverse reactions. The HDCV can be administered intramuscularly or intradermally. Administered in 5, 1-mL doses on days 0, 3, 7, 14, and 28. The World Health Organization recommends a sixth dose on day 90, but this is not universally accepted.
6. Other rabies vaccines—Rabies Vaccine Adsorbed (RVA) and Purified Chick Embryo Cell Vaccine (PCEC) are available as intramuscular preparations and may be used in lieu of HDCV or in addition to it when the former is unavailable in some

locales. They are considered equally safe and efficacious, but care must be taken for those allergic to chicken products for the PCEC vaccine. There is no change in efficacy when a series is completed with a second vaccine product, such as when encountered in travelers.

7. Quarantine of animals inflicting wounds—Ordinarily quarantine is withheld for domestic dogs and cats with normal behavior, and quarantined for 10 days, which is sufficient for the disease to manifest if the animal is infected. If no signs become apparent, the animal can be considered nonrabid. The principal indication for the initiation of prophylaxis is a bite wound by an uncaptured dog or cat in an endemic area, or a bite wound by an uncaptured bat or appropriate species of carnivore in an unprovoked attack.

8. State and local health department and animal control agencies should be notified—State or local officials should be consulted regarding the possibility of rabies in local dog or cat populations before decisions on initiating rabies prophylaxis are made. Both animal bites and rabies are reportable entities in all states. Animal bites should be reported to the local animal control unit or police departments so that appropriate animals can be captured or quarantined for observation in a timely fashion.

Rabies antibody titers are not recommended following the fifth dose on day 28 for healthy individuals, but are recommended for an incomplete immunization course of immunocompromised patients (particularly those on corticosteroids). Both HRIG and HDCV should be administered in the deltoid muscle rather than in the gluteal area or anterolateral area of the thigh in children due to vaccine failures at the gluteal site, unless the vaccine requires intradermal administration.

Adverse reactions following the use of HRIG are limited to local pain and low-grade fever, which are transient and can be treated with salicylates, acetaminophen, or nonsteroidal anti-inflammatory drugs (NSAIDs). HDCV can precipitate similar local reactions and may manifest mild headache, nausea, dizziness, and myalgias. Booster doses in recipients previously immunized have experienced an immune complex-like reaction. Rabies prophylaxis should not be stopped because of mild reactions.

Serious neuroparalysis or anaphylaxis during treatment poses a therapeutic dilemma. Postexposure assessment of the clinical risk of rabies must be weighed against the risks of treatment with continuation of therapy, switching to an alternative vaccine, pretreatment with antihistamine for hypersensitive patients, or discontinuation of treatment. Both the Centers for Disease Control and state or county health departments can provide assistance in the management of complications.

For further reading in *Emergency Medicine: A Comprehensive Study Guide,* 5th ed., see Chap. 140, "Tetanus," by Donna L. Carden; and Chap. 141, "Rabies," by David J. Weber, David Wohl, and William A. Rutala.

---

90 | Malaria

Rebecca S. Rich

With increased international travel, more Americans are contracting malaria. Malaria must be considered in any person returning from the tropics with an unexplained febrile illness. Four species of the protozoa *Plasmodium* infect humans: *P. vivax, P. ovale, P. malariae,* and *P. falciparum.* The organism is transmitted by a mosquito bite and goes first to the liver, where asexual reproduction occurs (exoerythrocytic stage). The liver cell ruptures, releasing merozoites, which invade erythrocytes (erythrocytic stage). In *P. vivax* and *P. ovale* infections, some intrahepatic forms remain dormant and can later activate, causing relapse. The clinical symptoms of malaria first appear in the erythrocytic stage. Eventually the red cells lyses, releasing more merozoites, continuing the infection. These cycles tend to occur at regular intervals, giving rise to the classic periodicity of symptoms. Malaria may also be transmitted by blood transfusion or passed transplacentally from mother to fetus.

Malaria transmission occurs in large areas of Central and South America, the Caribbean, sub-Saharan Africa, the Indian subcontinent, Southeast Asia, the Middle East, and Oceania. More than half of all U.S. cases of malaria, including most cases due to *P. falciparum*, arise from travel to sub-Saharan Africa. Resistance of *P. falciparum* to chloroquine and other drugs continues to spread. The Centers for Disease Control and Prevention has a 24 h hotline and fax back service (888-232-3228), which can provide the most recent information on resistance patterns. When in doubt, assume chloroquine resistance for initial treatment.

Clinical Features

The incubation period ranges from one to several weeks. Partial chemoprophylaxis or incomplete immunity can prolong the incubation period to months or even years. The hallmark of malaria is the recurring febrile paroxysm, which corresponds to hemolysis of infected erythrocytes. With *P. falciparum,* hemolysis can be severe, since red blood cells of all ages are affected. Infected red blood cells lose flexibility and obstruct the microcirculation, causing tissue anoxia. Patients develop a prodrome of malaise, myalgias, headache, and low-grade fever and chills. The early manifestations are nonspecific and may resemble viral illness, influenza, or hepatitis. Illness progresses to high fever, severe chills, orthostatic dizziness, and extreme weakness. The malarial paroxysm—rigor and fever followed by profuse diaphoresis and exhaustion—occurs at regular intervals that correspond to the length of the erythrocytic cycle. The paroxysms may not be present in *P. falciparum* malaria.

The findings on physical examination are also nonspecific. Most patients look acutely ill, with high fever, tachycardia, and tachypnea. Splenomegaly is common. In *P. falciparum* infections, hepatomegaly, edema, and icterus often occur. Laboratory features include normocytic normochromic anemia, hemolysis, and thrombocytopenia. The white blood cell count is normal or low.

Complications of malaria can occur rapidly, particularly with *P. falciparum.* All forms cause hemolysis and splenomegaly, and predispose to splenic rupture. Glomerulonephritis occurs most often in *P. malariae* infections. *P. falciparum* infections are especially virulent and can be fatal. Cerebral malaria, characterized by somnolence, coma, delirium, and seizures, has a mortality rate over 20 percent. Other life-threatening complications associated with *P. falciparum* include noncardiogenic pulmonary edema and metabolic abnormalities, including lactic acidosis and profound hypoglycemia. Blackwater fever is a severe renal complication seen almost exclusively in *P. falciparum* infections, associated with massive intravascular hemolysis, jaundice, hemoglobinuria, and acute renal failure.

Diagnosis and Differential

The definitive diagnosis is established by finding the parasite on Giemsa-stained thin and thick smears. In early infection, especially with *P. falciparum*, parasitemia may be undetectable initially. Para-

TABLE 90-1 Treatment Regimens for Malaria

Clinical setting	Drug	Dosage guidelines	
		Adults	Children
Uncomplicated infection with *Plasmodium vivax, P. ovale, P. malariae,* and chloroquine-sensitive *P. falciparum*	Chloroquine phosphate	1 g load (600 mg base), then 500 mg (300 mg base) in 6 h, then 500 mg (300 mg base) per day for 2 d (total dose 2.5 g)	10 mg/kg base to maximum of 600 mg load, then 5 mg/kg base in 6 h and 5 mg/kg base per day for 2 d
	plus		
	primaquine phosphate*	26.3 mg load (15 mg base) per day for 14 d upon completion of chloroquine therapy	0.3 mg/kg base for 14 d upon completion of chloroquine therapy
Uncomplicated infection with chloroquine-resistant *P. falciparum*	(a) Quinine sulfate	600–650 mg PO tid for 5–7 d	8.3 mg/kg PO tid for 5–7 d†
	plus		
	doxycycline	100 mg PO bid for 7 d	Contraindicated in children <8 years of age
	plus/minus		
	pyrimethamine-sulfadoxine‡	3 tablets (75 mg/1500 mg) PO single dose	Over 2 months old:
			>50 kg 3 tablets
	OR		30–50 kg 2 tablets
			15–29 kg 1 tablet
			10–14 kg ½ tablet
			4–9 kg ¼ tablet

	(b) Mefloquine	1250 mg PO single dose	1 tablet/10 kg PO single dose§
	plus		
	doxycycline¶	See above	See above
	or		
	Halofantrine#	500 mg 6 h apart for 3 doses (repeat again in 1 week)	8 mg/kg salt PO q6h for 3 doses (repeat again in 1 week)
Complicated infection with chloroquine-resistant *P. falciparum*	Quinidine gluconate *plus*	10 mg/kg load over 2 h, then 0.02 (mg/kg)/min continuous infusion until patient is stabilized and able to tolerate PO therapy (see above)	Same as adults**
	doxycycline	100 mg IV q12h until tolerating PO therapy (see above)	Contraindicated in children <8 years of age

*Terminal treatment for *P. vivax* and *P. ovale* only.

†If unable to administer with doxycycline due to patient's age, extend treatment to full 10 d.

‡Optional; of unlikely value if acquisition in area with pyrimethamine-sulfadoxine resistance.

§Not formally approved yet by Food and Drug Administration in this setting.

¶Optional; many experts feel comfortable with mefloquine alone.

#Halofantrine is not commercially available in the United States (contact Smith-Kline Beecham at 1-800-366-8900). It is becoming the drug of choice for self-treatment of presumptive malaria in Thai-Cambodian and Myanmar borders *if* access to medical care is not available. In these areas, treatment may need to be extended to 3 d instead of 1 d.

**Consult an expert in pediatric infectious disease immediately for guidance.

Abbreviations: bid, twice a day; IV, intravenous; PO, oral; q, every; tid, three times a day.

sitemia fluctuates over time and is highest during chills and as the fever is on the rise. Therefore, failure to detect parasitemia is not an indication to withhold therapy. If parasites are not visualized, repeated smears should be taken at least twice daily for 3 days to fully exclude malaria.

Once malaria is diagnosed, the smear reveals the degree of parasitemia, which correlates with prognosis, and whether *P. falciparum* is present. Most patients with *P. falciparum* should be hospitalized, as should any patient with more than 3 percent parasitemia.

Emergency Department Care and Disposition

If *P. falciparum* can be excluded, most patients can be treated as outpatients with close follow-up, including repeated blood smears. The drug of choice for treatment of infection due to *P. vivax, P. ovale*, and *P. malariae* is chloroquine. Table 90-1 summarizes recommended treatment regimens. With treatment, the parasite load should decrease significantly over the first 24 to 48 h. Chloroquine has no effect on the exoerythrocytic forms of *P. vivax* and *P. ovale*, which remain dormant in the liver. Unless treated with primaquine, relapse will occur. However, primaquine should be avoided in patients with glucose-6-phosphate dehydrogenase (G-6-PD) deficiency because of hemolysis. Patients with significant hemolysis or with underlying diseases that can be aggravated by high fevers or hemolysis are best hospitalized, as are infants and pregnant women. *P. falciparum* infections are best managed in the hospital. Unless one is certain that the patient could not have chloroquine resistance, based on geographic exposure, it is best to assume that the infection is resistant and treat with one of the regimens listed in Table 90-1.

Patients with complications due to *P. falciparum* or with high parasitemia but unable to tolerate oral medication should receive intravenous treatment. Exchange transfusions have been lifesaving in some patients with parasitemia over 10 percent, pulmonary edema, altered mental status, or renal complications. Quinidine is the intravenous drug of choice. Both parenteral quinidine and quinine can cause severe hypoglycemia. They are also myocardial depressants and are contraindicated in patients with heart disease. Cardiac monitoring is recommended during administration.

For further reading in *Emergency Medicine: A Comprehensive Study Guide,* 5th ed., see Chap. 142, "Malaria," by Jeffrey D. Band.

91 | Common Parasitic Infections

Rebecca S. Rich

In the United States, parasitic disease is becoming more common due to immigration from developing countries, travel abroad, and increased infection in immunosuppressed persons, especially those with HIV. This chapter reviews selected helminths and protozoa.

Clinical Features

In considering parasitic diseases, ask about travel to or immigration from high-risk areas. Parasites flourish in warm, moist climates with poor sanitation and nutrition. Children are more often infected than adults because of their poor hygiene, oral behavior, and inability to ward off arthropod vectors. Parasitic disease should be considered in any patient with fever, abdominal pain, diarrhea, skin rash, ulcers, or eosinophilia. Symptoms may be protean, as listed in Table 91-1. Also making the diagnosis difficult is the fact that the latent period between exposure and symptoms may be months to years. Certain specific geographic areas may implicate particular parasites. For example, Hmong tribesmen from Southeast Asia often harbor the lung fluke *Paragonimus*, whereas visitors to Leningrad or the Rockies may return with *Giardia*. Historical risk factors can also provide clues (Table 91-2).

Diagnosis and Differential

Parasites can produce many symptoms. Diarrhea is particularly common; testing the stool for ova and parasites is the best way to detect intestinal parasites. Other specialized tests include acid-fast staining of stool, useful for *Cryptosporidia*, *Isospora*, and *Cyclospora*. For pinworms, cellophane tape is the most useful test. Occasionally, *Giardia, Cryptosporidia*, and the larvae of *Strongyloides* may be detected via duodenal aspirate or having the patient swallow a string with a gelatin capsule (entero-test).

Emergency Department Care and Disposition

For care and disposition, see specific parasites, below.

HELMINTHS

Helminths are multicellular worms. Unlike protozoa, helminths usually induce eosinophilia, a helpful clue. Types of helminths include nematodes, trematodes, and cestodes.

TABLE 91-1 Common Symptoms of Parasitic Disease

Symptom	Possible cause
Urticaria	*Ascaris, Strongyloides, Dracunculus, Trichinella, Fasciola*
Diarrhea	Hookworm, *Strongyloides, Trichuris, Trichinella, Schistosoma, Fasciola, Fasciolopsis, Taenia, Hymenolepis, Entamoeba, Giardia, Dientamoeba, Balantidium, Leishmania donovani*
Abdominal pain	*Ascaris*, hookworm, *Trichuris, Schistosoma, Entamoeba, Clonorchis, Fasciola, Taenia, Hymenolepis, Diphyllobothrium, Giardia*
Pruritus	*Enterobius, Trichuris*, filariae (*Onchocerca volvulus*), *Dientamoeba, Leishmania*
Nausea and vomiting	*Ascaris, Trichuris, Trichinella, Taenia, Entamoeba, Giardia, Leishmania*
Skin ulcers	*Dracunculus*, hookworm (*Ancylostoma duodenale*), *L. donovani, Trypanosoma*
Splenomegaly	*Babesia, Toxoplasma, Plasmodium* species
Intestinal obstruction	*Ascaris, Strongyloides*, fluke (*Fasciolopsis buski*), *Taenia, Diphyllobothrium*
Eosinophilia	*Strongyloides*, hookworm, *Trichuris, Dracunculus, Fasciola, Toxocara, Ascaris, Trichinella*, filariae *(W. bancrofti, B. malayi) Hymenolepis, Schistosoma*, fluke *(P. westermani, C. sinensis, Fasciolopsis buski), Taenia*
Fever	*Ascaris, Toxocara*, hookworm, *Trichuris, Trichinella*, filariae *(W. bancrofti), Schistosoma*, fluke *(C. sinensis), Fasciola, Entamoeba, Giardia, Trypanosoma, L. donovani, Babesia, Plasmodium* species
Hepatomegaly	*Trypanosoma, L. Donovani, Toxocara, Schistosoma*, fluke *(C. sinensis, O. viverrini, Fasciola)*, tapeworm *(Echinococcus), Plasmodium* species

Nematodes

Nematodes are cylindrical elongated white worms. Humans are infected by egg ingestion *(Ascaris* and *Enterobius)*, skin penetration *(Necator)*, and insect bite *(Filaria)*. The intestinal nematodes include hookworm, roundworm, and whipworm, in which a soil

TABLE 91-2 Risk Factors for Parasitic Disease

Blood transfusion: *Plasmodium* species, *Trypanosoma*, *Babesia*, *Toxoplasma*

Intravenous drug use: *Plasmodium* species

Homosexuality: *Entamoeba* (often seen after colonic irrigation therapy), *Giardia*, *Cryptosporidium*

Immunocompromised host: *Toxoplasma*, *Pneumocystis*, *Strongyloides*, *Cryptosporidium*, *Microsporidium*, *Isospora*, and *Cyclospora*

Institutionalization: *Hymenolepis nana*, *Entamoeba histolytica*, *Giardia*

Day-care centers: *Giardia*, *Cryptosporidium*

Livestock workers: *Cryptosporidium*

Pica: *Toxocara* (visceral larva migrans), hookworm (*Necator Americanus)*

Consumption of raw food
  Sushi, sashimi, gefilte fish: *Diphyllobothrium*, *Anisakis*
  Pork: *Taenia solium*, *Trichinella*, *Sarcocystis*
  Beef: *Taenia saginata*, *Toxoplasma*, *Sarcocystis*

phase is needed for fecally passed eggs to develop. Thus, these infections usually occur in areas of poor sanitation. (Pinworm eggs are infectious when excreted; thus, person-to-person spread occurs.) The tissue nematodes include filariae, arthropod-borne worms that induce lymphatic, ocular, and skin disease. Tissue nematodes are rare in the United States and are not discussed here.

Ascaris *(Roundworm)*

After *Ascaris* eggs are ingested, the larvae migrate through the lungs; they are then swallowed and mature into worms in the small intestine. During the lung phase, patients may develop pulmonary infiltrates with fever, cough, dyspnea, and hemoptysis. Adult worms in the gut may be asymptomatic despite their large size (10 to 35 cm) but can cause intestinal obstruction in heavy infections, especially in children. Worm migration into the biliary tract can cause biliary obstruction and pancreatitis. Treatment is with oral (PO) **mebendazole** 100 mg bid for 3 d or 500 mg once, **albendazole** 400 mg PO once, or **pyrantel pamoate** 11 mg/kg PO once up to 1 g. Surgery may be needed for intestinal obstruction.

Enterobius *(Pinworm)*

Adult pinworms inhabit the small bowel after humans ingest the eggs. The gravid female migrates to the anus at night and deposits eggs, causing intense itching. Pinworms most often affect children. The diagnosis is confirmed by finding eggs on a cellophane tape swab of the anus. Eosinophilia is usually absent, unlike findings with *Ascaris* and *Necator*. Treat with **pyrantel pamoate** 11 mg/kg PO once up to 1 g, **mebendazole** 100 mg PO once, or **albendazole** 400 mg PO once. Repeat all regimens 2 weeks later. All close household contacts should be treated.

Strongyloides *(Threadworm)*

Because this worm enters the body through the skin, rash and itching can occur. Migration through the lungs can cause cough, dyspnea, and pneumonia. The intestinal phase produces diarrhea and abdominal pain. This worm is unique in its ability to reproduce in the host without reinfection, so *Strongyloides* may persist for decades. In immunosuppressed patients, the reproductive cycle may be magnified, leading to fatal hyperinfection. Diagnosis is made by finding larvae in the stool or duodenal contents. Treat with **ivermectin** 200 μg/kg/d PO for 1 to 2 d or **thiabendazole** 50 mg/kg/d in 2 doses to a maximum of 3 g for 2 d.

Necator americanus *(Hookworm)*

Hookworm is more common in the South, associated with use of human fertilizer and lack of shoes and latrines. Infection is via the skin and may induce rash. There may be pulmonary and gastrointestinal symptoms as worms migrate. This worm also ingests blood, leading to iron-deficiency anemia. Diagnosis is by stool testing for eggs. Treatment is the same as for *Ascaris* (above).

Trichuris trichiura *(Whipworm)*

This worm is also most common in the rural South, most often in children who play in the soil. If symptoms occur, they are usually gastrointestinal. *Trichuris* can cause rectal prolapse or colitis in children. Diagnosis is made by stool testing. Treat with **mebendazole** or **albendazole** (same doses as for *Ascaris,* above).

Trichinella spiralis

This parasite is acquired by eating infected pork. In the early (enteric) phase, gastrointestinal symptoms predominate. Later, larvae travel to muscle, where encystment starts 3 weeks after infection. Symptoms include periorbital edema, splinter and subconjunctival hemorrhages, myalgia, urticaria, headache, weakness, and fever. Although encystment occurs only in striated muscle, inflammation also occurs in the heart, lungs, and central nervous system (CNS), with myocarditis, pneumonia, and CNS disturbances. Laboratory clues include eosinophilia and muscle enzymes. The triad of periorbital edema, myalgias, and eosinophilia strongly suggests trichinosis. The diagnosis may be confirmed serologically. Biopsy of involved muscle may be helpful after the fourth week. Stool specimens are only helpful early. **Mebendazole** 200 to 400 mg PO tid for 3 d and then 400 to 500 mg PO tid for 10 d is indicated for the intestinal phase but may not be effective after encystment. Steroids are indicated for serious CNS disease and myocarditis, but not routinely. Most cases are mild and resolve without specific therapy.

Trematodes (Flukes)

Trematodes are leaflike flatworms that live in intermediate hosts such as snails, crabs, and fish in the tropics. *Clonorchis*, the liver fluke, is endemic in the Far East and causes biliary disease. *Paragonimus*, the lung fluke, produces hemoptysis and lung disease. The most common flukeborne disease is schistosomiasis. Freshter schistosomes penetrate the skin, inducing dermatitis. Acute disease includes fever, cough, hepatosplenomegaly, urticaria, and eosinophilia. Chronic disease occurs from egg deposition in the bladder, intestines, and liver, with resultant scarring. In *Schistosoma haematobium*, dysuria, hematuria, and bladder infection occur. With the other schistosomes, cirrhosis and portal hypertension result. The diagnosis is made by finding eggs in the urine or stool or by rectal biopsy. **Praziquantel** (dose varies for specific worms) 40 to 60 mg/kg/d PO for 2 to 3 doses is the recommended treatment.

Cestodes (Flatworms)

Commonly called tapeworms, cestodes grow by segmentation, producing new proglottids that can be detected in stool.

Hymenolepis nana

The most common tapeworm in the United States is the dwarf tapeworm, *Hymenolepis nana*, which often occurs in children and institutionalized patients. It is treated with **praziquantel** 25 mg/kg PO once.

Taenia

Taenia solium, the pork tapeworm, occurs occasionally in the United States in immigrants from Central America or the Middle

East. *Taenia saginata,* the beef tapeworm, is more common, seen in people who eat raw beef. Adult worms live in the small bowel. Infections may be asymptomatic or cause gastrointestinal distress, weight loss, and weakness. Eggs or proglottids may be identified in the stool, or eggs may be detected by perianal tape application. Praziquantel 5 to 10 mg/kg PO once is the treatment. *Taenia solium* can also cause a more serious disease, cysticercosis, in which eggs encyst in multiple organs, including the eye, heart, and brain, where seizures and hydrocephalus may result. X-rays show curvilinear calcifications characteristic of cysts. The cysts also show up on computed tomography (CT) scans of the head. For cysticercosis, **albendazole** 400 mg PO bid for 8 to 30 d or **praziquantel** 50 mg/kg/d PO in 3 doses for 15 d are recommended. Adjunctive surgery may also be necessary to remove cysts.

Diphyllobothrium

The fish tapeworm *Diphyllobothrium* occurs in people who eat raw fish (e.g., sushi, sashimi, and gefilte fish). Since the worm competes with the host for vitamin B_{12}, pernicious anemia may occur. Treatment is the same as for *Taenia.*

PROTOZOA

Amebiasis

Amebiasis, caused by *Entamoeba histolytica,* is spread by the fecal-oral route and associated with poor sanitation. Outbreaks have also occurred in institutions and in gay men. Amebae inhabit the cecum and ascending colon, where they cause inflammation and ulcers. An ameboma in the liver can present as an abscess. Half of all infected persons are asymptomatic. Symptoms include nausea, vomiting, diarrhea, fever, and abdominal pain. As with all protozoan infections, eosinophilia does not occur. The diagnosis is made by stool testing; serologic tests are helpful in cases of extraintestinal disease. Treat with **metronidazole** 500 to 750 mg PO tid for 10 d.

Giardia

This protozoan is the most common intestinal parasite in the United States. Cysts are ingested in fecally contaminated water and food. Water-borne outbreaks are increasingly common because cysts resist chlorination. Outbreaks by interpersonal spread have also occurred in day-care centers and institutions. Many infected persons are asymptomatic. Acute symptoms include watery diarrhea, cramps, nausea, vomiting, fever, burping, and flatus. Stools are greasy and malodorous. Chronic diarrhea with weight loss and malabsorption may occur. Diagnosis is by stool testing. Occasionally, duodenal aspiration, string testing, or small bowel biopsy may be needed. **Metronidazole** 250 mg PO tid for 5 d is the treatment of choice.

Trypanosoma

American trypanosomiasis (Chagas' disease) is spread by the reduvid (kissing) bug and, much less often, transfusion. A nodular swelling appears at the bite site. The acute phase lasts several months and includes fever, headache, conjunctivitis, rash, and, in severe cases, myocarditis or meningoencephalitis. Chronic infection can lead to heart failure, cardiac dysrhythmias, megacolon, and megaesophagus. During the acute phase, blood smear and serologic testing may be helpful. In the chronic phase, serologic testing or biopsy of liver, spleen, or bone marrow may be diagnostic. **Nifurtimox** 8 to 10 mg/kg/d PO divided tid to qid for 90 to 120 d is the recommended treatment.

Babesia

Babesia microti is spread by *Ixodes* ticks, which also transmit Lyme disease, but has also been spread by transfusion. Babesiosis is most common in the Northeast. Patients present with fevers, splenomegaly, hemolysis, and jaundice. Infection can be fatal in splenectomized patients. Diagnosis is by blood smear, but the organism may be mistaken for malaria. Lyme disease and Rocky Mountain spotted fever are also in the differential diagnosis. Treat with **clindamycin** 600 mg PO tid for 7 d or 1.2 g intravenously (IV) bid plus **quinine** 650 mg PO tid for 7 d.

Cryptosporidium

Previously regarded a disease of immunosuppressed patients, *Cryptosporidium* is now recognized as an important cause of diarrhea worldwide. Water-borne transmission is well documented. The organism can also affect cows, and dairy runoff can contaminate reservoirs. *Cryptosporida* alter small-bowel villi, causing profuse watery diarrhea without blood or leukocytes. There may be abdominal cramps, nausea, vomiting, and fever. In normal hosts, the disease lasts several days to weeks, but in immunocompromised persons the diarrhea can be protracted, leading to dehydration, malabsorption, and weight loss. Diagnosis is made by finding oocysts in the stool using an acid-fast stain. Infection is self-limited in normal hosts. In immunocompromised patients, treatment with many antimicrobial and antidiarrheal agents has not been very successful. **Paromomycin** is the recommended best treatment 25 to 35 mg/kg/d PO tid to qid; the required duration is unclear.

For further reading in *Emergency Medicine: A Comprehensive Study Guide,* 5th ed., see Chap. 143, "Common Parasitic Infections," by Harold H. Osborn.

---

92 | Infections from Animals

Gregory S. Hall

Zoonoses, or diseases that are transmitted from animals or arthropod vectors to humans, are still common in North America, where pets are often the primary reservoirs. These infections are caused by myriad organisms, including bacteria, viruses, *Rickettsia,* and parasites, and their prevalence continues to be underestimated in the United States. The high morbidity and mortality rates often associated with these diseases mandates their careful consideration in patients who present with fever and other nonspecific symptoms. In such cases, specific risk factors for zoonotic infection should always be sought, namely, exposure to household pets or nondomesticated animals; recent travel or residence in rural areas or underdeveloped countries; dressing, skinning, or handling animal skins or raw flesh; animal bites or scratches; or ingestion of animal or dairy products. In the United States, where most zoonoses have a higher incidence during spring and summer, ticks are the most prolific agent of disease transmission. Unfortunately many patients with tick acquired disease do not give a history of recent tick bite; hence, clinical suspicion should remain high for patients in endemic areas.

LYME DISEASE

Lyme disease remains the foremost vector-borne zoonotic infection in the United States, with reported cases in all 48 continental states (highest prevalence in the Northeast). The spirochete bacteria *Borrelia burgdorferi* is responsible for this disease via transmission by bite of *Ixodes* species ticks. Small mammals (e.g., rabbits and rodents) along with deer serve as host reservoirs in the wild. Less than one-third of affected patients can recall a tick bite.

Clinical Features

Lyme disease is a multiorgan infection that is typically divided into three distinct stages. Be aware that not all patients may suffer all three stages, stages may overlap, and there may be remissions between stages. The hallmark of stage I is erythema chronicum migrans (ECM), an annular, erythematous skin lesion with central clearing, which forms at the site of tick bite, usually 2 to 20 days after the bite. ECM is found in only 60 to 80 percent of cases and may be accompanied by (in decreasing order of frequency) generalized malaise and fatigue, headache, fever and chills, stiff neck, arthralgias, and other constitutional symptoms. Untreated, ECM and other symptoms usually remit spontaneously in 3 to 4 weeks.

Stage II corresponds to dissemination of the spirochete, resulting in multiple secondary annular skin lesions (similar to the first), fever, adenopathy, splenomegaly, and flulike constitutional symptoms. Approximately 10 percent of untreated stage II patients develop neurologic disease including headache, meningoencephalitis, and, most commonly, cranial neuritis—often a uni- or bilateral facial nerve palsy. In addition, other peripheral neuropathies can develop along with asymmetric oligoarticular arthritis, usually of the large joints. Some patients may develop first-, second-, or third-degree atrioventricular nodal block. Stage III represents chronic persistent infection, occurs years after stage I, and includes chronic arthritis, myocarditis, subacute encephalopathy, axonal polyneuropathy, and leukoencephalopathy. Chronic arthritis usually takes the form of brief recurrent episodes of migratory oligoarthritis most commonly affecting (in declining order of frequency) the knee, shoulder, temporomandibular joint, ankle, wrist, hip, and small joints of hands and feet.

Diagnosis and Differential

Diagnosis must rely on clinical features. A two-step serologic test, enzyme immunoassay, and western immunoblot test may be used for confirmation. *B. burgdorferi* can be cultured from ECM lesions, but culture requires special media, has a low sensitivity, and is not widely available.

Emergency Department Care and Disposition

Lyme disease generally responds well to antimicrobial therapy, especially if begun early in the course. A number of agents may be effective for early disease, but optimal therapy for the late stage remains unclear. Prophylactic treatment following a tick bite cannot be generally recommended, since fewer than 10 percent of tick bites actually transmit the disease and prophylactic antibiotics may actually depress the immune response to the infection. A vaccine is currently under investigation but not yet available.

1. For early Lyme disease (ECM), the first choice is oral (PO) **doxycycline** 100 mg PO bid for 10 to 21 d. Acceptable alternatives are **amoxacillin** 500 mg PO tid for 10 to 21 d, **cefuroxime** 500 mg PO bid for 21 d, and **clarithromycin** 500 mg PO bid for 21 d.
2. Bell's palsy, mild arthritis, or mild cardiac manifestations may be managed similarly to ECM, using oral doxycycline or amoxacillin (preferred in children).
3. Serious central nervous system (CNS) disease (e.g., meningitis, encephalitis, encephalopathy, or neuropathy), serious cardiac manifestations, or severe arthritis is probably best managed by hospital admission for supportive care and a 14- to 21-d course of intravenous (IV) ceftriaxone or penicillin G.
4. Timely consultation with an infectious disease expert as well as the patient's primary physician is highly recommended for any patient with suspected Lyme disease. Close follow-up is crucial for any patient who will be treated as an outpatient.

ROCKY MOUNTAIN SPOTTED FEVER

Rocky Mountain spotted fever (RMSF), one of the most frequently reported rickettsial zoonoses in the United States, is caused by *Rickettsia rickettsii*, a pleiomorphic obligate intracellular coccobacillus. *Dermacentor* species ticks serve as the primary vector, with deer, rodents, horses, cattle, cats, and dogs as the usual animal hosts. Ninety-five percent of cases reported occur between April 1 and September 30, with two-thirds of cases reported in children under 15 years old. The highest incidence of RMSF appears to occur in the mid-Atlantic states, but cases have been reported in the majority of continental states.

Clinical Features

RMSF affects multiple organ systems, and most patients develop moderate to severe symptoms unless treated early. A triad of fever, rash, and a history of tick exposure have classically defined

RMSF. Unfortunately, only about half of infected patients can recall a tick bite. The incubation period is usually 4 to 10 days, followed by abrupt or insidious onset of symptoms. Initial findings (which are nonspecific and may lead to misdiagnosis) include fever, malaise, severe headache, myalgias, nausea, vomiting, diarrhea, anorexia, abdominal pain, and photophobia. Other signs or symptoms that may develop are lymphadenopathy, hepatosplenomegaly, conjunctivitis, confusion, meningismus, renal and respiratory failure, and myocarditis.

Rash, the hallmark feature of RMSF, usually develops within the first 2 weeks of illness, often between the third and fifth day. Initially the rash is maculopapular and typically begins on the extremities around the wrists and ankles, often involving the palms and soles. The rash then spreads centripetally up the trunk, usually sparing the face. Rash may be absent in up to 17 percent of patients with so-called "spotless" RMSF; most often this occurs in African-Americans, the elderly, and severe fatal cases. Gastrointestinal symptoms are often prominent features and may precede the onset of rash, leading to a misdiagnosis of gastroenteritis or even acute abdomen. Pneumonitis, a common and potentially fatal complication of RMSF, typically presents with cough, dyspnea, pulmonary edema, and systemic hypoxia. Serious neurologic involvement may occur in 23 to 28 percent of cases, with symptoms including confusion, stupor, ataxia, coma, and seizures.

Diagnosis and Differential

Early recognition of RMSF is crucial because mortality rates are near zero for patients treated before day six of the illness, while untreated patients may suffer up to 25 percent mortality rates. Thus, a high index of clinical suspicion must be maintained, especially since the early symptoms are often nonspecific and the characteristic rash, which aids in the diagnosis, may be absent. Laboratory abnormalities are nonspecific and may include a normal or elevated white blood cell count, thrombocytopenia, elevated liver function test results, hyponatremia, and cerebrospinal fluid (CSF) pleocytosis with elevated protein levels. Serologic tests may help confirm RMSF, but since results do not become reliably positive for 6 to 10 days after onset of symptoms, the diagnosis must be made on clinical grounds in order to ensure correct early therapy. RMSF can be confirmed with a rise in antibody titer between acute and convalescent sera or via skin (rash) biopsy with immunofluorescent testing (but negative skin biopsy results do not exclude RMSF). The differential diagnosis includes viral illnesses (e.g., measles, rubella, hepatitis, mononucleosis, encephalitis, or enteroviral exanthem), gastroenteritis, acute abdomen, disseminated gonorrhea, meningitis (meningococcus), secondary syphilis, leptospirosis, pneumonia, typhoid fever, and streptococcal infection (pharyngitis with rash).

Emergency Department Care and Disposition

Early therapy with appropriate antimicrobials yields a dramatic reduction in mortality rates from RMSF.

1. Appropriate therapy for adults includes **doxycycline** 100 mg PO bid, **tetracycline** 500 mg PO qid, or **chloramphenicol** 50 to 75 mg/kg/d IV in 4 divided doses.
2. Appropriate therapy for children under 45 kg or 100 lb includes **doxycycline** 4.4 mg/kg/d PO in 2 divided doses on day 1, followed by 2.2 mg/kg/d PO in 2 divided doses thereafter. Alternatives include **tetracycline** 30 to 40 mg/kg/d PO in 4 divided doses for children over 8 years old and **chloramphenicol** 100 mg/kg/d (3 g maximum) IV in 4 divided doses. Doxycycline has been used for short courses in children without significant staining of the teeth, but these cosmetic risks must be balanced against the potentially serious adverse effects of chloramphenicol. It would be prudent to discuss these risks with the parents and primary care physician at the onset of therapy in order to reach a consensus on treatment. Informed consent for this therapy is highly recommended. Chloramphenicol has been advocated for therapy of pregnant patients.
3. Antimicrobial therapy is generally administered for 5 to 7 days, continuing until the patient is afebrile and clinically improving for at least 2 days.
4. Hospital admission for IV doxycycline, chloramphenicol, or tetracycline is strongly recommended for any patient with nausea, vomiting, or significant systemic disease. Patients with all but the most minor of symptoms of RMSF should be considered for hospital admission for observation and antimicrobial therapy. Seriously ill patients often require aggressive supportive care and careful attention to fluid and electrolyte imbalances. Those discharged should have close follow-up to ensure their clinical response.

TICK PARALYSIS

Tick paralysis, a relatively uncommon disease, is important to recognize because it is potentially fatal and yet easily cured. It is thought to be caused by a neurotoxic venom secreted from female tick salivary glands, which produces a conduction block at the motor end plate of peripheral nerves. *Dermacentor* species ticks have been the usual vector. Incidence is highest in spring to late summer, with children most commonly affected.

Clinical Features

Symptoms usually begin within 4 to 7 days after attachment by the female tick. An initial prodrome of malaise, irritability, restlessness, and paresthesias of the hand or foot is followed by a symmetric, ascending, flaccid paralysis similar to that of Guillain-Barré syndrome. Fever is generally absent. Loss of deep tendon reflexes, difficulty swallowing, and involuntary eye movements may also occur, but sensation remains intact. Poor coordination and ataxia may indicate cerebellar involvement. In severe, untreated cases, respiratory paralysis may lead to death.

Diagnosis and Differential

Recognition of clinical features along with discovery of an attached tick leads to a proper diagnosis. Carefully search the patient for a tick, being certain to check the scalp. The main differential diagnosis is Guillain-Barré syndrome.

Emergency Department Care and Disposition

Essential to proper treatment is the discovery of the causative tick and its prompt but careful removal. Most patients develop signs of spontaneous recovery within hours of tick removal and complete recovery within 48 to 72 h. Aggressive supportive care, especially ventilatory support, is indicated for patients with respiratory compromise prior to tick removal.

TULAREMIA

Tularemia (rabbit skinner's disease) is caused by *Francisella tularensis*, a small, gram-negative coccobacillus. Principal zoonotic vectors are ticks of the *Dermacentor* and *Amblyomma* species and the deerfly. Natural animal reservoirs include rabbits and hares, deer, muskrats, beavers, and some domestic animals. Although widely reported throughout the continental United States, the highest incidence of tularemia occurs in Arkansas, Missouri, and Oklahoma. Cases can occur year round but may be more common in early winter in adults and in early summer in children. Methods of transmission include arthropod bites; animal bites; inoculation of skin, conjunctiva, or oral mucosa by blood or tissue from an infected host; and handling or ingestion of contaminated soil, grain, hay, or water.

The average incubation period is 3 to 5 days, followed by sudden onset of fever, chills, headache, anorexia, malaise, and fatigue. Myalgias, cough, vomiting, pharyngitis, abdominal pain, and diarrhea may also develop. Fever often persists for several days, remits briefly, and then recurs. Clinical features at presentation depend on the route of inoculation. Ulceroglandular fever, the most common syndrome, follows tick bites or animal contact, and is characterized by a papule at the bite site, which evolves into a tender, necrotic ulcer with painful regional adenopathy. Glandular tularemia consists of tender regional adenopathy without a skin lesion. Oculoglandular tularemia results in a painful conjunctivitis along with periauricular, submandibular, and cervical adenopathy. Pharyngeal tularemia, acquired from ingestion of contaminated food or water, presents with exudative pharyngitis or tonsillitis. Typhoidal tularemia may occur with any form of transmission and includes multiorgan signs and symptoms, such as fever, headache, vomiting, diarrhea, myalgias, hepatosplenomegaly, cough, and pneumonitis. Tularemic pneumonitis can occur via inhalation of the organism, with either no signs and symptoms or a productive cough, pleuritic chest pain, rales, consolidation, and pleural rub.

Laboratory findings are nonspecific for all forms of tularemia, and the key to diagnosis rests on the clinical features coupled with a history of potential exposure. Serologic studies (ELISA) to determine acute and convalescent titers or culture from blood, wounds, lymph nodes, or sputum may confirm the diagnosis. The multiple clinical variations of tularemia lead to a broad differential diagnosis that must include such entities as pyogenic bacterial infection, syphilis, anthrax, plague, Q fever, psittacosis, typhoid, brucellosis, and rickettsial infection. Preferred therapy includes **streptomycin** 7.5 to 10 mg/kg every 12 h intramuscularly (IM) or IV for 7 to 14 d. The pediatric dose is 30 to 40 mg/kg IM in 2 divided doses for 7 d or **gentamicin** 3 to 5 mg/kg/d divided every 8 h IV for 7 to 14 d. Chloramphenicol may be added if meningitis is suspected. Patients should be admitted for close monitoring of response.

EHRLICHIOSIS

Ehrlichiosis is a zoonotic infection with two clinical subtypes, human granulocytic and human monocytic, which are thought to be caused by *Ehrlichia phagocytophila* or *Erlichia qui* and *Ehrlichia chaffeensis,* respectively. *Ehrlichia* are small, gram-negative coccobacilli that infect circulating leukocytes. Animal reservoirs include deer, dogs, and other mammals. *Ixodes* and *Amblyomma* species ticks serve as vectors of transmission. Most patients report a tick bite in the preceding 3 weeks, and the incubation period ranges from 1 to 21 days (median 7 days). The characteristic clinical features are consistent with a nonspecific febrile illness, including high fever, headache, nausea, vomiting, malaise, abdominal pain, anorexia, and myalgias. In a minority of cases a maculopapular or petechial rash develops, which may involve the palms or soles. Serious complications can include renal failure, respiratory failure, disseminated intravascular coagulopathy, cardiomegaly, encephalitis, and seizures. The diagnosis must be made on clinical grounds, but serologic tests may provide confirmation. Laboratory findings are most prominent at 5 to 7 days and may include leukopenia, absolute lymphopenia, thrombocytopenia, and elevated serum hepatic enzyme levels. Rarely, CSF pleocytosis is seen. The differential diagnosis includes the other rickettsial diseases and bacterial meningitis. Treat with **doxycycline** 100 mg PO or IV bid for 7 to 14 d. Tetracycline is an acceptable alternative. There is no current recommendation for children or pregnancy.

COLORADO TICK FEVER

Colorado tick fever is an acute viral illness caused by an RNA virus of the *Coltivirus* species, with *Dermacentor* species ticks serving as the vector. Most cases occur between late May and early July in the mountainous western regions of the United States. Symptoms begin suddenly 3 to 6 days after a tick bite and include fever, chills, severe headache, photophobia, and myalgias. Symptoms usually persist for 5 to 8 days and then spontaneously remit. Fifty percent of patients experience a secondary phase, with return of symptoms, usually 3 days after initial remission. The secondary phase lasts for 2 to 4 days and may be accompanied by a transient, generalized maculopapular or petechial rash. Diagnosis must be suspected by clinical features but may be confirmed with serologic studies or isolation of the virus from blood or CSF. Laboratory abnormalities may include leukocytosis and thrombocytopenia. The differential diagnosis includes meningitis and rickettsial infections. No specific therapy exists, and supportive care usually suffices. Recovery is spontaneous, typically within 3 weeks. Empiric antimicrobial therapy to cover other potential diagnoses (especially *Rickettsia* and meningitis) pending serologic confirmation would be prudent.

ANTHRAX

Anthrax, while extremely rare in North America, remains a significant threat, in part because of its potential as an agent of biological warfare. Anthrax is an acute bacterial infection caused by *Bacillus anthracis*, an aerobic gram-positive rod that forms central oval spores. (Oxygen is required for sporulation but not germination of the spores.) In nature, the disease is most commonly seen in domestic herbivores (cattle, sheep, horses, and goats) and wild herbivores. Human infection can result from inhalation of spores, inoculation of broken skin, arthropod bite (fleas), or ingestion of inadequately cooked infected meat.

Inhaled, or pulmonic, anthrax usually results from handling unsterilized, imported animal hides or imported raw wool. It results in a mediastinitis, rather than pneumonia, and is universally fatal. Initial presentation consists of flulike symptoms, which progress over 3 to 4 days to include marked mediastinal and hilar edema and respiratory failure. Cutaneous anthrax begins with a small red macule at the site of inoculation, which progresses (over a week's time) through papular, vesicular, or pustular forms to result in an ulcer with a black eschar and adjacent brawny edema. Once fully developed, it may be painless. Spontaneous healing occurs in a majority of cases, but a small minority of untreated patients develop rapidly fatal bacteremia. Gastrointestinal anthrax exhibits variable symptoms, such as fever, nausea, vomiting, abdominal pain, bloody diarrhea, ascites, pharyngitis, and tonsillitis.

Gram's stain, direct fluorescent antibody stain, or culture of skin lesions may establish the diagnosis. Blood cultures may also be positive. Laboratory abnormalities may include normal leukocyte counts in mild cases or leukocytosis in more severe cases. Sera may also be tested for antibody to *B. anthracis*. Treat with either **ciprofloxacin** 750 mg bid PO or 400 mg IV or **doxycycline** 100 mg bid PO or IV. Penicillin G or erythromycin is an alternative. A vaccine is available and is currently being given to active-duty U.S. military personnel. Although there is great concern for the potential use of anthrax as a terrorist warfare agent, the delivery system required to generate and distribute large volumes of cultured spores would not be easy to use in a large population center.

PLAGUE

Plague (*Yersinia pestis*) is a gram-negative aerobic bacillus of the Enterobacteriaceae family endemic to the United States. It is most often found in rock squirrels and ground rodents of the Southwest but may also be carried by cats and dogs. The rodent flea serves as the primary vector. Transmission to humans occurs through the bite of a flea from an infected animal host or through ingestion of infected rodents. Plague takes on three forms: bubonic or suppurative (most common), pneumonic, or septicemic. The incubation period ranges from 2 to 7 days after the flea bite, which some patients may not recall. Frequently an eschar develops at the initial bite wound, which is followed by development of a painful, sometimes suppurative, bubo (enlarged regional lymph nodes), often in the groin. Associated symptoms may include fever, headache, malaise, abdominal pain, nausea, vomiting, and bloody diarrhea. After the lymphatic system, the lung is the organ most commonly affected, with 10 to 20 percent of patients progressing to secondary pneumonia. This may include multilobar infiltrates, bloody sputum, and respiratory failure. The pneumonic form is highly contagious and can be transmitted from person to person via aerosolized respiratory secretions. Subclinical disseminated intravascular coagulation may also occur in a large number of patients. Untreated bubonic plague may proceed (without other organ systems involved) to generalized sepsis, hypotension, and death.

Diagnosis must be made based on clinical findings in a patient with possible contact with vector or host animal. Needle aspiration of a bubo with direct staining of the aspirate using Wayson's or Giemsa stain reveals bipolar, safety pin-shaped organisms. Fluorescent antibody staining or antibody titers of acute and convalescent sera may also confirm the diagnosis. Laboratory findings are nonspecific and may include leukocytosis, modest elevations of serum hepatic transaminase levels, and evidence of disseminated intravascular coagulation (i.e., thrombocytopenia, prolonged partial thromboplastin time, and fibrin degradation products). Chest x-ray may show infiltrates, frequently with pleural effusion. The differential diagnosis includes lymphogranuloma venereum, syphilis, staphylococcal or streptococcal lymphadenitis, or tularemia. Because plague is a rapidly progressive infection, therapy should begin immediately for any suspected case. Recommended antimicrobials are **gentamicin** 2.0 mg/kg IV load and then 1.7 mg/kg every 8 h IV or **streptomycin** 1.0 g every 12 h IV or IM. Alternatives include doxycycline or chloramphenicol. Hospital admission is recommended, and patients suspected of pneumonic plague should have strict respiratory isolation.

For further reading in *Emergency Medicine: A Comprehensive Study Guide,* 5th ed., see Chap. 145, "Infections from Animals," by John T. Meredith.

93 | Soft Tissue Infections

Chris Melton

Patients with soft tissue infections present frequently to the emergency department (ED). The management of these infections involves an understanding of appropriate antibiotic treatment, outpatient or inpatient, as well as an understanding of when surgical intervention is necessary.

GAS GANGRENE

Clinical Features

Gas gangrene, or clostridial myonecrosis, is a rapidly progressive life- and limb-threatening disease. Patients present with pain out of proportion to physical findings and a sense of heaviness in the affected part. Physical findings typically include a combination of edema, brownish skin discoloration, bullae, malodorous serosanguineous discharge, and crepitance. The patient frequently has a low-grade fever and a tachycardia out of proportion to the fever. Mental status changes, including delirium and irritability, may also accompany gas gangrene.

Diagnosis and Differential

Familiarity with the disease and an appreciation of the subtle physical findings are the most important factors in making the diagnosis of gas gangrene. Additional findings that may confirm the clinical suspicion include gas within soft tissue on plain radiographs, metabolic acidosis, leukocytosis, anemia, thrombocytopenia, myoglobinuria, and renal or hepatic dysfunction. The differential diagnosis includes other gas-forming infections, such as necrotizing fasciitis, streptococcal myositis, acute streptococcal hemolytic gangrene, and crepitant cellulitis. When crepitance is present, it should be differentiated from that caused by laryngeal or tracheal fracture, pneumothorax, and pneumomediastinum.

Emergency Department Care and Disposition

The patient with gas gangrene should be adequately resuscitated with crystalloid intravenous (IV) fluids as well as packed red blood cells if there is significant hemolysis and anemia. Urine output and central venous pressure readings should be used to assess volume status. Vasoconstrictors should be avoided in these patients because of compromised perfusion in the affected part.

1. Antibiotic therapy should be administered using **penicillin** G 10 to 40 million U/d in divided doses as well as either **vancomycin** 1 g IV every 12 h or a penicillinase-resistant penicillin, such as **nafcillin** 2 g IV every 4 h. In the penicillin allergic patient, **clindamycin** 900 mg IV every 6 h or **metronidazole** 15 mg/kg IV load and then 7.5 mg/kg IV every 6 h may be used.
2. Tetanus prophylaxis should be administered as indicated.
3. Surgical consultation for débridement should be obtained immediately, and the patient should be admitted for further antibiotics, surgical care, and hyperbaric oxygen therapy.

CELLULITIS

Cellulitis is a local soft tissue inflammatory response secondary to bacterial invasion of the skin. It is more common in the elderly, immunocompromised, and patients with peripheral vascular disease.

Clinical Features

Cellulitis presents as localized tenderness, erythema, and induration. Lymphangitis and lymphadenitis may accompany cellulitis and indicate a more severe infection. Patients may become bacteremic and have fever and chills.

Diagnosis and Differential

The clinical presentation is usually sufficient for diagnosis. In patients with underlying disease or signs of bacteremia, blood cultures and leukocyte counts are indicated. Otherwise, no further investigation is necessary. The differential diagnosis includes any erythematous skin condition. Cellulitis is sometimes complicated by deep venous thrombosis and may require venogram or Doppler studies for a complete evaluation.

Emergency Department Care and Disposition

Simple cellulitis can be treated in an outpatient setting using oral (PO) **dicloxacillin** 500 mg every 6 h, a macrolide such as **clarithromycin** 500 mg PO every 12 h, or **amoxicillin-clavulanate** 875 mg/ 125 mg PO every 12 h for 10 days. All patients discharged should have close follow-up to evaluate the patient's cellulitis and response to therapy. Patients with diabetes mellitus, alcoholism, evidence of bacteremia, or other immunosuppressive disorders and all patients with cellulitis involving the head or neck should be admitted for intravenous antibiotics. IV antibiotics, such as first-generation cephalosporin (**cefazolin** 1 g IV every 6 h) or a penicillinase-resistant penicillin (**nafcillin** 2 g IV every 4 h), may be used unless the patient has diabetes. In patients with diabetes, **ceftriaxone** 1 to 2 g/d IV can be used, or in severe cases **imipenem** 500 mg IV every 6 h is indicated.

ERYSIPELAS

Erysipelas is a superficial cellulitis with lymphatic involvement caused primarily by group A streptococcus. Infection is usually through a portal of entry in the skin.

Clinical Features

Onset is acute with sudden high fever, chills, malaise, and nausea. Over the next 1 to 2 days, a small area of erythema with a burning sensation develops. The erythema is sharply demarcated from the surrounding skin and is tense and painful. Lymphangitis and lymphadenitis are common. Purpura, bullae, and necrosis may accompany the erythema.

Diagnosis and Differential

The diagnosis is based primarily on physical findings. Leukocytosis is common. Cultures, ASO titers, and anti-DNAase B titers are of little use in the ED. Differential diagnosis includes other forms of local cellulitis. Some believe necrotizing fasciitis is a complication of erysipelas and should be considered in all cases.

Emergency Department Care and Disposition

Penicillin G 1 to 2 million U IV every 6 h may be used in nondiabetic patients. Penicillinase-resistant penicillins, such as **nafcillin** 2 g IV every 4 h, or parental second- or third-generation cephalosporins, such as **ceftriaxone** 1 to 2 g/d, should be used in diabetic patients and in those with facial involvement. **Imipenem** 500 mg IV every 6 h is indicated in severe cases. In patients allergic to penicillin, a macrolide may be used, such as **azithromycin** 500 mg/d IV for 2 d and then PO. Except for clearly mild cases, all patients should be admitted for IV antibiotics.

CUTANEOUS ABSCESSES

Cutaneous abscesses are the result of a breakdown in the cutaneous barrier, with subsequent contamination with resident bacterial flora. Incision and drainage (I & D) is usually the only necessary treatment.

Clinical Features and Emergency Department Care

Patients present with an area of swelling, tenderness, and erythema. The area of swelling is frequently fluctuant. Cutaneous abscesses are usually localized, although they may cause systemic toxicity in the immunosuppressed. Cutaneous abscesses should be closely inspected for predisposing injury and foreign bodies. Common specific abscesses are listed below.

1. *Bartholin's gland abscess* presents as unilateral painful swelling of the labia with a fluctuant 1 to 2 cm mass. *Neisseria gonorrhoeae* and *Chlamydia trachomatis* are commonly found in these abscesses. Cervical cultures should be done on all women with a Bartholin's abscess. Routine antimicrobial treatment is not necessary unless there is a strong suspicion of sexually transmitted disease. Treatment involves I & D along the vaginal mucosal surface of the abscess, followed by the insertion of a Word catheter.

2. *Hidradenitis suppurativa* is a recurrent chronic infection involving the apocrine sweat glands. These abscesses tend to occur in the axilla and in the groin. The causative organism is usually *Staphylococcus,* although *Streptococcus* may be present as well. The abscesses are typically multiple and in different stages of progression. ED treatment involves the I & D of any acute abscess, treating with antibiotics for any cellulitis that may be present, and referral to a surgeon for definitive treatment.

3. *Infected sebaceous cysts* may develop in the sebaceous glands, which occur diffusely throughout the skin. Cysts present with an erythematous, tender, cutaneous mass that is often fluctuant. I & D is the appropriate ED treatment, with wound rechecks in 2 to 3 days in the ED or surgeon's office.

4. *Pilonidal abscess* presents as a tender, swollen, and fluctuant mass along the superior gluteal fold. Treatment includes I & D with subsequent iodoform gauze packing. The patient should be rechecked in 2 to 3 days and the wound repacked. Surgical referral is usually necessary for definitive treatment. Antibiotics are not necessary unless there is an accompanying cellulitis.

5. *Staphylococcal soft tissue abscess.* Folliculitis is the inflammation of a hair follicle because of bacterial invasion and is usually treated with warm compresses. When deeper invasion occurs, the soft tissue surrounding the hair follicle becomes infected and a furuncle (boil) is formed. Warm compresses are usually enough to promote spontaneous drainage. If several furuncles coalesce, they may form a large area of interconnected sinus tracts and abscesses called a carbuncle. Carbuncles usually require surgical referral for wide excision.

See Chap. 10 for information on conscious sedation. In the healthy, immunocompetent patient routine use of antibiotics is not indicated unless there is a secondary infection. In the potentially immunocompromised patient, the threshold for antibiotic use should be lowered. Patients presenting with secondary cellulitis or systemic symptoms should be considered for antibiotic therapy. Abscesses involving the hands and the face should also be treated more aggressively with antibiotics. Appropriate choices if antibiotics are used include a first-generation cephalosporin, such as **cephalexin** 500 mg PO every 6 h; **clindamycin** 300 mg PO every 6 h; or **amoxicillin-clavulanate** 875 mg/125 mg PO every 12 h. Prophylaxis for endocarditis in patients with structural cardiac abnormalities should be considered. See Chap. 24 for information on those at risk.

SPOROTRICHOSIS

Sporotrichosis is caused by traumatic inoculation of the fungus *Sporothrix schenckii,* which is found on plants and in the soil.

Clinical Features

After a 3 week incubation period, three types of infection may occur. The fixed cutaneous type is at the site of inoculation and looks like a crusted ulcer or verrucous plaque. The local cutaneous type also remains at the site of inoculation but presents as a subcutaneous nodule or pustule. The surrounding skin may become erythematous. The lymphocutaneous type is the most common of the three. It presents as a painless nodule at the site of inoculation that develops subcutaneous nodules with migration that follows lymphatic channels.

Diagnosis and Differential

The diagnosis is based on the history and physical examination. Tissue biopsy cultures are often diagnostic but of limited use in the ED. The differential diagnosis includes tuberculosis, tularemia, cat-scratch disease, leishmaniasis, nocardiosis, and staphylococcal lymphangitis.

Emergency Department Care and Disposition

Itraconazole 100 to 200 mg/d PO for 3 to 6 months is highly effective when treating sporotrichosis. If disseminated, sporotrichosis may be treated with IV **amphotericin** B 0.5 mg/kg/d. Most cases of cutaneous sporotrichosis can be treated on an outpatient basis. Those patients who have systemic symptoms or who are acutely ill should be admitted for possible treatment with amphotericin B.

For further reading in *Emergency Medicine: A Comprehensive Study Guide,* 5th ed., see Chap. 146, "Soft Tissue Infections," by Steven G. Folstad.

---

94 | Common Viral Infections
David M. Cline

Viral illnesses are among the most common reasons that people come to an emergency department. This chapter focuses on the viral illness for which antiviral therapy has been developed. Treatment of primary herpes zoster and mononucleosis is discussed in Chap. 82, and genital herpes is discussed in Chap. 86. Treatment of HIV is covered in Chap. 88, and treatment of cytomegalovirus is discussed in Chap. 95.

INFLUENZA A AND B

Flu occurs worldwide, in the winter months, and sporadically year round in the tropics. Influenza is spread by droplets generated by coughing. After exposure, the incubation period is usually about 2 days.

Clinical Features

Classic flu symptoms include fever of 38.6° to 39.8°C (101° to 103°F), with chills or rigor, headache, myalgia, and generalized malaise. Respiratory symptoms include dry cough, rhinorrhea, and sore throat, frequently with bilateral tender, enlarged cervical lymph nodes. Almost half of affected children have gastrointestinal symptoms, but these are unusual in adults.

The fever generally lasts 2 to 4 days, followed by rapid recovery from most of the systemic symptoms.

Diagnosis and Differential

A clinical diagnosis of flu during a known outbreak has an accuracy of approximately 85 percent, but bacteremia should also be considered in patients with rigor and myalgia. Newer rapid antigen tests are becoming available that may change the approach to flulike illnesses. One commercially available test requires a little more than 1 h to perform and lists a sensitivity of 50 to 70 percent, with a specificity of 93 to 100 percent.

Emergency Department Care and Disposition

Two antiviral drugs—**amantadine** and **rimantadine**—are currently approved for the treatment of influenza A. For maximal effectiveness, both need to be started within 48 h of onset of symptoms and can reduce the duration of systemic symptoms by 1 to 2 days. The dose is 100 mg two times daily for 5 days for both drugs. Amantadine causes an increase in seizure activity in patients with a preexisting seizure disorder. Rimantadine has a significantly lower incidence of central nervous system (CNS) side effects than does amantadine but is seven times more expensive. Neither medicine should be used during pregnancy. A new medication, zanamavir, appears promising in clinical trials and has activity against both influenza A and B.

HERPES SIMPLEX VIRUS 1

Transmission of herpes simplex virus (HSV) is via contact of infected secretions (saliva or genital) with mucous membranes or with open skin.

Clinical Features

HSV-1 primarily causes oral lesions, but may cause genital infection. The primary infection of HSV-1 is often mild or asymptomatic. The lesions are distributed throughout the mouth; the lesions are raised, erythematous, and may not become vesicular. In children under age 5, it may present as a pharyngitis or gingivostomatitis associated with fever and cervical lymphadenopathy. The primary lesions generally last 1 to 2 weeks. The diagnosis is largely clinical.

Recurrent oral lesions occur in 60 to 90 percent of infected individuals and are usually milder and generally occur on the lower lip at the outer vermilion border. The recurrences are often triggered by local trauma, sunburn, or stress. Patients may have "tingling" prior to developing lesions. The lesions may begin as erythematous papules and then become vesicular.

Emergency Department Care and Disposition

Oral acyclovir has been shown to shorten the duration of symptoms in children if begun within the first 72 h of symptoms. Treatment of recurrent oral herpes labialis with oral **acyclovir** 400 mg five times per day in adults shortens duration of symptoms. Topical **pencyclovir** applied every 2 h for 4 days shortens duration of symptoms and has recently been approved for this indication.

HERPES ZOSTER

Herpes zoster (shingles) is the reactivation or latent herpes zoster virus infection. There is a lifetime incidence of almost 20 percent, with the majority of cases being among the elderly.

Clinical Features

The lesions of shingles are identical to those of chickenpox, but are limited to a single dermatome in distribution. Thoracic and lumbar dermatomes are most common. The cranial nerves may be affected as well, with the potential complications of herpes zoster ophthalmicus (HZO) and Ramsay Hunt syndrome (symptoms similar to Bell's Palsy). The disease begins with a prodrome of pain in the affected area for 1 to 3 days, followed by the outbreak of a maculopapular rash that quickly progresses to a vesicular rash. The course of the disease is usually around 2 weeks, but may persist for a full month.

Ocular involvement can be seen in the presence of only a slight rash on the forehead. HZO induces keratitis and may be followed by involvement of deeper structures. A dendriform corneal ulcer can often be identified with fluorescein staining.

The most common complication of shingles is postherpetic neuralgia (PHN). PHN occurs in 10 to 20 percent of all patients after an episode of acute zoster, but in up to 70 percent of patients aged 70 years or older. It generally resolves in 1 to 2 months, but may last greater than a year in some patients.

Emergency Department Care and Disposition

The treatment of herpes zoster in the normal host is aimed at decreasing the risk of PHN, as the antivirals have a clinically small, but statistically significant, effect on the duration of the acute disease. Treatment should begin as soon as possible, and within 72 h of disease onset for maximal benefit. There is a suggestion that both **famciclovir** (500 mg two times a day for 7 days) and **valacyclovir** (1000 mg three times a day for 7 days) may be more effective than **acyclovir** (800 mg five times a day for 7 days), but this has not been shown to be clinically significant.

Initial treatment of patients with PHN is typically systemic analgesia, often narcotics. Patients should be referred back to their primary care provider, because first-line agents often fail, and a trial of amitriptyline or carbamazepine may be tried as second-line therapy.

HZO or suspected HZO mandates an ophthalmologic consultation due to the threat to vision.

Newer Antiviral Medications

New antiviral medications are currently being developed. Pleconaril has been developed for the treatment of viral meningitis. The drug reduced headache and quickened return to work or school in one study. This drug may have benefits in patients with viral respiratory tract infections. It is too early to recommend its widespread use at this date. The success of antiviral medications predicts that newer drugs will be developed.

For further reading in *Emergency Medicine: A Comprehensive Study Guide,* 5th ed., see Chap. 150, "Common Viral Infections: Influenzaviruses and Herpesviruses," by Robert A. Brownstein.

---

95 | Management of the Transplant Patient
David M. Cline

Management of the transplant patient in the emergency department can be divided into two general areas—disorders specific to the transplanted organ and disorders common to all transplant patients due to their immunosuppressed state. Compromised response to infection and other side-effects of immunosuppressive medication are common to all transplant recipients. Disorders specific to the transplanted organ are manifestations of acute rejection, surgical complications specific to the procedure performed, and altered physiology (most important in cardiac transplantation). Also, the management of routine injuries or illnesses may be complicated by the patient's immunosuppressed state or medication. Before prescribing any new drug for a transplant recipient, discuss your treatment plan with a representative from the transplant team.

POSTTRANSPLANT INFECTIOUS COMPLICATIONS

Infections after transplantation are a common and feared complication. Predisposing factors include ongoing immunosuppression in all patients and the presence of diabetes mellitus, advanced age, obesity, and other host factors in some. Table 95-1 displays the broad array of potential infections and the time after transplant they are most apt to occur.

The most common infection in recipients of solid organs, especially in bone-marrow graft recipients, is cytomegalovirus (CMV). This infection may manifest with daily fever and malaise in its mildest form. Progressively more serious disease manifestations include leukopenia, hepatopathy (elevated transaminase enzymes), enteropathy (epigastric pain and diarrhea), and pneumonitis. Mortality associated with CMV pneumonitis exceeds 50 percent. A patient presenting with a febrile illness should have as part of their assessment a complete blood cell count, chest x-ray, and measurement of liver function. During active CMV infection, immunosuppression is maintained at the minimum possible level and, if liver, gut, or pulmonary involvement is documented, intravenous ganciclovir therapy, often in conjunction with immune globulin, is prescribed.

The initial presentation of a potentially life-threatening infectious illness may be quite subtle in transplant recipients. The transplant recipient receiving glucocorticoids may not mount an impressive febrile response. A nonproductive cough with little or no findings on physical examination may be the only clue to emerging *Pneumocystis carinii* pneumonia on CMV pneumonia. The threshold for obtaining chest x-rays for these patients should be low. Central nervous system (CNS) infections are more common in transplant recipients than in other patients. Common etiologies include *Listeria monocytogenes* and cryptococci. Complaints of recurrent headaches, therefore, with or without fever, should be investigated vigorously, first with a structural study to exclude a mass lesion (CNS lymphomas occur with increased frequency too), then with a lumbar puncture. Finally, a significant subset of renal transplant recipients have undergone intentional splenectomy to

TABLE 95-1 Infectious Complications of Whole-Organ Transplantation

First Month Post-Transplant

Bacterial
  Wound infection (*Staph. aureus, S. epidermidis* gram-negative bacilli)
  Pneumonia (gram-negative bacilli)
  Urinary tract infection (gram-negative bacilli, enterococcus)
  Line-related sepsis (*Staph. aureus, S. epidermidis,* gram-negative bacilli)
  Intraabdominal infections (liver transplant)

Viral
  HSV

Fungal
  Candidal pharyngitis, esophagitis, cystitis

Second to Sixth Month Post-Transplant

Bacterial
  Pneumonia: pneumococcal and other community acquired
  Meningitis (*Listeria monocytogenes*)
  Urinary tract infection
  Nocardial infection
  Listeriosis

Viral
  Cytomegalovirus, EBV, HSV, varicella zoster
  Adenovirus
  Hepatitis A, B, C

Fungal
  Aspergillosis
  Candidal pharyngitis, esophagitis, cystitis

Other opportunistic infection
  Pneumocystis carinii pneumonia, tuberculosis, toxoplasmosis

Beyond Sixth Month Post-Transplant

Bacterial
  Pneumonia: pneumococcal and other community acquired
  Urinary tract infection
  Listeriosis

Viral
  Cytomegalovirus chorioretinitis
  Varicella zoster
  Hepatitis C, B

Fungal
  Cryptococcal

Other opportunistic infection
  P. carinii pneumonia

Abbreviations: HSV, herpes simplex virus; EBV, Epstein-Barr virus.

improve allograft survival. Although this procedure is no longer routinely practiced, these patients, as in other postsplenectomy patients, are at particularly high risk for overwhelming sepsis caused by encapsulated bacteria such as pneumococci or meningococci.

Liver transplant patients are especially susceptible to intraabdominal infections during the first postoperative month. Lung transplant patients are especially prone to pneumonia during the first 3 postoperative months. Cardiac transplant patients may develop mediastinitis during the first postoperative month.

Management of Infection

Alternatives for therapy follow, however, drug choice, dose, and ultimate management should be accomplished in consultation with the transplant team.

1. For skin and superficial wounds, probable offending organisms are gram-positive cocci, especially *Staphylococcus aureus,* and treatment should be with a penicillinase-resistant penicillin (e.g., nafcillin or oxacillin) or a first-generation cephalosporin (e.g., cefazolin), unless there is a suspicion for methicillin-resistant organisms or sensitivity to β-lactams, in which case vancomycin should be used.
2. Nosocomial pneumonia is likely due to gram-negative organisms such as *Escherichia Coli, Enterobacter,* or *Pseudomonas* and should be treated with a broad-spectrum antibiotic (e.g., cefoxitin, cefotetan, cefotaxime, ceftriaxone, or ceftazidime). Community-acquired pneumonia should be treated as such, with the proviso that opportunistic infection may also be present.
3. Intraabdominal infection may be due to enterococci, gram-negative bacilli, or anaerobes and sometimes *S. aureus.* Triple coverage may be necessary empirically with ampicillin or vancomycin plus and an aminoglycoside to treat enterococci; a broad-spectrum penicillin or second- or third-generation cephalosporin to treat gram-negative organisms; and piperacillin, cefoxitin, cefotetan, clindamycin, or metronidazole to treat anaerobes. Penicillins with β-lactamase inhibitors (e.g., sulbactam and clavulanic acid) have broad coverage against gram-positive cocci, gram-negative bacilli, and anaerobes.
4. Meningitis is frequently due to *L. monocytogenes,* and patients with suspected meningitis should be treated with a third-generation cephalosporin and ampicillin.
5. The mainstay of fungal treatment has been amphotericin B. *Candida albicans* can be treated first with fluconazole.

6. Viral therapy depends on the disease syndrome and the offending agent. CMV disease is treated with ganciclovir, with a dose of 5 mg/kg intravenously twice daily. Varicella and herpes simplex virus are typically treated with acyclovir, which has renal excretion; the dose must be adjusted for renal insufficiency. Epstein-Barr virus (EBV) is typically treated with a reduction in the immunosuppression regimen.
7. Treatment of choice for *P. carinii* pneumonia is cotrimoxazole, with pentamidine reserved as an alternative therapy if cotrimoxazole is not tolerated. Toxoplasmosis is treated with pyrimethamine/sulfadiazine or clindamycin.
8. Urinary tract infections, invasive gastroenteritis (due to *Salmonella, Campylobacter,* and *Listeria*) and diverticulitis can be treated with the usual antimicrobial agents.

COMPLICATIONS OF IMMUNOSUPPRESSIVE AGENTS

Therapeutic immunosuppression is accompanied by a number of side effects and complications (Table 95-2). Combined toxicities

TABLE 95-2 Drug Side Effects

Cyclosporine
  Nephrotoxicity
  Neurotoxicity—tremors, seizures, headaches
  Hyperkalemia
  Hyperuricemia
  Hypertension
  Hypomagnesemia
  Anorexia
  Hyperbilirubinemia
  Glucose intolerance
  Cholestasis
  Gastric dysmotility

Prednisone
  Cushing's syndrome
  Osteoporosis
  Adrenal suppression
  Hypertension
  Hyperglycemia
  Peptic ulcer disease
  Myopathy
  Poor wound healing

Azathioprine (Imuran)
  Leukopenia
  Thrombocytopenia
  Cholestatic jaundice
  Alopecia

can produce or worsen preexisting renal insufficiency, hypertension, and hyperglycemia. Elevated cyclosporine levels cause renal arteriolar constriction, which reduces glomerular blood flow and stimulates the renin-angiotensin system, and elevated blood pressure. Glucocorticoids promote renal salt and water retention, which further aggravate hypertension. A headache syndrome often indistinguishable from migraine is common in transplant recipients and usually develops within the first 2 months of immunosuppression. An important differential must include infectious causes and malignancy when headache first presents and usually requires a head computed tomography (CT) scan with subsequent biochemical analysis of cerebrospinal fluid.

Recently, the newer immunosuppressive agents tacrolimus and mycophenolate mofetil have been used in place of cyclosporine and azathioprine, respectively. The most common side effects of tacrolimus are similar to cyclosporine. The most common side effects of mycophenolate mofetil are diarrhea, vomiting, leukopenia, and increased opportunistic infections, especially CMV.

Any illness that prevents transplant patients from taking or retaining their immunosuppressive therapy warrants hospital admission for intravenous therapy, preferably at a transplant center.

CARDIAC TRANSPLANTATION

Transplantation results in a denervated heart that does not respond with centrally medicated tachycardia in response to stress or exercise, but does respond to circulating catecholamines and increased preload. Patients may complain of fatigue or shortness of breath with the onset of exercise, which resolves with continued exertion as an appropriate tachycardia develops.

The donor heart is implanted with its sinus node intact to preserve normal atrioventricular conduction. The normal heart rate for a transplanted heart is 90 to 100 beats per minute. The technique of cardiac transplantation also results in the preservation of the recipient's sinus node at the superior cavoatrial junction. The atrial suture line renders the two sinus nodes electrically isolated from each other. Thus, electrocardiograms (ECGs) will frequently have two distinct P waves. The sinus node of the donor heart is easily identified by its constant 1:1 relationship to the QRS complex, whereas the native P wave marches through the donor heart rhythm independently.

Clinical Features

Because the heart is denervated, myocardial ischemia does not present with angina. Instead, recipients present with heart failure secondary to silent myocardial infarctions or with sudden death.

Transplant recipients who have new-onset shortness of breath, chest fullness, or symptoms of congestive heart failure (CHF) should be evaluated, in routine fashion with an ECG and serial cardiac enzyme levels, for the presence of myocardial ischemia or infarction.

Although most episodes of acute rejection are asymptomatic, symptoms can occur. The most common presenting symptoms are dysrhythmias and generalized fatigue. The development of either atrial or ventricular dysrhythmias in a cardiac transplant recipient (or CHF) must be assumed due to acute rejection until proved otherwise. In children, rejection may present with low-grade fever, fussiness, and poor feeding.

Emergency Department Care and Disposition

1. Consultation—Differentiating rejection from other acute illnesses in the transplant patient can be difficult. Treatment for rejection without biopsy confirmation is contraindicated except when patients are hemodynamically unstable.
2. Rejection—Management of acute rejection includes 1 g of methylprednisolone intravenously, after consultation with a representative from the transplant center.
3. Dysrhythmias—If patients are hemodynamically compromised by dysrhythmias, empiric therapy for rejection with methylprednisolone, 1 g intravenously, may be given after consultation. Atrial dysrhythmias may respond to treatment with digoxin or calcium channel blockers. Ventricular dysrhythmias may respond to lidocaine or other class I-C agents. Frequently dysrhythmias will be controlled only with antirejection therapy. Atropine has no effect on the denervated heart; isoproterenol is the drug of choice for bradydysrhythmias in these patients.
4. Hypotension—Low-output syndrome, or hypotension, should be treated with inotropic agents such as dopamine or dobutamine when specific treatment for rejection is instituted.
5. Hospitalization—Transplant patients suspected of having rejection or acute illness should be hospitalized, preferably at the transplant center, if stable for transfer.

LUNG TRANSPLANTATION

Clinical Features

Clinically, patients suffering rejection may have a cough, chest tightness, fatigue, and fever (>0.5°C above baseline). Acute rejection may be manifest with frightening rapidity, causing a severe decline in patient status in only a day. Isolated fever may be the only finding; in contrast, spirometry may show a 15 percent drop in FEV_1, and examination may reveal rales and adventitious sounds. Chest x-ray may demonstrate bilateral interstitial infiltrates, septal lines, and effusions. The chest x-ray may be normal, however, when rejection occurs late in the course. The longer period a patient is from transplant, the less classic a chest x-ray may appear for acute rejection. Infection, such as interstitial pneumonia, may present with a clinical picture similar to acute rejection. Diagnostically, bronchoscopy with transbronchial biopsy is usually needed not only to confirm rejection but to exclude infection.

Two late complications of lung transplant are obliterative bronchiolitis and posttranspalnt lymphoproliferative disease (PTLD). Obliterative bronchiolitis presents with episodes of recurrent bronchitis, small airway obliteration, wheezing, and eventually respiratory failure. PTLD is associated with Epstein-Barr virus and presents with painful lymphadenopathy and otitis media (due to tonsillar involvement), or may present with malaise, fever, and myalgia.

Evaluation of the lung-transplant patient should include chest x-ray, arterial blood gas analysis; complete blood cell count (CBC); serum electrolyte, creatinine, and magnesium levels; and, in some cases, a cyclosporine level.

Emergency Department Care and Disposition

1. Consultation—Communication should be made directly with the transplant center (often a nurse coordinator). Coordinators should have patients' current medication doses, recent infection history, and knowledge of complications for which patients may be at risk.
2. Rejection—If clinically indicated (i.e., infection is excluded), methylprednisolone 500 to 1000 mg intravenously should be given. Patients who have a history of seizures associated with the administration of high-dose glucocorticoids will also need concurrent benzodiazepines to prevent further seizure episodes.
3. Late complications—Obliterative bronchiolitis is treated with increased immunosuppression, whereas PTLD is treated with reduced immunosuppression. These decisions should be made by specialists from the transplant center.

RENAL TRANSPLANT

Clinical Features

Diagnosis and treatment of acute rejection is most critical. Without timely recognition and intervention, allograft function may deteriorate irreversibly in a few days.

Renal transplant recipients, when symptomatic from acute rejection, complain of vague tenderness over the allograft (in the left or right iliac fossa). Patients may also describe decreased urine output, rapid weight gain (from fluid retention), low-grade fever, and generalized malaise. Physical examination may disclose worsening hypertension, allograft tenderness, and peripheral edema. The absence of these symptoms and signs, however, does not exclude the possibility of acute rejection. With improved methods of maintenance immunosuppression, the only clue may be an asymptomatic decline in renal function. Even a change in creatinine levels from 1.0 mg/dL to 1.2 or 1.3 mg/dL may be important. When such changes in creatinine levels are reproducible, a careful workup consists of complete urinalysis, renal ultrasonography, and a trough level of cyclosporine, in addition to a careful history and examination. It is critical to interpret changes in renal function in the context of prior data (e.g., trends of recent serum creatinine levels, recent history of rejection, or other causes of allograft dysfunction). Evaluation should consider the multiple etiologies of decreased renal function in the renal transplant recipient. The two most common causes, apart from acute rejection causing an increase in creatinine, are volume contraction and cyclosporine-induced nephrotoxicity.

Emergency Department Care and Disposition

1. Consultation—Communication should be made directly with the transplant center (often a nurse coordinator). Coordinators should have patients' current medication doses, recent infection history, and a knowledge of complications for which patients may be at risk.
2. Rejection—Treatment of allograft rejection consists of high-dose glucocorticoids, typically methylprednisolone (250 to 500 mg intravenously).

LIVER TRANSPLANT

Clinical Features

Though frequently subtle in presentation, a syndrome of acute rejection includes fever, liver tenderness, lymphocytosis, eosinophilia, liver enzyme elevation, and a change in bile color or production. In the perioperative period, the differential diagnosis must include infection, acute biliary obstruction, or vascular insufficiency. Diagnosis can be made with certainty only by hepatic ultrasound and biopsy, which usually requires referral back to the transplant center for management and follow up.

Two possible surgical complications in liver transplant patients are biliary obstruction or leakage and hepatic artery thrombosis. Biliary obstruction follows three typical presentations. The most common is intermittent episodes of fever and fluctuating liver function tests. The second is a gradual worsening of liver function tests without symptoms. Finally, obstruction may present as acute bacterial cholangitis with fever, chills, abdominal pain, jaundice, and bacteremia. It can be difficult to distinguish clinically from rejection, hepatic artery thrombosis, CMV infection, or a recurrence of a preexisting disease, especially hepatitis.

If a biliary complication is suspected, all patients should have a CBC; serum chemistry levels; liver-function tests; amylase and lipase levels; cultures of blood, urine, bile, and ascites, if present; a chest x-ray; and abdominal ultrasound. Ultrasound rules out the presence of fluid collections, screens for the presence of thrombosis of the hepatic artery or portal vein, and identifies any dilatation of the biliary tree.

Biliary leakage is associated with 50 percent mortality. It occurs most frequently in the third or fourth postoperative week. The high mortality may be related to a high incidence of concomitant hepatic artery thrombosis, infection of leaked bile, or difficult bile repair where the tissue is inflamed. Patients most often have peritoneal signs and fever, but these signs may be masked by concomitant use of steroids and immunosuppressive agents. Presentation is signaled by elevated PT and transaminase levels and little or no bile production, but this complication may also present as acute graft failure, liver abscess, unexplained sepsis, or a biliary tract problem (leak, obstruction, abscess, or breakdown of the anastomosis).

Emergency Department Care and Disposition

1. Consultation—Communication should be made directly with the transplant center (often a nurse coordinator). Coordinators should have patients' current medication doses, recent infection history, and a knowledge of complications for which patients may be at risk.
2. Rejection—Acute rejection is managed with high-dose glucocorticoid bolus.
3. Surgical complications are best managed at the transplant center. Biliary obstruction is managed with balloon dilatation, and all patients should receive broad spectrum antibotics against gram-negative and gram-positive enteric organisms. Biliary

leakage is treated with reoperation, and hepatic artery thrombosis is treated with retransplantation.

For further reading in *Emergency Medicine: A Comprehensive Study Guide,* 5th ed., see Chap. 56, "Cardiac Transplantation," by Michael R. Mill and Michelle S. Grady; Chap. 66, "The Lung Transplant Patient," by Thomas P. Noeller; Chap. 86, "The Liver Transplant Patient," by Steven Kronick; and Chap. 96, "The Renal Transplant Patient," by Richard Sinert.

TOXICOLOGY

96	General Management of Poisoned Patients

Sandra L. Najarian

It is estimated that over 4 million poisonings occur in the United States annually. The poisoned patient requires a thorough, systematic evaluation. Poison centers are an invaluable resource. Prompt consultation can aid diagnosis and help ensure efficient and cost-effective management of the poisoned patient.

Clinical Features

A detailed medical history is essential. Every attempt should be made to ascertain the number of persons exposed, timing, type, amount, and route of exposure. Family members, witnesses, prehospital personnel on scene, and the patient's primary physician are important sources of information. They should be utilized to corroborate the patient's history. Details about the environment in which the patient was found (e.g., presence of pill bottles or empty containers, drug paraphernalia, unusual odors or smells, or presence of a suicide note) are important, since these may provide clues to identifying the poison (Table 96-1).

A thorough head-to-toe physical exam on a fully disrobed patient is necessary. Use caution when searching the patient's clothing for substances. Pay careful attention to vital signs, general appearance, skin, pupils, mucous membranes, heart, lung, gastrointestinal, and neurologic exams. Exposure to certain substances may result in specific toxidromes (Table 96-2). When the exposure is unknown, recognition of these toxidromes can assist the emergency physician in narrowing the differential diagnosis (Table 96-3).

Diagnosis and Differential

Diagnosis is based on history and clinical presentation. When there is a question of ingestion, having the actual container, remnant pills, or liquids is very important. Having family, friends, or emergency personnel retrieve these items is essential. Laboratory studies may be useful but often serve only to confirm the diagnosis.

TABLE 96-1 Nontoxic Ingestions

Only one substance is involved in the exposure.

The substance must be absolutely identified.

The substance's product label must not contain any consumer product safety commission signal words indicating a potential hazard of toxicity.

The exposure must have been unintentional.

The route of exposure must be known.

An approximate amount of the substance involved in the exposure must be known.

The exposed individual must be free of symptoms for the extent of the observation period.

Follow-up consultation must be easily available or a responsible parent or guardian must be present.

Note: All of the criteria listed must be fulfilled in order for an ingestion to be classified as nontoxic.

Source: Adapted from Mofenson and Grensher and Mofenson et al. *Emerg Med Clin North Am* 2:159, 1984.

Drug screens may be useful in unknown ingestions but rarely alter management. Acetaminophen and aspirin are common coingestions in suicide attempts, so consideration should be given to testing for these drugs. Other tests that may be useful include an electrocardiogram, arterial blood gas analysis, and electrolyte and glucose levels.

Emergency Department Care and Disposition

1. The **ABCs** always take precedence in managing the poisoned patient. Once the ABCs are secured, decontamination, elimination of the toxin, and administration of the antidote should take place.
2. Primary evaluation includes assessment of gag reflex and quality of respirations. Early intubation should be considered, especially if gastric lavage is indicated in any patient with a depressed level of consciousness. Respiratory status should be continuously monitored. Abnormalities in breathing are not usually the direct effect of a toxin, but rather a result of the patient's altered level of consciousness. Hypotension should be corrected with intravenous fluids. Pressors are rarely required. Ventricular dysrhythmias should be treated according to standard ACLS protocol unless treatment of a particular toxin dictates an alternative treatment. Atropine should be used for bradyarrhythmias; cardiac pacing may be necessary.

3. For those patients found unresponsive or with altered mental status, administration of **oxygen, naloxone** (0.4 to 2.0 mg IV in adults), **glucose** (50 mL 50% dextrose), and **thiamine** (100 mg) should be considered after taking into account the history, vital signs, and immediate laboratory data. Intravenous access must be secured. Routine use of flumazenil, a benzodiazepine antagonist, is not recommended. A Foley catheter should be placed in unconscious patients. Placing physical restraints prior to reversing opioid intoxication should be considered. Administration of naloxone, a competitive opioid antagonist, may precipitate acute withdrawal syndrome, especially if large doses are given.

4. Immediate treatment should be initiated for seizing patients and agitated patients. Seizures with benzodiazepines initially, followed by phenobarbital, if necessary. (Phenytoin is less useful for the poisoned patient.) Using physical and chemical restraints should be considered in the agitated patient. Short-acting benzodiazepines or haloperidol may be useful.

5. Decontamination of the poisoned patient is the mainstay of therapy. Gross (surface) decontamination is the initial step. The patient should be removed from the toxic substance; this includes undressing patients completely and washing the skin with copious amounts of water. Properly gowned staff should assist the patient in an isolated area so as to avoid contamination to other patients and staff. With ocular exposure, the eyes must be flushed immediately with irrigation solution until the pH of the eyes return to a physiologic range.

6. Gastric decontamination includes gastric emptying, adsorption of the toxin in the gut, and irrigation of the bowel. The method depends upon the toxin, timing of exposure, clinical status of the patient, and technical skills of the physician. **Gastric lavage** is the preferred method of gastric emptying. Ipecac is no longer recommended. Gastric lavage mainly benefits those obtunded patients presenting within 1 h of ingestion. Gastric lavage should be reserved for those patients with potentially life-threatening ingestions. If performed, a large-bore (36 to 40 Fr) orogastric tube with connections for infusion and drainage. Place the patient in a left lateral decubitus position with the head lower than the feet. Infusion of 250 mL aliquots of tap water should be prepared until return is clear. Prior to removing the tube, **activated charcoal** (1 g/kg) should be administered to help bind any remaining toxin. Activated charcoal may be given per nasogastric tube or in a slurry mixed with juice or soda when lavage is not indicated. **Osmotic cathartics** (1 g/kg of 70% sorbitol or 4 mg/kg of 10% magnesium citrate) may be given with activated

TABLE 96-2 Toxidromes

Toxidrome	Representative agent(s)	Most common findings	Additional signs and symptoms	Potential interventions
Opioid	Heroin Morphine	CNS depression, miosis, respiratory depression	Hypothermia, bradycardia Death may result from respiratory arrest, pulmonary edema	Ventilation or naloxone
Sympathomimetic	Cocaine Amphetamine	Psychomotor agitation, mydriasis, diaphoresis, tachycardia, hypertension, hyperthermia	Seizures, rhabdomyolysis, myocardial infarction Death may result from seizures, cardiac arrest, hyperthermia	Cooling, sedation with benzodiazepines, hydration
Cholinergic	Organophosphate insecticides Carbamate insecticides	Salivation, lacrimation, diaphoresis, nausea, vomiting, urination, defecation, muscle fasciculations, weakness, bronchorrhea	Bradycardia, miosis/mydriasis, seizures, respiratory failure, paralysis Death may result from respiratory arrest 2° to paralysis and/or bronchorrhea, seizures	Airway protection and ventilation, atropine, pralidoxime
Anticholinergic	Scopolamine Atropine	Altered mental status, mydriasis, dry/flushed skin, urinary retention, decreased bowel sounds, hyperthermia, dry mucous membranes	Seizures, dysrhythmias, rhabdomyolysis Death may result from hyperthermia and dysrhythmias	Physostigmine (if appropriate), sedation with benzodiazepines, cooling, supportive management

514

Salicylates	Aspirin Oil of wintergreen	Altered mental status, respiratory alkalosis, metabolic acidosis, tinnitus hyperpnea, tachycardia, diaphoresis, nausea, vomiting	Low-grade fever, ketonuria Death may result from pulmonary edema, cardiorespiratory arrest	MDAC, alkalinization of the urine with potassium repletion, hemodialysis, hydration
Hypoglycemia	Sulfonylureas Insulin	Altered mental status, diaphoresis, tachycardia, hypertension	Paralysis, slurring of speech, bizarre behavior, seizures Death may result from seizures, altered behavior	Glucose containing solution intravenously, and oral feedings if able, frequent capillary blood for glucose measurement
Serotonin syndrome	Meperidine/ dextromethorphan + MAOI, SSRI + TCA, SSRI/TCA/MAOI + amphetamine, SSRI overdose	Altered mental status, increased muscle tone, hyperreflexia, hyperthermia	"Wet dog shakes" (intermittent whole body tremor) Death may result from hyperthermia	Cooling, sedation with benzodiazepines, supportive management, theoretical benefit—cyproheptadine

Abbreviations: CNS, central nervous system; MDAC, multidose activated charcoal; MAOI, monoamine oxidase inhibitor; SSRI, selective serotonin reuptake inhibitor; TCA, tricyclic antidepressant.

TABLE 96-3 Agents that May Alter Presenting Signs or Symptoms[a]

Drugs	Seizures	Change in blood pressure	Change in ventilation	Change in heart rate	Temperature change
Alcohol withdrawal	✓	↓	↓	↓	↓
Amphetamines	✓	↓	↓	↓	↓
Anticholinergic	✓	↓	↓	↓	↓
Baclofen	✓	↑	↑	↑	↑
Caffeine	✓	↓	↓	↓	
Camphor	✓				
Cocaine	✓	↓	↓	↓	↓
Gyrometria esculenta (mushroom)	✓				
Isoniazid	✓				
Lithium	✓				
Methaqualone	✓	↓	↑	↓	
Serotonin syndrome	✓	↓	↓	↓	↓
Theophylline	✓	↓	↓	↓	
Tricyclic antidepressants	✓	↑	↑	↑	
β-adrenergic antagonists	✓	↑		↑	
Calcium channel blockers		↑		↑	
Clonidine		↑	↑	↑	↑

Agent[a]					
Ethanol		↓	↓	↓	↓
Phenothiazines		↓	↓	↓	↓
Opioids		↓	↓	↓	↓
Organophosphates	↘	↓	↓	↓	↓
Meprobamate	↘	↓	↓	↓	↓
Monoamine oxidase inhibitor overdose	↘	↑	↑	↑	↑
Phencyclidine	↘	↑	↑	↑	↑
Sedative hypnotic withdrawal		↑	↑	↑	↑
Phenylpropanolamine		↑	↑	↑	
Barbiturates		↓	↓	↓	↓
Ethchlorvynol		↓	↓	↑	
Glutethamide		↓	↓	↑	
Salicylates		↑	↑	↑	←
Nicotine	↘	↑	↑	↑	
Hydrocarbons		↓	↓	↑[b]	
Toxic alcohols	↘	↓	↓	↑	
Iron	↘	↓	↓	↑	←

[a]Listed are the most common or most classically seen with the agent.
[b]Halogenated and aromatic hydrocarbons.

charcoal to reduce transit time through the gastrointestinal tract. Multiple-dose activated charcoal is an option usually reserved for very large ingestions, toxins known to slow gut motility, or slow-release toxis. Whole bowel irrigation may be useful in eliminating sustained-release preparations, toxins not known to be adsorbed by activated charcoal, or packages of toxic drugs (body packers). Administration 2 L/h of **polyethylene glycol** is indicated in adults (500 mL/h in pediataric patients) until rectal effluent is clear.

7. Once decontamination is underway, specific antidotes or other special treatment may be given. Enhancing elimination of certain toxins may be indicated, such as urinary alkalization, hemoperfusion or hemodialysis for specific toxins, such as salicylates, methanol, lithium, or theophylline.

8. Disposition of patients depends on the nature of the exposure and underlying conditions. Consideration should be given to delayed effects and absorption of toxins. Psychiatric consultation should be obtained for all intentional overdoses. Poisonings in children over 5 years old should be considered suspicious and warrant social-work consult or law-enforcement involvement. Patients and families should be given instructions on prevention of poisonings.

For further reading in *Emergency Medicine: A Comprehensive Study Guide,* 5th ed., see Chap. 151, "General Management of Poisoned Patients," by Jason B. Hack and Robert S. Hoffman.

---

97 | Anticholinergic Toxicity

Keith L. Mausner

Anticholinergic toxicity is commonly seen in the emergency department. Table 97-1 lists the important anticholinergic agents and the classes to which they belong.

TABLE 97-1 Anticholinergic Substances

Antihistamines
  Ethanolamines
    Dimenhydrinate (Dramamine)
    Diphenhydramine (Benadryl)
  Ethylenediamines
    Triplennamine (Pyribenzamine)
  Alkylamines
    Chlorpheniramine (Teldrin)
  Piperazines
    Astemizole (Hismanal)
    Terfenadine (Seldane)
    Loratadine (Claritin)
    Cyclizine (Marezine)
    Meclizine (Antivert)
  Phenothiazines
    Prochlorperazine (Compazine)
    Promethazine (Phenergan)

Antiparkinsonian drugs
  Benztropine mesylate (Cogentin)
  Biperiden (Akineton)
  Ethopropazine (Parsidol)
  Trihexyphenidyl (Artane)
  Procyclidine (Kemadrin)

Antipsychotics
  Phenothiazines
    Chlorpromazine (Thorazine)
    Thioridazine (Mellaril)
    Perphenazine (Trilafon)
  Nonphenothiazines
    Clozaril (Clozapine)
    Molindone (Moban)
    Loxapine (Loxitane)

Antispasmodics
  Clidinium bromide (Quarzan, Librax)
  Dicyclomine (Bentyl)
  Methantheline bromide (Banthine)
  Propantheline bromide (Pro-Banthine)
  Tridihexethyl chloride (Pathilon)

Plants
  Deadly nightshade
  Mandrake
  Jimsonweed

(continued)

TABLE 97-1 Anticholinergic Substances (*Continued*)

Belladonna alkaloids, synthetic cogeners
  Atropine (Hyoscyamine)
  Belladonna alkaloid mixtures
  Glycopyrrolate (Robinul)
  Homatropine (Dia-Quel, Malcotran)
  Methscopolamine bromide (Pamine)
  Scopolamine hydrobromide (Hysocine)

Cyclic antidepressants
  Amitryptyline hydrochloride (Elavil, Ammitril, Endep)
  Desipramine hydrochloride (Norpramine, Pertofrane)
  Doxepin hydrochloride (Sinequan, Adapin)
  Imipramine hydrochloride (Tofranil, Pramine)
  Notriptyline hydrochloride (Aventyl, Pamelor)
  Protriptyline hydrochloride (Vivactil)
  Trimipramine (Surmontil)
  Maprotiline hydrochloride (Ludiomil)
  Zimelidine hydrochloride
  Fluoxetine (Prozac)
  Amoxapin (Asendin)

Ophthalmic products
  Atropine and scopolamine solutions
  Cyclopentolate hydrochloride (Cyclogyl)
  Tropicamide (Mydriacyl)

OTC medications (including antihistamines and belladonna alkaloids)
  Analgesics: Excedrin PM, Percogesic
  Cold remedies: Actifed, Allerest, Coricidin, Dristan, Flavihist, Romex, Sine-Off
  Hypnotics: Compoz, Sleep-Eze, Sominex
  Menstrual products: Pamprin, Premesyn PMS

Skeletal muscle relaxants
  Orphenadrine citrate (Norflex)
  Cyclobenzaprine hydrochloride (Flexeril)

Mushrooms
  Amanita muscaria
  Amanita pantherina

Other
Diphenidol (Cephadol, Vontrol)

Source: Adapted from Goldfrank LR (ed): *Goldfrank's Toxicologic Emergencies,* 6th ed. Stamford, CT, Appleton & Lange, 1998, with permission.

Clinical Features

Clinical findings include mydriasis, hypo- or hypertension, absent bowel sounds, tachycardia, flushed skin, disorientation, urinary retention, hyperthermia, dry skin and mucous membranes, and auditory and visual hallucinations. Sinus tachycardia is the most common electrocardiographic finding.

Diagnosis and Differential

Diagnosis is primarily clinical. In isolated anticholinergic toxicity, routine laboratory study results should be normal, and toxicology screening is of little value. The differential diagnosis includes delirium tremens, acute psychiatric disorders, and sympathomimetic toxicity.

Emergency Department Care and Disposition

Treatment is primarily supportive

1. Place the patient on a cardiac monitor and obtain intravenous (IV) access.
2. Gastric lavage may be useful within 1 h of ingestion. **Activated charcoal** may decrease drug absorption.
3. Hyperthermia is treated conventionally.
4. Hypertension usually does not require intervention but may be treated conventionally if necessary.
5. Standard antiarrhythmics are usually effective, but avoid class Ia. Dysrhythmias, a widened QRS complex, and hypotension from sodium-blocking agents (e.g., cyclic antidepressants) can be treated with IV bicarbonate.
6. Seizures can be treated with benzodiazepines and barbiturates.
7. Agitation can be treated with benzodiazepines. Avoid phenothiazines.
8. **Physostigmine** treatment is controversial. It is indicated only if conventional therapy fails to control seizures, agitation, unstable dysrhythmia, coma with respiratory depression, malignant hypertension, or hypotension. The initial dose is 0.5 to 2 mg IV over 5 min. Physostigmine may worsen cyclic antidepressant toxicity and is contraindicated in patients with cardiovascular or peripheral vascular disease, bronchospasm, intestinal obstruction, heart block, or bladder obstruction. The patient should be observed for cholinergic symptoms.

Patients with mild anticholinergic toxicity can be discharged after 6 h of observation if their symptoms are improving. Patients receiving physostigmine usually require at least 24-h admission.

For further reading in *Emergency Medicine: A Comprehensive Study Guide,* 5th ed., see Chap. 177, "Anticholinergic Toxicity," by Leslie R. Wolf.

---

98 | Psychopharmacologic Agents
C. Crawford Mechem

TRICYCLIC ANTIDEPRESSANTS

Tricyclic antidepressants (TCAs) are used to manage major depression, obsessive-compulsive disorder, and chronic pain. They are associated with significant toxicity and cause more drug-related deaths than any other class of prescription medication.

Clinical Features

Life-threatening symptoms usually occur with ingestion of more than 10 mg/kg in adults. Serious toxicity may be seen at lower doses, especially in coingestions and in children, the elderly, and patients with preexisting cardiac disease.

Serious toxicity manifests within 6 h of acute overdose, with hypotension, respiratory depression, cardiac conduction delays, dysrhythmias, dry mucosae, decreased bowel sounds, urinary retention, depressed mental status, seizures, and coma. Complications include aspiration pneumonia, pulmonary edema, hyperthermia, and rhabdomyolysis.

Diagnosis and Differential

Diagnosis is made on clinical grounds. The electrocardiogram (ECG) is helpful in assessing severity of toxicity. Abnormalities develop within 6 h of ingestion and include sinus tachycardia;

right-axis deviation (RAD); and prolongation of PR, QRS, and QT intervals. Life-threatening complications are more likely when the QRS interval is greater than 100 ms or with RAD of the terminal 40 ms greater than 120°. This is recognized by a positive terminal R wave in aV_R and a negative S wave in lead I.

The differential diagnosis includes toxicity due to carbamazepine, cyclobenzaprine, diphenhydramine, phenothiazines, class IA and IC antidysrhythmics, propranolol, propoxyphene, cocaine, lithium, and hyperkalemia.

Emergency Department Care and Disposition

The patient's respiratory and hemodynamic status should be stabilized. All patients need IV access, continuous cardiac monitoring, and an ECG. Appropriate laboratory studies include serum electrolytes determinations, renal function tests, determination of glucose level, arterial blood gas analysis, and determination of acetaminophen level.

1. All patients should receive **activated charcoal** 1 g/kg orally (PO) or per nasogastric (NG) tube.
2. Gastric lavage is indicated in the first 2 to 3 h after ingestion.
3. **Sodium bicarbonate** 1 to 2 mg IV is given for QRS interval greater than 100 ms, refractory hypotension, or ventricular dysrhythmias and repeated to achieve a serum pH of 7.50 to 7.55. An IV infusion is prepared by adding 2 ampules (50 meq/50 mL) to 1 L 5% dextrose in water (D_5W). Serum potassium levels should be closely monitored.
4. **Dextrose, thiamine,** and **naloxone** are warranted for altered mental status.
5. Seizures should be controlled with IV **lorazepam** or **diazepam.** Refractory cases are treated with **phenobarbital** at an initial loading dose of 18 mg/kg IV. Hypotension and respiratory depression should be anticipated.
6. **Crystalloid IV fluids** should be administered in increments of 10 mL/kg to treat hypotension and the patient closely watched for signs of pulmonary edema. **Norepinephrine** is the vasopressor of choice in refractory cases.

Patients who remain asymptomatic 6 h after ingestion may be medically cleared. All symptomatic patients should be admitted to a monitored setting.

NEWER ANTIDEPRESSANTS AND SEROTONIN SYNDROME

The newer antidepressants are used for the treatment of depression, panic disorder, and obsessive-compulsive disorder. They lack the cardiotoxicity and antimuscarinic effects of TCAs but can still cause serious toxicity, including serotonin syndrome.

Trazodone and Nefazodone

Clinical Features

Adverse effects due to trazodone include orthostatic hypotension, sedation, dry mouth, nausea, vomiting, dizziness, liver toxicity, and priapism. Cardiac dysrhythmias may include sinus bradycardia, atrial fibrillation, sinus arrest, atrioventricular (AV) blocks, premature ventricular contractions, and torsades de pointes. Nefazodone produces orthostatic hypotension, dry mouth, nausea, constipation, priapism, headache, drowsiness, weakness, tremor, and blurred vision. It can inhibit metabolism of terfenadine, astemizole, and cisapride, resulting in QT interval prolongation and torsades de pointes. It also potentiates central nervous system (CNS) depression caused by benzodiazepines.

In acute trazodone overdose, serious toxicity is rare at doses less than 2 g. Manifestations include CNS depression, orthostatic hypotension, vomiting, abdominal pain, muscle weakness, priapism, ataxia, seizures, and coma. Respiratory depression is rarely seen. On ECG, QT prolongation may be seen, rarely leading to torsades de pointes. In acute nefazodone overdose, somnolence, nausea, and vomiting have been reported.

Emergency Department Care and Disposition

In most trazodone or nefazodone overdoses, supportive care is sufficient. The patient should be assessed for respiratory or hemodynamic compromise from a coingestion, and an acetaminophen level should be obtained.

1. An IV line should be started and cardiac monitoring initiated in all patients.
2. **Activated charcoal** 1 g/kg should be administered. Gastric lavage is unnecessary unless there is a clear history of life-threatening coingestion.
3. Hypotension is best treated initially with **crystalloid IV fluids.** In refractory cases, **norepinephrine** is the vasopressor of choice.

Patients who remain asymptomatic 6 h after ingestion can be medically cleared. Symptomatic patients should be admitted to a monitored setting.

Bupropion

Clinical Features

Adverse effects include dry mouth, nausea, constipation, dizziness, headache, tremor, anxiety, confusion, blurred vision, and increased motor activity. It has been rarely associated with catatonia, hallucinations, psychosis, and paranoia.

Bupropion has a low toxic-to-therapeutic ratio. In acute overdose, toxicity may be seen at doses at or just above the maximum therapeutic dose of 450 mg/day. Findings include mild hyperthermia and hypertension, vomiting, lethargy, confusion, tremor, and seizures. Seizures usually develop within the first 4 h, often without associated signs of toxicity. Sustained-release preparations may cause seizures up to 14 h postingestion. ECG abnormalities include sinus tachycardia and QT-interval prolongation.

Emergency Department Care and Disposition

Seizures should be anticipated in all patients. Significant cardiotoxicity is unlikely except in mixed overdoses.

1. IV access should be established and the patient placed on a cardiac monitor.
2. Early gastric lavage and **activated charcoal** 1 g/kg PO or per NG tube are recommended.
3. Seizures should be controlled with **benzodiazepines** and **phenobarbital.**

Admission to a monitored setting is indicated for patients with sinus tachycardia, lethargy, or seizures. Patients who remain asymptomatic 8 h after ingestion of regular-release bupropion may be medically cleared. Ingestion of more than 450 mg of a sustained-release preparation warrants longer monitoring.

Mirtazapine

Clinical Features

Adverse effects include weight gain and somnolence. Mirtazapine has limited toxicity in acute overdose. The patient may present with sinus tachycardia, mild hypertension, sedation, and confusion. Respiratory depression or coma may be seen at higher doses or when combined with another CNS depressant.

Emergency Department Care and Disposition

Since experience with mirtazapine overdose is limited, early consultation with a poison control center is recommended. Supportive care is usually sufficient. **Activated charcoal** 1 g/kg should be administered. Gastric lavage may be indicated early after large overdoses or with serious coingestion. Symptomatic patients should be admitted to a monitored setting. Patients who remain asymptomatic 8 h postingestion may be medically cleared.

Selective Serotonin Reuptake Inhibitors

Clinical Features

The selective serotonin reuptake inhibitors (SSRIs) have a high toxic-to-therapeutic ratio. The most serious adverse effect is development of serotonin syndrome. Other effects include sedation, headache, insomnia, dizziness, fatigue, tremor, and seizures. Dystonic reactions, akathisia, and parkinsonism have been reported. Other adverse effects include vomiting, diarrhea, increased sweating, blurred vision, priapism, hyponatremia, and hypoglycemia.

In acute overdose, patients may present with sinus tachycardia, hypertension or hypotension, vomiting, diarrhea, mydriasis, sedation, tremor, or seizures. While cardiotoxicity is uncommon, citalopram may cause QRS widening and QT prolongation.

Emergency Department Care and Disposition

Pure SSRI overdoses are rarely associated with serious toxicity. However, the patient should be carefully observed for the development of seizures or serotonin syndrome.

1. All patients should have IV access and cardiac monitoring.
2. **Activated charcoal** 1 g/kg should be administered. Gastric lavage is indicated only in the setting of very large overdoses or mixed ingestions.
3. **Sodium bicarbonate** is used to treat QRS prolongation.

All patients should be observed for 6 h postingestion. Patients who continue to manifest symptoms should be admitted for further monitoring.

Venlafaxine

Clinical Features

Adverse effects are similar to those of SSRIs, including development of serotonin syndrome. Venlafaxine also produces hypertension in daily doses exceeding 225 mg.

In acute overdose, signs and symptoms include tachycardia, hypertension or hypotension, diaphoresis, mydriasis, tremor, CNS depression, and generalized seizures. ECG findings include sinus tachycardia, QRS widening, and QT interval prolongation.

Emergency Department Care and Disposition

Venlafaxine has greater toxicity in overdoses than SSRIs, and onset of symptoms may be precipitous.

1. All patients should have IV access and placed on a cardiac monitor.

2. Early gastric lavage should be strongly considered.
3. **Activated charcoal** 1 g/kg should be administered to all patients.
4. **Benzodiazepines** are the agents of choice for control of seizures.
5. **IV sodium bicarbonate** should be considered for QRS greater than 100 ms.
6. Patients should be observed for 6 h postingestion. Symptomatic patients should be admitted.

Serotonin Syndrome

Serotonin syndrome is a rare, idiosyncratic complication of antidepressant therapy characterized by cognitive impairment and autonomic and neuromuscular dysfunction. It may be caused by any drug or combination of drugs that increases central serotonin transmission. The majority of cases occur at therapeutic drug levels.

Clinical Features

The diagnosis is made on clinical grounds. Cognitive and behavioral findings include confusion, agitation, hallucinations, lethargy, coma, and seizures. Autonomic signs include hyperthermia, tachycardia, hypertension or hypotension, tachypnea, mydriasis, diaphoresis, flushed skin, and diarrhea. Neuromuscular findings include myoclonus, hyperreflexia, tremor, ataxia, nystagmus, opisthotonus, and trismus. Muscle rigidity, especially involving the lower extremities, is a reliable marker.

Emergency Department Care and Disposition

Therapy involves discontinuing all serotoninergic agents and providing supportive care.

1. Antiserotoninergic agents may have a role. Most experience has been with **cyproheptadine** 4 to 8 mg PO repeated in 2 h if no response is noted. Patients who respond are then given 4 mg PO every 6 h for 48 h.
2. **Benzodiazepines** may be used to relieve muscle rigidity and pain.

Patients should be closely monitored for development of acidosis and rhabdomyolysis. All patients should be admitted to the hospital.

MONOAMINE OXIDASE INHIBITORS

Monoamine oxidase inhibitors (MAOIs) have for the most part been replaced by safer antidepressants. However, they are still used for refractory cases. MAOIs decrease clearance of dietary biogenic amines, such as tyramine, and cause accumulation of neurotransmitters in presynaptic nerve terminals. They have a narrow therapeutic index, lead to potentially fatal food and drug interactions, and cause severe toxicity in overdose.

Food Interactions

Tyramine is a dietary amine found in aged meats, cheeses, and red wine. Coingestion with MAOIs results in release of norepinephrine, epinephrine, serotonin, and dopamine.

Clinical Features

Within 90 min of ingestion of tyramine, patients may develop hypertension, diaphoresis, headache, mydriasis, neck stiffness, neuromuscular excitation, palpitations, and chest pain. Symptoms generally resolve within 6 h but deaths, usually due to intracranial hemorrhage or myocardial infarction, have been reported.

Emergency Department Care and Disposition

Care is supportive. An ECG should be obtained on patients with chest pain and a head computed tomography (CT) scan in patients with neurologic findings.

1. **Phentolamine** 2.5 to 5 mg IV every 5 to 15 min or a **nitroprusside** infusion 1 to 4 μg/kg/min are used to treat hypertension.
2. β **blockers** are **contraindicated** due to unopposed α-receptor stimulation.
3. Patients with symptoms 6 h after onset should be admitted to a monitored setting.

Drug Interactions

MAOI use leads to many drug interactions. These include a hyperadrenergic state similar to the tyramine reaction when taken with sympathomimetics (Table 98-1). MAOIs inhibit the clearance of other drugs, including opiates and sedative-hypnotics. Tranylcypromine and phenelzine stimulate insulin secretion, leading to hypoglycemia in patients on sulfonylureas. Finally, serotonin syndrome has been reported, especially when combined with other serotonergic agents, such meperidine and dextromethorphan.

Acute Overdose

Clinical Features

Toxicity develops at doses less than 2 mg/kg. A dose of 4 to 6 mg/kg may be fatal. Signs and symptoms usually develop 6 to 12 h postingestion but may be delayed up to 24 h. Symptoms include

TABLE 98-1 Drugs Contraindicated with MAOIs*

Indirect Sympathomimetics	Miscellaneous Drugs
Benzphetamine	Beta blockers
Bretylium	Bupropion
Cocaine	Buspirone
Dexfenfluramine	Caffeine
Diethylpropion	Carbamazepine
Dopamine	Cyclobenzaprine
Ephedrine	Dextromethorphan
Fenfluramine	Disulfiram
Guanethidine	Ergot alkaloids
Isometheptene	Fentanyl
Mephentermine	Furazolidone
Metaraminol	Ketamine
Methamphetamine	Levodopa (L-dopa)
3,4-methylenedioxymethamphetamine (MDMA)	Lithium
Methyldopa	Meperidine
Methylphenidate	Mirtazapine
Pemoline	Oral hypoglycemic agents
Phentermine	Phenothiazines
Phencyclidine	Procarbazine
Phenylpropanolamine	St. John's wort
Propylhexedrine	Sumatriptan
Pseudoephedrine	Theophylline
Reserpine	Tramadol
Ritodrine	Tricyclic antidepressants
Tyramine	

*See additional list of drugs causing serotonin syndrome in *Emergency Medicine: A Comprehensive Study Guide,* 5th ed., Chap. 153, on newer antidepressants, Table 153-3.

headache, palpitations, nausea, agitation, and tremor. Signs include sinus tachycardia, hyperventilation, hypertension, hyperthermia, chest pain, diaphoresis, mydriasis, nystagmus, hyperreflexia, muscle rigidity, and confusion. Severe toxicity presents with bradycardia, severe hyperthermia, papilledema, seizures, coma, and cardiac arrest. Hypotension is associated with a poor prognosis.

Diagnosis and Differential

The diagnosis is a clinical one. Laboratory tests are used to detect complications such as hypoxia, rhabdomyolysis, renal failure, hyperkalemia, metabolic acidosis, hemolysis, and disseminated intravascular coagulation.

The differential diagnosis for MAOI toxicity includes all causes of a hyperadrenergic state, altered mental status, and muscle rigidity (Table 98-2).

Emergency Department Care and Disposition

Emergency department management involves supportive care and early identification and treatment of complications.

TABLE 98-2 Differential Diagnosis of Monoamine Oxidase Inhibitor Overdose

Intoxications	Medical conditions	Adverse drug reactions
Amphetamines	Heat stroke	Dystonic reactions
Antimuscarinics	Hypoglycemia	Malignant
Cathinone	Hyperthyroidism	hyperthermia
Clonidine (early)	Pheochromocytoma	Serotonin syndrome
Cocaine		Tyramine reaction
Lysergic acid		Spontaneous
diethylamide (LSD)		hypertensive crisis
Methylphenidate		Neuroleptic
MDMA*		malignant syndrome
Nicotine (early)		
Phencyclidine		
Phenylpropanolamine		
Strychnine		
Theophylline		
Tricyclic		
antidepressants (early)		
Withdrawal states	Infectious diseases	Psychiatraic
Ethanol (delirium	Encephalitis	Lethal catatonia
tremens)	Meningitis	
Sedative-hypnotics	Rabies	
Clonidine	Sepsis	
Beta blockers	Tetanus	

*3,4-Methylenedioxymethamphetamine.

1. All patients need IV access, cardiac monitoring, and supplemental oxygen.
2. Gastric lavage within 2 h of significant overdose is recommended.
3. A single dose of **activated charcoal** 1 g/kg should be administered.
4. **Phentolamine** 2.5 to 5 mg IV every 10 to 15 min is used to treat hypertension. **Sodium nitroprusside** starting at 1 μg/kg/min is an effective alternative.
5. Hypotension is treated with **crystalloid IV fluid** boluses of 10 to 20 mL/kg.
6. **Norepinephrine** is the preferred vasopressor in refractory hypotension.
7. **Lidocaine, procainamide,** and **phenytoin** are used to treat dysrhythmias. Bradycardia is treated with **atropine, isoproterenol,** and **dobutamine.**
8. **Benzodiazepines** are the agents of choice for seizure control. **Barbiturates** are alternatives but may precipitate hypotension and respiratory depression.
9. Hyperthermia is managed with cool mist sprays, fans, or ice baths. **Benzodiazepines** may be given to minimize muscle hyperactivity and associated heat production. **Nondepolarizing neuromuscular blockers** or **dantrolene** 0.5 to 2.5 mg IV every 6 h may be required for muscle relaxation in refractory cases.

With few exceptions, all patients with MAOI exposures should be monitored for at least 24 h. All intentional overdoses and accidental exposures of greater than 1 mg/kg should be admitted to an intensive care unit. Others can be admitted to a lower level setting.

ANTIPSYCHOTICS

Antipsychotics are used to manage schizophrenia and other psychoses; for chemical restraint; as antiemetics; and to control hiccups, migraines, and certain involuntary motor disorders. Older agents, referred to as typical antipsychotics, have numerous adverse effects. A new generation of atypical antipsychotics have a greater safety profile.

Clinical Features

Antipsychotics have a high therapeutic index. However, they have adverse effects related to their anticholinergic, antihistaminic, and antiadrenergic properties. They also can cause dystonic reactions, akathisia, bradykinesia, tardive dyskinesia, and neuroleptic malignant syndrome.

In acute overdose, patients present with tachycardia, hypotension, seizures, impaired thermoregulation, and depressed mental status. Cardiac conduction disturbances may develop, ranging from asymptomatic QT prolongation to ventricular dysrhythmias, including torsades de pointes. Fatalities in acute overdose are rare.

Emergency Department Care and Disposition

Management is supportive. All patients require an ECG and continuous cardiac monitoring.

1. Patients with altered mental status should receive **oxygen** and **naloxone,** and their blood glucose level should be determined at bedside.
2. Hypotension is treated with **crystalloid IV fluids.** If vasopressors are required, those with β-adrenergic properties (epinephrine, dopamine, and isoproterenol) should be avoided, since they could exacerbate the hypotension.
3. **Activated charcoal** 1 g/kg should be administered. Gastric lavage may be appropriate early after a large overdose.
4. Ventricular dysrhythmias are treated with class Ib antidysrhythmics (e.g., **lidocaine**); the class Ia agents (quinidine, procainamide, and disopyramide) should be avoided.
5. Seizures may be controlled with **benzodiazepines, phenobarbital,** or **phenytoin.**

Patients with altered mental status or cardiotoxicity should be admitted to an intensive care unit. All patients who have ingested thioridazine or mesoridazine should be monitored for at least 24 h. Other patients may be medically cleared if asymptomatic 6 h postingestion.

LITHIUM

Lithium is used to treat bipolar disorder and other medical and psychiatric conditions. The majority of patients on chronic lithium therapy develop some form of toxicity.

Clinical Features

The most common adverse effects are tremor, polyuria, and rash. Nephrogenic diabetes insipidus and renal tubular acidosis have been reported. Neurologic effects include memory loss, decreased concentration, ataxia, and dysarthria.

Toxicity results from acute or chronic overdose or decreased drug clearance. Patients with renal insufficiency or volume deficiency are at increased risk. In acute overdose, gastrointestinal symptoms are more common and include nausea, vomiting, diarrhea, and abdominal pain. Cardiac abnormalities include hypotension, conduction disturbances, and ventricular dysrhythmias. On

ECG there may be transient ST depression and T-wave inversion. Renal dysfunction is common and includes nephrogenic diabetes insipidus and acute renal failure. CNS findings are more common in chronic overdose and include muscle weakness, fasciculations, tremor, ataxia, lethargy, agitation, seizures, and coma.

Emergency Department Care and Disposition

Initial treatment includes cardiovascular and respiratory stabilization, continuous cardiac monitoring, and baseline laboratory studies and ECG.

1. **Activated charcoal** does not bind lithium but may be indicated for coingestions. Early gastric lavage or whole-bowel irrigation should also be considered.
2. Seizures may be controlled with **benzodiazepines** or **phenobarbital.**
3. **IV normal saline solution** is infused to correct sodium and volume deficits.
4. **Hemodialysis** is used in severe cases to reduce the serum lithium level to less than 1 meq/L. Indications include a level greater than 3.5 meq/L (4.0 meq/L in acute overdose), little change in a level of 1.5 to 3.5 meq/L after 6 h of hydration, an increasing level, renal failure, or ingestion of sustained-release preparations.
5. **Sodium polystyrene sulfonate** 15 g PO qid or 30 g rectally may be useful in clearing lithium in mild to moderate toxicity.

In acute overdose, patients who remain asymptomatic after 6 h may be medically cleared. While serum levels do not correlate well with symptoms, it is recommended that patients with levels greater than 1.5 meq/L be admitted, as should patients who have ingested sustained-release preparations. In chronic toxicity, patients with mild symptoms and no other risk factors may be hydrated for 4 to 6 h and discharged if their levels drop below 1.5 meq/L. Patients with more severe manifestations should be admitted.

For further reading in *Emergency Medicine: A Comprehensive Study Guide,* 5th ed., see Chap. 152, "Tricyclic Antidepressants"; Chap. 153, "Newer Antidepressants and Serotonin Syndrome"; and Chap. 154, "Monoamine Oxidase Inhibitors," by Kirk C. Mills; Chap. 155, "Antipsychotics," by Richard A. Harrigan and William J. Brady; and Chap. 156, "Lithium," by Sandra M. Schneider and Daniel J. Cobaugh.

99 | Sedative-Hypnotics

Keith L. Mausner

The sedative-hypnotics include barbiturates, benzodiazepines, and nonbenzodiazepine drugs such as gamma-hydroxybutyrate (GHB), chloral hydrate, ethchlorvynol, glutethimide, meprobamate, methaqualone, buspirone, and zolpidem. These drugs have numerous applications in anesthesia, neurology, and psychiatry, as well as significant potential for abuse. Overdose, either alone or in combination with other agents, may result in serious morbidity and mortality.

BARBITURATES

Clinical Features

The main effect of barbiturates is depression of activity in nerve and muscle cells. Mild-to-moderate intoxication resembles alcohol intoxication; drowsiness, disinhibition, ataxia, slurred speech, and confusion worsen with increasing dose. Stupor, coma, or complete neurologic unresponsiveness occur with severe intoxication. Respiratory depression and hypothermia may occur and are centrally mediated. Hypotension may occur from decreased vascular tone and venous pooling. Pulse rate is not diagnostic; and pupil size and reactivity, nystagmus, and deep tendon reflexes are variable. Gastrointestinal (GI) motility is slowed, delaying gastric emptying. Hypoglycemia may be seen.

Early death from barbiturate overdose is usually from cardiovascular collapse and respiratory arrest. Complications include aspiration pneumonia, noncardiogenic pulmonary edema, and adult respiratory distress syndrome. Severe poisoning can be assumed if more than 10 times the hypnotic dose is ingested at one time.

Diagnosis and Differential

Barbiturate serum levels may establish the diagnosis and are useful in distinguishing long- from short-acting barbiturates, since the treatment approach is different for each. Long-acting agents include barbital and phenobarbital (duration of action > 6 h). Amobarbital is an intermediate acting agent (3 to 6 h duration). Pentobarbital and secobarbital are short-acting agents (< 3 h duration), and thiopental and methohexital are ultrashort acting, with durations of action of 0.3 h. The differential diagnosis of barbiturate poisoning includes intoxication with other sedative-hypnotics or alcohol, as well as environmental hypothermia and other causes of coma. Barbiturates are more likely to produce coma and myocardial depression than benzodiazepines. Chloral hydrate is associated with cardiac dysrhythmias. Ethchlorvynol may produce a vinyl-like odor and prolonged coma. Glutethimide may cause fluctuating central nervous system (CNS) impairment and anticholinergic signs.

Emergency Department Care and Disposition

1. Emergent priorities remain **airway, breathing, and circulation.** Cardiac monitoring and an intravenous line should be instituted. Bedside glucose determination is indicated for all patients with altered levels of consciousness, as well as consideration of naloxone and thiamine administration. Laboratory studies should include electrolyte, blood urea nitrogen, creatinine, and glucose levels; complete blood cell count; toxicology screen, including acetaminophen to rule out coingestion; electrocardiogram (ECG); and chest x-ray. An arterial blood gas analysis may be useful.

2. Volume expansion with **isotonic saline** is the primary treatment for shock and hypotension. In elderly patients, or those with a history of congestive heart failure or renal failure, 200-mL boluses may be prudent. Dopamine or norepinephrine may be necessary if resuscitation with crystalloid is ineffective.

3. **Activated charcoal** (AC) decreases absorption. The physician should administer 1 to 2 g/kg AC; the addition of a cathartic such as sorbitol also may be beneficial. The airway should be secured first if patients are at significant risk for aspiration. Multiple dose AC every 4 h may decrease serum levels. There is no evidence of any benefit of gastric lavage over AC. Ipecac-induced emesis is potentially dangerous due to CNS depression and risk of aspiration and should be avoided.

4. Forced diuresis with saline and furosemide, titrating urine output to 4 to 6 mL/kg/h, is beneficial in phenobarbital poisoning.

5. **Urinary alkalinization** promotes the excretion of long-acting barbiturates. The physician should administer 1 to 2 meq/kg **sodium bicarbonate** intravenous bolus. Then 100 to 150 meq bicarbonate should be added to 1 L D_5W and the drip rate adjusted to maintain an arterial pH of 7.45 to 7.50, urinary pH of 8.0, and urine output of 2 mL/kg/h. Serum potassium must remain at least 4.0 meq/L for alkalinization to be effective. Electrolytes and effectiveness of therapy should be monitored every 2 to 4 h.

6. **Hemodialysis** and **hemoperfusion** are indicated for patients who deteriorate despite aggressive supportive care.

Close monitoring and documentation of neurologic and vital signs improvement may allow patients with mild-to-moderate toxicity to be discharged to psychiatric care or home. Severe toxicity requires admission, and toxicology consultation is recommended.

Barbiturate abstinence syndrome occurs with abrupt withdrawal in chronic users and produces minor withdrawal symptoms within 24 h and major life-threatening manifestations in 2 to 8 days. Short-acting agents produce more severe withdrawal than do long-acting agents. Clinical manifestations are similar to alcohol withdrawal. Minor findings include anxiety, depression, insomnia, anorexia, nausea, vomiting, muscle twitching, abdominal cramping, and sweating. Severe manifestations include psychosis, hallucinations, delirium, seizures, hyperthermia, and cardiovascular collapse. Treatment consists of aggressive supportive care and intravenous benzodiazepines or barbiturates, with subsequent tapering of dose.

BENZODIAZEPINES

Clinical Features

Isolated benzodiazepine overdose has a relatively low morbidity and mortality; serious toxicity usually occurs with coingestion of other agents or with parenteral administration. Fatal isolated benzodiazepine overdose is more likely with short-acting agents such as triazolam, alprazolam, or temazepam.

The most significant effects of benzodiazepines are on the CNS: drowsiness, dizziness, slurred speech, confusion, and cognitive impairment. Other reported effects include headache, nausea, vomiting, chest pain, arthralgias, diarrhea, and incontinence. Paradoxical reactions are rare but include rage and delirium. Respiratory depression and hypotension are more likely to occur with parenteral administration or with coingestants. The elderly are more susceptible to the adverse effects of benzodiazepines.

Diagnosis and Differential

Toxicology screening may be useful in establishing the diagnosis, but the laboratory may not routinely screen for all available benzodiazepines. It is, therefore, essential to know the laboratory's limitations. Serum benzodiazepine levels are not clinically useful in overdoses. The findings of benzodiazepine toxicity are nonspecific. See preceding section, "Diagnosis and Differential" of barbiturates, for findings that may help distinguish benzodiazepine toxicity from that of the other sedative-hypnotics.

Emergency Department Care and Disposition

1. Emergent priorities remain **airway, breathing, and circulation.** Cardiac monitoring and an intravenous line should be instituted.

Bedside glucose determination is indicated for all patients with altered level of consciousness, as well as consideration of naloxone and thiamine administration. Laboratory tests should include acetaminophen level (to rule out coingestion), toxicology screening, electrolytes, ECG, and other studies as clinically indicated.

2. **Activated charcoal** should be administered (same protocol as earlier for barbiturates).

3. Flumazenil, a benzodiazepine antagonist, is *not* indicated for empiric administration in poisoned patients. Seizures may occur in mixed ingestions, especially involving tricyclic antidepressants, and in patients chronically dependent on benzodiazepines or with underlying seizure disorders. Flumazenil is also contraindicated in suspected elevated intracranial pressure or head injury. Its primary use is in reversing the effects of benzodiazepines administered for diagnostic or therapeutic purposes, and due to its short half-life (approximately 1 h), it is mainly effective with short-acting agents such as midazolam. Flumazenil is administered 0.2 mg IV every minute to response or a total dose of 3 mg.

4. There is no role for forced diuresis or urinary alkalinization.

Care for benzodiazepine ingestions is primarily supportive. Hospital admission is indicated for significant alterations in mental status, respiratory depression, and hypotension. Psychiatric consultation is indicated for intentional overdoses.

Abrupt cessation of benzodiazepines in dependent individuals may produce a withdrawal syndrome similar to alcohol or barbiturate withdrawal. (See the preceding section on barbiturate abstinence syndrome.)

NONBENZODIAZEPINE SEDATIVE-HYPNOTICS

Gamma-Hydroxybutyrate

Gamma-Hydroxybutyrate (GHB) is used abroad as an anesthetic and in the treatment of narcolepsy and substance withdrawal. It has no approved clinical uses in the United States. It has been implicated in substance-induced rape. Effects are dose dependent and range from euphoria, nystagmus, ataxia, and dizziness, to coma, respiratory depression, apnea, seizure-like activity, and bradycardia. GHB toxicity may produce sudden onset of aggressive behavior followed by drowsiness, dizziness, euphoria, or coma, with rapid reawakening and amnesia.

Chloral Hydrate

Toxic doses produce severe CNS, respiratory, and cardiovascular depression, as well as resistant ventricular dysrhythmias, which are the leading cause of mortality in overdose. Clues to ingestion include a combination of a pearlike breath odor, hypotension, and dysrhythmias. It is also a GI irritant and overdose may be associated with GI bleeding. Chloral hydrate is radiopaque and abdominal x-rays may be useful in diagnosis.

Ethchlorvynol

CNS effects of overdose include nystagmus, lethargy, and prolonged coma. Hypothermia, hypotension, bradycardia, and noncardiogenic pulmonary edema may occur. A distinct vinyl-like breath odor may be a clue to diagnosis.

Glutethimide

The manifestations of glutethimide overdose are similar to barbiturate toxicity except for the presence of prominent anticholinergic findings, and a fluctuating, prolonged coma.

Meprobamate

The CNS manifestations of meprobamate toxicity are similar to other sedative-hypnotics. Hypotension is a common feature of serious overdose. Seizures, cardiac dysrhythmias, and pulmonary edema have been reported as well. Prolonged fluctuating coma may occur secondary to continued absorption from GI concretions of the drug.

Methaqualone

Methaqualone has similar CNS, respiratory, and cardiovascular effects to the other sedative hypnotics. However, unlike the others, it also causes hypertonicity, clonus, hyperreflexia, and muscle twitching. It often impairs judgment and impulse control, increasing risk of morbidity and mortality from trauma.

Buspirone

Buspirone is unrelated to the other sedative-hypnotics and does not appear to be addictive. Overdoses of up to 3 g (150 times the average anxiolytic dose) have produced no lasting ill effects. Symptoms of overdose include drowsiness and dysphoria. Rarely described findings include hypotension, bradycardia, seizures, GI upset, dystonia, and priapism. Hypertensive reactions may occur with coadministration of monoamine oxidase inhibitors.

Zolpidem

Zolpidem is used for the treatment of insomnia. Findings in overdose include drowsiness, vomiting, and rarely coma and respiratory depression. Flumazenil may reverse some of the effects of zolpidem, but its use is not recommended in most overdose situations for the reasons outlined in the section on benzodiazepines.

Emergency Department Care and Disposition

1. Emergent priorities remain **airway, breathing, and circulation.** Cardiac monitoring and an intravenous line should be instituted. Bedside glucose determination is indicated for all patients with altered level of consciousness, as well as consideration of naloxone and thiamine administration. Laboratory tests should include acetaminophen level (to rule out coingestion), toxicology screening, electrolytes, ECG, and other studies as clinically indicated. Serum levels are not usually clinically useful except in establishing diagnosis and may guide the decision to treat patients not responding to standard supportive therapy with hemoperfusion, which is more effective than hemodialysis.
2. Treatment for nonbenzodiazepine toxicity is primarily supportive.
3. Chloral hydrate-induced dysrhythmias may respond to **lidocaine** or **β-blockers. Overdrive pacing** may be necessary for ventricular tachycardia. β-adrenergic agents (epinephrine, isoproterenol, and dopamine) may worsen dysrhythmias. If a pressor is needed to treat hypotension, an α-acting agent such as norepinephrine should be used.
4. Because of meprobamate's tendency to form GI concretions, **whole bowel irrigation** using 2 L/h polyethylene glycol (40 mL/kg/h in children) until rectal effluent is clear may be beneficial. Forced diuresis is not useful in these agents due to limited renal excretion.

Most patients with overdoses of these substances should be admitted into the hospital, especially when there is any significant CNS or respiratory depression, hypotension, or dysrhythmias. Glutethimide and meprobamate are of special concern because of the potential for fluctuating or delayed manifestations.

For further reading in *Emergency Medicine: A Comprehensive Study Guide,* 5th ed., see Chap. 157, "Barbiturates," by Raquel M. Schears; Chap. 158, "Benzodiazepines," by George M. Bosse; and Chap. 159, "Nonbenzodiazepine Sedative-Hypnotics," by Raquel M. Schears.

100 | Alcohols
Michael P. Kefer

In discussing the toxicity of common alcohols, an understanding of the osmolal gap is important. The presence of an osmolal gap suggests the presence of a low-molecular-weight substance such as ethanol, isopropanol, methanol, or ethylene glycol.

· The Osmolal gap = Osmol measured − Osmol calculated
· Normal Osmol gap < 10 mosmol/L
· Osmol measured is determined in the laboratory by freezing-point depression.
· Osmol calculated = 2(Na) + BUN/2.8 + glucose/18

ETHANOL

Although acute ethanol intoxication may cause death directly from respiratory depression, morbidity and mortality are usually related to accidental injury from impaired cognitive function. Ethanol intoxication predisposes patients to trauma and complicates evaluation of the injured patient. On average, nondrinkers eliminate ethanol from the bloodstream at a rate of 15 to 20 mg/dL/h, and chronic drinkers at a ratio of 25 to 35 mg/dL/h.

Clinical Features

Signs and symptoms of ethanol intoxication include slurred speech, disinhibited behavior, central nervous system (CNS) depression, and altered coordination. Manifestations of serious head injury may be identical to, or clouded by, ethanol intoxication. Ethanol use is associated with abuse of other elicit drugs.

Emergency Department Care and Disposition

The mainstay of treatment is observation of the patient until clinically sober. A careful physical exam should be performed to evaluate for complicating injury or illness.

1. Hypoglycemia can be excluded by measuring finger-stick glucose levels. *Thiamine 100 mg* **IV** *or* **IM** should be administered. If required, intravenous fluids should contain 5% dextrose, as these patients are often glycogen-depleted.
2. Any deterioration or lack of improvement during observation should be considered secondary to causes other than ethanol

and managed accordingly. The patient can be discharged once intoxication has resolved to the extent that the patient does not pose a threat to self or others. Those who plan to operate a motor vehicle should have ethanol levels approaching 0.

ISOPROPANOL

Isopropanol is commonly found in rubbing alcohol, solvents, skin and hair products, paint thinners, and antifreeze. Its CNS depressant effects are twice as potent and twice as long-lasting as ethanol. Acetone is the principle metabolite.

Clinical Features

Clinically, isopropanol intoxication manifests similar to ethanol intoxication except the duration is longer and the CNS depressant effects are more profound. The smell of rubbing alcohol may be noted on the patient's breath. Severe poisoning is marked by early-onset coma, respiratory depression, and hypotension. Hemorrhagic gastritis is a characteristic finding, causing nausea, vomiting, and abdominal pain. Upper gastrointestinal (GI) bleeding may be severe. Other, less common complications include hepatic dysfunction, acute tubular necrosis, and rhabdomyolysis.

Laboratory investigation reveals ketonemia and ketonuria from the accumulation of acetone, without hyperglycemia or glycosuria. Mild acidosis may be present from acetone metabolism to acetate and formate.

Diagnosis and Differential

Diagnosis is based on clinical presentation and laboratory findings of ketonemia and ketonuria and an osmolal gap with or without a minimal metabolic acidosis. Diagnosis is confirmed by an elevated isopropanol level. Isopropanol intoxication is characteristically distinguished from that of other common alcohols by the significant osmolal gap without a significant anion gap metabolic acidosis and a negative ethanol level.

Emergency Department Care and Disposition

1. General supportive measures are indicated. As with any patient who has altered mental status, administration of glucose, thiamine, and naloxone should be considered. Laboratory evaluation includes levels of serum electrolytes, blood urea nitrogen (BUN), creatinine, glucose, and acetone. An isopropanol level is used mainly to confirm the diagnosis; it does not usually

influence management. Charcoal does not bind alcohols, so it is useful only if there is coingestion of an absorbable substance.
2. Hypotension usually responds to intravenous fluids. Severe hemorrhagic gastritis may require transfusion.
3. Hemodialysis is indicated for refractory hypotension or when the predicted peak level of isopropanol is >400 mg/dL. Hemodialysis removes both isopropanol and acetone.

Patients with prolonged CNS depression require admission. Those who are asymptomatic after 6 to 8 h of observation can be discharged or referred for psychiatric evaluation if indicated.

METHANOL AND ETHYLENE GLYCOL

Methanol (wood alcohol) is commonly found as a solvent in paint products, windshield-washing fluids, and antifreeze. Ethylene glycol is commonly used as a coolant and preservative and is found in polishes and detergents. Toxicity from these alcohols is due to formation of their toxic metabolites, which results in a high anion gap metabolic acidosis ($Na - [Cl + HCO_3] > 12 + 4$ mEq/L). Prognosis is related to the severity of the acidosis.

Clinical Features of Methanol

Methanol metabolism results in formation of formaldehyde and formic acid. Symptoms may not appear for 12 to 18 h after ingestion because these toxic metabolites must accumulate. Time or symptom onset may be longer if ethanol is consumed, as ethanol inhibits methanol metabolism.

Symptoms include CNS depression, visual disturbances (classically the patient complains of looking at a snowstorm), abdominal pain, nausea, and vomiting. The GI symptoms may be due to mucosal irritation or pancreatitis. On examination, CNS signs can vary from lethargy to coma. Fundoscopic exam may show retinal edema or hyperemia of the optic disk.

Laboratory investigation reveals a high anion gap metabolic acidosis with a high osmolal gap.

Clinical Features of Ethylene Glycol

Ethylene glycol poisoning often exhibits three distinct clinical phases after ingestion due to the toxic metabolites. First, within 12 h, CNS effects predominate. The patient appears intoxicated without the odor of ethanol on the breath. Second, 12 to 24 h after ingestion, cardiopulmonary effects predominate. Elevated heart and respiratory rate and blood pressure are common. Chronic heart failure, respiratory distress syndrome, and circulatory collapse are also noted. Third, 24 to 72 h after ingestion, renal effects predominate. Flank pain with costovertebral angle tenderness is noted. Acute tubular necrosis with acute renal failure occurs if appropriate treatment is not received.

Hypocalcemia may result from precipitation of calcium oxalate into tissues and may be severe enough to cause tetany and typical changes on the electrocardiogram. Calcium oxalate crystals are noted on urinalysis. Elevated creatine phosphokinase levels may be seen.

Diagnosis and Differential

The diagnosis of toxicity is based on the clinical presentation and laboratory findings of a high anion gap metabolic acidosis and a high osmolal gap. The diagnosis may be confirmed by elevated levels of methanol or ethylene glycol.

The differential diagnosis includes other causes of an anion gap metabolic acidosis, recalled by the acronym MUDPILES (see Table 126-1). Ethylene glycol poisoning differs from methanol poisoning in that visual disturbances and fundoscopic abnormalities are absent and calcium oxalate crystals are present in the urine.

Basic laboratory investigation includes a complete blood cell count; serum electrolytes, BUN, and creatinine levels, urinalysis, and levels of calcium, magnesium, ethanol, isopropanol, methanol, and ethylene glycol.

Emergency Department Care and Disposition

Treatment is based on preventing formation of the toxic metabolites and removing them from the body. General supportive measures are indicated including the administration of glucose, thiamine, and naloxone in the patient with altered mental status.

1. Charcoal does not bind the alcohols and is useful only if these is coingestion of an absorbable substance. Bicarbonate is administered to correct acidosis; large amounts may be required.
2. **Fomepazole 15 mg/kg intravenous load followed by 20 mg/kg every 12 h** for 4 doses is now favored over ethanol as the treatment of choice for ethylene glycol toxicity. It has been used for methanol poisoning but has not been FDA approved. Fomepazole is a potent inhibitor of alcohol dehydrogenase with 8000 times greater affinity than ethanol and with less side effects. Indications for fomepazole administration include strong clinical suspicion of ethylene glycol poisoning, ethylene glycol level >20 mg/dL, or presence of acidosis. Treatment with fomepazole does not affect indications for dialysis.

3. If fomepazole is not available, **ethanol** should be administered. Ethanol competitively inhibits metabolism of methanol and ethylene glycol by alcohol dehydrogenase. Because ethanol has 10 to 20 times greater affinity for alcohol dehydrogenase than methanol and 100 times that of ethylene glycol, formation of toxic metabolites is inhibited. Indications for ethanol treatment are the following: (a) suspected methanol or ethylene glycol poisoning; (b) the presence of an anion gap metabolic acidosis with an osmolal gap; (c) a methanol or ethylene glycol level >20 mg/dL; and (d) any patient requiring hemodialysis. Ethanol 0.6 g/kg intravenously should be administered as a loading dose, followed by a maintenance dose of 0.11 g/kg/h in the average drinker and 0.15 g/kg/h in the heavy drinker. The maintenance infusion is adjusted accordingly to keep the blood ethanol level at 100 to 150 mg/dL.

   If necessary, oral therapy with commercial alcoholic beverages can be initiated. The amount of ethanol contained in these is calculated by grams ethanol = mL beverage × 0.9 × (proof/200).

   Ethanol administration is continued until the methanol or ethylene glycol level is 0 and the acidosis has resolved. Hypoglycemia may be induced, especially in children.

4. **Dialysis** eliminates both methanol and ethylene glycol and their toxic metabolites. Indications for dialysis are the following: (a) signs or symptoms of significant toxicity; (b) methanol or ethylene glycol level > 20 to 25 mg/dL; (c) presence of a metabolic acidosis; and (d) signs of nephrotoxicity in ethylene glycol poisoning. Peritoneal dialysis is considered only when hemodialysis is not available.

   During dialysis, since ethanol is dialyzable, the maintenance rate of ethanol will need to be increased (doubled initially) and readjusted accordingly to maintain a blood alcohol level of 100 to 150 mg/dL. Dialysis and ethanol are continued until methanol and ethylene glycol levels are 0 and acidosis has resolved.

5. Vitamin therapy is thought to play an important role in treatment as well. In methanol poisoning, folate is a cofactor for the conversion of formic acid to carbon dioxide; therefore, **folate 50 mg IV should be administered every 4 h.** In ethylene glycol poisoning, pyridoxine and thiamine are cofactors for the conversion of toxic metabolites to nontoxic compounds. Therefore, **thiamine and pyridoxine 100 mg IV or intramuscularly should be administered every day.**

Any patient with serious signs or symptoms of toxicity should be admitted to the intensive care unit at a facility with hemodialysis capabilities. Asymptomatic individuals should be admitted for observation because of possible delayed onset of toxic symptoms.

For further reading in *Emergency Medicine: A Comprehensive Study Guide,* 5th ed., see Chap. 160, "Alcohols," by William A. Berk and Wilma V. Henderson.

---

101 | Drugs of Abuse
Judith A. Linden

Commonly abused psychoactive drugs include narcotics, cocaine, amphetamine-like drugs, and hallucinogens. While patients who ingest a single drug often present with typical signs and symptoms, multiple drug ingestions may confound the clinical picture. Withdrawal syndromes may be present with certain classes of drugs (i.e., opiates, cocaine, and amphetamines).

Opioids (Narcotics)

The most commonly available opiates are heroin, methadone, meperidine, morphine, codeine, oxycodone, hydrocodone, and hydromorphone. The classic triad of clinical features is miosis, respiratory depression, and depressed mental status. Other signs and symptoms include needle track marks, hypotension, ileus, nausea, vomiting, and occasionally non-cardiogenic pulmonary edema (NCPE). Propoxyphene may be associated with cardiac toxicity (ventricular dysrhythmias, bradydysrhythmias, and prolonged QT-syndrome) and seizures. Meperidine may cause seizures, which are unresponsive to naloxone therapy. The combination of meperidine or dextromethorphan with monoamine oxidase inhibitors (MAOIs) can precipitate serotonin syndrome (hyperthermia, confusion, muscular rigidity, and hypotension or hypertension). Opiate withdrawal is characterized by flu-like symptoms (myalgias, lacrimation, piloerection, yawning, abdominal cramping, vomiting, diarrhea, anxiety, and insomnia).

Treatment is primarily supportive. If respiratory or mental status depression is present, administer a naloxone (Narcan) test dose of 0.2 to 0.5 mg intravenously (IV), intramuscularly (IM), or by endotracheal tube. A test dose decreases the risk of violent withdrawal symptoms and agitation. Administer a larger dose of 2 mg IV as needed. Some opiates (e.g., fentanyl and propoxyphene) require larger doses of naloxone. The half-life of naloxone is 1 h, and it has a 2- to 3-h duration of action. Naloxone IV drip 2 mg/500 mL 5% dextrose in water (D_5W) may be administered at 0.4 mg/h if a longer-acting opiate (e.g., methadone or propoxyphene) has been ingested. NCPE may occur up to 24 h after serious heroin and methadone overdoses. Treatment is supportive (oxygen and respiratory support with positive end-expiratory pressure). Lasix and naloxone are ineffective.

Patients with severe toxicity, as manifested by initial respiratory arrest, pulmonary edema, persistent respiratory depression, or persistent hypotension, should be admitted. Patients who have overdosed on longer-acting drugs (e.g., meperidine, methadone, or propoxyphene) should be admitted. Most opiate overdoses can be managed by observing the patient for 4 to 8 h in the emergency department. Treatment of opiate withdrawal is supportive and with oral clonidine 0.1 to 0.2 mg.

Cocaine and Amphetamines

Cocaine intoxication presents with signs of adrenergic stimulation (tachycardia, tachypnea, hypertension, anxiety, diaphoresis, and hyperthermia). Common presenting symptoms include chest pain, abdominal pain, palpitations, shortness of breath, and headache. Psychiatric symptoms, such as paranoia, mania, agitation, and coma, may be present. Complications of cocaine use include myocardial, mesenteric, spinal cord, and cerebral ischemia or infarction; myocarditis; aortic dissection; seizure; stroke; pneumomediastinum; and rhabdomyolysis. Cocaine withdrawal symptoms include irritability and depression.

Amphetamines include illicit drugs such as methamphetamine (speed), MDMA (ecstasy), and methcathinone (ice). Over-the-counter medications, such as phenylpropanolamine and pseudoephedrine, may produce similar symptoms. Signs and symptoms of acute amphetamine intoxication are tachycardia, mydriasis, hypertension, hyperthermia, anxiety, restlessness, repetitive behavior, and paranoid psychosis. Complications include seizures and malignant hyperthermia. Amphetamine withdrawal symptoms include lethargy, depression, increased appetite, abdominal cramps, diarrhea, headache, and chills.

The treatments of cocaine and amphetamine toxicity are similar. Patients should be placed in a quiet room with dim lighting. They should undergo continuous cardiac monitoring and have IV access established. They should be administered lorazepam 1 to 2 mg IV or diazepam 2.5 to 5 mg IV titrated for adequate sedation. The initial treatment of choice for severe hypertension is benzodiazepines. If ineffective, nitroprusside 0.5 to 10 μg/kg/min IV or phentolamine 5 mg IV should be initiated. β blockers should not be administered because they can result in worsening hypertension secondary to unopposed alpha stimulation.

For patients who present with chest pain, an electrocardiogram (ECG) and chest radiograph should be obtained. The patient should be administered oxygen, benzodiazepines, and sublingual nitroglycerin. Seizures should be treated in standard fashion.

For patients who are psychotic, IV benzodiazepines or droperidol 2.5 to 5 mg IV are helpful. Hyperthermia should be treated in standard fashion. The efficacy of dantrolene 1 mg/kg, repeated if necessary to a maximum of 10 mg/kg, is controversial, but it may be used if other cooling measures fail. Patients who appear toxic or have unstable vital signs, mental status changes, persistent chest pain, ECG changes consistent with ischemia, or prolonged seizures should be admitted.

Body stuffers are patients who ingest poorly packaged drugs to destroy evidence. They should be treated with activated charcoal 1 g/kg or 50 g and observed for 6 to 8 h. Body packers are individuals who ingest large amounts of well-packed drugs for smuggling. They should be treated with whole-bowel irrigation (PEG or GOLYTELY) and admitted until the packets have passed. If there are signs of toxicity or bowel obstruction, surgical consultation is indicated.

Hallucinogens

Hallucinogens, which include lysergic acid diethylamide (LSD), phencyclidine (PCP), mescaline, certain mushrooms, anticholinergics, and some amphetamines, have the effect of creating a sensory experience that does not exist outside the mind. The hallucinations may be visual, auditory, or tactile. Clinical features and complications of intoxication are listed in Table 101-1. Other causes of hallucinations, such as hypoglycemia, drug and alcohol withdrawal, and infection, should be considered.

Treatment is primarily supportive, with quiet surroundings and benzodiazepines as needed for agitation. Droperidol 2.5 to 5.0 mg IV may be administered for extreme agitation. Multiple dose activated charcoal every 6 h is recommended for PCP intoxication.

TABLE 101-1 Clinical Features of Hallucinogens

Drug	Clinical features	Complications
PCP	Mild: vertical nystagmus, ataxia, emotional lability, violence Moderate: muscular rigidity, hypertension, tachycardia Severe: coma, hyperpyrexia	Seizures, muscular rigidity, rhabdomyolysis hyperthermia, flashbacks
LSD	Paranoia, anxiety, psychosis, mydriasis	Flashbacks, traumatic injuries
Peyote (mescaline)	Nausea and vomiting, abdominal pain, diaphoresis, headache	Rare
Hallucinogenic amphetamines	Excitement, confusion, anorexia	Muscular rigidity, seizures, coma, intracranial hemorrhage, hyperthermia, rhabdomyolysis vasculitis
Anticholinergics	Agitation, tachycardia, mydriasis, urinary retention, ileus	Supraventricular tachycardia, hypertension, seizures, hyperthermia
Marijuana	Euphoria, relaxation, decreased motor performance, paranoia, conjunctival injection	Rare
Nutmeg	Nausea and vomiting, mydriasis, abdominal pain, delirium, stupor	Rare

Note: Hallucinations may be present with all of the drugs listed.

Patients should be admitted for hyperthermia, cardiovascular instability, seizures, rhabdomyolysis, or metabolic abnormalities. Asymptomatic patients may be discharged after a short observation period. Patients with mild to moderate ingestions should be observed in the emergency department for 4 to 8 h.

GAMMA-HYDROXYBUTYRIC ACID

Gamma-hydroxybutyric acid (GHBA) is abused by weightlifters, ingested with alcohol, or utilized to drug a sexual assault victim.

Clinical features include agitation, hallucinations, seizures, coma, miosis, drowsiness, vomiting, dizziness, and hypotonia. Treatment is supportive, with most symptoms resolving in 2 to 8 h. Patients are often amnestic to events surrounding the ingestion. GHBA ingestion should be suspected in a patient who loses consciousness after minimal alcohol or drug intake, especially sexual assault victims.

In general, helpful laboratory tests for patients who have abused any of the abovementioned drugs include a serum glucose level, acetaminophen level, chemistry panel, creatine phosphokinase determination, and serum or urine toxicologic screening. Coagulation tests and liver enzyme tests should be ordered for hyperthermic patients. If GHBA ingestion is suspected, Hoffmann-LaRoche offers free drug testing (call 800-608-6540).

For further reading in *Emergency Medicine: A Comprehensive Study Guide,* 5th ed., see Chap. 161, "Opioids," by Suzanne Doyon; Chap. 162, "Stimulants, Cocaine, and Amphetamines," by Jeanmarie Perrone and Robert S. Hoffman; and Chap. 163, "Hallucinogens," by Karen N. Hansen.

---

102 | Analgesics
Keith L. Mausner

Salicylate and acetaminophen overdoses are potentially life-threatening and must be rapidly identified and treated. Nonsteroidal anti-inflammatory drug (NSAID) overdoses are rarely fatal and usually require only supportive care.

SALICYLATES

Clinical Features

The clinical manifestations of salicylate toxicity depend on the dose, whether exposure is acute or chronic, and the patient's age. Acute ingestion of less than 150 mg/kg usually produces mild toxicity with nausea, vomiting, and gastrointestinal (GI) irritation.

Acute ingestion of 150 to 300 mg/kg usually results in moderate toxicity with vomiting, hyperventilation, sweating, and tinnitus. In adults, these findings often coincide with salicylate levels about 30 mg/dL. There is usually a combined respiratory alkalosis and increased anion gap metabolic acidosis. However, coingestion of sedative drugs may impair the respiratory drive and result in respiratory acidosis.

Toxicity from ingestion of more than 300 mg/kg is usually severe. Uncommon manifestations of severe acute salicylate toxicity include fever, neurologic dysfunction, renal failure, pulmonary edema, and adult respiratory distress syndrome (ARDS). Rarely, rhabdomyolysis, gastric perforation, and GI hemorrhage occur. Fatality is more likely with advanced age. Unconsciousness, fever, severe acidosis, seizures, and dysrhythmias are also associated with increased mortality risk.

In children, acute salicylate overdoses generally present within a few hours of ingestion. Children under age 4 tend to develop metabolic acidosis (pH < 7.38), whereas children over age 4 usually have mixed acid-base disturbance as in adults.

Chronic salicylate toxicity (associated with long-term therapeutic use) is usually seen in elderly patients with underlying medical problems. It may present with hyperventilation, tremor, papilledema, agitation, paranoia, bizarre behavior, memory loss, confusion, and stupor. Chronic salicylism should be considered in any patient with unexplained nonfocal neurologic and behavioral abnormalities, especially with coexisting acid-base disturbance, tachypnea, dyspnea, or noncardiogenic pulmonary edema.

In children, chronic (repeated dose) salicylate toxicity is usually more serious than acute toxicity, and more likely to be lethal. It may take several days for symptoms to appear, and there may be an underlying illness that triggered the salicylate administration. Chronic salicylism may be mistaken for an infectious process. Children have hyperventilation, volume depletion, acidosis, marked hypokalemia, and central nervous system (CNS) disturbances. Fever indicates a worse prognosis. Renal failure is a severe complication. Pulmonary edema is rare in pediatric patients.

Additional significant laboratory abnormalities may occur in salicylism. Hypo- or hyperglycemia may be seen with severe acute or chronic toxicity. Elevated prothrombin time (PT) may occur in severe chronic toxicity.

Diagnosis and Differential

Clinical status is the key to diagnosis and treatment. Salicylate levels should be interpreted cautiously; severe toxicity may be present despite a "therapeutic" or declining level. The use of the Done nomogram, which was developed to predict toxicity after acute ingestion within a known time frame, may be misleading and is *not* recommended.

The differential diagnosis of salicylate toxicity includes theophylline toxicity, caffeine overdose, acute iron poisoning, Reye's syndrome, diabetic ketoacidosis, sepsis, and meningitis.

Emergency Department Care and Disposition

1. Emergent priorities remain **airway, breathing, and circulation.** Cardiac monitoring and an intravenous line should be instituted. Bedside glucose determination is indicated for altered level of consciousness or seizures. Laboratory studies should include electrolyte, glucose, blood urea nitrogen (BUN), and creatinine levels; complete blood cell count (CBC); PT; salicylate level; and acetaminophen level (to rule out coingestion), as well as an arterial blood gas analysis to determine acid-base status.

2. **Activated charcoal (AC)** 1 g/kg should be administered to minimize absorption and hasten elimination. Multiple doses are probably not beneficial. **Whole bowel irrigation** may be effective when toxicity is due to sustained release or enteric coated aspirin.

3. IV normal saline should be administered to patients with evidence of volume depletion. Except for the initial saline resuscitation, all subsequent fluids should contain at least 5% dextrose. Never administer plain 5% dextrose to children.

4. **Alkalinization of the serum and urine** enhances salicylate protein binding and urinary elimination. This may be accomplished with a second IV line concurrent with volume resuscitation. The physician should administer a bolus of 1 to 2 meq/kg of sodium bicarbonate. Then 100 to 150 meq (2 to 3 ampules) of sodium bicarbonate should be added to 1 L D_5W and infused at 1.5 to 2.0 times the patient's maintenance rate; adjust the infusion to maintain urine pH above 7.5. After urine output is established, administer 40 meq/L of potassium. Closely monitor serum electrolyte levels and volume status. Alkalinization decreases the serum potassium level; furthermore, alkalinization cannot be maintained unless the serum potassium level is at least 4.0 meq/L.

5. **Hemodialysis** is indicated for clinical deterioration despite supportive care and alkalinization, renal insufficiency or failure, severe acid-base disturbance, altered mental status, or ARDS.

6. Hemorrhage due to elevated PT is rarely seen, but may be treated with **fresh frozen plasma** and **vitamin K.**

7. Dysrhythmias should be treated by correcting metabolic abnormalities and with standard antidysrhythmics.

In significant ingestions, patients should be serially examined and salicylate levels checked every 2 h until the peak occurs, then every 4 to 6 h until the level is nontoxic. In severe ingestions, hourly levels correlated with clinical status are indicated. Except with ingestion of enteric-coated or sustained-release formulations (see later), patients may be discharged from the emergency department (ED) if there is progressive clinical improvement, no significant acid-base abnormality, and a decline in serial salicylate levels toward the therapeutic range. In deliberate overdoses, a psychiatric consultation should be obtained prior to discharge.

With enteric-coated and sustained-release salicylates, peak serum levels may not occur until 10 to 60 h after ingestion. In potentially large ingestions, admit and observe patients for at least 24 h to assure declining serial salicylate levels and improving clinical status. Enteric-coated aspirin may be visible on plain radiographs; however, a negative x-ray does not rule it out.

ACETAMINOPHEN

Clinical Features

Acute acetaminophen toxicity presents in four stages:

1. During the first day, patients may be asymptomatic or have nonspecific symptoms such as anorexia, nausea, vomiting, and malaise.
2. On days 2 to 3, nausea and vomiting may improve, but evidence of hepatotoxicity, such as right upper quadrant pain and tenderness with elevated transaminases and bilirubin, may be present.
3. On days 3 to 4, there may be progression to fulminant hepatic failure with lactic acidosis, coagulopathy, renal failure, and encephalopathy, as well as recurrent nausea and vomiting.
4. Those who survive hepatic failure will begin to recover over the next weeks with complete resolution of hepatic dysfunction.

Diagnosis and Differential

Acetaminophen toxicity may occur with acute ingestion of more than 140 mg/kg, or when more than 7.5 g are ingested by an adult in a 24-h period. The diagnosis of a significant ingestion depends on laboratory testing, since symptoms may initially be absent or nonspecific. An acetaminophen level should be measured in all patients presenting with any drug overdose, since acetaminophen is a common coingestant.

In a single large overdose, the Rumack-Matthew nomogram (Fig. 102-1) accurately predicts acetaminophen toxicity based on the serum acetaminophen level measured 4 to 24 h after the estimated time of ingestion. The nomogram is not useful outside of this 4- to 24-h window. A 4-h level greater than 150 μg/dL is usually toxic. After 24 h, a detectable acetaminophen level or the presence or elevated transaminases may predict toxicity.

When multiple ingestions have occurred over a period of time, assessment is problematic. One approach is to assume a single ingestion at the earliest possible point in time and use the Rumack-Matthew nomogram accordingly.

Clinical experience with Tylenol Extended Relief (Tylenol ER) ingestion is limited. Because of possible delayed peak serum levels, one approach is to add 2 h to the time from ingestion. Thus, at 4-h postingestion, the nomogram should be interpreted as if it were 6-h postingestion.

Time (hours post-ingestion)

FIG. 102-1. Rumack-Matthew nomogram. *Abbreviation: APAP, N-acetyl-p-aminophenol (acetaminophen).* (From Rumack BH, Matthew H: Acetaminophen poisoning and toxicity. *Pediatrics* 55:871, 1975, with permission.)

The differential diagnosis of acetaminophen toxicity includes viral and alcoholic hepatitis, other drug- or toxin-induced hepatitides, and hepatobiliary disease. Acute acetaminophen poisoning can often be distinguished from other forms of hepatitis by its acute onset, rapid progression, and markedly elevated transaminase levels.

Emergency Department Care and Disposition

1. Emergent priorities remain **airway, breathing, and circulation.** An acetaminophen level, drawn as soon as possible within 4 to 24 h of ingestion, will guide subsequent therapy and disposition. Other laboratory studies, including electrolyte, glucose, BUN, creatinine, and transaminases levels, CBC, and PT, should be drawn if clinically indicated or if the acetaminophen level falls in the toxic range on the Rumack-Matthew nomogram.
2. **Activated charcoal** 1 g/kg is indicated for GI decontamination and in case of coingestion of other drugs.
3. **N-acetylcysteine (NAC)** is the specific antidote. It effectively prevents toxicity if administered within 8 h of ingestion, significantly reduces hepatotoxicity if administered within 24 h of ingestion, and may be of value even after 24 h. If the acetaminophen level is not going to be available within 8 h of ingestion, NAC therapy should be initiated and continued if indicated based on the subsequent acetaminophen level.
4. NAC is administered orally or by nasogastric tube as a 140 mg/kg loading dose, followed by 70 mg/kg every 4 h for 17 additional doses. NAC may be administered immediately after activated charcoal; there is no evidence that this decreases NAC's effectiveness. NAC is safe in pregnancy.
5. Nausea and vomiting during NAC therapy may be reduced by diluting NAC in a beverage, and by administration of antiemetics such as metoclopramide or ondansetron.
6. IV NAC therapy is not approved in the United States, but may be used in consultation with a toxicologist for patients unable to tolerate or receive oral therapy.
7. Treatment of fulminant hepatic failure includes NAC therapy, correction of coagulopathy and acidosis, treatment of cerebral edema, and early referral to a liver transplant center.

Patients with nontoxic acetaminophen levels based on the Rumack-Matthew nomogram may be discharged from the ED if there is no evidence of other drug ingestion. In deliberate overdoses, a psychiatric evaluation should be obtained prior to discharge. All patients receiving NAC therapy should be admitted.

NONSTEROIDAL ANTI-INFLAMMATORY DRUGS

Clinical Features

Chronic NSAID toxicity associated with therapeutic use is more common than acute overdose. The most frequent problems are GI bleeding and renal insufficiency. CNS effects such as headache, mental status changes, and aseptic meningitis may be seen. Pulmonary manifestations such as bronchospasm and pneumonitis have been reported. Hepatic dysfunction may occur, especially in the elderly and in patients with autoimmune disease. Inhibition of platelet aggregation may lead to bleeding. Bone marrow suppression, including aplastic anemia, has been reported. In addition, NSAIDs account for approximately 10 percent of cutaneous drug reactions, ranging from benign rashes, to phototoxic reactions, to severe Stevens-Johnson's syndrome and toxic epidermal necrolysis. Fetal NSAID exposure may lead to premature closure of the ductus arteriosus, oligohydramnios, renal dysfunction, necrotizing enterocolitis, and CNS hemorrhage.

Acute NSAID overdose generally has low morbidity and usually becomes clinically apparent within 4 h of ingestion. Abdominal pain, nausea, and vomiting may occur. CNS manifestations include altered mental status, diplopia, nystagmus, headache, and rarely seizures. Hypotension and bradydysrhythmias have been reported. Renal failure may occur, with serum electrolyte abnormalities and volume overload.

Diagnosis and Differential

The manifestations of NSAID toxicity are nonspecific. NSAID levels are not readily available and are not clinically useful in assessing toxicity. Acetaminophen and salicylate levels will exclude coingestion of these agents.

Emergency Department Care and Disposition

1. Emergent priorities remain **airway, breathing, and circulation.** Laboratory evaluation should include electrolyte and glucose levels, renal and hepatic function, acetaminophen level, salicylate level, and CBC. Bedside glucose determination is indicated for altered mental status or seizures.
2. **Activated charcoal** 1 g/kg is indicated for GI decontamination.
3. **Volume resuscitation,** correction of acid-base and electrolyte disorders, and standard treatment of other complications such as seizures and renal failure are performed as indicated.

Patients with asymptomatic NSAID ingestions may be safely discharged from the ED after screening for coingestants and a 4- to 6-h observation period. In deliberate overdoses, a psychiatric consultation should be obtained prior to discharge.

For further reading in *Emergency Medicine: A Comprehensive Study Guide,* 5th ed. see, Chap. 164, "Salicylates," by Luke Yip and Richard C. Dart; Chap. 165, "Acetaminophen," by Oliver Hung and Lewis S. Nelson; and Chap. 166, "Nonsteroidal Anti-Inflammatory Drugs," by G. Richard Bruno and Wallace A. Carter.

---

103 | Xanthines

Mark B. Rogers

Theophylline and caffeine are the two most common xanthines. Caffeine is thought to be the most widely used drug worldwide.

Clinical Features

Theophylline toxicity can cause life-threatening cardiac, neurologic, and metabolic abnormalities. Even therapeutic levels of theophylline can cause significant side effects. Elderly patients with concomitant medical problems are more susceptible to life-threatening toxicity after chronic overmedication than younger patients after an acute overdose.

Cardiac side effects include sinus tachycardia, premature atrial contractions, atrial flutter, and atrial fibrillation. Premature ventricular contractions and ventricular tachycardia are seen, particularly in the elderly with chronic overdoses and levels of 40 to 60 μg/mL. Younger patients with acute ingestions may tolerate levels above 100 μg/mL. Hypotension may occur.

Neurologic side effects include agitation, headache, irritability, sleeplessness, tremors, and seizures. Seizures are seen in those with high serum levels and in those with a history of epilepsy. Hallucinations and psychosis may be seen.

Metabolic side effects include an increase in catecholamine, glucose, free fatty acid, and insulin levels. Hypokalemia may occur and be worsened by β-agonist therapy. Gastrointestinal (GI) side effects commonly include nausea and vomiting. GI bleeding and epigastric pain may occur.

Caffeine produces many of the same toxic effects as theophylline. Paroxysmal atrial tachycardia may occur but ventricular dysrhythmias are rare except for premature ventricular contractions. Central nervous system effects include agitation, seizures, and coma. GI effects include abdominal pain, nausea, and vomiting. Metabolic effects include rhabdomyolysis, hyperglycemia, leukocytosis, and metabolic acidosis.

Diagnosis and Differential

Therapeutic serum theophylline levels of 10 to 20 μg/mL may produce toxic effects. It is a common misnomer that the severity of symptoms is dependent on the serum level. Life-threatening effects may occur with little warning and before minor symptoms are evident. Theophylline's half-life is increased by smoking cessation, disease states such as congestive heart failure and chronic obstructive pulmonary disease, and medications such as cimetidine and erythromycin. With caffeine, toxicity is seen after 1 g doses in adults and 80 mg/kg in children.

Emergency Department Care and Disposition

The treatment of xanthine toxicity consists of initial stabilization, gastric decontamination and elimination, treatment of life-threatening toxic effects, and, in severe cases, hemoperfusion or dialysis. Patients should be observed on a cardiac monitor, noninvasive blood pressure device, and pulse oximeter. An intravenous line should be inserted.

1. **Gastric lavage** should be considered for acute ingestions of toxic doses within 2 to 4 h. Ipecac should not be used.
2. Multiple doses of oral **activated charcoal** (1 g/kg), mixed with a cathartic such as sorbitol, should be administered every 2 to 4 h in the first 24 h.
3. **Ranitidine** (50 mg IV) is useful for the nausea and vomiting associated with toxicity.

TABLE 103-1 Indications for Hemoperfusion Use

Clinical conditions	Recommendation
Life-threatening toxicity (i.e., seizures, tachydysrhythmias) not responsive to other therapy	Hemoperfusion or dialysis indicated
Acute overdose with level > 100 μg/mL	Hemoperfusion or dialysis possibly indicated
Chronic overdose with level > 60 μg/mL	Hemoperfusion or dialysis possibly indicated
Elderly patient with prolonged half-life, severe liver or severe cardiac disease, or level > 40 μg/mL	Hemoperfusion or dialysis controversial
Theophylline level < 30 μg/mL	Hemoperfusion or dialysis not indicated

4. Seizure activity may be treated with diazepam, phenobarbital, or phenytoin.
5. Hypotension initially should be treated with IV isotonic crystalloid. In patients unresponsive to IV fluids or who have life-threatening dysrhythmias, medications with a beta-blocker effect, such as labetalol or esmolol, may be cautiously administered. Diltiazem, lidocaine, phenytoin, and digoxin have been effective. Adenosine for supraventricular tachycardia may induce bronchospasm. Hypokalemia should be considered and treated.

Patients with seizures or ventricular dysrhythmias should be monitored until their levels normalize. Patients with mild symptoms or levels below 25 μg/mL do not require specific treatment or admission but their medication dosing should be decreased or discontinued. Patients with levels above 30 μg/mL should be treated with oral activated charcoal and monitored for toxic side effects. Indications for hemoperfusion and dialysis are listed in Table 103-1.

For further reading in *Emergency Medicine: A Comprehensive Study Guide,* 5th ed., see Chap. 167, "Xanthines," by Daniel J. Kranitz and Charles L. Emerman.

104 Cardiac Medications

C. Crawford Mechem

DIGITALIS GLYCOSIDES

Digitalis glycosides, found in plants including foxglove and oleander, are used to treat supraventricular tachydysrhythmias and congestive heart failure.

Clinical Features

Toxicity results from both acute overdose and from chronic use.
At increased risk are elderly patients and patients with underlying
medical conditions such as chronic obstructive pulmonary disease,
heart or renal disease, or electrolyte abnormalities such as hypokalemia. After *acute overdose,* symptoms include nausea, vomiting,
bradydysrhythmias, supraventricular dysrhythmias with atrioventricular block, and ventricular dysrhythmias. *Chronic toxicity* is
more common in elderly patients taking diuretics and presents with
gastrointestinal symptoms, weakness, seeing yellow-green halos
around objects, syncope, altered mental status, seizures, and ventricular dysrhythmias.

Diagnosis and Differential

Diagnosis requires a careful history, physical examination, and
laboratory studies. Hyperkalemia is often seen in acute poisoning
but may be absent in chronic toxicity. Serum digoxin levels are
neither sensitive nor specific for toxicity.

The differential diagnosis includes sinus node disease or overdose of calcium channel blockers, β blockers, quinidine, procainamide, clonidine, organophosphates, or cardiotoxic plants such
as rhododendron or yewberry.

Emergency Department Care and Disposition

Management includes supportive care, prevention of further absorption, treatment of complications, and antidote administration.
All patients require continuous cardiac monitoring and intravenous access.

1. **Activated charcoal,** 1 g/kg, then 0.5 g/kg every 4 to 6 h, is given
   to all patients.
2. **Atropine,** 0.5 to 2.0 mg IV, and cardiac pacing are used for
   bradydysrhythmias.

3. Ventricular dysrhythmias are treated with **phenytoin,** 15 mg/kg, infused no faster than 25 mg/min; **lidocaine,** 1 mg/kg; or **magnesium sulfate,** 2 to 4 g IV. Electrocardioversion may induce refractory ventricular dysrhythmias and should be considered only as a last resort. The initial setting should be 10 to 25 W/s.
4. Hyperkalemia is treated with **glucose followed by insulin, sodium bicarbonate, potassium-binding resin,** or **hemodialysis.** Calcium chloride should be avoided.
5. **Digoxin-specific Fab** is indicated for ventricular dysrhythmias, bradydysrhythmias with hypotension, and hyperkalemia greater than 5.5 meq/L (Table 104-1).

Patients who are asymptomatic after 12 h of observation may be medically cleared. Patients with signs of toxicity or with a history of a large overdose should be admitted to a monitored setting. Patients receiving Fab should be admitted to an intensive care unit.

β BLOCKERS

β blockers are used in the management of hypertension, tachydysrhythmias, and acute myocardial infarction. In an overdose, they may cause cardiac decompensation and death.

Clinical Features

Toxicity presents with bradycardia, QRS widening, hypotension, congestive heart failure, depressed consciousness, and seizures.

TABLE 104-1 Calculating Digoxin-Specific Fab Fragment Dosage

1) Calculate total body load
   Based on history of amount ingested:
   Total body load = amount ingested (mg) $\times$ 0.80 (bioavailability)
   Based on serum digoxin concentration:
   $$\text{Total body load} = \frac{\text{serum digoxin level} \times 5.6 \text{ L/kg} \times \text{Patient's wt (kg)}}{1000}$$

2) Calculate number of vials of digoxin-specific Fab fragments needed to neutralize the calculated total body load:
   It is assumed that an equimolar dose of Fab fragments is required for neutralization.
   One vial (40 mg) of Fab fragments binds 0.6 mg of digoxin.
   $$\text{Number of vials required} = \frac{\text{Total body load}}{0.6}$$

A simple and accurate variation of the above calculations:
   $$\text{Number of vials of Fab} = \frac{\text{serum digoxin level} \times \text{Patient's wt (kg)}}{100}$$

Sotalol may cause QT prolongation and ventricular tachycardia, torsades de pointes, and ventricular fibrillation.

Diagnosis and Differential

The differential diagnosis includes overdose of calcium-channel blockers, centrally acting α agonists, digoxin, organophosphates, plants such as oleander and rhododendron, and Chinese herbal preparations containing cardiac glycosides.

Emergency Department Care and Disposition

All patients require supportive care, continuous cardiac monitoring, and intravenous access.

1. **Activated charcoal,** 1 g/kg, should be administered to all patients.
2. **Glucagon** is a first-line agent, given as an IV bolus of 50 to 150 μg/kg, and repeated as needed or administered as a continuous infusion at 1 to 10 mg/h.
3. **Dopamine** or **norepinephrine** is used for refractory hypotension.
4. **Lidocaine, magnesium sulfate, isoproterenol,** and **overdrive pacing** are used to treat sotalol-induced ventricular dysrhythmias.

Patients who are symptom-free after 8 to 10 h with a normal repeat electrocardiogram (ECG) may be medically cleared. All others should be admitted to a monitored bed or intensive care unit.

CALCIUM CHANNEL BLOCKERS

Calcium channel blockers consist of phenylalkylamines (verapamil), benzothiazepines (diltiazem), and dihydropyridines (nifedipine). Acute overdose of calcium channel blockers cause several dozen deaths each year.

Clinical Features

Cardiac manifestations include sinus bradycardia with hypotension, conduction disturbances, and complete sinus arrest with ventricular escape rhythms. Patients also may present with hemiplegia, seizures, or altered mental status. Noncardiogenic pulmonary edema, hypokalemia, hyperkalemia, hypercalcemia, hyperglycemia, and lactic acidosis with compensatory tachypnea have been reported.

Diagnosis and Differential

Severe toxicity is recognized by slow junctional rhythm, hypoxemia, lactic acidosis, and decreased left ventricular ejection fraction on echocardiography.

Emergency Department Care and Disposition

Treatment is supportive. All patients require supplemental oxygen, cardiac monitoring, and at least one large-bore IV line.

1. **Crystalloid IV fluids** should be administered for hypotension.
2. **Activated charcoal,** 1 g/kg, is indicated for all patients.
3. Whole bowel irrigation has been advocated for sustained-release preparations.
4. Hypotension is treated with **calcium chloride** starting with 1 g in 100 mL normal saline run through a central venous line over 5 min followed by 20 to 50 mg/kg/h.
5. **Glucagon** is used for hypotension resistant to fluids or calcium chloride, starting at a dose of 0.1 mg/kg mixed in normal saline, followed by an infusion of 0.1 mg/kg/h.
6. **Dopamine,** 1 to 20 μg/kg/h, should be used for persistent hypotension.
7. Rescue therapies for persistent hypotension include **amrinone,** 750 μg/kg IV, followed by an infusion of 1 to 20 μg/kg/h; **insulin**, 1.0 U/kg over the first hour followed by 0.5 U/kg/h, with coadministration of 20 to 30 g/h glucose to maintain euglycemia; **4-aminopyridine,** infused at 10 to 50 μg/kg/h; or **cardiac pacing.**
9. Acidosis should be corrected with hyperventilation or **sodium bicarbonate.**

Patients who are asymptomatic after trivial ingestions can be observed for 6 h and medically cleared. Patients who have taken a sustained-release preparation require longer observation. Symptomatic patients should be admitted to a monitored setting or intensive care unit.

ANTIHYPERTENSIVES

Antihypertensives include diuretics, clonidine and other centrally-acting agents, angiotensin-converting enzyme (ACE) inhibitors, angiotensin II receptor antagonists, peripheral vasodilators, and ganglionic blockers.

Diuretics

Diuretics include thiazides (hydrochlorothiazide), loop diuretics (furosemide, bumetanide, and ethacrynic acid), potassium-sparing diuretics (spironolactone, triamterene, and amiloride), carbonic anhydrase inhibitors (acetazolamide), and osmotic agents (mannitol).

Clinical Features

Thiazides and loop diuretics Patients present with hypotension, tachycardia, altered mental status, hyponatremia, hypokalemia, hypolcalcemia, hypomagnesemia, and hypochloremic metabolic alkalosis.

Potassium-sparing diuretics Toxicity manifests with volume depletion, hyperkalemia, hyponatremia, and hypochloremia.

Carbonic anhydrase inhibitors Overdose results in volume depletion, electrolyte disturbances, and non-anion-gap metabolic acidosis.

Osmotic agents Signs of toxicity include volume depletion, electrolyte abnormalities, pulmonary edema, anaphylaxis, and acute renal failure.

Emergency Department Care and Disposition

Management is supportive and includes fluid resuscitation and correction of electrolyte and pH abnormalities. All patients require supportive care, continuous cardiac monitoring, and intravenous access.

1. **IV normal saline** is used to correct hypovolemia, hyponatremia, and alkalosis.
2. **Dopamine** is used for hypotension refractory to volume resuscitation.
3. Potassium abnormalities should be aggressively corrected.

Most asymptomatic patients can be medically cleared after therapy and observation. Patients with electrolyte abnormalities may require admission.

Clonidine and Other Centrally Acting Agents

Clonidine, guanabenz, and methyldopa are used for the management of hypertension. Clonidine is also used to mitigate the effects of opiate and ethanol withdrawal.

Clinical Features

Clonidine toxicity causes hypotension and bradycardia, leading to myocardial ischemia and congestive heart failure. Other findings include respiratory depression, hypothermia, mental status changes, and seizures. Guanabenz and methyldopa cause hypotension, bradycardia, and mental status changes.

Emergency Department Care and Disposition

Management is supportive, with special attention to correcting hypotension. Recurrent apnea, most commonly seen in children, may warrant endotracheal intubation. All patients require continuous cardiac monitoring and intravenous access.

1. **Crystalloid IV fluids** should be administered for hypotension.
2. **Dopamine** is used for hypotension refractory to fluid resuscitation.
3. **Naloxone** has been reported to be effective for cases of hypotension refractory to fluids and dopamine and for respiratory depression.
4. **Atropine** is indicated for management of symptomatic bradycardia.
5. Seizures are controlled with standard anticonvulsants.
6. Dialysis may be warranted in severe cases of guanabenz toxicity.

Symptoms of clonidine toxicity can persist for up to 72 h, so admission should be considered for any patient suspected of clonidine overdose.

Angiotensin-Mediated Antihypertensives

Antihypertensives acting on the renin-angiotension pathway include ACE inhibitors and angiotensin II receptor antagonist.

Clinical Features

Acute overdose of both ACE inhibitors and angiotensin II receptor antagonists causes profound hypotension. Angiotensin II receptor antagonists also cause bradycardia.

Emergency Department Care and Disposition

Care is supportive and is directed at the patient's respiratory and hemodynamic status. All patients require continuous cardiac monitoring and intravenous access.

1. **IV normal saline** is administered for hypotension.
2. **Dopamine** is warranted in refractory cases.
3. **Naloxone** has been reported to reverse hypotension caused by captopril.

Close observation is indicated for patients overdosing on one of these agents.

Peripheral Vasodilators and Ganglionic Blockers

These groups include prazosin, hydralazine, minoxidil, and sodium nitroprusside.

Clinical Features

Overdose of *prazosin, hydralazine,* and *minoxidil* may cause hypotension and tachycardia. Following minoxidil overdose, patients with renal insufficiency may also develop fluid retention and pericardial effusion. Acute toxicity due to *sodium nitroprusside* presents with hypotension and dysrhythmias. Thiocyanate and cyanide toxicity as well as methemoglobinemia have been reported after prolonged nitroprusside therapy.

Emergency Department Care and Disposition

All patients require supportive care, continuous cardiac monitoring, and intravenous access.

1. **Crystalloid IV fluids** are used to treat hypotension.
2. Vasopressors such as **dopamine** are indicated for refractory cases.
3. Beta blockers can be used judiciously for symptomatic tachycardia.
4. In cases of thiocyanate toxicity following sodium nitroprusside administration, dialysis may be warranted.

Symptomatic patients should be admitted to a monitored setting.

For further reading in *Emergency Medicine: A Comprehensive Study Guide,* 5th ed., see Chap. 168, "Digitalis Glycosides," by William H. Dribben and Mark A. Kirk; Chap. 169, "β-Blocker Toxicity," by William P. Kerns II; Chap. 170, "Calcium Channel Blockers," by Jeffrey A. Kline; and Chap. 171, "Antihypertensives," by Arjun Chanmugam.

105 | Phenytoin and Fosphenytoin

Mark B. Rogers

Intentional phenytoin overdose rarely leads to death, provided that adequate supportive care is administered. Most phenytoin-related deaths have been caused by rapid intravenous administration and hypersensitivity reactions.

Clinical Features

Phenytoin toxicity depends upon the duration of exposure, dosage taken, and most importantly, route of administration. An acute oral overdose is typically dose-related and usually presents with nystagmus, nausea, vomiting, ataxia, dysarthria, choreoathetosis, opisthotonos, and central nervous system (CNS) depression or excitation. Death from oral overdose alone is extremely rare. Life-threatening effects such as hypotension, bradycardia, and asystole can be seen with intravenous administration, and are secondary to the diluent of the intravenous preparation, propylene glycol. This morbidity can be avoided by slowing the rate of administration.

Recently, fosphenytoin (a prodrug of phenytoin) has been approved. It is more soluble and less irritating to tissues. Intravenous fosphenytoin can cause pruritis and hypotension. Blood pressure and cardiac monitoring are recommended when loading fosphenytoin intravenously but not intramuscularly. The adverse and toxic effects of fosphenytoin are the same as phenytoin, except the toxic effects of propylene glycol do not exist.

CNS toxicity begins with horizontal nystagmus; however, vertical, bidirectional, or alternating nystagmus may occur with severe intoxication. A depressed level of consciousness is common, with sedation, lethargy, ataxic gait, and dysarthria progressing to confusion, seizures, coma, and apnea in a large overdose. Depressed or hyperactive deep tendon reflexes, clonus and extensor toe responses may be noted. Acute dystonia and movement disorders, such as opisthotonus and choreoathetosis, may occur. Peripheral neuropathy and ataxia may persist for months.

Cardiovascular toxicity is usually seen with intravenous administration only. In an otherwise healthy patient, cardiac toxicity has never been reported after an oral overdose of phenytoin; when observed, this requires assessment for other causes. Cardiovascular toxocity includes hypotension, bradycardia, conduction delays (which may progress to complete atrioventricular nodal block), ventricular tachycardia, ventricular fibrillation, and asystole. Electrocardiographic changes include increased PR interval, widened QRS interval, and altered ST-wave and T-wave segments. Bradycardia, hypotension, and syncope in healthy volunteers have been reported after small intravenous doses. Most of these side effects are due to the propylene glycol.

Phenytoin causes significant soft tissue toxicity. Intramuscular injection can result in localized crystallization of the drug, hematoma, sterile abscess, and myonecrosis. Reported complications of extravasation after intravenous infusion have included skin and soft tissue necrosis, compartment syndrome, gangrene, and death. Fosphenytoin is well tolerated intramuscularly or intravenously.

Hypersensitivity reactions usually occur within 1 to 6 weeks of initiation of phenytoin therapy. Reactions can include systemic lupus erythematosus, erythema multiforme, toxic epidermal necrolysis, Stevens-Johnson syndrome, hepatitis, rhabdomyolysis, acute interstitial pneumonitis, lymphadenopathy, leukopenia, disseminated intravascular coagulation, and renal failure. Obtaining a history of previous hypersensitivity reactions is important.

Phenytoin is teratogenic and should never be initiated in a pregnant patient without consulting a neurologist and obstetrician.

Diagnosis and Differential

Therapeutic levels are between 10 to 20 μg/mL (40 to 80 μmol/L). Some patients require levels above 20 μg/mL for seizure control. Individual variation in toxicity depends on baseline neurologic status, response to the drug, and free drug fraction. Patients with underlying brain disease are predisposed to toxicity and may become toxic at low levels. Toxicity generally correlates with increasing plasma levels (Table 105-1). Due to erratic absorption, serial phenytoin levels should be obtained to ensure the level has peaked.

Almost any CNS-active drug, such as ethanol, carbamazepine, benzodiazepines, barbiturates, and lithium, can mimic phenytoin toxicity. Disease states that resemble phenytoin toxicity include hypoglycemia, Wernicke encephalopathy, and posterior fossa hemorrhage or tumor. Seizures caused by phenytoin toxicity are uncommon, and other causes should be investigated such as trauma or alcohol withdrawal.

Emergency Department Care and Disposition

The treatment of phenytoin toxicity consists of initial stabilization, activated charcoal, and observation. Patients should be placed on

TABLE 105-1 Correlation of Plasma Phenytoin Level and Side Effects

Plasma level (μ/mL)	Side effects
< 10	Usually none
10–20	Occasional mild nystagmus
20–30	Nystagmus
30–40	Ataxia, slurred speech, nausea, and vomiting
40–50	Lethargy, confusion
> 50	Coma, seizures

a cardiac monitor, noninvasive blood pressure device, and pulse oximeter. An IV line should be inserted.

1. Supplemental **oxygen** should be administered to maintain an adequate pulse-oximetry reading. Respiratory acidosis should be avoided.
2. Hypotension from IV administration of phenytoin should be treated with IV **isotonic crystalloid** and the discontinuation of the infusion.
3. For an acute oral overdose, multiple doses of oral **activated charcoal** (1 g/kg), mixed with a cathartic such as sorbitol, should be given every 2 to 4 h in the first 24 h due to the extended absorptive phase.
4. Bradydysrhythmias may require atropine or cardiac pacing.
5. Seizures may be treated with a benzodiazepine or phenobarbital.

Hemodialysis and hemoperfusion are of no benefit. Appropriate orthopedic or plastic surgery consultation should be obtained for any signs of local soft tissue toxicity.

Following an oral ingestion, patients with serious complications (e.g., seizures, coma, altered mental status, and ataxia) should be admitted. With mild symptoms, the patient may be treated with activated charcoal in the ED and discharged home if repeat serum levels return to normal and the patient is not actively suicidal. Patients with symptomatic chronic intoxication should be admitted for observation unless the toxic effects are minimal, adequate care can be obtained at home, and they are 8 to 12 h from their last dose. Phenytoin should be stopped and levels rechecked in 2 to 3 days.

Following IV administration of phenytoin, patients with significant or persistent complications should be admitted for observation. Those with transient effects can be discharged.

For further reading in *Emergency Medicine: A Comprehensive Study Guide,* 5th ed., see Chap. 172, "Phenytoin and Fosphenytoin Toxicity," by Harold H. Osborn.

---

106 | Iron

O. John Ma

Iron toxicity from an intentional or accidental ingestion is a common poisoning. When determining the amount of iron ingested, elemental iron must be used in calculations. Ferrous sulfate, ferrous fumarate, and ferrous gluconate contain about 20 percent, 33 percent, and 12 percent elemental iron, respectively.

Clinical Features

Based on clinical findings, iron poisoning can be divided into five stages. It is imperative to note that patients can die in any stage of iron poisoning.

The first stage develops within the first few hours after the ingestion. The direct irritative effects of iron on the gastrointestinal (GI) tract produce abdominal pain, vomiting, and diarrhea. Hematemesis is not unusual. The absence of these symptoms within 6 h of ingestion essentially excludes a diagnosis of significant iron toxicity.

During the second stage, which may continue for up to 24 h following ingestion, the patient's GI symptoms may resolve, thereby giving a false sense of security despite toxic amounts of iron being absorbed into the body. Patients may not be symptomatic but will still appear ill and may have abnormal vital signs and evidence of poor tissue perfusion.

The third stage may appear either early in poisonings or develop hours after the second stage. Shock and a metabolic acidosis develop. Iron-induced coagulopathy may worsen bleeding and hypovolemia. Hepatic dysfunction, heart failure, and renal failure also may occur.

The fourth stage develops 2 to 5 days after ingestion. It manifests as elevation of aminotransferase and may progress to hepatic failure.

The fifth stage, which occurs 4 to 6 weeks after ingestion, involves gastric outlet obstruction secondary to the corrosive effects of iron on the GI tract.

Diagnosis and Differential

The diagnosis of iron poisoning is based on the clinical picture and the history provided by the patient, significant others, or out-of-hospital care providers. Toxic effects have been reported following oral doses as low as 10 to 20 mg/kg elemental iron. Moderate toxicity occurs at doses of 20 to 60 mg/kg, and severe toxicity can be expected following doses of greater than 60 mg/kg.

Laboratory work should be sent for levels of serum electrolytes, blood urea nitrogen, and serum glucose; coagulation studies; complete blood count; and hepatic enzymes and serum iron levels. It is crucial to note that the determination of a single serum iron level does not reflect what iron levels have been previously, what direction they are going, or the degree of iron toxicity in the tissues.

Serum iron levels have limited use in directing management since excess iron is toxic intracellularly and not in the blood. In general, serum iron levels between 300 to 500 μg/dL correlate with mild systemic toxicity and iron levels between 500 to 1,000 μg/dL correlate with moderate systemic toxicity. Levels greater than 1000 μg/dL are associated with significant morbidity. A single low serum level does not exclude the diagnosis of iron toxicity. The total iron-binding capacity is now thought to have little value in the assessment of iron-poisoned patients because it becomes falsely elevated in the presence of elevated serum iron levels of deferoxamine.

A plain radiograph of the kidneys, ureters, and bladder may reveal iron in the GI tract; however, many iron preparations are not routinely detected so negative radiographs do not exclude iron ingestion.

Emergency Department Care and Disposition

Patients who have remained asymptomatic for 6 h after ingestion of iron and who have a normal physical examination do not require medical treatment for iron toxicity. Patients whose symptoms resolve after a short period of time and who have normal vital signs, usually have mild toxicity and require only supportive care. This subset of patients still requires an observation period.

Patients who are symptomatic or demonstrate signs of hemodynamic instability after iron ingestion should be managed aggressively in the ED.

1. Patients should receive supplemental **oxygen,** be placed on a **cardiac monitor,** and have two large-bore IV lines established.
2. Patients should receive **IV crystalloid infusion** to help correct hypovolemia and tissue hypoperfusion.
3. Patients who present within 2 h of ingestion should undergo **gastic lavage.** Activated charcoal does not bind iron salts and its use is not recommended.
4. Whole bowel irrigation with **polyethylene glycol** solution has been demonstrated to be efficacious. Administration of 250 to 500 mL/h in children and 2 L/h in adults via nasogastric tube may clear the GI tract of iron pills before absorption occurs.
5. Coagulopathy should be corrected with **vitamin K_1** (5 to 25 mg) or **fresh frozen plasma** (200 to 500 mL). Blood should be typed and screened or cross-matched, as necessary.
6. **Deferoxamine** is a chelating agent that can remove iron from tissues and can remove free iron from plasma. Deferoxamine combines with iron to form water-soluble ferrioxamine, which is excreted in the urine. Deferoxamine is safe to administer to children and pregnant women.

   Patients with mild iron toxicity may be treated with **deferoxamine 90 mg/kg IM,** up to 1 g in children and 2 g in adults. The dose may be repeated every 4 to 6 h, as clinically indicated.

   For patients with more severe iron toxicity, the preferred route of deferoxamine administration is as an IV infusion. Sinch hypotension is the rate-limiting factor for IV infusion, it is recommended to **begin with a slow IV infusion at 5 mg/kg/h.** The deferoxamine infusion rate can be increased to **15 mg/kg/h,** as tolerated. It is recommended not to exceed a total daily dose of 6 to 8 g. In a clinically ill patient with a known acute ingestion of iron, deferoxamine therapy should be initiated without waiting for the serum iron level results.

   Determination for the efficacy of deferoxamine involves evaluating serial urine samples. As ferrioxamine is excreted, the urine changes to the classic *vin rose* appearance.

7. Patients who remain asymptomatic after 6 h of observation and have a reliable history of an insignificant ingestion may be considered for discharge. Patients initially symptomatic who become asymptomatic should still be admitted since this may represent the second stage. Patients who receive deferoxamine therapy should be admitted to an intensive care setting. All patients should be assessed for suicide risk.

For further reading in *Emergency Medicine: A Comprehensive Study Guide,* 5th ed., see Chap. 173, "Iron," by Joseph G. Rella and Lewis S. Nelson.

---

107 | Hydrocarbons and Volatile Substances

Judith A. Linden

Hydrocarbons are a diverse group of organic compounds that include fuels, lighter fluids, paint strippers, spot removers, glues, lubricants, and degreasers. Exposure may be unintentional (e.g., occupational exposure to fumes) or recreational (e.g., glue sniffing, "huffing," or "bagging") in an attempt to get high.

Clinical Features

Toxicity depends on route of exposure (ingestion, inhalation, or dermal), physical characteristics (volatility, viscosity, and surface tension), chemical characteristics (aliphatic, aromatic, or hydrogenated), and the presence of toxic additives (e.g., lead or pesticides). Pulmonary and cardiac toxicity are the most common. Toxicity is discussed by organ system in Table 107-1.

Aspiration of highly volatile aliphatic substances, such as gasoline, kerosene, methane, or butane, may cause chemical pneumonitis, the most frequent pulmonary complication. Other complications include pneumomediastinum, pneumothorax, and pneumatocele. Common symptoms are coughing, dyspnea, choking,

TABLE 107-1 Chemical Toxicity

Chemical composition	Example	Commercial use	Toxicity

Aliphatic (open chain)	Short chain
	  Methane
	  Butane
			Pulmonary
			
			Negligible GI absorption

	Intermediate chain
	  Gasoline
	  Kerosene
	  Mineral seal oil
	Long chain
	  Tar
		Motor fuel
		Stove fuel
		Furniture polish
			Gas/kerosene hemolysis
			
			N-hexane, butyl ketone polyneuropathy

Aromatic (benzene ring)	Benzene Toluene Xylene	Gasoline Airplane glue Cleaning agent, degreaser	Dysrhythmias Benzene aplastic anemia, CML
Halogenated (substituted halogen group)	Carbon-tetrachloride Chloroform TCE, TCA	Refrigerant, propellant Solvent Spot remover, degreaser Typewriter correction fluid	Dysrhythmias Hepatic toxicity Acute renal failure TCE-hemolysis

Abbreviations: CML, chronic myelogenous leukemia; TCA, trichloroethylene; TCE, trichloroethane.

and gasping. Physical examination findings may include tachypnea, wheezing, grunting, and decreased breath sounds. Radiographic findings lag behind clinical signs and symptoms but are typically present within 4 to 6 h.

Central nervous system (CNS) toxicity is most common with volatile petroleum distillates [e.g., toluene and trichloroethane (TCE)]. Symptoms range from giddiness, slurred speech, ataxia, hallucinations, and seizures to lethargy, obtundation, and coma. Chronic exposure may cause cerebellar ataxia and mood lability.

Aromatic and halogenated hydrocarbons sensitize the myocardium to catecholamines and may cause serious dysrhythmias (ventricular tachycardia or fibrillation), decreased cardiac contractility, bradycardia, and heart blocks.

Some halogenated hydrocarbons (e.g., carbon tetrachloride and chloroform) cause hepatocellular injury. Liver enzyme levels may be elevated within 24 h, and right upper quadrant abdominal pain and jaundice develop within 48 to 96 h. Chronic exposure causes cirrhosis and hepatoma.

Gasoline, kerosene, and TCE can cause hemolysis. Chronic benzene abuse can cause aplastic anemia and hematologic malignancies.

Dermal toxicity includes rashes (erythema, papules, vesicles, or scarlatiniform rash), eczematous dermatitis, and burns.

Emergency Department Care and Disposition

1. All symptomatic patients should receive supplemental **oxygen** and undergo continuous cardiac monitoring. Consider **endotracheal intubation** if there is respiratory distress. Add positive end-expiratory pressure if necessary, but monitor closely for pneumothorax or pneumatocele.
2. The patient should undergo standard HAZMAT decontamination measures, preferably in the out-of-hospital setting.
3. Hypotension should be treated with **IV crystalloid fluids**. Except in cases of cardiac arrest, pressors should be avoided, since they may precipitate life-threatening dysrhythmias. Tachydysrhythmias should be treated with β blockers (IV propranolol 1 mg, may repeat if blood pressure is stable) or **lidocaine** 1 mg/kg IV (may repeat up to 3 mg/kg). Seizures should be managed using standard protocols.
4. Gastrointestinal (GI) decontamination should be performed for ingestion of hydrocarbons that are absorbed through the GI tract, such as CHAMP (camphor, halogenated hydrocarbons, aromatic hydrocarbons, metals, or pesticides) and wood distillate (e.g., turpentine or pine oil). Aliphatic hydrocarbons are poorly absorbed from the GI tract and have an increased risk of toxicity when aspirated during attempted decontamination; thus, their ingestion should not be treated with GI decontamination measures. Activated charcoal and cathartics are of no benefit.
5. **Hyperbaric oxygen** therapy may be beneficial in methylene chloride exposures with elevated carbon monoxide levels or mental status changes.
6. Useful laboratory and radiographic studies include arterial blood gas analysis, liver enzyme tests, blood urea nitrogen and creatinine determinations, hematocrit, carboxyhemoglobin level for methylene chloride exposure, chest x-ray, and a kidneys-ureter-bladder x-ray for radiopaque substances (e.g., chlorinated hydrocarbons).

7. Since most fatalities occur in the first 24 to 48 h, all symptomatic patients should be admitted. Asymptomatic patients may be discharged from the emergency department if they have a normal chest x-ray and remain asymptomatic after 4 to 6 h of observation.

For further reading in *Emergency Medicine: A Comprehensive Study Guide,* 5th ed., see Chap. 174, "Hydrocarbons and Volatile Substances," by Paul M. Wax.

---

108 | Caustic Ingestions

Judith A. Linden

Many industrial and household solutions contain caustics. Acids are present in solutions used in rust removal, photography, drain and toilet bowl cleaning, and fertilizers. Common acids include sulfuric acid, formic acid, nitric acid, phosphoric acid, acetic acid, and chromic acid. Hydrofluoric acid, used for metal etching, rust removal, jewelry cleaning, and petroleum distillation, is extremely invasive and corrosive and will penetrate the skin, causing extensive tissue necrosis, limb loss, and electrolyte abnormalities. Alkalies are used in drain and oven cleaners, household bleach, and batteries. Common alkalies include sodium hydroxide, lithium hydroxide, ammonium hydroxide, and sodium hypochlorite (household bleach).

Clinical Features

Acids are foul-tasting and malodorous. Acids cause coagulation necrosis and eschar formation, thus limiting tissue penetration. Signs and symptoms of acid ingestions include hematemesis, melena, and gastric perforation with peritonitis. Pooling in the gastric antrum causes pylorospasm and mucosal injury. Gastric outlet obstruction is a late complication.

Alkalies are relatively tasteless and odorless. Alkali ingestions typically present after larger quantities have been ingested. Alkaline chemicals cause liquifaction necrosis, which leads to extensive tissue penetration and full thickness esophageal burns with perforation. Alkali ingestions can present acutely with orofacial burns, drooling, vomiting and odynophagia (after esophageal and gastric injury), dyspnea, and hoarseness and stridor (after laryngeal and epiglottic injury). The oral mucosa may have burns or a soapy film appearance. The absence of visible oral lesions does not exclude significant gastrointestinal (GI) injury (10 to 30 percent have no lesions on presentation). Symptoms of chest pain suggest esophageal perforation with mediastinitis. Immediate injury is followed in 2 to 3 days by tissue sloughing, with an increased risk of perforation of 5 to 14 days.

Dermal exposures to acid and alkalies cause local irritation. One exception is hydrofluoric acid, which may cause extensive tissue penetration and life-threatening systemic absorption. Alkaline eye exposures may cause perforation and blindness, whereas acid exposures generally cause less ocular injury.

Diagnosis and Differential

The diagnosis is made by history. The product information insert or a poison control center should be consulted for unknown substances. Depending on the ingestion, helpful laboratory tests include arterial blood gas analysis (in acid ingestions); complete blood cell count; liver profile; levels of electrolytes, calcium, magnesium, BUN (blood urea nitrogen), and creatinine; type and crossmatch, and coagulation studies. An upright chest x-ray should be obtained to evaluate for aspiration, abdominal free air, and pneumomediastinum.

Emergency Department Care and Disposition

1. **Oxygen** should be administered and the airway stabilized with early **endotracheal intubation** if there is stridor or drooling. Cricothyrotomy is indicated if there is extensive upper airway edema. Two large-bore IV catheters should be secured and crystalloid should be infused if the patient is hypotensive.
2. For patients with chest pain or signs of peritonitis, **urgent surgical consultation** should be obtained. A chest and abdominal computed tomography scan should be ordered for the hemodynamically stable patient.
3. Nasogastric (NG) tube placement is controversial. Insertion of a small NG tube for significant acid ingestions should be

considered but insertion of one for alkali ingestions should be avoided because of the increased risk of aspiration.

4. **Sodium bicarbonate** should be administered for serum pH < 7.1.

5. For ocular exposures, **copious irrigation** with at least 2 to 3 L (up to 10 L) of normal saline should be administered and continued until the pH is 7.4 to 7.6 (see Chap. 145, "Ocular Emergencies").

6. Hydrofluoric acid dermal exposures should be treated with copious irrigation of the skin. **Benzylalkonium chloride** or **calcium gluconate paste** (surgilube mixed with calcium gluconate powder, 2.5% wt/vol) should be applied to the exposed skin. Pain relief is the endpoint for successful treatment. Other therapy include **intradermal calcium gluconate** (not greater than 0.5 mL/cm$_2$) and **intraarterial calcium gluconate** (10 mL of 10% calcium gluconate in 40 mL normal saline over 4 h, or until pain-free) for distal extremity exposures not responding to standard treatment. Oral ingestions should be treated with NG tube aspiration and irrigation and oral magnesium citrate (300 mL).

7. All patients with significant acid and alkali ingestions should be admitted. Early endoscopy (12 to 24 h) will determine the extent of injury in alkali ingestions. Delayed endoscopy increases the risk of perforation. Treatment of severe burns with systemic steroids (methylprednisolone 2 mg/kg per 24 h for 2 to 3 weeks) and antibiotics (if steroids are used) is controversial, and should be administered in consultation with the GI specialist.

8. Chemical exposures that require specialized treatment include ingestions of Clinitest tablets and button batteries. Clinitest tablets, used in urine ketone testing, are solid and can cause extensive mucosal burns. **Dilution** (with water or milk) is recommended if no stridor or drooling is present. For a button-battery ingestion, chest and abdominal radiographs are helpful in determining the location of the battery. A battery lodged in the esophagus requires **endoscopy** for removal, whereas one that has passed beyond the gastroesophageal junction can be followed with stool checks and serial abdominal radiographs. After a battery ingestion, should signs of obstruction or perforation develop, immediate surgical removal of the battery is mandated.

For further reading in *Emergency Medicine: A Comprehensive Study Guide,* 5th ed., see Chap. 175, "Caustics," by G. Richard Bruno and Wallace A. Carter.

109 | Pesticides

Charles J. Havel, Jr.

Pesticides are divided into the target-based groupings of insecticides, herbicides, and rodenticides. Insecticides include organophosphates, carbamates, organochlorine compounds (DDT and lindane), and pyrethrins. Herbicides are represented by chlorphenoxy (dioxins and furans), bipyridyl (paraquat and diquat), and urea-substituted compounds. Rodenticides include a heterogeneous group of agents classified as high toxicity compounds (SMFA, MNFA, strychnine, heavy metal agents, and yellow phosphorous), moderate toxicity compounds, and low toxicity compounds, including the superwarfarins.

Pesticides are responsible for a large number of accidental, occupational, and intentional exposures each year. Mass poisoning may be seen with organophosphates in the setting of terrorist activity or chemical warfare. Pesticide toxicity can be associated with oral, dermal, conjunctival, gastrointestinal (GI), or respiratory contact. Acute exposure may result in a class-specific toxidrome within 12 to 24 h; however, early presentation, high lipid solubility, the presence of other inactive ingredients, and chronic low-grade poisoning may all contribute to less than clear clinical features in individual cases. Poison center consultation is suggested in deciding management strategies.

Clinical Features

Nonsystemic symptoms of insecticide exposure include dermatitis, eye, and mucous membrane irritation with topical exposure and wheezing with inhalational exposure. Organophosphates induce cholinergic excess derived from the inhibition of cholinesterase resulting in muscarinic, nicotinic, and central nervous system (CNS) effects. Muscarinic overstimulation results in bradycardia, bronchorrhea, respiratory distress, visual disturbance, and the *SLUDGE* syndrome (*S*alivation, *L*acrimation, *U*rination, *D*efecation, *G*astrointestinal, and *E*mesis). Pronounced nicotinic activity may override the bradycardia characteristic of muscarinic activity, causing tachycardia and hypertension. Additionally, muscle fasciculations with weakness or paralysis may be seen. CNS effects include headache and altered mental status, ranging from anxiety to lethargy and coma; this often predominates in pediatric patients. Carbamates produce a similar cholinergic toxidrome to that of organophosphates but of shorter duration and with less CNS symptomatology. Acute poisoning with organochlorine compounds produces fever associated with predominately neurologic symptoms that include headache, fatigue, hyperexcitability, myoclonus, and seizures. Pyrethrins most commonly cause hypersensitivity responses to include bronchospasm and anaphylaxis. They may produce dermal, pulmonary, GI, and neurologic findings.

Herbicide toxicity leads to a wide variety of symptoms generally based upon which organ system has been exposed. Topical exposure causes local irritation, ingestion results in nausea, vomiting and diarrhea, and inhalation causes pulmonary edema and respiratory distress. Chlorphenoxy compounds may cause tachycardia, dysrhythmias, and hypotension, and muscle toxicity manifested by muscle pain, fasciculations, and rhabdomyolysis. Paraquat is especially toxic with caustic effects resulting in severe dermal, corneal, and mucous membrane burns, including that of respiratory and GI epithelium. Cardiovascular collapse may occur early, especially in the case of large ingestions, and results in pulmonary edema, renal failure, hepatic necrosis, and multi-system organ failure. Urea-substituted compounds are much less toxic than other herbicides and generally cause few systemic effects other than methemoglobinemia.

The clinical signs of rodenticide poisoning vary widely, and specific features are associated with individual agents. SMFA and related compounds typically demonstrate delayed toxicity until metabolites take their effect in blocking aerobic metabolic pathways. Patients exhibit nausea and anxiety followed by respiratory depression, cardiovascular collapse, altered mental status, and seizures. Strychnine toxicity causes inhibition of spinal motor neuron function and results in facial grimacing, muscle twitching, severe extensor spasms, and opisthotonos; it eventually may lead to medullary paralysis and death. Exposure to thallium sulfate initially causes GI hemorrhage followed by a latent period, in turn succeeded by the development of neurologic symptoms, respiratory failure, and dysrhythmias. Zinc phosphide ingestion results in the liberation of phosphine gas which subsequently causes GI irritation, hepatocellular toxicity, direct pulmonary injury (if the gas is inhaled), cardiovascular collapse, altered mental status, seizures, and noncardiogenic pulmonary edema. Yellow phosphorous causes severe topical burns to areas of contact and also may cause jaundice, seizures, and cardiovascular collapse. Arsenic presents as a syndrome similar to other heavy metal poisonings. As for the moderate toxicity rodenticides, ANTU exhibits primarily pulmonary effects with dyspnea, pleuritic chest pain, and noncardiogenic pulmonary edema, while cholecalciferol causes the typical symptoms of vitamin D excess. Red squill poisoning is a low toxicity rodenticide that presents as severe GI distress and cardiac dys-rhythmias. The most common low toxicity agent poisoning occurs with superwarfarins and related compounds. Exposures most commonly come to attention on a delayed basis with symptoms of an unexplained coagulopathy.

Diagnosis and Differential

The diagnosis of pesticide poisoning is made on the basis of the history and physical examination in the overwhelming majority of cases. In the case of organophosphate poisoning, an assay of both serum and red blood cell cholinesterase activity can be obtained for diagnosis and to guide treatment, though results seldom become available for decision making in the emergency department (ED). Qualitative and quantitative assays of blood and urine for paraquat may at times be clinically useful. In the case of superwarfarin ingestion, determination of the prothrombin time at 24 and 48 h is recommended. Other routine laboratory testing is nondiagnostic but may reveal any one or a combination of hyperglycemia, electrolyte abnormalities and metabolic acidosis, leukocytosis, hyperamylasemia, liver enzyme abnormalities, and abnormalities on urinalysis. In cases involving severe respiratory distress, a chest x-ray may show signs of pulmonary edema. Electrocardiographic findings are variable and include tachydysrhythmia, ventricular blocks, or bradydysrhythmia.

The differential diagnosis of pesticide poisoning is exceedingly wide and, in patients with significant exposures, includes any of the causes of respiratory insufficiency, cardiac dysrhythmia, cardiovascular collapse, altered neurologic function, coma, or GI dysfunction. Patients with mild exposures may have nonspecific symptoms suggesting a viral illness. However, the cholinergic toxidrome associated with organophosphate and carbamate toxicity is generally distinctive. In these cases the differential is narrower and includes exposure to pilocarpine, mushrooms (specifically *Amanita muscaria*), betel nut, and carbachol. Nicotinic effects can be seen with tobacco toxicity and black widow spider envenomation.

Emergency Department Care and Disposition

1. The mainstay of treatment for pesticide exposure is identification of the specific agent involved and **supportive monitoring and treatment.** Continuous cardiac and pulse-oximetry monitoring, noninvasive blood pressure monitoring, and intravenous access are essential. Symptomatic patients require attention to airway protection and ventilation with supplemental **oxygen** to maintain saturation to $\geq 95\%$. **Tracheal intubation** and **mechan-**

ical ventilation with high oxygen concentrations may be necessary in severe poisoning. Maintenance of intravascular volume and urine output should be assured. Cardiac dysrhythmias should be treated in standard fashion. Meticulous attention to **patient decontamination** (dermal, ocular, or GI) is important as is **prevention of absorption** by patients and caretakers involved in patient care. **Benzodiazepines** (e.g., lorazepam 1 to 2 mg intravenously) are generally the first choice for seizures. Administration of a specific antidote may be appropriate for selected individual agents (see Table 109-1).

2. Disposition depends upon the pesticide involved in the exposure. Asymptomatic patients with a history of contact with a pesticide may require decontamination and a 6 to 8 h observation period only. Close follow-up should be arranged for patients with exposure to rodenticides that produce symptoms on a delayed basis. A low threshold for admission should be maintained for patients with intentional ingestions. Any patient

TABLE 109-1 Pesticides and Specific Antidotes

Pesticide	Antidote	Dosing
Organophosphates	Atropine	0.5 mg/kg up to 2–4 mg IV q 5–15 min—consider IV infusion and titrate to effect (drying secretions)
	2-PAM	20–40 mg/kg up to 1 g IV—may repeat in 1–2 h, then every 6–8 h for 48 h
Carbamates	Atropine 2-PAM	As for organophosphates Use is controversial and may be contraindicated
Urea-substituted Herbicides	Methylene blue	As for treatment of methemoglobinemia
Zinc phosphide	NaHCO$_3$	Used for intragastric alkalinization
Yellow Phosphorous	K Permanganate or H$_2$O$_2$	Used for gastric lavage
Arsenic	Heavy metal chelators	As for heavy metal poisoning
Red Squill	Antidysrhythmics, Fab fragments	As for digoxin toxicity
Superwarfarins	Vitamin K	Up to 20 mg IV, repeated, and titrated to effect

with a history of paraquat or diquat exposure should be admitted because of the extreme lethality of these compounds. Consideration for admission to the intensive care unit is an individual one based upon the specific toxin involved and the overall clinical picture.

For further reading in *Emergency Medicine: A Comprehensive Study Guide*, 5th ed., see Chap. 176, "Insecticides, Herbicides, Rodenticides," by Walter C. Robey III and William J. Meggs.

---

110 | Carbon Monoxide and Cyanide

Charles J. Havel, Jr.

CARBON MONOXIDE

Carbon monoxide (CO) is a colorless, odorless, nonirritating gas that displaces oxygen from hemoglobin, resulting in tissue hypoxia. Sources of exposure to CO include the incomplete combustion of organic fuels, tobacco smoke, the metabolism of methylene chloride (contained in the vapors of paint removers), and the low-grade physiological exogenous production of CO.

Clinical Features

The clinical picture at the site of poisoning often corresponds to the severity of poisoning and to on-scene carboxyhemoglobin levels (Table 110-1). However, patients treated with high-flow oxygen during transport to the emergency department (ED) may demonstrate significant clinical changes upon arrival. Moreover, vague or nonspecific symptoms may suggest a variety of conditions further confusing patient assessment (Table 110-2). Fetuses and neonates are particularly susceptible to the toxic effects of the gas due to the presence of fetal hemoglobin and an oxygen dissociation curve that is already shifted to the left. Children are frequently affected and make up almost 40 percent of patients treated with hyperbaric oxygen therapy.

TABLE 110-1 Symptoms and Signs at Various
Carboxyhemoglobin Concentrations

COHb Level (%)	Symptoms and signs
0	Usually none
10	Frontal headache
11	Throbbing headache, dyspnea with exertion
12	Impaired judgment, nausea, dizziness, visual disturbances, fatigue
40	Confusion, syncope
50	Coma, seizures
60	Hypotension, respiratory failure
≥70	Death

Diagnosis and Differential

The primary key to the diagnosis is maintaining a high degree of clinical suspicion. The most useful laboratory test is the determination of the blood carboxyhemoglobin level (COHb). Psychometric testing can detect subtle deficits in mental status and assess for indications for hyperbaric oxygen therapy. Adjunctive testing may include other toxicologic assays and assessment of acid-base status. In cases of symptomatic exposure, electrocardiogram (ECG) and cardiac enzyme determinations are suggested. Chest radiographs are generally obtained for fire victims, and other pulmonary function testing may be helpful as well. Computed tomography scan or magnetic resonance imaging may identify specific lesions or generalized cerebral edema.

The differential diagnosis is extremely wide and includes a wide variety of toxins, infectious agents, and cardiac and pulmonary diseases, as well as the host of causes for altered mental status. Particularly in colder months, patients with headache, nausea, weakness, fatigue, difficulty in concentrating, dizziness, chest pain, and abdominal pain must be evaluated with CO toxicity in mind. Victims of house fires with appropriate symptoms and signs must be evaluated specifically for CO poisoning.

Emergency Department Care and Disposition

1. Initially, patients must be removed from the source of exposure with close attention to the ABCs. **100% oxygen** should be administered with a tight-fitting mask and reservoir and **cardiac monitoring** instituted. Intravenous access and frequent noninvasive blood pressure monitoring are also required. (Table 110-3 outlines appropriate treatment guidelines for CO poisoning.)

TABLE 110-2 Complications and Symptoms and Signs of Carbon Monoxide Poisoning

System involved	Manifestation
Neuropsychiatric	Coma, seizures, agitation, leukoencephalopathy, cerebral edema, behavioral disorders, decreased cognitive ability, Tourette-like syndrome, mutism, fecal and urinary incontinence, parietal lobe dysfunction, ataxia, muscular rigidity, parkinsonism, gait disturbance, peripheral neuropathy, psychosis, memory impairment, abnormal EEG, personality changes
Cardiovascular	Angina, tachycardia, ST-segment changes, hypotension, dysrythmias, heart block, myocardial infarction
Pulmonary	Pulmonary edema and hemorrhage, unilateral diaphragmatic paralysis
Ophthalmologic	Flame-shaped retinal hemorrhages, decreased light sensitivity, decreased visual acuity, cortical blindness, retrobulbar neuritis, papilledema, pancentral scotomata
Vestibular and auditory	Central hearing loss, tinnitus, vertigo, nystagmus
Gastrointestinal	Vomiting, diarrhea, hepatic necrosis, hematochezia, melena
Dermatologic	Bullae, alopecia, sweat gland necrosis, cherry-red skin color, edema, cyanosis, pallor, erythematous patches
Hematologic	Leukocytosis, disseminated intravascular coagulation, thrombotic thrombocytopenic purpura
Musculoskeletal	Rhabdomyolysis, myonecrosis, compartment syndrome
Renal	Acute renal failure secondary to myoglobinuria, proteinuria
Metabolic	Lactic acidosis, hyperglycemia, nonpancreatic hyperamylasemia, diabetes insipidus, hypocalcemia
Fetal	Death, cerebral atrophy, microcephalus, low birth weight, psychomotor retardation, seizures, spasticity

Abbreviation: EEG, electroencephalogram.

TABLE 110-3–Carbon Monoxide Poisoning Treatment Guidelines

Mild poisoning	
Criteria	COHb levels < 30%
	No symptoms or signs of impaired cardiovascular or neurologic function
	May have complaint of headache, nausea, vomiting
Treatment	100% oxygen by tight-fitting non-rebreathing mask until COHb level remains < 5%
	Admission for COHb level of > 25%
	Admission for patients with underlying heart disease regardless of COHb level
Moderate poisoning	
Criteria	COHb levels 30–40%
	No symptoms or signs of impaired cardiovascular or neurologic function
Treatment	100% oxygen by tight-fitting non-rebreathing mask until COHb level remains < 5%
	Cardiovascular status followed closely even in asymptomatic patients, consider ECG and cardiac enzymes
	Determination of acid-base status (will be corrected by high-flow oxygen)
	Admission for observation and cardiovascular monitoring
Severe poisoning	
Criteria	COHb levels > 40%
	or
	Cardiovascular or neurologic impairment at any COHb level
Treatment	100% oxygen by tight-fitting non-rebreathing mask
	Cardiovascular function monitoring
	Determination of acid-base status
	Admission
	or
	Transfer to a HBO facility immediately if available, or if no improvement in cardiovascular or neurologic function within 4 h

Abbreviations: COHb, carboxyhemoglobin; ECG, electrocardiogram; HBO, hyperbaric oxygen therapy.

2. **Hyperbaric oxygen therapy** (HBO) is indicated for severe poisoning based upon clinical findings and the COHb level. The goal of treatment is not only amelioration of the acute event but also prevention of delayed neuropsychiatric sequelae. HBO should be carefully considered especially for patients at the extremes of age and in pregnancy.

CYANIDE

Cyanide is a naturally occurring and potent cellular toxin. Acute poisoning results from accidental occupational exposures, accidental or suicidal exposure to substances converted to cyanide (e.g., burning wool, silk, polyurethane, or vinyl), ingestion of plants or foods containing naturally occurring cyanogenic glycosides, or iatrogenic toxicity due to prolonged nitroprusside therapy.

Clinical Features

The hallmark of cyanide poisoning is apparent hypoxia without cyanosis. Metabolic acidosis is prominent with high lactate levels due to failed oxygen utilization. Awake patients complain of breathlessness and anxiety. In more severe cases, loss of consciousness (often with seizures) and tachydysrhythmias are apparent, which may proceed on to bradycardia and apnea and, finally, to asystolic cardiac arrest. Other clues to cyanide toxicity are bright red retinal blood vessels, oral burns from ingestions, the smell of bitter almonds on the patient's breath, and high peripheral venous oxygen saturations (acyanosis). Absorption of cyanide gas is immediate, and ingestion of cyanide salts may cause symptoms within minutes. At the other end of the spectrum, ingestion of cyanogenic compounds may not take effect for hours.

Diagnosis and Differential

The diagnosis of cyanide toxicity always should be considered in the poisoned patient with profound metabolic acidosis. Further support for the diagnosis is any finding suggesting decreased oxygen utilization. Laboratory testing has a limited role in diagnosing cyanide poisoning. Whole blood levels can be obtained but results generally will not be available for decisfiion making. Arterial blood gas assays can identify acid-base disturbances and the presence of an oxygen saturation gap, while serum lactate levels may provide additional supporting evidence.

The differential diagnosis includes other cellular toxins such as carbon monoxide, hydrogen sulfide, and simple asphyxiants. In the setting of an ingestion, other possibilities are methanol, ethylene glycol, iron, and salicylates. Severe isoniazid or cocaine poisoning may mimic the effects of cyanide, causing severe metabolic acidosis and seizures.

Emergency Department Care and Disposition

1. All patients should have frequent blood pressure and continuous cardiac monitoring, administration of **100% oxygen**, and intravenous access. Those with altered mental status must be considered for **IV-glucose**, **thiamine**, and **naloxone** administration. **Gastric lavage** and administration of **activated charcoal** are standard for cyanide ingestion; dermal contacts require skin decontamination and inhalational exposures require removal from the source.
2. Specific treatment with **nitrite-thiosulfate antidote therapy** in the form of a kit from Taylor Pharmaceuticals must be considered (Table 110-4). Asymptomatic patients or those with mini-

TABLE 110-4 Treatment of Cyanide Poisoning

	Children	
1. 100% oxygen.		
2. Administration of IV sodium nitrite and sodium thiosulfate:		
Hb (g/100 mL)	3% $NaNO_2$ (mL/kg)	25% $Na_2S_2O_3$ (mL/kg)
7	0.19	1.65
8	0.22	1.65
9	0.25	1.65
10	0.27	1.65
11	0.30	1.65
12	0.33	1.65
13	0.36	1.65
14	0.39	1.65

3. May repeat once at half dose if symptoms persist.

4. Monitor methemoglobin to keep level less than 30%.

Adults

1. 100% oxygen.

2. Amyl nitrite; crack and inhale 30 s/min.*

3. Sodium nitrite: 10 mL IV (10 mL ampule of 3% solution = 300 mg).

4. Sodium thiosulfate: 50 mL IV (50 mL ampule of 25% solution = 12.5 g).

5. May repeat once at half dose if symptoms persist.

*Administration of amyl nitrite is only necessary if venous access has not been obtained.

mal symptoms should be observed and treated only if clinical deterioration is noted. Severely toxic patients with a clear history of exposure demand full and immediate treatment. Due to the potential side effects of hypotension and induction of methemoglobinemia, hypotensive acidotic patients without clear cyanide toxicity or with smoke inhalation are best served by administration of IV **sodium thiosulfate** only.

For further reading in *Emergency Medicine: A Comprehensive Study Guide,* 5th ed., see Chap. 198, "Carbon Monoxide Poisoning," by Keith W. Van Meter; and Chap. 182, "Cyanide," by Kathleen A. Delaney.

---

111 | Heavy Metals

Todd C. Rothenhaus

Acute metal and metalloid toxicity, while rare, result in significant morbidity and mortality if unrecognized or improperly treated. Metal toxicity manifests itself on the body's enzymatic systems, resulting primarily in neurologic, gastrointestinal, hematologic, and renal impairment. Chelation therapy is the mainstay of treatment.

LEAD

Lead is the most common cause of chronic metal poisoning and the second leading cause of acute metal toxicity. Elevated blood lead levels have detrimental effects on intellectual development, and lead remains a major public health concern. Elevated levels are most common in children less than 5 years of age and have been linked with poverty, urban dwelling, and African-American race.

Clinical Features

Lead poisoning results in a number of nonspecific signs and symptoms that tend to be more severe in young children. Patients may present with central nervous system (CNS) symptoms (coma, seizures, delirium, or memory problems) and abdominal symptoms (colic or pain) as well as hematologic manifestations (hemolytic anemia). The combination of abdominal pain, neurologic symptoms, and hemolytic anemia should raise particular suspicion for lead toxicity.

Diagnosis and Differential

A history of lead exposure (occupational, hobby, environmental, or retained bullet) is the most important clue to making the diagnosis. Dietary history (pica), social history, or previous history of elevated lead levels are particularly helpful in making the diagnosis. Lead toxicity should be considered in all cases of encephalopathy, as well as in patients with vague neurologic or abdominal complaints. Diagnosis rests on demonstrating an elevated blood lead (PbB) level. However, this test is rarely available in the emergency department. Clues to the diagnosis include a normocytic or microcytic anemia, basophilic stippling of red blood cells (RBCs) on peripheral smear, lead bands on longbone radiographs, and radiopaque material or retained bullets on plain radiographs.

Emergency Department Care and Disposition

1. Patients with encephalopathy should begin chelation therapy as soon as possible with **dimercaprol (BAL)** 3 to 5 mg/kg IM, followed in 4 h with **CaNa$_2$-EDTA** 1500 μg/m^2 every 24 h via continuous IV infusion. Symptomatic patients without encephalopathy should be treated with BAL 3 mg/kg and CaNa$_2$-EDTA 1000 μg/m^2.
2. The approach to asymptomatic patients is somewhat controversial, and experience with newer chelating agents (e.g., **DMSA** [Succimer] and **d-penicillamine**) is becoming more widespread. Consultation with a poison control center is recommended. Admission is indicated for symptomatic patients, asymptomatic children with PbB levels greater than 70 μg/dL, and patients with suspected toxicity when returning to the home environment poses a risk for additional exposure.

ARSENIC

Arsenic, a nearly tasteless, odorless metal, is the most common cause of acute metal poisoning and the second leading cause of chronic metal toxicity. Arsenic is found in insecticides, herbicides, wood preservatives, homeopathic remedies, and contaminated well water, and is used in mining and smelting operations.

Clinical Features

Symptoms from acute exposure usually occur within a few hours and include nausea, vomiting, and severe diarrhea. Patients may also complain of a metallic taste. Subacute and chronic toxicity usually manifests as weakness, malaise, morbilliform skin rash, and a stocking-glove sensory/motor peripheral neuropathy that can progress to ascending paralysis. Mees' lines (1 to 2 mm wide transverse white lines on the nails) may be seen 4 to 6 weeks after an acute exposure.

Diagnosis and Differential

Arsenic toxicity should be considered in patients with unexplained hypotension, especially after a bout of severe gastroenteritis, and in patients with peripheral neuropathy, skin changes, or recurrent diarrhea. Definitive diagnosis rests on demonstrating elevated 24-h urine arsenic levels. Other laboratory clues to the diagnosis include eosinophilia or basophilic stippling of RBCs. A prolonged QT interval may be seen.

Emergency Department Care and Disposition

1. Death from arsenic toxicity results from hypotension and dysrhythmias. **Volume resuscitation** and cardiopulmonary monitoring should be instituted and inotropic support provided as necessary. Dysrhythmias are best treated with **lidocaine** and **bretylium**. Drugs that prolong the QT interval should be avoided.
2. **Gastric lavage** should be considered in acute ingestions, since arsenic is poorly adsorbed by activated charcoal. Chelation with **BAL** 3 to 5 mg/kg every 4 h should be instituted as soon as possible. Experience with **DMSA (Succimer)** is becoming more widespread and may be an acceptable alternative. However, *d*-penicillamine is not effective.

MERCURY

Mercury occurs in both inorganic and organic forms. While all forms are toxic, they differ in clinical effects and response to therapy.

Clinical Features

Clinical toxicity of mercury depends upon its form and route of exposure. The short-chained alkyl compounds (methyl, dimethyl, and ethyl mercury) as well as elemental mercury primarily affect the CNS. Erethism describes a constellation of neuropsychiatric abnormalities including anxiety, depression, irritability, mania, excessive shyness, and memory loss. Tremor, paresthesias, ataxia, spasticity, and hearing or visual impairment also have been described. Acrodynia is an immune-mediated condition, characterized by generalized rash, fever, irritability, hypotonia, and splenomegaly, seen in children exposed to all forms of mercury except the short-chained alkyl compounds. Acute mercury inhalation results in severe pneumonitis, acute respiratory distress syndrome, and pulmonary fibrosis.

Diagnosis and Differential

A history of exposure (e.g., occupational or environmental) is invaluable in making the diagnosis. The differential diagnosis includes causes of encephalopathy (e.g., metabolic or endocrine disorders, drug overdose, or carbon monoxide poisoning), tremor (e.g., Parkinson's disease, drug withdrawal, or cerebellar disease), and all causes of corrosive gastritis (e.g., acid, alkali, arsenic, phosphorous, or iron). For all forms of mercury except the short-chained alkyls, an elevated 24-h urinary measurement of mercury is required to make the diagnosis. Short-chained alkyl mercurials are excreted primarily via the bile, and whole-blood mercury levels, while less reliable for diagnosing mercury toxicity in general, must be employed to make the diagnosis.

Emergency Department Care and Disposition

Ingestion of mercury salts should be treated with aggressive gastrointestinal decontamination, including **gastric lavage** and **instillation of egg whites and charcoal** to bind mercury. **BAL** (3 to 5 mg/kg every 4 h) should be administered. Experience with DMSA is increasing, and it may become the treatment of choice for short-chained alkyl compounds.

For further reading in *Emergency Medicine: A Comprehensive Study Guide,* 5th ed., see Chap. 178, ''Metals and Metalloids,'' by Marsha D. Ford.

112 | Hazardous Materials Exposure
Todd C. Rothenhaus

A hazardous material is any substance that poses a risk to health, safety, property, or the environment. Well over a one-half million potentially toxic compounds have been produced, including industrial chemicals as well as nuclear, biologic, and chemical agents, also known as weapons of mass destruction. The incidence of serious hazardous material exposure is greater now than in any point in history, occurring at industrial sites, during transportation of materials, or resulting from malicious (terrorist) activity. Exposure to hazardous materials results not only in direct toxicity, but is frequently associated with trauma, burns, inhalation injury, and ocular injury.

General Principles

Hazardous materials incidents, while rare, can quickly overwhelm a medical facility, especially when mass casualities are involved. Prior planning is essential to coordinate resources, minimize loss of life, and prevent secondary contamination of health care workers.

Hazardous Material Information

Data about involved chemicals are essential. Sources include regional poison centers, material safety data sheets, transportation specific markings (DOT placards, shipping papers, and bills of lading), private agencies (CHEMTREC), government agencies (National Regulatory Commission, Center for Disease Control, Environmental Protection Agency, and ATSDR), computer databases (Poisindex, Safetydex, Tomes Plus, ToxNet), and the Internet.

Triage

Triage occurs outside the hospital where both urgency of care and adequacy of decontamination are assessed. *Under no circumstances is a patient allowed into the hospital unless fully decontaminated.* Medical stabilization prior to decontamination is limited to opening the airway, cervical spine stabilization, oxygen administration, ventilatory assistance, and application of direct pressure to arterial bleeding.

Decontamination

The goal of decontamination is to decrease further exposure to the victim and to prevent secondary contamination of health care workers. Decontamination is performed in three "zones." The *hot zone* is the area at the scene or *outside the hospital*, where patients with no prior decontamination are held. The *warm zone* is the area outside (or physically isolated from) the hospital where decontamination occurs. The *cold zone* is where fully decontaminated victims are transferred. There should be no movement of personnel between zones. Access to the hot and warm zones is restricted to personnel with suitable protective clothing (including, but not limited to, a chemical-resistant suit and self-contained breathing apparatus when the highest level of protection is needed).

Decontamination is begun by removing all clothing and brushing away gross particulate matter. Whole body irrigation is then initiated with copious amounts of water and mild soap or detergent, except in cases where water reactive substances (lithium, potassium, sodium, calcium, lime, calcium carbide, and others) may be involved. The hands and face are generally the most contaminated areas; decontamination should begin at the head and work downward, taking care to avoid runoff onto other body parts. Decontamination should continue for at least 3 to 5 min. Patients should then be wrapped in clean blankets and transfered to the cold zone.

SPECIFIC MEDICAL MANAGEMENT

Inhaled Toxins

Inhaled toxins include gases, dusts, fumes, and aerosols, and generally result in either upper airway damage or pulmonary toxicity. Specific agents include *phosgene*, *chlorine*, *ammonia*, and *riot control agents* (mace and pepper spray). Patients may have cough, wheezing, and stridor, but may also be initially asymptomatic. Administration of **100% oxygen** should be given first with **bronchodilators** next, followed by examination of the upper airway for signs of compromise. Patients should be intubated if they develop respiratory distress or airway edema. Consider carbon monoxide and cyanide toxicity if a history of combustion is present. Riot control agents [including CS, used by law enforcement, and CN (Mace), sold as self-protection] result in self-limited irritation of exposed mucous membranes and skin.

Neurotoxins

Five organophosphate compounds are recognized as nerve agents: tabun (GA), sarin (GB), soman (GD), GF, and VX. These agents inhibit acetylcholinesterase, resulting in build-up of acetylcholine at brain synapses (causing seizures and coma), motor endplates (causing weakness, paralysis, and respiratory insufficiency) and the autonomic nervous system (causing salivation, lacrimation, urination, diarrhea, bronchorrhea, and miosis). Treatment consists of complete decontamination, oxygen administration, administration of a combination of **atropine 2 mg** and **pralidoxime (2-PAMCl) 600 mg** IV or IM, and supportive care.

Dermal Toxins

Dermal toxins include *alkalines* (sodium hydroxide and cement), *phenol*, *hydrofluoric acid*, and *vesicants* [mustard (sulfur mustard; H; HD)], *Lewisite* (L), and *phosgene oxime* (CX)]. These agents may also cause significant pulmonary and ocular toxicity. Skin decontamination with deluge volumes of water is the mainstay of treatment. Hydrofluoric acid burns may result in systemic toxicity and should be treated with intravenous **calcium** or **magnesium** as well as topical **calcium gluconate gel**.

Ocular Exposures

Ocular exposures demand **immediate irrigation** with large volumes of water. In stable patients, immediate *prehospital* irrigation for up to 20 min prior to transport is recommended. Gross particulate matter should be brushed from around the eye, and contact lenses should be removed. Absence of pain may not indicate cessation of ocular damage, and irrigation should continue until ocular pH returns to 7.4.

Biologic Weapons

Biologic weapons include microbes (anthrax, plague, tularemia, Q fever, and viruses), mycotoxins (trichothecene), and bacterial toxins (ricin, staphylococcal enterotoxin B, botulinum, and *shigella*). Biological agents used as weapons are almost invariably delivered via droplet (aerosol) spread, resulting in fulminant infectious complications after a variable incubation period. 0.5% sodium hypochlorite solution (household bleach diluted 1:9 with water) is effective at neutralizing most biohazard materials and should be used for patient decontamination. Contact and respiratory isolation should be instituted, and empiric antibiotic therapy against suspected pathogens initiated. Detection is difficult and often relies upon isolation in a specialized laboratory.

For further reading in *Emergency Medicine: A Comprehensive Study Guide*, 5th ed., see Chap. 181, "Hazardous Materials Exposure," by Suzanne R. White and Col. Edward M. Eitzen, Jr.

113 | Dyshemoglobinemias

Howard E. Jarvis III

The dyshemoglobinemias are a group of disorders in which the hemoglobin molecule is structurally altered and prevented from carrying oxygen. The most relevant of these are carboxyhemoglobinemia, methemoglobinemia, and sulfhemoglobinemia. Carboxyhemoglobinemia follows carbon monoxide exposure (see Chap. 110). Both acquired methemoglobinemia and sulfhemoglobinemia are typically caused by exposures to various drugs and chemicals, which cause an oxidant stress.

Clinical Features

The clinical suspicion of methemoglobinemia should be raised when the patient's pulse oximetry approaches 85 percent, there is no response to supplemental oxygen, and brownish-blue skin and "chocolate-brown" blood discoloration is noted. Exposure to known causes, such as nitrates (in well-water and vegetables) and certain medications, should raise concern. Medications that may precipitate this condition include phenazopyridine (for symptomatic treatment of urinary tract infections), benzocaine (a topical anesthetic), and dapsone (an antibiotic often used in HIV-related therapy). There may be significant time delays from exposure to symptoms with some agents.

   Patients with normal hemoglobin concentrations do not develop clinically significant effects until methemoglobin levels rise in 15% of the total hemoglobin. They may seek evaluation for cyanosis that occurs with methemoglobin levels of 1.5 g/dL. This is approximately 10% of total hemoglobin in normal individuals. Patients with anemia require a higher percentage as it is the absolute concentration (1.5 g/dL) that determines cyanosis. When levels reach 15 to 30%, symptoms include anxiety, headache, weakness, and light-headedness. Tachypnea and sinus tachycardia may occur. Methemoglobin levels of 50 to 60% impair oxygen delivery to vital tissues, causing myocardial ischemia, dysrhythmias, depressed mental status (including coma), seizures, and lactate-related cyanosis. Levels above 70% are largely incompatible with life. Patients with anemia and those with preexisting disease that impairs oxygen delivery (e.g., chronic obstructive pulmonary disease and congestive heart failure) may be symptomatic at lower concentrations of methemoglobin.

Sulfhemoglobinemia is caused by many of the same agents that cause methemoglobinemia, though it is clinically less concerning. Cyanosis may occur at levels of 0.5 g/dL due to increased pigmentation.

Diagnosis and Differential

The diagnosis of methemoglobinemia must be considered in any cyanotic patient, particularly if the cyanosis is unresponsive to oxygen. The blood has a "chocolate-brown" color, analogous to the chocolate-brown agar used to plate gonococcus. Pulse oximetry must be interpreted with caution since it cannot properly differentiate oxyhemoglobin from methemoglobin. It may be normal with moderate methemoglobinemia and may trend toward 85% in those with severe methemoglobinemia. Definitive identification of methemoglobin relies on cooximetry, which is a widely available test and requires only venous blood (though arterial blood can be used). It can differentiate oxyhemoglobin, deoxyhemoglobin, carboxyhemoglobin, and methemoglobin species. The oxygen saturation obtained from an arterial blood gas analyzer also will be falsely normal since it is calculated from dissolved oxygen tension, which is appropriately normal. Sulfhemoglobin is differentiated from methemoglobin by the addition of cyanide to the laboratory cooximetry sample. Failure to eliminate the methemoglobin peak with the addition of cyanide confirms the diagnosis of sulfhemoglobinemia.

Emergency Department Care and Disposition

Patients with methemoglobinemia required optimal supportive measures to ensure oxygen delivery.

1. The efficacy of gastric decontamination is limited due to the substantial time interval from exposure to development of methemoglobin. If an on-going source of exposure exists, a single dose of oral **activated charcoal** is indicated.
2. Antidotal therapy with **methylene blue** is reserved for those patients with documented methemoglobinemia or a high clinical suspicion of disease. Unstable patients should receive methylene blue, but may require blood transfusion or exchange transfusion for immediate enhancement of oxygen delivery. The initial dose of methylene blue is 1 to 2 mg/kg IV, and its effect should be seen within 20 min. If necessary, repeat dosing of methylene blue is acceptable, but high doses (> 7 mg/kg) may actually induce methemoglobin formation.

3. Treatment failures occur in some groups, which include glucose-6-phosphate dehydrogenase (G6PD) deficiency and other enzyme deficiencies, and may occur with hemolysis. Hemolysis is seen with some precipitants of methemoglobinemia, such as chlorates. Agents with long half-lives, such as dapsone, may require serial dosing of methylene blue.
4. Patients with the clinically indistinguishable sulfhemoglobinemia will not respond to methylene blue and are treated supportively. They may require blood transfusions in cases of severe toxicity. Likewise, those with methemoglobinemia unresponsive to methylene blue should be treated supportively. If clinically unstable, the use of blood transfusions or exchange transfusions is indicated. If newly administered red blood cell hemoglobin undergoes oxidation, it will likely respond to methylene blue.

For further reading in *Emergency Medicine: A Comprehensive Study Guide,* 5th ed., see Chap. 183, "Dyshemoglobinemias," by Sean M. Rees and Lewis S. Nelson.

ENVIRONMENTAL INJURIES

114 | Frostbite and Hypothermia

Kent N. Hall

Frostbite and hypothermia constitute a spectrum of illness. Frostbite and its related entities, chilblains and trench foot, are localized skin damage caused by cold injury with or without associated factors. Hypothermia is defined as a core temperature less than 35°C (95°F).

Clinical Features

Clinical entities in the spectrum of focal cold-related injuries include chilblains, trench foot, and frostbite. Chilblains (or pernio) consists of painful, inflamed skin lesions (usually on the hands, ears, lower legs, and feet) caused by chronic, intermittent exposure to damp, nonfreezing ambient temperatures. Manifestations include edema, erythema, cyanosis, plaques, nodules, ulcerations, vesicles, or bullae that develop up to 12 h after acute exposure. Patients often complain of burning paresthesias and pruritis. Blue nodules may develop upon rewarming and may last for several days.

Trench foot results from cooling of soft tissues, is accelerated by wet conditions, and takes hours to days to develop. At first, tingling and numbness develop in the affected area. Initially the area appears pale and mottled, and is anesthetic, pulseless, and immobile. A hyperemic phase occurs hours after rewarming and is associated with a severe burning sensation and return of sensation in the proximal area. Edema and bullae develop in the area over the next 2 to 3 days. Anesthesia of the area may be permanent. In severe cases gangrene may develop. Long-term hyperhidrosis and cold sensitivity are common.

Frostbite can occur on any skin surface but is usually limited to the exposed skin. The spectrum of injuries from frostbite appears in Table 114-1. Frostnip is a less severe form of frostbite, associated with discomfort that resolves with rewarming and no tissue loss.

TABLE 114-1 Classification of Cold Injury According to Severity

Classification	Symptoms
Superficial	
First degree: partial skin freezing Erythema, edema, hyperemia No blisters or necrosis Occasional skin desquamation (5–10 d later)	Transient stinging and burning Throbbing and aching possible May have hyperhidrosis
Second degree: full-thickness skin freezing Erythema, substantial edema, vesicles with clear fluid Blisters that desquamate and form blackened eschar	Numbness, followed by aching and throbbing Vasomotor disturbances in severe cases
Deep	
Third degree: full-thickness skin and subcutaneous freezing Violaceous/hemorrhagic blisters Skin necrosis Blue-gray discoloration of skin	Initially no sensation Patient states it "feels like block of wood" Later, shooting pains, burning, throbbing, aching
Fourth degree: full-thickness skin, subcutaneous tissue, muscle, tendon, and bone freezing Little edema Initially mottled, deep red, or cyanotic Eventually dry, black, mummified	Possible joint discomfort

First- and second-degree frostbite injuries have an excellent prognosis. The prognosis for third degree frostbite is often poor, while that for fourth degree is extremely poor.

In "mild" hypothermia, defined as a body temperature between 32°C and 35°C (90°F and 95°F), heart rate and blood pressure rise, and shivering occurs. When body temperature falls below 32°C, shivering ceases and the heart rate and blood pressure begin to fall. Below 30°C (86°F) the patient is prone to ventricular dysrhythmias, the incidence increasing as body temperature falls. Typically, the heart rhythm progresses from sinus bradycardia to atrial fibrillation with a slow ventricular response to ventricular fibrillation to asystole as the body temperature drops. The classic electrocardiogram (ECG) finding of hypothermia is the Osborn (J) wave, a slow positive deflection at the end of the QRS complex.

Pulmonary effects of hypothermia include initial tachypnea, followed by progressive decrease in respiratory rate and tidal volume. Bronchorrhea and loss of the cough and gag reflex also occur. Hypothermia causes a depression of the central nervous system, initially manifested by incoordination, followed by confusion, lethargy, and coma. Renal effects include a "cold diuresis," which can cause significant volume loss, exacerbated by a plasma shift to the extravascular space. This can result in hemoconcentration, intravascular thrombosis, and disseminated intravascular coagulation.

Emergency Department Care and Disposition

1. Management of the patient with chilblains and trench foot is supportive. Affected skin should be rewarmed, bandaged, and elevated. **Nifedipine** 20 mg tid, topical corticosteroids, and sometimes oral prednisone have been shown to be helpful in ameliorating the symptoms of chilblains. Affected areas are more prone to reinjury. With trench foot, the best therapy is preventive. Changing socks several times a day and never sleeping in wet socks and boots are the best preventive measures. Once symptoms develop, keep feet warm, dry, and elevated.

2. **Rapid rewarming** is the most important aspect of frostbite therapy. Placement of the involved extremity in gently **recirculating water** at a temperature of 40°C to 42°C (104°F to 108°F) for 10 to 30 min results in complete thawing. Rewarming with dry air should be avoided. Severe pain is associated with rewarming, and **parenteral narcotics** should be administered and titrated to effect. Current recommendations are to débride or aspirate all clear blisters, leaving hemorrhagic blisters intact. All blisters should be treated with topical aloe vera every 6 h. Affected digits should be wrapped separately with dry, sterile cotton bandages. Use of topical **aloe vera** and oral **ibuprofen** 12 mg/kg/d help to blunt the arachidonic acid cascade and limit tissue damage. Prophylactic use of **penicillin G 500,000 U** every 6 h for 48 to 72 h has been beneficial, according to some published protocols. Early surgical intervention is not indicated and, in fact, may result in greater tissue loss. Limited, early escharotomy may be indicated in cases where range of motion or circulation is compromised. All patients with more than isolated and superficial frostbite lesions should be admitted to the hospital. Transfer to a tertiary care center should be considered for severe cases.

3. Management of the patient with hypothermia includes both supportive measures and specific rewarming techniques (Table 114-2). Supportive measures include attention to the ABCs of resuscitation (airway, breathing, and circulation). If indicated for oxygenation, gentle endotracheal intubation rarely results in complications. **Oxygen and intravenous fluids should be warmed**. The patient's core body temperature should be monitored using an electronic or glass thermometer capable of recording in the severe hypothermic (below 32°C, or 89.6°F) range. Most rhythm disturbances in the severely hypothermic patient are not immediately life-threatening. Ventricular fibrillation, when present, is usually refractory to therapy until the patient's core temperature is above 30°C (86°F). Current American Heart Association guidelines recommend countershock three times if ventricular fibrillation occurs. If these attempts are unsuccessful, cardiopulmonary resuscitation is begun and rapid rewarming instituted.

4. **Rewarming techniques** include passive external, active external, and active core (Table 114-2). Passive rewarming uses the patient's endogenous heat production for rewarming and is the most physiologic. When intrinsic thermoregulatory mechanisms

---

TABLE 114-2 Rewarming Techniques

Passive rewarming
  Removal from cold environment
  Insulation

Active external rewarming
  Warm water immersion
  Heating blankets
  Heated objects (water bottles, etc.)
  Radiant heat
  Forced air

Active core rewarming
  Inhalation rewarming
  Heated intravenous fluids
  Gastrointestinal tract lavage
  Bladder lavage
  Peritoneal lavage
  Pleural lavage
  Extracorporeal rewarming
  Mediastinal lavage via thoracotomy

---

are not intact, metabolic heat production does not occur, and passive rewarming will not work.

5. Active external rewarming provides exogenous heat to the body and includes the use of **warm water immersion, heating blankets, heated objects**, or **radiant heat**. Core temperatures may continue to drop after rewarming has begun. This "core temperature afterdrop" is clinically insignificant. "Rewarming shock" is seen secondary to peripheral vasodilation and venous pooling when active external rewarming is used. Washout of lactic acid from the periphery into the central circulation may increase demands on the circulatory system with no reserve, further increasing tissue hypoxia and acidosis.

6. Active core rewarming allows the heart to be preferentially warmed, decreasing myocardial irritability and returning cardiac function. **Inhalation rewarming** (using warmed, humidified oxygen by mask or endotracheal tube) and use of **warmed intravenous fluids** provide for only a small amount of heat transfer but should be used on every moderately or severely hypothermic patient. Lavage of the stomach and bladder is simple, and large volumes of warmed fluid may be used rapidly.

7. **Peritoneal and pleural lavage** have been shown to be effective in animal studies and human cases, and can be instituted quickly in emergency department with readily available material. In the case of peritoneal lavage, potassium free saline solution is warmed to 42°C (107.6°F) and instilled in the peritoneal cavity through a peritoneal dialysis or DPL catheter. Similar fluid can be instilled into the left chest through a thoracostomy tube placed in the second left intercostal space at the midclavicular line. An effluent tube placed in the fifth or sixth intercostal space at the midaxillary line allows the fluid to drain.

8. Rewarming through an **extracorporeal circuit** is the method of choice in the severely hypothermic patient in cardiac arrest. This requires placement of bypass catheters, usually in the femoral vessels. Rapid rewarming rates, circulatory support, and oxygenation are achieved with this technique. Unfortunately, specialized equipment and personnel are required.

9. A general approach to rewarming takes into account the degree of hypothermia and the patient's cardiovascular status. If endogenous heat production mechanisms are functional, gradual rewarming without active modalities is usually sufficient. When the patient has severe hypothermia but a stable cardiac rhythm, active external rewarming in conjunction with inhalational and heated intravenous fluids may be attempted, although some

authorities recommend active core rewarming in this setting. In the presence of cardiovascular insufficiency, rapid rewarming is required, and active core techniques should be used.

For further reading in *Emergency Medicine: A Comprehensive Study Guide,* 5th ed., see Chap. 185, "Frostbite and Other Localized Cold-Related Injuries," by Mark B. Rabold; and Chap. 186, "Hypothermia," by Howard A. Bessen.

---

115 | Heat Emergencies

Todd C. Rothenhaus

Heat emergencies represent a continuum of disorders, ranging from minor syndromes, such as *prickly heat, heat cramps,* and *heat exhaustion,* to the life-threatening disorder known as *heat stroke.* Heat-related illness is most prevalent in the elderly and in patients under 4 years of age. Although seen most commonly during summer heat waves, heat emergencies can occur during milder temperatures, especially in patients with chronic medical conditions, drug abuse, mental illness, occupational exposure to high temperatures, or insufficient acclimatization.

HEATSTROKE

Clinical Features

Patients with heat stroke have an alteration in mental status and an elevated body temperature ($> 45°C$). A history of environmental or occupational heat exposure can usually be discerned. Neurologic abnormalities include ataxia, confusion, bizarre behavior, agitation, seizures, and coma. Anhidrosis, although classically described, is not invariably present, and the presence of perspiration in no way rules out the diagnosis.

Diagnosis and Differential

Heatstroke is a diagnosis of exclusion, and should be considered in any patient with an elevated body temperature and altered mental status. The differential diagnosis includes infection (sepsis, meningitis, encephalitis, malaria, tetanus, typhoid fever, and brain abscess), toxins (anticholinergics, phenothiazines, salicylates, PCP, cocaine, amphetamines, and alcohol withdrawal), metabolic and endocrinologic emergencies (thyrotoxicosis and DKA), primary central nervous system disorders (status epilepticus and intracranial hemorrhage), neuroleptic malignant syndrome, and malignant hyperthermia.

Laboratory studies should include a complete blood cell count; electrolytes, blood urea nitrogen, and creatinine levels; hepatic panel; and coagulation studies. Creatinine kinase (CK) levels should be taken to evaluate patients for possible rhabdomyolysis, and cardiac isoenzymes levels should be considered in patients at risk for coronary artery disease. An arterial blood gas analysis, urinalysis, chest radiograph, and pregnancy test should also be obtained. A computed tomography (CT) scan of the head and lumbar puncture should be considered in evaluating for CNS pathology.

Emergency Department Care and Disposition

Heatstroke is a true medical emergency. Failure to rapidly lower core body temperature can lead to further end-organ damage and multiple organ dysfunction syndrome.

1. Assess **ABCs:** High-flow supplemental oxygen should be provided. Patients with significantly altered mental status, hypoxia, or inadequate gag reflex should be intubated.
2. **Monitoring**: Cardiac monitor, pulse oximeter, and time-cycled blood pressure cuff should be applied. Continuous core temperature monitoring should be initiated with a rectal or bladder probe. More invasive hemodynamic monitoring (central venous pressure and pulmonary artery catheter) should be considered if the patient is hemodynamically unstable.
3. IV fluids: Isotonic fluid resuscitation should be intiated with either normal saline or Ringer's lactate solution. Patients with evidence of volume depletion should receive up to 2 L of crystalloid (20 mL/kg). Patients should be monitored closely for signs of volume overload.
4. Cooling: **Evaporative cooling** is the most efficient and practical means of cooling patients in the emergency department (ED). Patients must be completely disrobed with their entire skin wet with room temperature water and placed in front of cooling fans. Cold water or ice packs applied to patients may cause shivering and should be avoided. Cooling efforts should be discontinued when the core temperature drops below 40°C to avoid iatrogenic hypothermia. Cardiopulmonary bypass may be considered if standard cooling methods fail. Shivering should

be treated with benzodiazepines (midazolam 2 mg IV) or **phenothiazines** (Thorazine 25 mg IM). Antipyretics are of no benefit in patients with heatstroke.

5. Disposition: Patients with true heat stroke should be observed for development of further end-organ damage. Patients should be admitted to an intensive care unit or monitored bed as appropriate.

MINOR HEAT ILLNESSES

Heat exhaustion is a clinical syndrome resulting from heat exposure characterized by any or all of the following: headache, weakness, dizziness, nausea, vomiting, myalgias, diaphoresis, tachypnea, tachycardia, or orthostatic hypotension. Core body temperature is frequently elevated, but may be normal. Although patients may complain of neurologic symptoms, the patient's sensorium and neurologic examination should be normal. Treatment consists of rest, evaporative cooling, and administration of intravenous normal saline or oral electrolyte solution, depending upon severity. Laboratory studies should be considered, especially creatinine kinase to rule out rhabdomyolysis, in more severe cases. Patients should be observed until symptoms resolve.

Heat syncope results from volume depletion, peripheral vasodilation, and decreased vasomotor tone and occurs most commonly in elderly and poorly acclimatized individuals. Postural vital signs may or may not be demonstrable on presentation to the ED. Patients should be thoroughly evaluated for injury resulting from a fall, and all cardiac, neurologic, or other potentially serious causes for syncope should be considered. Treatment consists of rest and oral or intravenous rehydration.

Heat cramps are characterized by painful muscle spasms, especially in the calves, thighs, and shoulders. Especially common during athletic events, they are thought to result from dilutional hyponatremia as individuals replace evaporative losses with free water, but not salt. Core body temperature may be normal or elevated. Treatment consists of rest and administration of oral electrolyte solution or intravenous normal saline. Patients should be instructed to replace future fluid losses with a balanced electrolyte solution.

Heat rash (prickly heat) is a maculopapular eruption, most commonly found over clothed areas of the body, resulting from inflammation and obstruction of sweat ducts. Early stages present with a pruritic, erythematous eruption best treated with antihistamines and chlorhexidine cream or lotion. Continued blockage of pores results in a nonpruritic, nonerythematous, whitish, papular rash known as the *profunda stage* of prickly heat, best treated with oral antibiotics that combat *Staphylococcus aureus* and application of 1% salicylic acid to affected areas three times daily.

Heat edema results when cutaneous vasodilation and pooling of increased interstitial fluid in dependent extremities lead to swelling of the hands and feet. It is self-limited and rarely lasts more than a few weeks. Treatment consists of elevation of the extremities, and, in severe cases, application of compressive stockings. Administration of diuretics may exacerbate volume depletion and should be avoided.

For further reading in *Emergency Medicine: A Comprehensive Study Guide,* 5th ed., see Chap. 187, "Heat Emergencies," by James S. Walker and S. Brent Barnes.

---

116 | Bites and Stings

Burton Bentley II

HYMENOPTERA (WASPS, BEES, AND STINGING ANTS)

Wasps, bees, and stinging ants are members of the order Hymenoptera. Both local and generalized reactions may occur in response to an encounter.

Clinical Features

Local reactions consist of edema at the sting site. Although it may involve neighboring joints, local reactions cause no systemic symptoms. Severe local reactions increase the likelihood of serious systemic reactions if the patient is exposed again at a later time. *Toxic reactions* are a nonantigenic response to multiple stings. They have many of the same features that are seen in true systemic (allergic) reactions, but there is a greater frequency of gastrointestinal disturbance, while bronchospasm and urticaria do not occur. *Systemic* or *anaphylactic reactions* are true allergic reactions that range from mild to fatal. In general, the shorter the interval between the sting and the onset of symptoms, the more severe the reaction. Initial symptoms usually consist of itching eyes, urticaria, and cough. As the reaction progresses, patients may experience respiratory failure and cardiovascular collapse. *Delayed reactions* may appear 10 to 14 days after a sting. Symptoms of delayed reactions resemble serum sickness and include fever, malaise, headache, urticaria, lymphadenopathy, and polyarthritis.

Emergency Department Care and Disposition

1. The treatment for all Hymenoptera encounters is the same. First, **any bee stinger remaining in the patient should be removed immediately,** and the wound should be cleansed. Ice packs and elevation may reduce the degree of swelling. Erythema and swelling seen in local reactions may be difficult to distinguish from cellulitis. As a general rule, infection is present in a minority of cases. For minor local reactions, oral antihistamines and analgesics may be the only treatment needed.
2. More severe reactions, such as chest constriction, nausea, presyncope, or a change in a mental status require treatment with **1:1000 epinephrine subcutaneously; 0.3 mL to 0.5 mL for an adult and 0.01 mL/kg for a child** (0.3 mL maximum). Some patients may require a second epinephrine injection in 10 to 15 min. **Parenteral H_1 and H_2 receptor antagonists** (e.g., diphenhydramine and ranitidine) and **steroids** (e.g., methylprednisolone) should be rapidly administered. Bronchospasm responds to courses of **inhaled β-agonists** (e.g., albuterol). Hypotension should be treated aggressively with **crystalloid,** though **dopamine** and **epinephrine** infusions may be required. Patients with minor symptoms who respond well to conservative measures may be discharged after monitoring for several hours. Severe reactions require admission to the hospital. All patients with Hymenoptera reactions should be referred to an allergist for further evaluation and possible immunotherapy.

ANTS (*FORMICIDAE*)

There are several species of fire ants (Solenopsis) in the United States, and their venom may cross-react in individuals sensitized to other Hymenoptera stings. Fire ants swarm during an attack and each sting results in a papule that evolves to a sterile pustule over 6 to 24 h. Local necrosis and scarring, as well as systemic reactions, can occur. Treatment is the same as for other Hymenoptera stings, and appropriate referral should be made for desensitization therapy.

ARACHNIDA (SPIDERS, SCABIES, CHIGGERS, AND SCORPIONS)

Brown Recluse Spider (*Loxosceles reclusa*)

Clinical Features

The *L. reclusa* bite causes a mild, erythematous lesion that may become firm and heal over several days to weeks. Occasionally, a severe reaction with immediate pain, blister formation, and bluish discoloration may occur. These lesions often become necrotic over the next 3 to 4 days and form an eschar from 1 to 30 cm in diameter. Loxoscelism is a systemic reaction that may occur 1 to 2 days after envenomation. Symptoms include fever, chills, vomiting, arthralgias, myalgias, petechiae, and hemolysis; severe cases progress to seizure, renal failure, disseminated intravascular coagulation, and death. The diagnosis of *L. reclusa* envenomation may need to be made on clinical grounds since the bite is often unwitnessed. There is no lab result that specifically confirms *L. reclusa* poisoning, but all patients with suspected envenomation should have the following tests performed: Complete blood cell count (CBC); blood urea nitrogen, creatinine and electrolytes; coagulation profile; and urinalysis for hemoglobinuria.

Emergency Department Care and Disposition

Treatment of the brown recluse spider bite includes the usual supportive measures. Currently, there is no commercially available antivenin. Tetanus prophylaxis, analgesics, and antibiotics may be offered when appropriate. Surgery is reserved for lesions greater than 2 cm and is deferred for 2 to 3 weeks following the bite. The role of **dapsone** (50 to 200 mg/d) and **hyperbaric oxygen** have been challenged but may prevent some ongoing local necrosis. Patients with systemic reactions and hemolysis must be hospitalized for consideration of blood transfusion and hemodialysis.

Black Widow Spider (*Latrodectus mactans*)

Clinical Features

Black widow bites are initially painful, and within one hour, the patient may experience erythema (often "target" shaped), swelling, and diffuse muscle cramps. Large muscle groups are involved, and painful cramping of the abdominal wall musculature can mimic peritonitis. Severe pain may wax and wane for up to 3 days, but muscle weakness and spasm can persist for weeks to months. Serious acute complications include hypertension, respiratory failure, shock, and coma.

Emergency Department Care and Disposition

1. Initial therapy includes local wound treatment and supportive care. **Analgesics** and **benzodiazepines** will relieve pain and cramping, and some patients may benefit from intravenous **calcium gluconate.**
2. An **antivenin** derived from horse serum is effective for severe envenomation. If the patient tolerates placement of a standard cutaneous test dose, the usual intravenous dose is 1 to 2 vials over 30 min. Major complications including anaphylaxis have occurred with this therapy.

Scabies (*Sarcoptes scabiei*)

Clinical Features

Scabies bites are concentrated in the web spaces between fingers and toes. Other common areas include the penis, children's faces and scalps, and the female nipple. Transmission is typically by direct contact. The distinctive feature of scabies infestation is intense pruritus with "burrows." These white, threadlike channels form zigzag patterns with small gray spots at the closed end where the parasite rests. Undisturbed burrows can be traced with a hand lens, and the female mite is easily scraped out with a blade edge. Associated vesicles, papules, crusts, and eczematization may obscure the diagnosis.

Emergency Department Care and Disposition

Adult treatment of scabies infestation consists of a thorough application of **permethrin** (Elimite) from the neck down; infants may require additional application to the scalp, temple, and forehead. The patient should first bathe in warm soapy water, apply the medication, then bathe again in 12 h. Reapplication is necessary only if mites are found 2 weeks following treatment, though the pruritus may last for several weeks after successful therapy.

Chiggers (*Trombiculidae*)

Clinical Features

Chiggers are tiny mite larvae that cause intense pruritus when they feed on host epidermal cells. Itchiness begins within a few hours, followed by a papule that enlarges to a nodule over the next 1 to 2 days. Single bites can also cause soft tissue edema while infestation has been associated with fever and erythema multiforme. Children who have been sitting on lawns are prone to chigger lesions in the genital area. The diagnosis of chigger bites can be made on the basis of typical skin lesions in the context of a known outdoor exposure.

Emergency Department Care and Disposition

Treatment consists of symptomatic relief with antihistamines, though topical or oral steroids may be required in more severe cases. Annihilation of the mites requires **lindane** (Kwell), **permethrin** (Elimite), or **crotamiton** (Eurax) topical applications. The package insert provides techniques for proper application.

Scorpion (*Scorpionidae*)

Clinical Features

Of all North American scorpions, only the bark scorpion (*Centruroides exilicauda*) of the western United States is capable of producing systemic toxicity. *C. exilicauda* venom causes immediate burning and stinging although no local injury is visible. Systemic effects are infrequent, and mainly occur at the extremes of patient age. Findings may include tachycardia, excessive secretions, roving eye movements, opisthotonos, and fasciculations. The diagnosis may be elusive if the scorpion is not seen, though roving eye movements are pathognomonic. A positive "tap test" (i.e., exquisite local tenderness when the area is lightly tapped) is also suggestive.

Emergency Department Care and Disposition

Treatment is supportive, including local wound care. Reassurance is also important since many patients harbor misconceptions about the lethality of scorpion stings. Patients with pain in the absence of other toxic symptoms may be briefly observed before they are discharged home with analgesics. The **application of ice** often provides immediate relief of local pain. Muscle spasm and fasciculations respond promptly to **benzodiazepines.** Severe toxicity may warrant **scorpion antivenin,** a product available only in Arizona. One to two vials of this goat-derived product affords immediate symptomatic resolution.

Fleas (*Siphonaptera*)

Flea bites are frequently found in zigzag lines, especially on the legs and waist. They are intensely pruritic lesions with hemorrhagic puncta, surrounding erythema, and urticaria. Discomfort is relieved with **starch baths** (1 kg starch in a tub of water), **calamine lotion,** and oral **antihistamines.** Severe irritation may require topical steroid creams. Patients may develop impetigo and other local infections from scratching. Fingernails should be cut short, and infections should be treated in the standard manner.

Lice (*Anoplura*)

Body lice concentrate on the waist, shoulders, axillae, and neck. Their bites produce red spots that progress to papules and wheals. They are so intensely pruritic that linear scratch marks are suggestive of infestation. The white ova of head lice are adherent to the hair shaft, and can therefore be distinguished from dandruff. Pubic lice are spread by sexual contact. They cause intense pruritus, and their small white eggs (nits) are visible on hair shafts. Reactions to lice saliva and feces may cause fever, malaise, and lymphadenopathy. As with scabies, **permethrin** is the primary treatment for body lice infestation. Treatment of any hair-borne infestation requires a thorough application of **pyrethrin with piperonyl butoxide** (RID Lice Killing Shampoo) with mandatory reapplication in 10 days. A fine-toothed comb will aid in removal of dead lice and nits. Clothing, bedding, and personal articles must be sterilized in hot ($> 52°C$) water to prevent reinfestation.

KISSING BUG, PUSS CATERPILLAR, AND BLISTER BEETLE

Kissing Bug (*Triatoma sp.*)

Cone-nose or kissing bugs feed on blood and commonly attack the exposed surface of a sleeping victim. Proper identification is difficult if the insect is not recovered. The initial bite is painless, and the victim may be unaware of the attack. Bites are often multiple and result in wheals or hemorrhagic papules and bullae. Anaphylaxis commonly occurs in the sensitized individual. Treatment consists of local wound care and analgesics. **Allergic reactions must be treated as previously outlined for Hymenoptera envenomation.** Hypersensitive individuals should be referred to an allergist for immunotherapy.

Puss Caterpillar (*Megalopyge opercularis*)

The puss caterpillar has stinging spines on its body that provoke immediate, intense, and rhythmic pain. Local edema and pruritus with vesicles, red blotches, and papules may follow. Infrequently, fever, muscle cramps, anxiety, and shocklike symptoms may occur. Lymphadenopathy with local desquamation may develop in a few days. Treatment consists of **immediate spine removal with cellophane tape.** Intravenous **calcium gluconate, 10 mL of a 10% solution,** is effective in relieving pain. Mild cases may respond to an

antihistamine, such as tripelennamine (PBZ; 25 to 50 mg every 4 to 6 h in adults, or 5 mg/kg/d in divided doses for children).

Blister Beetle (*Coleoptera*)

Blister beetles produce local irritation and blistering within hours of contact, though they provoke intense gastrointestinal disturbances if ingested. Treatment consists of an occlusive dressing to protect the bullae from trauma. Large bullae should be drained and covered with a topical antibiotic ointment. Application of steroid creams may also speed recovery.

RATTLESNAKE BITES

There are approximately 8000 venomous snake bites each year in the United States, but only about 10 deaths result. In fact, 25% of bites are "dry strikes" with no effect from the venom. Except for imported species, the only venomous North American snakes are the pit vipers (e.g., rattlesnakes, copperhead, water moccasin, and massasauga) and coral snakes. Pit vipers are identified by their two retractable fangs and by the heat-sensitive depressions ("pits") located bilaterally between each eye and nostril.

Clinical Features

The effects of envenomation depend on the size and species of snake, the age and size of the victim, the time elapsed since the bite, and the characteristics of the bite itself. Since the degree of poisoning following an encounter is variable, bites that seem innocuous at first may rapidly become severe. The hallmark of pit viper envenomation is fang marks with local pain and swelling, but there are three classes of criteria that determine the severity of a rattlesnake bite:

1. Degree of local injury (swelling, pain, and ecchymosis)
2. Degree of systemic involvement (hypotension, tachycardia, and paresthesia)
3. Evolving coagulopathy (thrombocytopenia, elevated INR, and hypofibrinogenemia). Abnormalities in *any* of these three areas indicate that envenomation has occurred. Conversely, the absence of any clinical findings after 8 to 12 h effectively rules out venom injection.

Diagnosis and Differential

In general, all affected patients have swelling within 30 min, though some may take up to 12 h. The diagnosis is based on the clinical findings, and corroborating laboratory data as described earlier, while the envenomation itself is graded on an evolving continuum. *Minimal* envenomation describes cases with *local swelling,* no systemic signs, and no laboratory abnormalities. *Moderate* envenomation causes increased swelling that spreads from the site. These patients may also have systemic signs such as nausea, paresthesia, hypotension, and tachycardia. Coagulation parameters may be abnormal, but there is no significant bleeding. *Severe* envenomation causes extensive swelling, potentially life-threatening systemic signs (hypotension, altered mental status, and respiratory distress), and markedly abnormal coagulation parameters that may result in hemorrhage.

Emergency Department Care and Disposition

1. All patients bitten by a pit viper must be evaluated at a medical facility. **Consultation with a specialist familiar with snake bite is recommended for all but the simplest cases; one resource is the Arizona Poison Control Center at (520) 626-6016.** The patient should minimize physical activity, remain calm, and immobilize any bitten extremity in a neutral position below the level of the heart.

2. Intravenous access should be established, the patient should be resuscitated aggressively per ACLS protocols, and specimens for a CBC, INR, partial thromboplastin time, urinalysis, and blood typing should be obtained. Local wound care and tetanus immunization should be given, but prophylactic antibiotics and steroids have no proven benefit. Limb circumference at several sites above and below the wound should be checked every 30 min, and the border of advancing edema should be marked.

3. Any patient with progressive local swelling, systemic effects, or coagulopathy should immediately receive **equine-derived Antivenin (Crotalidae) Polyvalent.** An intradermal skin test (0.03 mL of 1:10 diluted antivenin) must be placed before the patient is treated; a 10-mm wheal within 30 min is considered positive. A positive skin test warrants a risk-benefit analysis before any antivenin is administered; these cases should be discussed with a toxicologist at once. **The starting dose of antivenin is 10 vials intravenously; severe cases require 20 vials.** Dosing regimens are exactly the same for both children and adults, though the amount of fluid in which the antivenin is mixed will need to be adjusted accordingly. The antivenin package insert will guide in administration, and the physician must be prepared to treat severe allergic and anaphylactic reactions. The endpoint of antivenin therapy is the arrest of progressive

symptoms and coagulopathy. Laboratory determinations are repeated every 4 h or after each course of antivenin, whichever is more frequent. **Additional 10-vial doses of antivenin are repeated if the patient's condition worsens or if the coagulopathy increases.**

4. *Compartment syndromes* may occur secondary to envenomation. If suspected, determine the compartment pressure. Pressures over 30 mmHg require limb elevation and **mannitol** (1 to 2 g/kg intravenously over 30 min) if no contraindications exist. **Repeated dosing of antivenin** is the most effective therapy for elevated compartment pressures. An additional 10 to 15 vials over 60 min should be given and the pressure reassessed. Persistently elevated pressures may require consultation for emergent **fasciotomy.**

5. All patients with a pit viper bite must be observed for at least 8 h. Patients with severe bites and those receiving antivenin must be admitted to the intensive care unit. Patients with mild envenomation who have completed antivenin therapy may be admitted to the general ward. Patients with no evidence of envenomation after 8 to 12 h may be discharged. All patients who receive antivenin should also be counseled about serum sickness since this occurs in nearly all patients at 7 to 14 days following therapy.

CORAL SNAKE BITE

Coral snakes are brightly colored with a pattern of black, red, and yellow bands. All true coral snakes have their yellow bands directly touching the red bands; nonpoisonous impostors have an intervening black band. Only the bite of the eastern coral snake (*Micrurus fulvius fulvius*) requires significant treatment; the bite of the Sonoran (Arizona) coral snake is mild and only needs local care. Eastern coral snake venom is neurotoxic causing tremor, salivation, respiratory paralysis, seizures, and bulbar palsies (dysarthria, diplopia, and dysphagia).

Emergency Department Care and Disposition

Patients with possible envenomation must be admitted to the hospital for 24 to 48 h of observation. The toxic effects of coral snake venom may be preventable, but they are not easily reversed. Therefore, **all patients who have potential envenomation should receive 3 vials of Antivenin (*Micrurus fulvius*)**. Additional doses are required if symptoms appear, and these patients must be admitted to an intensive care unit.

GILA MONSTER BITE

Gila monster bites result in pain and swelling. Systemic toxicity is rare, but may consist of diaphoresis, paresthesia, weakness, and hypertension. The bite may be tenacious, and the reptile should be removed as soon as possible. If the reptile is still attached, it may loosen its bite when placed on a solid surface, which no longer suspends it in mid-air. Other techniques include submersion of the animal, use of a cast spreader, and local application of an irritating flame. Once removed, standard wound care should be performed, including a search for implanted teeth. No further treatment is required.

For further reading in *Emergency Medicine: A Comprehensive Study Guide,* 5th ed., see Chap. 188, "Arthropod Bites and Stings," by Richard F. Clark, and Chap. 189, "Reptile Bites," by Richard C. Dart, Hernan F. Gomez, and Frank F.S. Daly.

---

117 | Trauma and Envenomation from Marine Fauna

Keith L. Mausner

Exposure to hazardous marine fauna occurs primarily in tropical areas, but dangerous marine animals are seen as far north as 50° N latitude. Exposure also may occur in home aquariums.

Clinical Features

Marine animals reported in attacks include sharks, great barracudas, moray eels, giant groupers, sea lions, seals, crocodiles, alligators, needle fish, wahoos, piranhas, and triggerfish. Injuries include abrasions, puncture wounds, lacerations, and crush injuries.

Coral cuts are the most common underwater injury and cause local stinging pain, erythema, and pruritus. This may progress to cellulitis with ulceration and tissue sloughing, lymphangitis, and reactive bursitis.

Ocean water contains many potentially pathogenic bacteria, including *Aeromonas hydrophila, Bacteroides fragilis, Chromobacterium violaceum, Clostridium perfringens, Erysipelothrix rhusopathiae, Escherichia coli, Mycobacterium marinum, Salmonella enteritidis, Staphylococcus aureus, Streptococcus* species, and *Vibrio* species. *Vibrio vulnificus* and *Vibrio parahaemolyticus* may cause severe cellulitis, myositis, or necrotizing fasciitis. *V. vulnificus* is also associated with sepsis in chronically ill patients, especially those with liver disease; it has 60 percent mortality rate. *A. hydrophila* can cause rapidly developing cellulitis or necrotizing myositis.

Numerous invertebrate and vertebrate marine species are venomous. The invertebrates include five phyla: Cnidaria, Porifera, Echinodermata, Annelida, and Mollusca. Cnidaria include fire corals, Portuguese men-of-war, jellyfish, sea nettles, and anemones. Most of these organisms have tentacles with nematocysts that release venom upon contact. Most reactions are localized, with pain, erythema, and other cutaneous manifestations. The anemones, jellyfish, and men-of-war may produce severe systemic manifestations that occur in minutes to hours. Indo-Pacific box jellyfish envenomation has a 15 to 20 percent mortality rate.

Porifera are sponges that produce allergic dermatitis. In addition, spicules of silica or calcium carbonate carried by the sponge become embedded in the skin and also cause dermatitis. In severe cases, erythema multiforme with systemic manifestations may occur.

Echinodermata include starfish, sea urchins, and sea cucumbers. Sea urchin spines produce immediate pain, followed by erythema, myalgia, and local swelling. Severe envenomation may cause nausea, paresthesia, paralysis, abdominal pain, syncope, respiratory distress, and hypotension. Starfish spines cause pain, bleeding, and edema; severe envenomation may cause nausea, vomiting, paresthesia, and paralysis. Sea cucumbers produce mild contact dermatitis, but eye exposure may result in a severe reaction.

Annelida include bristleworms, which embed bristles in the skin, causing pain and erythema. Mollusca include cone shells and octopuses. Mild cone shell envenomation is similar to a bee sting. Severe reactions produce muscle paralysis and respiratory failure. Octopus bites may produce paresthesia, paralysis, and respiratory failure.

The stingray has a venomous spine and is the most common vertebrate involved in envenomations. The spine produces a puncture or laceration, and may be retained in the wound, causing an intense local painful reaction. Systemic manifestations may include weakness, nausea, vomiting, diarrhea, syncope, seizures, paralysis, hypotension, and dysrhythmias. The venomous spines of scorpionfish may produce paralysis of skeletal, smooth, and cardiac muscle. Other spined venomous fish include catfish, weeverfish, surgeonfish, horned sharks, toadfish, ratfish, rabbitfish, stargazers, and leatherbacks.

Sea snake venom contains a paralyzing neurotoxin and a myotoxin. Myalgia, ophthalmoplegia, ascending paralysis, and respiratory failure may occur, as well as myoglobinuria and elevated liver enzyme levels. Death is commonly due to respiratory failure.

Emergency Department Care and Disposition

1. Attend to **airway**, **breathing**, **circulation**, treatment of life-threatening injuries, and correction of hypothermia.
2. **Copiously irrigate lacerations**, explore for foreign matter, and débride devitalized tissue. Soft tissue radiographs may help locate foreign bodies. Most wounds should undergo delayed primary closure. Tetanus prophylaxis is indicated if the patient is not immunized.
3. Prophylactic antibiotics are not indicated for minor wounds in healthy patients. Immunocompromised patients and those with grossly contaminated or extensive lacerations require **antibiotic prophylaxis**; in high-risk patients the initial dose should be parenteral. Infected wounds may have retained foreign bodies. Send aerobic and anaerobic cultures; alert the laboratory, since special media may be needed. Always cover for *Staphylococcus* and *Streptococcus* species, and in ocean-related infections also cover for *Vibrio* species with a third-generation cephalosporin, trimethoprim-sulfamethoxazole, doxycycline, a fluoroquinolone, an aminoglycoside, or chloramphenicol. Imipenem may be useful for severe infections or sepsis.
4. In Cnidaria envenomation, **rinse with saline solution**; avoid fresh water, which may cause further envenomation. **Acetic acid** (vinegar, 5%) or **isopropyl alcohol** (40 to 70%) inactivate the venom; apply for 30 min or until pain is resolved. Remove the deactivated nematocyst by applying shaving cream or talcum powder and shaving with a razor. Corneal envenomation should be irrigated and then treated with topical steroids. Observe patients with systemic symptoms for at least 8 h. There is an antivenin for box jellyfish venom. Sponge-induced dermatitis is treated with gentle drying of the skin and removal of spicules with adhesive tape. Acetic acid or isopropyl alcohol may be helpful. Apply topical steroids only after acetic acid treatment.
5. Echinodermata envenomation is treated by removing spines and with **hot water immersion** (45°C, or 113°F) for 30 to 90

min. In Annelida envenomation, remove bristles with tape or forceps. Acetic acid or isopropyl alcohol may be helpful in sea cucumber and Annelida envenomation. Mollusca envenomations are treated with supportive and wound care.

6. With stingray, scorpionfish, and other vertebrate envenomations, immerse the affected area in **hot water**, remove spines, and explore and débride the wound as necessary. Observe the patient for 4 h to rule out systemic toxicity. With sea snake bites, keep the injured area immobilized and dependent; the application of local pressure, for example, with an elastic bandage, may help sequester the venom. Incision and suction are not recommended. Sea snake antivenin is indicated for symptomatic patients and may be beneficial up to 36 h after envenomation; tiger snake or polyvalent Elapidae antivenin may be used if sea snake antivenin is not available. **Hemodialysis** also may be beneficial. If no symptoms develop after 8 h, envenomation did not occur.

For further reading in *Emergency Medicine: A Comprehensive Study Guide,* 5th ed., see Chap. 190, "Trauma and Envenomation from Marine Fauna," by Paul S. Auerbach.

---

118 | High Altitude Medical Problems

Keith L. Mausner

High altitude syndromes are primarily due to hypoxia; the rapidity and height of ascent influence the risk of occurrence.

Clinical Features

Acute mountain sickness (AMS) is usually seen in unacclimated people making a rapid ascent to over 2000 m (6600 ft) above sea level. The earliest symptoms are light-headedness and mild breathlessness. Symptoms similar to a hangover may develop within 6 h after arrival at altitude but may be delayed as long as

1 day. These include bifrontal headache, anorexia, nausea, weakness, and fatigue. Worsening headache, vomiting, oliguria, dyspnea, and weakness indicate progression of AMS. There are few specific physical findings. Postural hypotension and peripheral and facial edema may occur. Localized rales are noted in 20 percent of cases. Fundoscopy reveals tortuous and dilated veins; retinal hemorrhages are common at altitudes over 5000 m.

High altitude cerebral edema (HACE) is an extreme progression of AMS and is usually associated with pulmonary edema. It presents with altered mental status, ataxia, stupor, and progression to coma. Focal neurologic signs such as 3rd and 6th cranial nerve palsies may be present.

High altitude neurologic syndromes distinct from HACE include high altitude syncope, cerebrovascular spasm (migraine equivalent), cerebrovascular thrombosis, transient ischemic attack, and cerebral hemorrhage. These syndromes typically have more focal findings than HACE. Previously asymptomatic brain tumors may be unmasked by ascent to high altitude. Underlying epilepsy may be worsened by hyperventilation, which is part of the normal acclimatization response.

High altitude pulmonary edema (HAPE) is the most lethal of the high altitude syndromes. Risk factors include heavy exertion, rapid ascent, cold exposure, excessive salt intake, use of sleeping medications, and previous history of HAPE. Table 118-1 summarizes the classification, symptoms, and findings in the different stages of HAPE; early recognition, descent, and treatment are essential to prevent progression. Low-grade fever is common and may make it difficult to distinguish HAPE from pneumonia.

High altitude may adversely affect chronic obstructive pulmonary disease (COPD), heart disease, sickle cell disease, and pregnancy. COPD patients may require supplemental O_2, or an increase in their usual O_2 flow rate. Patients with atherosclerotic heart disease do surprisingly well at high altitude, but there may be a risk of early onset of angina and worsening of congestive heart failure. Ascent to 1500 to 2000 m may cause a vasoocclusive crisis in individuals with sickle cell disease or sickle thalassemia. Individuals with sickle cell trait usually do well at altitude, but splenic infarction has been reported during heavy exercise. Pregnant long-term high altitude residents have an increased risk of hypertension, low-birth-weight infants, and neonatal jaundice, but no increase in pregnancy complications has been reported in visitors to high altitude who engage in reasonable activities.

Diagnosis and Differential

The differential diagnosis of the high altitude syndromes includes hypothermia, carbon monoxide poisoning, pulmonary or central

TABLE 118-1 Severity Classification of HAPE

Grade	Symptoms	Signs*	Chest film
1 Mild	Dyspnea on exertion, dry cough, fatigue while moving uphill	HR (rest) < 90–100, RR (rest) < 20, dusky nail beds, localized rales, if any	Minor exudate involving less than one-fourth of one lung field
2 Moderate	Dyspnea, weakness, fatigue on level walking, raspy cough, headache, anorexia	HR 90–100, RR 16–30, cyanotic nail beds, rales present, ataxia may be present	Some infiltrate involving 50% of one lung or smaller area of both lungs
3 Severe	Dyspnea at rest, productive cough, orthopnea, extreme weakness, stupor, coma, blood-tinged sputum	Bilateral rales, HR > 110, RR > 30, facial and nail bed cyanosis, ataxia	Bilateral infiltrates > 50% each lung

*HR, heart rate; RR, respiratory rate.

Source: Hultgren HN: High altitude pulmonary edema, in Staub NC (ed): *Lung Water and Solute Exchange.* New York, Marcel Dekker, 1978, pp 437–469.

nervous system infections, dehydration, and exhaustion. HACE may be difficult to distinguish in the field from the other high altitude neurologic syndromes. HAPE must be distinguished from pulmonary embolus, cardiogenic pulmonary edema, and pneumonia. A key to diagnosis is the clinical response to treatment.

Field and Emercency Department Care and Disposition

1. Mild AMS usually improves or resolves in 12 to 36 h if further ascent is delayed and acclimatization is allowed. A decrease in altitude of 500 to 1000 m may provide prompt relief of symptoms. **Oxygen** relieves symptoms, and nocturnal low-flow O_2 (0.5 to 1 L/min) is helpful. Patients with mild AMS should not ascend to a higher sleeping elevation. Descent is indicated if symptoms persist or worsen. Immediate descent and treatment is indicated if there is a change in the level of consciousness, ataxia, or pulmonary edema. Gradual ascent is effective at preventing AMS. A reasonable recommendation for sea-level dwellers is to spend a night at 1500 to 2000 m before sleeping at altitudes above 2500 m. High altitude trekkers should allow 2 nights for each 1000 m gain in sleeping altitude starting at 3000 m. Eating a high carbohydrate diet and avoiding overexertion, alcohol, and respiratory depressants may also help prevent AMS.

2. **Acetazolamide** causes a bicarbonate diuresis, leading to a mild metabolic acidosis. This stimulates ventilation and pharmacologically produces an acclimatization response. It is effective in prophylaxis and treatment. Specific indications for acetazolamide are the following: (*a*) prior history of altitude illness; (*b*) abrupt ascent to over 3000 m (10,000 ft); (*c*) treatment of AMS; and (*d*) symptomatic periodic breathing during sleep at altitude. The adult dose is 125 to 250 mg twice a day and is continued until symptoms resolve or for 3 to 4 days as a prophylaxis. It should be restarted if symptoms recur.

3. **Dexamethasone** (4 mg PO, IM, or IV every 6 h) is effective in moderate-to-severe AMS. Tapering of the dose over several days may be necessary to prevent rebound. Aspirin or acetaminophen may improve headache. **Prochlorperazine** (5 to 10 mg IM or IV) may help with nausea and vomiting. Diuretics may be useful for treating fluid retention, but should be used with caution to avoid intravascular volume depletion.

4. HACE mandates **immediate descent or evacuation. Oxygen** should be administered. **Dexamethasone** should be started (8 mg PO, IM, or IV, then 4 mg every 6 h). **Furosemide** (40 to 80 mg) may help reduce brain edema. **Mannitol** should be

considered in severe cases not responding to treatment. **Intubation and hyperventilation** are necessary in severe cases. Carefully monitor arterial blood gas analysis to prevent excessive lowering of pCO_2 (below 25 to 30 mmHg), which may cause cerebral ischemia.

5. HAPE should also be treated with **immediate descent. Oxygen** may be life-saving if descent is delayed. The patient should be kept warm and exertion minimized. Drugs are second-line treatment after descent and oxygen. **Nifedipine** (10 mg PO every 4 to 6 h, or 30 mg extended release every 12 h), as well as morphine and furosemide, may be effective. These patients are usually volume-depleted, and care should be taken to avoid precipitating drug-induced hypotension. An expiratory positive airway pressure mask may be useful in the field and, without supplemental O_2, can increase oxygen saturation by 10 to 20 percent. Portable fabric-inflatable hyperbaric chambers may be effective in the field when immediate descent is not possible.

For further reading in *Emergency Medicine: A Comprehensive Study Guide,* 5th ed., see Chap. 191, "High Altitude Medical Problems," by Peter H. Hackett and Mark B. Rabold.

---

119 Dysbarism

Keith L. Mausner

Dysbarism is commonly encountered in scuba divers and refers to complications associated with changes in environmental ambient pressure and with breathing compressed gases.

Clinical Features

Barotrauma is the most common diving-related affliction and is caused by the direct mechanical effects of pressure. Middle-ear squeeze, or barotitis media, is the most frequently seen form of barotrauma and occurs secondary to eustachian tube dysfunction during descent. The diver complains of ear fullness or pain. If the dive is not aborted or pressure is not equalized, the eardrum may rupture, and the diver may have a sensation of escaping air bubbles from the ear, with nausea and vertigo. On physical examination there may be blood around the ear and mouth, mild conductive hearing loss, and tympanic membrane (TM) hemorrhage or perforation. External ear squeeze is less common and occurs when the external canal is occluded by cerumen, debris, or ear plugs. Sinus squeeze most commonly affects the frontal and maxillary sinuses. Squeeze may also affect the conjunctiva, sclera, and periorbital areas if a diver does not exhale into his mask and equalize pressure during descent. The most rare ear affliction is inner ear barotrauma, which usually occurs after an overly forceful valsalva maneuver, or with very rapid descent. This may lead to inner ear damage including hemorrhage, fistula formation, or rupture of Reissner's membrane. Inner ear barotrauma may present with tinnitus, vertigo, and sensorineural hearing loss, as well as a feeling of ear fullness, nausea, and vomiting.

Barotrauma during ascent is due to expansion of gas in body cavities. Although rare, "reverse squeeze" may affect the ear or sinuses during ascent. Alternobaric vertigo (ABV) can occur during ascent due to unbalanced vestibular stimulation from unequal middle-ear pressures. Tooth squeeze may be noted during ascent from air-filled dental cavities. Gastrointestinal barotrauma presents with abdominal fullness, colicky abdominal pain, belching, and flatulence; symptoms are usually relieved by venting bowel gas during ascent, but severe cases causing syncope, shocklike states, or, rarely, bowel rupture, may be seen.

Pulmonary overpressurization syndrome (POPS) may occur during ascent, resulting in mediastinal and subcutaneous emphysema. After the dive these patients may have gradual onset of increasing hoarseness, neck fullness, substernal chest pain, dyspnea, and dysphagia. In severe cases, syncope and pneumothorax may also be seen.

Air embolism is the most severe form of pulmonary barotrauma. Gas bubbles may enter the systemic circulation through ruptured pulmonary veins and occlude distal circulation. This typically presents immediately on surfacing in a diver who ascends too rapidly. Cardiac arrest and dysrhythmias may occur. The neurologic picture may be consistent with stroke affecting multiple areas of cerebral circulation. Multiplegias, sensory disturbances, confusion, vertigo, seizures, or aphasia may be seen.

Decompression sickness (DCS) is not a form of barotrauma. It is due to gas bubble formation as inert gas comes out of solution in blood and tissues, if the ascent is too rapid without adequate time for decompression. In conventional compressed-air diving, nitrogen is the culprit. DCS is a multiorgan system disorder, due to the direct effects of nitrogen bubbles on circulation and cells, as well as to secondary inflammatory responses and activation of clotting mechanisms. Severe, aching joint pain is a common symptom. Numerous neurologic complications can occur, and common findings are bladder dysfunction and lower extremity paraplegia, paraparesis, and paresthesias. Chest pain, cough, dyspnea, pulmonary edema, and shock also may occur. Risk factors for DCS include advanced age, obesity, dehydration, recent alcohol intake, cold water diving, vigorous underwater exercise, and multiple repetitive dives.

Nitrogen narcosis is due to the anesthetic effect of nitrogen, similar to that of alcohol, at elevated partial pressures, and becomes evident in most divers at a depth of 90 to 100 ft of seawater (fsw). Impairment is usually severe at 200 fsw, and unconsciousness occurs at depths over 300 to 350 fsw. Nitrogen narcosis resolves with ascent, but it is a common precipitating factor in diving accidents and may result in amnesia of the circumstances concerning the accident.

Diagnosis and Differential

The time of symptom onset in relation to the dive and descent and ascent may assist in diagnosis. During descent, the most common maladies are the squeeze syndromes. Breathing-gas problems, such as carbon monoxide poisoning or hypoxia, are also more likely to present early during descent. During the 'at-depth phase,' the most likely problems are mechanical trauma and encounters with marine fauna, as well as nitrogen narcosis. During the ascent phase, barotrauma or ABV are most likely to occur. DCS, if severe, may become symptomatic during ascent.

Onset of severe symptoms within 10 min of surfacing is an air embolism until proved otherwise. Onset of symptoms after 10 min is DCS until proved otherwise. Most cases of DCS become symptomatic 1 to 6 h after surfacing, but may be delayed up to 48 h. Mild POPS and other forms of barotrauma may also present in the immediate hours after a dive.

Emergency Department Care and Disposition

1. Airway, breathing, circulation, and immediately life-threatening injuries should be attended to first. High-flow **oxygen** should

be administered. Evaluation and treatment for hypothermia should then follow. **If air embolism is suspected, the patient should be placed in a supine position;** Trendelenburg and left lateral decubitus positions are no longer recommended because of concerns about interference with breathing and worsening cerebral edema.

2. If air embolism or DCS is suspected, **recompression-chamber therapy** should be initiated as quickly as possible. Aeromedical transport should be at an altitude of less than 1000 ft, or in an aircraft that can be pressurized to 1 atm. Most DCS patients are volume-depleted; **IV fluids** should be administered, if not otherwise contraindicated.

3. Patients with middle-ear and other squeeze syndromes should stop diving until symptoms resolve. **Decongestants** and **antihistamines** may be helpful. **Antibiotics,** such as amoxicillin, are indicated if the TM is ruptured, and diving is contraindicated until it has healed. Sinus squeeze is treated similarly to middle-ear squeeze; antibiotics are usually indicated for frontal-sinus squeeze. External ear squeeze is treated by keeping the canal dry; antibiotics should be administered if there is evidence of infection or TM rupture. Inner ear barotrauma usually mandates ENT consultation since surgical repair may be indicated; these patients should avoid straining and be at bed rest with the head elevated.

4. POPS may require **needle thoracostomy** and a **chest tube** if a pneumothorax occurs. POPS usually resolves with rest and supplemental oxygen and rarely requires recompression therapy.

For assistance in treating diving-related conditions and for the location of the nearest recompression unit, the National Diving Alert Network at Duke University can be called, 24 h a day, at (919) 684-8111. For you to facilitate consultation, history should include the type of equipment and any special gas mixtures used and the number, depth, bottom time, and surface interval between repetitive dives for all dives in the 72 h preceding symptom onset.

For further reading in *Emergency Medicine: A Comprehensive Study Guide,* 5th ed., see Chap. 192, "Dysbarism," by Kenneth W. Kizer.

120 | Near Drowning
Stephen W. Meldon

Drowning often occurs in young, healthy individuals. Although prevention is the most important way to reduce the associated morbidity and mortality, once near drowning has occurred, the patient's prognosis is dependent on early rescue and resuscitation.

Clinical Features

Respiratory failure and hypoxic neurologic injury dominate the clinical course. Initial hypoxemia results from alveolar flooding and impairment of gas exchange or laryngospasm and glottal closure. Aspiration of water leads to surfactant loss, atelectasis, ventilation perfusion mismatch, and alveolar capillary membrane damage. Noncadiogenic pulmonary edema results. A metabolic acidosis from poor perfusion and hypoxemia is common. Respiratory insufficiency may be indicated by dyspnea, tachypnea, or use of accessory muscles of respiration. Physical examination may reveal wheezing, rales, or rhonchi. Neurologic status may range from full alertness to coma. Hypothermia is common and may occasionally be severe, with core temperatures of less than 30°C.

Diagnosis and Differential

The diagnosis of near drowning is usually known because of the history or evidence of submersion. Evidence of other injuries should be sought, especially cervical spine injuries, which are associated with diving accidents. Essential diagnostic tests include a chest x-ray and arterial blood gas (ABG) analysis. The chest x-ray may show generalized pulmonary edema, perihilar infiltrates, and other patterns or be normal. Since the chest x-ray may not correlate with the arterial PO_2, an ABG analysis to assess oxygen saturation and metabolic acidosis is important. Complete blood cell count, electrolytes, and renal function should be measured, although abnormalities are seldom significant. Regarding the differential diagnosis, occasionally an acute cardiovascular (e.g., dysrhythmia or myocardial infarction) or neurologic event (e.g., hypoglycemia or seizure) may precipitate submersion and near drowning.

Emergency Department Care and Disposition

ED care should emphasize initial resuscitation, treatment of respiratory failure, and evaluation of associated injuries.

1. **Airway, ventilation, and oxygenation** should be assessed. **Stabilization and evaluation of the patient's cervical spine** may be indicated, especially if the mechanism of injury includes diving or surfing.
2. All patients should receive supplemental **oxygen.** An IV line, cardiac monitoring, and continuous pulse oximetry should be established.
3. **Intubation and mechanical ventilation** should be instituted for patients with continuing hypoxemia (PaO_2, less than 60 mmHg in adults or 80 mmHg in children) despite high-flow oxygen (40 to 50%). Positive end-expiratory pressure (PEEP) is generally required and neuromuscular paralysis may be needed in some patients.
4. A nasogastric and Foley catheter should be placed and a core body temperature should be measured.
5. Standard therapy for bronchospasm, seizures, dysrhythmias, and hypothermia should be instituted as needed. Prophylactic antibiotics and steroids are not indicated.

Need for cardiotonic medications, cardiopulmonary resuscitation (CPR), or unreactive pupils indicate a poor prognosis. However, up to 24 percent of children admitted to the intensive care unit, after experiencing cardiac arrest, survive with intact neurologic function. Since survival and neurologic outcome may be unpredictable, all patients requiring CPR should have advanced life support and resuscitation initiated. Patients with severe hypoxia, the need for mechanical ventilation and severe neurologic deficits require admission to the intensive care unit. Patients with mild-to-moderate hypoxemia corrected by supplemental oxygen should be admitted and monitored closely. Those with minimal or no symptoms and a normal chest x-ray and ABG analysis or pulse oximetry should be observed in the ED for several hours and then discharged if stable.

For further reading in *Emergency Medicine: A Comprehensive Study Guide,* 5th ed., see Chap. 193, "Near Drowning," by Bruce E. Haynes.

121 | Thermal and Chemical Burns
Stephen W. Meldon

THERMAL BURNS

Approximately 1.25 million patients present to EDs with burn injuries each year, and about 50,000 are hospitalized. Risk of burns is highest in the 18 to 35 year old group; scalds are more common in the very young (1 to 5 years) and in the elderly. While the overall mortality is only 4 percent, the death rate in patients over 65 years of age is much higher.

Clinical Features

Burns are defined by their size and depth. Burn size is quantified as a percentage of body surface area (BSA) involved. The most common method of approximating the percentage of BSA burned is the "rule of nines." A more precise estimation, especially in infants and children is to use a Lund Browder burn diagram (Fig. 121-1). Smaller burns can be estimated by using the area of the back of the patient's hand as approximately 1 percent of the BSA. Burn depth is classified as superficial partial-thickness, deep partial-thickness, and full-thickness. Superficial partial-thickness burns have blistering exposed dermis that is red and moist with intact capillary refill and are very painful to touch. They heal in 14 to 21 days and scarring is minimal. Deep partial-thickness burns extend into the deep dermis. The exposed dermis is white to yellow and does not blemish. Capillary refill and pain sensation are absent. Healing takes 3 weeks to 2 months, and scarring is common. Skin grafting may be necessary. Full-thickness burns involve the entire skin thickness. The skin is charred, pale, painless, and leathery. Skin grafting is necessary, and significant scarring results. Burns may also be associated with smoke inhalation injuries. Signs of pulmonary injury, which can have a delayed presentation for 12 to 24 h, include cough, wheeze, and respiratory distress. Thermal injury to the upper airway can occur and result in hoarseness, stridor, and rapidly occurring upper airway edema. Carbon monoxide poisoning should be suspected in all patients with smoke inhalation. Clinical signs include headache, vomiting, confusion, lethargy, and coma.

Relative Percentages of Areas Affected by Growth (Age in Years)

	0	1	5	10	15	Adult
A: half of head	$9\frac{1}{2}$	$8\frac{1}{2}$	$6\frac{1}{2}$	$5\frac{1}{2}$	$4\frac{1}{2}$	$3\frac{1}{2}$
B: half of thigh	$2\frac{3}{4}$	$3\frac{1}{4}$	4	$4\frac{1}{4}$	$4\frac{1}{2}$	$4\frac{3}{4}$
C: half of leg	$2\frac{1}{2}$	$2\frac{1}{2}$	$2\frac{3}{4}$	3	$3\frac{1}{4}$	$3\frac{1}{2}$

Second degree _____ and

Third degree _____ =

Total percent burned ___

FIG. 121-1 Lund and Browder diagram to estimate percentage of pediatric burn.

Diagnosis and Differential

Burns also can be diagnosed as major, moderate, or minor. An example of major burns include full-thickness burns greater than 10 percent BSA or partial-thickness burns greater than 10 percent BSA. Burns involving the face, hands, feet, or perineum are also major. Minor burns include partial-thickness burns less than 10 or 15 percent BSA or full-thickness burns less than 2 percent BSA. Moderate burns are those not meeting criteria for either major or minor burns. The diagnosis of smoke inhalation is suggested by the history of a fire in an enclosed space. Physical signs include soot in the mouth or nose, carbonaceous sputum, and respiratory symptoms. Chest x-ray may be normal initially. Bronchoscopy may be helpful in determining the extent of injury. Carboxyhemoglobin levels should be obtained if carbon monoxide poisoning is suspected.

Emergency Department Care and Disposition

Attention to the ABCs, appropriate fluid resuscitation, and accurate burn assessment are critical.

1. Administeration of **100% oxygen** is performed initially. If there are signs of airway compromise, then the patient should be intubated. An arterial blood gas analysis should be obtained as well as a carboxyhemoglobin level and a chest x-ray.
2. IV lines should be established. Initial **fluid resuscitation** is 2 to 4 mL/kg per %BSA per 24 h. Half the calculated amount is given in the first 8 h following the burn, and the remainder over the next 16 h. **Lactated Ringer's** solution is appropriate. A Foley catheter should be placed. Resuscitation should be monitored by assessment of the patient's urinary output (0.5 to 1.0 mL/kg/h) and other signs of perfusion.
3. The burn should be assessed and evidence of other trauma investigated. Small burns should be covered with moist saline dressing and large burns with a sterile drape. **Narcotic analgesia** and a **tetanus booster** should be administered.
4. Patients who require admission (Table 121-1) should generally be transferred to a hospital with a burn unit.
5. Outpatient management of minor burns is appropriate. Burns should be cleansed and covered with a **topical antibiotic** (e.g., bacitracin) and sterile dressing. Dressings should be changed daily. Oral analgesics (e.g., ibuprofen) should be prescribed. Initial follow-up should be in 24 h.

TABLE 121-1 American Burn Association Criteria for Transfer to a Burn Unit

1. Partial- or full-thickness burns involving greater than 10 percent of body surface area (BSA) in patients under 10 or over 50 years of age.

2. Partial- or full-thickness burns of greater than 20 percent of BSA in other age groups.

3. Partial- or full-thickness burns with the threat of functional or cosmetic impairment that involve face, hands, feet, genitalia, perineum, or major joints.

4. Full-thickness burns of greater than 5 percent of BSA in any age group.

5. Electrical burns, including lightning injury.

6. Chemical burns with the threat of functional or cosmetic importance.

7. Inhalation injury with burns.

8. Circumferential burns of the extremities or chest.

9. Burn injury in patients with preexisting medical disorders that could complicate management, prolong recovery, or affect mortality.

10. Any burn patient with concomitant trauma, such as fracture.

11. Hospitals without qualified personnel or equipment for the care of children should transfer burned children to a burn center with these capabilities.

Source: From American Burn Association: Hospital and prehospital resources for optimal care of patients with burn injury: Guidelines for development and operation of burn centers. *J Burn Care Rehab* 11:98, 1990, Reprinted by permission.

CHEMICAL BURNS

Chemical burns can occur in a variety of settings, including the home, industry, and school or research laboratories. More than 25,000 products are capable of producing chemical burns.

Clinical Features

Clinical features of chemical burns depend on the agent, concentration, and duration of exposure. Acids generally result in coagulation necrosis of the involved area. Superficial to full-thickness burns may result. An exception is hydrofluoric acid (HF), which rapidly penetrates intact skin causing severe pain and progressive, deep tissue damage. The involved skin may develop a blue-gray appearance with surrounding erythema. However, signs and symptoms may not develop until 12 to 24 h after exposure. Oxalic acid may result in hypocalcemia and renal impairment. Alkalies generally cause liquefaction necrosis and deeper tissue destruction.

Soft, gelatinous brownish eschars often result. Wounds that initially appeared superficial may progress to full-thickness burns. Pepper mace exposure causes mucous membrane, ocular, and upper airway irritation. Bronchospasm may occur. Chemical burns to the eyes results in redness, pain, and tearing. Corneal edema and ulceration may occur. Last, systemic toxicity may result. Hypocalcemia, acidosis, hypotension, and renal and hepatic necrosis can occur depending on the agents involved.

Diagnosis and Differential

The diagnosis is usually made by a history of exposure to a chemical agent. Acids with a pH less than 2 and alkalies with a pH greater than 12 are considered strong corrosives. Careful questioning regarding possible exposures (especially in the home setting) and type of agents involved is important. For ocular exposures, pH paper can determine the presence of alkali. Chemical burns should be considered in all cases of pain and irritation to the skin. This is especially true with HF acid burns, where skin findings may be minimal. Acetic and (< 40%) solutions used in hair products are a common cause of chemical burns to the scalp.

Emergency Department Care and Disposition

The first priority is to stop the burning processes. Hydrotherapy is the corner stone of the initial treatment for chemical burns. Dry chemical particles should be brushed away before irrigation. Treatment ideally should begin at the scene of the accident.

1. Remove the offending chemical, including contaminated garments.
2. Copious irrigation is indicated for alkalies, acids, and pepper mace exposure. For eye irrigation, 1 to 2 L of normal saline should be used for a minimum of 1 h continuous irrigation.
3. Exceptions to irrigation include: the elemental metals (sodium, lithium, and magnesium), which should be covered with **mineral oil** or extinguished with a class D fire extinguisher; and phenol, which should be decontaminated with **PEG300, glycerol,** or **isopropyl alcohol**.
4. HF acid burns often require additional treatment. **Calcium gluconate** can be used topically if mixed with DMSO. **Subcutaneous** and **intradermal injections** of a **5 to 10% solution** into the affected skin is recommended. A maximum dose of 0.5 mL of 10% calcium gluconate per square centimeter of burned skin is recommended.

5. Cardiac monitoring and evaluation of electrolytes, renal functions, and calcium levels are indicated in significant HF, chromic, and oxalic acid burns.
6. After initial specific measures, treatment should be as a thermal burn, with IV fluid replacement, analgesics, and tetanus prophylaxis. Checking the conjunctival pH (normal 7.3 to 7.7) may be helpful in determining whether ocular burns need further irrigation. All significant ocular burns require an ophthalmology consult.

For further reading in *Emergency Medicine: A Comprehensive Study Guide,* 5th ed., see Chap. 194, "Thermal Burns," by Lawrence R. Schwartz and Chenicheri Balakrishnan, and Chap. 195, "Chemical Burns," by Fred P. Harchelroad, Jr., and J. Michael Ballester.

---

122 | Electrical and Lightning Injuries
Howard E. Jarvis III

ELECTRICAL INJURIES

Electrical injuries present with a wide spectrum of damage, from superficial skin burn to multisystem injury and death. It is important to suspect occult injury to tissue and organs in the current's path. Most electrical injuries occur in young children, adolescent males, and workers exposed to electrical hazards.

Clinical Features

Electricity causes damage by direct effects of current upon cells and by thermal damage from the heat generated by the resistance of tissues. Energy is greatest at the contact point; thus the skin often has the greatest observable damage. The exit wound is often larger than the entrance site. As current flows through the body, the greatest damage is sustained by nerves, blood vessels, and muscles. This may result in coagulation necrosis, neuronal death, and damage to blood vessels. As a result, the overall picture often resembles a crush injury more than a thermal burn. Since the size of the skin injury does not correlate well with the underlying damage, a careful search for deeper injuries is necessary. Traumatic injuries frequently accompany electrical injuries. Specific complications are summarized in Table 122-1.

Diagnosis and Differential

Diagnosis of electrical injury is usually based on history. The type of current (high-tension wires produce the greatest injury) and surrounding circumstances, such as falls and intoxication, should be noted. In unclear cases, characteristic skin lesions or oral lesions in children may be helpful. A thorough examination to exclude occult injuries is essential. Examine bones for fractures and dislocations even without a history of trauma. The absence of findings on the initial examination does not exclude serious injury. Laboratory studies should include a complete blood cell count (CBC); electrolytes; calcium; blood urea nitrogen (BUN); creatinine level profile; coagulation arterial blood gas (ABG) analysis; myoglobin (MB); creatinine kinase and CK-MB values. The CK-MB may be elevated without myocardial damage due to extensive muscle injury. Urinalysis should include a myoglobin screen. Liver function studies and amylase levels are indicated for suspected abdominal injury. Blood should be typed and cross-matched for those with severe injuries. An electrocardiogram (ECG) should be performed. Radiographic studies of sites with suspected injuries should also be performed. Cranial computed tomography (CT) scanning is indicated for those with severe head injury, coma, or those with unresolving mental status changes.

Emergency Department Care and Disposition

The airway, breathing, and circulation should be stabilized. Cervical spine immobilization should be instituted for any unwitnessed events or when there is a potential for cervical spine injury. Patients should have continuous cardiac monitoring, pulse oximetry, noninvasive blood pressure monitoring and preferably two large-bore IV lines.

Treatment should include the following:

1. High-flow **oxygen** should be administered by face mask.
2. Ventricular fibrillation, asystole, or ventricular tachycardia should be treated by standard ACLS protocols. Other dysrhythmias are usually transient and do not need immediate therapy.
3. **Intravenous crystalloid fluid** should be given with an initial bolus of 20 to 40 mL/kg. Fluid requirements are generally higher than those of thermal burn patients. Urine output should be maintained at 1.0 mL/kg/h. A Foley catheter for urine output measurement is useful in severely injured patients.

TABLE 122-1 Complications of Electrical Injuries

Type of involvement	Complication
Cardiovascular	Sudden death (ventricular fibrillation, asystole), chest pain, dysrhythmias, ST-T segment abnormalities, bundle branch block, myocardial damage, ventricular dysfunction, myocardial infarction (rare), hypotension (volume depletion), hypertension (catecholamine release)
Neurologic	Altered mental status, agitation, coma, seizures, cerebral edema, hypoxic encephalopathy, headache, aphasia, weakness, paraplegia, quadriplegia, spinal cord dysfunction (may be delayed), peripheral neuropathy, cognitive impairment
Cutaneous	Electrothermal contact injuries, noncontact arc and "flash" burns, secondary thermal burns (clothing ignition, heating of metal—e.g., watches, rings)
Vascular	Thrombosis, coagulation necrosis, intravascular hemolysis, delayed vessel rupture, compartment syndrome
Pulmonary	Respiratory arrest (central or peripheral—e.g., muscular tetany), aspiration pneumonia, pulmonary edema, pulmonary contusion
Renal/Metabolic	Acute renal failure (due to heme pigment deposition and hypovolemia), myoglobinuria, metabolic (lactic) acidosis, hypokalemia, hypocalcemia, hyperglycemia
Gastrointestinal	Paralytic ileus, perforation, intramural esophageal hemorrhage, hepatic necrosis, pancreatic necrosis, GI bleeding
Muscular	Myonecrosis, compartment syndrome, clostridial myositis
Skeletal	Vertebral compression fractures, long bone fractures, shoulder dislocations (anterior and posterior), scapular fractures, aseptic necrosis, periosteal burns, bony matrix destruction, osteomyelitis
Infectious	Sepsis, wound infections, clostridial myonecrosis, cellulitis, pneumonia, osteomyelitis
Ophthalmologic	Corneal burns, delayed cataracts, intraocular hemorrhage or thrombosis, uveitis, retinal detachment, orbital fracture
Auditory	Hearing loss, tinnitus, tympanic membrane perforation (rare)
Oral Burns	Delayed labial artery hemorrhage, scarring and facial deformity, delayed speech development, impaired mandibular/dentition development
Fetal	Spontaneous abortion, fetal death, oligohydramnios, intrauterine growth retardation, hyperbilirubinemia

4. If evidence of rhabdomyolysis is present, urinary alkalization should be accomplished by giving 50 meq of **sodium bicarbonate** per liter of IV fluids. Blood pH should be maintained at 7.45 and urinary output at 1.5 to 2.0 mL/kg/h. Administration of mannitol should be avoided in patients with thermal burns.
5. **Tetanus** prophylaxis should be given.
6. Prophylactic antibiotics are not necessary initially unless large open wounds are present.
7. Seizures are treated with standard therapy.
8. Fractures should be reduced and splinted as appropriate.

It is appropriate to consult a general surgeon if there is evidence of systemic or deep tissue injury. These patients may require formal wound exploration, debridement, or fasciotomy and long-term care. Children with oral injuries should be evaluated by an ENT specialist or plastic surgeon. Those with severe electrical injuries should be admitted to a regional burn or trauma center. Table 122-2 summarizes admission criteria.

Disposition of patients with brief exposures to low-intensity current is controversial, but it appears that asymptomatic patients with a normal ECG, urinalysis, and no evidence of significant electrothermal burns may be discharged after 6 to 8 h of observation. Patients with an unclear history of exposure or degree of

TABLE 122-2 Admission Criteria for Patients with Electrical Injuries

High voltage > 600 V
Symptoms suggestive of systemic injury *Cardiovascular:* chest pain, palpitations *Neurologic:* loss of consciousness, confusion, weakness, headache, paresthesias *Respiratory:* dyspnea *Gastrointestinal:* abdominal pain, vomiting
Evidence of neurologic or vascular injury to a digit or extremity
Burns with evidence of subcutaneous tissue damage
Dysrhythmia or abnormal ECG
Suspected foul play, abuse, or suicidal intent
High-risk exposures
Associated injuries requiring admission
Comorbid diseases (cardiac, renal, neurologic)

ECG, electrocardiogram.

injury should be admitted. Children with isolated oral injuries can usually be discharged.

LIGHTNING INJURIES

There are about 1500 lightning injuries reported each year in the United States, with about 25 percent being fatal. Unlike the preceding electrical injuries, extensive tissue damage and renal failure are rare, though as many as 75 percent of survivors sustain significant morbidity and permanent sequelae.

Clinical Features

Lightning injuries can vary in severity depending on the circumstances of the strike. Minor injuries produce a stunned patient. These people appear well. Their vital signs will be normal, or they will exhibit a mild tachycardia or hypertension. They may have signs of confusion, amnesia, and short-term memory problems. Other symptoms include headache, muscle pain, paresthesias, and temporary visual or auditory problems. Most patients with minor lightning injuries have a gradual improvement and little long-term sequelae. Complications associated with lightning injuries are summarized in Table 122-3.

Diagnosis and Differential

The diagnosis of lightning injury is based on history and should be considered in patients found unconscious or in arrest who were outside during appropriate weather conditions. Ruptured tympanic membranes or fernlike erythematous skin markings should alert the physician to potential lightning injury. A careful examination should assess neurologic status, otologic and ophthalmologic injuries, and blunt trauma. Diagnostic tests should include an ECG in all patients, and a CBC, urinalysis with myoglobin, and a CK-MB level in most patients. For those with more severe injuries, tests should include an ABG; electrolytes, calcium, magnesium, BUN, and creatinine levels; coagulation studies; and myoglobin levels. Consider cranial CT scanning, chest radiograph, and cervical spine films. Common misdiagnoses include stroke or intracranial hemorrhage, seizure disorder, and cerebral, spinal cord, or other neurologic trauma. Other considerations are Stokes-Adams attacks, toxic ingestion or envenomation, myocardial infarction, dysrhythmias, and physical assault.

Emergency Department Care and Disposition

Unlike other trauma, priority is given to people who appear dead when there are multiple victims. Aggressive resuscitation measures

TABLE 122-3 Complications Associated with Lightning Injuries

System affected	Early injury	Late injury
Cardiovascular	Dysrhythmias (asystole, ventricular fibrillation, premature ventricular contractions, ventricular tachycardia), electrocardiogram changes	Myocardial infarction
Pulmonary	Respiratory arrest, pulmonary edema, contusion, hemorrhage	Pulmonary infarction, pneumonia
Central nervous	Loss of consciousness, confusion, amnesia, intracranial hemorrhage, respiratory center paralysis, cerebral edema, cerebral infarction	Hemiplegia, amnesia, neuritis, decreased reflexes, seizures, parkinsonian syndrome, progressive muscular atrophy, amyotrophic lateral sclerosis, progressive cerebellar syndrome, myelopathy
Peripheral nerves	Transient paralysis, paresthesias, mottling, intense vasomotor spasm	Neuritis, neuralgia
Cutaneous	Burns (first to third degree)	Scars and contractures
Ophthalmologic	Corneal lesions, uveitis, iridocyclitis, vitreous hemorrhage, diplopia, chorioretinitis, retinal detachment, hyphema	Cataracts, macular degeneration, optic atrophy
Otologic	Tympanic membrane rupture, cerebrospinal fluid otorrhea, hemotympanum, temporary deafness	Hearing loss, chronic otitis
Renal	Myoglobinuria, hemoglobinuria, renal failure (rare)	None
Gastrointestinal	Gastric atony, ileus, intestinal perforation	None
Psychiatric	Hysteria, anxiety	Sleep disturbance, depression, anxiety, storm phobia, cognitive dysfunction
Miscellaneous	Secondary blunt trauma, muscular compartment syndrome, disseminated intravascular coagulation	

are indicated, as survival has been reported after prolonged respiratory arrest. Cervical spine immobilization should be used in unwitnessed events or when there is potential cervical spine injury. Continuous cardiac monitoring, pulse oximetry, noninvasive blood pressure monitoring, and at least one large-bore IV should be utilized.

Treatment, particularly in moderate-to-severe cases, should include the following:

1. High-flow **oxygen** should be administered by face mask.
2. Ventricular tachycardia or fibrillation and asystole should be treated with standard ACLS protocols.
3. Fluid resuscitation is usually unnecessary.
4. **Tetanus** prophylaxis should be given.
5. Seizures may be treated with standard therapy.
6. Fractures and dislocations should be splinted and reduced as appropriate.

Extensive wound debridement is rarely necessary. Those with moderate or severe injuries should be admitted to a critical care unit with appropriate consultation. Most patients with minor injuries should be admitted for close monitoring of cardiac and neurologic statuses. All pregnant patients should be admitted and undergo fetal monitoring.

For further reading in *Emergency Medicine: A Comprehensive Study Guide,* 5th ed., see Chap. 196, "Electrical Injuries," by Ann S. Chinnis, Janet M. Williams, and Kimberly N. Treat; and Chap. 197, "Lightning Injuries," by Kimberly N. Treat, Janet M. Williams, and Ann S. Chinnis.

---

123 | Radiation Injuries

Keith L. Mausner

Use of radioactive isotopes is widespread in power plants, industry, and medicine; there is also a growing potential for terrorism involving nuclear weapons. Emergency physicians should have a basic understanding of radiation injuries, and all hospitals are required to have a management plan for radiation accidents.

Clinical Features

X-rays, gamma rays, neutrons, and alpha and beta particles are forms of ionizing radiation that damage tissue at the cellular level. In addition, neutron irradiation can render matter radioactive; this would most likely occur at nuclear power plants, weapons facilities, or particle accelerators or from a nuclear explosion. High-level ionizing radiation exposure may cause direct cell death; lower level exposure may interfere with cell division. Cells with high turnover rates, such as those of the hematopoietic, gastrointestinal, and reproductive systems, are more vulnerable than slowly dividing cells of the central nervous system (CNS) and musculoskeletal system.

The radian (rad) and gray (Gy) are units of absorbed dose; they measure the amount of energy imparted by radiation as it passes through matter. The rem equals the dose in rads multiplied by a factor that accounts for biological destructiveness; the sievert (Sv) has the same relationship to the gray. Rad and rem for x-rays, gamma rays, and beta particles are equivalent. However, 1 rad of alpha particles may be 20 times more destructive and represent an exposure of 20 rem. A Geiger-Müller (GM) instrument detects gamma and x-rays; dosage can be directly measured only if the victim was wearing a dosimeter at the time of exposure. A GM instrument can also detect contamination with beta-particle-emitting matter. A special probe is required to detect alpha particles.

Exposure may involve either external or internal contamination, or external irradiation. External contamination can spread to the local environment, leading to internal contamination of the victim or others. Internal contamination occurs through inhalation, ingestion, or absorption through mucous membranes or abraded skin. An internally deposited radioisotope will continue to irradiate local tissue until it decays to a stable isotope or is biologically eliminated. Alpha and beta particle emitters are primarily of concern as sources of internal and external contamination. The most likely causes of this type of exposure are radioactive iodine, plutonium, cesium, and tritium. Beta radiation penetrates millimeters into tissue, and external contamination can result in a local skin dose. Alpha radiation does not penetrate intact skin and is a significant hazard only when internalized. Iodine 131 is the predominant internal contaminant from nuclear accidents and weapons tests, and exposure carries significant risk of thyroid cancer or hypothyroidism.

Damage from external irradiation depends on a number of factors. A quickly delivered dose causes more harm than does a protracted exposure. The time from exposure to symptom onset is inversely related to dose. Acute radiation syndrome is most likely due to whole-body gamma or x-ray exposure. Table 123-1 summarizes clinical syndromes associated with increasing doses. In addition, doses of 800 to 900 rad may cause pneumonitis, pulmonary fibrosis, and interstitial edema. Local radiation injury primarily involves the skin and rarely causes systemic manifestations. High local doses can cause severe injury resembling a third-degree burn.

Diagnosis and Differential

Exposure dosage and prognosis can be estimated from clinical and laboratory data. Nausea and vomiting are sensitive clinical indicators and are seldom seen with exposures under 100 rad. At 24 h after exposure, a lymphocyte count above 1200/mL indicates

TABLE 123-1 Acute Radiation Syndrome

Approximate dose	Onset of prodrome	Duration of latent phase	Manifest illness
> 2 Gy (200 rad)	Within 2 days	1–3 weeks	Hematopoietic syndrome with pancytopenia, infection, and hemorrhage.
> 6 Gy (600 rad)	Within hours	<1 week	GI syndrome with dehydration, electrolyte abnormalities, GI bleeding, and fulminate enterocolitis.
> 30 Gy (3000 rad)	Within minutes	None	CV/CNS syndrome with refractory hypotension and circulatory collapse. Fatal within 24–72 h.

TABLE 123-2 Commonly Treated Forms of Internal Contamination

Radionuclide	Primary route of intake	Principal hazard	Treatment mechanism	Agent	Usual administration*
I-131	Inhalation Ingestion Percutaneous absorption	Thyroid	Block thyroid uptake	KI	Oral: 390 mg a day for 7 to 14 days
Pu-239	Inhalation Ingestion Absorption through wounds	Bone Liver Lung	Chelation Increase excretion	DTPA	1 g/day for 5 days IV: 1 g in 250 cc NS or D_5W over 30 min Aerosol: 1 g in nebulizer; inhale over 15 to 20 min
H-3	Inhalation Ingestion Percutaneous absorption	Whole-body dose	Isotopic dilution Increase excretion	Water	Oral: 3–4 liters a day for 2 wks
Cs-137	Inhalation Ingestion	Whole-body dose	Mobilization Decrease GI uptake	Ferric Ferrocyanide (Prussian blue)	Oral: 1 g in 100–200 cc water tid for several days

*Duration of therapy is based on dose estiminations from radiochemical measurements of urine and fecal samples.

a good prognosis; a count less than 500/mL predicts a severe clinical course. If lymphocytes are depleted within 6 h, death is likely.

Emergency Department Care and Disposition

Hospitals should have an emergency department radiation accident protocol addressing prehospital care, notification of appropriate authorities, maintenance of appropriate supplies, and HAZMAT procedures, including isolation and decontamination.

1. The first priority in all radiation accident victims is to address airway, breathing, circulation, and other potential life threats, including thermal burns or internal injuries.
2. Isolation techniques should be employed and victims scanned with radiation detection devices for contamination. Stable patients can be decontaminated prior to treatment. Critical patients can be triaged to an isolated area and resuscitated. Personnel can leave this area only if they have passed a contamination survey.
3. Table 123-2 summarizes the common forms of internal contamination and their treatments. The treatment for acute radiation syndrome from whole-body irradiation is primarily supportive. Bone marrow transplantation is considered for exposures above 800 to 900 rad. Treatment of local radiation injury is also supportive, with burn and surgical care as needed. Local injuries can also have delayed cutaneous manifestations from 1 to 5 weeks of postexposure. Long-term observation for neoplastic changes is also needed. Injuries to a fetus generally occur with exposures greater than 10 to 20 rad. However, fetal dosage above 500 millirad, especially between 8 to 15 weeks gestation, may increase the risk of CNS damage and growth defects; counseling from an individual with appropriate expertise is recommended in such cases.

For assistance and additional information, the Radiation Emergency Assistance Center/Training Site (REACTS), Oak Ridge, TN, can be contacted 24 h a day at 423-481-1000.

For further reading in *Emergency Medicine: A Comprehensive Study Guide*, 5th ed., see Chap. 199, "Radiation Injuries," by Pamela L. Piggott.

124 | Poisonous Plants and Mushrooms

Sandra L. Najarian

Plants and mushrooms have evolved a diverse array of metabolites that are harmful to humans. Chemicals applied to cultivated plants also may cause toxicity. Mushroom ingestion can lead to morbidity and even mortality among amateur foragers and recreational drug users, with the *Amanita* species responsible for most fatalities.

Clinical Features

Signs and symptoms of plant toxicity are highly variable, often depending on which part of the plant is ingested or contacted. In most cases, patients are asymptomatic or have mild gastrointestinal (GI) symptoms. Nausea, vomiting, hematemesis, abdominal pain, and diarrhea (at times bloody) may follow ingestion of Actaea (baneberry), Abrus, aloe, Cicuta macualta (water hemlock), Conium (poison hemlock), Convallaria (lily of the valley), Daphne, Euphorbia (poinsettia), Ilex (holly), Phytolacca (pokeweed), rhododendron, Ricinus, Solanum (nightshades), and Taxus (yews). Fatalities can occur from electrolyte abnormalities.

Direct irritation and chemical burns to the oropharynx have been reported after ingestion of Actaea, Abrus (rosary pea), Capsicum (ornamental peppers), Daphne, Dieffenbachia, and rhododendron. Capsicum, Laportea, Toxidendron, and Urtica also can cause a contact dermatitis. Cardiovascular symptoms, including hypotension, dysrhythmias, and conduction defects, have been reported after ingestion of Convallaria, Taxus, rhododendron, and oleander.

Ingestion of Datura (jimson weed) seeds or smoking its leaves may cause hallucinations. These can be attributed to the plant's anticholinergic properties. Hallucinations have been reported with Actaea ingestion. Seizures may be seen after ingestion of Conium, Actaea, and Ricinus. Amygdalin, found in the pits of peaches, apricots, pears, crab apples, and hydrangea, is metabolized to hydrocyanic acid and can lead to acute cyanide poisoning if ingested in sufficient quantities. Poisonous mushrooms can be divided into eight groups based on their clinical toxicity and onset of symptoms. Amatoxin poisoning presents with nausea, vomiting, diarrhea, and abdominal pain 6 to 48 h after ingestion. Dehydration, hypotension, tachycardia, and oliguria may result. Patients may develop manifestations of hepatic failure, intestinal necrosis, and renal failure 1 to 3 days after ingestion.

Gyromitrin poisoning also presents with delayed onset of GI symptoms usually 6 to 24 h after ingestion. Hepatitis leading to hepatic failure may ensue. Severe headache and altered mental status also may be observed. Methemoglobinemia is another complication. Development of GI symptoms 1 to 3 days after ingestion is characteristic of orellanine and orelline poisoning. Patients may subsequently develop renal failure, which often becomes symptomatic between 3 to 20 days after ingestion.

Ingestion of ethanol after consuming coprine-containing mushrooms results in a disulfiram-like reaction, with nausea and vomiting, diaphoresis, facial flushing, chest tightness, palpitations, hypotension, dysrhythmias, and weakness.

Mushrooms containing ibotenic acid and muscimol are generally consumed for their mind-altering effects. Toxicity develops within 2 h and includes vomiting, severe headache, lethargy, ataxia, euphoria, delirium, visual hallucinations, and psychosis. Muscle fasciculations and cholinergic and anticholinergic manifestations may be seen.

Muscarinic poisoning begins within 15 min to 2 h of ingestion. Manifestations of SLUDGE syndrome are apparent. In addition, patients can present with diaphoresis, muscle fasciculations, miosis, bradycardia, and bronchorrhea.

Psilocybin- and psilocin-containing mushrooms also are consumed for their mind-altering effects. Symptoms begin within 60 min and include ataxia, confusion, headache, visual hallucinations, aggressive or suicidal behavior, paresthesias, and weakness. Physical signs include hyperreflexia, pulse and blood pressure abnormalities, and miosis.

Miscellaneous unidentified toxins are generally associated with early onset of GI symptoms, lasting up to 48 h. Less common complaints include bloody diarrhea, chills, diaphoresis, dyspnea, headache, myalgias, light-headedness, carpopedal spasm, paresthesia, and weakness.

Diagnosis and Differential

Diagnosis of plant and mushroom poisoning is mainly clinical. Most patients are asymptomatic or have mild GI symptoms, which could be attributed to gastroenteritis. Patients at risk should be routinely asked about plant or mushroom ingestion. The type and quantity consumed should be ascertained. The time between ingestion and onset of symptoms should be determined. This is most important in mushroom poisoning. Early onset of symptoms (less than 6 h) generally indicates a benign ingestion of ibotenic acid and muscimol, muscarine, psilocin and psilocybin, or miscellaneous unidentified toxins. Delayed onset of symptoms (greater than 6 h) suggests a more toxic ingestion with amatoxin, gyromitrin, or orellanine and orelline. Mushroom ingestion and alcohol consumption, especially 2 to 72 h after ingestion, suggests coprine toxicity.

Physical examination should include mental status assessment and hydration status. It is important to search for evidence of cholinergic, anticholinergic, or sympathetic nervous system stimulation. The pharynx and skin should be examined for signs of irritation. Any jaundice should be noted. A complete cardiopulmonary examination is important, especially in those individuals at risk for dysrhythmias or cardiac conduction defects.

Laboratory studies are rarely helpful in identifying the type of plant ingested and should be used only if clinically indicated. With mushroom poisonings, however, laboratory studies may have a higher yield and should include a complete blood cell count; electrolytes; blood urea nitrogen, creatinine, and glucose levels; and urinalysis. If symptoms are suggestive of ingestion of a cytotoxic mushroom, serum amylase level, liver function tests, and coagulation studies should be obtained. An electrocardiogram is appropriate for patients with hemodynamic compromise. If available, a sample of the mushroom or plant should be sent to a botanist or mycologist for identification.

Emergency Department Care and Disposition

1. Initial treatment is mainly supportive. Airway management, ventilation, and fluid resuscitation with isotonic saline take priority. Assessment for hypoglycemia should be made in patients with altered mental status. Standard cooling measures for hyperthermia should be used.
2. Benzodiazepines should be administered to control seizures and agitation.
3. Any acid-base and electrolyte abnormalities should be corrected.
4. The GI tract should be decontaminated. **Activated charcoal** (1g/kg orally or per nasogastric (NG) tube) should be administered along with a cathartic such as sorbitol. Consideration should be given to whole bowel irrigation (0.5 to 2 L/h of **Golytely** orally or per NG tube) in patients suspected of ingesting cytotoxic mushrooms and presenting within 24 h.
5. Those patients with potential amatoxin, gyromitrin, or orellanine/orelline poisoning, or those with refractory symptoms should be admitted and monitored for at least 48 h. Other

patients may be discharged if symptom-free after 4 to 6 h of observation or treatment. They should be instructed to return at once if they develop vomiting, abdominal pain, diarrhea, or hallucinations.

6. For amatoxin poisoning, **hemodialysis** and **charcoal hemoperfusion** are standard therapy. Forced diuresis is often advocated, but no clinical trials have shown efficacy. **Penicillin G** (0.3 to 1 million units/kg/d) in divided doses inhibits liver uptake of amatoxin and increases renal excretion of the toxin. It is the most effective therapy and should be initiated as soon as amatoxin ingestion is suspected. High-dose **cimetadine** (10 g/d) has been shown to be useful in humans. Silymarin (silybinin), a free radical scavenger which acts by interrupting the enterohepatic circulation of amatoxin when given orally, has been used successfully in Europe, but is not available in the United States. Fab monoclonal antibodies have been developed against amatoxin and may be proved to be effective in eliminating the toxin when used with plasmapheresis.

7. For gyromitrin poisoning, **pyridoxine** (25 mg/kg IV over 15 to 30 min) may reverse neurologic toxicity. Benzodiazepines may be used for controlling agitation and neuromuscular hyperactivity. Normal urine output must be maintained to help prevent hemolysis-induced renal dysfunction. **Methylene blue** (0.1 to 0.2 mL/kg of a 1% solution IV) should be used to treat methemoglobinemia.

8. For orellanine/orelline toxicity, fluid and electrolyte support and hemodialysis are the mainstay treatment. Aggressive fluid resuscitation and pressor support may be necessary in patients suffering from coprine-ethanol reactions. Beta blockers, such as **propranolol,** should be used to control tachydysrhythmias. Neuromuscular hyperactivity and seizures due to ibotenic acid/muscimol poisoning should be treated with benzodiazepines and barbiturates. **Physostigmine** (1–2 mg IV in adults, 0.5 mg in children) should be considered in those patients with severe anticholinergic symptoms. Continuous cardiopulmonary and blood pressure monitoring are essential during administration. **Atropine** (0.5 to 1.0 mg in adults, 0.01 mg/kg in children) should be administered to those with severe muscarinic symptoms. Repeat the dose as necessary to control bronchorrhea, hypotension, or bradycardia. Consider administration of inhaled bronchodilators and antihistamines.

9. Patients with psilocin/psilocybin poisoning should be placed in a quiet environment and provided with reassurance and sedation as necessary.

10. In patients with miscellaneous unidentified mushroom toxins, supportive care should be administered.

For further reading in *Emergency Medicine: A Comprehensive Study Guide,* 5th ed., see Chap. 200, "Mushroom Poisoning," by Sandra M. Schneider and Anne F. Brayer; and Chap. 201, "Poisonous Plants," by Mark A. Hostetler and Sandra M. Schneider.

ENDOCRINE EMERGENCIES

125 | Diabetic Emergencies

Michael P. Kefer

HYPOGLYCEMIA

Since glucose is the main energy source of the brain, severe hypoglycemia can cause brain damage and death. Diabetics on insulin or oral hypoglycemic therapy are especially at risk. Also at risk are patients on beta blockers, barbiturates, or salicylates, and patients with alcoholism, sepsis, adrenal insufficiency, hypothyroidism, or malnutrition.

Hypoglycemic agents are the mainstays of treatment for diabetics. Overdose of these agents, intentional or accidental, is a common cause of hypoglycemia.

Insulin comes in various forms. The duration of action ranges from 6 (regular) to 36 h (ultralente). Since sulfonylureas have long half-lives, they can lead to recurrent episodes of hypoglycemia (see Table 125-1).

Biguanides include phenformin and metformin. Phenformin is not available in the United States due to its association with fatal lactic acidosis. Metformin rarely causes lactic acidosis. Patients on metformin should not receive radiographic intravenous contrast agents due to the risk of acute renal failure. Metformin alone does not cause hypoglycemia. Troglitazone reduces insulin resistance and lowers plasma glucose levels in combination with either insulin or a sulfonylurea. Acarbose decreases *gastrointestinal* absorption of carbohydrates. It does not cause hypoglycemia.

Clinical Features

Typical symptoms include sweating, shakiness, anxiety, nausea, dizziness, confusion, slurred speech, blurred vision, headache, lethargy, and coma. Other major neurologic manifestations noted are cranial nerve palsies, hemiplegia, seizure, and decerebrate postur-

TABLE 125-1 Characteristics of Hypoglycemia Agents

Class and name	Duration of action, h	Metabolism
	INSULIN	
Ultra–short acting		
Lispro	< 5	Hepatic
Short acting		
Regular	6–8	Hepatic
Semilente	12–16	Hepatic
Intermediate acting		
Lente	24	Hepatic
NPH	24	Hepatic
Mixtard	24	Hepatic
Long acting		
PZI	24–36	Hepatic
Ultralente	> 36	Hepatic
	SULFONYLUREAS	
First generation		
Acetohexamide	12–24	Renal
Chlorpropamide	24–72	Renal
Tolazamide	12–24	Renal
Tolbutamide	6–12	Renal
Second generation		
Glipizide	10–16	Renal
Glyburide	24	Renal, hepatic

ing. Unsuspected hypoglycemia can easily be misdiagnosed as a primary neurologic, psychiatric, or cardiovascular condition.

Diagnosis and Differential

The actual blood glucose level that defines hypoglycemia is arbitrary. Some people with low glucose levels are asymptomatic, and some with normal levels are symptomatic. Therefore, the diagnosis is based on the glucose level in conjunction with the clinical presentation. The history usually gives important clues to the cause of hypoglycemia. For example, consider the patient who presents with hypoglycemia and depression that is, or has a family member, being treated with an oral hypoglycemic agent.

Emergency Department Care and Disposition

Treatment is glucose administration, oral or IV, as the patients condition warrants. Often, diabetics with insulin reactions will require a continuous infusion of a **5%, 10%, or 20% glucose**

solution to maintain a blood glucose level greater than 100 mg/dL. If there is not a prompt response to glucose infusion, **hydrocortisone 100 mg** and **glucagon 1 mg** should be added to each additional liter of glucose solution. Glucagon 0.5 to 2.0 mg IV, IM, or subcutaneously (SQ) is used in select cases.

Hypoglycemia secondary to the sulfonylureas may require adjunctive treatment with **diazoxide 300 mg IV** over 30 min every 4 h as needed.

Most diabetics with insulin reactions respond rapidly. They can be discharged with instructions to continue oral intake of carbohydrates and closely monitor their finger stick glucose level. All patients with sulfonylurea-induced hypoglycemia should be admitted due to the prolonged half-life of and, therefore, risk of recurrence from these agents.

DIABETIC KETOACIDOSIS

Diabetic ketoacidosis (DKA) results from a relative insulin deficiency and counterregulatory hormone excess causing hyperglycemia and ketonemia. DKA is precipitated by noncompliance with insulin therapy, infection, stroke, myocardial infarction, trauma, pregnancy, and many other physiologic stresses.

Clinical Features

Clinical manifestations are directly related to metabolic derangements. Hyperglycemia causes an osmotic diuresis with dehydration, hypotension, and tachycardia. Ketonemia causes an acidosis with myocardial depression, vasodilation, and compensatory Kussmaul's respiration. Nausea, vomiting, and abdominal pain and tenderness are also common. Since inappropriate normothermia is seen, infection must be excluded by other means.

Laboratory investigation reveals elevated levels of serum glucose and ketones and decreased levels of sodium, chloride, calcium, phosphorus, and magnesium from osmotic diuresis. Pseudohyponatremia is common; for each 100-mg/dL increase in the blood glucose level, the sodium level decreases by 1.6 meq/L. Serum potassium levels may be low from osmotic diuresis, and vomiting normal or high from acidosis. It is important to note that, in acidosis, potassium is driven extracellularly. Therefore, the acidotic patient with a normal or low potassium level has marked depletion of total body potassium.

An anion gap metabolic acidosis results from formation of ketone bodies. Acetone, formed from oxidation of ketone bodies, causes the characteristic fruity odor of the patient's breath. In DKA, formation of β-hydroxybutyrate from acetoacetate is favored. Therefore, the patient may have low levels of acetoacetate and high levels of β-hydroxybutyrate. If the nitroprusside test is used to detect serum or urine ketones, results may be falsely low or negative, since it detects only acetoacetate and not β-hydroxybutyrate.

Diagnosis and Differential

Diagnosis of DKA is suspected based on clinical presentation and a glucose level greater than 300 mg/dL, a HCO_3 level less than 15 meq/L, and a pH less than 7.3.

Differential diagnosis includes other causes of an anion gap metabolic acidosis, which are easily recalled by the acronym *MUD-PILES* (see Table 126-1). Hypoglycemia and nonketotic hyperosmolar coma are two other causes of metabolic coma that should be considered in a diabetic patient.

Emergency Department Care and Disposition

Basic laboratory investigation consists of determination of serum glucose, electrolyte, blood urea nitrogen (BUN), creatinine, phosphorus, and magnesium levels; a complete blood count; urinalysis (and pregnancy test if indicated); electrocardiogram; and chest x-ray to assess the severity of DKA and search for the underlying cause. The goal of treatment is to correct the volume deficit, acid-base imbalance, and electrolyte abnormalities; administer insulin; and treat the underlying cause.

1. **Isotonic fluid resuscitation** is the most important initial step in restoring intravascular volume and tissue perfusion. The average patient in DKA has a body water deficit of 5 to10 L. The first liter is administered over 30 to 60 min. Once intravascular volume is restored, or if the serum sodium level is greater than 155 meq/L, hypotonic solution is infused to provide free water for intracellular volume replacement. Patients with heart disease may need invasive monitoring to avoid congestive heart failure.
2. **Insulin** is required to shut off ketosis and restore cellular glucose stores. Low dose IV insulin has the advantage of allowing close control of the amount of insulin given compared to IM or SQ administration, where absorption may be erratic or delayed in an unstable patient. The half-life of regular insulin given IV is 5 min; it is 2 h when given IM or SQ. Continuous IV infusion of insulin at 0.1 U/(kg/h) is recommended with or without a loading dose of 0.1 U/kg IV bolus. If there is no response within the first hour of treatment, insulin resistance is suggested, and

the infusion rate is doubled each hour until a response is obtained. Hyperglycemia is controlled much more rapidly with insulin than is ketoacidosis. To reverse ketoacidosis, insulin treatment must continue despite decreasing serum glucose levels. Therefore, to prevent hypoglycemia, glucose infusion will be necessary when the serum glucose level falls to 250 mg/dL.

3. **Potassium** is administered to maintain normal serum levels during the acute phase of treatment. Upon initiating treatment for DKA, potassium levels will fall due to dilution from volume replacement, correction of acidosis, renal excretion, and the insulin effect of driving potassium intracellularly. To avoid the dangerous effects of hypokalemia, potassium replacement should begin early. If the urine output is adequate, potassium chloride 20 meq may be added to each liter of IV fluid as required by close monitoring of serum potassium. Potassium phosphate 20 meq may be used if phosphorus supplementation is also required.

4. **Phosphorus** has an important role in energy production (ATP), oxygen delivery (2,3-DPG), and enzymatic reactions. Acute deficiency has been associated with all types of muscle dysfunction. Phosphorus replacement is recommended if the serum level is less than 1 mg/dL. Potassium phosphate 20 meq IV may be used if the patient still requires potassium.

5. **Magnesium** is administered if levels are low or the patient has symptoms of hypomagnesemia.

6. **Bicarbonate therapy** remains controversial as to when the benefits of correcting the effects of acidosis (vasodilation, depression of cardiac contractility and respiration, and central nervous system depression) outweigh the risks of bicarbonate treatment (paradoxical cerebrospinal fluid acidosis, hypokalemia, impaired oxyhemoglobin dissociation, rebound alkalosis, and sodium overload). However, current recommendations favor administration of bicarbonate when the pH is less than 6.9.

All patients on an insulin infusion will require close monitoring to avoid complications of treatment. Development of cerebral edema during treatment is a continual problem, predominately in young patients. The blood glucose, anion gap, potassium, and bicarbonate should be monitored every 1 to 2 h until recovery is well established.

HYPEROSMOLAR HYPERGLYCEMIC NONKETOTIC SYNDROME

The term *hyperosmolar hyperglycemic nonketotic syndrome* is preferred to *nonketotic hyperosmolar coma,* which better describes an extreme and relatively rare presentation of the former. This condition is distinguished from DKA by the absence of ketosis. It is a relatively common presentation of new-onset diabetes. Similar to DKA, precipitating factors include noncompliance, myocardial infarction, cerebrovascular accident, infection, and trauma. Drugs such as thiazide diuretics, beta blockers, and steroids also predispose to this condition.

Clinical Features

Typically, patients have a history of type 2 diabetes, present with complaints of weakness and mental status changes, and have preexisting renal or heart disease. Metabolic changes occur over days to weeks, and symptoms may not be obvious.

Physical examnation reveals signs of dehydration with orthostasis, dry skin and mucous membranes, and altered mental status. Kussmaul's respiration and the smell of acetone on the breath are not present. Mental status changes range from confusion to coma. Focal deficits and focal or generalized seizures also occur.

Defining laboratory parameters are a glucose level above 400 mg/dL, serum osmolality greater than 315 mosmol/kg, pH greater than 7.3, and absence of ketones. Pseudohyponatremia is more prominent. Serum and urine ketones are absent. However, metabolic acidosis may be present secondary to hypovolemia, which can cause lactic acidosis and/or azotemia.

Diagnosis and Differential

Diagnosis is based on clinical and laboratory findings. This condition is distinguished from DKA by laboratory investigation. Typically, in addition to the absence of ketones, the degree of acidosis is less and the degree of hyperglycemia may be marked.

Emergency Department Care and Disposition

Treatment is aimed at correction of volume deficit, electrolyte imbalance, and hyperosmolality as well as the underlying cause.

1. **Intravenous fluid therapy** consists of first restoring intravascular volume and then providing free water with hypotonic fluids to restore intracellular volume. The average fluid deficit is 8 to12 L. One-half the deficit is replaced over 12 h, the other half over the next 24 h. Along with large volume losses are sodium and potassium losses. As with DKA, potassium replacement should be initiated as soon as renal function is determined adequate. Glucose should be added to IV fluids when the blood glucose

level approaches 250 mg/dL. Rapid lowering below this level poses an increased risk of cerebral edema.
2. An **insulin drip 0.1 U**/kg/h can be initiated. In less severe cases, the patient will correct with fluids alone, or the patient may only require a bolus dose or two of regular insulin 0.1 U/kg in conjunction with fluid therapy.

For further reading in *Emergency Medicine: A Comprehensive Study Guide,* 5th ed., see Chap. 184, "Hypoglycemic Agents," by Joseph G. Rella and Lewis S. Nelson; Chap. 202, "Hypoglycemia," by William J. Brady and Richard A. Harrigan; Chap. 203, "Diabetic Ketoacidosis," by Michael E. Chansky and Cary L. Lubklin; and Chap. 205, "Hyperosmolar Hyperglycemic Nonketotic Syndrome," by Charles S. Graffeo.

---

126 | Alcoholic Ketoacidosis
Michael P. Kefer

Alcoholic ketoacidosis results from heavy alcohol intake, either acute or chronic, and minimal or no food intake. Alcohol and body fat metabolism generate ketoacids, with a resultant anion-gap metabolic acidosis.

Clinical Features

Patients with alcoholic ketoacidosis typically complain of nausea, vomiting, orthostasis, and abdominal pain 24 to 72 h after the last alcohol intake. Physical examination reveals the patient to be acutely ill and dehydrated with a tender abdomen. Abdominal tenderness is either diffuse and nonspecific or is a result of other causes associated with the use of alcohol, such as gastritis, hepatitis, or pancreatitis. Furthermore, the presentation may be confounded by other common complications of alcoholism, such as infection or alcohol withdrawal.

Laboratory investigation reveals an anion-gap $[Na^+ - (Cl^- + HCO_3)] > 12 \pm 4$ meq/L] metabolic acidosis. However, the serum pH may be low, normal, or high, as these patients often have mixed acid-base disorders such as a metabolic acidosis from alcoholic ketoacidosis and a metabolic alkalosis from vomiting and volume depletion. Blood glucose ranges from low to mildly elevated. The alcohol level is usually low or 0 as vomiting and abdominal pain limit intake. Serum ketones, acetoacetate and β-hydroxybutyrate, are elevated. Serum and urine ketones are measured by the nitroprusside test, which detects acetoacetate but not β-hydroxybutyrate. Although serum ketones are usually detected in significant amounts, the redox state may be such that most or all acetoacetate is reduced to β-hydroxybutyrate, resulting in a falsely negative or falsely low estimate of the severity of ketoacidosis.

Diagnosis and Differential

The diagnosis of alcoholic ketoacidosis is established in the patient with a history of recent heavy alcohol consumption, decreased food intake, vomiting, abdominal pain, and laboratory findings of an anion-gap metabolic acidosis, a positive nitroprusside test for ketones, and a low to mildly elevated glucose.

The differential diagnosis includes other causes of anion-gap metabolic acidosis, commonly recalled by the acronym MUD-PILES (Table 126-1). These can be excluded by clinical and laboratory data.

TABLE 126-1
Differential Diagnosis of
an Anion-Gap Metabolic Acidosis

Methanol

Uremia

Diabetic ketoacidosis

Paraldehyde

Iron, Isoniazid, Inhalants

Lactic acidosis

Ethanol, Ethylene glycol

Salicylates

Emergency Department Care and Disposition

1. Treatment of alcoholic ketoacidosis consists of infusion of a crystalloid solution containing glucose. The **crystalloid** solution restores intravascular volume. **Glucose** administration stimulates insulin release, which inhibits ketosis. **Thiamine** (50 to 100 mg IV) should also be given.
2. Unlike treatment for diabetic ketoacidosis, insulin administration is not necessary, as endogenous insulin secretion occurs normally with restoration of volume and glucose administration. Sodium bicarbonate administration is controversial but is considered when the pH < 7.1. Reversal of alcoholic ketoacidosis usually occurs in 12 to 18 h but may occur sooner or later depending on the severity.

For further reading in *Emergency Medicine: A Comprehensive Study Guide,* 5th ed., see Chap. 204, "Alcoholic Ketoacidosis," by William A. Woods and Debra G. Perina.

---

127 | Thyroid Disease Emergencies
Stephen W. Meldon

THYROID STORM

Thyroid storm is a rare, life-threatening condition due to hyperthyroidism. It is most often seen in patients with antecedent Graves' disease and is usually precipitated by infection or some other stressful event.

Clinical Features

The clinical presentation is explained by enhanced sympathetic nervous system activity. The earliest signs are fever, tachycardia, diaphoresis, and emotional lability. Clues to the diagnosis include a history of Graves' disease, exophthalmos, a widened pulse pressure, and a palpable goiter. Central nervous system (CNS) disturbance occurs in 90 percent of patients and includes confusion, delirium, seizure, and coma. Cardiovascular abnormalities are seen in 50 percent of patients, with sinus tachycardia most common. Other dysrhythmias include atrial fibrillation and premature ventricular contractions. Gastrointestinal symptoms, such as diarrhea and hyperdefecation, occur in most patients. Apathetic thyrotoxicosis is a distinct presentation seen in elderly patients, in which the characteristic symptoms are absent, and lethargy, slowed mentation, and apathetic facies are seen. Goiter, weight loss, and proximal muscle weakness are present. Atrial fibrillation and congestive heart failure may occur.

Diagnosis and Differential

Thyroid storm is a clinical diagnosis, since no laboratory tests distinguish it from thyrotoxicosis. Diagnostic criteria include a temperature higher then 37.8°C (100.4°F); tachycardia out of proportion to fever; dysfunction of the CNS, the cardiovascular system, or the gastrointestinal systems; and exaggerated peripheral manifestations of thyrotoxicosis. In this clinical setting, an elevated L-thyroxine (T_4) level and a suppressed thyroid-stimulating hormone (TSH) level confirm the diagnosis. The differential diagnosis includes sepsis, pulmonary or enteric infections, and meningitis; other causes of congestive heart failure; cerebrovascular accident; complications of diabetes [e.g., diabetic ketoacidosis (DKA) or hypoglycemia]; heat stroke; delirium tremens; and sympathomimetic drug overdose. The diagnosis is complicated by the fact that any of these entities may precipitate thyroid storm.

Emergency Department Care and Disposition

The importance of early treatment of thyroid storm based upon the clinical impression must be emphasized. Therapeutic goals can be divided into five areas: general supportive care, inhibition of thyroid hormone synthesis, retardation of thyroid hormone release, blockade of peripheral thyroid hormone effects, and identification and treatment of precipitating events.

1. Supplemental **oxygen, intravenous (IV) fluids,** and cardiac monitoring are indicated. Fever should be controlled by the use of acetaminophen and a cooling blanket. Intravenous glucocorticoids, such as **dexamethasone** 10 mg IV, should be given.
2. Adrenergic blockade is a mainstay of therapy. **Propranolol** 1 mg IV every 10 min to a total dose of 10 mg is the drug of

choice. The lowest possible dose required to control the cardiac and psychomotor symptoms should be used and can be repeated every 3 to 4 h as needed. Propranolol should be used with caution in the setting of severe bronchospastic disease, heart block, or congestive heart failure. **Guanethidine** 1 to 2 mg/kg orally per day and **reserpine 1 to 5 mg IM** followed by 1 to 2.5 mg every 4 to 6 h are alternatives to propranolol.

3. The antithyroid drugs **propylthiouracil (PTU)** and **methimazole** act by blocking thyroid hormone synthesis. They must be given orally or by nasogastric tube. The initial loading dose of PTU is 600 to 1000 mg orally, followed by 200 to 250 mg orally every 4 h. Oral methimazole 40 mg given initially, followed by 25 mg orally every 6 h, is an acceptable alternative.

4. **Iodide** retards thyroid release of stored hormones. Iodide should be administered 1 h after PTU. The dose is 5 drops of potassium iodide every 4 to 6 h, or sodium iodide 0.5 to 1.0 g every 12 h by slow IV infusion.

5. Precipitating causes should be sought. Appropriate cultures and antibiotics may be indicated. Congestive heart failure may be refractory to standard therapy.

All patients should be monitored closely and admitted to the intensive care unit. Despite treatment, mortality rates remain high (20 to 50 percent).

HYPOTHYROIDISM AND MYXEDEMA COMA

Myxedema coma is a rare, life-threatening expression of severe hypothyroidism. It is most often seen during the winter months in elderly women with undiagnosed or undertreated hypothyroidism. Precipitating events include pulmonary infections, congestive heart failure, and exposure to a cold environment.

Clinical Features

The typical symptoms of hypothyroidism include fatigue, weakness, cold intolerance, constipation, weight gain, and deepening of voice. Cutaneous signs include dry, scaly, yellow skin; nonpitting, waxy edema of the face and extremities (myxedema); and thinning eyebrows. Cardiac findings include bradycardia, enlarged heart, and low-voltage electrocardiogram. Paresthesia, ataxia, and prolongation of the deep tendon reflexes are characteristic neurologic findings. A thyroidectomy scar may be present, but a goiter is uncommon. The patient with myxedema coma will present with several additional findings: hypothermia (in 80 percent of cases), altered mental status, hyponatremia, hypotension and bradycardia, and a paralytic ileus or megacolon. Respiratory failure with hypoventilation, hypercapnia, and hypoxia is common. Delusions and psychosis (myxedema madness) may occur.

Diagnosis and Differential

The diagnosis of myxedema coma must be suspected based upon the clinical presentation and characteristic laboratory abnormalities previously mentioned. Confirmatory thyroid tests will typically show low free T_4 levels and elevated with a low-reading thermometer, arterial blood gases, chest x-ray, electrocardiogram, and serum electrolytes. Differential diagnosis includes coma secondary to respiratory failure, hyponatremia, hypothermia, congestive heart failure, stroke, or drug overdose.

Emergency Department Care and Disposition

Patients with myxedema coma are critically ill, and initial treatment must be supportive. Specific treatment requires large doses of thyroid hormone, which could be fatal to a euthyroid, comatose patient. Other causes of coma must be considered and excluded.

1. All patients require **dextrose-containing IV fluids,** cardiac monitoring, and Foley and nasogastric catheters. Respiratory failures should be treated with supplemental **oxygen** and **mechanical ventilation,** if needed.
2. Hypothermic patients should be gradually **rewarmed.** Hyponatremia may require **hypertonic saline solution** and **furosemide** in addition to fluid restriction. **Vasopressors** are usually ineffective in this setting and should be used only for severe hypotension. Sedating drugs, such as phenothiazines, generally should be avoided. Antibiotics are indicated for underlying infection. Other precipitating causes should be sought and treated. In addition, **hydrocortisone** 100 mg IV every 8 h should be given.
3. Thyroid hormone is the most critical and specific therapy for myxedema coma. Intravenous **levothyroxine** in an initial dose of 300 to 500 μg should be given by slow infusion; this is followed by 50 to 100 μg IV daily. Alternative treatment consists of L-**triiodothyronine (T$_3$)** 25 μg IV or orally every 8 h. T_3 dosage should be halved in patients with cardiovascular disease. Patients should be admitted to a monitored setting. Overall clinical improvement should be seen in 24 to 36 h with either regimen.

For further reading in *Emergency Medicine: A Comprehensive Study Guide,* 5th ed., see Chap. 206, "Hyperthyroidism and Thyroid Storm," and Chap. 207, "Hypothyroidism and Myxedema Coma," by Horace K. Liang.

128 | Adrenal Insufficiency and Adrenal Crisis

Michael P. Kefer

Adrenal insufficiency may be acute or chronic and results when the physiologic demand for glucocorticoids and mineralocorticoids exceeds the supply from the adrenal cortex. The hypothalamus secretes corticotropin releasing factor (CRF). CRF stimulates the pituitary to secrete adrenocorticotropic hormone (ACTH). ACTH stimulates the adrenal cortex to secrete cortisol (and aldosterone to a minor degree). Cortisol has negative feedback on the pituitary. Adrenal insufficiency is described as primary, secondary, or tertiary based on whether the insufficiency occurs at the level of the adrenal glands, pituitary, or hypothalamus, respectively.

Clinical Features

Clinical features of *adrenal insufficiency* vary in number and severity depending on the etiology and duration of onset. Manifestations of *primary adrenal insufficiency* are due to cortisol and aldosterone deficiency and include weakness, dehydration, hypotension, anorexia, nausea, vomiting, weight loss, abdominal pain (that may present as an acute abdomen), and increased pigmentation of both exposed and nonexposed skin and mucous membrane. Laboratory investigation reveals varying degrees of hyponatremia, hyperkalemia, hypoglycemia, and prerenal azotemia. Electrocardiogram (ECG) changes are either nonspecific or typical of hyperkalemia, if present.

    Secondary and tertiary adrenal insufficiency differ from primary in that manifestations are due to cortisol and adrenal androgen deficiency. Hypoglycemia is a prominent feature. Aldosterone levels are not significantly affected because of regulation through the renin angiotensin system. Therefore, the hyperpigmentation, hyponatremia, hyperkalemia, and volume depletion of primary adrenal insufficiency are not seen.

Adrenal crisis is an acute, life-threatening condition due to cortisol and aldosterone deficiency. Clinical features are as described earlier, but to the extreme, with shock and altered mental status.

All patients with adrenal insufficiency have low baseline plasma cortisol levels. In primary adrenal insufficiency, the diseased adrenal cortex will not increase cortisol levels upon stimulation with exogenous ACTH. In secondary and tertiary adrenal insufficiency, the adrenal cortex remains responsive to ACTH and will increase cortisol levels.

Diagnosis and Differential

The diagnosis of adrenal insufficiency may be difficult because the typical clinical features are nonspecific. The diagnosis can be made in the emergency department (ED) based on the presence of the clinical features discussed and after performing a cosyntropin (synthetic ACTH) stimulation test. This test is performed by drawing a baseline cortisol level, then administering cosyntropin 0.25 mg IM or IV. After 30 to 60 min a repeat cortisol level is drawn. This repeat level should be double the baseline. Definitive diagnosis requires prolonged testing outside the scope of ED care.

The most common cause of adrenal insufficiency and adrenal crisis is adrenal suppression from prolonged steroid use with subsequent abrupt withdrawal or exposure to increased stress (e.g., injury, illness, surgery, etc.). Adrenal suppression occurs with steroids given by any route: oral, topical, intrathecal, or inhaled. In general, there is no adrenal suppression regardless of the dose of steroids, if given for less than 3 weeks, and regardless of the duration of steroids, if the dose is less than 10 mg a day (unless the dose is taken at night). It may take up to 1 year for recovery of the hypothalamic-pituitary-adrenal gland axis to recover following prolonged suppression with steroid treatment.

Other causes of adrenal insufficiency include autoimmune and idiopathic disorders, metastatic cancer, infection, or bilateral adrenal hemorrhage associated with meningococcemia (Waterhouse-Friderichsen's syndrome) or heparin therapy.

Emergency Department Care and Disposition

1. Treatment of primary adrenal insufficiency requires cortisol, aldosterone, and estrogen replacement. A typical regimen is

prednisone 5 mg orally every morning and 2.5 mg orally every evening for glucocorticoid replacement, **fludrocortisone** 0.05 to 0.2 mg orally every day for mineralocorticoid replacement and, in women, **fluoxymesterone** 2 to 5 mg orally every day for estrogen replacement. Treatment of secondary and tertiary adrenal insufficiency is similar except that mineralocorticoid replacement is not necessary as aldosterone levels are not significantly affected (as discussed in clinical features).

2. Treatment of adrenal crisis includes resuscitation with fluids, glucocorticoids, and mineralocorticoids to correct volume, glucose, and sodium deficits. Intravenous **D₅NS** is the fluid of choice and a bolus should be initiated immediately. **Hydrocortisone** 100 mg IV bolus and 100 mg added to the IV solution provides adequate glucocorticoid and mineralocorticoid activity. If a cosyntropin stimulation test is being performed during resuscitation, then **dexamethasone** 4 mg IV should be substituted for hydrocortisone so as not to give a false-positive test. In refractory cases, **additional hydrocortisone or vasopressors** may be necessary to support patients. Clearly, all patients with severe symptoms will require admission for additional treatment and monitoring. Once stabilized, oral maintenance therapy is initiated.

For further reading in *Emergency Medicine: A Comprehensive Study Guide,* 5th ed., see Chap. 208, "Adrenal Insufficiency and Adrenal Crisis," by Gene Ragland.

HEMATOLOGIC AND ONCOLOGIC EMERGENCIES

129 | Evaluation of Anemia and the Bleeding Patient

Sandra L. Najarian

Patients with anemia are encountered daily in the emergency department (ED). Anemia may be chronic and unrelated to the chief complaint, or it may result from acute blood loss as seen in trauma, gastrointestinal (GI) bleeding, or other acute hemorrhage. Underlying bleeding disorders must be suspected in patients with spontaneous bleeding from multiple sites, bleeding from nontraumatized sites, delayed bleeding several hours after injury, or bleeding into deep tissues or joints.

Clinical Features

The rate of the development of the anemia, the extent of the anemia, and the ability of the cardiovascular system to compensate for the decreased oxygen-carrying capacity determine the severity of the patient's symptoms and clinical presentation. Patients may complain of palpitations, dizziness, feelings of postural faintness, exertional intolerance, and tinnitus. Patients may have pale conjunctiva, skin, and nail beds. Tachycardia, hyperdynamic precordium, and systolic murmurs may be present. Tachypnea at rest and hypotension are late signs. Use of ethanol, prescription drugs, and recreational drugs may alter the patient's ability to compensate for the anemia.

Patients with bleeding may or may not have an obvious site of hemorrhage. When suspecting an underlying bleeding disorder, the emergency physician should inquire about the presence of excessive or abnormal bleeding in the patient and other family members, a history of liver disease and the use of ethanol, aspirin, nonsteroidal anti-inflammatory agents, warfarin, antibiotics, and aspirin-containing products.

Mucocutaneous bleeding (including petechiae, ecchymoses, purpura, and epistaxis) and GI, genitourinary, or heavy menstrual bleeding are features of those patients with qualitative or quantitative platelet disorders. Patients with deficiencies of coagulation factor often have delayed bleeding, hemarthrosis, or bleeding into potential spaces such as between fascial planes and into the retroperitoneum. Patients with combination abnormalities of platelets and coagulation factor, such as disseminated intravascular coagulation, have both mucocutaneous and deep space bleeding.

Diagnosis and Differential

Presence of decreased red blood cell (RBC) count, hemoglobin level, and hematocrit are diagnostic for anemia. Determining the exact etiology of the anemia is not essential in the ED, except in the face of acute hemorrhage. The initial evaluation of newly diagnosed anemia should include a Hemoccult examination, complete blood cell count (CBC), reticulocyte count, review of RBC indices, and examination of the peripheral blood smear (Table 129-1).

Laboratory studies used to diagnose bleeding disorders can be divided into the following three categories: (a) those that test the initial formation of a platelet plug (primary hemostasis); (b) those that assess the formation of cross-linked fibrin (secondary hemostasis); and (c) those that test the fibrinolytic system, which is responsible for limiting the size of the fibrin clots formed. These tests are detailed in Table 129-2. A CBC with platelet count, prothrombin time, and partial thromboplastin time are the initial studies needed in patients with suspected bleeding disorders. The clinical situation can guide any further laboratory testing.

Emergency Department Care and Disposition

Management of anemia depends on the etiology of the anemia and clinical status of the patient.

1. Stabilizing the airway, assisting ventilation, providing circulatory support, and controlling direct hemorrhage takes priority.
2. **Blood should be typed and cross-matched** in those patients with anemia and ongoing blood loss so that it is available for transfusion if necessary.
3. Immediate **transfusion** of packed RBCs should be considered in symptomatic patients who are hemodynamically unstable and have evidence of tissue hypoxia or have limited cardiopulmonary reserve.
4. Patients with anemia and ongoing blood loss should be admitted

TABLE 129-1 Initial Laboratory Evaluation of Anemia

Test	Interpretation	Normal value	Clinical correlation
RBC indices:			
MCV	Reflects average RBC size	80–95 fL	*Decreased MCV* (microcytosis)—chronic iron deficiency, thalassemia, anemia of chronic disease *Increased MCV* (macrocytosis)—decreased level of vitamin B_{12} or folate, chronic ethanol ingestion, chronic liver disease, reticulocytosis, phenytoin, HIV drugs
MCH	Reflects weight of hemoglobin in average RBC	28–32 pg	The MCH and MCHC do not provide much additional information for the classification of anemia.
MCHC	Reflects concentration of hemoglobin in average RBC	32–36 g/dL	
Reticulocyte count	These RBCs of intermediate maturity are an index of the production of mature RBCs by the bone marrow, reported as a percent of total RBCs	0.5–1.5%	*Decreased reticulocyte count* reflects impaired RBC production; seen with low levels of iron, vitamin B_{12}, folate, bone marrow failure *Elevated reticulocyte count* reflects accelerated erythropoiesis, the normal marrow response to anemia; seen with blood loss and hemolytic anemia
Peripheral blood smear	Used for the evaluation of: 1. Overall size of the RBCs; example: normocytic, microcytic, macrocytic 2. Amount of hemoglobin in the RBCs; example: hypochromic 3. Look for abnormal shapes such as sickled cells or schistocytes (evidence of hemolysis) 4. Examination of white blood cells and platelets		

RBC, red blood cell; MCV, mean cellular volume; MCH, mean cellular hemoglobin; MCHC, mean cellular hemoglobin concentration; RBC, red blood cell.

TABLE 129-2 Tests of Hemostasis

Screening tests	Normal value	Measures	Clinical correlations
Platelet count	150,000–300,000/mm³	Number of patelets per mm³	Decreased platelet count (thrombocytopenia) Bleeding usually not a problem until platelet count <50,000; high risk of spontaneous bleeding including CNS with count <10,000/mm³. Causes: Decreased production—viral infections (measles); marrow infiltration; drugs (thiazides, ETOH, estrogens, interferon-α) Increased destruction—viral infections (mumps, varicella, EBV, HIV); ITP; TTP, DIC, HUS; drugs heparin, protamine Splenic sequestration (hypersplenism, hypothermia) Loss of platelets (hemorrhage, hemodialysis, extracorporeal circulation) Pseudothrombocytopenia—platelets are clumped but not truly decreased in number, examine blood smear to recognize this Elevated platelet count (thrombocytosis)—commonly reactive to inflammation or malignancy, or in polycythemia vera; can be associated with hemorrhage or thrombosis
Bleeding time (BT)	2.5–10 min (template BT)	Interaction between platelets and the subendothelium	Prolonged BT caused by: Thrombocytopenia (platelet count <50,000/min³) Abnormal platelet function (vWD, ASA, NSAIDs, uremia, liver disease) Collagen abnormalities (congenital abnormality or prolonged use of steroids)

Prothrombin time (PT)	10–12 s, but laboratory variation	Extrinsic system and common pathway—factors VII, X, V, prothrombin, and fibrinogen	*Prolonged PT*—most commonly caused by: Use of coumadin/warfarin (inhibits vitamin K-dependent factors II, VII, IX and X) Liver disease with decreased factor synthesis Antibiotics, some cephalosporins, (moxalactam, cefamandole, cefotaxime, cefoperazone) that inhibit vitamin K-dependent factors
Activated partial thromboplastin time (aPTT)	Depends on type of thromboplastin used; "activated" with kaolin	Intrinsic system and common pathway including factors XII, XI, IX, VIII, X, V, prothrombin, and fibrinogen	*Prolongation of aPTT* most commonly caused by: Heparin therapy Factor deficiencies; factor levels have to be < 30% of normal to cause prolongation **Note:** high doses of heparin or warfarin can cause prolongation of both the PT and aPTT due to their activity in the common pathway.
Thrombin clotting time (TCT)	10–12 s	Conversion of fibrinogen to fibrin monomer	*Prolonged TCT* caused by: Low fibrinogen level (DIC) Abnormal fibrinogen molecule (liver disease) Presence of heparin, FDPs or a paraprotein (multiple myeloma); these interfere with the conversion Very high fibrinogen level (acute phase reactant)
"Mixes"	Variable	Performed when one or more of the above screening tests is prolonged; the patients plasma ("abnormal") is mixed with "normal" plasma and the screening test is repeated	If the "mix" *corrects* the screening test, one or more factor deficiencies are present. If the "mix" *does not correct the screening test*, an inhibitor is present.

TABLE 129-2 Tests of Hemostasis (*Continued*)

Screening tests	Normal value	Measures	Clinical correlations
			OTHER HEMOSTATIC TESTS
Fibrin degradation products and D-dimer (evaluate fibrinolysis)	Variable	*FDPs* measure breakdown products from fibrinogen and fibrin monomer; *D-Dimer* measures breakdown products of cross-linked fibrin	Levels of these are elevated in DIC, thrombosis, pulmonary embolus, liver disease.
Factor level assays	60–130% (0.60–1.30 units/mL)	Measures the percent activity of a specified factor compared to normal	Used to identify specific factor deficiencies and in therapeutic management of patients with deficiencies
Inhibitor screens	Variable	Verifies the presence or absence of antibodies directed against one or more of the coagulation factors	*Specific inhibitors*—directed against one coagulation factor, most commonly against factor VIII; can be in patients with congenital or acquired deficiency. *Nonspecific inhibitors*—directed against more than one of the coagulation factors; example is lupus-type anticoagulant

Abbreviations: ASA, aspirin; CNS, central nervous system; DIC, disseminated intravascular coagulation; EBV, Epstein-Barr virus; ETOH, ethanol; FDPs, fibrin degradation products; HIV, human immunodeficiency virus; HUS, hemolytic uremic syndrome; ITP, idiopathic thrombocytopenic purpura; NSAIDs, nonsteroidal anti-inflammatory drugs; TTP, thrombotic thrombocytopenic purpura; vWD, von Willebrand disease.

for further evaluation. Patients with chronic anemia or newly diagnosed anemia with unclear etiology require admission if they are hemodynamically unstable and hypoxic and have acidosis or ongoing cardiac ischemia.

5. Hematology consultation should be considered to assist in evaluation of those patients with anemia of unclear etiology, anemic patients with concomitant abnormalities of platelets and white blood cell counts, and patients with suspected bleeding disorders.

For further reading in *Emergency Medicine: A Comprehensive Study Guide,* 5th ed., see Chap. 210, "Evaluation of Anemia and the Bleeding Patient," by Mary E. Eberst.

---

130 | Acquired Bleeding Disorders
John Sverha

Acquired bleeding disorders can be caused by platelet abnormalities, coagulation factor deficiencies, drugs, systemic illness, and endogenous anticoagulants. Early recognition of these disorders is required for prompt, etiology-specific treatment.

BLEEDING DUE TO PLATELET ABNORMALITIES

Acquired platelet abnormalities include both qualitative and quantitative platelet defects. Quantitative platelet disorders can be caused by decreased platelet production (i.e., marrow infiltration, aplastic anemia, viral infections, and drugs), increased platelet destruction (i.e., idiopathic thrombocytopenic purpura (ITP), thrombotic thrombocytopenic purpura (TTP), hemolytic uremic syndrome, disseminated intravascular coagulation (DIC), and viral infection), increased platelet loss (i.e., hemorrhage and hemodialysis), and splenic sequestration. Qualitative platelet disorders result in excessive bleeding regardless of the platelet count. Common causes of qualitative platelet disorders include uremia, liver disease, DIC, drugs, and antiplatelet antibodies.

Emergency Department Care and Disposition

1. Platelet transfusion is warranted in all patients with a platelet count $< 10,000/\mu L$, regardless of etiology.
2. Most patients with a platelet count of $< 50,000/\mu L$, and active bleeding should receive platelet transfusion. However, hematologic consultation should be obtained as some conditions, such as DIC and TTP, may actually be worsened by platelet transfusion.

BLEEDING DUE TO WARFARIN USE OR VITAMIN K DEFICIENCY

Vitamin K is a necessary cofactor in the production of coagulation factors II, VII, IX, and X, as well as proteins C and S. Sodium warfarin is a vitamin K antagonist used widely as an anticoagulant. Patients with liver disease, those with vitamin K deficiency due to poor nutrition or malabsorption, and patients taking warfarin are at increased risk of bleeding.

Emergency Department Care and Disposition

1. Treatment of bleeding in patients taking warfarin depends on the severity of the bleeding. Patients with a prolonged prothrombin time (PT) but no active bleeding may only need temporary discontinuation of warfarin.
2. Fresh frozen plasma (FFP) rapidly replenishes coagulation factors and should be used to treat serious bleeding.
3. Vitamin K (10 mg SQ or IM) also may be used to treat active bleeding although it takes approximately 24 h to take effect and prevents anticoagulation with warfarin for about 2 weeks.

BLEEDING IN LIVER DISEASE

Patients with liver disease are at increased risk for bleeding for multiple reasons including decreased synthesis of coagulation factors, vitamin K deficiency, thrombocytopenia, and increased fibrinolysis.

Emergency Department Care and Disposition

1. All patients with liver disease and active bleeding should receive vitamin K (10 mg SQ or IM), although this may take 24 h to take effect.
2. Patients with severe bleeding should receive FFP to rapidly replace coagulation factors.

3. Platelet transfusion can be used in severe bleeding with associated thrombocytopenia.
4. Desmopressin (DDAVP) (0.3 μg/kg SQ or IV) may shorten bleeding time in some patients.

BLEEDING IN RENAL DISEASE

The bleeding tendency exhibited by patients in renal disease is related to the degree and duration of uremia. It is caused by uremic degradation products, chronic anemia, platelet dysfunction, deficiency of coagulation factors, and thrombocytopenia.

Emergency Department Care and Disposition

1. Transfusion of packed red blood cells (RBCs) to maintain a hematocrit between 26 and 30 optimizes platelet function.
2. Hemodialysis improves platelet function transiently for 1 to 2 days.
3. DDAVP (0.3 μg/kg SQ or IV) shortens bleeding time in the majority of patients.
4. Conjugated estrogens improve bleeding time in most patients by an unknown mechanism.
5. Platelet transfusions and cryoprecipitate are indicated for life-threatening bleeding only and are to be used in conjunction with the other therapies listed earlier.

BLEEDING DUE TO HEPARIN USE OR THROMBOLYTIC THERAPY

Bleeding is the most common side effect when using heparin or thrombolytic therapy. Major bleeding complications (defined as those requiring packed RBC transfusion) occur in approximately 1 to 2 percent of patients receiving these drugs.

Emergency Department Care and Disposition

1. Heparin or thrombolytic therapy should be discontinued at any sign of significant bleeding.
2. Protamine can be used to neutralize heparin at a dose of 1 mg IV per 100 U of infused heparin. Protamine is also effective in reversing the effects of low-molecular-weight heparin.
3. Massive bleeding associated with thrombolytic use should be treated with cryoprecipitate (10 U IV). If bleeding persists, treat with FFP (2 U IV). Further treatment should be in con-

junction with a hematologist but may include platelet transfusion or aminocaproic acid administration.

BLEEDING IN DISSEMINATED INTRAVASCULAR COAGULATION

DIC results from the activation of both the coagulation and fibrinolytic systems. The most common trigger of DIC is the liberation of tissue factor from the extravascular space. The most common causes of DIC are in the clinical settings of infection, carcinoma, acute leukemia, trauma, shock, liver disease, pregnancy, vascular disease, envenomation, acute respiratory distress syndrome (ARDS), and transfusion reactions.

Clinical Features

DIC results in both bleeding and thrombotic complications, although in an individual patient, one usually predominates. Bleeding occurs in up to 7 percent of patients and typically occurs in the skin and mucous membranes. The skin may show signs of petechiae or ecchymoses. Bleeding from several sites, including venipuncture sites and surgical wounds, is common. Gastrointestinal, urinary tract, and central nervous system bleeding also may occur. Other patients show primarily thrombotic symptoms. Depending on the site of the thrombosis, patients may exhibit focal ischemia of the extremities, mental status changes, oliguria, or symptoms of ARDS. Purpura fulminans develops when there is widespread thrombosis resulting in gangrene of the extremities and hemorrhagic infarction of the skin.

Diagnosis and Differential

The diagnosis of DIC is based on the clinical setting and characteristic laboratory abnormalities that are listed in Table 130-1.

Emergency Department Care and Disposition

1. Hemodynamic stabilization should be provided through IVF or packed RBC transfusion.
2. The underlying medical or surgical illness should be treated.
3. If bleeding predominates and the PT is elevated more than 2 s, replacement of coagulation factors is indicated. FFP is infused 2 U at a time. Cryoprecipitate is used to replace fibrinogen. It is typically infused 10 bags at a time. If the platelet count is $< 50,000/\mu L$ with active bleeding or $< 20,000/\mu L$ without bleeding, platelet transfusion should be initiated. All patients

TABLE 130-1 Laboratory Abnormalities Characteristic of Disseminated Intravascular Coagulation

Studies	Result
	MOST USEFUL
PT	Prolonged
Platelet count*	Usually low
Fibrinogen level†	Low
	HELPFUL
aPTT	Usually prolonged
TCT‡	Prolonged
Fragmented RBCs§	Should be present
FDPs and D-dimers‖	Elevated
Specific factor assays#	
Factor II	Low
Factor V	Low
Factor VII**	Low
Factor VIII††	Low, normal, high
Factor IX	Low (decreases later than other factors)
Factor X	Low

Abbreviations: PT, prothrombin time; aPTT, activated partial thromboplastin time; RBCs, red blood cells; FDPs, fibrin degradation products; DIC, disseminated intravascular coagulation; TCT, thrombin clot time.
*Platelet count usually low, most important that it is falling if it started at an elevated level.
†Fibrinogen level correlates best with bleeding complications; it is an acute phase reactant so it may actually start out at an elevated level; fibrinogen level <100 mg/dL correlates with severe DIC.
‡Not a sensitive test, prolonged by many abnormalities.
§Fragmented RBCs and schistocytes are not specific for DIC.
‖Levels may be chronically elevated in patients with liver or renal disease.
#The factors in the extrinsic pathway are most affected (VII, X, V, and II).
**Factor VII is usually low early because it has the shortest half-life.
‡‡Factor VIII is an acute phase reactant so its level may be normal, low, or elevated in DIC.

with bleeding due to DIC should also receive vitamin K (10 mg SQ or intramuscularly) and folate (1 mg IV).
4. If thrombosis predominates, heparinization should be considered, although this is controversial. Heparin is most likely to be beneficial if the underlying medical condition is carcinoma,

acute promyelocytic leukemia, or retained uterine products, or if patients exhibit signs of purpura fulminans.

BLEEDING DUE TO CIRCULATING ANTICOAGULANTS

Circulating anticoagulants are antibodies directed against one or more of the coagulation factors. The two most common circulating anticoagulants are factor VIII inhibitor (a specific inhibitor directed only against factor VIII) and lupus anticoagulant (a nonspecific inhibitor directed against several of the coagulation factors).

Clinical Features

Patients with factor VIII inhibitor have massive spontaneous bruises, ecchymoses, and hematomas. Patients with the lupus anticoagulant may have thromboses or recurrent fetal loss. Bleeding abnormalities are rare in patients with lupus anticoagulant.

Diagnosis and Differential

Laboratory studies in patients with factor VIII inhibitor reveal a normal PT, normal thrombin clot time (TCT), and a greatly prolonged activated partial thromboplastin time (aPTT) that does not correct with "mixing." A factor VIII specific assay will show that the factor VIII activity is very low. Patients with lupus anticoagulant will have a normal or slightly prolonged PT, a normal TCT, and a moderately prolonged aPTT that also does not correct with mixing. Factor specific assays will show a decrease in all factor levels.

Emergency Department Care and Disposition

1. Patients with factor VIII inhibitor and active bleeding should be managed in conjunction with a hematologist. Treatment options include high doses of factor VIII concentrate, prothrombin complex concentrates, and recombinant factor VIIa.
2. Patients with lupus anticoagulant and thrombosis should be treated with long-term anticoagulation using either warfarin (venous thrombosis) or aspirin (arterial thrombosis).

For further reading in *Emergency Medicine: A Comprehensive Study Guide,* 5th ed., see Chap. 211, "Acquired Bleeding Disorders," by Mary E. Eberst.

131

Hemophilias and Von Willebrand's Disease

John Sverha

HEMOPHILIAS

Clinical Features

The most common hemophilias are due to the deficiency of either factor VIII (hemophilia A) or factor IX (hemophilia B). Both hemophilia A and B are recessive X-linked disorders. The clinical classification of hemophilia patients is based on the severity of their factor deficiency. Patients are classified as having mild disease if they have between 6 and 60 percent of normal factor VIII or IX activity, moderate disease if they have between 1 and 5 percent of normal factor activity, and severe disease if there is less than 1 percent of factor activity. Bleeding in hemophilic patients is characterized by deep hematomas and hemarthroses that occur spontaneously or with minimal trauma. Spontaneous or traumatic bleeding into the neck, pharynx, or retropharynx can result in airway compromise. Retroperitoneal bleeding can occur and presents with back, thigh, groin, or abdominal pain. Central nervous system (CNS) bleeding may cause a new headache or other neurologic symptoms. In general, hemophilic patients do not have problems with minor cuts or abrasions.

Diagnosis and Differential

Laboratory tests in patients with hemophilia typically reveal a normal prothrombin time (PT), a normal thrombin clot time (TCT), and a prolonged activated partial thromboplastin time (aPTT). If patients have mild disease, with a factor activity level > 30 percent, the aPTT may be normal. The only way to distinguish hemophilia A and B is by specific factor assays for factors VIII and IX. About 10 percent of patients with hemophilia will develop an inhibitor, which is an antibody against the missing factor. An inhibitor can be diagnosed if the plasma from patients with hemophilia and prolonged aPTT is mixed 50-50 with the plasma from a normal control and the aPTT does not correct. The quantity of inhibitor that is present is measured by the Bethesda inhibitor assay (BIA) and is reported in BIA units.

Emergency Department Care and Disposition

The management of hemophiliac bleeding depends on the site and severity of the bleeding, the type and severity of the hemophilia, and the presence or absence of inhibitor. Life-threatening bleeding can occur in the CNS, neck, oropharynx, and retroperitoneum. When hemophilic patients have symptoms of bleeding at any of these sites, they should receive immediate factor replacement. Diagnostic imaging and lab tests can then be performed.

1. If patients have mild or moderate hemophilia A and no inhibitor, they may be able to be treated with **desmopressin (DDAVP).** DDAVP can raise the factor VIII activity level threefold. It is helpful to know if patients have been successfully treated with DDAVP previously, as not all patients will respond to this treatment. The usual dose is 0.3 μg/kg IV or SQ with a 30 μg maximum dose. DDAVP also can be administered intranasally at a dose of 150 μg for patients weighing less than 50 kg and 300 μg for patients weighing 50 kg or more. A response in the factor VIII level should be seen within 1 h.

2. If patients have moderate or severe hemophilia A, no inhibitor, and significant bleeding, they will require **factor VIII replacement.** Table 131-1 lists the desired factor VIII activity levels to be achieved after treatment. The desired activity levels vary from 30 to 100 percent depending on the severity of the bleeding. The formula for determining the initial dose of factor VIII to be infused follows:

Factor VIII units = (weight in kg/2) $\times$ (% activity level desired $-$ % intrinsic activity)

(Recommendations for dosing intervals and duration of treatment can be found in Table 131-1.) Ideally, all patients requiring factor VIII replacement should receive recombinant factor to eliminate the risk of viral transmission. If this is not available and life-threatening bleeding is present, **fresh frozen plasma (FFP)** or **cryoprecipitate** may be used. Each milliliter of FFP contains 1 U of factor VIII. Each bag of cryoprecipitate contains about 100 U of factor VIII. Ancillary therapies (often used in dental bleeding) include the use of antifibrinolytic agents such as **aminocaproic acid** and **tranexamic acid.**

3. If patients have moderate-to-severe hemophilia A inhibitor present and significant bleeding, the treatment is guided by the inhibitor titer (measured in BIA units) and the type of response patients have had to factor VIII concentrates. Table 131-2 outlines the various treatment options. If patients have moderate-to-severe hemophilia B, no inhibitor, and significant bleeding, they will require **factor IX replacement.** Table 131-3 lists the desired factor IX activity levels to be achieved after treatment. The desired activity levels vary from 20 to 100 percent de-

TABLE 131-1 Factor VIII Replacement Therapy for Patients with Hemophilia A (No Inhibitor)

Type of hemorrhage	Factor VIII level required for hemostasis, % of normal	Factor VIII dose in U/kg (initial dose)	Dosing interval, h*	Duration of therapy, days
Minor				
Hemarthroses	30–50	15–25	24	1–2
Superficial muscular or soft tissue	30–50	15–25	24	1–2
Moderate				
Epistaxis	30–50	15–25	12	Until resolved
Dental extractions	50	25	12–24	1–2
Muscular or soft tissue with dissection	50–100	25–50	12	Variable
GI bleeding	50–100	25–50	12	7–10
Hematuria	50–100	25–50	12	Until resolved
Life-threatening				
CNS	75–100	50	12	10–14
Retropharynx/pharynx	75–100	50	12	10–14
Retroperitoneum	75–100	50	12	10–14
Surgery	75–100	50	12	Variable

Abbreviations: GI, gastrointestinal; CNS, central nervous system.

*Continuous infusion of factor VIII concentrate may be used in hospitalized patients; a typical dose after the loading dose is 150 U/h; this is adjusted based on factor VIII levels.

TABLE 131-2 Replacement Therapy for Hemophilia A Patients with Inhibitors

Type of product (trade names)	Used for	Dose	Frequency, h	Comments
Factor VIII concentrates	Inhibitor titer less than 5–10 BIA units	5000–10,000 U bolus	Continuous infusion at about 1000 U/h	If patient is a "high responder," in about 3 days the inhibitor titer will rise
PCCs PCCs contain factors II, VII, IX, X (Bebulin VH, Proplex T, Profilnine HT, and Konyne-80)	Inhibitor titer >10 units; known good response to these products	75–100 U/kg of body-weight	Repeat dose q8–12 h	Complications of use include development of thromboembolic disease, DIC, very low risk of hepatitis transmission
Activated PCCs aPPCs contain factors II, VII, IX, and X with variable amounts of activated factors VII$_a$, IX$_a$, and X$_a$ (Autoplex, FEIBA)	Patients who do not respond to PCCs	Same as with PCCs	Repeat dose q12–24 h	Same as with PCCs
Porcine factor VIII	Patients with high inhibitor titers not responsive to the above products	Variable	Variable	Patients will often develop an inhibitor to the porcine product
Recombinant factor VII$_a$	Not yet commercially available	Variable	Variable	Less thrombogenic risk than PCCs and no risk of viral transmission

Abbreviations: BIA, Bethesda inhibitor assay; PCCs, prothrombin complex concentrates; aPTT, activated partial thromboplastin time.

TABLE 131-3 Factor IX Replacement Therapy for Patients with Hemophilia B

Type of hemorrhage	Factor IX level required for hemostasis, % of normal	Initial factor IX dose in U/kg	Duration of therapy, days
Minor			
Hemarthroses	20–30	20–30	1–2
Superficial muscular or soft tissue	20–30	20–30	1–2
Moderate			
Epistaxis	25–50	25–50	Until resolved
Dental extractions	25–50	25–50	2–7
Muscular or soft tissue bleeds with dissection	25–50	25–50	Until resolved
Hematuria	25–50	25–50	Until resolved
GI bleeding	50	50	5–10
Life-threatening*			
CNS	50	50	7–10
Retropharynx/pharynx	50	50	7–10
Retroperitoneum	50	50	7–10
Surgery	50	50	7–10

Abbreviations: GI, gastrointestinal; CNS, central nervous system.
*Factor IX levels higher than 50 percent may be necessary and are safely obtained using the highly purified factor IX concentrates.

pending on the severity of the bleeding. The formula for determining the initial dose of factor IX to be infused follows:

$$\text{Factor IX units} = (\text{weight in kg}) \times (\%\ \text{activity level desired} - \%\ \text{intrinsic activity})$$

(Recommendations for dosing intervals and duration of treatment can be found in Table 131-3.) Ideally, all patients requiring factor IX replacement should receive recombinant factor to eliminate the risk of viral transmission. If this is not available and life-threatening bleeding is present, FFP may be used. In an average-sized person, 1 U of FFP should raise the factor IX level by 3 percent.

4. If patients have moderate-to-severe hemophilia B inhibitor present and significant bleeding, treatment is guided by the inhibitor titer (measured in BIA units) and the type of response the patient has had to factor IX concentrates. Table 131-4 outlines the various treatment options.

TABLE 131-4 Products Used for Replacement Therapy in Patients with Hemophilia B with Inhibitors

Type of product	Used for	Initial dose
Highly purified factor IX concentrates	Bethesda inhibitor titer < 10 U	Variable
PCCs	Bethesda inhibitor titer < 10 U	75 U/kg
aPPCs	Bethesda inhibitor titers > 10 U or unresponsive to the above	Variable, about 75 U/kg
Recombinant factor VII$_a$	Not yet commercially available	Variable

Abbreviations: PCCs, prothrombin complex concentrates; aPCC, activated prothrombin-complex concentrates.

5. Indications for admitting patients with hemophilia include any potentially life-threatening bleed involving the CNS, neck, pharynx, retropharynx, or retroperitoneum, or any potential compartment syndrome. Patients should also be admitted if incapable of administering replacement factor at home, if treatment will be required for several days, or if patients require parenteral pain control.

VON WILLEBRAND'S DISEASE

Clinical Features

Von Willebrand's disease (vWD) is caused by a deficiency or abnormality of von Willebrand's factor (vWF). The normal function of vWF is to allow platelets to adhere to damaged endothelium and to carry factor VIII in the plasma. There are three major types of vWD. They differ in the molecular defect present in the vWF molecule and vary tremendously in their clinical severity. Of patients with vWD, 80 percent have type I disease. Bleeding in type I vWD tends to be mild with symptoms such as epistaxis, easy bruising, menorrhagia, bleeding after dental extractions, and gastrointestinal (GI) bleeding. Less than 10 percent of patients with vWD have type III disease. These patients have a severe bleeding diathesis and symptoms such as spontaneous hematomas and hemarthroses as seen in severe hemophilia.

Diagnosis and Differential

Patients with vWD typically have a normal PT, TCT, and aPTT. Moderate or severe vWD may cause a prolongation in the aPTT.

Other findings in vWD include a prolonged bleeding time, a low vWF antigen level, a low vWF activity level, and a low or normal factor VIII activity level. vWD can be very difficult to distinguish from mild hemophilia A.

Emergency Department Care and Disposition

Treatment of vWD depends on the type of disease and the severity of the bleeding.

1. Patients with type I vWD can usually be treated with **DDAVP**. The usual dose is 0.3 μg/kg IV or SQ with a 30 μg maximum dose. DDAVP can also be administered intranasally at a dose of 150 μg for patients weighing less than 50 kg and 300 μg for patients weighing less 50 kg or more. Bleeding due to dental procedures can sometimes be managed with antifibrinolytic agents such as **aminocaproic acid** and **tranexamic acid.** Women with vWD are often treated with hormonal agents (estrogens and progesterones) which cause an increase in the vWF activity.
2. Patients with type II or type III vWD usually require infusion of factor VIII concentrates such as **Humate-P** or **Koate-HS.** If these are not available, cryoprecipitate may be used. Each bag of cryoprecipitate contains about 100 U of vWF activity. Its use is associated with a small risk of viral transmission.

For further reading in *Emergency Medicine: A Comprehensive Study Guide,* 5th ed., see Chap. 212, "Hemophilias and Von Willebrand's Disease," by Mary E. Eberst.

---

132 Hemolytic Anemias

Sandra L. Najarian

Hemolytic anemias are divided into hereditary and acquired types. Hereditary anemias include sickle cell anemia and its variants, glucose-6-phosphate dehydrogenase deficiency and hereditary spherocytosis. Acquired anemias may be antibody-mediated or result from fragmentation, direct toxicity, mechanical injury, or hypersplenism.

HEREDITARY HEMOLYTIC ANEMIAS

Sickle Cell Disease

Clinical Features

Patients with sickle cell disease (SCD) have a wide variety of symptoms, which can involve nearly every organ system. As a result of this chronic hemolytic anemia, patients may have flow murmurs, congestive heart failure, cardiomegaly, cor pulmonale, lower extremity ulcerations, icterus, and hepatomegaly. Patients may have pulmonary manifestations such as pleuritic chest pain, fever, sudden decrease in pulmonary function, and hypoxia. Neurologic manifestations include cerebral infarction in children, cerebral hemorrhage in adults, transient ischemic attacks, headache, seizure, and coma.

Painful vasoocclusive crises are the most common reason for emergency department (ED) visits. Common precipitants include cold exposure, dehydration, high altitude, and infections, particularly with encapsulated organisms such as *Haemophilus influenzae* or pneumococcus. Patients may have joint, muscle, or bone pain or diffuse abdominal pain.

Hematologic crises present with weakness, dyspnea, fatigue, worsening chronic heart failure (CHF), or shock, in the setting of a precipitous drop in hemoglobin. Acute splenic sequestration of blood and bone marrow suppression (aplastic crisis) are two types of hematologic crisis.

Other clinical presentations of SCD include priapism; swelling of hands or feet due to vasoocclusion (dactylitis); and infarction of the renal medulla, with flank pain and hematuria.

Diagnosis and Differential

The clinical presentation guides the ED evaluation. For patients suffering an acute crisis, a drop in hemoglobin by 2 g/dL from the patient's baseline suggests hematologic crisis or blood loss. A reticulocyte count is necessary in these patients. A count less than the baseline of 5 to 15 percent may reflect aplastic crisis. A leukocytosis, along with a left shift, should raise the suspicion of infection. Electrolytes should be checked in patients with evidence of dehydration. A urinalysis should be obtained in patients with urinary symptoms. Liver enzymes are indicated in patients with abdominal pain. Arterial blood gas analysis is warranted in patients with respiratory complaints and evidence of hypoxia on pulse oximetry. Those with SCD may have a mild-to-moderate hypoxia; however, a Pao$_2$ of less than 60 suggests an acute problem. Radiographic studies may include chest radiograph for patients with pulmonary symptoms, abdominal computed tomography (CT) scan or ultrasound for patients with acute abdominal findings on physical examination, head CT scan for patients with neurologic deficits, and plain radiographs for patients with focal bone pain.

Differential diagnosis for complaints related to SCD is extensive and includes osteomyelitis, acute arthritides, pancreatitis, hepatitis, pelvic inflammatory disease, pyelonephritis, pneumonia, pulmonary embolus, and meningitis.

Emergency Department Care and Disposition

Management is primarily supportive, with close attention to possible precipitants of acute crises.

1. Patients with evidence of dehydration or acute pain should receive oral rehydration, if they can tolerate fluids or **IV fluids,** such as 0.45 normal saline or normal saline at 1$\frac{1}{3}$ times maintenance.
2. **Narcotics** should be promptly administered for severe pain. Patients who present to the ED frequently will benefit from a protocol treatment plan.
3. Supplemental **oxygen** should be administered to patients with demonstration of hypoxia on pulse oximetry.
4. Cardiac monitoring is appropriate for patients with cardiopulmonary symptoms.
5. Patients with symptoms of acute infections or with temperatures > 38°C should have the appropriate cultures drawn. **Broad-spectrum antibiotics,** such as cefuroxime or ceftriaxone, should be administered.
6. Patients with significant cardiopulmonary decompensation, an acute CNS event, or priapism, should receive exchange transfusions.
7. Patients with priapism require hydration, analgesia, and urgent urologic consultation.
8. Patients with acute bone pain suggestive of possible osteomyelitis should have cultures drawn and receive antibiotic therapy to cover *Staphylococcus aureus* and *S. typhimurium.*

Admission criteria include pulmonary, neurologic, aplastic, or infectious crises; splenic sequestration; unremitting pain crisis; persistent nausea and vomiting; or patients with uncertain diagnoses. Discharged patients should receive oral analgesics, close follow-up, and instructions to return immediately for fever $> 38°C$ or worsening symptoms.

Sickle Cell Trait

The most common variant of SCD is sickle cell trait. These carriers have minimal complications, and sickling is not seen except in conditions of extreme hypoxia. These patients are generally asymptomatic and have normal life expectancy. Mild-to-moderate hemolytic anemia, mild reticulocytosis, and splenomegaly may be seen in those with sickle cell–hemoglobin C disease. Most patients usually have mild complications, whereas others can have painful crises and complications similar to those patients with SCD. Presentation and complications from sickle cell–β-thalassemia disease depends on the type of β-thalassemia gene that is inherited. Presentations can range from mild-to-severe hemolytic anemia and vasoocclusive crises.

Glucose-6-Phosphate Dehydrogenase (G-6-PD) Deficiency

African-American males are most commonly affected and may have acute hemolytic crises, hemoglobinuria, and vascular collapse due to infections, exposure to oxidant drugs, metabolic acidosis and ingestion of fava beans. The diagnosis is made by decreased G-6-PD activity on quantitative assay. There is no specific treatment; prevention involves early treatment of infection and avoidance of oxidant stress.

Hereditary Spherocytosis

Hereditary spherocytosis (HS) is seen in people of northern European descent and is characterized by mild hemolytic anemia, splenomegaly, and intermittent jaundice. Laboratory features include mild anemia, spherocytes on peripheral smear, a normal mean cellular volume, and an increased mean cellular hemoglobin concentration ($> 36\%$). Splenectomy is the treatment of choice.

ACQUIRED HEMOLYTIC ANEMIAS

Clinical Features

Antibody-mediated hemolytic anemias include warm and cold antibody types. The warm type is more common in elderly, female patients with underlying medical conditions. In children, it may develop after acute infections or immunizations. Patients may have mild anemia and splenomegaly to life-threatening anemia, splenomegaly, pulmonary edema, mental status changes, and venous thrombosis.

Cold antibody hemolytic anemia presents in two forms. Cold agglutinin disease may present as an acute disease in younger people following infections such as *Mycoplasma pneumoniae.* The anemia is usually mild. The chronic form is seen in elderly patients with underlying lymphoid neoplasms and involves hemolysis in parts of the body exposed to cold. Paroxysmal cold hemoglobinemia is another acute form found in patients with untreated syphilis or viral illnesses and presents with fever, chills, hemoglobinuria, and pain involving the back, legs, and abdomen.

Autoimmune hemolytic anemia also can be drug-induced, involving α-methyldopa, penicillin, sulfa drugs, and quinidine. Hemolysis ceases after discontinuation of the drug.

Microangiopathic hemolytic anemia (MAHA) results from fragmentation hemolysis. This includes damage to red blood cells (RBCs) from passage through artificial heart valves, calcified aortic valves, or through arterioles and microcirculation damaged by thrombotic thrombocytopenia purpura (TTP), hemolytic uremic syndrome (HUS), pregnancy, vasculitis, malignant hypertension, and certain malignancies.

TTP more commonly affects women and presents with fever, neurologic changes, hemorrhage, and renal insufficiency. HUS is a disease of early childhood and presents with fever, acute renal failure, and neurologic deficits following a prodromal infection. Fragmentation hemolysis in pregnancy is seen in preeclampsia, eclampsia, and abruption.

Direct toxic effects causing hemolysis may result from infection, copper exposure, and the venom of bees, wasps, certain spiders, and cobras. Oxidative hemolysis of RBCs results from methemoglobin-producing drugs, such as lidocaine and sulfonamides.

Mechanical damage to RBCs can result in hemolysis and hemoglobinuria. Etiologies include extensive burns and strenuous physical activity. Patients who have been on cardiopulmonary bypass can develop hemolysis, fever, and leukopenia, known as postperfusion syndrome. The passage of blood through the oxygenator activates complement, leading to acute intravascular hemolysis. Hemolysis as a result of sequestration and destruction of RBCs in the spleen, or hypersplenism, is most commonly seen in portal hypertension, infiltrative disease, and infections.

Diagnosis and Differential

Diagnosis is based on recognition of clinical signs and symptoms and obtaining appropriate laboratory studies. Compelete blood cell count will reveal anemia. Thrombocytopenia is present in TTP with platelet counts often < 20,000. Patients with HUS will have thrombocytopenia, though not to the degree of those with TTP. An elevated reticulocyte count is the best indicator of a normal bone marrow in the setting of hemolysis and may be as high as 30 to 40 percent. Review of the peripheral blood smear is vital and often will give keys to the diagnosis. Schistocytes—fragmented RBCs—are seen in MAHA and are the result of direct trauma. Spherocytes are evidence of warm antibody immune hemolysis and hereditary spherocytosis. Other laboratory abnormalities include elevations in lactic acid dehydrogenase and indirect bilirubin. The direct Coombs' test is positive in those patients with immune-mediated hemolysis. Elevated blood urea nitrogen and creatinine levels are seen in HUS and TTP. Patients with HELLP syndrome demonstrate hemolysis, elevated LFTs, and low platelets in the setting of preeclampsia.

Emergency Department Care and Disposition

Treatment is directed at stabilization of vital signs and correction of the underlying disease process.

1. **Prednisone** (1.0 mg/kg/d) is the initial treatment for warm antibody hemolytic anemia and TTP. **Azathioprine** and **cyclophosphamide** are occasionally utilized, and splenectomy may be required for those who fail or cannot tolerate steroids.
2. **Plasma exchange transfusion** is the foundation of therapy for TTP. If unavailable, **fresh frozen plasma** should be infused while arranging transfer to a tertiary-care center. Platelet transfusions should be avoided because they can aggravate the thrombotic process. Antiplatelet therapy consisting of aspirin or dipyridamole also should be initiated. Immunotherapy may also be initiated for patients who are refractory to treatment.
3. **Transfusion of RBCs** is indicated for angina, CHF, mental status changes, or hypoxia.
4. Patients with cold antibody hemolytic anemia should be kept in a **warm environment.**
5. Early **dialysis** should be considered in the management of HUS.
6. Prompt delivery of the infant followed by supportive care is mandatory for patients with HELLP syndrome.
7. Iron and folate should be given to patients with traumatic hemolysis due to artificial heart valves. If hemolysis is severe, the defective valve may need replacement.
8. Methemoglobin levels greater than 20 to 30% of total hemoglobin are treated with **methylene blue** (1 to 2 mg/kg in a 1% solution IV over 5 min).

For further reading in *Emergency Medicine: A Comprehensive Study Guide,* 5th ed., see Chap. 213, "Hereditary Hemolytic Anemias," and Chap. 214, "Acquired Hemolytic Anemias," by Mary E. Eberst.

133 | Blood Transfusions and Component Therapy

Keith L. Mausner

This chapter reviews blood and component therapy, complications of transfusions, emergency transfusion, and massive transfusion.

WHOLE BLOOD

Whole blood provides both volume and oxygen-carrying capacity. However, this is better achieved using packed red blood cells (PRBCs) and crystalloid solution. Disadvantages of whole blood include low levels of clotting factors; frequently elevated levels of potassium, hydrogen ion, and ammonia; the presence of a large number of antigens; and the potential for volume overload before the needed components are replaced. A unit of whole blood contains about 500 mL of blood plus a preservative-anticoagulant, usually citrate phosphate dextrose adenine (CPDA-1).

PACKED RED BLOOD CELLS

One unit of PRBCs raises an adult's hemoglobin by 1 g/dL or the hematocrit by 3 percent. The decision to transfuse depends on the underlying cause and rate of blood loss, and the patient's health status and cardiopulmonary reserve. The major indications for PRBC transfusion include the following: (*a*) acute hemorrhage: blood loss greater than 25 to 30 percent blood volume (1500 mL) in otherwise healthy adults usually requires transfusion of PRBCs to replace oxygen-carrying capacity and crystalloid infusion to replace volume; (*b*) surgical blood loss greater than 2 L usually requires transfusion of PRBCs and crystalloid; and (*c*) in chronic anemia, transfusion may be indicated for symptomatic patients, those with underlying cardiopulmonary disease, and those with hemoglobin levels less than 7 g/dL.

RBCs are available as leukocyte poor, frozen, or washed. Leukocyte-poor RBCs have up to 85 percent of the leukocytes removed and are indicated for transplant recipients or candidates and for patients with a history of febrile nonhemolytic transfusion reactions. Frozen RBCs are a source of rare blood types and provide reduced antigen exposure. Washed RBCs are for patients who have hypersensitive reactions to plasma, for neonatal transfusions, and for those with paroxysmal nocturnal hemoglobinuria.

PLATELETS

One unit contains about 4×10^{11} platelets in a volume of 250 to 350 mL. Platelets are usually transfused 6 U at a time, which raises the platelet count about 50,000/mL. ABO- and Rh-compatible platelets are preferable. The platelet count should be checked 1 and 24 h after infusion. Transfused platelets survive 3 to 5 days unless there is platelet consumption.

Principles for platelet transfusions in adults include the following: (a) if the platelet count is above 50,000/mL, bleeding from thrombocytopenia is unlikely unless there is platelet dysfunction; (b) maintain the platelet count greater than 50,000/mL in patients undergoing major surgery or with significant bleeding; (c) a platelet count between 10,000 and 50,000/mL increases the risk of bleeding with trauma or invasive procedures, and patients with platelet dysfunction (e.g., renal or liver disease) may have spontaneous bleeds with these counts; and (d) a platelet count below 10,000/mL presents a high risk of spontaneous bleeding, and prophylactic transfusion is indicated; however, in immune thrombocytopenia (due to platelet destruction) transfusion may have little effect.

FRESH-FROZEN PLASMA

One bag of fresh-frozen plasma (FFP) contains 200 to 250 mL, 1 U/mL of each coagulation factor, and 1 to 2 mg/mL of fibrinogen. FFP should be ABO compatible. A typical starting dose is 8 to 10 mL/kg, or 2 to 4 bags of FFP. FFP is indicated for (a) acquired coagulopathy with active bleeding or before invasive procedures when there is greater than 1.5 times prolongation of the prothrombin time (PT) or activated partial thromboplastin time (aPTT), or a coagulation factor assay less than 25 percent of normal; (b) congenital isolated factor deficiencies when specific virally safe products are not available; (c) thrombotic thrombocytopenic purpura (TTP) patients undergoing plasma exchange; (d) patients receiving massive transfusion who develop coagulopathy and active bleeding, and (*e*) antithrombin III deficiency when antithrombin III concentrate is not available.

CRYOPRECIPITATE

Cryoprecipitate is derived from FFP; one bag contains 80 to 100 U factor VIIIC, 80 U von Willebrand factor, 200 to 300 mg fibrinogen, 40 to 60 U factor XIII, and variable amounts of fibronectin. The usual dose is 2 to 4 bags per 10-kg body weight (10 to 20 bags); ABO compatible bags are preferable. Indications for cryoprecipitate are (1) fibrinogen level less than 100 mg/dL associated with disseminated intravascular coagulation (DIC) or congenital fibrinogen deficiency; (2) von Willebrand disease with active bleeding when desmopressin (DDAVP) is not effective and factor VIII concentrate containing von Willebrand factor is not available; (3) hemophilia A when virally inactivated factor VIII concentrates are not available; (4) use as fibrin glue surgical adhesives; and (5) fibronectin replacement.

ALBUMIN

Albumin is available as 5 and 25% solutions in saline solution. Albumin does not transmit viral diseases. Albumin infusion is controversial and is currently used infrequently.

IMMUNOGLOBULINS

Indications for intravenous immunoglobulins (IVIg) include treatment of primary and secondary immunodeficiency, and treatment of immune or inflammatory disorders such as immune thrombocytopenia and Kawasaki syndrome. Several cases of hepatitis C have been documented from IVIg.

ANTITHROMBIN III

Antithrombin III (ATIII) is a serum protein that inhibits coagulation factors, thrombin, and activated factors IX, X, XI, and XII. Deficiency can be congenital or acquired. ATIII is mainly used for prophylaxis of thrombosis or to treat thromboembolism in patients with hereditary ATIII deficiency.

SPECIFIC FACTOR REPLACEMENT THERAPY

Table 133-1 outlines therapy for congenital coagulation factor deficiencies.

TABLE 133-1 Replacement Therapy for Congenital Factor Deficiencies

Coagulation factor	Incidence*	Replacement therapy
Factor I (fibrinogen)	150 cases	Cryoprecipitate
Factor II (prothrombin)	>30 cases	FFP for minor bleeding episodes Prothrombin complex concentrate† for major bleeding
Factor V	150 cases	FFP
Factor VII	150 cases	FFP for minor bleeding episodes Prothrombin complex concentrates for major bleeding Recombinant factor VII$_a$ (experimental)
Factor VIII‡	1 in 10,000 males	Factor VIII concentrates (cryoprecipitate or FFP if not available) DDAVP for those with mild hemophilia
von Willebrand disease	up to 1 in 100 persons	DDAVP (or some factor VIII concentrates or cryoprecipitate)
Factor IX‡	1 in 30,000 males	Factor IX concentrates
Factor X	1 in 500,000	FFP for minor bleeding episodes Prothrombin complex concentrates for major bleeding
Factor XI§	3 in 10,000 Ashkenazi Jews 1 in 1,000,000 in general	FFP
Factor XII	Several hundred cases	Replacement not required
Factor XIII	>100 cases	FFP or cryoprecipitate

Abbreviations: DDAVP, desmopressin; FFP, fresh-frozen plasma.
*Incidence as of 1998.
†See Chap. 212 in *Emergency Medicine: A Comprehensive Study Guide,* 5th ed., for details concerning prothrombin complex concentrates.
‡See Chap. 212 in *Emergency Medicine: A Comprehensive Study Guide,* 5th ed., for detailed management recommendations for patients with hemophilia A and hemophilia B.
§Factor XI levels correlate poorly with bleeding complications; many patients have low levels, but no bleeding complications.

COMPLICATIONS OF TRANSFUSIONS

Adverse reactions occur in up to 20 percent of transfusions and are usually mild. Transfusion reactions can be immediate or delayed. Table 133-2 summarizes the types of immediate reaction as well as recognition, management, and evaluation.

DELAYED TRANSFUSION REACTIONS

1. Infection may result from transfusion. There is a small risk of transmission of HIV, hepatitis B and C, cytomegalovirus, parvovirus, and human T-cell lymphotropic viruses I and II. Other rare but reported pathogens include Epstein-Barr virus, syphilis, malaria, babesiosis, toxoplasmosis, and trypanosomiasis.
2. Delayed hemolytic reactions can occur 7 to 10 days after transfusion.
3. Hypothermia may occur from rapid transfusions of refrigerated blood.
4. Noncardiogenic pulmonary edema may be caused by incompatible passively transferred leukocyte antibodies and usually occurs within 4 h of transfusion. Clinical findings are respiratory distress, fever, chills, tachycardia, and patchy infiltrates on chest x-ray without cardiomegaly. There is no evidence of fluid overload. The majority of cases resolve with supportive care.
5. Electrolyte imbalance may occur. Citrate is part of the preservative solution and chelates calcium. Significant hypocalcemia even with massive transfusion is rare because patients with normal hepatic function readily metabolize citrate into bicarbonate. Hypokalemia can occur with large transfusions due to the metabolism of citrate to bicarbonate, leading to alkalosis, which drives potassium ions to the intracellular space. Hyperkalemia can occur in patients with renal failure or in neonates.
6. Graft-versus-host disease, fatal in greater than 90 percent of cases, occurs when nonirradiated lymphocytes are inadvertently transfused into an immunocompromised patient.

EMERGENCY TRANSFUSIONS

Use of type O or type-specific incompletely cross-matched blood may be lifesaving but carries the risk of life-threatening transfusion reactions. Limit its use to the early resuscitation of patients with severe hemorrhage without adequate response to crystalloid infusion. Before transfusing, obtain blood for baseline laboratory tests

TABLE 133-2 Acute Transfusion Reactions: Recognition, Management, Evaluation

Reaction type	Sign and Symptoms	Management	Evaluation
Acute intravascular hemolytic reaction	Fever, chills, low back pain, flushing dyspnea, tachycardia, shock, hemoglobinuria	Immediately stop transfusion IV hydration to maintain diuresis; diuretics may be necessary Cardiorespiratory support as indicated Can be life-threatening	Retype and crossmatch Direct and indirect Coombs' tests CBC, creatinine, PT, aPTT Haptoglobin, indirect bilirubin, LDH, plasma free hemoglobin Urine for hemoglobin
Acute extravascular hemolytic reaction	Often have low-grade fever but may be entirely asymptomatic	Stop transfusion Rarely causes clinical instability	Hemolytic workup as above to rule out the possibility of intravascular hemolysis
Febrile nonhemolytic transfusion reaction	Fever, chills	Stop transfusion Manage as in intravascular hemolytic reaction as above because cannot initially distinguish between the two Can treat fever and chills with acetaminophen and meperidine Usually mild but can be life-threatening in patients with tenuous cardiopulmonary status Consider infectious work-up	Hemolytic workup as above because initially cannot distinguish the etiology

| Allergic reaction | If mild, urticaria, pruritus
If severe, dyspnea, bronchospasm, hypotension, tachycardia, shock | Stop transfusion
If mild reaction, can treat with diphenhydramine; if symptoms resolve, can restart transfusion
If severe, may require cardiopulmonary support; do not restart transfusion | For mild symptoms that resolve with diphenhydramine, no further workup is necessary, although blood bank should be notified
For severe reaction, do hemolytic workup as above because initially will be indistinguishable from a hemolytic reaction |
| Hypervolemic | Dyspnea, tachycardia, hypertension, headache, jugular venous distention, pulmonary rales, hypoxia | Stop transfusion or decrease rate to 1 mL/kg/h
Diuresis
Can be difficult to distinguish from a hemolytic reaction; if cannot distinguish, stop transfusion and treat as if intravascular hemolytic reaction | If clearly hypervolemic, no further evaluation is needed; CXR may be helpful
If hemolytic reaction is a possibility, do hemolytic workup as above |

Abbreviations: IV, intravenous; CBC, complete blood count; PT, prothrombin time; aPTT, activated partial thromboplastin time; LDH, lactate dehydrogenase; CXR, chest radiograph.

and type and cross matching. Type-specific blood can be available in 15 min and fully cross-matched blood in 30 to 60 min. Rh-negative blood is preferable when it is not fully cross-matched. Only PRBCs are available for emergency transfusion; plasma products contain too many antigens.

MASSIVE TRANSFUSION

Massive transfusion is the replacement of a patient's blood volume within a 24-h period. Complications include bleeding, citrate toxicity, and hypothermia. Bleeding may result from thrombocytopenia, platelet dysfunction, DIC, or coagulation factor deficiencies. Platelet transfusions are indicated only if there is thrombocytopenia with bleeding, and FFP is indicated only if there are documented coagulopathy and bleeding. Patients receiving more than 5 U of whole blood, those with liver disease, and neonates are at risk of hypocalcemia from citrate toxicity. The QT interval is not a reliable indicator in this setting; an ionized calcium level is necessary. Treat hypocalcemia with 5 to 10 mL of IV calcium gluconate slowly. Beware of hypothermia when administering 3 U or more of blood rapidly.

BLOOD ADMINISTRATION

Always ensure correct identification of the patient and the unit to be transfused. A 16-gauge or greater IV catheter is preferred, to prevent hemolysis and to permit rapid infusion; micropore filters should be used to filter out microaggregates of platelets, fibrin, and leukocytes. Normal saline solution is the only crystalloid compatible with PRBCs. Warmed saline solution (39° to 43°C, or 102.2° to 109.4°F) may be given concurrently or a blood warmer used to prevent hypothermia; the blood itself will hemolyze if warmed to greater than 40°C (104°F). Rapid infusion may be facilitated by the use of pressure infusion devices. Patients at risk of hypervolemia should receive each unit over 3 to 4 h.

For further reading in *Emergency Medicine: A Comprehensive Study Guide,* 5th ed., see Chap. 215, "Blood Transfusions and Component Therapy," by Mary E. Eberst.

134 | Exogenous Anticoagulants and Antiplatelet Agents

Keith L. Mausner

This chapter reviews the major antithrombotic agents, their indications, and complications of therapy.

ANTITHROMBOTIC AGENTS

Oral Anticoagulant

Warfarin inhibits vitamin K–dependent clotting factors. Dosing is guided by the international normalized ratio (INR), derived from the prothrombin time (PT); the desired INR is usually between 2.0 and 2.5. Onset of anticoagulation occurs after 3 to 4 d. Warfarin also affects proteins C and S, and for 24 to 36 h there may be a hypercoagulable effect; this is minimized by a starting dose of 5 mg/d. In situations where immediate anticoagulation is critical, a heparin product should be used until an adequate INR is achieved. Warfarin is contraindicated in pregnancy.

Parenteral Anticoagulants

Unfractionated heparin forms a complex with antithrombin III (ATIII), which inhibits factors IXa and Xa. It is administered subcutaneously (SC) or intravenously (IV). The SC route is adequate only for prophylaxis. Body weight–based IV dosing is recommended, typically 70 to 80 U/kg IV bolus, followed by IV infusion at 15 to 18 U/kg/h. Therapy is monitored by the activated partial thromboplastin time (aPTT); the therapeutic range is 1.5 to 2.5 times the normal value. Low-molecular-weight (LMW) heparin fractions (enoxaparin, dalteparin, and ardeparin) are derived from unfractionated heparin. These agents are effective when administered SC once to twice daily. LMW heparin is used for both prophylaxis and treatment. Enoxaparin is U.S. Food and Drug Administration (FDA) approved for deep venous thrombosis (DVT) prophylaxis, and for treatment of DVT with or without pulmonary embolism (PE), non–Q-wave myocardial infarction (MI), and unstable angina. Dalteparin is FDA approved for DVT prophylaxis and for treatment of non–Q-wave MI and unstable angina. Dalteparin is used in Europe and Canada for DVT and PE treatment as well. For DVT, PE, and unstable angina, enoxaparin 1 mg/kg SC bid or dalteparin 100 IU/kg SC bid may be used. Lower doses of these agents are used for prophylaxis. Danaparoid works similarly to the LMW heparins and is used in DVT prophylaxis (750 U SC bid). The heparins and danaparoid may be used in pregnancy. LMW heparins and danaparoid produce minimal elevation in PT or aPTT; laboratory monitoring is not routinely necessary, except in renal failure, where anti-Xa activity can be measured. Hirudin analogues work by binding to thrombin, and are used in patients with heparin associated thrombocytopenia.

Blockers of Platelet Activation

Aspirin blocks the enzyme cyclooxygenase, which results in inhibition of platelet activation. Dose is 81 to 162 mg/d.

Blockers of Platelet Aggregation

Platelet aggregation involves binding of fibrinogen to the platelet glycoprotein IIb-IIIa receptor. Platelet-membrane-altering agents ticlopidine 250 mg bid and clopidogrel 75 mg/d render the receptor ineffective and block aggregation. These agents are generally used in patients who are intolerant of or have failed aspirin therapy. Glycoprotein IIb-IIIa inhibitors (abciximab, eptifibatide, and tirofiban) have been found beneficial in acute myocardial infarction (AMI), unstable angina, and patients undergoing percutaneous angioplasty.

Fibrinolytic Agents

Fibrinolytics work by activating plasminogen to plasmin, which then dissolves the fibrin in thrombi. Streptokinase (SK) is usually administered 1.0 to 1.5 million U over 60 min. Anistreplase (APSAC) is derived from and has a similar effect to SK but can be administered as a slow bolus (typically 30 mg over 5 min). Tissue plasminogen activator (tPA) in theory produces less systemic fibrinolysis and is more "clot specific." In AMI, a front-loaded regimen is commonly used: 15-mg bolus, then 0.75 mg/kg over 30 min (maximum 50 mg), and then 0.50 mg/kg over 60 min (maximum 35 mg). Reteplase, a derivative of tPA, is administered as a double bolus (10 U bolus, repeated in 30 min). SK and APSAC are more antigenic than are tPA or reteplase and therefore are more likely to produce allergic reactions.

INDICATIONS FOR ANTITHROMBOTIC THERAPY

Acute Myocardial Infarction

Fibrinolytic therapy should be initiated within 30 min or angioplasty within 60 min of arrival at the emergency department.

Criteria for fibrinolytic therapy include (*a*) presentation within 12 h of symptom onset; (*b*) ST-segment elevation in two or more contiguous leads or new-onset left bundle branch block; and (*c*) absence of contraindications (Table 134-1). Angioplasty is preferred over fibrinolysis in cardiogenic shock. Rapid initiation of fibrinolytic therapy is more important than the specific agent used. However, tPA is the agent of choice with a history of the following: (*a*) allergy to SK or APSAC, (*b*) treatment with SK in the previous 6 months or with APSAC in the previous 12 months, (*c*) streptococcal infection in the previous 12 months, or (*d*) hemodynamic instability. Aspirin should be administered immediately. Unfractionated heparin is given to patients who received tPA and continued for at least 72 h.

TABLE 134-1 Contraindications to Fibrinolytic Therapy

ABSOLUTE
Active or recent internal bleeding ($\leq$14 d)
CVA < 2–6 months or hemorrhagic CVA
Intracranial or intraspinal surgery or trauma $\leq$2 months
Intracranial or intraspinal neoplasm, aneurysm, or arteriovenous malformation
Known severe bleeding diathesis
On anticoagulants (warfarin, PT > 15 s, heparin, increased aPTT)
Uncontrolled hypertension (i.e., blood pressure > 185/100 mmHg)
Suspected aortic dissection or pericarditis
Pregnancy
RELATIVE
Active peptic ulcer disease
Cardiopulmonary resuscitation > 10 min
Hemorrhagic opthalmic conditions
Puncture of noncompressible vessel < 10 d
Advanced age > 75 years
Significant trauma or major surgery > 2 weeks and < 2 months
Advanced kidney or liver disease

Abbreviations: CVA, cardiovascular accident; PT, prothrombin time; aPTT, activated partial thromplastic time.
*Concurrent menses is *not* a contraindication
†In ischemic CVA, symptoms > 3 h, severe hemispheric stroke, platelets < 100/mL, and glucose < 50 or > 400 mg/dL are additional contraindications.

Deep Venous Thrombosis or Pulmonary Embolism

Treatment of DVT or PE can be initiated with either unfractionated or LMW heparin. Selected patients may benefit from fibrinolytic therapy followed by heparin.

Ischemic Stroke

Tissue plasminogen activator may benefit some patients if given within 3 h of symptom onset, although there is an increased risk of intracranial hemorrhage.

COMPLICATIONS OF ANTICOAGULATION AND ANTITHROMBOTIC THERAPY

The risk of warfarin-related bleeding is reduced by careful monitoring of the INR. Warfarin anticoagulation may be reversed by vitamin K_1, fresh-frozen plasma (FFP), and coagulation factor concentrates. Warfarin has many potential drug interactions, especially with antibiotics as well as drugs that affect the cytochrome P450 system; the most serious interactions can markedly increase the PT and lead to bleeding complications. Another warfarin complication is skin necrosis, which primarily affects individuals with protein C deficiency.

Heparin-associated bleeding is first treated by stopping the infusion. In severe cases protamine 1 mg IV per 100 U of heparin in previous 4 h reverses the effect of heparin. LMW heparins cause less bleeding than does unfractionated heparin. Reversal of LMW heparins by protamine is compound specific; enoxaparin is only partially reversed. Heparin-induced thrombocytopenia (HIT) is a potentially deadly complication that affects 3 percent of patients on unfractionated heparin and fewer patients on LMW heparins. HIT is antibody mediated, causing platelet activation, thrombocytopenia, and thrombosis; onset is usually 5 to 12 days into treatment. Heparin therapy is stopped as soon as HIT is recognized. Platelet counts usually recover in 4 to 6 days.

Aspirin-related life-threatening gastrointestinal bleeding is uncommon. Severe hemorrhage may respond to transfusion of functional platelets to increase the platelet count by 50,000/mL (6 U of platelets).

Fibrinolytic-therapy-related bleeding can be minimized by avoiding administration to patients with absolute contraindications. External bleeding can be controlled by local pressure. Stop any heparin infusion and reverse with protamine. Monitor airway, breathing, and circulation; resuscitate as needed. Major hemorrhage mandates coagulation factor replacement. Administer 10 U cryoprecipitate, and repeat this dose if the fibrinogen level is less than 100 mg/dL. If bleeding persists, administer 2 U FFP. If bleeding then persists, administer an antifibrinolytic agent (aminocaproic acid or tranexamic acid). If there is continued bleeding, the bleeding time is also checked, and if it is more than 9 min, administer 6 to 12 U platelets. Intracranial hemorrhage requires rapid and simultaneous administration of the abovementioned measures and immediate neurosurgical consultation.

For further reading in *Emergency Medicine: A Comprehensive Study Guide,* 5th ed., see Chap. 216, "Exogenous Anticoagulants and Antiplatelet Agents," by Stephen D. Emond, John R. Cooke, and J. Stephan Stapczynski.

---

135 | Emergency Complications of Malignancy

John Sverha

The emergency physician must be able to recognize and treat a wide range of oncologic emergencies. Emergency complications of malignancy can generally by classified as related to local tumor compression, electrolyte abnormality, endocrine abnormality, circulatory disorder, or infection.

ACUTE SPINAL CORD COMPRESSION

Clinical Features

Symptoms of spinal cord compression include leg weakness or numbness, urinary retention, and difficulty walking. Virtually all patients with spinal cord compression caused by metastases also have back pain. The pain usually has been continuously present for weeks to months and is progressive in its severity. An exception is patients with cord compression due to lymphoma who typically have little pain unless lytic bone lesions are present.

Diagnosis and Differential

The emergency physician must have a high suspicion of metastatic disease in patients with persistent unexplained neck or back pain and a history of cancer. Spinal cord compression is most commonly caused by carcinoma of the breast or lung and multiple myeloma. Patients with back pain and a history of cancer should receive a thorough neurologic exam that includes testing of sensory and motor function, reflexes, rectal tone, and gait. There may be tenderness to percussion over the involved vertebrae. Patients with back pain and new neurologic deficits in whom spinal cord compression is suspected should receive magnetic resonance imaging or myelography for definitive diagnosis.

Emergency Department Care and Disposition

Patients with spinal cord compression due to malignancy should receive immediate administration of **dexamethasone** 10 mg IV or **methylprednisolone** 30 mg/kg IV. Consultation with specialists in oncology, radiation oncology, and neurosurgery should be initiated to determine the need for **radiation therapy** or **surgical decompression**.

UPPER AIRWAY OBSTRUCTION

Clinical Features

Upper airway obstruction due to malignancy is an insidious process that usually occurs over weeks to months. It is often accompanied by a change in the quality of the patient's voice. It is a late complication of a variety of tumors arising in the oropharynx, neck, and superior mediastinum. Acute compromise can occur when an existing stricture is obstructed by new bleeding, secretions, or infection.

Diagnosis and Differential

Other causes of airway obstruction to be considered include foreign bodies and oropharyngeal infections. Soft tissue neck radiographs and fiberoptic laryngoscopy can aid in the diagnosis.

Emergency Department Care and Disposition

Patients with impending airway obstruction due to malignancy require immediate intervention to **create a secure and patent airway**. Ideally, this is performed in the operating room after urgent otolarnygologic consultation. **Heliox** therapy may be an effective temporizing measure in patients who exhibit respiratory distress.

Otherwise, orotracheal intubation or cricothyroidotomy should be performed.

MALIGNANT CARDIAC EFFUSION

Clinical Features

A pericardial effusion can cause chest pain, dizziness, and shortness of breath. The severity of patients' symptoms depends on the size of the effusion and how quickly it accumulates. Common causes of malignant pericardial effusions are breast carcinoma, lung carcinoma, and malignant melanoma.

Diagnosis and Differential

Patients with pericardial effusion may have jugular venous distention and muffled heart tones on physical exam. If patients are also hypotensive, pericardial tamponade may be present. An electrocardiogram (ECG) may show low QRS voltages, and a chest x-ray may show an enlarged cardiac silhouette without evidence of congestive heart failure. Definitive diagnosis is obtained through echocardiography.

Emergency Department Care and Disposition

Patients with signs and symptoms of pericardial tamponade should have immediate percutaneous **pericardiocentesis** performed. The care of patients with malignant pericardial effusions who are not in extremis should be discussed with an oncologist.

SUPERIOR VENA CAVA SYNDROME

Clinical Features

Patients presenting to the emergency department with symptoms of superior vena cava (SVC) syndrome often do not have a previous diagnosis of cancer. Patients with mild obstruction of blood flow through the SVC complain of headache, edema of the face and arms, or a vague feeling of head congestion. As venous pressure rises, so does intracranial pressure, and syncope may occur.

Diagnosis and Differential

Physical exam may reveal neck and upper chest vein distention, edema of the face or arms, facial telangiectasia, and sometimes a palpable supraclavicular mass. Papilledema on fundoscopic exam indicates critically high intracranial pressure. A chest x-ray may show an enlarged mediastinum or an isolated lung nodule. Definitive diagnosis is obtained with contrasted chest CT scan or venography.

Emergency Department Care and Disposition

Prompt administration of **furosemide** 40 mg IV, and **methylprednisolone** 120 mg IV may help reduce venous pressure. Patients should be admitted, and **chemotherapy and radiation therapy** initiated after the specific tumor type is determined.

HYPERCALCEMIA OF MALIGNANCY

Clinical Features

Symptoms of hypercalcemia include nausea, vomiting, anorexia, and lethargy. Altered mental status occurs with rapid elevation in serum calcium level or severe hypercalcemia. The ECG may reveal shortening of the QT interval. Elevated ionized calcium can cause neuromuscular dysfunction. Malignancies known to cause hypercalcemia include multiple myeloma, carcinoma of the breast, squamous cell carcinoma of the lung, lymphoma, and renal cell carcinoma.

Emergency Department Care and Disposition

Patients with malignancy associated hypercalcemia should be treated with 1 to 2 L of IV **normal saline** and **furosemide** 80 mg IV. Assuming patients have normal renal function, this will provide a rapid calcium diuresis. Other therapies have a slower onset and should be discussed with an oncologist before being initiated. They include **phosphate** (oral or IV), **prednisone**, and **mithramycin**.

SYNDROME OF INAPPROPRIATE ADH

Clinical Features

The symptoms of the syndrome of inappropriate antidiuretic hormone (SIADH) are those of hyponatremia. Depending on the degree of hyponatremia, patients may develop nausea, vomiting, weakness, confusion, seizures, and coma. Malignancies associated with SIADH include primary and metastatic brain cancer, small cell lung carcinoma, pancreatic adenocarcinoma, and prostate carcinoma.

Diagnosis and Differential

Patients with SIADH will have a low serum sodium, less than maximally dilute urine, excessive urine sodium excretion (> 30 meq/L), and decreased serum osmolarity, all in the setting of euvolemia, absence of diuretic therapy, and normal renal, adrenal, and thyroid function.

Emergency Department Care and Disposition

Patients with mild or moderate hyponatremia can be treated with **water restriction** (0.5 to 1 L/d). Patients with serum sodium levels less than 115 meq/L or central nervous system symptoms should be treated more aggressively. **Furosemide** 40 mg IV can be given with 1 L of normal saline IV fluid to promote a free water diuresis. **Normal saline** or **hypertonic saline infusion** (3%) may be started at 1 to 2 mL/kg/h and then adjusted based on urinary output and urinary sodium. Correction of the serum sodium level should be done at a rate of 1 meq/L/h or less to avoid central pontine myelinolysis.

HYPERVISCOSITY SYNDROME

Clinical Features

Marked elevations in serum proteins can cause an increase in serum viscosity. This can produce sludging of blood flow and a reduction of microcirculatory perfusion. The most common cause of hyperviscosity syndrome is macroglobulinemia due to multiple myeloma. Early symptoms include fatigue, headache, and somnolence. As viscosity increases, microthromboses occur and patients may develop visual disturbances, deafness, seizures, or coma.

Diagnosis and Differential

Emergency physicians must suspect this syndrome in patients with unexplained stupor or coma. The most specific physical exam findings are in the ocular fundi and include "sausage-linked" retinal vessels, hemorrhages, and exudates. A clue may be provided if the laboratory is unable to run chemistry tests due to "too thick" blood. Patients often are anemic with rouleau formation noted on peripheral blood smear. Measurement of serum viscosity and protein electrophoresis are diagnostic.

Emergency Department Care and Disposition

Initial therapy is IV **normal saline** (1 to 2 L) and **emergency plasmapheresis.** When coma is present and the diagnosis has been rapidly established, **phlebotomy** (2 U) with saline infusion and replacement of patients' red blood cells may be used as a temporizing measure until plasmapheresis can be performed.

ADRENAL INSUFFICIENCY AND SHOCK

Clinical Features

Adrenal insufficiency (also see Chap. 128) in oncology patients may be caused by adrenal gland replacement by metastatic tumor or by adrenal suppression by therapeutic glucocorticoid administration. Adrenal insufficiency typically becomes apparent when patients are stressed by infection, dehydration, surgery, or trauma. Patients typically develop hypotension that is resistant to intravenous fluid administration.

Diagnosis and Differential

Other more common causes of hypotension in oncology patients, such as sepsis, dehydration, and blood loss, must be considered. Laboratory clues as to the possible presence of adrenal insufficiency include hyponatremia, hyperkalemia, mild hypoglycemia, and eosinophilia. A definitive diagnosis is made if patients have an abnormally low serum cortisol or, ideally, an abnormal cosyntropin stimulation test.

Emergency Department Care and Disposition

Patients with suspected acute adrenal insufficiency should be treated empirically with **hydrocortisone** (100 to 300 mg IV). A serum cortisol level may be drawn prior to treatment, but treatment should not be delayed in waiting for the results.

POLYCYTHEMIA AND LEUKOCYTOSIS

Clinical Features

Occasionally, the emergency physician may encounter a dramatically elevated hematocrit or white blood cell count (WBC) that produces symptomatic hyperviscosity. An elevated hematocrit (polycythemia) can be due to primary overproduction of red blood cells by the bone marrow (polycythemia vera) or as a paraneoplastic syndrome associated with renal cell carcinoma and hepatomas, among others. At levels > 60 percent, patients can develop symptoms such as headache, fatigue, blurred vision, and thrombotic complications such as stroke or mesenteric ischemia. Both acute and chronic leukemias can produce WBCs, $>100,000/\mu L$. Leukocytosis to this degree can impair circulation and cause symptoms such as headache, confusion, and dyspnea.

Emergency Department Care and Disposition

The treatment of choice in patients with symptomatic polycythemia is **phlebotomy** (approximately 500 mL). Treatment of symptomatic leukocytosis is by **emergent leukapheresis** and **chemotherapy**.

GRANULOCYTOPENIA, IMMUNOSUPPRESSION, AND INFECTION

Clinical Features

Oncology patients are at increased risk of infection for many reasons including impaired host defense mechanisms and the myelosuppression and immunosuppression caused by chemotherapy. Infections in these patients can be severe, rapidly progressive, and life-threatening. Both the frequency of infection and the mortality rate increase when the granulocyte count is $< 1,500/\mu L$.

Diagnosis and Differential

Patients are at risk of infection from typical microorganisms as well as viruses and fungi. Sometimes, the source of the fever is the malignant process itself. Febrile oncology patients should have a complete evaluation including complete blood cell count with differential, chest x-ray, and cultures of blood, urine, and sputum. Any focal complaint should prompt a thorough evaluation and cultures appropriate to the site.

Emergency Department Care and Disposition

Patients with an absolute neutrophil count $< 500/\mu L$ and a fever $> 38°C$ (100.4°F) constitute a true medical emergency. These patients should be treated empirically with antibiotics after cultures are obtained. Currently, monotherapy with a third-generation cephalosporin such as **ceftazidime** (1 to 2 g IV) or **cefepime** (1 to 2 g IV) is considered adequate coverage. **Vancomycin** (1 g IV) may be added on the basis of clinical suspicion or local institutional bacterial sensitivities.

BONE MARROW TRANSPLANTS

Emergency physicians can expect to care for increasing numbers of bone marrow transplant(BMT) patients due to the rising prevalence and survivability of this procedure. BMT patients are at increased risk of infection long after their transplant occurs. Even with a normal neutrophil count, BMT patients have a residual cellular and humoral immunodeficiency that persists for 12 to 24 months following transplantation. Any fever in BMT patients should be taken seriously, and a treatment plan should be developed in conjunction with patients' hematologists. A complication unique to BMT patients is graft-versus-host disease. This is caused by immunogically competent donor cells attacking target antigens in the recipient. Patients develop a rash, diarrhea, and an elevated serum bilirubin. Treatment is with **immunosuppressants**. Another unusual complication of BMT is hepatic venoocclusive disease. This typically occurs within 30 days of transplantation and causes jaundice, tender hepatomegaly, and ascites.

For further reading in *Emergency Medicine: A Comprehensive Study Guide,* 5th ed., see Chap. 217, "Emergency Complications of Malignancy," by John J. Sverha and Marc Borenstein.

136 | Headache and Facial Pain

Kent N. Hall

HEADACHE

Headache is a ubiquitous complaint, accounting for up to 4 percent of all emergency department (ED) visits. Headaches are generally classified according to whether they are primary headache syndromes or secondary to other phenomena (Table 136-1).

Evaluation beyond the history and physical examination of the patient with headache in the ED is warranted if there is an atypical history, a substantial change from prior headache patterns, or other high-risk features (Table 136-2). Patients thought to have malignant secondary causes of headache should undergo complete evaluation and have treatment begun in the ED. Patients thought to have benign or reversible secondary causes of headache should have diagnostic tests if suggested and have treatment initiated and appropriate follow-up arranged prior to ED discharge. Patients with benign primary headache syndromes may have a workup initiated in the outpatient setting, with appropriate therapy started in the ED.

Clinical Features

The clinical features of headache depend on the cause. Migraine headaches can occur with or without aura, the latter being more common. Table 136-3 lists the criteria to be met for an individual headache to be classified as a migraine. Because migraine headaches are recurrent phenomena, the patient must have at least two attacks before the diagnosis of migraine with aura is made, and five before the diagnosis of migraine without aura is made. Less common forms of migraine include ophthalmoplegic, childhood periodic syndromes (recurrent abdominal pain or nausea with or without headache), and migrainous infarction.

TABLE 136-1 Primary and Secondary Causes of Headache

Primary headache syndromes	Secondary headache syndromes (continued)
Migraine	Other CNS
Tension type	Tumor (benign or malignant)
Cluster	Pseudotumor cerebri
Secondary headache syndromes	Ophthalmic
Vascular	Glaucoma
Subarachnoid hemorrhage	Iritis
Intraparenchymal hemorrhage	Optic neuritis
Subdural or epidural hematoma	Drug-related and toxic or metabolic
Ischemic (stroke, transient ischemic attack)	Nitrates and nitrites
Cavernous sinus thrombosis	Chronic analgesic use and abuse
Arteriovenous malformation	Hypoxia or high altitude
Temporal arteritis	Hypercapnea
Carotid or vertebral artery dissection	Hypoglycemia
CNS infection	Monosodium glutamate
Meningitis (bacterial, viral, other)	Carbon monoxide poisoning
Encephalitis	Alcohol withdrawal
Cerebral abscess	Miscellaneous
Non-CNS infection	Malignant hypertension
Focal or systemic	Preeclampsia
Sinusitis	Fever
Herpes zoster of face or scalp	Post–lumbar puncture
	Dental (referred)

Cluster headache is relatively uncommon, predominantly affects men, and has its onset in the late twenties. There is no associated aura. Peak pain occurs 10 to 15 min after onset and lasts 45 to 60 min. Pain is unilateral (often felt behind the eye and in the temple), excruciating, penetrating, and nonthrobbing. Associated findings include ipsilateral lacrimation, conjunctival injection, nasal stuffiness or rhinorrhea, and facial swelling. Ptosis and miosis may occur.

Tension-type headache is the most common type of headache. To be diagnosed as a tension-type headache, the headache should have most of the following qualities: (*a*) bilateral location, (*b*) mild or moderate intensity, (*c*) no associated nausea or vomiting, and (*d*) no aggravation by mild physical activity. Associated symptoms may include anorexia, photophobia, and phonophobia. Pain usually progresses throughout the day.

Postlumbar puncture headache occurs in 10 to 36 percent of patients receiving a lumbar puncture. It occurs within hours of

TABLE 136-2 High-Risk Features of Headache Pain

History	
Headache pattern	First, severe headache; worst headache ever; headache that began days earlier and progressively worsened; significant change from prior headaches
Onset	Sudden-onset headache, especially during exercise
Associated symptoms	Syncope, altered level of consciousness, confusion, neck pain or stiffness, persistent visual disturbance, fever, seizures
Other history	Medications (MAOIs, nitrates, anticoagulants), remote history of trauma, toxic exposures (CO_2), coagulopathy, HTN
Family history	SAH
Physical examination	
Vital signs	Fever, marked HTN
General examination	Sinuses, temporal artery, TMJ, eyes with fundoscopy
Neurologic examination	Mental status, cranial nerves, motor and sensory examination, reflexes, gait, cerebellar function

TABLE 136-3 Diagnosis of Migraine Headache

For a headache to be classified as a migraine headache, the following must be present:
Duration of 4-72 h (without treatment)

And at least two of the following:
1. Unilateral position
2. Pulsating quality
3. Moderate or severe intensity (inhibits or prohibits daily activities)
4. Aggravation by walking stairs or similar routine physical activity

And at least one of the following:
1. Nausea, vomiting, or both
2. Photophobia and phonophobia

In addition, to be classified as a migraine with aura, the following must be satisfied:
1. One or more fully reversible aura symptoms indicating brain dysfunction
2. At least one aura symptom developing gradually over more than 4 min or two or more symptoms occuring in succession
3. No single aura symptoms lasting more than 60 min
4. Headache following aura with a free interval of less than 60 min

the procedure, lasts 1 to 2 days, and is bicranial, pulsatile, and exacerbated by the upright position. Usually the pain is cervical and suboccipital in location.

Clinical features of secondary headache syndromes appear in Table 136-4.

Diagnosis and Differential

The most important tool in making the diagnosis in the patient with headache is the history. The differential diagnosis of the patient with headache is shown in Table 136-4, along with associated historical and physical findings. A thorough physical examination, especially the neurologic examination, can rule out significant underlying pathologic conditions in the majority of patients with headache. Areas to concentrate on include the fundoscopic examination; palpation of the temporal region, sinuses, teeth, and distribution of the fifth cranial nerve; stiffness of the neck; and unilateral "drift" in an outstretched, supinated arm.

Available modalities for further evaluation of the headache patient in the ED include computed tomography (CT) scanning, lumbar puncture, and magnetic resonance imaging (MRI). For a patient with a worrisome history or physical examination, a CT scan of the head without contrast is usually the next step. Contrast increases the cost and potential morbidity without significantly increasing the yield of the CT scan and so is not routinely recommended. Lumbar puncture is required for suspected cases of meningitis and clinical suspicion of subarachnoid hemorrhage (SAH) with a negative CT scan. MRI is limited in the ED by its restricted availability and expense. Its primary utility is in diagnosing diffuse axonal injury. It is no better than CT scanning for diagnosing SAH.

Emergency Department Care and Disposition

1. Care of the patient with migraine headache consists of general comfort measures, abortive medications, and prophylactic therapy. General comfort measures include placing the patient in a darkened, quiet room and providing a cool, damp cloth for the forehead. Abortive medications used in the treatment of the patient with migraine headache include **dihydroergotamine mesylate (DHE), sumatriptan, and phenothiazine derivatives**. Doses and considerations in the use of these agents are shown in **Table 136-5**.

2. For cluster headaches, inhaled **oxygen** at 5 to 8 L/min for 10 min may be effective in up to 70 percent of patients. Four percent **intranasal lidocaine** in the ipsilateral nostril can also be used.

TABLE 136-4 Differential Diagnosis of the Patient with Headache

Type of headache	History/physical findings
Migraine headache	Young at onset; lasts longer than 60 min; unilateral, pulsating, throbbing; with or without visual aura; nausea and vomiting; precipitated by foods, drugs, alcohol, exercise or orgasm; positive family history
Cluster headache	Onset in twenties; predominantly male; brief episodes of pain (45–60 min); orbital/retroorbital pain; periodic and seasonal (spring/autumn); nasal congestion and conjunctival injection/tearing associated; negative family history
Tension-type headache	Onset at any age; dull, nagging, persistent pain; progressively worse throughout day
Subarachnoid headache	Sudden onset, "worst headache ever"; loss of consciousness; meningismus; vomiting; occipitonuchal location
Hypertensive headache	Throbbing, occipital
Meningitis	Entire head; fever; meningismus
Mass lesions	
Subdural hematoma	Depressed mental status; variable-quality headache
Epidural hematoma	History of trauma, consciousness with headache followed by unconsciousness; fracture across groove of middle meningeal artery
Brain tumor	Pain on awakening or with Valsalva maneuver; new headache associated with nausea and/or vomiting
Brain abscess	Findings similar to those of mass lesions; fever
Sinusitis	Stabbing or aching pain, worse by bending or coughing, decreased in supine position
Toxic/metabolic headache	Bicranial; headache remits after removal from offending agent/environment
Postconcussion headache	History of trauma within hours to days; vertigo, nausea, vomiting, mood alterations, concentration difficulty associated
Pseudotumor cerebri	Obese, young female; irregular menstrual cycles/amenorrhea; papilledema
Acute glaucoma	Nausea, vomiting, orbital pain; edematous/cloudy cornea; mid-position pupil; conjunctival injection; increased intraocular pressure

TABLE 136-5 Agents Used in the ED Management of
Migraine Headache

Agent	Route	Considerations
Ergotamine	Inhalation, rectal	Contraindicated in coronary artery disease, hypertension, pregnancy
Chlorpromazine	0.1 mg/kg IV	May cause extrapyramidal effects, excellent antiemetic
Prochlorperazine	10 mg IV	May cause extrapyramidal effects, excellent antiemetic
Metoclopramide	10–20 mg IV	May cause extrapyramidal effects, excellent antiemetic
DHE	0.75–1.0 mg IV over 2 min	Contraindicated in coronary artery disease, hypertension, pregnancy
Sumatriptan	6 mg SC	Contraindicated in coronary artery disease, hypertension, pregnancy
Ketorolac	60 mg IM	Moderately effective only

3. Tension headaches usually require only mild analgesics, such as acetaminophen, aspirin, and other **nonsteroidal anti-inflammatory drugs (NSAIDs)**. However, severe tension-type headaches may be treated with the medications listed in Table 136-5 with excellent results.
4. The best treatment of post–lumbar puncture headache is preventive. Patients should avoid lifting for 3 days. Medications that have been successful include simple analgesics, narcotic analgesics, ergots, barbiturates, and caffeine. If these fail, an **epidural blood patch** can be placed.

Discharge instructions should include avoidance of machinery use and driving for patients who have received mentation-altering medications. Referral to a primary care physician is important, since headache is often a chronic problem requiring ongoing care that is not best delivered in an ED. Discharge with analgesics that combine different mechanisms of action, thus leading to a lower dose of both analgesics, is recommended. These combination analgesics include acetaminophen or aspirin plus butalbital with or without caffeine. This combination is also available with or without codeine. Ergotamine is available sublingually and may be used if not contraindicated.

Admission for management of pain associated with headache is rare. Reasonable indications for admission include

1. migraine lasting for days associated with vomiting and dehydration
2. headache complicated by overuse of abortive medications
3. chronic headache unresponsive to outpatient therapy
4. headache secondary to suspected intracranial pathology (SAH, tumor, meningitis, etc.)
5. Underlying significant medical or surgical pathology
6. Intractable cluster headache
7. Headache that significantly interferes with activities of daily living

FACIAL PAIN

Temporal Arteritis

Temporal arteritis is a vasculitis affecting branches of the external carotid artery. Women are affected four times more frequently than men. It usually occurs in individuals over 50 years of age and is often associated with polymyalgia rheumatica. The pain is usually unilateral. The artery is tender on palpation. Systemic signs and symptoms may be present and include fever, malaise, weight loss, anorexia, diplopia, blurred vision, and polymyalgia. The differential diagnosis includes other causes of headache mentioned above. This condition is distinguished by the tenderness over the involved artery, and elevated erythrocyte sedimentation rate (usually above 50 mm/h), and the frequently associated systemic signs and symptoms. Biopsy of the artery is diagnostic. Emergency treatment includes **prednisone** 40 to 60 mg/d to prevent blindness secondary to ischemic papillitis. NSAIDs are beneficial in relieving the associated pain. Close follow-up is required and should be arranged prior to discharge from the ED. Prednisone can be vision saving, even if the patient has already lost vision in the ipsilateral eye, since vision in the contralateral eye is at risk without this therapy.

Temporomandibular Disorder

Patients with temporomandibular disorder present with unilateral or bilateral pain in the temporomandibular joint or joints. The area may be tender to palpation, and clicking or sticking of the joint with limitation of opening of the mouth may be seen. Other symptoms may include bruxism and tongue, lip, or cheek biting. Deviation of the mandible to the affected side may be present, as may a sense of fullness, popping, and tinnitus in the ear. Differential diagnosis includes temporal arteritis, trigeminal neuralgia, cluster headache, and pain of dental origin. The history and physical examination should effectively exclude these diagnoses. Treatment with NSAIDs, with appropriate referral to a dentist or oral surgeon at the time of discharge from the ED, is usually all that is required. Definitive treatment consists of an occlusal splint or bite guard.

Trigeminal Neuralgia

Trigeminal neuralgia, or tic douloureux, is characterized by brief, intermittent pains that often have an "electric-like" quality. There is no pain between paroxysms. Inciting maneuvers include eating, talking, washing the face, or applying cosmetics. Conditions included in the differential diagnosis are postherpetic neuralgia, dental and maxillary sinus problems, cluster headaches, and atypical facial pain. Findings upon physical examination, including neurologic examination, are normal. ED treatment consists of starting or restarting carbamazepine or other chronic medications (e.g., phenytoin and baclofen). Discharge instructions should include close follow-up with the primary care physician or referral to a neurologist for intractable symptoms despite appropriate medical therapy.

For further reading in *Emergency Medicine: A Comprehensive Study Guide,* 5th ed., see Chap. 219, "Headache and Facial Pain," by Michael Schull.

---

137 | Stroke Syndromes
Kent N. Hall

Stroke is the third leading cause of death and is a major cause of disability in the United States. It affects 700,000 Americans annually and costs $30 billion a year in medical costs and lost wages.

Clinical Features

Stroke is the result of any process that causes disruption of blood flow to a particular part of the brain. There are two main mechanisms of stroke: (*a*) blood vessel occlusion leading to neuronal ischemia and death (80 to 85 percent of all strokes) and (*b*) blood vessel rupture leading to hemorrhage, direct cell trauma, mass effect, elevated intracranial pressure, and release of biochemical toxins (15 to 20 percent of all strokes).

Ischemic strokes are most often caused by large-vessel thrombosis, although embolism or systemic hypoperfusion may also cause them. Causes of thrombosis include atherosclerotic disease, vasculitis, dissection, polycythemia, hypercoagulable states, and infectious diseases (e.g., HIV, syphilis, tuberculosis, and trichinosis). Signs and symptoms of thrombotic stroke usually develop over minutes to hours, often with waxing and waning characteristics. Similar, short-lived episodes, transient ischemic attacks (TIAs), often precede thrombotic strokes. Embolic strokes account for 20 percent of all strokes in the United States. Common sources of emboli in embolic strokes are the heart (valvular vegetations, mural thrombi, paradoxical emboli, and cardiac tumor) and major vessels.

Hemorrhagic strokes have a 30-day mortality rate of 30 to 50 percent, occur in a younger patient population than ischemic strokes, and are divided into intracerebral (ICH) and subarachnoid hemorrhages (SAH). Risk factors for an ICH include hypertension, older age, race (higher incidence in blacks and Asians), tobacco and alcohol abuse, and prior stroke. Bleeding diathesis, vascular malformations, and cocaine use can cause ICH. Most SAHs are due to berry aneurysm rupture and arteriovenous malformations.

Diagnosis and Differential

In obtaining a history, it is important to ask whether there is any history of TIA-like symptoms. Aspects of the stroke itself, including timing of onset, presence of headache, nausea, vomiting, and recent neck trauma are important. Young patients are more likely to have stroke from arterial dissection, cardioembolic events, migraines, air embolism, and substance abuse. Pregnant patients, especially in the peripartum and postpartum periods, are also at increased risk for stroke.

The general physical examination should include a complete evaluation of the skin, fundi, heart, and lungs, as well as listening for carotid and other vascular bruits.

The neurologic examination is done to assess the patient's baseline level of function and to localize the brain lesion. The seven areas of the neurologic examination are (*a*) level of consciousness, (*b*) visual assessment, (*c*) motor function, (*d*) sensation and neglect,

TABLE 137-1 Neurologic Examination

Level of consciousness	Level of alertness, ability to answer simple questions, ability to follow simple commands
Visual assessment	Visual fields and extraocular movements
Motor function	Pronator drift, leg strength
Sensation and neglect	Pinprick testing, graphesthesia, double-simultaneous extinction test
Cerebellar function	Gait, finger-to-nose testing, heel-to-shin testing
Language	Dysarthria (slurred speech); aphasia (difficulty in processing language), either receptive or expressive
Cranial nerves	Individual testing of all twelve cranial nerves important, noting whether ipsilateral or contralateral to motor weakness

TABLE 137-2 Stroke Syndromes

Ischemic stroke syndromes
  Transient ischemic attack: resolves within 24 h (most within 30 min), 5–6% risk of stroke per year
  Dominant hemispheric infarct: contralateral weakness or numbness, contralateral visual field cut, gaze preference, dysarthria, aphasia
  Nondominant hemispheric infarct: contralateral weakness or numbness, visual field cut, constructional apraxia, dysarthria
  Anterior cerebral artery infarct: contralateral weakness or numbness (leg more than arm), dyspraxia, speech perseveration, slow responses
  Middle cerebral artery infarct: most common area involved, contralateral weakness or numbness (arm or face more than leg)
  Posterior cerebral artery infarct: often go unrecognized by patient, minimal motor involvement, light-touch and pinprick sensation significantly affected
  Vertebrobasilar syndrome: dizziness, vertigo, diplopia, dysphagia, ataxia, cranial nerve palsies, bilateral limb weakness, crossed neurologic deficits
  Basilar artery occlusion: quadriplegia, coma, locked-in syndrome
  Cerebellar infarct: "drop attack" associated with vertigo, headache, nausea, vomiting, and/or neck pain, cranial nerve abnormalities
  Lacunar infarct: pure motor or sensory deficits
  Arterial dissection: often associated with severe trauma, headache and neck pain hours to days prior to onset of neurologic symptoms

Hemorrhagic stroke syndromes
  Intracerebral hemorrhage: similar to cerebral infarction with lethargy, headache, nausea, vomiting, significant hypertension
  Cerebellar hemorrhage: dizziness, vomiting, truncal ataxia, inability to walk, rapidly progress to coma, herniation and death
  Subarachnoid hemorrhage: severe headache, vomiting, decreased level of consciousness

(*e*) cerebellar function, (*f*) language, and (*g*) cranial nerves (Table 137-1). These areas are incorporated in the National Institutes of Health stroke scale, which is used to monitor the patient's progress over time.

Integration of information from the history and physical examination allows the physician to determine the area of brain involvement. Specific stroke syndromes are listed in Table 137-2. Table 137-3 lists the differential diagnosis of patients with stroke syndromes.

Emergency Department Care and Disposition

1. Patients should receive supplemental **oxygen**, be placed on a cardiac monitor, and have intravenous access established. Diagnostic tests that should be immediately obtained include a blood glucose determination, noncontrast head computed tomography scan, and electrocardiogram. Other tests that may be helpful include laboratory tests (a complete blood count, coagulation studies, toxic screening, and cardiac enzyme determinations), echocardiogram, magnetic resonance imaging (MRI) or magnetic resonance angiography, and carotid duplex scanning.

TABLE 137-3 Differential Diagnosis of Acute Stroke

Hypoglycemia

Postictal paralysis (Todd's paralysis)

Bell's palsy

Hypertensive encephalopathy

Epidural or subdural hematoma

Brain tumor or abscess

Complicated migraine

Encephalitis

Diabetic ketoacidosis

Hyperosmotic coma

Meningoencephalitis

Wernicke's encephalopathy

Multiple sclerosis

Meniere's disease

Drug toxicity (lithium, phenytoin, carbamazepine)

Emergency MRI should be considered if a dural sinus thrombosis or posterior circulation lesion is considered.

2. Patients with stroke syndromes and sickle cell anemia (SSA) should be evaluated as other patients with potential stroke syndromes. However, in addition to the abovementioned laboratory testing, a reticulocyte count and type and crossmatch should be obtained. In patients with SSA and ischemic stroke, immediate **simple or exchange transfusion** should be initiated to reduce the hemoglobin S concentration to below 30%. Use of hyperosmotic contrast solutions should be delayed until the hemoglobin S concentration is below 30%.

3. *Acute ischemic stroke.* The NINDS trial showed that patients who received rt-PA within 3 h of symptom onset had a significantly lower morbidity rate. This study resulted in U.S. Food and Drug Administration approval of rt-PA for this indication in selected individuals (Table 137-4). Total dose of rt-PA is 0.9 mg/kg, with a maximum dose of 90 mg. Ten percent of the dose should be administered as an initial bolus, followed by an infusion of the remainder over 60 min. rt-PA is not indicated if the exact time of onset of symptoms cannot be ascertained. No aspirin or heparin therapy is given within the first 24 h of treatment. Admission to an intensive care unit setting is recommended. Worsening of neurologic symptoms should suggest ICH and warrants intensive investigation and management, including administration of coagulation products and immediate neurosurgical consultation.

4. *Subacute ischemic stroke.* Patients with embolic stroke and minor deficits should be anticoagulated with **heparin**, as should patients with TIAs, if they have known high-grade stenosis, a cardioembolic source, increasing frequency of TIAs (crescendo TIAs), or TIAs despite antiplatelet therapy. Heparin anticoagulation should be withheld for 3 to 4 d in patients with large cardioembolic stroke. Treatment for stable thrombotic stroke is supportive. Anticoagulation is not indicated. However, **aspirin** 300 mg/d is beneficial. Avoid glucose-containing solutions because of increased neuronal damage in hyperglycemia. Only severe hypertension (systolic blood pressure above 220 mmHg or diastolic blood pressure above 120 mmHg) should be treated. Hypotension should be treated with fluid therapy and vasopressors if needed. Early neurosurgical consultation is needed for patients with cerebellar infarction.

5. *Hemorrhagic stroke.* Patients with intracerebral hemorrhage and hypertension should have their blood pressure lowered only if their systolic blood pressure is above 220 mmHg or their diastolic blood pressure is above 120 mmHg. **Labetalol**

TABLE 137-4 Criteria for Use of rt-PA in Acute Ischemic Stroke and Management of Patients Following Use of rt-PA

Inclusion	Exclusion
Age 18 or over	Minor stroke syndromes
Clinical diagnosis of ischemic stroke	Rapidly improving neurologic signs
Well-established time of onset <3 h	Prior intracranial hemorrhage Blood glucose <50 or >400 Seizure at onset of stroke Gastrointestinal or genitourinary bleeding within preceding 21 days Recent myocardial infarction Major surgery within 14 days Pretreatment SBP >185 mmHg or DBP >110 mmHg Previous stroke or head injury within 90 days Current use of oral anticoagulants Use of heparin within preceding 48 h Platelet count 100,000 mL Suspected aortic or vascular dissection or LP

Management

Monitor arterial blood pressure during the first 24 h after starting treatment, every 15 min for 2 h after starting infusion, then every 30 min for 6 h, and then every 60 min for 24 h total.

If SBP is 180–230 mmHg or DBP is 105–120 mmHg for two or more readings 5–10 min apart:
  Give IV labetalol 10 mg over 1–2 min. The dose may be repeated or doubled every 10–20 min up to a total dose of 150 mmHg.
  Monitor blood pressure every 15 min during labetalol treatment and observe for hypotension.

If SBP > 230 mmHg or if DBP is 121–140 mmHg for two or more readings 5–10 min apart:
  Give IV labetalol 10 mg over 1–2 min. The dose may be repeated or doubled every 10–20 min up to a total dose of 150 mmHg.
  Monitor blood pressure every 15 min during labetalol treatment and observe for hypotension.
  If no satisfactory response, infuse sodium nitroprusside 0.5–1.0 μg/kg/min; continuous arterial pressure monitor is advised.

If DBP > 140 mmHg for two or more readings 5–10 min apart:
  Infuse sodium nitroprusside 0.5–1.0 μg/kg/min; continuous arterial pressure monitor is advised.

Abbreviations: DBP, diastolic blood pressure; IV, intravenous; SBP, systolic blood pressure.

or **nitroprusside** is the agent of choice. Therapy to lower blood pressure should extend over 12 to 24 h. The desired endpoint is the prehemorrhage level of blood pressure, if it is known. Mannitol and furosemide are recommended if increased intracranial pressure is suspected.

6. To prevent rebleeding, patients with SAH should have their blood pressure maintained at prehemorrhage levels (if known), or the mean arterial pressure should be maintained at 110 mmHg. **Nimodipine** 60 mg every 6 h should be given to prevent vasospasm related to the SAH. **Prophylactic phenytoin** should be given to all patients with SAH, and nausea and vomiting should be treated promptly.

7. Patients with new-onset strokes should be admitted to the hospital, as should patients with new-onset TIAs unless high-grade stenosis of the carotid arteries can be ruled out. Patients with a prior history of anterior circulation stroke who present with a completed (greater than 24 h old) stroke and have reliable support may be discharged home after appropriate consultation and with follow-up within 48 h. Clear instructions to return for worsening symptoms should be emphasized to the patient and family.

For further reading in *Emergency Medicine: A Comprehensive Study Guide,* 5th ed., see Chap. 220, "Stroke, Transient Ischemic Attack, and Other Central Focal Conditions," by Phillip A. Scott and William G. Barsan.

---

138 | Altered Mental Status and Coma

C. Crawford Mechem

Mental status is the clinical state of a person's emotional and intellectual functioning. Causes of altered mental status frequently encountered in emergency department (ED) patients include delirium, dementia, and coma.

DELIRIUM

Delirium is an acute, transient confusional state with associated impairment of attention and cognition. Thinking is disorganized, wake-sleep cycles may be disturbed, and level of consciousness fluctuates. It is important to remember that delirium is secondary to another process that may or may not be related to the central nervous system (CNS) and may be readily treatable (Table 138-1).

TABLE 138-1 Common Medical Causes of Altered Mental Status/Sensorium

Infection*	Meningitis/encephalitis
	Sepsis
	Urinary tract infection
	Pneumonia
Toxic	Drug toxicity (including alcohol)
	Drug withdrawal (example alcohol)
	Environmental exposure (example carbon monoxide)
Metabolic	Electrolyte disturbance (e.g., hyper/hyponatremia, hypercalcemia)
	Endocrine disorders (e.g., hyper/hypo: -glycemia, -adrenal, -thyroid)
	Hepatic encephalopathy
	Uremia
	Environmental exposure (example hypothermia)
Hypoxemia/hypercarbia	(examples: CHF, PE, COPD)
Cerebrovascular	Trauma related (example subdural hematoma)
	CVA (bland, hemorrhagic)
	CNS vasculitis
	Hypertensive encephalopathy
CNS (other)	Trauma (diffuse injury with increased ICP)
	Space occupying lesions
	Seizure and postictal states
Psychiatric†	Functional psychosis
	Severe depression

Abbreviations: CHF, congestive heart failure; PE, pulmonary embolism; COPD, chronic obstructive pulmonary disease; CVA, cerebrovascular accident; CNS, central nervous system; ICP, intracranial pressure.

*Seemingly minor infections (urinary tract, pneumonia) may alter sensorium in the elderly.

†Other etiologies should be considered before a psychiatric etiology becomes the working diagnosis.

Clinical Features

By definition, symptoms of delirium are present for days or weeks, never more than a month, and may be intermittent. Thinking and memory are distorted and alertness reduced. Activity level may be increased, decreased, or variable, with the patient rapidly fluctuating from hyper- to hypoactive states. The wake-sleep cycle is often disrupted, with increased somnolence during the day and agitation at night, referred to as "sundowning." Other signs and symptoms may include tachycardia, hypertension, diaphoresis, emotional outbursts, and delusions. Hallucinations may be present in up to 40 percent of cases, with visual hallucinations predominating.

Diagnosis and Differential

Diagnosis is based on history and physical exam. Family members should be queried on the acuity of onset of symptoms and whether the patient's level of confusion fluctuates. A thorough medication history, including over-the-counter products, must be taken. Physical exam is directed at identifying a precipitant, such as infection, and carefully documenting the patient's presenting mental status. Special attention should be given to level of consciousness, orientation, mood, affect, dress, situational behavior, and speech content and process. Appropriate diagnostic studies may include basic chemistries, urinalysis, blood cultures, chest x-ray, head computed tomography (CT) scan, and cerebrospinal fluid (CSF) analysis, as determined by the individual case.

The differential diagnosis for delirium includes dementia and psychiatric psychoses (Table 138-2). The distinction can often be made based on the time course of onset and assessment of the patient's mental status.

Emergency Department Care and Disposition

Treatment of delirium involves supportive care while efforts are made to identify and treat the underlying cause. It also should be emphasized that identification of one possible etiology does not exclude the presence of another, such as hypoxia, hypoglycemia, or infection.

Useful adjuncts to management include adequate lighting and psychosocial support to help the patient interpret the surroundings correctly. Restraints should be used for patient safety when necessary, in accordance with institutional guidelines. Sedation may be needed to relieve agitation.

TABLE 138-2 Features of Delirium, Dementia, and Psychiatric Psychosis

Characteristic	Delirium	Dementia	Psychiatric psychoses
Onset	Sudden	Insidious	Sudden
Course over 24 h	Fluctuating	Stable	Stable
Consciousness	Reduced or clouded	Alert	Alert
Attention	Disordered	Normal	May be disordered
Cognition	Disordered	Impaired	May be impaired
Orientation	Impaired	Often impaired	May be impaired
Hallucinations	Usually visual	Often absent	Usually auditory
Delusions	Transient, poorly organized	Usually absent	Sustained
Movements	Asterixis, tremor may be present	Often absent, it presents usually unrelated	Absent

Source: Modified from Lipowski Z: Delirium in the elderly patient. N Engl J Med 320:578, 1989.

1. **Haloperidol,** 1 to 5 mg, may be given orally or parenterally and repeated every 20 to 30 min as needed. It should be avoided in patients at risk for developing seizures or hypotension.
2. **Lorazepam,** 1 to 2 mg, may be used in combination with haloperidol. The dose should be guided by the patient's age and degree of agitation.

Delirium is associated with a high mortality rate, especially in the elderly, due to the underlying etiology. Therefore, unless a readily reversible precipitant is identified and the patient's condition rapidly resolves, the majority of patients should be admitted for further diagnostic workup and management.

DEMENTIA

Dementia is a chronic state of reduced cognitive ability with a slow and insidious onset. The etiology for most cases is either idiopathic (Alzheimer's disease) or vascular. A smaller number of cases have a potentially reversible cause, which must be aggressively sought (Table 138-3).

TABLE 138-3 Mnemonic for Potentially Treatable/Reversible
Causes of Dementia

D	Drugs (anticholinergic, narcotic, sedatives, phenothiazines, others)
E	Electrolytes, eye or ear problems (partial blindness or deafness)
M	Metabolic disturbances (thyroid disease, hepatic failure, others)
E	Emotional (depression, schizophrenia)
N	Nutritional (B_{12}, folate deficiency, Wernicke-Korsakoff) Normal pressure hydrocephalus
T	Trauma, Tumor (includes subdural hematoma)
I	Inflammation (SLE, others) Infections (chronic meningitis, syphilis, Lyme, HIV)
A	Alcohol*

Abbreviations: HIV, human immunodeficiency virus; SLE, systemic lupus erythematosus.
*Chronic effects of alcohol are not easily reversible, however, with abstinence and proper nutrition, even severely affected (ex-) alcoholics may show improvement.
Source: Modified from Tueth MJ: Dementia: Diagnosis and emergency behavioral complications. *J Emerg Med* 13:519, 1995.

Diagnosis and Differential

Diagnosis is based on history and physical exam, with judicious use of diagnostic studies in an attempt to identify treatable causes. Memory problems are usually slowly progressive. The patient or caretakers may describe memory loss or problems naming items. As the condition progresses, the patient may lose reading ability, show decreased performance in social situations, and get lost easily. Late in the course, the patient may be profoundly disoriented, have difficulty performing self-care tasks, and exhibit marked personality changes. Abrupt deterioration in the course suggests a vascular etiology. Family history is contributory in that it may be positive for inheritable dementing illnesses such as Huntington's disease.

Findings on physical exam are usually nonspecific or normal. Focal neurologic signs may indicate a vascular etiology or mass lesion. Increased motor tone, rigidity, or movement disorders may suggest Parkinson's disease.

Recommended laboratory studies include complete blood cell count; serum electrolyte, calcium, glucose, blood urea nitrogen (BUN) and creatinine levels; liver function tests, thyroid functions, serum B_{12}, and serology for syphilis. Optional tests include sedimentation rate, serum folate level, HIV testing, chest x-ray, and urinalysis. Head CT or magnetic resonance imaging (MRI) should be considered for all patients. The need for CSF analysis is case-specific.

Emergency Department Care and Disposition

Management is directed at correcting any treatable underlying etiologies, such as subdural hematoma or normal pressure hydrocephalus. However, in the majority of cases, no acute intervention in the ED is required. Caretakers may be counseled on long-term-care issues after consultation with the primary care physician. Hallucinations, delusions, repetitive behaviors, and depression are common in these patients. Associated psychotic and nonpsychotic behavior may be managed with antipsychotics, but adverse effects may limit the efficacy of these agents. Control of hypertension in patients with vascular dementia may slow progression.

The decision to admit or discharge a patient brought to the ED for evaluation of dementia will depend on the patient's social support system and whether an identifiable and treatable etiology can be identified. The existence of coexisting medical conditions, a rapidly progressive course, or an unsafe or uncertain home environment should prompt consideration for admission. If the patient is to be discharged from the ED, environmental and psychosocial interventions may be suggested to help the patient better cope with his or her impaired cognitive function.

COMA

Coma is an eyes-closed state with inappropriate responses to environmental stimuli. Wakefulness, self-awareness, language, reasoning, spatial relationship integration, and emotions are all affected.

Clinical Features

Findings on exam are, in part, dependent on the etiology and may help to distinguish a structural lesion from diffuse CNS dysfunction due to a toxic or metabolic etiology. Diffuse CNS dysfunction is associated with nonlocalizing findings on exam. Movements and reflexes, when present, are symmetric. Pupillary reflexes are intact, and pupils tend to be small and reactive. If extraocular movements are present, they too are symmetric.

Coma due to hemispheric lesions or supratentorial masses may present with progressive hemiparesis and asymmetry of muscle tone and reflexes. Eyes may be conjugately deviated to the side of the lesion. In the case of a large mass lesion with elevated intracranial pressure, lateralizing signs may be absent. In severe cases, the Cushing reflex, a combination of hypertension and bradycardia, may be noted.

Expanding posterior fossa or infratentorial lesions may cause abrupt coma, extensor posturing, loss of pupillary reflexes, and loss of extraocular movements. Early brainstem compression with loss of brainstem reflexes may develop rapidly. Pontine hemorrhage may present with pinpoint pupils. Vertebrobasilar occlusion by thrombosis or embolism may cause coma by affecting the reticular activation system. Cranial nerve deficits and hemi- or paraparesis may be noted. Severe cases may lead to the "locked-in" syndrome or death.

Pseudocoma or psychogenic coma are occasionally encountered. Careful observation of the patient and lack of consistent findings on neurologic exam should provide evidence of nonphysiologic or feigned unresponsiveness.

Diagnosis and Differential

Diagnosis is based on a careful history and physical exam. The main objective is identification of a treatable cause (Table 138-4). The history must be obtained from caregivers, bystanders, EMS personnel, or old medical records. The rate of onset of coma is highly suggestive of an etiology. Abrupt onset may be due to head trauma, catastrophic stroke, seizures, or cardiac pathology. A gradual onset is more consistent with brain tumor, subdural hematoma, or metabolic causes such as hyperglycemia or other hyperosmolar states.

Physical exam of the comatose patient may be difficult and unrewarding. Vital signs and oxygen saturation require close attention. A general exam may reveal signs of trauma. A toxidrome, such as small pupils and hypoventilation from opioid overdose, may also be detected. Because the patient is unable to cooperate with a traditional neurologic exam, the focus should be placed on pupillary exam, corneal reflexes, oculovestibular reflexes, muscle tone, and deep tendon reflexes. Asymmetry suggests a focal lesion. Flexor or extensor posturing are nonspecific findings but indicate profound CNS dysfunction.

Diagnostic studies are similar to those used for evaluating dementia. Bedside serum glucose determination and assessment for hypoxia should be performed early in the evaluation. Head CT readily detects acute hemorrhage, mass lesions, and midline shift.

Emergency Department Care and Disposition

Care involves stabilization of the airway, breathing, and circulatory status while searching for a treatable etiology (Table 138-5). Em-

TABLE 138-4 Differential Diagnosis of Coma

COMA FROM CAUSES AFFECTING THE BRAIN DIFFUSELY
  Encephalopathies
    Hypoxic
    Metabolic
      Hypoglycemia
      Diabetic ketoacidosis
      Hyperosmolar state
      Other electrolyte abnormalities
      Organ system failure
        Hepatic encephalopathy
        Uremia/renal failure
        Endocrine
    Hypertensive encephalopathy
  Toxins and drug reactions
    CNS sedatives
    Alcohols
    Carbon monoxide, other inhalants
    Neuroleptic malignant syndrome
  Environmental causes—hypothermia, hyperthermia
  Deficiency state: Wernicke's encephalopathy

COMA FROM PRIMARY CNS DISEASE OR TRAUMA
  Direct CNS trauma
  Vascular disease
    Intraparenchymal hemorrhage
      Hemispheric
      Basal ganglia
      Brainstem
      Cerebellar
    Infarction
      Hemispheric
      Brainstem
    Subarachnoid hemorrhage
  CNS infections
  Neoplasms
  Seizures
    Nonconvulsive status epilepticus
    Postictal state

Abbreviation: CNS, central nervous system.

phasis should be placed on distinguishing a toxic or metabolic cause from a structural lesion. If physical exam or neuroimaging suggests elevated intracranial pressure, steps should be taken to correct this. The intubated patient may be hyperventilated to a $PaCO_2$ of approximately 30 mmHg to decrease cerebral blood volume and intracranial pressure (ICP). Chemical paralysis and

TABLE 138-5 Management Steps for the Comatose Patient

I. History—utilize all resources

II. Initial assessment
  A. Primary survey
    1. Establish unresponsiveness/protect cervical spine
    2. *A*—manage airway, *B*—assess breathing, *C*—circulation
  B. Resuscitation/lifesaving intervention
    1. Oxygen supplementation
    2. Establish intravenous access/draw initial blood sample
    3. Cardiac monitor
    4. Pulse oximetry monitor
    5. Thiamine: 100 mg IV (adults only)
    6. Glucose: 50 mL of 50% dextrose solution or glucose test
    7. Naloxone: administer 2 mg IV or SQ (or more)
  C. Secondary assessment
    1. Complete vital signs and general physical exam
    2. Neurologic examination
      a. Respiratory pattern
      b. Observation of posture and movements
      c. Verbal and motor response to stimulation
      d. Cranial nerve examination
      e. Reflexes
      f. Assignment to rating system/serial exams
    3. Other monitoring
      a. Arterial blood gas analysis
      b. ECG monitor

III. Laboratory evaluation
  A. Routine labs: electrolytes, CBC, ABG
  B. Additional labs in selected patients
    1. COHgb, toxicologic screen, hepatic, CSF, thyroid, cortisol

IV. Radiologic evaluation tailored to patient. C-spine, CXR, cranial CT

V. Definitive care
  A. Supportive, monitoring
  B. Treatment
    1. Specific treatment if possible in emergency department
    2. Nonspecific treatment in selected cases
      a. Osmotic agents or loop diuretics
      b. Steroids
      c. Hyperventilation, head position
  C. Appropriate consultation

Abbreviations: IV, intravenous; SQ, subcutaneous; ECG, electrocardiogram; CBC, complete blood cell count; ABG, arterial blood gas analysis; COHgb, carboxyhemoglobin; CSF, cerebrospinal fluid; CXR, chest x-ray; CT, computed tomography.

sedation should be employed to minimize ICP elevation due to patient movement or agitation.

1. **Mannitol,** 0.5 to 1 mg/kg, will decrease intravascular volume and brain water, thereby decreasing ICP.
2. Steroids, such as **dexamethasone,** will reduce brain edema over several hours. Choice of agent and dosage may be made in discussion with consultants.

Patients with readily reversible causes of coma, such as insulin-induced hypoglycemia, may be discharged after treatment and a period of observation. Adequate home support and close follow-up are mandatory. All other patients should be admitted for further evaluation and management.

For further reading in *Emergency Medicine: A Comprehensive Study Guide,* 5th ed., see Chap. 221, "Altered Mental Status and Coma," by J. Stephen Huff.

---

139 | Gait Disturbances

C. Crawford Mechem

Ataxia is the failure to produce smooth, intentional movements. Gait disturbances include ataxia as well as other conditions. Ataxia and gait disturbances are symptoms of underlying disease and must be viewed in the context of the overall clinical picture.

Clinical Features

Diagnosis requires a careful history and physical exam. How the symptoms began and their rate of progression determine acuity. Associated headache, nausea, fever, weakness, or paresthesias should be sought and may help guide evaluation. An effort should be made to determine if the ataxia is sensory or motor in origin, and whether the primary process is systemic or within the central nervous system (CNS). Patients should be asked about ethanol use, prescription medications such as anticonvulsants or sedative-hypnotics, or heavy metal exposure. In children, it is important to exclude musculoskeletal pathology, metabolic disorders such as pyruvate decarboxylase deficiency, recent immunizations, or viral illnesses including varicella.

A thorough neurologic exam should be performed, including gait testing. Patients should be observed sitting upright, rising to a standing position, walking, and turning. A *cerebellar* or *motor ataxic* gait is wide-based with unsteady, irregular steps. The gait of sensory ataxia results from loss of proprioception and involves abrupt movement of the legs and slapping impact of the feet. An *apraxic* gait is one in which patients have seemingly lost the ability to initiate the process of walking, although motor function is intact. This is seen in right or nondominant hemisphere lesions, frontal lobe disease, or normal pressure hydrocephalus. An *equine* (high-stepping) gait is characterized by footdrop due to peroneal nerve weakness. A *festinating* gait is narrow-based with small, shuffling steps that become more rapid and is common in Parkinson's disease. A *senile* gait is slow with a short stride and wide base and is commonly seen in the elderly. It also may be seen in neurodegenerative disorders. A *functional* gait is one in which patients are seemingly unable to walk steadily despite normal sensory, motor, and cerebellar function. This is usually a manifestation of conversion disorder.

The cerebellum is tested by having patients perform smooth, voluntary and rapidly alternating movements. Abnormalities include *dysmetria,* characterized by inaccurate fine movements. *Dyssynergia* is the breakdown of movements into parts and is assessed by finger-to-nose testing. *Dysdiadochokinesia* is characterized by clumsy rapid movements and is identified by having patients pat their thighs with their palms, then the back of the hand in rapidly alternating movements. This should be performed on both sides. The heel-to-shin test also assesses cerebellar function. In cerebellar disease, there is an action tremor and the knee is initially overshot. In posterior column disease, there is difficulty locating the knee and the heel weaves from side to side or falls off the shin.

Romberg's test assesses sensation and distinguishes sensory from motor ataxia. Patients stand upright with feet close together, arms outstretched, and eyes open. Inability to maintain a steady posture confirms the presence of ataxia. Patients are then asked to close the eyes. If the ataxia worsens, the test is positive, suggesting a sensory ataxia. If there is little or no change with eye closure (Romberg's test negative), a motor ataxia is suggested with possible localization to the cerebellum.

Sensory exam should include position or vibration testing (posterior columns) and sensation to pinprick. Testing deep tendon reflexes may demonstrate asymmetry or spasticity suggestive of an alternative diagnosis. Abnormal nystagmus suggests that the disorder arises from the CNS, rather than the spinal cord or peripheral nervous system.

Diagnosis and Differential

Diagnosis is usually made on the basis of history and physical exam. Laboratory studies may be appropriate in select cases looking for hyponatremia or anticonvulsant or heavy metal toxicity. If a mass lesion is suspected, a neuroimaging study should be obtained. Children with ataxia may require a more extensive workup, including lumbar puncture if an infectious etiology is suspected.

Emergency Department Care and Disposition

Patients with acute gait failure over hours to days need thorough evaluation in the emergency department, consultation, and possible admission. Patients whose symptoms develop over weeks or months may be referred for outpatient follow-up, assuming the safety of the home environment is assured.

For further reading in *Emergency Medicine: A Comprehensive Study Guide,* 5th ed., see Chap. 222, "Ataxia and Gait Disturbances," by J. Stephen Huff.

---

140 | Vertigo and Dizziness
Gary L. Swart

Dizziness is a common but nonspecific complaint in the emergency department. Patients may use the term *dizziness* to refer to symptoms ranging from weakness or fatigue to dysequilibrium (a sensation of imbalance) to vertigo (a perception of movement where none exists) to presyncope or syncope. The clinician must first clarify the patient's symptoms in order to determine the presence of vertigo and then consider the associated factors such as age, setting, and associated signs and symptoms, as well as comorbidities, in order to properly manage the patient with dizziness.

Clinical Features

Sensations of weakness, fatigue, and dysequilibrium are differentiated from true vertigo by the presence of a perception of movement. So-called room-spinning dizziness, or the sensation one may recall from childhood of spinning around and then attempting to run, describes true vertigo. Presyncope and syncope refer, respectively, to a graying-out or total loss of consciousness. Syncope may or may not be postural and may be associated with emotional upset at best, or focal neurologic deficits, chest pain, palpitations, or sudden-onset headache at worst.

Vertigo is classified by etiology as either peripheral or central, referring to the structures causing vertigo (Table 140-1). Peripheral vertigo involves the balance organs peripheral to the brainstem (eighth cranial nerve and vestibular apparatus). Although the

TABLE 140-1 Classification of Vertigo

	Peripheral	Central
Onset	Sudden	Slow
Severity of vertigo	Intense spinning	Ill-defined, less intense
Pattern	Paroxysmal, intermittent	Constant
Aggravated by position/ movement	Yes	No
Associated nausea/ diaphoresis	Frequent	Infrequent
Nystagmus	Rotatory-vertical, horizontal	Vertical
Fatigue of symptoms/signs	Yes	No
Hearing loss/tinnitus	May occur	Does not occur
Abnormal tympanic membrane	May occur	Does not occur
CNS symptoms/signs	Absent	Usually present

causes of peripheral vertigo are not typically life-threatening, the onset of peripheral vertigo is abrupt and intense. It is typically exacerbated by movement, particularly of the head, and frequently associated with a sense of being thrown through space. Waves of nausea and vomiting also occur. Tinnitus and hearing loss are associated with some peripheral causes of vertigo.

Conversely, the causes of central vertigo (involving the brainstem and cerebellum) are more serious. The onset of symptoms, however, is more gradual with a poorly defined sense of vertigo and no positional exacerbation. Other neurologic findings are commonly associated with central vertigo, but hearing loss and tinnitus are rare.

Diagnosis and Differential

Most patients with vertigo have a peripheral etiology. The most common of these is benign paroxysmal peripheral vertigo (BPPV). BPPV may occur at any age, but is most common in patients greater than 50 years of age and is more common in women. The commonly accepted etiology is canalolithiasis in which freefloating particulate aggregates in the posterior semicircular canal result in aberrant stimulation. Episodes of BPPV are associated with position change (with a latency of 1 to 5 s between movement and symptoms), subside in less than 1 min, and fatigue over the course of the day. The episodic vertigo in BPPV typically resolves spontaneously after days to weeks. Tinnitus and hearing loss do not occur. A benign paroxysmal vertigo in children less than 3 years old also may occur, but has been related to migraine syndrome.

Meniere's disease may be caused by excess endolymph and, like BPPV, is associated with episodic vertigo. Unlike BPPV, however, episodes typically last hours and may be days apart. Roaring tinnitus and a sense of fullness and diminished hearing in the affected ear are typical.

Perilymph fistula causes vertigo when an opening in the round or oval window allows pneumatic changes to be transmitted to the vestibule. Trauma, including barotrauma, and infection may cause a perilymph fistula, and symptoms are typically associated with situations resulting in pneumatic fluctuation such as flying, diving, or sneezing.

Vestibular neuronitis is characterized by the sudden onset of severe vertigo that is often incapacitating. Hearing loss and tinnitus may occur. Episodes may last for days, after which the patient recovers rapidly. A viral etiology is suspected, and patients may have concurrent symptoms of upper respiratory infection. Labyrinthitis of infectious etiology also causes vertigo with hearing loss. Although commonly viral, bacterial labyrinthitis may occur with otitis media, meningitis, and mastoiditis.

Tumors of the eighth cranial nerve and cerebellopontine angle such as meningioma, acoustic neuroma, and acoustic schwannoma also may present as vertigo with hearing loss. These tumors may be associated with ipsilateral facial weakness and impaired corneal reflexes and cerebellar signs.

Vertigo may occur following closed head injury due to direct labyrinthine trauma or dislodgment of canaliths leading to BPPV. In the former, the onset is typically immediate and may be constant and associated with nausea and vomiting. The vertigo tends to resolve over weeks. Posttraumatic vertigo may be associated with basilar skull fracture.

Ototoxicity from a multitude of drugs and chemicals may induce vertigo and hearing loss. Common offenders causing peripheral toxicity include aminoglycosides, cytotoxic agents, quinidine, and quinine-related antimalarial agents. Anticonvulsants, antidepressants, neuroleptics, hydrocarbons, alcohol, and phencyclidine may cause centrally mediated vertigo.

Cerebellar hemorrhage or infarction is a central cause of vertigo. As is characteristic of central vertigo, the vertigo is of moderate intensity and may or may not be associated with nausea and vomiting. Truncal ataxia is typical, with abnormal Romberg and gait-testing apparent.

Lateral medullary infarction of the brainstem, or Wallenberg's syndrome, causes vertigo along with ipsilateral facial numbness, loss of the corneal reflex, Horner's syndrome and pharyngeal and laryngeal paralysis. Contralateral loss of pain and temperature sensation in the extremities also occurs.

Vertebrobasilar insufficiency (VBI) may result in vertigo due to brainstem transient ischemic attacks in patients with the typical risk factors for cerebrovascular disease. The vertigo may be sudden in onset and last minutes to hours, but should not last more than 24 h. Associated focal brainstem signs are also likely to be present, as may syncope. Unlike other causes of central vertigo, VBI may be induced by movement of the head resulting in decreased vertebral artery blood flow.

Central vertigo also can be associated with migraine syndrome as a part of the aura, associated with the headache or the migraine equivalent. Basilar migraine is defined as a migraine that has an aura with symptoms similar to VBI.

Other causes of central vertigo include multiple sclerosis with demyelination of isolated areas of the brainstem and fourth ventricular neoplasms.

The physical examination in patients with vertigo should include an assessment of hearing, a complete neurologic examination, and the Dix-Hallpike (or Nylen-Barany) position test. Hearing loss typifies peripheral vertigo, whereas focal neurologic findings are found in central vertigo. The Dix-Hallpike position test may help to differentiate BPPV from central causes of vertigo. In this maneuver, the patient begins seated with the head straight. The patient is assisted rapidly to a supine position with the head over the edge of the bed an additional 30° to 45°. The maneuver is then repeated twice more with the head turned 45° to either side. Patients with peripheral vertigo will exhibit a latent and short-lived nystagmus with the rapid component toward the affected ear. This may reverse upon resuming an upright position.

Emergency Department Care and Disposition

The major concern in the care and disposition of patients with vertigo is to determine a peripheral versus central cause.

1. In patients with peripheral vertigo, management of symptoms is the major concern (Table 140-2). Although the mechanism of action of these drugs in vertigo is not known, vestibular suppression is commonly ascribed to their **anticholinergic** effects and **antihistaminic** properties. Benzodiazepines exhibit vestibular suppression, but also inhibit central vestibular compensation and are not recommended. Patients with BPPV may benefit from canalith-repositioning exercises (Epley's maneuver). Imaging studies are usually not necessary in peripheral vertigo as long as there is no suspicion of eighth nerve or cerebellopontine angle tumor. The majority of patients with peripheral vertigo may be discharged home with primary care follow-up. Patients with perilymph fistula, labyrinthitis of sus-

TABLE 140-2 Pharmacotherapy of Acute Peripheral Vertigo

Anticholinergics	Scopolamine	0.5 mg transdermal patch q 3–4 days (behind ear)
Antihistamines	Dimenhydrinate	50–100 mg IM or PO q 4 h
	Diphenhydramine	25–50 mg IM or PO q 6 h
	Cyclizine	50 mg PO q 4 h (not to exceed 200 mg/24 h)
	Meclizine	25 mg PO q 8–12 h
Antiemetics	Hydroxyzine	25–50 mg q 6 h
	Promethazine	25–50 mg q 6–8 h

pected bacterial etiology, and Meniere's disease may benefit from follow-up with an ENT specialist. Patients with intractable symptoms may require admission for bed rest.

2. Patients with central vertigo often require imaging studies and specialty referral. Posterior fossa hemorrhage is a neurosurgical emergency for which immediate consultation must be obtained. Similarly, suspected tumors should have urgent neurosurgical consultation and appropriate imaging studies. Other ischemic cerebrovascular incidents, suspected multiple sclerosis, and vertiginous migraine should have neurologic consultation for either inpatient or outpatient workup. Treatment for vertiginous migraine may be initiated in the emergency department with antihistamines, as earlier, as well as prophylactic beta or calcium channel blockers.

3. In all cases, it must be remembered that antivertigo medications can have undesirable anticholinergic side effects such as drowsiness and urinary retention. In patients without true vertigo, these medications may exacerbate the dizziness experienced by the patient.

For further reading in *Emergency Medicine: A Comprehensive Study Guide,* 5th ed., see Chap. 223, "Vertigo and Dizziness," by Brian Goldman.

---

141 | Seizures and Status Epilepticus in Adults

C. Crawford Mechem

A seizure is an episode of neurologic dysfunction caused by abnormal electrical discharge of brain neurons. Generalized seizures are caused by near simultaneous activation of the entire cerebral cortex, with associated loss of consciousness. Partial seizures are due to electrical discharges beginning in a localized region of the cortex. Consciousness may or may not be affected. Status epilepticus is defined as two or more seizures without full recovery of consciousness between attacks or continuous seizure activity for 30 min or more. It has a mortality rate of 1 to 10 percent and can cause permanent neurologic sequelae in survivors. Therefore, a presumptive diagnosis should be made and appropriate therapy instituted for all continuous seizures lasting more than 10 min.

Clinical Features

Generalized seizures consist of tonic-clonic (grand mal) seizures and absence (petit mal) seizures. Patients with grand mal seizures present with abrupt body rigidity, extension of the trunk and extremities, and loss of consciousness and postural tone. Patients are often apneic and profoundly cyanotic and may urinate or defecate. As the rigid (tonic) phase subsides, the patient develops symmetric, rhythmic (clonic) jerking of the trunk and extremities, which usually lasts 60 to 90 s. Consciousness gradually returns but may be accompanied by a postictal period of confusion lasting several hours.

Absence seizures occur in children and are characterized by sudden loss of consciousness without loss of postural tone, accompanied by staring and twitching of the eyelids. Episodes last only a few seconds, during which the patient does not respond to voice or other stimuli. The patient then returns to preseizure activity without postictal confusion.

Partial seizures are subdivided into simple partial, in which consciousness remains intact, and complex partial, in which consciousness is affected. Simple partial seizures may be accompanied by auras attributable to the area of the brain affected, including flashing lights, visual distortion, or olfactory or gustatory hallucinations. Complex partial seizures usually originate in the temporal lobe and may be accompanied by epigastric discomfort, automatism, memory disturbances, distorted perception, and affective disorders. These symptoms are often misinterpreted as evidence of psychiatric illness.

Diagnosis and Differential

Diagnosis requires a careful history to determine whether, in fact, the patient has had a seizure. A physical description of the attack should be obtained from the patient or bystanders. Important points to ascertain include abrupt or gradual onset, presence of aura, whether the activity was focal or generalized, progression of motor activity, or loss of bowel or bladder control. A history of seizure disorder should be sought, as well as a history of compliance with anticonvulsant medications.

Factors that may precipitate seizures should be determined, including sleep deprivation, head trauma, illicit drug use, electrolyte abnormalities, anticoagulation, febrile illnesses, HIV infection, pregnancy, and alcohol abuse (Table 141-1). In HIV-infected patients, causes of seizures include encephalopathy, meningitis, neurosyphilis, central nervous system (CNS) tuberculosis, and intracranial mass lesions due to toxoplasmosis and lymphoma. Seizures during pregnancy may be a manifestation of a preexisting seizure disorder. When combined with edema, proteinuria, and hypertension, they are diagnostic of eclampsia. Patients with a history of alcohol abuse may develop alcohol withdrawal seizures, usually within 6 to 48 h of reduction or cessation of alcohol consumption. Alcoholics also may develop seizures as a result of head trauma or infection.

The physical examination should be directed at determining

TABLE 141-1 Causes of Secondary Seizures

Intracranial hemorrhage (subdural, epidural, subarachnoid, intraparenchymal)

Structural abnormalities
  Vascular lesion (aneurism, arteriovenous malformation)
  Mass lesions (primary or metastatic neoplasms)
  Degenerative diseases
  Congenital abnormalities

Trauma (recent or remote)

Infection (meningitis, encephalitis, abscess)

Metabolic disturbances
  Hypo- or hyperglycemia
  Hypo- or hypernatremia
  Hyperosmolar states
  Uremia
  Hepatic failure
  Hypocalcemia, hypomagnesemia (rare)

Toxins and drugs (many)
  Cocaine, lidocaine
  Antidepressants
  Theophylline
  Alcohol withdrawal
  Drug withdrawal

Eclampsia of pregnancy (may occur up to eight weeks postpartum)

Hypertensive encephalopathy

Anoxic-ischemic injury (cardiac arrest, severe hypoxemia)

both a cause of seizures and any sequelae. Temperature should be noted. Fever may suggest underlying infection. The patient should be examined for signs of head or cervical spine trauma, tongue lacerations, posterior shoulder dislocation, or aspiration. A directed neurologic examination should be performed and the patient's mental status closely followed. Steady improvement is reassuring, whereas deterioration mandates aggressive diagnostic testing.

The need for laboratory studies is determined by the specific case. Patients with a known seizure disorder may only need determination of anticonvulsant levels and serum glucose level. Patients with a first-time seizure require more extensive studies, including serum glucose, electrolyte, calcium, and magnesium determinations; renal function tests; creatine phosphokinase determination to assess for rhabdomyolysis; pregnancy test; toxicology screening; and cerebrospinal fluid analysis.

The use of radiographic studies following seizures is controversial and should be individualized. Patients with a febrile seizure or a seizure typical of their usual seizure pattern do not need radiographic imaging. Patients with a first-time seizure warrant a head computed tomography scan or magnetic resonance imaging to identify a structural lesion. Patients who have recovered from a seizure, have normal neurologic examination findings, are not anticoagulated, and have no electrolyte abnormalities may have imaging performed on an outpatient basis after consultation with the neurologist who will be assuming their care. All other patients should have imaging performed as part of their emergency department evaluation.

The differential diagnosis for seizures includes syncope, pseudoseizures, hyperventilation syndrome, movement disorders, migraines with aura, narcolepsy, and cataplexy. Features that suggest a seizure include abrupt onset and cessation, lack of recall, associated purposeless movements, and a postictal period of confusion.

Emergency Department Care and Disposition

Basic management principles apply to patients who are seizing or postictal. A patent airway must be ensured and vital signs stabilized. Patients who are actively seizing should be protected from injury and turned to one side to prevent aspiration. Intravenous (IV) access should be obtained, the serum glucose level determined at bedside; and oxygen, pulse oximetry, and cardiac monitor applied. Intubation should be considered for patients with prolonged seizures, those requiring gastrointestinal decontamination, and those being transferred to another facility. Patients should be assessed for trauma and any metabolic abnormalities corrected. Following stabilization, a careful search should be made for a precipitant and appropriate therapy initiated. While emergent drug therapy is usually not required for routine seizures, in the setting of eclampsia or status epilepticus early intervention is mandatory to minimize death or long-term disability (Table 141-2).

1. **Thiamine** 100 mg IV and **glucose** 25 to 50g IV should be given to any patient with suspected or confirmed hypoglycemia.
2. **Benzodiazepines** are administered to control seizures before more specific agents can be given. Typical doses are **lorazepam** 2 mg/min IV up to 0.1 mg/kg or **diazepam** 5 mg IV every 5 min up to 20 mg.
3. **Phenytoin** is loaded IV at a dose of 18 to 20 mg/kg at a rate of 25 to 50 mg/min. If seizures continue, a second dose of 5 to

TABLE 141-2 Guidelines for Management of Status Epilepticus

	Time Frame
Establish/maintain airway ↓	
IV, oxygen, monitor ↓	
Dextrose 25–50 g IV if indicated ↓	0–5 min
Consider thiamine 100 mg IV and magnesium 1–2 g IV for alcoholic or malnourished patients ↓	
Lorazepam 2 mg/min IV up to 0.1 mg/kg (or diazepam 5 mg IV q 5 min up to 20 mg) ↓	
Phenytoin 20 mg/kg IV at 50 mg/min or fosphenytoin 20 mg/kg PE IV at 150 mg/min ↓	10–20 min
Additional phenytoin 5–10 mg/kg IV or additional fosphenytoin 5–10 mg/kg PE IV ↓	
Phenobarbital up to 20 mg/kg IV at 50–75 mg/min IV ↓	
Additional phenobarbital 5–10 mg/kg IV ↓	30 min
General anesthesia with Midazolam 0.2 mg/kg slow IVP then 0.75–10 μg/kg/min or propolol 1–2 mg/kg IV then 1–15 mg/kg/h or pentobarbital 10–15 mg/kg IV over 1 h then 0.5–1.0 mg/kg/h	

Source: Adapted from Lowenstein DH, Alldredge BK: Status epilepticus. *N Engl J Med* 338(14):970, 1998, with permission.

10 mg IV may be administered. Phenytoin reaches therapeutic levels in 1 to 2 h. It also may be administered orally but will not reach therapeutic levels for 2 to 24 h.

4. **Fosphenytoin** is a prodrug of phenytoin given as an IV loading dose of 15 to 20 phenytoin equivalents (PE)/kg infused at 100 to 150 PE/min.

5. **Phenobarbital** is considered a second-line agent for seizures refractory to benzodiazepines and phenytoin. The loading dose is 20 mg/min IV infused at 50 to 75 mg/min. A second dose of 5 to 10 mg/kg may be given if seizures continue. Respiratory depression and hypotension are common, especially when used in conjunction with benzodiazepines.

6. Seizures refractory to the abovementioned interventions are treated with IV infusions of **midazolam, propofol, thiopental,** or **pentobarbital** to induce general anesthesia, with continuous electroencephalographic (EEG) monitoring.

7. **Neuromuscular blocking agents**, such as **succinylcholine, pancuronium,** or **vecuronium,** may facilitate patient management. However, their use mandates **continuous EEG monitoring** to assess the effectiveness of anticonvulsant therapy.

8. **Magnesium sulfate** is used to treat seizures in eclampsia, starting with a 4- to 6-g bolus, followed by a 1- to 2-g/h infusion. Definitive therapy is delivery of the fetus.

Patients with an underlying seizure disorder who present with a seizure may be discharged after returning to their baseline mental status and their anticonvulsant serum level has been checked. If the level is subtherapeutic, a loading dose should be administered prior to discharge. If loaded with oral phenytoin, patients should be warned that their level may not be therapeutic for up to 24 h. Whether patients with a first-time seizure should be discharged on an anticonvulsant is case specific and should be discussed with the patient and the physician who will be assuming care in follow-up. All patients should be advised to avoid swimming unattended, operating machinery, working at heights, and driving a motor vehicle. Patients with status epilepticus, persistently altered mental status, underlying CNS infection or mass lesion, or clinically significant hypoxia, hypoglycemia, hyponatremia, or dysrhythmias should be admitted.

For further reading in *Emergency Medicine: A Comprehensive Study Guide,* 5th ed., see Chap. 224, "Seizures and Status Epilepticus in Adults," by Christina Catlett Viola.

142 | Acute Peripheral Neurologic Lesions
Howard E. Jarvis III

A systematic approach to evaluating acute neurologic symptoms includes (*a*) differentiating acute from chronic symptoms, (*b*) separating peripheral from central causes, (*c*) assessing reflexes, and (*d*) arranging close follow-up.

DISORDERS OF THE NEUROMUSCULAR JUNCTION

Botulism is caused by *Clostridium botulinum* toxin and occurs in three forms: food-borne, wound, and infantile. In the United States, the principal source is improperly prepared or stored food. In infantile botulism, organisms arise from ingested spores, often in honey, and produce a systemically absorbed toxin. Wound botulism should be considered in patients with a wound or a history of intravenous (IV) drug use and progressive, symmetric descending paralysis. Clinical features appear 1 to 2 d following ingestion and may be preceded by nausea, vomiting, and diarrhea. Early complaints commonly involve the eye or bulbar musculature, and progress to descending weakness and respiratory insufficiency. Absent light reflex is a diagnostic clue, and mentation is normal. Infants may present with poor sucking, listlessness, constipation, regurgitation, and weakness. Treatment includes respiratory support, **gastrointestinal and wound decontamination**, **botulinum antitoxin** (in consultation with an infectious disease specialist), and admission.

Myasthenia gravis is discussed in Chap. 143.

ACUTE PERIPHERAL NEUROPATHIES

Guillain-Barré syndrome usually follows an acute febrile episode, upper respiratory infection, or acute metabolic problem by days or weeks. It may be rapidly progressive. Although numerous variants exist, extremity weakness, more pronounced initially in the legs, is typical. Bulbar musculature may be involved. Respiratory failure and lethal autonomic fluctuations may occur. Objective sensory deficits are rare. The absence of deep tendon reflexes is classic. Cerebrospinal fluid findings typically reveal a high protein level and a normal glucose level and cell count. Differential diagnosis includes diptheria, botulism, lead poisoning, tick paralysis, cord compression, and porphyria. Emergency department (ED) treatment includes respiratory support, admission to a monitored setting, and neurologic consultation.

Acute intermittent porphyria is a rare autosomal dominant disorder involving the triad of weakness, psychosis, and abdominal pain. Occasionally they occur together, but each may occur independently. Seizures may be seen. Certain medications may trigger flares, such as phenytoin, barbiturates, sulfonamides, and estrogen. Neurologic findings include weakness and diminished reflexes, particularly in the legs. Sensory abnormalities may occur. The differential diagnosis includes causes of pain and lower extremity weakness, such as spinal cord compression (brisk reflexes and up-going toes) and aortic aneurysm or dissection. ED treatment includes discontinuation of the offending drug, supportive care, **glucose** infusions, **vitamin B₆**, and **hematin** 4 mg/kg/d for 1 to 2 weeks.

MYOPATHIES

Polymyositis is an inflammatory myopathy with multiple causes characterized by rapidly evolving weakness, muscular pain, arthralgias, dysphagia, fever, and Raynaud's phenomenon. Sensation is normal, as are reflexes, except with very severe weakness. Laboratory studies may reveal an elevated erythrocyte sedimentation rate and creatine kinase level, and leukocytosis. Differential diagnosis includes Eaton-Lambert syndrome, endocrinopathies, toxic myopathies, dermatomyositis, and others. Admission is usually warranted to monitor the airway and clinical progression and to complete the evaluation. Treatment includes steroids and methotrexate but should be administered in consultation with a neurologist.

Dermatomyositis has similar laboratory findings and clinical manifestations, with the addition of a violaceous rash, often on the face and hands. Treatment is aimed at immunosuppression. Numerous other causes of myopathy include environmental (e.g., alcohol), occupational, drugs (e.g., steroids, AZT, and cholesterol lowering agents), and infection (e.g., trichinosis and viral agents).

ENTRAPMENT NEUROPATHIES

Carpal tunnel syndrome is discussed in Chap. 177. Other common nerve entrapments include ulnar (mimicking C8 radiculopathy), deep peroneal (causing footdrop and numbness between the first and second toes), and meralgia paresthetica (entrapment of the lateral cutaneous nerve of the thigh). The latter may follow weight loss or pelvic or gynecologic surgery and causes lateral thigh numbness. These and other entrapments often cause numbness and weakness, and require referral to a specialist.

PLEXOPATHIES

Brachial neuritis causes severe shoulder, back, or arm pain followed by weakness in the arm or shoulder girdle, and is bilateral in up to one-third of cases. Patients have weakness in various distributions of the brachial plexus. Sensory deficits are less profound, and reflexes in the involved arm are diminished. Differential diagnosis includes multiple radiculopathies, pancoast tumors, and neoplastic or inflammatory infiltration of the plexus, although a history of pain followed by weakness that plateaus in 1 to 2 weeks makes other diagnoses unlikely. A chest x-ray should be done to screen for mass lesions involving the plexus. ED treatment consists of conservative management, and close neurologic follow-up is indicated. If other causes are excluded, admission is elective.

Lumbar plexopathy, or diabetic amyotrophy, presents in diabetics with acute back pain followed within days by ipsilateral progressive leg weakness. Decreased strength (and possibly reflexes) in a variety of patterns, with relatively symmetric sensation, is found. Bowel and bladder functions are not affected. Plain films and magnetic resonance imaging (MRI) are ultimately needed. The differential diagnosis includes cauda equina and conus medullaris syndromes and arteriovenous malformation compression. Abdominal computed tomography (CT) scanning aids in excluding aortic aneurysm. Patients should be admitted for further evaluation of the weakness.

HIV-ASSOCIATED PERIPHERAL NEUROLOGIC DISEASE

HIV and its complications and treatments cause a variety of peripheral nerve disorders. The most common, drug-induced and HIV neuropathies, are chronic and do not cause acute symptoms. Patients with HIV have a higher rate of mononeuritis multiplex and a myopathy resembling polymyositis. In early infection, they are more prone to Guillain-Barré syndrome. In the latter stages of AIDS, they may develop cytomegalovirus radiculitis, with acute weakness, primarily lower extremity involvement, and variable bowel or bladder dysfunction. Primarily lower extremity weakness and hyporeflexia, as well as sensory deficits, are seen. Rectal tone may be decreased. MRI (indicated to exclude mass lesion) shows swelling and clumping of the cauda equina. Admission is required for therapy with IV **gancyclovir** 5 mg/kg every 12 h for 14 d.

OTHER CONDITIONS

Mononeuritis multiplex is caused by a vasculitis and involves multiple deficits in a stepwise fashion, usually involving both sides of the body. For example, a left footdrop may follow a right wristdrop. This must be differentiated from multiple compression neuropathies, and it requires urgent referral to a neurologist, with treatment usually in collaboration with a rheumatologist.

Bell's palsy causes seventh cranial nerve dysfunction, and patients may complain of facial weakness, articulation problems, or difficulty keeping an eye closed. Physical examination findings reveal weakness of one side of the face, including the forehead, and no other focal neurologic findings. The differential diagnosis includes stroke, Lyme disease, parotid tumors, middle ear lesions, cerebellopontine angle tumors, eighth cranial nerve lesions, HIV, and vascular disease. The ear should be inspected for ulcerations caused by cranial herpes zoster activation (Ramsey-Hunt syndrome), which should be treated with oral acyclovir. If muscle strength is retained in the forehead and upper face, the lesion is most probably central (i.e., in the brainstem or above); this would exclude Bell's palsy, and CT scanning of the head is indicated. Treatment is controversial, but most neurologists favor a short course of **prednisone** 50 mg/d for 7 d. Steroids are withheld if paresis has been present for greater than a week. Recent data suggest that adding **acyclovir** 200 mg 5 times daily for 10 d may be beneficial. Patients should use **lacrilube** in order to prevent corneal drying and scarring. Close follow-up with a neurologist or otolaryngologist is indicated.

For further reading in *Emergency Medicine: A Comprehensive Study Guide,* 5th ed., see Chap. 225, "Acute Peripheral Neurologic Lesions," by Michael M. Wang.

---

143 | Chronic Neurologic Disorders

Mark B. Rogers

An awareness of chronic neurologic disorders and their treatments are necessary to address certain complications, most notably respiratory failure.

AMYOTROPHIC LATERAL SCLEROSIS

Clinical Features

Amyotrophic lateral sclerosis (ALS) is caused by both upper and lower motor neuron degeneration, leading to rapidly progressive muscle wasting and weakness. Upper motor neuron dysfunction causes limb spasticity, hyperreflexia and emotional lability. Lower neuron dysfunction causes limb muscle weakness, atrophy, fasciculations, dysarthria, dysphagia, and difficulty in mastication. Symptoms are often *asymmetric* and more prominent in the upper extremities. Patients may initially have cervical or back pain consistent with an acute compressive radiculopathy. Respiratory muscle weakness progresses from dyspnea on exertion to dyspnea at rest, eventually leading to respiratory distress and failure.

Diagnosis and Differential

Most patients with ALS will go to the emergency department (ED) with the diagnosis established. The clinical diagnosis is suggested by symptoms of both upper and lower motor neuron dysfunction without other central nervous system (CNS) dysfunction. Other illnesses that should be considered include myasthenia gravis, diabetes, dysproteinemia, thyroid dysfunction, vitamin B_{12} deficiency, lead toxicity, vasculitis, and CNS and spinal cord tumors.

Emergency Department Care and Disposition

Emergency care is required for acute respiratory failure, aspiration pneumonia, choking episodes, or trauma from falls. The treatment goal is to **optimize pulmonary function,** which may require nebulizer treatments, steroids, antibiotics, or endotracheal intubation. Admission is indicated for impending respiratory failure, pneumonia, inability to handle secretions, and worsening disease process that may require long-term placement.

MULTIPLE SCLEROSIS

Clinical Features

Multiple sclerosis (MS) is due to multifocal areas of CNS demyelination that cause motor, sensory, visual, and cerebellar dysfunction. Deficits associated with MS are described as a heaviness, weakness, stiffness, or extremity numbness. Lower extremity symptoms are usually more severe. Lhermitt's sign is described as an electric shock sensation, a vibration, or dysesthetic pain going down the back into the arms or legs from neck flexion. Physical exam may show decreased strength, increased tone, hyperreflexia, clonus, decrease in vibration sense and joint proprioception, and reduced pain and temperature sense. Increases in body temperature, associated with exercise, hot baths, or fever, may worsen symptoms.

Rarely, acute transverse myelitis may occur. Cerebellar lesions may cause an intention tremor, saccadic dysmetria, and truncal ataxia. Brainstem lesions may cause vertigo. Cognitive and emotional problems are common, including dementia, poor motivation, and mood disorders.

In up to 30 percent of cases, optic neuritis is the first presenting symptom and may cause an afferent pupillary defect (Marcus Gunn pupil). Acute or subacute central vision loss occurs over several days and is usually unilateral. Retrobulbar or extraocular muscle pain usually precede vision loss. The pain usually resolves in days; however, visual disturbances may last months. Fundoscopy is usually normal, but the optic disc may be pale. Visual acuity may worsen with increased body temperature. Other visual disturbances include nystagmus, diplopia, and internuclear ophthalmoplegia (INO). INO causes abnormal adduction and horizontal nystagmus, often bilaterally. Acute bilateral INO is highly suggestive of MS.

Dysautonomia causes vesicourethral gastrointestinal (GI) tract, and sexual dysfunction. Urinary retention, urgency, frequency, detrusor-external sphincter dyssynergia, and stress or overflow incontinence can occur. Constipation or fecal incontinence may be seen.

Diagnosis and Differential

The diagnosis of MS is clinical and is suggested by two or more episodes, lasting days to weeks, causing neurologic dysfunction that implicates different sites in the white matter. Magnetic resonance imaging of the head may demonstrate various abnormalities, including discrete lesions in the supratentorial white matter or periventricular areas. Cerebrospinal fluid (CSF) protein and gammaglobulin levels are often elevated.

The differential diagnosis includes systemic lupus erythematosus, Lyme disease, neurosyphilis, and HIV disease.

Emergency Department Care and Disposition

Treatment is directed at addressing the complications of acute MS exacerbations.

1. Those with severe motor or cerebellar dysfunction may be treated with **steroids.** A short-term (up to 5 days), high-dose

(1 g) course of pulsed IV methylprednisolone, followed by oral prednisone tapered over 2 to 3 weeks, may be beneficial.
2. Fever must be reduced to minimize deficits. A careful search for a source of infection should be initiated. Respiratory infections and distress must be aggressively managed. With any MS exacerbation, patients should be evaluated for acute cystitis and pyelonephritis, and any infection associated with postvoiding residuals greater than 100 mL requires intermittent catheterization. Admission is indicated for those at risk for further complications, respiratory compromise, depression with suicidal ideation, and those requiring IV antibiotics or steroid therapy. For subtle new-onset symptoms, referral to a neurologist for further evaluation is essential.

MYASTHENIA GRAVIS

Clinical Features

Myasthenia gravis (MG) is an autoimmune disease caused by antibody destruction of the acetylcholine receptors (AChR) at the neuromuscular junction, which results in variable muscle weakness. Most MG patients have generalized weakness, specifically of the proximal extremities, neck extensors, and facial or bulbar muscles. Ptosis and diplopia are the most common symptoms. Around 10 percent of patients will have ocular muscle weakness only, but most will develop dysarthria, dysphagia, and limb weakness. Symptoms usually worsen as the day progresses or with muscle use (e.g., prolonged chewing or reading) and then improve with rest. There is usually no deficit in sensory, reflex, and cerebellar function. Elderly MG patients may be misdiagnosed with ischemic stroke with new-onset facial weakness.

Extreme weakness in the respiratory muscles may cause respiratory failure. This life-threatening condition, termed *myasthenic crisis,* may be seen prior to the diagnosis of MG.

Diagnosis and Differential

MG should be considered based on clinical findings, such as ocular, bulbar, proximal limb muscle weakness, that worsen during the day and improve with rest. The diagnosis is confirmed through administration of edrophonium (an acetylcholinesterase inhibitor), electromyogram, and serum testing for AChR antibodies.

Performed at the bedside, the edrophonium (Tensilon) test not only confirms the diagnosis but can differentiate inadequate treatment from overmedication (cholinergic crisis). Edrophonium is preferred because of rapid onset (30 s) and short duration (5 to

10 min). First, a test dose of 1 to 2 mg IV is given and, if symptoms such as muscle weakness or respiratory depression worsen (cholinergic crisis), then the test is stopped. Emergent intubation may be necessary. Otherwise, up to 10 mg IV of edrophonium is administered and, if symptoms improve transiently (10 min), then the test is considered positive, indicating myasthenic crisis. Edrophonium rarely causes heart block.

The differential diagnosis includes Eaton-Lambert syndrome, drug-induced disorders (e.g., penicillamines, aminoglycosides, and procainamide), ALS, botulism, thyroid disorders, and other CNS disorders (intracranial mass lesions).

Emergency Department Care and Disposition

MG is treated with aggressive airway management, acetylcholinesterase inhibitors, and high-dose steroids with plasmapheresis or IV immunoglobulins.

1. With myasthenic crisis, supplemental **oxygen** should be administered. If the patient is unable to handle secretions or is in respiratory failure, the airway should be secured via **endotracheal intubation.** Depolarizing paralytic agents (e.g., succinylcholine) and long-acting nondepolarizing agents should be avoided.
2. If the Tensilon test is positive (myasthenic crisis), **neostigmine** can be given (0.5 to 2 mg IV or SQ, or 15 mg orally), effective within 30 min and lasting 4 h. Any severe MG patients should receive **high-dose steroid therapy,** which mandates admission to an intensive care unit due to possible increased weakness. MG patients treated for other conditions should receive their usual cholinergic inhibitors (usually pyridostigmine 60 to 90 mg orally every 4 h). A neurologist should always be consulted for disposition, admission, and arrangement of plasmapheresis.

PARKINSON'S DISEASE

Clinical Features

Parkinson's disease (PD) presents with four classic signs: resting tremor, cogwheel rigidity, bradykinesia or akinesia, and impaired posture and equilibrium. Other signs include facial and postural changes, voice and speech abnormalities, depression, and fatigue. Initially, most complain of a unilateral resting arm tremor, described as "pill rolling," which improves with intentional movement.

Diagnosis and Differential

The diagnosis is clinical and based on the four classic clinical signs. Inquiries should be made concerning family history of neurologic disorders, medications, and exposure to toxins or street drugs. "Parkinsonism" can result from street drugs, toxins, neuroleptic drugs, hydrocephalus, head trauma, and other rare neurologic disorders. Drug-induced PD most commonly presents with akinesia. No laboratory test or neuroimaging study is pathognomonic.

Emergency Department Care and Disposition

Most patients with PD will go to the ED with the diagnosis established. They will be on medications that increase central dopamine (e.g., levodopa, carbidopa, and amantadine), anticholinergics (e.g., bromocriptine), and dopamine receptors (e.g., bromocriptine). Medication toxicity includes psychiatric or sleep disturbances, cardiac dysrhythmias, orthostatic hypotension, dyskinesias, and dystonia. With significant motor or psychiatric disturbances (e.g., hallucinations or frank psychosis) or decreased drug efficacy, a **"drug holiday"** for 1 week should be initiated.

POLIOMYELITIS AND POSTPOLIO SYNDROME

Clinical Features

Poliomyelitis is caused by an enterovirus that causes paralysis via motor neuron destruction and muscle denervation and atrophy. Most symptomatic patients have only a mild viral syndrome and no paralysis. Symptoms include fever, malaise, headache, sore throat, and GI symptoms. Spinal polio results in *asymmetric* proximal limb weakness and flaccidity, absent tendon reflexes, and fasciculations; sensory deficits are usually not seen. Maximal paralysis occurs within 5 days and is followed by muscle wasting. Autonomic dysfunction is common. Paralysis will resolve within the first year in nearly all patients. Other sequelae include bulbar polio (speech and swallowing dysfunction) and encephalitis.

Postpolio syndrome is the recurrence of motor symptoms after a latent period of several decades. Symptoms may include muscle fatigue, joint pain, or weakness of new and previously affected muscle groups. These patients may have new bulbar, respiratory, or sleep difficulties.

Diagnosis and Differential

Polio should be considered in patients with an acute febrile illness, aseptic meningitis, and asymmetric flaccid paralysis with loss of deep tendon reflexes and normal sensation. CSF may reveal an elevated white blood cell count (mostly neutrophils) and positive cultures for poliovirus. Throat and rectal swabs are even higher yield tests. The diagnosis of postpolio syndrome is based on a prior history of paralytic polio with recovery, and presentation with new symptoms not attributable to other causes.

The differential diagnosis includes Guillain-Barré syndrome, peripheral neuropathies (e.g., mononucleosis, Lyme disease, or porphyria), abnormal electrolyte level, toxins, inflammatory myopathies, and other viruses (e.g., Coxsackie, mumps, echo, and various enteroviruses).

Emergency Department Care and Disposition

Treatment is supportive. With severe cases of postpolio syndrome, problems such as dyspnea, respiratory dysfunction, sleep disorders, and psychiatric disorders need to be addressed. Disposition should be made in consultation with a neurologist.

For further reading in *Emergency Medicine: A Comprehensive Study Guide,* 5th ed., see Chap. 226, "Chronic Neurologic Disorders," by Edward P. Sloan.

---

144 | Meningitis, Encephalitis, and Brain Abscess

O. John Ma

MENINGITIS

The primary goal in the emergency department management of bacterial meningitis is prompt recognition and empiric treatment.

Clinical Features

In classic and fulminant cases of bacterial meningitis, the patient presents with fever, headache, stiff neck, photobia, and altered mental status. Seizures may occur in up to 25 percent of cases. The presenting picture, however, may be more nonspecific, particularly in the very young and elderly. Confusion and fever may be signs of meningeal irritation in the elderly. It is important to inquire about recent antibiotic use, which may cloud the clinical picture in a less florid case. Physical examination must include assessment for meningeal irritation with resistance to passive neck flexion, Brudzinski's sign (flexion of hips and knees in response to passive neck flexion), and Kernig's sign (contraction of hamstrings in response to knee extension while hip is flexed). The skin should be examined for the purpuric rash characteristic of meningococcemia. Paranasal sinuses should be percussed and ears examined for evidence of primary infection in those sites. Focal neurologic deficits, which are present in 25 percent of cases, should be documented. Fundi should be assessed for papilledema, indicating increased intracranial pressure.

Diagnosis and Differential

When the diagnosis of bacterial meningitis is entertained, performing a lumbar puncture (LP) is mandatory. At a minimum, cerebrospinal fluid (CSF) should be sent for Gram's stain and culture, cell count, and protein and glucose determinations. Typical CSF results for meningeal processes are listed in Table 144-1. Additional studies to be considered are latex agglutination or counterimmune electrophoresis for bacterial antigens in potential partially treated bacterial cases, India ink and latex agglutination assay for fungal antigen in cryptococcal meningitis, acid-fast stain

TABLE 144-1 Typical Spinal Fluid Results for Meningeal Processes

Parameter (Normal)	Bacterial	Viral	Neoplastic	Fungal
OP (<170 mm CSF)	>300 mm	200 mm	200 mm	300 mm
WBC (<5 mononuclear)	>1000/μL	<1000/μL	<500/μL	<500/μL
% PMNs (0)	>80%	1–50%	1–50%	1–50%
Glucose (>40 mg/dL)	<40 mg/dL	>40 mg/dL	<40 mg/dL	<40 mg/dL
Protein (<50 mg/dL)	>200 mg/dL	<200 mg/dL	>200 mg/dL	>200 mg/dL
Gram stain (−)	+	−	−	−
Cytology (−)	−	−	+	+

Abbreviations: OP, opening pressure; PMNs, polymorphonuclear cells; and WBC, white blood cell.

Source: From Greenlee JE: Approach to diagnosis of meningitis: Cerebrospinal fluid evaluation. *Infect Dis Clin North Am* 4:83, 1990.

and culture for mycobacteria in tuberculous meningitis, *Borrelia* antibody determination for possible Lyme disease, and viral cultures for suspected viral meningitis. Other laboratory tests should include a complete blood count, blood cultures, and partial thromboplastin and prothrombin times, as well as serum glucose, sodium, and creatinine determinations.

The differential diagnosis includes subarachnoid hemorrhage, meningeal neoplasm, brain abscess, viral encephalitis, and cerebral toxoplasmosis.

Emergency Department Care and Disposition

1. Emergent respiratory and hemodynamic support are given top priority.
2. Upon presentation of the patient with suspected bacterial meningitis, LP should be performed expeditiously if the patient has no focal neurologic deficits or evidence of intracranial mass and coagulopathy on clinical grounds. Antibiotic therapy should be initiated as preparations for LP are made. Antiobiotic therapy administered up to 2 h prior to LP will not decrease the diagnostic sensitivity if CSF bacterial antigen assays are obtained along with CSF cultures. However, if the patient has focal neurologic deficits or papilledema, a head computed tomography (CT) scan should be performed prior to LP in order to determine the possible risks for transtentorial or tonsillar herniation associated with LP. In these cases, antibiotic therapy must be initiated prior to patient transport to the radiology suite for CT scanning. Antibiotic therapy should *always* be initiated in the emergency department and never be delayed for CT scanning or other studies.
3. Currently, the antibiotic therapy of choice is a third-generation cephalosporin, such as **ceftriaxone** or **cefotaxime.** A dose of 2 g intravenously (IV) should be administered and will cover the most common organisms (*Streptococcus pneumoniae, Haemophilus influenzae, Neisseria meningitidis*). In addition, it is recommended that **ampicillin** 2 g IV be administered to cover for *Listeria monocytogenes.* **Vancomycin** should be added if *S. pneumoniae* resistance is possible. For the patient who is severely penicillin allergic, the combination of **chloramphenicol** and **trimethoprim-sulfamethoxazole** is recommended. Steroid therapy (**dexamethasone** 0.15 mg/kg IV) is controversial in adults and, if initiated, should be given prior to the first dose of antibiotics.
4. Other general management measures also are important. Hypotonic fluids should be avoided. Serum sodium levels should be

monitored to detect the syndrome of inappropriate antidiuretic hormone or cerebral salt wasting. Hyperpyrexia should be treated with **acetaminophen**. Coagulopathy need to be corrected using specific replacement therapies. Seizures should be treated with **benzodiazepines** and, if needed, **phenytoin** loading. Evidence of marked intracranial pressure should be treated with **hyperventilation**, **head elevation**, and **mannitol**.

5. Viral meningitis without evidence of encephalitis can be managed on an outpatient basis, provided the patient is nontoxic in appearance, can tolerate oral fluids, and has reliable follow-up. However, it remains a diagnosis of exclusion; unless the diagnosis of viral meningitis is obvious, admission is warranted.

ENCEPHALITIS

Viral encephalitis is a viral infection of brain parenchyma producing an inflammatory response. It is distinct from but often coexists with viral meningitis.

Clinical Features

Encephalitis should be considered in patients presenting with any or all of the following features: new psychiatric symptoms, cognitive deficits (e.g., aphasia, amnestic syndrome, or acute confusional state), seizures, and movement disorders. Signs and symptoms of headache, photophobia, fever, and meningeal irritation may be present. Assessment for neurologic findings and cognitive deficits is crucial. Motor and sensory deficits are not typical. Encephalitides may show special regional trophism. Herpes simplex virus (HSV) involves limbic structures of the temporal and frontal lobes, with prominent psychiatric features, memory disturbance, and aphasia. Some arboviruses predominantly affect the basal ganglia, causing chorea athetosis and parkinsonism. Involvement of the brainstem nuclei leads to hydrophobic choking characteristic of rabies encephalitis.

Diagnosis and Differential

Emergency department diagnosis can be suggested by findings on magnetic resonance imaging (MRI) and LP. MRI not only excludes other potential lesions, such as brain abscess, but may display findings highly suggestive of HSV encephalitis if the medial temporal and inferior frontal gray matter are involved. On LP, findings of aseptic meningitis are typical.

The differential diagnosis includes brain abscess; Lyme disease; subarachnoid hemorrhage; bacterial, tuberculous, fungal, or neoplastic meningitis; bacterial endocarditis; postinfectious encephalomyelitis; toxic or metabolic encephalopathies; and primary psychiatric disorders.

Emergency Department Care and Disposition

1. The patient suspected of suffering from viral encephalitis should be admitted. Of the viruses causing encephalitis, only HSV has been shown by clinical trial to be responsive to antiviral therapy. The agent of choice is **acyclovir** 10 mg/kg IV.
2. Potential complications of encephalitis–seizures, disorders of sodium metabolism, increased intracranial pressure, and systemic consequences of a comatose state–should be handled in standard ways.

BRAIN ABSCESS

A brain abscess is a focal pyogenic infection. It is composed of a central pus-filled cavity ringed by a layer of granulation tissue and an outer fibrous capsule.

Clinical Features

Since patients typically are not acutely toxic, the presenting features of brain abscess are nonspecific. For this reason, the initial diagnosis can be difficult in the ED. Presenting signs and symptoms include headache, neck stiffness, fever, vomiting, confusion, or obtundation. Meningeal signs and focal neurologic findings, such as hemiparesis, seizures, and papilledema, are present in fewer than half the cases.

Diagnosis and Differential

Classically, brain abscess can be diagnosed by a CT scan of the head with contrast, which demonstrates one or several thin, smoothly contoured rings of enhancement surrounding a low-density center and in turn surrounded by white matter edema. LP is contraindicated when brain abscess is suspected and after the diagnosis has been established. Other studies, such as routine laboratory work and electroencephalogram, are nonspecific. Blood cultures should be obtained.

The differential diagnosis includes cerebrovascular disease, meningitis, brain neoplasm, subacute brain hemorrhage, and other focal brain infections, such as toxoplasmosis.

Emergency Department Care and Disposition

1. Decisions on antibiotic therapy for brain abscess should depend on the likely source of the infection. In a suspected otogenic

case, initial therapy should consist of a third-generation cephalosporin, such as **ceftriaxone** or **cefotaxime**, or **trimethoprim-sulfamethoxazole with chloramphenicol or metronidazole**. In a suspected sinogenic or odontogenic case, initial therapy should consist of **high-dose penicillin with chloramphenicol or metronidazole**. In a suspected cardiac case, initial therapy should consist of **vancomycin with chloramphenicol or metronidazole**. When communication with the exterior is suspected, as in penetrating trauma or following a neurosurgical procedure, initial therapy should consist of **vancomycin** or **nafcillin**. **Ceftazidime** should be added if gram-negative aerobes are suspected. Finally, in cases where no clear etiology exists, initial empiric therapy should consist of a third-generation cephalosporin and metronidazole.

2. Neurosurgical consultation and admission are warranted, since many cases will require surgery for diagnosis, bacteriologic study, and, often, definitive treatment.

For further reading in *Emergency Medicine: A Comprehensive Study Guide,* 5th ed., see Chap. 227, "Meningitis, Encephalitis, and Brain Abscess," by Keith E. Loring, David C. Anderson, and Alan J. Kozak.

EYE, EAR, NOSE, THROAT, AND ORAL EMERGENCIES

145 | Ocular Emergencies

| *Burton Bentley II*

INFECTIONS

Stye (External Hordeolum)

A stye is an acute infection of a oil gland at the lid margin that appears as a pustule. **Warm compresses** and **erythromycin ointment** bid for 7 to 10 d will allow the lesion to express itself and resolve.

Chalazion (Internal Hordeolum)

A chalazion is an acute or chronic inflammation of the eyelid secondary to meibomian gland blockage in the tarsal plate. It appears as a red papule at the lid margin or within the lid itself. Chalazions are prone to periods of quiescence with periodic flares. Treatment is approached in the same manner as a stye, but refractory lesions may improve with a 2- to 3-week course of **doxycycline**. A recurrent or persistent chalazion should be referred to an ophthalmologist for incision and curretage.

Conjunctivitis

Bacterial conjunctivitis presents as monocular or binocular eyelash matting, mucopurulent discharge, and conjunctival inflammation. The cornea should appear clear without fluorescein staining. Treatment consists of topical antibiotic drops. **Sulfacetamide 10%** is preferred in infants. Adults may use **trimethoprim-polymyxin B**

drops, sulfacetamide 10% drops, tobramycin ointment, or **erythromycin ointment**. All agents are dosed tid or qid for 5 to 7 d. Extremely purulent conjunctivitis should prompt Gram-staining, culture, and possible treatment for *Neisseria gonorrhea*. Gonorrhea is always suspected when gram-negative intracellular diplococci are seen. **Intramuscular (IM) ceftriaxone** 1 g , topical tetracycline drops, frequent saline solution washes, and ophthalmologic consultation are required. Contact lens wearers with conjunctivitis are presumed to have a *Pseudomonas* infection and require empiric treatment with a **fluoroquinolone** or an **aminoglycoside**. The lens should be discarded and not replaced until the infection has completely resolved.

The majority of patients who present with "pink eye" have viral conjunctivitis, often with a concurrent viral upper respiratory infection. The patient may complain of excessive tearing (epiphora) and discomfort. Conjunctival injection and edema (chemosis) with preauricular adenopathy is often found. Epidemic keratoconjunctivitis (EKC) is a particularly contagious viral infection that causes greater pain and redness, often with photophobia and eventual contralateral involvement. On slit-lamp examination, EKC may show subepithelial corneal infiltrates that may significantly reduce the patient's visual acuity. All viral conjunctivitis is self-limited in about 10 d, but EKC may last up to 3 weeks. Since mild bacterial conjunctivitis can appear viral initially, it is not unreasonable to treat all cases with a topical antibiotic. This strategy also may prevent bacterial superinfection. Alternatively, if the diagnosis is clear, then symptomatic treatment alone should suffice. **Cool compresses** and **naphazoline/pheniramine (Naphcon-A) drops** (1 drop tid as needed for inflammation) provide some relief. Ophthalmologic consultation for topical steroids in severe EKC may be considered. All cases of viral conjunctivitis are extremely contagious, and appropriate precaution against transmission must be taken.

This is a noninfectious conjunctivitis that causes stringy white discharge, redness, chemosis, and intense pruritus. Symptoms may occur seasonally or following a direct allergen exposure. Treatment includes **topical antihistamine-decongestant combinations**, such as **naphazoline/pheniramine** one drop qid. Cool compresses and avoidance of contact lens wearing will promote comfort.

Newborns with conjunctivitis require a careful history and examination to rule out maternal transmission of herpes simplex virus type II (HSV-II), *Chlamydia*, or *N. gonorrhea*. Herpes and *N. gonorrhea* infections typically present within the first 3 d of life, whereas *Chlamydia*, *Haemophilus*, *Staphylococcus aureus*, and *Streptococcus pneumoniae* often present 5 to 10 d post-partum. A Gram's stain is immediately useful to differentiate gonorrheal infections from more common staphylococcal and streptococcal involvement, but a culture is still required. *N. gonorrhea* is treated with **erythromycin ointment** and **parenteral ceftriaxone**. HSV-II is treated with topical **trifluridine (Viroptic)** every 2 h, and additional parenteral **acyclovir** may be required. If either of these infections is suspected, immediate ophthalmologic consultation is required. *Chlamydia* is treated with **topical and oral erythromycin**; the clinician must also be aware that the neonate is at risk for chlamydial pneumonia. *Haemophilus* responds to **topical and oral erythromycin**; staphylococcal and streptococcal infections require **topical erythromycin only**.

Herpes Simplex Virus

HSV infection may involve the eyelids, conjunctiva, or cornea, and the latter two are often infected concurrently (i.e., herpes simplex keratoconjunctivitis). The classic "dendrite" of herpes keratitis appears as a linear, branching epithelial defect with terminal bulbs that stains brightly with fluorescein dye during slit-lamp examination. An initial outbreak of HSV involving only the eyelids and conjunctiva may be treated with oral **acyclovir (Zovirax)** or **famciclovir (Famvir)**. Trifluiridine drops five times daily are also required. If keratitis is diagnosed, then **trifluridine** must be increased to nine times daily and topical erythromycin should be added to prevent secondary infection. All treatment should be performed in consultation with an ophthalmologist.

Herpes Zoster Ophthalmicus

Shingles in a trigeminal distribution with ocular involvement is termed herpes zoster ophthalmicus (HZO). Photophobia and pain secondary to iritis are often present. Slit-lamp examination may show a "pseudodendrite," a poorly staining mucous plaque without epithelial erosion. Treatment requires acyclovir therapy and topical erythromycin to prevent secondary infection. The associated iritis responds to topical steroids and cycloplegics. Since topical steroid use in patients with herpes simplex keratoconjunctivitis may be catastrophic, it is imperative that this herpes simplex is not mistaken for HZO. For this reason, and because patients with HZO may require hospital admission for parenteral acyclovir, all cases require ophthalmologic consultation.

Periorbital Cellulitis (Preseptal Cellulitis)

Periorbital cellulitis is a superficial infection of the eyelids that does not extend past the orbital septum. The eyelids become warm, indurated, and erythematous, but the eye itself is not involved. Periorbital cellulitis in children less than 5 years old may be associated with bacteremia and meningitis; a complete septic evaluation, including intravenous (IV) antibiotics, is required. All other cases may be treated with oral antibiotics. The most important step in managing periorbital cellulitis is to rule out orbital cellulitis (see below). This is done by documenting that there is no restriction of ocular motility, no proptosis, no painful eye movement, and no impairment of pupillary function. Simple periorbital cellulitis in adults and children older than 5 years of age is treated with oral **amoxicillin-clavulanate** 40 mg/kg divided tid in children or 500 mg tid in adults. For complex cases or children less than 5 years of age, hospital admission for **ceftriaxone** and **vancomycin** may be required.

Orbital Cellulitis (Postseptal Cellulitis)

Orbital cellulitis is a serious ocular infection deep to the orbital septum that often spreads from the paranasal sinuses. Orbital cellulitis is suspected whenever findings of periorbital cellulitis are accompanied by fever, toxicity, proptosis, painful ocular motility, or limited ocular excursion. Orbital and sinus thin-slice computed tomography (CT) imaging is immediately required; if findings are negative, a CT with contrast may demonstrate subperiosteal abscess. Ophthalmologic consultation and hospital admission for IV **cefuroxime** is required.

Corneal Ulcer

A corneal ulcer is a serious infection of corneal stroma itself. It may result from dessication, trauma, direct invasion, or contact lens use (particularly if left in overnight or for extended periods of time). The typical ulcer causes pain, redness, and photophobia. Slit-lamp examination reveals a staining corneal defect with a surrounding hazy infiltrate. In advanced cases, a hypopyon (i.e., purulent anterior chamber infection) may be seen. All corneal ulcers require aggressive management to avert corneal destruction. **Topical ofloxacin** or **ciprofloxacin** should be instilled hourly. Topical cycloplegics, such as **1% cyclopentolate** 1 drop tid, aid in pain relief. Eye patching is absolutely contraindicated in any eye infection, but particularly in corneal ulcers. Ophthalmologic follow-up is required within 24 h.

TRAUMA

Corneal Abrasion

Traumatic abrasions may cause superficial or deep epithelial defects resulting in tearing, blepharospasm, and severe pain. A topical anesthetic (proparacaine or tetracaine) will facilitate the examination. A small amount of fluorescein instilled into the tear film will cause dye uptake (green color) wherever epithelial cells are disrupted. Consider providing patients with a cycloplegic **(1% cyclopentolate** or **5% homatropine** 1 drop every 8 h) unless the patient is at risk for narrow-angle glaucoma; cycloplegia relaxes ciliary spasm to provide lasting pain relief. Simple, clean abrasions are treated with a layer of **topical erythromycin, tobramycin,** or **bacitracin-polymyxin** ointment applied tid. Placement of a light-pressure eye patch is optional, but contraindicated in dirty abrasions and cases with a high potential for infection. Such patients must be left unpatched while being treated with antibiotic drops every 4 h while awake. Broad-spectrum choices include **ciprofloxacin, ofloxacin,** or **tobramycin.** All abrasions caused by contact lenses are at risk for *Pseudomonas* infection and should be treated with **ofloxacin** or **ciprofloxacin** drops qid. Abrasions caused by contact lenses should never be patched, since this may promote *Pseudomonas* keratitis. Patients may be discharged with oral analgesics or cycloplegics, but topical anesthetics are absolutely contraindicated, since repeated use may cause permanent corneal damage. All but the simplest of abrasions should be reexamined in 24 h when the patch is removed.

Conjunctival Foreign Bodies

Foreign bodies of the conjunctiva are removed under topical anesthesia using a moistened sterile swab. Eversion of the upper lid is performed to rule out foreign matter in the superior conjunctival fornix.

Corneal Foreign Bodies

Superficial foreign bodies of the cornea are removed under topical anesthesia using a slit lamp. They may be approached with a moistened sterile swab, fine needle tip, or special eye spud. Any corneal foreign body located deep within the corneal stroma or in the central visual axis should be removed by an ophthalmologist. Metallic foreign bodies often leave an epithelial "rust ring," which may be removed immediately with an eye burr. Since more rust may appear the next day even if a thorough job is done initially, it is not necessary to aggressively remove all rust during the first day. In fact, it may be easier to remove rust at the follow-up appointment if it is allowed to soften for 1 to 2 d. All patients with residual rust or deeper stromal involvement should be referred to an ophthalmologist within 2 d. A corneal abrasion will result from foreign body removal and is treated in the standard manner.

Lid Lacerations

All eyelid and adnexal lacerations require meticulous evaluation to rule out ocular and nasolacrimal injury. Lid margin lacerations require closure under magnification by an ophthalmologist. For medial lid lacerations, injury to the lacrimal canaliculi and puncta must be excluded. Fluorescein instilled into the tear layer that appears in an adjacent laceration confirms the injury. All suspected or proven nasolacrimal injuries require ophthalmologic evaluation. Upper lid lacerations that involve the levator mechanism and all through-and-through lid lacerations must be repaired in the operating room.

Subconjunctival Hemorrhage

This injury represents a disruption of blood vessels within the normally clear conjunctiva and will resolve spontaneously. It may occur traumatically or from sneezing, gagging, and the Valsalva maneuver. A dense, circumferential subconjunctival hemorrhage ("bloody chemosis") requires exploration to rule out occult globe rupture.

Traumatic Iritis and Iridocyclitis

Mild inflammation of the iris (iritis) or iris and ciliary body (iridocyclitis) is commonly seen after blunt trauma to the eye. Symptoms include a deep, aching pain with photophobia. Signs include injection at the corneoscleral limbus ("ciliary flush") as well as white blood cells and protein in the anterior chamber ("cell and flare"). Treatment consists of topical cycloplegics (**cyclopentolate 1%** or **homatropine 5%** applied tid) and topical steroids **(Pred-Forte**, 1 drop qid). Ophthalmologic consultation should be obtained within 24 h.

Traumatic Miosis and Mydriasis

The ciliary body may respond to blunt trauma with either mydriasis (pupillary dilation) or miosis (constriction). Small triangular defects at the pupillary margin result from tears of the sphincter. None of these injuries requires specific treatment, but they should be followed by an ophthalmologist.

Iridodialysis

Blunt trauma may cause iridodialysis, a separation of the iris peripherally at the ciliary body. This serious injury creates a lentiform defect ("accessory pupil") at the limbus, and there is often an associated hyphema. Ophthalmologic consultation must be obtained.

Hyphema

Hyphema is blood in the anterior chamber that occurs either spontaneously or following trauma. The volume ranges from minimal amounts seen only with a slit lamp to massive amounts filling the entire chamber. Rebleeds often occur between 2 and 5 d following the initial injury and are associated with a high rate of complication. Management consists of a Fox shield to prevent further injury, placement of the patient at 45° to keep red cells from staining the cornea and clogging the trabecular meshwork, and emergent ophthalmologic consultation to consider various treatment options. It is useful for the ophthalmologist to know the extent of the hyphema, since bleeds involving less than one-third of the anterior chamber may be carefully managed on an out-patient basis. Patients with sickle cell disease tolerate hyphema poorly, and emergent consultation should be sought.

Orbital Blowout Fractures

Orbital blowout fractures commonly involve the inferior wall (maxillary sinus) and medial wall (ethmoid sinus). Inferior wall fractures are associated with maxillary sinus clouding or an air-fluid level on the Water's view radiograph. The "teardrop sign," a teardrop-shaped opacity within the maxillary sinus from extruded orbital contents, also suggests fracture. Entrapment of the inferior rectus muscle may cause restriction of upward gaze with a resultant diplopia. Medial wall fractures may produce subcutaneous emphysema, particularly when sneezing or blowing the nose. Isolated blowout fractures, with or without entrapment, require referral to a facial surgeon within 3 to 10 d; immediate surgery is not required. Because of the high incidence of associated ocular trauma, all cases should be referred to an ophthalmologist for reexamination. Antibiotic prophylaxis (e.g., oral **cephalexin** 250 mg qid for 10 d) may be considered.

Penetrating Ocular Trauma and Ruptured Globe

Globe penetration or rupture is a catastrophic injury that must be immediately identified. Suggestive findings include teardrop-shaped pupil, bloody chemosis, extrusion of globe contents, hyphema, shallow anterior chamber, or a significant reduction in visual acuity. A bright-green streaming appearance to fluorescein instilled into the tear layer (Seidel's test) is pathognomonic, but it may be absent if the wound has sealed. Once identified, any further manipulation of the eye must be avoided. A Water's view radiograph and orbital thin-slice CT imaging are helpful in confirming intraocular foreign bodies. Magnetic resonance imaging also may be used, but it is absolutely contraindicated if a ferromagnetic foreign body is suspected. Place a **Fox shield** over the eye to protect it from direct pressure, update the patient's tetanus status, start broad-spectrum antibiotics (e.g., **cefazolin** 1 g IV), and consult an ophthalmologist emergently.

Chemical Ocular Trauma

All corrosive burns, whether acid or alkali, are managed in a similar manner. The eye should be **immediately flushed** at the scene, and at least 1 to 2 L additional normal saline solution should be continued in the emergency department. A topical anesthetic and a Morgan lens will facilitate flushing. Inspect the fornices for retained matter and continue irrigation until the pH is between 6 and 8. The pH may be checked with an appropriate litmus paper or the pH square on a urine dipstick. Wait 10 min and recheck the pH to make sure that no additional corrosive is leaching out from the tissues. Record intraocular pressures, especially in alkali burns. Apply a cycloplegic (**cyclopentolate 1%** or **homatropine 5%**) to alleviate ciliary spasm, and coat the eye with a broad-spectrum antibiotic ointment. Most patients will need generous pain medications. An ophthalmologist should be consulted to arrange immediate follow-up, particularly if corneal clouding is seen. Chemical conjunctivitis (i.e., inflamed, edematous bulbar conjunctiva) is a common sequelae that is treated in the same manner as all other chemical ocular exposures. Ophthalmologic referral for isolated chemical conjunctivitis should be within 48 h.

Cyanoacrylate Glue Removal

Cyanoacrylate glue (e.g., Super-Glue or Krazy-Glue) readily adheres to the eyelids and corneal surface but usually causes no permanent damage. The lids and ocular surface should be irrigated for 15 min with warm water. Initial débridement should be limited to easily removable pieces. **Erythromycin** will further soften the glue until the patient can be seen by an ophthalmologist within 48 h.

Ultraviolet Keratitis and Laser-Induced Scotomas

Ultraviolet keratitis is a "corneal sunburn," which may result from tanning booths, welding flashes, or prolonged sun exposure. Severe pain and photophobia take 4 to 8 h to develop. Conjunctival hyperemia and punctate corneal fluorescein uptake are easily identified. Treatment consists of cycloplegia (**cyclopentolate 1%** or **homatropine 5%**), **antibiotic ointment**, **eye patching**, and **pain medication**. No permanent sequelae should be anticipated. Conversely, laser light that strikes the retina has the potential to permanently scar the tissue and cause a scotoma. There is no treatment for this injury.

ACUTE ALTERATIONS IN VISION

Central Retinal Artery Occlusion

A sudden, painless, monocular loss of vision always suggests central retinal artery occlusion (CRAO). Occlusion of the central retinal artery itself will cause complete visual loss; branch obstruction will cause loss only in the involved field. CRAO is often preceded by episodes of amaurosis fugax, which is a transient, monocular ischemic attack caused by an embolic event involving the retinal artery or arterioles. It causes a painless graying or blurring of the visual field often described as a descending "nightshade." Focal arteriole obstructions are occasionally seen with the ophthalmoscope. A thorough evaluation to uncover the embolic source is required.

In CRAO, the physical examination confirms the visual loss and may show an afferent pupillary defect, narrowed arterioles with segmented flow ("boxcars"), and a bright red macula ("cherry-red spot"). This is a true ophthalmologic emergency, and treatment must begin instantaneously once the diagnosis is suspected. The goal of treatment is to reduce the size of the ischemic insult by dislodging the central embolus into a peripheral branch. A moderate pressure massage is applied to the globe for 15 s, rapidly released for 5 s, and then repeated as necessary for the next 30 min. Breathing a 95:5 mixture of O_2 and CO_2 (**Carbogen**) for 10 min every hour may also promote vasodilation and relief; paper bag rebreathing may be attempted if Carbogen is not available. Intraocular pressures should be lowered with a single drop of **timolol (Timoptic)** 0.5% and 500 mg of IV **acetazolamide (Diamox)**. An ophthalmologist should be consulted immediately to consider surgical decompression and anticoagulation.

Central Retinal Vein Occlusion

Central retinal vein occlusion (CRVO) causes acute, painless visual loss, but not quite as abruptly as in CRAO. Examination reveals retinal hemorrhages, cotton wool spots, and edema in a dramatic pattern described as "retinal apoplexy." There is no immediate treatment for CRVO, but ophthalmologic follow-up is required and aspirin therapy may be considered.

Acute Angle Closure Glaucoma

Shallow anterior chambers may block aqueous outflow and predispose the patient to an attack of acute angle closure glaucoma (AACG). In severe episodes, patients may present with ocular injection, corneal haziness, iritis, a minimally reactive or nonreactive pupil, and an intraocular pressure (IOP) of 40 to 70 mmHg (normal range 10 to 20 mmHg). Intense orbital pain with nausea and blurry vision is common. Treatment to decrease the IOP must be started emergently. Multiple agents are used simultaneously in order to decrease aqueous production, facilitate aqueous outflow, and directly decrease IOP. Topical **timolol** (Timoptic 0.5%) directly lowers IOP and may facilitate the action of pilocarpine; use 1 drop in the affected eye immediately. **Pilocarpine 2%** is a miotic that promotes aqueous outflow; use 1 drop every 15 min in the affected eye and 1 drop every 6 h on the contralateral side for prophylaxis. **Apraclonidine (Iopidine 0.1%)** is an α_2 agonist that acts primarily by decreasing aqueous production. Place 1 drop in the affected eye immediately. Carbonic anhydrase inhibitors decrease aqueous formation; use **acetazolamide (Diamox)** 500 mg IV. Hyperosmotic agents also may be initiated. Oral regimens include **glycerol 50%** 1 mL/kg or 220 mL **isosorbide 45%**. Alternatively, **mannitol 20%** 1 to 2 g/kg may be given IV. All cases require immediate and concurrent ophthalmologic consultation.

Optic Neuritis

Optic neuritis (ON) is inflammation at any point along the optic nerve. The primary causes are infection (often viral), demyelination (frequently the presenting symptom of multiple sclerosis), and autoimmune disorders. ON results in a reduction or "dimness" of vision, often with poor color perception. Over half of patients have pain, mainly during extraocular movement. Visual field cuts with an afferent pupillary defect are the usual findings. Color vision is more adversely affected than is visual acuity, and the effects can be identified by the red desaturation test. To perform this test, have the patient use one eye to look at a dark-red object; then test the other eye. The affected eye will see the object as pink or light red. In anterior ON, the optic disc appears swollen (papillitis); there are no ophthalmoscopic findings in retrobulbar cases. Evaluation and treatment should be directed by an ophthalmologist. Oral steroids are contraindicated, but IV steroids may be considered.

OTHER OCULAR EMERGENCIES

Retinal Injury

Traction on the retina is painless and causes a sensation of flashing lights as the retina is stimulated. Detachment of the retina may occur acutely, but it is sometimes delayed by months to years. Depending on the location of the injury, a visual field defect may be identified and the actual billowy gray detached retina may be seen. Urgent consultation is required.

Vitreous Hemorrhage

Hemorrhage into the vitreous often results in "floaters," clumps of red blood cells that are seen by the patient as specks or strands floating in the visual field. Vitreous hemorrhage requires ophthalmologic referral. Patients should avoid antiplatelet medications and excessive straining.

Episcleritis

Episcleritis is a benign, self-limited inflammation of the tissue at the junction of the conjunctiva and sclera, known as the episclera. Patients present with discomfort, localized hyperemia, and swelling. **Topical decongestants** (e.g., naphazoline), **topical steroids**, and **oral nonsteroidal anti-inflammatory drugs** may help but should be used in consultation with an ophthalmologist.

Uveitis and Iritis

Uveitis is inflammation of the iris, ciliary body, and choroid. Most commonly, anterior uveitis is seen, and this is known as iritis. This disorder may result from traumatic, infectious, and autoimmune causes. Symptoms may include blurred vision, deep orbital aching, photophobia, and redness. Slit-lamp examination will identify cells in the anterior chamber ("cell"), with suspended proteins causing a fogginess of the slit-lamp beam ("flare"). Treatment consists of **topical steroids**, **topical cycloplegics**, and ophthalmologic consultation.

For further reading in *Emergency Medicine: A Comprehensive Study Guide,* 5th ed., see Chap. 230, "Ocular Emergencies," by John D. Mitchell.

146	Ear, Nose, and Facial Disorders
	Burton Bentley II

OTOLOGIC EMERGENCIES

Tinnitus

Tinnitus is the perception of sound without any external stimulation. It may be constant, pulsatile, variably pitched, ringing, hissing, or clicking. Since many drugs can cause tinnitus, the patient's medication list should be reviewed for any ototoxic agents. The most common offenders are aspirin, nonsteroidal anti-inflammatory agents (NSAIDs), antibiotics (particularly aminoglycosides), and chemotherapeutic agents. Once drug side effects have been ruled out, referral to an otolaryngologist is required for further evaluation. Antidepressant medications may relieve tinnitus when no underlying cause has been uncovered.

Hearing Loss

Hearing loss is categorized as either conductive or sensory. *Conductive* deficits occur when sound waves are not conducted to the inner ear. This may occur in the context of cerumen impaction, foreign body obstruction, external otitis, tympanic membrane (TM) perforation, tympanosclerosis, disruption of the ossicular chain, or middle-ear fluid. *Sensorineural* deficits are a consequence of disruption of the neural pathway and may result from viral neuronitis, acoustic neuroma, Ménière's disease, autoimmune disorders, or idiopathic causes.

The two forms of hearing loss are categorized by Weber's and Rinne's tests. For Weber's test, a tuning fork is held on the forehead while the patient notes in which ear the sound is heard the loudest. In cases of sensorineural hearing loss, sound lateralizes to the normal ear; in conductive loss, sound lateralizes to the abnormal ear. For Rinne's test, a tuning fork is first held on the mastoid until the sound is inaudible. It is then held near the ear canal where it should again be audible to a normal patient, but inaudible if there is a conductive deficit.

Bilateral hearing loss (normal Weber and Rinne with decreased hearing) suggests noise or ototoxin exposure. Ototoxicity has been reported with certain antibiotics (aminoglycosides, erythromycin, and vancomycin), NSAIDs, antimalarials, antineoplastics, and loop diuretics (furosemide and ethacrynic acid). Once life-threatening illnesses are excluded, all cases of acute hearing loss require ENT evaluation.

Otitis Externa

Otitis externa (OE) and malignant otitis externa (MOE) are diseases at the extremes of a spectrum progressing from dermatitis of the external auditory canal (EAC), to cellulitis, chondritis, and, finally, osteomyelitis of the temporal bone and base of the skull. OE occurs frequently in swimmers (i.e., "swimmer's ear"), and MOE occurs primarily in those with diabetes and immunocompromised patients. Any elderly, diabetic, or immunocompromised patient with OE, or any patient with OE refractory to 2 to 3 weeks of treatment, should be suspected of having MOE.

Patients with OE have ear pain exacerbated by movement of the pinna or tragus. The EAC may be erythematous or may be suppurative with edema, exudate, and debris that may completely obstruct the EAC and cause a conductive hearing loss. In MOE, the disease spreads to involve the pinna and periauricular structures. Malignant external otitis is not a neoplastic process. It is, therefore, more correctly known as *necrotizing otitis externa (NOE)*, if it is limited to soft tissues and cartilage, or as skull-base osteomyelitis (SBO) if it spreads to the temporal bone or skull base. As MOE progresses, patients may develop trismus, fever, sepsis, cranial nerve palsies, meningitis, or brain abscess. The diagnosis of OE and MOE is strictly clinical, though osteomyelitis in MOE may be confirmed by a nuclear bone scan or radiographic imaging. MOE may be suggested by otalgia that is out of proportion to routine OE, or by granulation tissue on the floor of the EAC.

OE is treated with **hydrocortisone and neomycin mixed with either polymyxin B (Cortisporin Otic)** *or* **colistin sulfate (Coly-Mycin S Otic)**. Cortisporin Otic *solution* is preferred over the *suspension,* but it may irritate the middle ear if the TM is perforated. **If the TM is perforated or not visualized, the suspension should be used**. The EAC should first be cleansed of debris with light suction, irrigation, or curettage. A gauze wick will facilitate antibiotic penetration for EACs with moderate obstruction. Four drops of medication should be placed in the ear 4 times daily until the OE resolves. If the TM is not visualized, the patient should be treated empirically with additional oral antibiotics for concurrent otitis media. Patients with only mild erythema of the pinna who are not at risk for MOE may be closely followed as outpatients. Patients with MOE require urgent ENT consultation, hospital admission, and treatment with either an **antipseudomonal cephalosporin** or an **antipseudomonal penicillin plus an aminoglycoside**.

Otitis Media

Otitis media (OM) is a common infection often heralded by acute otalgia. Fever frequently occurs, but findings may be much less specific, especially in infants. The diagnosis requires direct visualization of the TM, which may appear erythematous if inflamed, or white to yellow if middle-ear secretions are present. The TM is often bulging, though it may be retracted. In *otitis media with effusion,* an air-fluid level or bubbles may be seen. The normal TM is freely mobile, and loss of mobility on insufflation during pneumatic otoscopy is a sensitive sign of OM. *Bullous myringitis* is a particularly painful variant of OM that includes blood-filled or serous blisters on the TM. The causative organisms are often the same, though some cases of bullous myringitis are secondary to *Mycoplasma.*

Patients with OM are prescribed a **10-day course of antibiotic therapy** with outpatient follow-up at the completion of treatment. **Antipyretics** and **analgesics** may also be required. Antibiotic treatment is usually started with **amoxicillin; trimethoprim-sulfamethoxazole (Bactrim)** or **erythromycin-sulfisoxazole (Pediazole)** may be used for penicillin-allergic patients. Unresponsive OM should be treated with one of the alternate drugs for the same time period. Macrolides effective against *Mycoplasma* are the best choice for patients with bullous myringitis. Failure to respond to 2 to 3 days of therapy warrants an antibiotic change to include coverage of β-lactamase-producing species; appropriate choices include **amoxicillin-clavulanate (Augmentin)** or **cefaclor (Ceclor)**. Complications of OM may include TM perforation, cholesteatoma, hearing loss, mastoiditis, meningitis, or brain abscess.

Mastoiditis and Lateral Sinus Thrombosis

Mastoiditis is a serious complication of inadequately treated otitis media and occurs most often in the pediatric age group. Frequently, there is a history of otitis media, antibiotic use, persistent otalgia, or otorrhea. Clinical deterioration in the otitis media patient should always prompt concern for suppurative complications, including mastoiditis.

The diagnosis of mastoiditis is suspected on clinical findings that may include mastoid tenderness and erythema, loss of the postauricular crease, inferolateral displacement of the pinna, or local fluctuance. The TM is often erythematous, edematous, or perforated, though 10 percent of TMs may be normal. **All patients should have a computed tomography (CT) scan** to help confirm the diagnosis and to rule out other intracranial processes. **Emergent ENT consultation for surgical drainage** is required. Antibiotic therapy should be started with either **cefuroxime (Zinacef)**, **ampicillin-sulbactum (Unasyn)**, **ceftriaxone (Rocephin)** and **metronidazole (Flagyl)**, or **imipenem-cilastatin (Primaxin)**. Complications of mastoiditis may include facial palsies, extension of the abscess into the neck, meningitis, intracranial abscess, or septic thrombophlebitis.

Lateral sinus thrombosis (LST) is a rare complication of OM that arises from extension of the infection into the lateral and sigmoid sinuses. Headache is the most common symptom, though some patients may have papilledema, vertigo, or a sixth nerve palsy. ENT consultation, magnetic resonance imaging, and immediate antibiotic therapy are required. A combination of **nafcillin, ceftriaxone,** and **metronidazole** is recommended.

Trauma

A hematoma of the ear presents as a firm, painful swelling of the auricle. This may occur immediately after trauma or within several hours. If treated improperly, the injury may result in an auricular deformity known as a "cauliflower ear." The goal of treatment is to protect the cartilage by draining the hematoma and preventing reaccumulation. Utilizing sterile technique, a small semicircular incision is made in a position that provides the best positioning with the least exposure. The clot is then evacuated, and the wound is sutured closed. A through-and-through stitch is then used to fasten dental rolls or sterile pledgets as a compressive dressing on both sides of the ear. ENT consultation in 24 h is needed to assure that there is no recurrent hematoma.

Thermal injury to the auricle may be caused by either excessive heat or cold. Superficial injury of either type is treated with cleansing, topical non-sulfa-containing antibiotic ointments, and a light dressing. *Frostbite* is treated with rapid rewarming using saline-soaked gauze at 38° to 40°C. The rewarming process may be quite painful and necessitate the use of analgesics or conscious sedation. Any second-degree or third-degree burn requires immediate ENT or burn center consultation. All cold-induced injuries require immediate ENT referral.

Foreign Bodies in the Ear

On examination, the foreign body (FB) is usually visualized, and signs of infection or TM perforation should be sought. *Live insects* are particularly distressing to the patient and should be immediately immobilized with **2% lidocaine instilled into the ear canal** prior to removal. Patient cooperation is essential, and both **sedation** and **restraint** may be required to avoid lodging the FB more medially.

Options for removal depend on the size and composition of the FB. **Irrigation** is often useful for small objects, though organic matter may absorb the water and swell. Small FBs may be **grasped with microforceps,** whereas larger objects may be **hooked from behind** and removed with traction. A specially made **suction-cup catheter** is useful for round objects. **Cyanoacrylate glue** on the tip of a probe may allow the probe to be attached to a hard, smooth FB for removal.

ENT consultation is required in cases of TM perforation, ossicular damage, caustic substances, or if an impacted FB cannot be safely and easily removed.

Tympanic Membrane Perforations

Perforation of the TM may result from several diverse causes, including trauma, infection, or lightning. The patient may have slight hearing loss and pain. Vertigo and deafness signifies injury to the ossicles, labyrinth, or temporal bone and requires urgent consultation. Antibiotics are not useful in uncomplicated TM perforation, but standard antibiotics are used when there is coexistent otitis media. The patient must be instructed to protect the ear canal from water. **All perforations require ENT follow-up**.

OTHER FACIAL EMERGENCIES

Masticator Space Abscess

The masticator space consists of four contiguous spaces bounded by the muscles of mastication. Abscesses in this space often extend from infections in the buccal, submandibular, and sublingual areas. Signs and symptoms vary depending on the location of the abscess and may include trismus, facial swelling, pain, erythema, fever, dysphagia, or sepsis. Radiographs may show mandibular osteomyelitis, and CT scanning may define the extent of the abscess, but neither is required for the management of the stable patient. Masticator abscesses must also be distinguished from parotitis. With simple parotitis, the patient generally has no trismus and the pain has a cyclical relationship to eating.

Well-appearing patients with only minimal symptoms, slight trismus, and no palpable abscess are candidates for outpatient treatment. Therapy includes **analgesics, oral antibiotics** (e.g., penicillin, erythromycin, or clindamycin), and **follow-up** in 24 h. Patients with significant trismus, airway compromise, palpable abscess, diffuse cellulitis, or sepsis require **parenteral antibiotics** and **emergent ENT consultation** for operative drainage.

Ludwig's Angina

Ludwig's angina is an extensive bilateral cellulitis of the submandibular space that commonly evolves from infection of the lower molars. Patients have a febrile illness and painful edema of the submandibular area. Neck motion is restricted, and there may be drooling, trismus, dysphagia, dysphonia, or displacement of the tongue in a posterior and superior direction. Severe cases may have progressive respiratory distress with complete airway obstruction, involvement of the carotid artery and jugular vein, and mediastinitis. Direct laryngoscopy can provoke laryngospasm and should be avoided. Lateral neck radiographs are extremely useful and frequently show airway narrowing, soft tissue swelling, and subcutaneous emphysema. CT scanning is diagnostic, though it is often impossible to perform in the stridorous patient who is unable to lie supine.

Treatment consists of **parenteral antibiotics** and **emergent ENT consultation** for possible operative drainage. Antibiotic choices include penicillin, clindamycin, or erythromycin. Equipment for airway control must be readily available, and all patients must be admitted to an intensive care unit.

SALIVARY GLAND PROBLEMS

Sialoadenitis refers to inflammation of the parotid, sublingual, or submandibular salivary glands. *Mumps* is one cause of painful parotid swelling in the pediatric age group. Symptoms progress from fever and malaise to increasing pain with parotid swelling. Bilateral parotitis occurs in 70 percent of patients, though there is no discharge from Stenson's duct. The diagnosis is clinical, and the treatment is symptomatic. Several other viruses, including HIV, can cause parotitis.

Suppurative parotiditis sometimes occurs in people with a decreased flow of saliva. This includes the elderly, debilitated patients, postoperative patients, and those patients taking anticholinergic medications. The parotid is swollen and tender with pus expressed at Stenson's duct, with 25 percent of cases bilateral. Progression is heralded by fever, trismus, and involvement of the face and neck. Treatment consists of **hydration, massage, local heat, sialogogues** (e.g., lemon drops), and **β-lactamase-resistant antibiotics,** such as amoxicillin-clavulanate (Augmentin) or ampicillin-sulbactum (Unasyn). Severe cases and treatment failures require ENT consultation. Suppurative sialoadenitis may involve other glands, but the treatment and course is the same.

Salivary calculi (i.e., sialoliths) present with unilateral pain and swelling, most commonly involving the submandibular glands. The stone is often palpable and visible on intraoral radiographs. Treatment consists of **analgesics** and **sialogogues;** antibiotics are given if an infection is present. Easily located calculi may be milked from the duct. Persistently retained calculi, complicated cases, and intraglandular sialoliths require ENT referral.

NASAL EMERGENCIES AND SINUSITIS

Epistaxis

Epistaxis is classified as either anterior or posterior. *Anterior epistaxis* arises from the anterior nasal septum, and the site of hemorrhage is often easily visualized. *Posterior epistaxis* arises from more posterior locations and usually requires endoscopic instruments for localization. Posterior epistaxis is suspected when one of the following occurs:

1. An anterior source is not identified once bleeding has stopped.
2. Bleeding occurs from both nares.
3. Blood is seen draining into the posterior pharynx after anterior sources have been controlled.

Both anterior and posterior epistaxis require an initial evaluation to identify and control the source:

1. A quick history should determine the duration and severity of the hemorrhage, as well as contributing factors (trauma, anticoagulant use, infection, bleeding diathesis, etc.).
2. The patient should be seated while leaning forward with the head inclined anteriorly.
3. The patient should blow his or her nose to dislodge any clots.
4. A quick inspection should be made to identify obvious anterior sources. A Frazier suction catheter will help keep the passage clear.
5. Cotton swabs or pledgets moistened with a topical anesthetic or vasoconstrictor should be inserted into the nasal cavity with bayonet forceps. Excellent results are provided by **4% lidocaine** when mixed with **1:1000 epinephrine, 1% phenylephrine (Neo-Synephrine)**, or with **0.05% oxymetazoline (Afrin)**.
6. Direct external pressure should then be applied for 5 to 10 min. Active bleeding into the pharynx despite direct pressure suggests either inadequate pressure, drainage from a clot in the posterior nasal cavity, or true posterior epistaxis.
7. Following compression, the pledgets should be removed and the nasal cavity inspected with a speculum. If anterior hemorrhage is controlled and the site of mucosal disruption is identified, then the area may be locally cauterized. If anterior bleeding

continues, direct pressure should be attempted two more times. If this fails, an anterior pack should be placed (see later). If the anterior pack fails to control bleeding, then the diagnosis of posterior epistaxis should be considered and the nasal cavity should be packed both anteriorly and posteriorly. At this point, an intravenous line should be started and blood sent for complete blood cell count, prothrombin time, partial thromboplastin time, and typing. Close monitoring is required, and an ENT physician must be consulted.

Chemical cautery with silver nitrate is the standard of care for emergency department cautery of anterior epistaxis; thermal techniques are no longer recommended. After hemostasis is achieved, the mucosa should be cauterized by firmly rolling the tip of a silver nitrate applicator over the area until it turns silvery-black. A small surrounding area should also be cauterized to control local arterioles. Overzealous use of cautery is discouraged since it may cause septal perforation and unintended local tissue necrosis, and both thermal and electrocautery should be avoided.

Anterior nasal packing may be performed either with gauze or with newer commercial devices. There are several commercial nasal packs that have nearly the same efficacy as standard gauze packs but are more comfortable and easier to use. These devices should, therefore, be considered first-line treatments. One popular device is the **Merocel nasal sponge** (Merocel Corp., Mystic, CT), a compact, dehydrated sponge available in several lengths to control both anterior and/or posterior epistaxis. The sponge is rapidly inserted along the floor of the nasal cavity and will expand upon contact with blood or secretions. A film of antibiotic ointment applied to the sponge will ease insertion and reduce chances of infection. After insertion, expansion is hastened by rehydrating the sponge with sterile water from a catheter-tipped syringe after the sponge has been inserted. A mixture of lidocaine and a topical vasoconstrictor also may be used to hydrate the sponge while providing topical anesthesia and vasoconstriction. The longer sponges used to control posterior hemorrhages have been associated with some morbidity and should only be used when indicated; they are not indicated for the control of isolated anterior epistaxis. All nasal packs should be removed in 2 to 3 days by an ENT physician. Antibiotic prophylaxis is required while the pack is in place.

If a nasal tampon fails to control hemorrhage, a standard gauze pack should be utilized. The technique for placement of a standard gauze pack requires skill and experience; an improperly placed pack is a frequent cause of treatment failure. A single, long strip of petrolatum-impregnated gauze is utilized for this purpose:

1. First, hemorrhage should be maximally controlled as outlined earlier.
2. Using a nasal speculum and bayonet forceps, the physician inserts a loop of the gauze all the way into the posterior limit of the nasal cavity while the end of the strip is left outside the nostril.
3. The speculum should then be withdrawn and replaced such that the packing is firmly pressed against the nasal floor.
4. Using the bayonet forceps, the physician grabs another loop of gauze that is layered in an accordion fashion onto the first layer.
5. The process of using the forceps to place the next layer and then reintroducing the speculum to compress the preceding layer should be repeated until the entire nasal cavity is tightly packed. When applied correctly, the folded end of each layer will be visible at the nostril, both ends of the strip will extend from the nostril for easy removal of the pack, and anterior bleeding will be controlled. Generally, the pack is removed in 2 to 3 days at a follow-up appointment with an ENT physician. Rehydration with water allows for easy pack removal.

Posterior epistaxis may be treated with either a dehydrated posterior sponge pack (Merocel) as outlined earlier or with a commercial balloon tamponade device. The balloon devices use independently inflatable anterior and posterior balloons to quickly control refractory epistaxis at these sites; the instructions for insertion are included in the balloon kit. To protect against potentially serious complications, all patients with posterior packs require ENT consultation for possible hospital admission. Posterior packs are also removed in 2 to 3 days after placement. As with anterior packs, antibiotic prophylaxis is required while the pack is in place.

Complications of nasal packing include dislodgment of the pack, recurrent bleeding, sinusitis, and toxic shock syndrome. All patients with nasal packs should be administered antibiotic prophylaxis with either **cephalexin (Keflex)** or **amoxicillin-clavulanate (Augmentin)**. Penicillin-allergic patients may be given **clindamycin (Cleocin)** or **trimethoprim-sulfamethoxazole (Bactrim DS)**.

Nasal Fractures

A nasal fracture is a clinical diagnosis that should be suspected in all cases of facial trauma. Suggestive findings may include swelling, tenderness, crepitance, gross deformity, periorbital ecchymosis, epistaxis, or rhinorrhea. Radiographs are generally not indicated in the emergency department, though they may be obtained at a follow-up appointment.

A simple, nondisplaced nasal fracture requires only oral analgesics, protection from further injury, decongestant sprays if necessary, and elevation of the head with local ice therapy to reduce swelling. Uncomplicated anterior epistaxis may require a nasal pack. ENT referral is not mandatory unless there is nasal congestion or cosmetic deformity after the swelling diminishes in 2 to 5 days. When soft tissue swelling is severe, it may be impossible to acutely determine if a displaced fracture exists. These patients are treated in the same manner as patients with nondisplaced fractures, but they require follow-up with a specialist in 2 to 5 days. This time period allows the swelling to resolve so that the nasal bones can be reevaluated and reduced if necessary.

Perhaps the most important step in the evaluation of nasal trauma is to rule out serious associated injuries, particularly septal hematoma and fracture of the cribriform plate. A *septal hematoma* is a collection of blood beneath the perichondrium of the nasal septum and is easily identified on physical examination by the presence of a bluish, fluid-filled sac overlying this location. If left untreated, a septal hematoma may result in abscess formation or necrosis of the nasal septum. The treatment is local incision and drainage with placement of an anterior nasal pack to prevent reaccumulation of blood. A *fracture of the cribriform plate* may violate the subarachnoid space and cause cerebrospinal fluid (CSF) rhinorrhea. This injury should be suspected in any patient who has clear nasal drainage following facial trauma, even if the trauma occurred days to weeks earlier. The most accurate method to diagnose CSF rhinorrhea is with a highly specialized procedure known as metrizamide CT cisternography (MCTC). Bedside tests include glucose reagent strip testing (a glucose level of greater than 30 mg/dL suggests CSF) and the "halo" test (a clear "halo" surrounds a central blood stain when a drop of bloody CSF is placed on a piece of filter paper). If any tests are positive, or if a cribiform plate injury is suspected clinically, then a CT scan and immediate neurosurgical consultation must be obtained.

Nasal Foreign Bodies

Nasal FBs may present with a straightforward history, but they should be suspected in any case of unilateral nasal obstruction, foul rhinorrhea, or persistent unilateral epistaxis. They are often directly visible, but radiographs will occasionally demonstrate radiopaque FBs that are not otherwise seen. In cooperative children, nasal foreign bodies may be removed in the emergency department as follows:

1. The nasal mucosa should be prepared with a topical spray containing both a vasoconstrictor and an anesthetic agent; 0.25% phenylephrine (Neo-Synephrine) mixed with 4% lidocaine is an effective combination.
2. Using a nasal speculum, the object should be directly visualized.
3. Loose objects may be removed with a suction catheter. Small, irregular objects may be grasped with bayonet or alligator forceps.
4. Small or round objects may be removed if a small hooked instrument is passed behind them, rotated, and withdrawn. Care must be exercised to avoid lodging the object further into the nasopharynx.
5. Difficult objects may also be withdrawn once a #4 Fogarty vascular catheter is passed behind them. The balloon should then be inflated and the object withdrawn. Alternatively, the balloon may act as a buttress while frontal approaches are tried again.

An alternative method of FB removal involves the **positive pressure technique**. Following topical vasoconstrictors, the patient's caregiver gives a puff of air into the child's mouth while occluding the uninvolved nostril. The foreign body is then expelled onto the cheek of the caregiver.

If unsuccessful, ENT consultation is required. Immediate consultation is sought for ill-appearing children and for those whose FBs are at risk of aspiration; all other patients may be seen in 24 h.

Sinusitis

Maxillary sinusitis presents with pain in the infraorbital area, whereas *frontal sinusitis* causes pain in the supraorbital and lower forehead regions. *Ethmoid sinusitis,* which is especially serious in children because of its tendency to spread to the central nervous system, often produces a dull, aching sensation in the retroorbital area. *Sphenoid sinusitis* is extremely uncommon and has vague signs and symptoms. *Chronic sinusitis* often produces local discomfort and a chronic, purulent exudate.

Unfortunately, the physical findings of sinusitis are neither sensitive nor specific. They may include local erythema and warmth, tenderness to palpation and percussion, swollen nasal mucosa with purulent discharge, and diminished transillumination. Radiographs may show sinus opacification, air-fluid levels, or mucosal thickening of at least 6 mm, but they are generally not required in the emergency department.

Treatment of sinusitis includes nasal decongestant sprays such as **oxymetazoline (Afrin)** or **phenylephrine (Neo-Synephrine)** used twice daily for no longer than 3 days. Antibiotic choices for a 14- to 21-day regimen include **ampicillin, amoxicillin-clavulanate (Augmentin)**, or **cephalexin (Keflex)**. Penicillin-allergic patients may use **azithromycin (Zithromax), clarithromycin (Biaxin), doxycycline,** or **trimethoprim-sulfamethoxazole (Bactrim-DS)**. Cool-mist vaporizers, warm facial compresses, and analgesic medications may help to alleviate symptoms. Toxic patients, and those with spread of the infection beyond the sinus cavity, require admission. Treated patients whose symptoms last more than 7 days and those with chronic sinusitis require follow-up with their physician or ENT specialist.

For further reading in *Emergency Medicine: A Comprehensive Study Guide,* 5th ed., see Chap. 231, "Common Disorders of the External, Middle, and Inner Ear," by Anne Urdaneta and Michael Lucchesi; Chap. 232, "Face and Jaw Emergencies," by W. F. Peacock IV; and Chap. 233, "Nasal Emergencies and Sinusitis," by Thomas A. Waters and W.F. Peacock IV.

---

147 | Oral and Dental Emergencies
Burton Bentley II

ORAL PAIN

Tooth Eruption

Eruption of the primary teeth in infants and children may be associated with pain, low-grade fever (37.9°C), diarrhea, and refusal to eat. Other processes should be ruled out, however, before these symptoms are attributed simply to dental eruption. Adequate hydration along with oral analgesics (e.g., acetaminophen) or topical anesthetics (e.g., benzocaine) will usually control the symptoms. Adults may experience pain and local inflammation (i.e., pericoronitis) with the eruption of the third molars. Oral antibiotics (e.g., penicillin or erythromycin) and frequent rinsing of the mouth will temporize symptoms until an oral surgeon can remove the teeth in 1 to 2 days. Superficial incision and drainage is required for abscesses.

Dental Caries

The most common cause of toothache is a carious tooth. Examination sometimes finds a grossly decayed tooth, though frequently there is no visible pathology. Localization is easily accomplished by percussing individual teeth with a tongue blade. Treatment includes oral analgesics and referral to a dentist. Fluctuant oral abscesses from infected teeth require local incision and drainage, oral antibiotics, frequent saline rinses, and follow-up within 24 h.

Postextraction Pain

Pain experienced within 24 h of a tooth extraction, termed *periosteitis,* responds well to analgesics. Severe pain with foul odor and taste 2 to 3 days after an extraction is termed *alveolar osteitis* ("dry socket"). Treatment consists of irrigation of the socket followed by packing the socket with medicated dental packing or 1 in. of iodoform gauze dampened with eugenol (oil of cloves). Dental anesthesia may be required during packing, and antibiotics should be given in severe cases. The patient may be referred to a dentist within 24 h.

Periodontal Abscess

A *periodontal abscess* results from plaque and debris entrapped between the tooth and gingiva. Most cases resolve with oral antibiotics, analgesics, and saline irrigation. Appropriate antibiotic choices include **penicillin VK** 500 mg qid, **clindamycin** 300 mg qid, or **erythromycin** 500 mg qid. Larger abscesses may require incision and drainage. All patients need analgesics and prompt dental referral.

Acute Necrotizing Ulcerative Gingivitis

Acute necrotizing ulcerative gingivitis (ANUG or "trench mouth") is the only periodontal disease in which bacteria actually invade nonnecrotic tissue. It occurs mainly in emotionally stressed adolescents and young adults, but it also presents in malnourished children, HIV-positive adults, and patients with a prior history of ANUG. Examination finds regional lymphadenopathy with edematous and inflamed gingiva, though the hallmark is ulceration and blunting of the interdental papilla with a gray pseudomembrane. Gingival pain, bleeding gums, halitosis, fever, and malaise are associated signs and symptoms. Treatment requires oral **metronidazole** (Flagyl, 250 mg tid) and **chlorhexidine oral rinses** twice daily. Oral analgesics or 2% viscous lidocaine will provide pain relief. Symptomatic improvement is dramatic within 24 h, but dental follow-up is required.

SOFT TISSUE LESIONS OF THE ORAL CAVITY

Oral Candidiasis

Candidal organisms are harbored by 60 percent adults. Actual tissue invasion and clinical manifestations are required for the diagnosis of a candidal infection. Risk factors include extremes of age, immunocompromised states (e.g., AIDS), use of intraoral prosthetic devices, concurrent antibiotic use, and malnutrition. The appearance is typically that of white, curd-like plaques. Treatment is with oral antifungal agents such as **nystatin oral suspension** (500,000 U qid) or **fluconazole** (Diflucan 200 mg bid).

Aphthous Stomatitis

Aphthous stomatitis is a common pattern of intraoral ulceration triggered by cell-mediated immunity. These painful lesions, which are frequently multiple, involve the labial and buccal mucosa and measure from 2 mm to several centimeters in diameter. Treatment consists of topical steroids such as betamethasone syrup or 0.01% dexamethasone elixir used as a mouth rinse. Resolution is often complete within 2 days.

Herpes Gingivostomatitis

Herpes gingivostomatitis causes acute painful ulcerations of the gingiva and mucosal surfaces. Fever, lymphadenopathy, and prodromal tingling often precede the eruption of numerous vesicles which then rupture and form ulcerative lesions. The treatment is palliative, though **antiviral medications** (e.g., acyclovir 400 mg tid; or, valacyclovir 500 mg bid) initiated during the early or prodromal stage may lessen the severity of the lesions.

Herpangina

Herpangina occurs in the summer and autumn and is marked by the sudden onset of a high fever, sore throat, headache, and malaise followed by a diffuse vesicular eruption. The tiny vesicles rapidly rupture to leave painful, shallow ulcers. The soft palate, uvula, and tonsillar pillars are typically affected, while the buccal mucosa, tongue, and gingiva are spared. The course lasts 7 to 10 days and is distinguished from herpes by the lack of gingival involvement.

Hand, Foot, and Mouth Disease

Coxsackievirus infection, predominantly type A16, causes this classic eruption called hand, foot, and mouth disease. Initially, vesicles form on the soft palate, gingiva, tongue, and buccal mucosa. The vesicles then rupture leaving painful ulcers surrounded by red halos. Lesions may also appear on the lateral and dorsal aspects of the fingers and toes, as well as the palms, soles, and buttocks. The rash lasts 5 to 8 days before spontaneous resolution. No specific treatment is required.

Lesions of the Tongue

Erythema Migrans

Erythema migrans, or *geographic tongue,* is a common benign finding marked by multiple, sharply circumscribed zones of erythema predominantly on the tip and lateral borders of the tongue. The lesions are typically asymptomatic, but some may have a burning sensation. No specific treatment is required, though symptomatic lesions may respond to topical fluocinonide gel applied several times daily.

Black Hairy Tongue

Black, hairy tongue, a brown discoloration of unknown etiology, affects only the dorsum of the tongue anterior to the circumvallate papillae. Treatment consists of frequent tongue brushing and avoidance of tobacco, strong mouthwashes, and antibiotics. Symptomatic resolution is usually spontaneous.

OROFACIAL INJURIES

Dental Fractures

In all cases of tooth fracture, lacerated adjacent tissue should be palpated for missing tooth fragments and radiographed if necessary. Regardless of how minor a dental injury may appear, all patients with dental trauma should be warned that there may be an occult injury to the neurovascular supply and that the tooth may subsequently be lost. A painless dental injury may suggest this neurovascular disruption. The Ellis system is used to classify the anatomy of fractured teeth.

Ellis Class 1 fractures involves only the enamel of the tooth. These injuries may be smoothed with an emery board or referred to a dentist for cosmetic repair.

Ells Class 2 fractures expose the underlying pale yellow dentin and provoke thermal and air sensitivity. These are serious fractures, particularly in patients less than 12 years old, since incorrect management increases the chances of infecting the dental pulp. The exposed dentin must be thoroughly dried and promptly covered with either a glass ionomer cement or calcium hydroxide paste (Dycal). The area should then be covered with gauze, aluminum foil, or adhesive-backed dental foil. All patients should avoid extremes of temperature and seek dental care within 24 h. In patients under the age of 12, the protective dentinal layer is thin. A visible blush of pulp under this thin dentinal layer thus indicates that the pulp is at risk and should be treated like an Ellis Class 3 fracture.

Ellis Class 3 fractures expose the dental pulp and are true dental emergencies. They are identified by a red blush of the dentin or a drop of frank blood. If a dentist or maxillofacial surgeon is not immediately available, the tooth may be temporarily covered with either a glass ionomer cement or calcium hydroxide paste until the follow-up visit. Oral analgesics may be needed, but topical anesthetics are contraindicated since they may cause sterile abscesses. Referral to a dentist is needed immediately.

Subluxed, Intruded, and Avulsed Teeth

Dental trauma may result in the loosening of a tooth, termed *subluxation.* Blood in the gingival crevice is also a subtle indicator of trauma. Minimally subluxed teeth heal well in 1 to 2 weeks if the patient maintains a soft diet. Grossly mobile teeth require stabilization by a dentist. The patient may gently bite on gauze to stabilize the tooth while awaiting further evaluation.

Dental *intrusion* occurs when a tooth is forced below the gingiva. Intruded primary ("baby") teeth are allowed to erupt for 6 weeks before considering repositioning. Intruded permanent teeth require surgical repositioning. Failure to diagnose dental intrusion may result in infection and cosmetic deformity.

Dental *avulsion* describes a tooth that has been completely removed from the socket; this is a true dental emergency. If the missing tooth is not located, radiographs must be obtained to rule out dental intrusion or aspiration. *Primary (deciduous) teeth* in children are not replaced since they may ankylose and cause facial deformity. *Permanent teeth* that have been avulsed for less than 3 h must be immediately reimplanted. A percentage point for successful reimplantation is lost for each minute that the tooth is out of the socket. If a patient with an avulsed tooth is being transported, the tooth should be held only by the crown, gently rinsed under running water, and replaced into the socket. If reimplantation is not possible, the best transport medium is Hank's solution, available commercially in the "Save-A-Tooth" kit. Other options, in descending order of preference, include placing the tooth in the patient's mouth to bathe in saliva, placing the tooth in a glass of milk, or wrapping the tooth in wet gauze. Once in the emergency department, the tooth should be gently rinsed; scrubbing damages the delicate periodontal ligaments. If available, the tooth should be placed in Hank's solution for 30 min to restore cell viability. As soon as possible, the socket should be gently cleaned with irrigation to remove clots and the tooth reimplanted using firm pressure. Once replaced, the patient may gently bite on gauze until seen by a dentist who will perform permanent stabilization. It should be noted that even improper reimplantation holds a higher success rate than delayed reimplantation while waiting for an oral surgeon. Alternatively, the tooth may be left in Hank's solution, and the patient can be referred directly to a dentist or oral surgeon.

Oral Lacerations

Lacerations of the lips, oral mucosa, and gingiva are often associated with dentoalveolar trauma. Since stabilization of the dental injury will often require stretching of the soft tissues, it is preferable to repair soft tissues *after* repair of the dental injury. All oral lacerations require adequate tetanus prophylaxis. Prophylactic use of short courses of penicillin or erythromycin may also be considered, though they are not generally required.

Intraoral mucosal lacerations tend to heal poorly and become infected if they are gaping open. Smaller lacerations (< 1 cm) may be left alone. The wound should be inspected for foreign matter (including tooth fragments), debrided as necessary, irrigated, and closed with 4-0 chromic sutures. Laceration of the *maxillary frenulum* does not usually require repair. Lacerations of the *lingual frenulum,* however, often require repair because of vascularity. *Tongue lacerations* greater than 1 cm should be closed with 4-0 silk or chromic sutures. During tongue repairs, care must be taken to carefully approximate the wound edges since failure to do so may lead to a cleft requiring future revision.

P*alate lacerations* may involve the soft or hard palate. Soft palate injuries occur commonly in children who fall with a pointed object in their mouth. These may be treated as puncture wounds and left open to drain. Gaping edges should be loosely approximated, and injuries to the retropharynx and neighboring vascular structures must be considered. Lacerations of the hard palate are difficult to close since the tissue is not very mobile. Closure may be attempted with 4-0 chromic or silk suture on a fine needle. Abrasions will heal by granulation, but a dental emollient (e.g., Orabase) may be prescribed for comfort.

Lip lacerations require meticulous closure. The subcutaneous tissues must be closed with absorbable deep sutures to prevent premature separation when the superficial sutures are removed in 4 to 5 days. The skin is then closed with a 6-0 monofilament material. Failure to exactly reapproximate the edges of the lip at the vermilion border will lead to a noticeable cosmetic deformity. Therefore, when the vermilion border has been lacerated, the first suture should be meticulously placed to align its edges. Lip wounds should be cleansed daily with dilute hydrogen peroxide and covered with antibiotic ointment.

HEMORRHAGE SECONDARY TO EXTRACTION AND SURGERY

Bleeding following dental extraction is usually controlled by direct pressure applied by biting on gauze. Negative pressure from smoking, spitting, and use of straws will increase the amount of hemorrhage.

If bleeding persists, the socket should be suctioned free of clots and direct pressure should be tried again. Biting on a used tea bag may also aid hemostasis because of the effect of tannic acid. If this is unsuccessful, 2% lidocaine with epinephrine should be locally infiltrated into the area of the socket and gingiva followed by reapplication of pressure. A small absorbable gelatin sponge (Gel-Foam) can also be packed into the socket and sutured with a 3-0 silk suture. Failure of the preceding measures warrants a screening coagulation profile and consultation with an oral surgeon. Bleeding following *periodontal* surgery requires immediate consultation with the periodontist since incorrect placement of periodontal packs can result in treatment failure.

For further reading in *Emergency Medicine: A Comprehensive Study Guide,* 5th ed., see Chap. 234, "Oral and Dental Emergencies," by Ronald W. Beaudreau.

148 | Disorders of the Neck and Upper Airway

Burton Bentley II

PHARYNGITIS

Inflammation of the pharynx may be caused by bacteria, viruses, or fungi. Group A beta-hemolytic streptococcus (GABHS) infections account for 15 percent of cases and may result in the nonsuppurative sequelae of acute rheumatic fever and poststreptococcal glomerulonephritis. Sore throat, painful swallowing, and fever are the classic symptoms of GABHS infection. Headache, vomiting, and abdominal pain are commonly associated symptoms. Classic cases demonstrate erythematous tonsils, pharyngeal exudate, and tender anterior cervical lymph nodes. Empiric antibiotic therapy may be commenced when there is a high clinical suspicion of GABHS. Alternatively, a rapid antigen test or throat culture may be used to guide therapy. **Benzathine penicillin (Bicillin LA)** 1.2 million U or oral (PO) **penicillin** 250 mg qid for 10 d] is still the first-line drug of choice, while cephalosporins, macrolides, and clindamycin are appropriate alternatives.

ACUTE UPPER AIRWAY OBSTRUCTION

Airway foreign bodies (FBs) may present in a straightforward manner, or they may have an insidious presentation, such as progressive stridor or recurrent pneumonia. Upper airway FBs may cause stridor and odynophagia with subsequent respiratory arrest. Lower airway FBs, commonly on the right side, may present as cough, wheezing, dyspnea, pneumonia, or respiratory distress.

The stable patient is a candidate for direct inspection of the oropharynx, possibly aided by a laryngoscope and topical anesthesia. Soft tissue radiographs and endoscopy are further diagnostic adjuncts. Equipment for definitive management of the airway and emesis must be available, and extreme care is taken to avoid destabilizing a partial obstruction. Unstable patients may have had the Heimlich maneuver performed in an out-of-hospital setting, but once in the emergency department, a quick attempt at removal with direct laryngoscopy is indicated. Failure at removal may require a surgical airway or a deeply placed double-lumen endotracheal tube to attempt unilateral ventilation of the unaffected lung while preparation is made for emergent bronchoscopy.

LARYNGEAL TRAUMA

Laryngeal injuries may result from blunt or penetrating trauma and have significant morbidity and mortality rates. Patients may present with hoarseness, hemoptysis, dyspnea, dysphagia, aphonia, stridor, or respiratory distress. Physical examination signs include laryngeal swelling, tenderness, anterior neck contusion, altered laryngeal contour, tracheal deviation, or subcutaneous emphysema.

Emergent otolaryngolic consultation is warranted for all patients with signs and symptoms consistent with laryngeal injury. Initially minor laryngeal injuries may progress due to edema and expanding hematomas, and close observation is required. Stable patients may be placed on humidified oxygen while awaiting otolaryngolic consultation. The unstable patient requires aggressive airway management with tracheostomy. If this cannot be performed, gentle endotracheal intubation or cricothyroidotomy may be required; however, these approaches may be extremely difficult due to swelling and subcutaneous emphysema. Antibiotics active against respiratory flora (e.g., **ampicillin-sulbactam**) are given when there is mucosal violation or subcutaneous emphysema. The examination of choice in the stable patient is flexible fiberoptic nasopharyngolaryngoscopy, but computed tomography (CT) scanning also may be utilized. In the case of massive trauma, immediate tracheostomy and neck exploration will be required.

EPIGLOTTITIS

Epiglottitis is an acute life-threatening supraglottic infection occurring in all age groups, but predominantly in children ages 1 to 5. Pediatric epiglottitis progresses over a 12- to 24-h period and may include fever, anxiety, sore throat, dysphagia, drooling, toxic appearance, or respiratory arrest. Adult epiglottitis often presents with hours to days of dysphagia and throat pain that is out of proportion to the clinical examination findings.

In unstable patients, especially children, all diagnostic procedures are deferred until the patient is in the operating room with an otolaryngologist. Cooperative, stable patients with suspected epiglottitis should undergo indirect laryngoscopy; on occasion, the epiglottis of a calm child can be visualized with a tongue blade alone. A soft tissue lateral neck radiograph may show an edematous ("thumbprint") epiglottis with ballooning of the hypopharynx and loss of the vallecula.

Treatment consists of **oxygen**, **aggressive airway management**, and antibiotics. Parenteral antibiotic choices include **cefotaxime**, **ceftriaxone**, or **ampicillin-sulbactam**. Aztreonam or chloramphenicol can be used in penicillin-allergic patients. If there is any contact in the household less than 4 years old, all nonpregnant household members must receive rifampin prophylaxis. Steroids are controversial but may treat airway edema. The stable pediatric patient is treated with endotracheal intubation in the operating room. Stable adults are often treated in the same manner, but selected cases may be managed in the intensive care unit without intubation. The unstable patient may be temporized with a bag-valve mask, but a definitive airway will be required. This is preferably performed in the operating room, and an endotracheal tube that is 0.5 to 1.0 mm smaller than usual is used. If endotracheal intubation is unsuccessful, children under 8 years of age may require needle cricothyroidotomy, and those over 8 may require standard, open cricothyroidotomy. An otolaryngologist must be consulted for emergent tracheostomy.

PERITONSILLAR ABSCESS

Peritonsillar abscess occurs predominantly in teenagers and young adults and is often preceded by a throat infection. Presenting symptoms may include fever, sore throat, drooling, muffled voice, trismus, dysphagia, otalgia, or foul breath. Classic physical examination signs include a unilaterally enlarged tonsil with swelling of the anterior tonsillar pillar and contralateral deviation of the uvula. Advanced cases may have airway obstruction, pulmonary aspiration, or mediastinitis.

In stable patients, needle aspiration is both diagnostic and therapeutic, and provides resolution of trismus and odynophagia. These patients are then discharged home on broad-spectrum antistaphylococcal antibiotics such as amoxicillin-clavulanate. The procedure must be performed only by individuals skilled in the technique, and therefore most cases require immediate otolaryngologic consultation. Patients who are toxic, uncooperative, or unable to be successfully aspirated require parenteral antibiotics and drainage under general anesthesia. Ampicillin-sulbactam, clindamycin, or cefotaxime plus metronidazole are the antibiotics of choice.

RETROPHARYNGEAL ABSCESS

Retropharyngeal abscess is a disease predominantly of children less than 5 years old, but it also occurs in adults. Signs include fever, odynophagia, neck swelling, drooling, torticollis, meningismus, and possibly stridor. The lateral neck radiograph frequently shows prevertebral soft tissue swelling that exceeds one-half the width of the adjacent vertebral body. CT scanning with contrast is useful in differentiating cellulitis from abscess and in defining the extent of the infection.

Emergency department treatment consists of meticulous airway management and parenteral antibiotics. Emergent otolaryngologic consultation for operative drainage is required.

PARAPHARYNGEAL ABSCESS

The parapharyngeal space extends lateral to the pharynx from the base of the skull to the hyoid. Abscesses in this area may result from local infection, trauma, or dental procedures. Presenting complaints may include fever, pain on neck movement, sore throat, dysphagia, or drooling. Physical examination often finds cervical adenopathy, pharyngitis, torticollis, and bulging of the pharyngeal wall. Lateral neck radiographs may show retropharyngeal swelling, and CT scanning helps to confirm involvement of the parapharyngeal area.

All patients require parenteral broad-spectrum antibiotics, such as **ampicillin-sulbactam**. Emergent otolaryngologic consultation is mandatory for possible operative drainage. Patients in respiratory distress should be orally intubated with extreme care, and it is preferable to establish a surgical airway in the operating room.

For further reading in *Emergency Medicine: A Comprehensive Study Guide,* 5th ed., see Chap. 235, "Disorders of the Neck and Upper Airway," by Theresa A. Hackeling and Rudolph J. Triana, Jr.

DISORDERS OF THE SKIN

149 | Dermatologic Emergencies

William J. Brady

EXFOLIATIVE DERMATITIS

Exfoliative dermatitis—a cutaneous reaction to a drug, chemical, or underlying disease state—occurs when most or all of the skin is involved with a scaling erythema leading subsequently to exfoliation. Etiologies responsible for exfoliative dermatitis include (in decreasing order of incidence) generalized flares of preexisting skin disease (e.g., psoriasis, atopic and seborrheic dermatitides, lichen planus, pemphigus foliaceus, etc.), contact dermatitis, malignancy, and medications or chemicals.

Clinical Features

Patients may present with either acute, acute on chronic, or chronic disease. The acute form is encountered most often in cases involving medications, contact allergens, or malignancy while the chronic variety usually is related to an underlying cutaneous disease. Patients may complain of pain, pruritus, tightening of the skin, a chilling sensation of the skin, fever, nausea, vomiting, weight loss, and fatigue. The physical examination may show generalized warmth and erythroderma, scaling with desiccation, and exfoliation of the skin, as well as fever and other signs of systemic toxicity. High-output congestive heart failure (CHF) may be noted due to extensive cutaneous vasodilation in poorly compensated individuals. Chronic findings include dystrophic nails, thinning of body hair, alopecia, and hypo- or hyperpigmentation. Acute complicating factors include fluid and electrolyte losses, secondary infection, and excessive heat loss with hypothermia.

Diagnosis and Differential

Diffuse erythema with desiccation or exfoliation must be considered exfoliative dermatitis until proven otherwise. The diagnosis is confirmed with dermatologic consultation and skin biopsy. A careful search for etiologic factors is mandatory. Dermatologic syndromes to consider in the differential include acute generalized exanthematous pustulosis, toxic epidermal necrolysis, primary blistering disorders, and the toxic infectious erythemas as well as the general ichthyoses (dry skin conditions).

Emergency Department Care and Disposition

1. Emergency department management includes attention to the ABCs with appropriate correction of any life-threatening abnormality. After resuscitation is completed, treatment of secondary infection, correction of electrolyte disorders, control of body temperature, and management of CHF are clinical issues to address.
2. Dermatologic treatment includes **oral antihistamines, steroids** (topical or systemic), oatmeal baths, and bland lotions. For patients with a new presentation of or a significant recurrence of exfoliative dermatitis, admission with dermatologic consultation is advised. For patients with chronic disease with mild recurrence who are not systemically ill, outpatient treatment with prompt dermatologic follow-up is reasonable.

ERYTHEMA MULTIFORME

Erythema multiforme (EM) is an acute inflammatory skin disease with significant associated morbidity and mortality. EM presents across a spectrum of disease, ranging from a mild papular eruption (EM minor) to the severe vesiculobullous form with mucous membrane involvement and systemic toxicity (EM major or the Stevens-Johnson's syndrome). EM strikes all ages with the highest incidence in young adults, affects males twice as often as females, and occurs commonly in the spring and fall. Etiologies include infection, drugs, malignancy, rheumatologic disorders, physical agents, and pregnancy. Medications (adults) and infections (children) are the major etiologic factors.

Clinical Features

Symptoms include malaise, arthralgias, myalgias, fever, diffuse pruritus, and a generalized burning sensation, which may be noted many days prior to skin abnormalities. Signs noted on exam primarily involve the skin and mucosal surfaces, including erythematous papules and maculopapules, target (iris) lesion, urticarial plaques, vesicles, bullae, vesiculobullous lesions, and mucosal (oral, conjunctival, respiratory, and genitourinary) erosions. Significant systemic toxicity also may be noted on initial presentation. Patients are at risk for significant fluid and electrolyte deficiencies as well as secondary infection. Recurrence is noted especially involving cases where infection or medication were involved.

Diagnosis and Differential

The diagnosis of EM is based upon the simultaneous presence of lesions with multiple morphologies at times with mucous membrane involvement. The target lesion is highly suggestive of EM. Urticarial plaques are frequently misdiagnosed as allergic reactions. The differential diagnosis includes herpetic infections, vasculitis, toxic epidermal necrolysis, primary blistering disorders, and toxic infectious erythemas.

Emergency Department Care and Disposition

1. Patients may present in extremis; as such, attention to the standard resuscitative therapies is required.
2. Patients with localized papular disease without systemic manifestation and mucous membrane involvement may be managed as outpatients with dermatologic consultation. **Topical steroids** to noneroded skin as well as oral **analgesics** and **antihistamines** are recommended.
3. For patients with extensive disease or systemic toxicity, inpatient therapy in a critical care setting with immediate dermatologic consultation is advised. Paverterol analgesics and antihistamines are required in addition to intensive management of potential fluid, electrolyte, infectious, nutritional, and thermoregulatory issues. Systemic steroids are recommended by some authorities. **Diphenhydramine and lidocaine rinses** are useful for painful oral lesions; cool **Burrow's solution** (aqueous aluminum sulfate and calcium acetate) compresses are applied to blistered regions. Ophthalmologic care is advised if any eye complaints or findings are noted.

TOXIC EPIDERMAL NECROLYSIS

Toxic epidermal necrolysis (TEN) is an explosive, potentially fatal, inflammatory skin disease, striking all age and gender groups equally. Potential etiologies include medications, chemicals, infections, and immunologic factors. Medications are by far the major etiologic group; infectious triggers are much less commonly involved compared to EM.

Clinical Features

Patients may complain of malaise, anorexia, myalgias, arthralgias, fever, painful skin, and upper respiratory infection symptoms; these symptoms may be present prior to the development of the skin abnormality. Physical examination findings include a warm, tender erythema, flaccid bullae, a positive Nikolsky's sign, erosions with exfoliation, mucous membrane (oral, conjunctival, respiratory, and genitourinary) lesions, and systemic toxicity. Acute and chronic complications are similar to those encountered in EM major patients.

Diagnosis and Differential

The clinical diagnosis is often possible at presentation based on the following features: diffuse, tender erythema; mucous membrane involvement; areas of denuded skin with adjacent large bullous lesions; a positive Nikolsky's sign; and systemic toxicity. Ultimate diagnosis is made via skin biopsy. The differential includes toxic-infectious erythemas, exfoliative drug eruptions, primary blistering disorders, Kawasaki's syndrome, and EM major (Stevens-Johnson's syndrome).

Emergency Department Care and Disposition

Management of all patients with TEN is best performed in a critical care setting such as a burn unit. Attention to adequate cardiorespiratory function is essential; correction of fluid, electrolyte, and infectious complications are early treatment considerations. Immediate dermatologic consultation is required.

TOXIC INFECTIOUS ERYTHEMAS

A number of infectious syndromes caused by toxigenic bacteria with toxin-mediated dermatologic manifestations have been described, including toxic shock syndrome (TSS), streptococcal toxic shock syndrome (STSS), and staphylococcal scaled-skin syndrome (SSSS). TSS is a multisystem illness presenting with fever, shock, and erythroderma followed by desquamation associated with toxigenic *Staphylococcus aureus*. STSS, a syndrome caused by *Streptococcus* organisms, is characterized by multiple organ systems with fever, hypotension, and skin findings. The majority of cases of STSS are associated with soft-tissue infections—cellulitis, myositis, and fasciitis were the most common presenting diagnoses. SSSS develops in previously healthy children usually aged < 2 years of age in both outbreaks as well as the sporadic case. The toxin exfoliatin is responsible for the erythroderma and desquamation, while the patient's immune response to the antigenic toxin results in fever and irritability.

Clinical Features

The manifestations of TSS range from a mild, trivial disease, often misdiagnosed as a viral syndrome, to a rapidly progressive, potentially fatal, multisystem illness. Criteria for the diagnosis of TSS are defined in the case definition.

Major Criteria

1. Fever: Temperature > 38.5°C (102°F)
2. Rash: Erythroderma (localized or diffuse) followed by peripheral desquamation
3. Mucous membrane: Hyperemia of oral and vaginal mucosa and of conjunctiva
4. Hypotension: History of dizziness, orthostatic changes, or hypotension.

Multisystem Manifestations

1. CNS: Altered mentation without focal neurologic signs
2. Cardiovascular: Distributive shock, CHF, dysrhythmias
3. Pulmonary: Adult respiratory distress syndrome
4. Gastrointestinal: Vomiting and diarrhea
5. Hepatic: Elevations in bilirubin, alkaline phosphatase, and the transaminases
6. Renal: Blood urea nitrogen (BUN) and/or creatinine elevations, abnormal urinary sediment, oliguria
7. Hematologic: Thrombocytopenia or thrombocytosis, anemia, leukopenia or leukocytosis
8. Musculoskeletal: Myalgias, arthralgias, rhabdomyolysis
9. Metabolic: Hypocalcemia, hypophosphatemia
10. Absence of other etiological agent

The diagnosis of TSS requires the presence of all four major criteria and three or more indications of multisystem involvement. TSS is also identified by its sudden, violent onset and rapid progression to multisystem dysfunction.

The clinical presentation of STSS is similar to that of TSS; in fact, similar criteria may be used for the diagnosis. The majority of STSS cases have associated soft tissue infection (in contrast to TSS); an exhaustive search for the site of infection is warranted.

The presentation of SSSS can be divided into three phases: (*a*) initial and erythroderma, (*b*) exfoliative, and (*c*) desquamation and recovery. Initially, there is a sudden appearance of a tender erythroderma, usually diffuse, although localized disease is noted. The involved skin may have a sandpaper texture similar to the rash of scarlet fever. The exfoliative stage begins on the second day of the illness with a wrinkling and peeling of the previously erythematous skin; Nikolsky's sign is found. Large, flaccid, fluid-filled bullae and vesicles then appear. These lesions easily rupture and are shed in large sheets; the underlying tissue resembles scalded skin and rapidly desiccates. During the exfoliative phase, the patient is often febrile and irritable. After 3 to 5 days of illness, the involved skin desquamates, leaving normal skin in 7 to 10 days.

Diagnosis and Differential

For TSS and STSS, fever and hypotension with associated erythroderma should suggest the diagnosis. The differential diagnosis is broad and includes scarlet fever, Rocky Mountain spotted fever, leptospirosis, rubeola, meningococcemia, SSSS, Kawasaki's disease, TEN, Stevens-Johnson's syndrome, gram-negative sepsis, and exfoliative drug eruptions. Infants and toddlers with fever and diffuse erythroderma suggest SSSS. The differential diagnosis for SSSS includes TEN, TSS, exfoliative drug eruptions, staphylococcal scarlet fever, and localized bullous impetigo.

Emergency Department Care and Disposition

1. Management of patients with TSS and STSS is dictated by the severity of their illness. As in any patient presenting in extremis, the emergency physician must perform a rapid, thorough review of the ABCs, insuring a stable airway and ventilatory status, as well as an adequate hemodynamic state.
2. After patient stabilization, the next management goal involves identification and removal of any potential source of infection and associated toxin; **broad-spectrum antibiotic therapy** is indicated.
3. Last, patients must be monitored closely for evidence of organ system dysfunction. The vast majority of patients with TSS requires hospital admission; patients who are critically ill are best managed in the intensive care setting.
4. Management of patients with SSSS includes fluid resuscitation and correction of electrolyte abnormalities, as well as identification and treatment of the source of the toxigenic *Staphylococcus* with the appropriate antistaphylococcal antibiotic, preferably a **penicillinase-resistant penicillin.** Most patients, with the exception of neonates, do not require topical therapies. The newborn may be treated with topical sulfadiazine or its equivalent. Wet dressings are not recommended. A select few patients are treated on an outpatient basis with oral antibiotics, providing a motivated caretaker is involved and close medical follow-up is arranged.

BULLOUS DISEASES

Pemphigus vulgaris (PV) is a generalized, mucocutaneous, autoimmune, blistering eruption with a grave prognosis characterized by intraepidermal acantholytic blistering. Bullous pemphigoid (BP) is a generalized mucocutaneous blistering disease of the elderly, with an average age of 70 years at the time of initial diagnosis. Both PV and BP are characterized by the presence of unique antigen and autoantibody systems.

Clinical Features

The primary lesions of PV are vesicles or bullae that vary in diameter from < 1 cm to several centimeters, commonly first affecting the head, trunk, and mucous membranes. The blisters are usually clear and tense, originating from normal skin or atop an erythematous or urticarial plaque. Within 2 to 3 days, the bullae become turbid and flaccid with rupture soon following, producing painful, denuded areas. These erosions are slow to heal and prone to secondary infection. Nikolsky's sign is positive in PV and absent in other autoimmune blistering diseases. Mucous membranes are affected in 95 percent of PV patients. BP is characterized by tense blisters (up to 10 cm in diameter) arising from either normal skin or from erythematous or urticarial plaques; frequent sites of involvement include intertriginous and flexura areas. Ulceration with tissue loss follows blister formation. Lesions of the oral cavity occur in BP in 40 percent of cases, but with less consistency and severity than in PV. Because the blisters in the oral cavity rupture very easily and heal without scarring, involvement in the mouth is often overlooked.

Diagnosis and Differential

Diagnosis is suspected with the appearance of the blistering lesions and confirmed by skin biopsy and immunofluorescence testing. The differential diagnosis of PV and BP includes all of those diseases that can present with primary skin blistering, including TEN, EM, other autoimmune blistering diseases, burns, severe contact dermatitis, bullous diabeticorum, and friction blisters.

Emergency Department Care and Disposition

1. Initial care of patients with PV should be performed on an inpatient basis with early dermatologic consultation; initiation of high-dose systemic steroid and other immunosuppressive therapies is best performed on elderly patients in the hospital.
2. The cutaneous surfaces involved with blisters or eroded areas should be treated as burns with the application of **silver sulfadiazine cream** or antibiotic ointments with clean dressings; pain originating from oral lesions may be partially relieved with

soothing mouth washes (1:1 mixture of diphenhydramine elixir with Mylanta) or with viscous lidocaine; and oral hygiene should be maintained via frequent mouth washes with normal saline or chlorhexidine gluconate. Close observation and rapid treatment with appropriate antibiotics for superficial infection is imperative.

3. Treatment with **corticosteroids** results in the complete recovery of some PV patients and control of the disease in others if the therapy is continued. BP is also managed by **systemic steroids.** Mild disease, arbitrarily defined as less than 20 lesions, usually responds to lower doses of steroids (20 to 40 mg of prednisone daily), while more widespread illnesses require higher doses of steroids.

For further reading in *Emergency Medicine: A Comprehensive Study Guide,* 5th ed., see Chap. 241, "Generalized Skin Disorders," by William J. Brady and Daniel J. DeBehnke.

---

150 | Other Dermatologic Disorders

William J. Brady

PHOTOSENSITIVITY

Patients with *sunburn* may have minimal discomfort or be in extreme pain with extensive blistering. A tender, warm erythema is seen in sun-exposed areas; vesiculation may result, representing a second-degree burn injury. Diagnosis is suspected in patients who have frequented outdoors with significant ultraviolet (UV) light exposure. Sunburns are treated symptomatically with tepid baths, oral analgesics, and burn wound care including topical antibiotics to blisters.

Exogenous photosensitivity results from either the topical application or the ingestion of an agent that increases the skin's sensitivity to UV light. The topical photosensitizers usually result in a cutaneous eruption at the site of application once UV light is applied. Furocoumarins—lime juice, various fragrances, figs, celery, and parsnips when *topically applied*—are the most common group of agents causing photoeruptions; other topical photosensitizers include para-aminobenzoic acid (PABA) esters and topical psoralens. Numerous medications also can result in eruption, which frequently involves all sun-exposed areas. The exogenous photoeruption is similar to a severe sunburn reaction, often with blistering. A linear appearance of the rash suggests an externally applied substance. The diagnosis is based on identifying the offending agent. Initial management is similar to the sunburn reaction, including the avoidance of the sun until the eruption has cleared. The causative agent should be discontinued, if clinically feasible.

CONTACT DERMATITIS

Contact dermatitis may be a primary irritant reaction or an allergic-mediated event. Certain allergens may be applied to facial skin either via an aerosolization or direct physical contact. Agents capable of causing an aerosolized reaction include rhus (poison ivy and oak) when the plant has been burned. Examples of directly applied agents include nickel, nail polishes, toothpaste, preservatives in cosmetics, contact lens solutions, eyeglasses, and hair care products.

Allergic contact dermatitis resulting from an aerosolized allergen presents with erythema or scaling, at times accompanied by blistering. The involvement is diffuse with upper and lower eyelids affected. Direct application of the allergen produces similar findings on the most sensitive skin areas, such as the eyelids. For therapy, **corticosteroids** (topical or oral depending upon the severity) are often required. Only low-potency topical corticosteroids (hydrocortisone 2.5%) should be used on the face; creams or ointments should be used initially. Often times, extensive and severe periocular involvement requires oral prednisone. Oral **antihistamines** are also useful in reducing pruritus.

ALOPECIA

The causes of hair loss are numerous and are typically divided into scarring and nonscarring alopecia. The causative syndromes include the nonscarring (secondary syphilis, alopecia areata, contact dermatitis, and thyroid and medication-related disorders) and scarring (tinea capitis, zoster infection, discoid lupus, sarcoidosis, scleroderma, malignancy) syndromes.

Tinea capitis is a dermatophyte infection of the scalp and is most commonly seen in children. Areas of alopecia with broken hair shafts with peripheral scaling are noted; the alopecia is patchy and usually nonscarring. Areas of boggy, tender, indurated plaques with superficial pustules and overlying alopecia may be noted. Diagnosis is based on a KOH preparation or positive fungal culture. After a diagnosis is established, current therapy includes oral **griseofulvin** (15 mg/kg/d two times daily for 6 weeks) as the first-line agent; topical treatment alone is not effective. Patients should be reevaluated after 6 weeks of treatment. **Nizoral shampoo** at least three times per week is recommended in addition to griseofulvin. Other family members, especially children, should be evaluated as well.

Alopecia areata presents with a patchy alopecia; loose round patches of hair are lost leaving behind a normal scalp that lacks scaling or scarring. Any hair-bearing area may be affected, but the scalp is the most common site of involvement. Diagnosis is based on clinical examination. Alopecia areata usually resolves spontaneously within 2 to 6 months, particularly if the initial involvement is mild; extensive disease is less likely to resolve. If the disease is extensive, rapidly progressive, or of significant cosmetic concern, patients should be referred to a dermatologist for treatment. No specific emergency-department-based therapy is available.

PARONYCHIA

Paronychia, an inflammation of the nail folds, may be acute or chronic in nature. Acute paronychia (AP) results from trauma to the cuticle or nail fold (allows bacteria or yeast to enter) combined with excessive, prolonged water exposure. The most frequent organisms found in the acute version are *Staphylococcus* and *Streptococcus*. Chronic paronychia (CP) results from continued water exposure, which prevents the reforming of the cuticle, thus providing an environment for colonization of the area with bacteria or yeast.

AP presents with rapid swelling, tenderness, and erythema of the nail fold; an abscess may develop with expressible pus. Cellulitis may be seen adjacent to the nail with streaking. CP is less abrupt in onset; the associated swelling, tenderness, and erythema will wax and wane. Retraction of the cuticle is prominent in chronic paronychia, and the nail plate usually has horizontal ridging.

In AP, an abscess is usually present; early treatment includes **drainage** of the affected area as follows: (*a*) a number 15 scalpel blade is inserted between the nail plate and the cuticle (no incision through the nail fold); (*b*) the nail fold is then gently massaged to aid in drainage; and (*c*) a gauze wick may be inserted between the nail plate and the cuticle to aid in drainage (must be removed in 24 to 48 h). Warm tap water soaks for 10 to 15 min should be performed three times a day for 1 to 2 days. In acute cases with related cellulitis, oral antibiotics such as **cephalexin** or **dicloxacillin** should be administered. After drainage, the chronic case should be kept as dry as possible; drying agents are the treatment of choice (2 to 4% thymol in absolute ethanol solution can be applied four times daily). Topical antifungal solutions, such as **clotrimazole,** can be used two times daily as well; in recalcitrant cases, CP may require oral antifungal therapy with **fluconazole** or **itraconazole** with referral to a dermatologist. In both acute and chronic forms, patients should be counseled on the avoidance of all trauma to the nail area, as well as prolonged exposure to moisture.

TINEA INFECTIONS

Tinea pedis is a fungal infection of the feet, also known as "athlete's foot." *Tinea manuum,* a dermatophyte infection of the hand, is often unilateral and frequently associated with tinea pedis. Tinea pedis may present in several distinct forms. The most common form is the interdigital presentation, manifested by maceration and scaling in the web spaces between the toes; ulcerations may be present in severe cases with secondary infection. The second type, which is the form seen in tinea manuum, is characterized by chronic, dry scaling with minimal inflammation on the palmar or plantar surfaces; it often extends to the medial and lateral aspects of the feet but not the dorsal surface. Maceration between the toes is common. Onychomycosis may be present. The third type of fungal infection presents as an acute, painful, pruritic vesicular eruption on the palms or soles; erythema is a prominent feature while the nails and web spaces are usually spared.

Identification of fungal elements on a potassium hydroxide preparation or with fungal culture may be required if the diagnosis in uncertain. Nonbullous tinea pedis and manuum can be treated with topical antifungal agents, such as **clotrimazole**, **miconazole**, **ketoconazole**, **or econazole**. Treatment should be continued for 1 week after clearing has occurred. Nail infections also should be treated with oral antifungal agents (**itraconazole**, **fluconazole**, or **terbinafine**) as well. Bullous tinea pedis often does not respond to topical treatment; oral antifungal treatment is necessary.

Tinea cruris, a fungal infection of the groin commonly called "jock itch," is very common in males. Erythema with a peripheral annular, scaly edge is seen. The rash extends onto the inner thighs and the buttocks and spares the penis and scrotum—a feature that is important in distinguishing tinea cruris from other eruptions in the groin, as most other eruptions will affect the scrotum. The diagnosis is established by a positive KOH examination. Antifungal creams such as **clotrimazole, ketoconazole, or econazole** two times daily is the initial treatment of choice. Antifungal powders should be used on a daily basis to prevent recurrences.

CANDIDA INTERTRIGO

Candidal infections of the skin favor moist, occluded areas of the body. Although any skin fold may be involved, superficial candida infections are commonly seen in the diaper area of infants, the vulva and groin of women, the glans penis (balanitis) in uncircumcised males, and the inframammary and pannus folds of obese patients. Antibiotic therapy, systemic corticosteroid therapy, urinary or fecal incontinence, immunocompromised states, and obesity are predisposing factors. Women with vulvar or inner thigh involvement will often have vaginal candidiasis as well.

Clinical Features

The typical presentation is erythema and maceration with surrounding small erythematous papules or pustules; the satellite pustules are a characteristic finding in differentiating between candida intertrigo and other inflammatory disorders affecting the skin folds. Patients will complain of burning or itching.

Diagnosis and Differential

The rim of satellite pustules helps to distinguish candida intertrigo from other eruptions of the skin folds. A KOH preparation of the pustules or a leading edge scale may demonstrate short hyphae and spores; however, these may be difficult to find in cases with just erythema and maceration.

Emergency Department Care and Disposition

Astringent solutions such as **aluminum acetate** assist in drying wet, inflamed eruptions. A topical antifungal cream such as **clotrimazole, ketoconazole, or econazole** should be applied two times daily. The addition of **hydrocortisone 1% cream** two times daily can speed symptomatic relief and healing. Patients should be instructed to keep the involved areas dry and cool. Follow-up care with a primary care provider or dermatologist should be arranged.

For further reading in *Emergency Medicine: A Comprehensive Study Guide,* 5th ed., see Chap. 238, "Disorders of the Face and Scalp"; Chap. 239, "Disorders of the Hands, Feet, and Extremities;" and Chap. 240, "Disorders of the Groin and Skin Folds," by Lisa May.

TRAUMA

151 | Initial Approach to the Trauma Patient

Charles J. Havel, Jr.

Trauma is the leading cause of death up to the age of 44 years. All emergency physicians must be skilled in trauma resuscitation and initiating a team approach to patient management in concert with the emergency department (ED) staff and the surgeon on call.

Clinical Features

Trauma patients sustain infinite types and combinations of injuries. Many will present with obviously abnormal vital signs, neurologic deficit, or other gross evidence of trauma. These signs must prompt a thorough search for the specific underlying injuries and rapid interventions to correct the abnormalities. Nonspecific signs such as tachycardia, tachypnea, or mild alterations in consciousness must similarly be presumed to signify serious injury until proven otherwise, and these aggressively evaluated and treated. Furthermore, without signs of significant trauma, the mechanism of injury may suggest potential problems and these also should be pursued assiduously.

Diagnosis and Differential

The diagnosis in trauma begins with a history that includes the mechanism and sites of apparent injury. Other pertinent details are the blood loss at the scene and damage to any vehicles or types of weapons involved. The primary survey (A-B-C-D-E), including the assessment of a complete set of vital signs, is then initiated, characterized by the orderly identification and concomitant treatment of the most lethal injuries. First, *A*irway patency and *B*reathing is assessed by means of examination of the head and neck for gag reflex, airway obstruction, tracheal deviation, quality of breath sounds, flail chest, crepitation, sucking chest wounds, and fractures of the sternum. Problems such as tension pneumothorax, pneumothorax, hemothorax, and misplacement of the endotracheal tube are identified and immediately treated before proceeding further. Circulatory status is evaluated via vital signs and cardiac monitoring. Sites of obvious bleeding, indications of shock, and signs of cardiac tamponade (Beck's triad of hypotension, muffled heart sounds, and elevated venous pressure) are all identified. Finally, the primary survey concludes with a brief neurologic examination for Disability using the Glasgow Coma Scale, pupil size and reactivity, and motor function assessment. The patient is then completely Exposed and prepared for the secondary survey.

The secondary survey is a rapid but thorough head-to-toe examination to identify all injuries and to set priorities for care. Resuscitation and frequent monitoring of vital signs continue throughout this process. Evidence for significant head injury, e.g., skull and facial fractures, is sought, and the pupils rechecked. The neck, chest, and abdominal examinations are completed and the stability of the pelvis assessed. Following this, x-rays of the lateral cervical spine, chest, and pelvis are ordered, as appropriate for the scenario. The genitourinary system is evaluated by external inspection, a rectal examination done, and a urethrogram ordered for suspected urethral injury (meatal blood present or the prostate displaced); otherwise, a urinary catheter is placed and the urine obtained, checked for blood, and a pregnancy test ordered for female patients of childbearing age. Vaginal blood on a bimanual exam is an indication for a speculum examination. Patients must be log-rolled, while maintaining cervical spine stabilization, for examination of the back. Extremities are checked for soft tissue injury and fracture. A more thorough neurologic examination is completed.

After the secondary survey, laboratory studies are ordered as needed. Additional radiologic studies such as a cystogram, intravenous pyelogram, aortogram, or computed tomography (CT) scan of the head or abdomen are considered. Diagnostic peritoneal lavage is preferred over the CT scan to evaluate the hemodynamically unstable patient for intraabdominal bleeding. In some centers, the Focused Abdominal Sonogram for Trauma (FAST) is used for the rapid bedside identification of free intraperitoneal fluid. This includes examination for pericardial fluid collections. If fluid resuscitation has not been achieved at this time by crystalloid or blood administration, transfer to the operating room for exploration should be considered.

Emergency Department Care and Disposition

1. The ED management of trauma patients begins before patient arrival. A team captain and assistants with defined roles are assigned, a prehospital history is acquired, and at least 2 U of O-negative blood are obtained. Equipment for monitoring,

airway management, IV fluid administration, and laboratory evaluation should be ready.

2. At the outset of the primary survey, *A*irway patency is assured. A **chin lift** may initially help in opening the airway; **suctioning** may remove foreign material, blood, loose tissue, or avulsed teeth. Nasopharyngeal or oropharyngeal **airways** can be useful adjuncts. **Tracheal intubation** using a rapid sequence technique is indicated for patients with altered mental status including severe agitation or those who for any reason are unable to maintain an open airway on their own. In cases of extensive facial trauma or when tracheal intubation is indicated but cannot be accomplished in another way, **cricothyrotomy** or another advanced technique may be the airway management procedure of choice.

3. During the evaluation of *B*reathing, **100% oxygen** is administered by mask or endotracheal tube. Suspected tension pneumothorax is treated immediately with **needle decompression** followed by **tube thoracostomy.** For large hemothoraces, consideration may be given to **autotransfusion** and **immediate operative exploration** for initial chest tube output of ≥ 1500 mL of blood. For intubated patients who are noted to have unilateral (especially right-sided) decreased or absent breath sounds, proper tube placement must be confirmed or reestablished. The presence of a flail chest may mandate **tracheal intubation** to ventilate patients adequately. Sucking chest wounds require placement of an **occlusive dressing** followed by **chest tube placement.**

4. Management of *C*irculation requires placement of at least **2 peripheral large-bore intravenous lines**, with central lines initially used only if adequate peripheral access cannot be accomplished. **Two liters of warm crystalloid** is administered as rapidly as possible to treat shock followed by **O-negative or type specific blood** as required. Severe external hemorrhage should be managed with **compression** at the bleeding site.

5. Patients with *D*isability and evidence for intracranial injury on examination may benefit from **tracheal intubation** for airway protection. *E*xposure of patients facilitates the remainder of the management providing that measures to prevent hypothermia are taken.

6. Interventions are undertaken during the secondary survey to control problems as they are discovered. Bleeding from scalp lacerations can be controlled with **Raney clips**. Tamponade of severe epistaxis may be achieved with **balloon compression devices**. **Reduction of fractures** may prevent distal neurovascular compromise; all fractures should be **splinted**. A **gastric tube** should be inserted (orally in the setting of facial fractures)

and a **urinary catheter** placed, if not contraindicated. **Tetanus prophylaxis** must be assured; an antibiotic such as **cefotetan** 2 g IV is indicated for possible ruptured abdominal viscus, vaginal, or rectal lacerations; open skeletal fractures treated with **cephalexin** 2 g IV or similar coverage with consideration given to the addition of extra coverage for particularly contaminated injuries. Intravenous **mannitol** 0.5 to 1.0 mg/kg should be available and considered for acute neurologic deterioration. Potential closed spinal cord injuries are treated with **methylprednisolone** 30 mg/kg IV bolus over 15 min, followed 45 min later by an infusion of 5.4 mg/kg/h for 24 to 48 h. Patients with pelvic fractures and signs of persistent hemorrhage may benefit from **pelvic arteriography and embolization.**

7. Upon completion of the secondary survey, options for disposition of patients are to move to the operating room, admit to the hospital, or transfer to another facility. Ideally, the trauma surgeon or surgeon on-call is present for the secondary survey and can at that point assume primary responsibility. If transfer is to be made, the resuscitating physician must relay all pertinent information to the accepting physician. Complete records including flow sheets documenting vital signs, intake and output, and neurologic status, laboratory study results, and x-rays should be sent with patients. Advanced life-support personnel must accompany patients during transport.

For further reading in *Emergency Medicine: A Comprehensive Study Guide,* 5th ed., see Chap. 243, "Initial Approach to Trauma," by Edward E. Cornwell III.

---

152 | Pediatric Trauma
Charles J. Havel, Jr.

Trauma is the most common cause of death and disability in children more than 1 year of age. While trauma management priorities are similar to those for adults, important differences in anatomy, physiology, and psychology dictate some modification to the evaluation and treatment of injured pediatric patients. An additional factor to be considered in the evaluation of these patients is the possibility of nonaccidental trauma (child abuse).

Clinical Features

Emergency physicians must be aware of subtle variations in the presentation of injured children. As obligate nose breathers, infants less than 6 months of age with facial trauma or bleeding into the nasopharynx will have significant respiratory distress. A difference in the mechanics of breathing in children results in the early appearance of tachypnea and accessory muscle use in dyspneic patients. Nasal flaring, grunting, and retractions are also signs that should be noted. The physiology of shock in children causes tachycardia to be the most sensitive and earliest sign of volume loss; conversely, hypotension is a late and, therefore, ominous finding. Other important signs of hemorrhage are increased capillary refill time, decreased level of responsiveness, decreased urine output, narrowed pulse pressure, and decreased skin temperature. The ratio of surface area to mass is greater than in adults, putting pediatric patients at greater risk for hypothermia following injury. Signs of spinal cord injury may be subtle or transient, especially in the case of spinal cord injury without radiographic abnormality (SCIWORA). Complete development of symptoms may not be fully appreciated for a matter of hours subsequent to injury.

Diagnosis and Differential

The process of evaluation for adult and pediatric trauma patients is the same; the primary survey (A-B-C-D-E) and the secondary survey are completed in a systematic fashion. Airway patency and adequacy of Breathing are assessed. Definitive airway management and treatment of pneumothorax or hemothorax are accomplished before continuing further. The Circulatory status is evaluated, hemodynamic and cardiac monitoring initiated, vascular access secured, and fluid resuscitation initiated. A brief neurologic examination for Disability must include modification of the Glasgow Coma Score based upon age and examination of the fontanelle in infants for indications of changes in intracranial pressure. To complete the primary survey, the patient is Exposed in preparation for the secondary survey, vital signs recorded, and response to fluid administration noted.

The secondary survey proceeds from head to toe while resuscitation and monitoring of vital signs continue. The head and neck are examined for signs of injury, specifically for evidence of basilar skull fracture, facial bone fractures, and cervical spine fracture. Evaluation of the chest is performed recognizing that, due to the more compliant chest wall of the child, serious intrathoracic injury may exist without obvious external signs. As a corollary to this principle, external evidence of trauma, such as a rib fracture, is a sensitive indicator of serious underlying injury. The abdomen, pelvis, and perineum are examined, and a rectal examination is performed. Cervical spine, chest, and pelvis x-rays are then obtained, a naso- or orogastric tube placed to decompress the stomach, and a urinary catheter inserted. Patients must be log-rolled to examine the back, and the extremities checked for soft tissue injury and fractures. Last, a thorough neurologic examination is done in the context of the appropriate developmental stage of the patient and considering the typically heightened apprehension of pediatric patients.

On completion of the secondary survey, additional diagnostic studies are ordered. Routine laboratory determinations include a complete blood cell count; electrolyte, blood urea nitrogen, and creatinine levels; urinalysis; and liver enzymes (in abdominal trauma), along with a type and cross-match for blood products. The imaging modality of choice for evaluation of head injury is the CT scan; indications for ordering this test include significant loss of consciousness, deteriorating level of consciousness, neurologic deficits, apparent skull fracture on the physical examination, persistent nausea and vomiting, and seizure. A high clinical suspicion must be maintained for SCIWORA and a high cervical spine injury in the younger child. Physical findings consistent with spinal cord injury or abnormalities on spine x-rays are strong indications for CT scanning or standard tomography. In the evaluation of abdominal injury in pediatric patients, the physical examination has both a high false-positive and relatively high false-negative rate. Therefore, either CT scanning or diagnostic peritoneal lavage (primarily for hemodynamically unstable patients) is utilized frequently. CT is also indicated for patients with genitourinary trauma demonstrating as few as 20 red blood cells per hpf. Burn patients must have accurate documentation of the depth and extent of the injury, recognizing that the Rule of Nines may be inaccurate in estimating burn surface area (BSA). Consideration also must be given to evaluating these patients for carbon monoxide poisoning.

Emergency Department Care and Disposition

Many problems identified in pediatric trauma patients during the primary and secondary surveys are managed in a similar fashion to that in adult patients.

1. Airway management in children can be particularly challenging. Anatomic differences responsible for this include a relatively larger tongue and more cephalad location of the larynx. All patients initially should be administered **100% oxygen**. Suctioning, jaw thrust, or chin lift maneuvers and placement of either a nasal or an oral airway are other measures to be considered. The indications for **endotracheal intubation** are essentially the same as those for adults. The oral route for intubation is preferred; nasotracheal intubation should be avoided due to the cephalad location of the glottis and the propensity to traumatize the upper airway with this approach. In children less than 8 years of age, the narrowest portion of the airway is subglottic and a tube that fits through the vocal cords may not pass through this region. Choosing an appropriate endotracheal tube size is achieved by using the following formula:

Internal Diameter (in mm) = (16 + age of patient in years)/4

Patients in this age range should have an uncuffed endotracheal tube placed. **Rapid sequence intubation**, using pretreatment with **100% oxygen**, **lidocaine** at 1.0 mg/kg IV, **atropine** at 0.02 mg/kg IV (minimum dose 0.1 mg, maximum dose 1.0 mg), and appropriate sedation (e.g., **midazolam** 0.1 mg/kg IV). Pharmacologic paralysis may be achieved by using either **succinylcholine** 1.0 to 1.5 mg/kg IV or a nondepolarizing paralytic agent (e.g., **rocuronium** at a dose of 1 mg/kg IV). Securing an airway in the setting of severe facial trauma may be achieved by **transtracheal catheter ventilation**. Cricothyrotomy is not recommended in small children since identification of the cricothyroid membrane can be difficult and the cricoid cartilage is easily damaged. After establishing transtracheal catheter placement through the cricoid membrane, a tracheostomy tube or shortened endotracheal tube can be inserted over a guidewire using the catheter in a Seldinger-type procedure.

2. Vascular access can be difficult in children, especially with accompanying hypotension. Strong consideration must be given to early use of **interosseous cannulation**, particularly in young children and infants. Resuscitative fluids should be administered in **20 mL/kg boluses of crystalloid**; if there is no improvement or deterioration occurs after an initial response, **10 mL/kg boluses of packed red blood cells** or whole blood are indicated. Fluids should be warmed and used in conjunction with warming lights to prevent hypothermia. Burn patients should be resuscitated according to a standard burn formula, such as the **Parkland formula**.

3. For head and spinal cord injuries, evaluation of mental status may be difficult due to developmental stage and a heightened level of anxiety. Consequently, more liberal use of sedation using **midazolam** 0.1 mg/kg IV or another suitable agent in children is appropriate after completion of the neurologic examination. Children tend to recover better from head injury than adults, but aggressive treatment of hypoxia and hypotension is important to facilitate a good outcome. Severe head injury should be treated with **tracheal intubation and hyperventilation, elevation of the head of the bed to 30°**, and maintenance of the head and neck in a neutral position. Intravenous **mannitol** at 0.5 to 1.0 g/kg and **furosemide** at 1.0 mg/kg may be useful in treating cerebral edema. Posttraumatic seizures are more common in children than in adults and consideration is warranted for prophylaxis with **fosphenytoin** loading at 17 mg/kg (PE equivalents). In the setting of potential spinal trauma, immobilization must be achieved in infants and younger children allowing for their relatively larger head by placement of padding behind the shoulders. Steroids should be administered within 8 h in the setting of neurologic deficit attributable to spinal cord injury. Dosing consists of a bolus of **methylprednisolone** 30 mg/kg IV over 15 min, followed 45 min later by an IV infusion at a rate of 5.4 mg/kg/h.

4. Disposition of pediatric trauma patients can be challenging. Pediatric patients should be admitted to the hospital if they have sustained skull fractures or evidence of intracranial

TABLE 152-1 Indications for Transfer to a Pediatric Trauma Center

Mechanism of injury	Ejected from a motor vehicle
	Prolonged extrication
	Death of other occupant in motor vehicle
	Fall from greater distance than 3 times the child's height
Anatomic injury	Multiple severe trauma
	More than 3 long bone fractures
	Spinal fractures or spinal cord injury
	Amputations
	Severe head or facial trauma
	Penetrating head, chest, or abdominal trauma

injury on the CT scan, spinal trauma, significant chest trauma, abdominal trauma with evidence of internal organ injury, or significant burns. Suggested guidelines for referral to a pediatric trauma center appear in Table 152-1. Social services involvement and reporting to child protective services are indicated if there is any suspicion for nonaccidental trauma (see Chap. 182).

For further reading in *Emergency Medicine: A Comprehensive Study Guide,* 5th ed., see Chap. 244, "Pediatric Trauma," by William E. Hauda II.

---

153 | Geriatric Trauma

O. John Ma

With the rapid growth in the size of the elderly population, the incidence of geriatric trauma is expected to increase as well. Emergency physicians need to stay abreast with many of the unique injury mechanisms and clinical features associated with geriatric trauma patients, and apply special management principles when caring for them.

Clinical Features

Falls are the most common accidental injury in patients over 75 years of age and the second most common injury in the 65 to 74 age group. Syncope has been implicated in many cases, and this may be secondary to dysrhythmias, venous pooling, autonomic derangement, hypoxia, anemia, and hypoglycemia. Motor vehicle-related injuries rank as the leading mechanism of injury that brings elderly patients to a trauma center in the United States. Violent assaults account for 4 to 14 percent of trauma admissions in this age group. Just as in pediatric trauma cases, emergency physicians should have a heightened suspicion for elder or parental abuse in the geriatric trauma patient.

Since elderly patients may have a significant past medical history that impacts their trauma care, obtaining a precise history is vital. Often, the time frame for obtaining information about the traumatic event, past medical history, medications, and allergies is quite short. Family members, medical records, and the patient's primary physician may be helpful in gathering information regarding the traumatic event and the patient's previous level of function.

On physical examination, early assessment and frequent monitoring of vital signs is essential. Emergency physicians should be wary of a "normal" heart rate in the geriatric trauma victim. A normal tachycardic response to pain, hypovolemia, or anxiety may be absent or blunted in the elderly trauma patient. Medications such as β blockers may mask tachycardia and delay appropriate resuscitation.

Special attention should be paid to anatomic variation that may make airway management more difficult. These include the presence of dentures, cervical arthritis, or temporomandibular joint arthritis. A thorough secondary survey is essential to uncover less serious injuries. These injuries, which include various orthopedic and "minor" head trauma, may not be severe enough to cause problems during the initial resuscitation, but cumulatively may cause significant morbidity and mortality. Seemingly stable geriatric trauma patients can deteriorate rapidly and without warning.

Diagnosis and Differential

Head Injury

When evaluating the elderly patient's mental status during the neurologic examination, it would be a grave error to assume that alterations in mental status are due solely to any underlying dementia or senility. Elderly persons suffer a much lower incidence of epidural hematomas than the general population. There is, however, a higher incidence of subdural hematomas in elderly patients. More liberal indications for computed tomography (CT) scanning are justified.

Cervical Spine Injuries

The pattern of cervical spine injuries in the elderly is different than in younger patients, as there is an increased incidence of C-1 and C-2 fractures with the elderly. When the elderly trauma patient has neck pain, emergency physicians need to place special emphasis on maintaining cervical immobilization until the cervical spine is properly assessed. Because underlying cervical arthritis may obscure fracture lines, the elderly patient with persistent neck pain and negative plain radiographs should undergo CT scanning of the neck.

Chest Trauma

In blunt trauma, there is an increased incidence of rib fractures due to osteoporotic changes. The pain associated with rib fractures, along with any decreased physiologic reserve, may predispose patients to respiratory complications. More severe thoracic injuries, such as hemopneumothorax, pulmonary contusion, flail chest, and cardiac contusion, can quickly lead to decompensation in elderly individuals whose baseline oxygenation status may already be diminished. Arterial blood gas analysis may provide early insight into elderly patients' respiratory function and reserve.

Abdominal Trauma

The abdominal examination in elderly patients is notoriously unreliable compared to that given in younger patients. Even with an initially benign physical examination, emergency physicians must have a high index of suspicion for intraabdominal injuries in patients who have associated pelvic and lower rib cage fractures. For elderly patients, the adhesions associated with previous abdominal surgical procedures may increase the risk of performing diagnostic peritoneal lavage in the emergency department (ED). Therefore, the trauma ultrasound examination may assist in evaluating for hemoperitoneum and the need for exploratory laparotomy in hemodynamically unstable patients. For patients who are stable, CT scanning with contrast is a valuable diagnostic test. It is important to ensure adequate hydration and baseline assessment of renal function prior to the contrast load for the CT scan. Some patients may be volume depleted due to medications, such as diuretics. This hypovolemia coupled with contrast administration may exacerbate any underlying renal pathology.

Orthopedic Injuries

Hip fractures occur primarily in four areas: intertrochanteric, transcervical, subcapital, and subtrochanteric. Intertrochanteric fractures are the most common, followed by transcervical fractures. Emergency physicians must be aware that pelvic and long bone fractures are not infrequently the sole etiology for hypovolemia in elderly patients. Timely orthopedic consultation, evaluation, and treatment with open reduction and internal fixation should be coordinated with the diagnosis and management of other injuries.

Long bone fractures of the femur, tibia, and humerus may produce a loss of mobility with a resulting decrease in the independent lifestyle of elderly patients. Early orthopedic consultation for intramedullary rodding of these fractures may result in increased early mobilization.

The incidence of Colles's fractures and humeral head and surgical neck fractures in elderly patients are increased by falls on the outstretched hand or elbow. Localized tenderness, swelling, and ecchymosis to the proximal humerus are characteristic of these injuries. Early orthopedic consultation and treatment with a shoulder immobilizer or surgical fixation should be arranged.

Emergency Department Care and Disposition

As in all trauma patients, the primary survey should be assessed expeditiously.

1. The main therapeutic goal is aggressively maintaining adequate **oxygen** delivery. **Prompt tracheal intubation** and use of mechanical ventilation should be considered in patients with more severe injuries, respiratory rates greater than 40 breaths per minute, or when the Pa_{O_2} is < 60 mmHg or Pa_{CO_2} > 50 mmHg. While nonventilatory therapy helps to prevent respiratory infections and is always desirable, early mechanical ventilation may avert the disastrous results associated with hypoxia.
2. Geriatric trauma patients can decompensate with overresuscitation just as quickly as they can with inadequate resuscitation. Elderly patients with underlying coronary artery disease and cerebrovascular disease are at a much greater risk of suffering the consequences of ischemia to vital organs when they become hypotensive after sustaining trauma. During the initial resuscitative phase, crystalloid, while the primary option, should be administered judiciously since elderly patients with diminished cardiac compliance are more susceptible to volume overload. Strong consideration should be made for early and more liberal use of **red blood cell transfusion.** This practice early in the resuscitation would enhance oxygen delivery and help minimize tissue ischemia.
3. **Early invasive monitoring** has been advocated to help physicians assess the elderly's hemodynamic status. One study found that urgent invasive monitoring provides important hemodynamic information early, aids in identifying occult shock, limits hypoperfusion, helps prevent multiple organ failure, and improves survival. Survival was improved because of enhanced oxygen delivery through the use of adequate volume loading and inotropic support.

4. If the insertion of invasive monitoring lines is impractical in the ED, every effort should be made by emergency physicians to expedite care of elderly trauma patients and prevent unnecessary delays. In the ED evaluation of blunt trauma patients, the chest radiograph, cervical spine series, and pelvic radiographs are necessary diagnostic tests during the secondary survey. While it is vital to be thorough in the diagnosis of occult orthopedic injuries, expending a great deal of time in the radiology suite may compromise patient care. Only a few radiologic studies, such as emergent head and abdominal CT scans, should take precedence over obtaining vital information from invasive monitoring. Elderly trauma patients will benefit most from an expeditious transfer to the intensive care unit for invasive monitoring so that their hemodynamic status can be further assessed. Invasive monitoring in the intensive care environment may provide clues to subtle hemodynamic changes which may compromise geriatric patients with limited physiologic reserve.

Emergency physicians, in consultation with the trauma surgeon, should have a low threshold for having geriatric patients who have experienced significant traumatic events, admitted for further evaluation and observation.

For further reading in *Emergency Medicine: A Comprehensive Study Guide,* 5th ed., see Chap. 245, "Geriatric Trauma," by O. John Ma and Daniel J. DeBehnke.

---

154 | Trauma in Pregnancy

C. Crawford Mechem

Trauma is the leading cause of nonobstetric mortality in pregnant women and is associated with an increased risk of preterm labor, placental abruption, fetal-maternal hemorrhage, and miscarriage. An injured pregnant woman presents two patients requiring timely and effective evaluation, stabilization, and definitive care.

Clinical Features

Physiologic changes of pregnancy make determination of the severity of injury problematic. Heart rate typically increases 10 to 20 beats per minute during the second trimester, blood pressure drops 10 to 15 mmHg, and blood volume increases by up to 50%. It may be difficult to determine if tachycardia or hypotension is caused by ongoing blood loss or normal physiologic changes. In addition, patients may lose 30 to 35% of circulating blood volume before manifesting clinical signs of shock. By then, however, blood flow to the fetus may already be jeopardized.

Abdominal trauma can affect both mother and fetus. Splenic injury is the leading cause of intraabdominal hemorrhage. Lower abdominal viscera are protected by the enlarging uterus. However, uterine irritability and preterm labor can develop. Upward displacement of intestines may result in complex injuries in penetrating trauma to the upper abdomen. Uterine rupture, most commonly seen during the second and third trimester, is uncommon. It is diagnosed by loss of palpable uterine contour, ease of palpation of fetal parts, or radiologic evidence of abnormal fetal location.

Maternal death is the leading cause of fetal death. This is followed by placental abruption, which presents with abdominal pain, vaginal bleeding, uterine contractions, and signs of disseminated intravascular coagulation (DIC). For up to 12 weeks gestation the fetus is protected by the bony pelvis, making injury uncommon. Later in pregnancy, fetal injuries tend to involve the head. Fetal-maternal hemorrhage occurs in over 30 percent of cases of significant trauma and may result in Rh-isoimmunization of Rh-negative women. Fetal hemorrhage may also cause fetal hypovolemia, distress, and death.

Diagnosis and Differential

Appropriate laboratory evaluation includes the complete blood count, blood type and Rh determination, and coagulation studies. The Kleihauer-Betke test for maternal blood is useful to quantify the degree of fetal-maternal hemorrhage.

Intraabdominal injury may be detected using abdominal computed tomography (CT) scan, the trauma ultrasound examination, or diagnostic peritoneal lavage, which is performed using a supraumbilical approach. The indications for emergent laparotomy remain unchanged. While efforts should be made to limit radiographic studies to those that are clinically mandatory, studies should not be withheld out of concern for the fetus. Adverse fetal effects from radiation are greatest during the first 8 weeks of gestation and are negligible from doses less than 10 rad. Abdominal CT delivers between 2 and 5 rad. This can be reduced by decreasing the number of slices obtained. Standard trauma radiographs deliver substantially less than 1 rad. Fetal exposure can be further limited by judicious shielding of the uterus. MRI and ventilation-perfusion scanning have not been associated with adverse fetal outcome.

Emergency Department Care and Disposition

The best care for the fetus is proper resuscitation of the mother. Establishment of a patent airway, adequate ventilation, and large-bore vascular access are paramount. A trauma surgeon and an obstetrician should be involved early on in the care of any significantly injured pregnant patient.

1. The airway should be secured, and supplemental **oxygen** administered. Early passage of a nasogastric or orogastric tube decreases the risk of aspiration.
2. **Crystalloid IV fluids** should be administered to treat hypovolemia.
3. Any obvious source of hemorrhage should be controlled.
4. The patient should be kept in the left lateral decubitus position where feasible to minimize hypotension due to inferior vena cava compression by the gravid uterus.
5. **Vasopressors** impair uterine blood flow and should only be considered after aggressive fluid resuscitation.
6. **Rh immune globulin (RhoGAM),** 300 μg IM, should be administered to all Rh-negative patients with abdominal trauma beyond 12 weeks gestation. One dose protects against 30 mL of fetal blood. The Kleihauer-Betke test can be used to determine the need for additional doses.
7. **Tetanus prophylaxis** should be administered as indicated by the individual case.
8. The use of **tocolytic agents** for increased uterine contractility should be individualized, as they may interfere with the diagnosis of maternal and fetal injuries.

A detailed secondary survey with careful attention to the abdomen should be performed. The uterus should be assessed for tenderness or contractions and a sterile pelvic examination performed, inspecting for injuries or vaginal bleeding. Rupture of amnionic membranes is indicated by the presence of clear fluid of pH 7 in the vaginal canal that produces "ferning" when dried on a microscope slide.

Fetal assessment starts with determination of the fetal heart rate. Fetal viability is directly related to the presence of fetal heart sounds. When absent on patient arrival, resuscitation should be directed solely at the mother. Normal fetal heart rate is 120 to 160 beats per minute. Bradycardia suggests hypoxia, often due to maternal hypotension, hypothermia, respiratory compromise, or abruption. Tachycardia may result from hypoxia or hypovolemia. Bedside ultrasound can be used to determine fetal heart rate, as well as gestational age, fetal activity, placental location, and amnionic fluid volume. Ultrasound has not been shown useful in diagnosing placental abruption or uterine rupture.

External fetal monitoring should be initiated early. A minimum of 4 h of monitoring is predictive of immediate adverse outcome. After 20 weeks gestation, the presence of more than 8 contractions per hour is predictive of placental abruption. Beyond the viable gestational age of 23 weeks, fetal tachycardia, late decelerations, or lack of beat-to-beat variability may be indications for emergent cesarean section.

Should the pregnant trauma patient die, perimortem cesarean section may be considered if fetal heart tones are detected on patient arrival and the gestation is determined to be beyond 23 weeks. Resuscitation of the mother should be continued during the procedure. Infant outcome is excellent when performed within 5 min of maternal death.

The decision to admit or discharge the pregnant trauma patient is dictated on an individual basis, often after consultation with trauma surgeons and obstetricians. Patients who display evidence of fetal distress or increased uterine irritability during the initial observation should be admitted.

For further reading in *Emergency Medicine: A Comprehensive Study Guide,* 5th ed., see Chap. 246, "Trauma in Pregnancy," by Nelson Tang.

---

155 Head Injury

O. John Ma

Head injuries account for approximately half of all trauma-related deaths. An initial impact injury to the brain produces varying degrees of mechanical neuronal and axonal injury. Secondary brain injury occurs from potentially treatable factors, such as intracranial hemorrhage, cerebral edema, ischemia, hypoxia, hypotension, anemia, and increased intracranial pressure (ICP). Optimal emergency department management is paramount in helping to minimize secondary brain injury, thus decreasing the overall mortality and morbidity rates.

Clinical Features

Traumatic brain injury (TBI) results from either direct or indirect forces to the brain. Direct injury is caused by the force of an object striking the head or a penetrating injury. Indirect injuries result from acceleration-deceleration forces that result in the movement of the brain within the skull.

TBI can be classified as mild, moderate, and severe. Mild TBIs include patients with a Glasgow Coma Scale (GCS; see Table 155-1) of 14 or greater. Approximately 3 percent of patients presenting with mild TBI may "talk and deteriorate" within 48 h postinjury. Patients may be asymptomatic, with only a history of head trauma, or may be confused and amnestic of the event. Patients with high-risk physical examination findings include those with a skull fracture, large subgaleal swelling, focal neurologic findings, distracting injuries, or intoxication.

Moderate TBI (GCS 9 to 13) accounts for approximately 10 percent of all patients with head injuries. Overall, 40 percent of moderate TBI patients have a positive computed tomography (CT) scan, and 8 percent require neurosurgical intervention. Roughly 10 percent of these patients will deteriorate and progress to severe TBI.

Severe TBI (GCS less than 9) accounts for approximately 10 percent of head injury patients. The mortality rate of severe TBI approaches 40 percent.

Out-of-hospital medical personnel often may provide critical parts of the history, including mechanism and time of injury, presence and length of unconsciousness, initial mental status, seizure activity, vomiting, verbalization, and movement of extremities. For an unresponsive patient, family and friends should be contacted to gather key information, including past medical history, medications (especially anticoagulants), and recent use of alcohol or drugs.

Clinically important features of the neurologic examination include assessment of the mental status and GCS; pupils for size, reactivity, and anisocoria; cranial nerve function; motor, sensory, and brainstem function; deep tendon reflexes; and any development of decorticate or decerebrate posturing.

Clinical features of specific injuries are addressed below.

TABLE 155-1 The Glasgow Coma Scale for All Age Groups

	4 yrs to Adult	Child <4 yrs	Infant
EYE OPENING			
4	Spontaneous	Spontaneous	Spontaneous
3	To speech	To speech	To speech
2	To pain	To pain	To pain
1	No response	No response	No response
VERBAL RESPONSE			
5	Alert and oriented	Oriented, social, speaks, interacts	Coos, babbles
4	Disoriented conversation	Confused speech, disoriented, consolable, aware	Irritable cry
3	Speaking but nonsensical	Inappropriate words, inconsolable, unaware	Cries to pain
2	Moans or unintelligible sounds	Incomprehensible, agitated, restless, unaware	Moans to pain
1	No response	No response	No response
MOTOR RESPONSE			
6	Follows commands	Normal, spontaneous movements	Normal, spontaneous movements
5	Localizes pain	Localizes pain	Withdraws to touch
4	Movement or withdrawal to pain	Withdraws to pain	Withdraws to pain
3	Decorticate flexion	Decorticate flexion	Decorticate flexion
2	Decerebrate extension	Decerebrate extension	Decerebrate extension
1	No response	No response	No response
3–15			

GCS reporting should be modified for intubated and paralyzed patients.

Skull Fractures

Isolated linear nondepressed fractures with an intact scalp are common and do not require treatment. However, life-threatening intracranial hemorrhage may result if the fracture causes disruption of the middle meningeal artery or a major dural sinus. Depressed skull fractures are classified as open or closed, depending on the integrity of the overlying scalp. Although basilar skull fractures can occur at any point in the base of the skull, the typical location is in the petrous portion of the temporal bone. Findings associated with a basilar skull fracture include hemotympanum, otorrhea or rhinorrhea, periorbital ecchymosis ("raccoon eyes"), and retroauricular ecchymosis (Battle's sign).

Brain Concussion

Concussion is a diffuse head injury, usually associated with transient loss of consciousness, that occurs immediately following a nonpenetrating blunt impact to the head. It generally occurs when the head, while moving, strikes or is struck by an object. The duration of unconsciousness is typically brief (seconds to minutes). Symptoms of amnesia and confusion are clinical hallmarks. Complete recovery is typical, although persistent headache and problems with memory, anxiety, insomnia, and dizziness can continue in some patients for weeks after the injury.

Brain Contusion and Intracerebral Hemorrhage

Common locations for contusions are the frontal poles, the subfrontal cortex, and the anterior temporal lobes. Contusions may occur directly under the site of impact or on the contralateral side (contrecoup lesion). The contused area is usually hemorrhagic with surrounding edema, and occasionally associated with subarachnoid hemorrhage. Neurologic dysfunction may be profound and prolonged, with patients demonstrating mental confusion, obtundation, or coma. Focal neurologic deficits are usually present. Combination of parenchymal hemorrhage and contusion can produce an expanding mass lesion; when present in the anterior temporal lobe, uncal herniation can occur without a diffuse increase in ICP.

Epidural Hematoma

An epidural hematoma results from an acute collection of blood between the inner table of the skull and the dura. In approximately 80 percent of cases, it is associated with a skull fracture that lacerates a meningeal artery, most commonly the middle meningeal artery. Underlying injury to the brain may not necessarily be severe. In a classic scenario (20 percent of cases), the patient experiences loss of consciousness after a head injury. The patient may present to the ED with clear mentation, signifying the "lucid interval," and then begin to develop mental status deterioration in the ED. A fixed and dilated pupil on the side of the lesion and contralateral hemiparesis are classic late findings.

Subdural Hematoma

A subdural hematoma (SDH), a collection of venous blood between the dura matter and the arachnoid, results from tears of the bridging veins that extend from the subarachnoid space to the dural venous sinuses. A common mechanism is sudden acceleration-deceleration. Patients with brain atrophy, such as alcoholics or the elderly, are more susceptible to SDH. In acute SDH, patients present between 3 and 14 days, and most become symptomatic within 24 h of injury. After 2 weeks, patients are defined as having a chronic SDH. Symptoms may range from a headache to lethargy or coma. It is important to distinguish between acute and chronic SDH by history, physical examination, and CT scan.

Herniation

Diffusely or focally increased ICP can result in herniation of the brain at several locations. *Transtentorial (uncal) herniation* occurs when a SDH or temporal lobe mass forces the ipsilateral uncus of the temporal lobe through the tentorial hiatus into the space between the cerebral peduncle and the tentorium. This results in compression of the oculomotor nerve and parasympathetic paralysis of the ipsilateral pupil, causing it to become fixed and dilated. The cerebral peduncle is simultaneously compressed, resulting in contralateral hemiparesis. The increased ICP and brainstem compression result in progressive deterioration in the level of consciousness. Occasionally the contralateral cerebral peduncle is forced against the free edge of the tentorium on the opposite side, resulting in paralysis ipsilateral to the lesion, a false localizing sign. The posterior cerebral artery can be compressed against the free edge of the tentorium, resulting in infarction of the occipital lobe. If the herniation continues untreated, there is progressive brainstem deterioration, leading to hyperventilation, decerebration, and then apnea and death. *Cerebellotonsillar herniation* through the foramen magnum occurs much less frequently. Resultant medullary compression causes bradycardia, respiratory arrest, and death. *Cingulate or subfalcial herniation* occurs when one cerebral hemisphere is displaced underneath the falx cerebri into the opposite supratentorial space. This is rarely clinically diagnosed.

Penetrating Injuries

Gunshot wounds and penetrating sharp objects can result in penetrating injury to the brain. The degree of neurologic injury depends on the energy of the missile, whether the trajectory involves a single or multiple lobes or hemispheres of the brain, the amount of scatter of bone and metallic fragments, and whether a mass lesion is present.

Diagnosis and Differential

Approximately 5 percent of patients suffering a severe TBI have an associated cervical spine fracture. Cervical spine radiographs should be obtained on all patients who present with altered mental status, neck pain, intoxication, neurologic deficit, severe distracting injury, or a mechanism of injury deemed serious enough to potentially produce cervical spine injury.

All patients with moderate or severe TBI should undergo an emergent head CT scan without contrast after stabilization. Patients with mild TBI should undergo a CT scan if they experienced loss of consciousness, nausea or vomiting, posttraumatic seizure, or amnesia, or have a history of coagulopathy or intoxication without significant improvement after a period of observation. Other indications for CT scan include clinical neurologic deterioration during observation, persistent focal neurologic or mental status deficit, and skull fractures in the vicinity of the middle meningeal artery or major venous sinuses.

Routine skull radiographs are not indicated. Anteroposterior and lateral skull radiographs may be obtained for penetrating wounds of the skull or for suspected depressed skull fracture. Skull radiographs may help localize the position of a foreign body within the cranium and may determine the amount of bony depression. If a CT scan of the head is to be performed, bone windows can be obtained, eliminating the need for skull films.

Laboratory work for patients with significant head injury should include type and crossmatching; complete blood count; electrolyte, glucose, arterial blood gas, and directed toxicologic studies; prothrombin and partial thromboplastin times; platelet determinations; and DIC panel.

Emergency Department Care and Disposition

Standard protocols for evaluation and stabilization of trauma patients should be initiated (see Chap. 151). A careful search for other significant injuries should be made, since up to 60 percent of patients with severe TBI have associated major injuries.

1. Administer **100% oxygen**, and secure cardiac monitoring and two intravenous (IV) lines. For patients with severe TBI, **endotracheal intubation** to protect the airway and prevent hypoxemia is the top priority. Orotracheal rapid sequence intubation should be utilized. When properly performed, it assists in preventing increased ICP and has a low complication rate. When performing rapid sequence intubation, it is imperative to provide adequate cervical spine immobilization and use a sedation-induction agent.
2. Since hypotension can lead to depressed cerebral perfusion pressure, restoration of an adequate blood pressure is vital. Resuscitation with IV **crystalloid fluid** is indicated. Once an adequate blood pressure is maintained, IV fluids should be administered cautiously to prevent cerebral edema. Hypotonic and glucose-containing solutions should be avoided.
3. Once a positive head CT scan has been identified, immediate neurosurgical consultation is indicated.
4. All patients who demonstrate signs of increased ICP should have the **head of their bed elevated 30°** (provided the patient is not hypotensive), adequate volume resuscitation to a mean arterial pressure greater than 90 mmHg, and maintenance of adequate arterial oxygenation. **Mannitol** 0.25 to 1.0 g/kg IV should be administered. Hyperventilation is no longer recommended as an intervention to lower ICP because of its potential to cause cerebral ischemia. Hyperventilation should be reserved as a last resort for decreasing ICP; if used, it should be implemented as a temporary measure and the pCO_2 monitored closely.
5. For posttraumatic seizures, prophylactic phenytoin use for patients with severe TBI is recommended. Seizures should be treated with benzodiazepines, such as **lorazepam** or **diazepam**, and **phenytoin** at a loading dose of 18 mg/kg IV infused at a rate no faster than 50 mg/min.
6. Patients with an initial GCS of 15 that is maintained, normal serial neurologic examination results, and a normal CT scan may be discharged home. Those with a positive CT scan require neurosurgical consultation and admission. Patients with an initial GCS of 14 and a normal CT scan should be observed in the ED for at least 6 h. If their GCS improves to 15 and they remain completely neurologically intact, they can be discharged home. All patients who experience a head injury should be discharged home with a reliable companion who can observe

the patient for at least 24 h, carry out appropriate discharge instructions, and follow the head injury sheet instructions.

For further reading in *Emergency Medicine: A Comprehensive Study Guide,* 5th ed., see Chap. 247, "Head Injury," by Thomas D. Kirsch, Salvatore Migliore, and Teresita M. Hogan.

---

156 | Spinal Injuries
Charles J. Havel, Jr.

Spinal cord injury (SCI) causes catastrophic sequelae both in human terms and in health care dollars expended. The majority of patients are young, with a male-to-female ratio of 4:1. Close to 90 percent of SCIs are related to blunt trauma, with cervical spine, thoracolumbar junction, thoracic spine, and lumbosacral spine injured in order of decreasing frequency.

Clinical Features

Not all patients with SCI have an obvious neurologic deficit; unstable bony injury may exist without actual spinal cord or nerve root trauma. Some patients may voice complaints of paresthesias, dysesthesias, or other sensory disturbances, with or without specific physical findings. More severely injured patients will have findings of an obvious neurologic deficit on physical examination. Patients with severe acute SCI typically have "spinal shock"; that is, flaccid hemiplegia or quadriplegia, areflexia, and mild hypotension. The hypotension is neurogenic in origin and due to a loss of sympathetic tone. As opposed to hypovolemic shock, neurogenic shock is characterized by warm, pink, dry skin; adequate urine output; and relative ("paradoxical") bradycardia. Other signs of autonomic dysfunction may accompany spinal shock, such as gastrointestinal ileus, urinary retention, fecal incontinence, priapism, and loss of the normal ability to regulate body temperature.

Diagnosis and Differential

The history is useful in defining the mechanism of SCI allowing the clinician to anticipate specific potential injuries (Table 156-1). Any neurologic complaints from the patient even if transitory, must raise suspicion for a SCI. As part of a complete primary and secondary survey, the evaluation for a potential SCI should focus on examination of the spine itself and the neurologic examination. The neurologic examination should include the following assessments: pain perception, light touch and proprioception (to evaluate the posterior columns), motor strength and tone, reflexes, rectal tone, perianal sensation and wink, and bulbocavernosus reflex.

Patients with any one of the following characteristics must have (at the least) plain film radiography of the traumatized portion of their spine: (*a*) midline bony spinal tenderness, crepitus, or step-off; (*b*) physical findings of a neurologic deficit; (*c*) altered mental status of any etiology; (*d*) presence of additional painful or distracting injuries; and (*e*) complaint of paresthesias or numbness.

As for cervical spine x-rays, a minimum of three views (lateral, odontoid, and anteroposterior (AP) is required to evaluate for

TABLE 156-1 Mechanism of Injury and Related Cervical Spine Injury

Flexion	Anterior subluxation (hyperflexion sprain)
	Simple wedge compression fracture
	Flexion tear-drop fracture
	Bilateral interfacetal dislocation
	Clay-shoveler fracture
Flexion-rotation	Unilateral interfacetal dislocation
Hyperextension	Hyperextension dislocation
	Hyperextension fracture-dislocation
	Avulsion fracture of anterior arch of atlas
	Fracture of posterior arch of atlas
	Extension tear-drop fracture of axis
	Laminar fracture
	Traumatic spondylolisthesis (Hangman's fracture)
Extension-rotation	Pillar fracture
Lateral flexion	Uncinate process fracture
Vertical compression	Jefferson's burst fracture of atlas
	Burst fracture
Diverse or imprecisely understood mechanism	Atlantooccipital disassociation
	Odontoid fracture

fracture or other bony abnormality. A complete and systematic survey of the radiograph includes the following:

1. Determination that all 7 cervical vertebral bodies and the superior margin of T-1 are visible
2. Check for alignment of the four lordotic curves: the anterior longitudinal line, the posterior longitudinal line, the spinolaminar line, and the tips of the spinous processes
3. Check for abrupt angulation of greater than 11° at a single interspace
4. Check for fanning of spinous processes
5. Check of each vertebra for fracture
6. Examination of the atlantooccipital relation for dislocation
7. Determination of the width of the predental space; greater than 3 mm in adults or 4 mm in children may suggest cruciform ligament instability
8. Check of the AP diameter of the spinal canal
9. Examination of the width of the prevertebral soft tissues
10. Look for fracture of the odontoid on the open mouth view
11. Examination of the AP film for alignment of the spinous processes or any other sign of rotation

Plain radiography of the thoracic and lumbar spine is the initial technique used to image these levels. Discovery of a spine injury at one level must prompt imaging of the remainder of the spine. Additional imaging modalities may be indicated for patients with positive findings on initial plain films at any level or in those in whom spinal injury is still suspected despite a negative initial x-ray. These studies include flexion and extension views (of the cervical spine) that allow the physician to look for ligamentous instability, standard tomography, computed tomography (CT) scan with or without contrast myelography, or magnetic resonance imaging (for evaluation of neural elements).

Once a bony abnormality is identified, a key part of the differential is the degree of stability associated with that particular type of injury (Table 156-2). Apart from the cervical fractures listed, thoracic and lumbosacral fractures have differing degrees of stability depending on the type. Wedge or compression fractures may be unstable if there is loss of greater than 50 percent of vertebral body height and failure of the posterior ligaments. Burst fractures result from axial loading and may be responsible for retropulsion of fragments causing spinal cord compression. Distraction fractures are associated with motor vehicle collisions; a severe and unstable variant is the Chance fracture with horizontal fracture from the spinous process through the vertebral body. Thoracolumbar fracture-dislocations are grossly unstable and have a significant incidence of associated

TABLE 156-2 The Spectrum of Acute Instability in Cervical Spine Injuries

Most unstable
 Rupture of transverse atlantal ligament
 Fracture of odontoid
 Burst fracture with posterior ligamentous disruption (flexion teardrop)
 Bilateral facet dislocation (or equivalent posterior disruption)
 Burst fracture of vertebral body without posterior ligamentous disruption
 Hyperextension fracture-dislocation
 Hangman's fracture
 Extension teardrop fracture (stable in flexion)
 Jefferson's fracture (burst fracture of C1)
 Unilateral facet dislocation (or equivalent posterior disruption)
 Anterior subluxation
 Simple wedge compression fracture without posterior disruption
 Pillar fracture
 Fracture of the posterior arch of C1
 Spinous process fracture

Least unstable

SCI. Only occasionally do sacral fractures result in a neurologic deficit, usually related to sacral nerve impingement.

For patients with obvious SCI, the differential includes complete lesions and a number of incomplete lesions or syndromes. The difference between complete and incomplete lesions is crucial; the prognosis for complete injuries is poor, while patients with incomplete cord syndromes can be expected to improve to at least some degree. *Anterior cord syndromes* involve the loss of motor function, and pain and temperature sensation distal to the level of injury with preservation of crude touch, vibration, and proprioception. Hyperextension injuries in older patients typically produce the *central cord syndrome,* with motor weakness more prominent in the arms than legs and with variable sensory loss. The *Brown-Sequard syndrome* most often results from penetrating trauma and is caused by hemisection of the spinal cord. The findings in this instance are ipsilateral loss of motor function, proprioception, and vibratory sensation, and contralateral loss of pain and temperature sensation. The *cauda equina syndrome* is less of a spinal cord lesion than a peripheral nerve injury, and presents with variable motor and sensory loss in the lower extremities, sciatica, bowel or bladder dysfunction, and "saddle anesthesia." Entities peculiar to the pediatric patient are those injuries due to child abuse and spinal cord injury without radiographic abnormality (SCIWORA).

Emergency Department Care and Disposition

Blunt and penetrating injuries to the spine are treated with similar goals in mind. There are three priorities in the care of patients with potential spinal injury:

1. Standard protocols for evaluation and stabilization of trauma patients should be initiated (see Chap. 151). Airway management involves **in-line stabilization** (not traction), **cricoid pressure,** and **appropriate intubation** for patients unable to ventilate adequately or protect their own airway. **Fluid resuscitation** also facilitates spinal cord resuscitation; obvious bleeding must be controlled and occult hemorrhage ruled out. Strong consideration should be given to CT, ultrasound (FAST), or DPL to exclude significant abdominal injury, especially in hypotensive patients. As other injuries are treated, a thorough neurologic examination must be completed identifying the level and type of deficit present.
2. Stabilization of the injured spine is crucial, which prevents secondary injury and preserves residual spinal cord function. Patients must have constant **full spine immobilization**, including cervical stabilization with a **hard collar and sandbags** or other similar device. Though initially these patients should be **immobilized in the field on a hard backboard,** it is now routine to remove the board as quickly as possible (a reasonable goal being within 2 h) in order to prevent skin breakdown and pressure sores.
3. Treatments should be initiated to promote the highest possible chance for spinal cord recovery. Besides adequate fluid resuscitation and oxygenation, spinal shock often responds well to low-dose **dopamine** at 5 to 10 μg/kg/min. Closed SCIs are treated with IV high-dose **methylprednisolone.** Current recommendations are a loading dose of 30 mg/kg over 15 min followed by initiation of an IV drip 45 min later at 5.4 mg/kg/h for 23 h.

For patients evaluated and able to be discharged home, nonsteroidal anti-inflammatory drugs, cold packs, and relative rest are reasonable first-line therapy. Follow-up should be arranged within 2 weeks for a reevaluation specifically to look for signs of subacute instability, particularly for patients with cervical trauma. Any patient with an unstable spine, nerve root injury, uncontrollable pain, or intestinal ileus (common with lumbar fractures) should be admitted to the hospital. Patients with significant vertebral or cord trauma should be managed at a regional trauma or spinal cord injury center.

For further reading in *Emergency Medicine: A Comprehensive Study Guide,* 5th ed., see Chap. 248, "Spinal Cord Injuries," by Bonnie J. Baron and Thomas M. Scalea.

157 | Maxillofacial Trauma

C. Crawford Mechem

Despite the risk of cosmetic sequelae, the greatest concern in patients with maxillofacial trauma is airway compromise. Management requires a coordinated approach by emergency physicians and surgical specialists to ensure a favorable outcome.

Clinical Features and Diagnosis

Diagnosis is based on history, physical examination, and radiographs. Important historical points include mechanism of injury, loss of consciousness, visual changes, diplopia, paresthesias, or malocclusion. Physical examination should include inspection of the face from the front and above. The muscles of facial expression should be assessed. Ecchymoses around the eyes or over the mastoids suggest basilar skull fracture, while deviation of the jaw suggests a mandibular fracture or dislocation. Facial sensation should be tested. Anesthesia of the upper lip, nasal mucosa, lower lid, or maxillary teeth suggests ipsilateral infraorbital nerve damage due to a blowout or orbital rim fracture.

Next, the entire face should be palpated. Subcutaneous air suggests a sinus or nasal fracture. LeFort fractures are diagnosed by grasping the maxillary arch and rocking it while feeling the central face for movement with the opposite hand. In *LeFort I,* a transverse fracture separates the hard palate from the lower portion of the pterygoid plate and nasal septum. With stress of the maxilla, the hard palate and upper teeth move. A pyramidal fracture of the central maxilla and the palate defines a *LeFort II.* Facial tugging moves the nose but not the eyes. *LeFort III,* or cranial-facial disjunction, occurs when the facial skeleton separates from the skull. The entire face shifts with tugging.

The distance between the medial canthi, normally 35–40 mm, should be measured. Widening, or *telecanthus,* suggests serious orbital injury. An eye exam should be performed, including visual acuity. This is followed by a swinging light test to check for a Marcus Gunn pupil, which initially dilates (rather than constricts) when first illuminated, indicating damage to the retina or optic nerve. The eyes are checked for hyphema or subconjunctival hemorrhage, and the pupils are assessed for alignment, reactivity, and shape. A tear-drop shape may suggest globe rupture or penetration. The eyelids should be examined. Penetrating trauma to the medial third of the lids may cause damage to the lacrimal apparatus. Extraocular muscles are tested. Diplopia, especially on upward gaze, may be due to fractures of the zygomatic arch or orbital floor.

The nasoethmoidal-orbital complex (NEO) should be examined for injury, suggested by telecanthus or medial canthus tenderness. The mouth should be inspected for lacerations, malocclusion, tooth tenderness, or anesthesia, often due to fracture-induced nerve injury. To assess for mandibular fracture, the physician may have the patient bite down on a tongue blade, then twist it in an attempt to break it. Patients with a mandible fracture will open their mouth, whereas those with an intact mandible will break the tongue blade. The nose should be examined for deformity, crepitus, or subcutaneous air. Septal hematoma may be observed, appearing as a bluish, bulging mass on a widened septum. Cerebrospinal fluid (CSF) rhinorrhea is suggested by clear nasal drainage mixed with blood that forms a double ring or *halo sign* when dropped on a paper towel or bed sheet. Finally, the ears should be examined for subperichondral hematoma and the canals inspected for lacerations, CSF leak, hemotympanum, or tympanic membrane rupture.

Timing of radiographs depends on the stability of the patient. Patients who are stable, reliable, and have access to close follow-up may have facial radiographs done as an outpatient. Plain films are excellent as screening studies. Facial computed tomographies (CTs) are often used to make the definitive diagnosis and to plan surgical intervention.

Emergency Department Care and Disposition

Initial management emphasizes airway and hemorrhage control. A chin lift or jaw thrust without neck extension often restores airway patency. Severe mandible fractures may cause posterior displacement of the tongue. To prevent airway obstruction, the tongue may be pulled forward with a gauze pad, towel clips, or a large suture passed through the tip. Once the cervical spine has been cleared, the patient should be allowed to sit up and use a tonsil-tip suction catheter.

1. When **endotracheal intubation** is required, the oral route is preferred because of the risks of nasocranial intubation or severe epistaxis with the nasal route. Rapid-sequence intubation carries the risk of being unable to ventilate the patient if intubation is unsuccessful. Alternative strategies include awake intubation or the use of sedatives, such as benzodiazepines, with minimal respiratory depressant effect. If patients are given paralytics, equipment for emergent cricothyroidotomy should be at the bedside.

2. Hemorrhage may be controlled with **direct pressure.** Blind clamping should be avoided because of the risk of damaging the facial nerve or parotid duct. Pharyngeal bleeding may require packing around a cuffed endotracheal tube. In LeFort fractures, bleeding may be controlled by manually realigning the fragments. Severe epistaxis requires direct pressure to the nares or **nasal packing.** In massive nasopharyngeal bleeding, passing a Foley catheter along the floor of the nose and inflating the balloon may be life-saving.

Care of Specific Facial Fractures

Frontal Sinus and Frontal Bone Fractures

Frontal sinus and frontal bone fractures are frequently associated with intracranial injury and may warrant early consultation with a neurosurgeon. Antibiotics covering sinus pathogens are often administered, including **first-generation cephalosporins, amoxicillin-clavulanate,** or **trimethoprim-sulfamethoxazole.** Depressed fractures or posterior wall involvement warrant admission for intravenous antibiotics. Those with isolated fractures of the anterior wall may be treated as outpatients.

Orbital and NEO Fractures

Blowout fractures are the most common orbital fracture. Once diagnosed clinically or radiographically, a CT scan should be obtained to determine the surface area of the broken floor. Indications for surgery include enophthalmos or persistent diplopia. Antibiotics covering sinus pathogens are often recommended. Patients with NEO injuries warrant early consultation with a maxillofacial surgeon.

Nasal Fractures

A fractured nose is usually of little medical concern. Nasal films are rarely ordered, as they do not change ED management. A septal hematoma is treated by local anesthesia with benzocaine or cocaine, followed by **incision of the inferior border with a no.**

11 blade, allowing it to drain. Packing the nose will prevent reaccumulation.

Zygomatic Fractures

Patients with *tripod fractures,* which involve the infraorbital rim, a diastasis of the zygomatic-frontal suture, and disruption of the zygomatic-temporal junction at the arch, require admission for open reduction and internal fixation. Those with fractures of the arch can have elective outpatient elevation and repair.

Mandibular Fractures and Temporomandibular Joint Dislocation

Patients with open fractures require admission and IV antibiotics. **Penicillin, clindamycin,** or a **first-generation cephalosporin** is recommended. Many patients with closed fractures may be managed as outpatients. To reduce a temporomandibular joint dislocation, the physician should stand behind the seated patient and press downward and backward on the posterior molars or the mandibular ridge using thumbs wrapped in gauze. A Barton bandage, an ace wrap placed around the jaw and head, should be applied and the patient discharged on a liquid diet with close follow-up.

For further reading in *Emergency Medicine: A Comprehensive Study Guide,* 5th ed., see Chap. 249, "Maxillofacial Trauma," by Stephen A. Colucciello.

---

158 | Neck Trauma

Charles J. Havel, Jr.

Blunt and penetrating neck trauma have the potential to result in significant morbidity and mortality. Deep vital structures at risk include the airway, major blood vessels, a variety of neural elements including the cervical spinal cord, and the upper portion of the gastrointestinal (GI) tract.

Clinical Features

Patients with neck trauma may demonstrate a variety of clinical presentations from nearly asymptomatic to full cardiopulmonary arrest. Both blunt and penetrating laryngeal or pharyngeal trauma can cause dysphonia, stridor, hemoptysis, hematemesis, dysphagia, neck emphysema, and dyspnea progressing to respiratory arrest. Acute hemorrhage may be visible externally or occur internally, leading to hematoma formation with tracheal deviation or bleeding into the pharynx. In both situations, tachycardia, hypotension, and other signs of shock indicate significant blood loss; airway compromise may result from the mass effect of an expanding hematoma. Neurologic symptoms and signs range from complaints of pain or paresthesias to hemiplegia, quadriplegia, and coma. GI injury initially may be asymptomatic, though patients may complain of dysphagia and hematemesis may be observed. Strangulation may cause petechiae of the skin above the site of ligature and in the subconjunctivae.

Diagnosis and Differential

Penetrating wounds are classified by the zone of injury (Table 158-1) and evaluated for possible violation of the platysma muscle. No further probing of such wounds is warranted in the emergency department; full exploration awaits surgical consultation and the capacity for proximal and distal vascular control in the operating room.

Laboratory testing (e.g., complete blood cell count and blood type and cross-matching) is indicated for all patients in whom there is even the suspicion of serious injury. Plain film radiographs can identify cervical spine injury, the presence of any penetrating foreign body, air in the soft tissues, and soft tissue swelling. A chest x-ray is warranted for any suspected thoracic cavity penetration. Additional diagnostic procedures to be considered, in conjunction with surgical consultation, include arteriography or duplex sonography for suspected arterial injury, computed tomography (CT) scanning of the larynx or cervical spine, endoscopy of the airway and esophagus, or contrast studies of the esophagus.

TABLE 158-1 Zones of the Neck

Zone I	Base of the neck to the cricoid cartilage
Zone II	Cricoid cartilage to the angle of the mandible
Zone III	Angle of the mandible to the base of the skull

The differential diagnosis relates to the various structures at risk for injury. Airway injury may be encountered in cases involving blunt trauma as well as penetrating mechanisms of injury. Vascular injury is most common with penetrating trauma, although major vessel injury can occur due to blunt trauma and may simulate an acute stroke. Neurologic injuries include generalized brain ischemia (seen primarily with strangulation), spinal cord trauma, nerve root damage, and peripheral nerve damage. Cervical spine injury initially may present without neurologic deficit, but the spine can be cleared clinically in selected blunt trauma and gunshot wound victims. The remainder of patients must have their cervical spine cleared by plain films, CT, or, in some cases, magnetic resonance imaging. GI injuries are often occult and generally require evaluation by endoscopy or contrast radiography.

Emergency Department Care and Disposition

1. Standard protocols for evaluation and stabilization of trauma patients should be initiated (see Chap. 151). Hemodynamic and cardiac monitoring, IV access, and **100% oxygen** with pulse oximetry are required initially for all patients.
2. Airway management is made critical by the potential for direct injury and resulting potential for airway compromise. **Tracheal intubation** is indicated for patients unable to maintain airway patency secondary to structural disruption, edema, secretions, bleeding, enlarging hematoma, or impending respiratory arrest. In cases where oral or nasal intubation is not possible or is contraindicated, **cricothyrotomy** or **transtracheal jet insufflation** may be performed.
3. The chest must be evaluated for pneumothorax and hemothorax secondary to vascular injury, primarily in the setting of penetrating trauma. **Needle decompression** is done to relieve tension pneumothorax, and **tube thoracostomy** is performed for pneumothorax and hemothorax.
4. External hemorrhage is controlled with **direct pressure;** blind clamping of bleeding vessels is contraindicated due to the complex vital anatomy compressed into a relatively small space and the danger of causing further injury with a misguided surgical instrument. Fluid resuscitation should begin with **crystalloid,** followed by **blood products** if needed.
5. The cervical spine is secured and cleared clinically or radiographically, as appropriate.
6. The full extent of the injuries is assessed in the secondary survey and additional diagnostic studies ordered, depending on what specific injuries are suspected.

7. Penetrating wounds that do not violate the platysma muscle require only standard meticulous wound care and closure. After a period of observation, asymptomatic patients with these injuries often can be discharged home with close follow-up, presuming their medical condition otherwise makes this feasible. Wounds that violate the platysma muscle mandate surgical consultation. These patients are admitted for surgical exploration or for further diagnostic evaluation of any significant deep structure injury.

8. Patients with blunt neck trauma initially may present with subtle signs of injury and may develop significant symptoms on a delayed basis, particularly those with a strangulation mechanism. After a period of observation, asymptomatic patients may be discharged with close follow-up, although a low threshold for admission should be maintained. Hoarseness, dysphagia, and dyspnea are indications for more extensive evaluation. Any initial symptoms of airway, vascular, or neurologic injury demand evaluation and stabilization along with urgent surgical consultation and admission.

For further reading in *Emergency Medicine: A Comprehensive Study Guide,* 5th ed., see Chap. 250, "Penetrating and Blunt Neck Trauma," by Bonnie J. Baron.

---

159 | Thoracic Trauma

Kent N. Hall

Thoracic trauma is directly responsible for 25 percent of trauma deaths. Patients with isolated chest trauma have a relatively low mortality rate of 5 percent. Penetrating injuries routinely result in pneumothorax or hemothorax. Blunt trauma to the chest causes organ damage by compression, direct trauma, or acceleration-deceleration forces.

GENERAL PRINCIPLES AND CONDITIONS

The first step is to evaluate the patient's effort to breathe. No effort indicates a possible central nervous system problem, such as head trauma, drugs, or spinal cord injury. Significant effort signals an airway obstruction, most commonly a foreign body (including the tongue) in the hypopharynx, larynx, or trachea. If a laryngeal injury is suspected, careful endoscopic evaluation in the operating room should be performed as soon as possible. If the patient is attempting to breath and the airway is clear, thoracic injuries (flail chest, hemopneumothorax, diaphragmatic injury, or parenchymal lung damage) should be considered. In all cases of significant respiratory distress, the airway should be secured and adequate oxygenation and ventilation provided. Indications for ventilatory support are listed in Table 159-1.

The most frequent symptoms associated with thoracic trauma are chest pain and shortness of breath. Physical examination begins with inspection of the chest wall, looking for open ("sucking") chest wounds, flail segments, and contusions. The neck is examined for the presence of distended neck veins, which are associated with pericardial tamponade, tension pneumothorax, air embolus, and cardiac failure. Swelling and cyanosis of the face and neck often signal a superior mediastinal injury resulting in superior vena cava blockage. Subcutaneous emphysema from a bronchial injury or pulmonary laceration can result in severe swelling of the face

TABLE 159-1 Indications for Ventilatory Support

Impaired ventilation in spite of an open airway
Shock
Multiple injuries
Coma
Flail chest
Hypoxia ($Po_2 < 50$ mmHg on room air)
Drainage of hemopneumothorax
Preexisting pulmonary disease
Respiratory rate > 30 beats/min
Relief of chest wall pain
Multiple transfusions required
Elderly

and neck. Palpation of the trachea to determine its normal position, of the chest to localize areas of tenderness or crepitation, and of the abdomen for the position of abdominal contents is important. Auscultation should be done systematically and thoroughly. The quality and equality of breath sounds should be documented. The presence of bowel sounds in the chest may be the first indication of a diaphragmatic injury. Inequality of breath sounds may suggest a pneumothorax, hemothorax, or an improperly inserted endotracheal tube. Conditions that should be recognized and treated during the initial survey include tension pneumothorax, cardiac tamponade, massive hemothorax, open pneumothorax, and flail chest.

CHEST WALL INJURIES

Clinical Features and Diagnosis and Differential

Simple rib fractures should be suspected in the patient with point tenderness over a rib. The goal of evaluating these injuries is to look for complications, such as pneumothorax, pulmonary contusion, or major vascular injury. Suspicion of a pneumothorax that is not corroborated by chest x-ray may require inspiratory and expiratory radiographic views for detection. Pain from rib fractures can decrease ventilation, possibly resulting in atelectasis or pneumonia. First and second rib fractures not due to direct trauma may be associated with significant underlying injuries, including myocardial contusions, pulmonary contusions, bronchial tears, and major vascular injuries. Multiple rib fractures, especially the ninth, tenth, and eleventh, may be associated with intraabdominal injuries. Hypotension may indicate the presence of tension pneumothorax or hemothorax.

Segmental fractures of three or more adjacent ribs produce a flail segment of the chest, which can increase the work of breathing. Flail chest is recognized by paradoxical movement of the segment during the respiratory cycle (outward during expiration, inward during inspiration). In the case of an open pneumothorax ("sucking chest wound"), the wound is often obvious, although it can be obscured by the patient's position or clothing. Open chest wounds indicate invasion into the pleural space and can act as one-way valves, potentially creating a tension pneumothorax.

Traumatic asphyxia, caused by an inability to breath due to added weight on the chest wall, results in subconjunctival hemorrhage or petechiae and vascular engorgement, edema, and cyanosis of the head, neck, and upper extremities. Neurologic impairment is often temporary, and long-term conditions are primarily due to associated injuries.

Emergency Department Care and Disposition

1. Bleeding from chest wall injuries is best controlled by **direct pressure.** Probing of these wounds is not recommended. When subcutaneous emphysema is present, an underlying pneumothorax should be presumed. If the patient is to be intubated for any reason, a chest tube should be inserted.

2. For rib fractures, adequate **analgesia** and **pulmonary toilet** are the mainstays of therapy. Patients with multiple rib fractures should be admitted for 24 to 48 h if they cannot cough and clear secretions, are elderly, or have preexisting pulmonary disease.

3. Sternal fractures should alert the physician to the possible presence of underlying soft tissue injuries, especially of the heart and great vessels. Therapy for these fractures includes adequate analgesia and pulmonary toilet. Admission based solely on the presence of sternal fractures is controversial.

4. For flail chest, management consists of **stabilizing the flail segment,** either externally by using sandbags or internally by endotracheal intubation and mechanical ventilation. Nonventilatory management includes adequate analgesia, chest physiotherapy, and restriction of intravenous (IV) fluids. Indications for ventilatory support of a patient with a flail chest are (1) presence of shock, (2) three or more associated injuries, (3) severe head injury, (4) comorbid pulmonary disease, (5) fracture of eight or more ribs, and (6) age over 65. Patients with a flail chest should be suspected of having an underlying pulmonary contusion.

5. Open ("sucking") chest wounds should be covered with a **sterile, occlusive dressing** while a **chest tube** is inserted simultaneously at a separate site. If a tension pneumothorax develops, the occlusive dressing should be removed until the chest tube is inserted.

LUNG INJURIES

Clinical Features and Diagnosis and Differential

Pulmonary contusions are usually seen as opacifications of the lung on chest x-ray within 6 h of injury.

Pneumothorax is a collection of air in the pleural space. It does not usually cause significant symptoms unless a tension pneumothorax develops, the pneumothorax occupies more than 40 percent of a hemithorax, or the patient has preexisting shock or cardiopulmonary disease. Pneumothoraces are readily seen on expiratory chest x-rays. Clinical signs and symptoms of a tension pneumothorax include dyspnea, hypoperfusion, distended neck veins, deviated trachea, and decreased or absent breath sounds on the affected side.

Hemothorax should be considered in the severely traumatized patient with unilateral decreased breath sounds and dullness to percussion. Volumes of blood as low as 200 to 300 mL are usually visualized on upright chest x-rays. However, volumes in excess of 1 L of blood may be missed on supine chest x-rays because of its appearance as diffuse haziness without a distinct air-fluid level.

Subcutaneous emphysema in the neck and a "crunching" sound during systole (Hamman's sign) should raise the suspicion of pneumomediastinum. The major significance of pneumomediastinum is the possibility of associated injuries to the larynx, trachea, major bronchi, pharynx, or esophagus.

Emergency Department Care and Disposition

1. Treatment of pulmonary contusions involves maintenance of **adequate ventilation,** with the use of **mechanical ventilation** and **positive end-expiratory pressure** to optimize ventilation-perfusion matching. Mechanical ventilation is often required if more than 28 percent of lung volume (estimated by chest x-ray) is involved. With severe unilateral lung injury, synchronous independent lung ventilation through a double-lumen endobronchial catheter prevents overinflation of the normal lung and provides better overall oxygenation.

2. If a tension pneumothorax is suspected, a large bore needle or IV catheter (14 gauge) should be inserted in the second intercostal space at the midclavicular line for **needle decompression.** Emergent management should not be delayed while a chest x-ray is obtained. A chest tube can be inserted for definitive treatment later.

3. If a hemothorax or nontension pneumothorax is suspected in a patient with *severe* respiratory distress, a **chest tube** should be inserted prior to obtaining a chest x- ray. Small pneumothoraces that have not expanded on serial chest x-rays taken 6 to 12 h apart do not usually require chest tube insertion. Admission of these patients for observation and serial examinations is important. An "occult pneumothorax" [i.e., one seen on computed tomography (CT) scan but not on plain x-rays] does not require chest tube insertion unless the patient is on a ventilator. Insertion of a small (24 or 28F) chest tube is adequate if no hemothorax is present. A chest x-ray should be obtained in all patients after insertion of a chest tube. Persistent air leakage and failure of the lung to completely expand is an indication for thoracotomy.

4. With a massive hemothorax, the blood should be evacuated with a large bore (38F or larger) **chest tube.** Prophylactic antibiotics, while controversial, have led to a clear reduction in pneumonia and empyema. Serial examinations of the chest, including chest x-rays, and monitoring of ongoing blood loss through the chest tube are important. The decision to perform a thoracotomy should be made by an appropriately qualified surgeon taking into account available resources. A conservative approach is to perform a thoracotomy if ongoing blood loss from the chest tube exceeds 600 mL in 6 h. Also, if vital signs deteriorate as a large amount of blood is being evacuated from a chest tube, the tube should be clamped and the patient should undergo thoracotomy.

5. While adequate ventilation is being ensured, restoration of adequate tissue perfusion should be achieved. Management of patients in shock includes the insertion of two large bore IV catheters with rapid infusion of large volumes of crystalloid or blood. If peripheral veins are not accessible, subclavian catheterization on the same side as the injury is recommended.

TRACHEOBRONCHIAL INJURY

Injuries to the lower trachea and bronchi are usually caused by severe deceleration forces. Common presenting signs and symptoms include dyspnea, hemoptysis, subcutaneous emphysema, Hamman sign's, and sternal tenderness. On chest x-ray, a large pneumothorax, pneumomediastinum, deep cervical emphysema, or an endotracheal tube balloon that appears round all suggest tracheobronchial injury.

Management includes ensuring **adequate ventilation** and referral for immediate **bronchoscopy** to fully evaluate and treat the injury. Intrathoracic tracheal injury is usually associated with other intrathoracic injuries and is almost invariably fatal. Injuries of the cervical trachea usually occur at the junction of the trachea and cricoid cartilage and are caused by direct trauma, such as from a steering wheel. Inspiratory stridor is common in these patients and indicates a 70 to 80 percent obstruction. Oral intubation, preferably over a bronchoscope, should be attempted. If *gentle* intubation is not possible, a formal tracheostomy should be performed.

DIAPHRAGMATIC INJURY

The majority of diaphragmatic injuries are caused by penetrating trauma. Most series report that diaphragmatic injury associated with blunt injury is usually left sided. The diagnosis of diaphragmatic injury in penetrating trauma is often made intraoperatively due to the paucity of physical findings. An entrance wound in the abdomen with the missile located in the chest cavity should alert the physician of a probable injury to the diaphragm. In the setting of blunt trauma, any abnormality of the diaphragm or lower lung fields on chest x-ray should raise the suspicion of diaphragmatic injury. Many diaphragmatic injuries can be difficult to diagnose, and special techniques may be necessary for complete evaluation.

PENETRATING INJURY TO THE HEART

Clinical Features and Diagnosis and Differential

All patients with hypotension and penetrating chest injury any-where near the heart should be considered to have a cardiac injury until proven otherwise. Patients without signs of life in the field are not considered candidates for resuscitation. Beck's triad (distended neck veins, hypotension, and muffled heart tones) suggests a pericardial tamponade, although most patients with this type of injury do not have distended neck veins until volume resuscitation has occurred. In addition, the breath sounds are audible bilaterally and the trachea is usually midline.

Chest x-rays are rarely helpful in diagnosing acute cardiac injury, and electrocardiographic (ECG) changes are usually nonspecific. Transthoracic echocardiography is a sensitive test for the detection of pericardial fluid. Transesophageal echocardiography (TEE) in experienced hands is a sensitive, efficient diagnostic tool, especially if the patient is already intubated. Pericardiocentesis has limited value in the evaluation of the patient with possible cardiac injury due to the high incidence of false positive and false negative aspirates. In the hemodynamically stable patient, when echocardiography is not available, a subxiphoid pericardial window can be performed.

Emergency Department Care and Disposition

1. Management of the patient with cardiac injury includes attention to the airway, assurance of breathing, and adequate fluid resuscitation. Two large bore IV lines should be placed, with one flowing into the venous system draining into the inferior vena cava. Patients in shock who do not respond to adequate fluid resuscitation and who are suspected of having a cardiac injury should undergo **emergent thoracotomy.**
2. The patient with penetrating thoracic trauma who loses vital signs just prior to arriving at or in the emergency department (ED) may require emergent **pericardiocentesis** or **ED thoracot-**

omy. For ED thoracotomy, an incision is made at the fifth intercostal space on the affected side. The pericardium is opened vertically, with care to avoid the phrenic nerve. The heart, lung hilum, and aorta are inspected for injuries that can be repaired primarily. Patients with blunt traumatic arrest, penetrating abdominal or head injuries, or prolonged arrest times receive little if any benefit from ED thoracotomy.

BLUNT INJURY TO THE HEART

Clinical Features and Diagnosis and Differential

The most common mechanism of injury causing cardiac trauma is a deceleration injury, such as with a high-speed motor vehicle crash. In addition, compression between the sternum and vertebrae, a sudden increase in intrathoracic pressure, abdominal compression forcing abdominal contents against the heart, or strenuous cardiac massage, can all cause cardiac injury. Blunt trauma to the heart can result in multiple types of injuries, including rupture of an outer chamber wall, septal rupture, valvular injuries, direct myocardial injury, laceration of a coronary artery, or pericardial injury. Any history or physical examination finding suggestive of moderate to severe chest or upper abdominal trauma should raise the suspicion of cardiac injury.

Blunt myocardial injury (BMI) is the term currently in use to describe injuries previously termed myocardial concussions and myocardial contusions. The most common clinical features associated with a significant BMI are tachycardia out of proportion to blood loss, dysrhythmias (especially premature ventricular contractions and atrial fibrillation) and conduction defects. The chest x-ray is most useful in detecting associated injuries. Cardiac enzymes, including creatine phosphokinase-MB and the troponins, have been found to be nonspecific in making the diagnosis of significant BMI. Echocardiography does not seem to be very useful in evaluating the patient with suspected BMI, although it is the most widely used modality. It is currently recommended for patients who have cardiac dysrhythmias or dysfunction, and some authors recommend it on all patients with suspected BMI.

BMIs cause death very rarely, and the incidence of clinically significant dysrhythmias and other cardiac complications is low. Management of the patient with a significant BMI calls for the administration of supplemental oxygen and analgesics, treatment of significant cardiac dysrhythmias, and the administration of fluids or inotropes for hypotension.

Cardiac rupture results in immediate death in 80 to 90 percent of cases. Patients with cardiac rupture who arrive at the hospital alive usually have a right atrial tear. Shock out of proportion to the degree of recognized injury and shock that persists despite control of hemorrhage elsewhere and volume expansion should raise suspicion of cardiac rupture. Immediate left anterior thoracotomy may be lifesaving in such cases. Septal defects and valve injuries are rare after blunt trauma but should be considered if a murmur exists in the setting of possible cardiac damage. Signs of a ventricular septal defect include severe early hypoxemia with a relatively normal chest x-ray, heart murmur, and an injury pattern on ECG. Rupture of the aortic valve is the most common valvular lesion, followed by rupture of the papillary muscle or chordae tendinae of the mitral valve.

PERICARDIAL INJURY

A pericardial effusion may develop acutely or over time. The rate of fluid collection influences the onset and severity of symptoms. Evidence of acute pericardial injury is usually seen on the ECG as diffuse ST-segment elevation. Most patients are asymptomatic, and no specific therapy is required. A tear of the parietal pericardium at the apex of the heart may result in sudden severe shock and cardiac arrest if the heart herniates through the hole.

POSTPERICARDIOTOMY SYNDROME

Postpericardiotomy syndrome is seen in patients 2 to 4 weeks after heart surgery or trauma. Classically, patients have chest pain, fever, and pleural or pericardial effusions. Friction rubs, arthralgia, and pulmonary infiltrates may also be seen. The ECG will often show diffuse ST-T wave changes consistent with pericarditis. Management is symptomatic, with salicylates and rest often the only therapy required. Occasionally glucocorticoids are required. Rarely drainage of pericardial fluid is necessary.

PENETRATING TRAUMA TO THE GREAT VESSELS OF THE CHEST

Clinical Features and Diagnosis and Differential

Only 5 to 15 percent of patients with penetrating trauma who require hospital admission will need a thoracotomy, but 25 percent of these will have injury to a great vessel. When a stab wound causes injury, survival is generally much higher than when injury is caused by a gunshot wound. Simple lacerations of the great vessels can lead to exsanguination, tamponade, hemothorax, air embolism, or development of an arteriovenous (AV) fistula or false aneurysm.

Specific historical facts about the injury can be very helpful. If the patient did not have "signs of life" in the field, then no resuscitative efforts are warranted. However, if the patient "lost vital signs" immediately prior to arriving in the ED, then emergent ED thoracotomy is indicated. This procedure is undertaken based solely on the history. Information such as the amount of time the patient spent at the scene and in transit; the size, depth, and angle of penetration of the weapon; and the number of gunshots heard should be sought. It is important to thoroughly inspect the chest, remembering to look in the axilla, in thick chest hair, and in skin folds for possible occult entrance and exit wounds. In general, these wounds should not be probed. Assessment of bilateral upper extremity pulses for equality is important, since a large mediastinal hematoma may compress the subclavian vessels. The entire chest should be auscultated for bruits that may indicate a false aneurysm or AV fistula.

Radiographic evaluation starts with plain chest x-rays. In addition to evaluation for pneumothoraces, widening of the upper mediastinum may indicate injury to brachiocephalic vessels. A "fuzzy" foreign body may indicate motion artifact caused by a foreign body located within or adjacent to pulsatile structures. CT scans are rarely performed immediately for chest-penetrating wounds. However, in the stable patient, a CT scan can help localize hematomas adjacent to great vessels. The use of IV contrast helps further evaluate these structures and may demonstrate a vascular defect or false aneurysm. The major role of CT scans is to screen for great vessel injury. Arteriograms are most helpful in identifying major intrathoracic vascular injuries within hematomas, especially those resulting from penetrating injury to the lower neck. Contrast swallows using gastrografin may be performed on stable patients to evaluate the integrity of the esophagus. Endoscopy is sometimes used in hemodynamically stable patients with penetrating wounds of the chest or lower neck. Recently, use of TEE has been advocated, especially when the CT scan or aortogram is equivocal for injury to the aorta.

Emergency Department Care and Disposition

Early **endotracheal intubation** should be performed in patients with penetrating injuries to the thoracic inlet to avoid the problems associated with expanding hematomas distorting the airway. The patient in severe shock (systolic blood pressure less than 60 mmHg) should have **immediate surgery,** with aggressive fluid resuscitation waiting until after major bleeding sites are controlled. If the systolic blood pressure is 60 to 90 mmHg, 2 to 3 L of crystalloid should be given rapidly. If the patient remains hypotensive, then immediate surgery is required. Emergency thoracotomy is required if the patient loses vital signs in the ED. Indications for thoracotomy in the stable patient are based on chest tube output and other clinical indicators. Bullets that enter great vessels can embolize to distant sites and should be sought using multiple x-rays or fluoroscopy.

BLUNT TRAUMA TO THE GREAT VESSELS OF THE CHEST

Clinical Features and Diagnosis and Differential

Ninety percent of patients with injury to great vessels from blunt trauma who arrive at the hospital alive have an injury at the isthmus of the aorta (between the left subclavian artery and the ligamentum arteriosum). Other common sites of injury are the innominate or left subclavian artery at their origins, or a subclavian artery over the first rib.

Such injuries can occur even when no external signs of trauma exist. Therefore, they should be suspected in any patient with a high-speed deceleration mechanism of injury or high-speed impact from the side. Patients complain primarily of their associated injuries. Retrosternal or interscapular pain, often described as a "tearing" sensation, may be the only initial indication. Dysphagia, stridor, dyspnea, and hoarseness are reported less often.

One-third of patients with blunt trauma to the aorta have no external evidence of thoracic injury. Findings that suggest an aortic injury include a difference in blood pressure or pulse amplitude between the upper and lower extremities, acute-onset upper extremity hypertension, or a harsh systolic murmur across the precordium or in the interscapular area. Findings associated with traumatic rupture of the aorta on plain chest x-ray are shown in Table 159-2. The most frequent radiologic finding is mediastinal widening. Many unnecessary angiograms are performed because of technically poor chest x-rays that make the mediastinum appear wide. The best chest x-ray is an upright posteroanterior chest x-ray taken from 72 in and with the patient leaning forward 10 to 15°. The most specific radiographic sign of traumatic aortic rupture is deviation of the esophagus more than 1 to 2 cm to the right of the spinous process of T4. To see this, a nasogastric tube should be inserted prior to obtaining the chest x-ray. Up to one-third of patients with traumatic aortic rupture will have a normal chest x-ray initially.

TEE is a highly sensitive diagnostic modality to evaluate for traumatic aortic rupture. It can be used at the bedside while the resuscitation is ongoing and yields results that are at least as good as those of aortography. It visualizes the aortic isthmus and de-

TABLE 159-2 Chest Radiographic Findings Associated with Traumatic Rupture of the Aorta

Superior mediastinal widening > 8.0–8.5 cm

Deviation of esophagus and/or trachea at T4

Obscuration of aortic knob and/or descending aorta

Displacement of left mainstem bronchus > 40° below horizontal

Obscuration of medial aspects of left upper lobe

Widening of the paratracheal stripe

Displacement of the paraspinal lines (either left or right)

Fracture of first or second rib

Apical cap

scending aorta very well, and defines the pericardial cavity, cardiac valves, pulmonary veins, and regional wall motion.

Late generation helical CT scans of the chest have been recommended as a tool to screen for traumatic aortic rupture in selected patients. Patient selection guidelines include patients with an equivocal history and equivocal radiograph who have a low probability for injury to the other great vessels, are hemodynamically stable, are capable of tolerating two dye loads (one for the CT scan and one for an aortogram, if necessary). The presence of a mediastinal hematoma is an indication for aortography. Magnetic resonance imaging cannot be recommended as a tool in the evaluation of patients with suspected traumatic aorta rupture, primarily because it requires long periods in an isolated setting. Aortography is the traditional gold standard for diagnosing aortic rupture.

Injury to the ascending aorta usually results in immediate death. Such injuries tend to occur within the pericardium and result in cardiac tamponade. If there is an associated valvular injury, a murmur of aortic insufficiency may be heard. Chest x-ray shows a widened superior mediastinum with or without obscuring the aortic knob. The aortogram shows a pseudoaneurysm, possibly with aortic insufficiency.

Injuries to the innominate artery are associated with rib fractures, flail chest, hemopneumothorax, fractured extremities, head injuries, facial fractures, and abdominal injuries. The diagnosis is difficult because there are no characteristic physical findings except for some decrease in the right radial or brachial pulse. Findings on chest x-ray are similar to those found with traumatic rupture of the aorta except that the mediastinal hematoma is usually higher and the esophagus is pushed to the left. Aortography is generally required to establish the diagnosis.

Subclavian artery injuries are most often caused by fractures to the first rib or clavicle. Absence of a radial pulse on the affected side is the most important sign. A pulsatile mass or bruit at the base of the neck is suggestive of this injury. Associated injury to the brachial plexus occurs in 60 percent of patients, and complete neurologic evaluation of the upper extremity on the involved side is indicated. A Horner's syndrome may occur on the affected side as well. Chest x-ray may show a widened superior mediastinum without obscuring of the aortic knob.

Emergency Department Care and Disposition

Management of the patient with suspected traumatic aortic rupture requires attention to the ABCs (airway, breathing, and circulation), keeping the systolic blood pressure below 120 mmHg, and avoidance of Valsalva maneuvers. Sedatives, analgesics, vasodilators, and β blockers may be required to control the patient's blood pressure. Insertion of a nasogastric tube is important but must be done with extreme care to avoid the patient's gagging. Thoracotomy is the accepted standard of treatment. Delayed repair may be more appropriate in patients who have an extremely high operative risk or when conditions for surgery are not optimal. Most repairs are done under partial cardiopulmonary bypass.

ESOPHAGEAL AND THORACIC DUCT INJURIES

Injuries to the esophagus and thoracic duct are rare. If an esophageal injury is suspected, an esophagram should be performed. Most radiologists recommend gastrografin as the contrast agent because it causes a less inflammatory reaction than does barium. However, the false negative rate with gastrografin is as high as 25 percent. Flexible esophagoscopy can also be performed but carries a false negative rate of 20 percent. Thoracic duct injuries result in a chylothorax in the right hemithorax.

For further reading in *Emergency Medicine: A Comprehensive Study Guide,* 5th ed., see Chap. 251, "Thoracic Trauma," by William M. Bowling, Robert F. Wilson, Gabor D. Kelen, and Timothy G. Buchman.

160 | Abdominal Trauma

O. John Ma

The primary goal in the evaluation of abdominal trauma is to promptly recognize conditions that require immediate surgical exploration. A prolonged examination to pinpoint specific injuries is potentially detrimental to the patient. The most critical mistake is to delay surgical intervention when it is needed.

Clinical Features

Solid Visceral Injuries

Injury to the solid organs can cause morbidity and mortality primarily as a result of acute blood loss. The spleen is the most frequently injured organ in blunt abdominal trauma and is commonly associated with other intraabdominal injuries. The liver also is commonly injured in both blunt and penetrating injuries. Tachycardia, hypotension, and acute abdominal tenderness are the primary physical examination findings. Kehr's sign, representing referred left shoulder pain, is a classic finding in splenic rupture. Lower left rib fractures should heighten clinical suspicion for splenic injury. It is important to note that patients with solid organ injury occasionally may present to the emergency department with minimal symptoms and nonspecific findings on physical examination. This is especially true when the injury is associated with distracting injuries, head injury, or intoxication.

Hollow Visceral Injuries

Hollow visceral injuries produce symptoms by the combination of blood loss and peritoneal contamination. Perforation of the stomach, small bowel, or colon is accompanied by blood loss from a concomitant mesenteric injury. Gastrointestinal contamination will produce peritoneal signs over a period of time. As with solid visceral injuries, patients with head injury, distracting injuries, or intoxication may not exhibit peritoneal signs initially.

Small bowel and colon injuries are most frequently the result of penetrating trauma. However, a deceleration injury can cause a bucket-handle tear of the mesentery or a blowout injury of the antimesenteric border.

Retroperitoneal Injuries

The diagnosis of retroperitoneal injuries can be difficult. Signs and symptoms may be subtle or absent upon initial presentation to the emergency department. Duodenal injuries are most often associated with high-speed vertical or horizontal decelerating trauma. Clinical signs of duodenal injury are often slow to develop. Duodenal injuries may range in severity from an intramural hematoma to an extensive crush or laceration. Duodenal ruptures are usually contained within the retroperitoneum. Patients may present with abdominal pain, fever, nausea, and vomiting, but these symptoms may take hours to become clinically obvious.

Pancreatic injury is most common with penetrating trauma. It also occurs after a severe crush injury. The classic case is a blow to the midepigastrium from a steering wheel or the handlebar of a bicycle. Following blunt trauma, patients with pancreatic injuries can present with subtle signs and symptoms, making the diagnosis elusive. With the proper mechanism of injury, a high index of suspicion must be maintained for these injuries.

Urologic injuries are discussed in Chap. 162, "Genitourinary Tract Trauma."

Diaphragmatic Injuries

Presentation of diaphragmatic injuries is often insidious. Only occasionally is the diagnosis obvious, when bowel sounds can be auscultated in the thoracic cavity. On chest x-ray, with herniation of abdominal contents into the thoracic cavity, the diagnosis is confirmed. In most cases, however, there is no herniation, and the only finding on chest x-ray is blurring of the diaphragm or an effusion. This injury is diagnosed most often on the left.

Diagnosis and Differential

Plain Radiographs

For blunt trauma, routine use of plain abdominal radiographs is not a cost-effective and prudent method for evaluating the trauma patient. A chest radiograph is helpful in evaluating for herniated abdominal contents in the thoracic cavity and for evidence of free air under the diaphragm. An anteroposterior pelvis radiograph is important for identifying pelvic fractures, which can produce significant blood loss and be associated with intraabdominal visceral injury.

Diagnostic Peritoneal Lavage

Diagnostic peritoneal lavage (DPL) remains an excellent screening test for evaluating abdominal trauma. Its advantages include its sensitivity, availability, the relative speed with which it can be performed, and low complication rate. Disadvantages include the potential for iatrogenic injury, its misapplication for evaluation of retroperitoneal injuries, and its lack of specificity.

For blunt trauma, indications for DPL include (1) patients who are too hemodynamically unstable to leave the ED for CT scanning or who have physical examination findings that are unreliable secondary to drug intoxication or central nervous system injury and (2) unexplained hypotension in patients with equivocal physical examination findings.

In penetrating trauma, DPL should be performed when it is not clear that exploratory laparotomy should be performed. DPL is useful in evaluating patients sustaining stab wounds where local wound exploration indicates that the superficial muscle fascia has been violated. Also, it may be useful in confirming negative physical examination findings when tangential or lower chest wounds are involved.

The DPL is considered positive if more than 10 mL of gross blood is aspirated immediately, the red blood cell count is greater than 100,000 cells/μL, the white blood cell count is greater than 500 cells/μL, bile is present, or vegetable matter is present.

The only absolute contraindication to DPL is when surgical management is clearly indicated, in which case the DPL would delay patient transport to the operating room. Relative contraindications include patients with advanced hepatic dysfunction, severe coagulopathies, previous abdominal surgeries, or a gravid uterus.

Ultrasonography

Recent literature has demonstrated that the focused assessment with sonography for trauma (FAST), like DPL, is an accurate screening tool for abdominal trauma. Both emergency physicians and surgeons have demonstrated that they can reliably perform the FAST examination to accurately identify the presence of free intraperitoneal fluid in trauma patients. Many more trauma centers have begun to use the FAST examination to replace DPL. Advantages of the FAST examination are that it is accurate, rapid, noninvasive, repeatable, and portable. Another advantage of the FAST examination is that it is capable of evaluating for free pericardial fluid and free pleural fluid. Disadvantages include its inability to determine the exact etiology of the free intraperitoneal fluid and that it is operator dependent. Indications for FAST are the same as for DPL.

Computed Tomography

The abdominal CT scan has a greater specificity than DPL and ultrasonography, thus making it the initial diagnostic test of choice at most trauma centers. Oral and intravenous (IV) contrast material should be given to provide optimal resolution.

Advantages of CT scanning include its ability to precisely locate intraabdominal lesions preoperatively, to evaluate the retroperitoneum, and to identify injuries that may be managed nonoperatively, as well as its noninvasiveness. The disadvantages of CT scanning are the expense, time required to perform the study, need to transport the trauma patient to the radiology suite, and use of contrast materials.

Emergency Department Care and Disposition

1. Standard protocols for evaluation and stabilization of trauma patients should be initiated (see Chap. 151).
2. Administer **100% oxygen,** and secure cardiac monitoring and two IV lines.
3. For hypotensive abdominal trauma patients, resuscitation with **IV crystalloid fluid** is indicated. **Transfusion with O-negative or type-specific pRBCs** should be considered in addition to crystalloid resuscitation.

TABLE 160-1 Indications for Laparotomy

	Blunt		Penetrating
Absolute	Anterior abdominal injury and hypotension Abdominal wall disruption Peritonitis Free air on chest x-ray CT-diagnosed injury requiring surgery (e.g., pancreatic transection, duodenal rupture)	Absolute	Injury to abdomen, back, and flank with hypotension Abdominal tenderness Gastrointestinal evisceration Positive DPL High suspicion for transabdominal trajectory (GSW) CT-diagnosed injury requiring surgery (e.g., ureter or pancreas)
Relative	Positive DPL or FAST in stable patient Solid visceral injury in stable patient Hemoperitoneum on CT without clear source	Relative	Positive local wound exploration (SW)

4. Laboratory work for patients with abdominal trauma should be based on the mechanism of injury (blunt versus penetrating); it may include type and crossmatching; complete blood count; electrolyte, arterial blood gas, and directed toxicologic studies; prothrombin and partial thromboplastin times; and platelet, hepatic enzyme, and lipase evaluations.

5. Table 160-1 lists the indications for exploratory laparotomy. When a patient presents to the emergency department with an obvious high-velocity gunshot wound to the abdomen, DPL or the FAST examination should not be performed, since it will only delay transport of the patient to the operating room. If organ evisceration is present, it should be covered with a moist, sterile dressing prior to surgery.

6. For an equivocal stab wound to the abdomen, surgical consultation for **local wound exploration** is indicated. If the wound exploration demonstrates no violation of the anterior fascia, the patient can be discharged home safely.

7. For the hemodynamically stable blunt trauma patient with positive FAST examination results, further evaluation with CT scan may be warranted prior to admission to the surgical service.

For further reading in *Emergency Medicine: A Comprehensive Study Guide,* 5th ed., see Chap. 252, "Abdominal Injuries," by Thomas M. Scalea and Sharon Boswell.

---

161 | Flank and Buttock Trauma
Stephen W. Meldon

PENETRATING TRAUMA TO THE FLANK

Penetrating trauma to the flank is a distinct subcategory of penetrating torso trauma. The organs most commonly injured by penetrating trauma to this area include the liver, kidney, colon, duodenum, and pancreas. The diagnosis of these injuries, however, may be difficult because of the apparent absence of physical findings.

Clinical Features

The importance of obtaining a complete history and performing a thorough physical examination must be emphasized. Mechanism of injury, description of the wounding object, and time elapsed since injury are important to the evaluation. Both the chest and abdomen must be evaluated. Specific organ injuries are covered in the chapters on abdominal trauma (Chap. 160) and genitourinary tract trauma (Chap. 162).

Diagnosis and Differential

In the hemodynamically stable patient with no obvious visceral injury, adjunctive diagnostic tests such as wound exploration, diagnostic peritoneal lavage (DPL), computed tomography (CT), or portable ultrasound (US) are useful. Wound exploration should generally be reserved for superficial stab wounds with low probability of visceral injury. Sterile technique, adequate anesthesia, good exposure and hemostasis are key. Exploration of injuries that extend through fascia or muscle is not recommended. DPL is highly accurate for detecting intraperitoneal injuries, but poor in detecting retroperitoneal injuries. DPL may be indicated when injury to the diaphragm or hollow viscus is suspected. CT scanning can be accurate in detecting solid viscus intraperitoneal and retroperitoneal injuries. Oral, intravenous, and rectal contrast (for suspected rectal injuries) are necessary for an optimal study. Portable US is sensitive and specific for determining free intraperitoneal fluid which, in the unstable patient, is sufficient to recommend operative intervention. A chest x-ray should be obtained to rule out intrathoracic involvement.

Emergency Department Care and Disposition

All patients with penetrating trauma should be evaluated and resuscitated according to routine trauma protocol, as outlined in Chap. 151.

1. Two large-bore intravenous lines, supplemental oxygen, cardiac monitoring, and nasogastric and Foley catheters should be placed.
2. A baseline complete blood cell count (CBC), type and crossmatch, urinalysis, and rectal examination should be performed on all patients.
3. Trauma team involvement or early surgical consultation should be obtained. Selective management with early CT scanning results in fewer nontherapeutic laparotomies with no increase in untoward outcomes, and is now advocated. Exploratory lapa-

rotomy is indicated for patients with hemodynamic instability, evisceration, peritonitis, intraperitoneal free air, or transabdominal missile path. Selective management is also appropriate in stable patients with stab wounds. Appropriate patient management is directed by the findings. All patients should be admitted, with the exception of those patients with clearly defined superficial wounds.

PENETRATING BUTTOCK INJURIES

Penetrating trauma to the buttock has the potential to injure multiple organ systems, including gastrointestinal (GI), genitourinary (GU), and neurologic (sciatic and femoral nerves) systems. Significant morbidity and mortality may occur if such injuries are missed.

Clinical Features

The clinical features will vary depending on which organ system has been injured. Blood within the rectum signifies distal colon or rectal injuries. GU trauma can present with hematuria and scrotal or penile hematomas. Vascular injuries should be suspected when an enlarging hematoma, bruit, or change in peripheral pulses is present. Neurologic injuries will present with paresthesias, sensory loss, or motor weakness.

Diagnosis and Differential

Baseline laboratory evaluation should include a CBC, type and cross-match, and urinalysis. A careful rectal examination should be performed. Routine proctosigmoidoscopy will identify rectal and sigmoid colon injuries. Hematuria should be investigated with retrograde urethrogram and cystogram. Routine pelvic x-rays will reveal bony injury and suggest possible missile path. CT scan of the pelvis may reveal colon, urinary tract, or vascular injury. Angiography may be indicated in the evaluation of suspected vascular injury.

Emergency Department Care and Disposition

Initial resuscitation should be followed as noted earlier.

1. If a urethral injury is suspected, a Foley catheter should not be placed.
2. **Broad-spectrum antibiotics** (i.e., Zosyn 3.375 g IV) are indicated for rectal injuries.
3. Hemodynamic instability, peritonitis, or blood within the GI

tract are indications for operative therapy. Significant vascular or nerve injuries (sciatic or femoral nerves) usually require early operative intervention.
4. Trauma team evaluation or early surgical consultation should be obtained. All patients should be admitted for further evaluation and monitoring.

For further reading in *Emergency Medicine: A Comprehensive Study Guide,* 5th ed., see Chap. 253, "Penetrating Trauma to the Flank and Buttock," by Alasdair K. T. Conn.

---

162   Genitourinary Trauma

C. Crawford Mechem

Injuries to the genitourinary system occur in 2 to 5 percent of adult trauma patients, usually in the setting of blunt trauma. Although rarely life-threatening in themselves, they are often associated with more serious injuries and require prompt and thorough management.

Clinical Features

History and physical examination should raise suspicion for genitourinary injuries. Patients with any abdominal trauma, including penetrating trauma in the vicinity of genitourinary structures, are at risk. High-velocity deceleration predisposes to renal pedicle injuries, including lacerations and thromboses of the renal artery and vein. Fractures of the lower ribs or lower thoracic or lumbar vertebrae are often associated with renal or ureteral injuries, while pelvic fractures and straddle injuries are associated with urethral or bladder trauma.

Because genitourinary trauma is rarely life-threatening, the initial evaluation should focus on more emergent injuries. However, during the secondary survey, a careful abdominal and genitourinary examination should be performed. Flank ecchymoses, tenderness, or masses suggest renal injuries. The perineum should be inspected for blood or lacerations. The presence of a penile, scrotal, or perineal hematoma or blood at the penile meatus suggests urethral injury. If blood at the meatus is present, a urethral catheter should not be passed out of concern for converting a partial urethral laceration into a complete transection. A rectal examination should be performed, assessing sphincter tone, checking for blood, and determining the position of the prostate. A high-riding prostate suggests injury to the membranous urethra. The scrotum should be examined, looking for ecchymoses, lacerations, or testicular disruption. In females, the labia should be carefully assessed for injuries and a bimanual examination performed to check for vaginal lacerations.

Diagnosis and Differential

The approach to evaluation depends on whether the mechanism of injury is blunt or penetrating, the patient's age and hemodynamic stability, whether there is hematuria, and, if so, whether it is gross or microscopic. Microscopic hematuria is defined as > 5 red blood cells (RBCs) per high power field (hpf). Generally, the urine should be evaluated for hematuria before passage of a urinary catheter is considered. If placement of a catheter is urgent and injury to the urethra has not been excluded, the suprapubic approach may be employed. Trauma survey x-rays should be obtained, including an anteroposterior view of the pelvis.

Analysis of the first-voided urine may help localize the injury. Initial hematuria suggests injury to the urethra or prostate, while terminal hematuria is associated with bladder neck trauma. Continuous hematuria is often due to injury to the bladder, ureter, or kidney. In blunt trauma, the degree of hematuria does not correlate with severity of injury. However, in hemodynamically stable patients, isolated microscopic hematuria rarely represents significant injury. Exceptions to this include associated transient hypotension, a rapid deceleration mechanism with renal pedicle injury, or pediatric cases. In stable children, injury is unlikely if the urine contains < 50 RBCs/hpf.

The choice of imaging study will be dictated by the hemodynamic stability of patients and suspicion for associated injuries. Patients of blunt trauma with microscopic hematuria and associated injuries or patients with gross hematuria should undergo abdominal computed tomography (CT) scan, which has the advantage of simultaneously imaging other organs. However, it should only be performed on hemodynamically stable patients. Patients who are unstable should undergo a one-shot intravenous pyelogram (IVP), either in the emergency department or operating room. If the patient's systolic blood pressure is 70 mmHg or less, dye-induced nephrotoxicity may result. IVP also can be used in stable patients if CT is unavailable, but the resolution is poor. IVP remains the mainstay of diagnosing ureteral injuries, identified by extravasation of contrast dye. However, in many centers spiral CTs are also being used for this purpose and have the advantage of visualizing the entire retroperitoneal space.

In penetrating trauma, there is no correlation between the degree of hematuria and the severity of injury. Therefore, penetrating trauma patients with the potential for genitourinary injury should be imaged by IVP prior to exploratory laparotomy.

Cystography is commonly used to diagnose bladder injuries in patients with gross hematuria. It is performed by instilling contrast media retrograde into the bladder and looking for extravasation, preferably under fluoroscopy. Urethral injuries also are investigated by retrograde cystography. An unlubricated urinary catheter is passed 2 to 3 cm into the distal urethra, the balloon inflated with 1 to 3 mL water, and 20 to 30 mL contrast material injected. An oblique film is obtained, looking for extravasation. Urethral injuries should not be investigated in the case of pelvic trauma until it is certain that pelvic angiography or embolization is not required.

Emergency Department Care and Disposition

Standard protocols for evaluation and stabilization of trauma patients should be initiated (see Chap. 151). Emphasis should be placed on identifying life-threatening injuries. Patients with isolated microscopic hematuria and no other injuries may be discharged with repeat urinalysis in 2 to 3 weeks.

MANAGEMENT OF SPECIFIC INJURIES

Kidney

Contusions account for 92 percent of renal injuries, with renal lacerations, pedicle injuries, and shattered kidneys making up the rest. Renal injuries are graded according to severity (Table 162-1). Grades 1 and 2 injuries are usually managed nonoperatively. In the absence of other injuries, these patients may be discharged with repeat urinalysis in 2 to 3 weeks. Patients with grades 3 and 4 injuries should be admitted. Many of these patients have associated injuries requiring surgical repair. However, in the

TABLE 162-1 Grading of Renal Injuries

Grade	Injury
I	Contusion (microscopic or gross hematuria, with normal urologic study results) Subscapsular, nonexpanding hematoma without laceration
II	Parenchymal laceration <1.0 cm depth limited to cortex, no extravasation Nonexpanding hematoma, confined to retroperitoneum
III	Parenchymal laceration >1 cm depth with extravasation or collecting system rupture
IV	Laceration extending through to collecting system Vascular pedical injury, hemorrhage contained
V	Shattered kidney Avulsed hilum (devascularized kidney)

Source: From Moore EE, Shackford SR, Pachter HL, et al: Organ injury scaling: Spleen, liver, kidney. *J Trauma* 29:1664, 1989, with permission.

case of isolated injury, patients may be managed nonoperatively with frequent reassessment. They should be put at bed rest, kept well hydrated, have frequent hematocrit determinations, and frequent urinalysis to assess degree of hematuria. Patients with grade 5 injuries require operative repair, as do any patients with uncontrolled hemorrhage, multiple kidney lacerations, a pulsatile or expanding hematoma on abdominal exploration, or penetrating injuries.

Ureter

Ureteral injuries are the rarest of the genitourinary injuries and usually result from penetrating trauma. If the ureter is completely transected, hematuria may be absent. Ureter injuries should be managed operatively.

Bladder

Bladder contusions are treated expectantly. Incomplete bladder lacerations may be managed by catheter placement and observation. Bladder rupture is either intra- or extraperitoneal. Intraperitoneal rupture usually results from a burst injury of a full bladder and is managed operatively. Extraperitoneal rupture is often associated with a pelvic ring fracture. Symptoms include abdominal pain and tenderness, hematuria, and inability to void. Management involves urethral catheter drainage alone. Penetrating bladder injuries are managed operatively.

Urethra

Urethral injuries in males involve the posterior (prostatomembranous) urethra and the anterior (bulbous and penile) urethra. Posterior injuries are associated with pelvic fractures. Anterior injuries result from direct trauma or instrumentation. In females, urethral injuries are often associated with pelvic fractures and commonly present with vaginal bleeding. Anterior contusons are managed conservatively, with or without a urethral catheter. Partial anterior urethral lacerations are managed with an indwelling catheter or with suprapubic cystotomy. Complete lacerations are repaired with end-to-end anastomosis. Partial lacerations of the posterior urethra are managed with urethral or suprapubic drainage. Complete lacerations are managed either surgically or with suprapubic drainage alone.

Testicles and Scrotum

Blunt testicular injuries consist of contusions or rupture. Testicular ultrasound can help to determine the type and extent of injury. Contusions may be managed conservatively, whereas rupture or penetrating trauma require operative repair to improve outcome.

Penis

Lacerations and amputations require operative debridement and reconstruction. A fractured penis, due to traumatic rupture of the corpus cavernosum, is managed by immediate surgical drainage of blood clot and repair of the torn tunica albuginea and any associated urethral injuries.

For further reading in *Emergency Medicine: A Comprehensive Study Guide,* 5th ed., see Chap. 254, "Genitourinary Trauma," by Gabor D. Kelen.

163 | Penetrating Trauma to the Extremities

C. Crawford Mechem

While rarely life-threatening, penetrating extremity trauma can result in long-term morbidity if not treated appropriately. Emergency physicians play a crucial role in the management of these injuries through early diagnosis and prompt initiation of care is important to limb survival.

Clinical Features

After the initial trauma resuscitation is complete, patients should be asked about past medical history, including any preexisting vascular or neuromuscular deficits. The mechanism of injury should be determined, such as the type of weapon used. A careful physical examination of the affected extremity should then be performed. The size and shape of any wounds should be noted. The affected extremity should be examined for evidence of underlying soft tissue injury, retained foreign body, compartment syndrome, fracture, or neurovascular compromise. Penetrating trauma near a joint warrants a careful search for damage to the joint capsule.

Prompt recognition of arterial injury is one of the fundamental goals of management. "Hard signs" of vascular injury, seen in fewer than 6 percent of cases, include absent or diminished distal pulses, obvious arterial bleeding, an expanding or pulsatile hematoma, audible bruit, palpable thrill, or evidence of distal ischemia. "Soft signs," which are more common, include a small, stable hematoma; injury to an anatomically related nerve; unexplained hypotension; a history of hemorrhage that has now stopped; proximity of the injury to a major vessel; or a complex fracture.

The color, temperature, and capillary refill time in the affected extremity may provide clues to subtle vascular injury. The presence and quality of pulses distal to the injury should be noted and compared with the unaffected side. Ankle-brachial indices (ABI) should be calculated. To accomplish this, patients are placed in a supine position and the systolic blood pressure measured in all four extremities using a Doppler device. To measure an ankle systolic pressure, a standard adult blood pressure cuff should be snugly wrapped around the ankle just above the malleoli and the signal from the posterior or anterior tibial artery monitored. An ABI is then calculated by dividing the ankle systolic blood pressure by the greater of the two upper extremity systolic blood pressures. An ABI > 1.0 is normal. An ABI of 0.5 to 0.9 is indicative of injury to a single arterial segment. An ABI < 0.5 is indicative of severe arterial injury or injury to multiple arterial segments. A difference > 20 mmHg between the upper extremity blood pressures is indicative of upper extremity arterial injury.

A careful neurologic examination should be performed, testing both sensory and motor function (Table 163-1). While arterial hemorrhage is the most dramatic result of extremity trauma, injur-

TABLE 163-1 Clinical Examination of the Nerves of the Extremities

Nerve	Text of motor function	Test for sensation
Axillary (C5-6)	Arm abduction Arm internal, external rotation	Lateral aspect of shoulder
Musculocutaneous (C5-6)	Forearm flexion	Lateral forearm
Radial (C5-8)	Forearm, wrist, and finger extension	Dorsoradial hand, thumb
Median (C6-T1)	Wrist flexion, finger adduction	Volar aspect of thumb and index finger
Ulnar (C7-T1)	Finger abduction	Volar aspect of little finger
Femoral (L1-L4)	Knee extension	
Obturator (L2-L4)	Hip adduction	
Superior gluteal (L4-S1)	Hip abduction	
Sciatic (L4-S3)	Knee flexion	
Deep peroneal (L4-S1)	Ankle and great toe dorsi flexion	
Superficial peroneal (L5-S1)		
Tibial (L5-S2)	Ankle plantar flexion	
Posterior tibial (L5-S2)	Great toe plantar flexion	
Spinal L4		Medial calf
Spinal L5		Dorsal foot
Spinal S1		Lateral plantar foot

ies to major nerves are the most likely to lead to long-term disability. Fortunately, 70 percent of peripheral nerve injuries recover completely within 6 months.

Diagnosis and Differential

Plain radiographs should be obtained in all cases, including the joints above and below the injury, looking for evidence of fracture, foreign bodies, or joint space penetration. *Computed tomography* may be valuable in certain cases before definitive orthopedic care. *Angiography* is used to delineate the extent, nature, and location of vascular injury. It is especially helpful in the setting of shotgun wounds, multiple or severe fractures, thoracic outlet wounds, extensive soft tissue injury, or in patients with underlying vascular disease. Angiography for the evaluation of wounds in close proximity to a major artery without "hard signs" of injury identifies abnormalities in 10 to 20 percent of cases, with only 2 percent of these requiring surgical repair. When "hard signs" are present, preoperative angiography may be appropriate to help plan operative care. However, some cases warrant immediate surgery without further evaluation. *Duplex ultrasonography* has a diagnostic accuracy of 96 to 98 percent and can image extremity vessels with as much resolution as contrast angiography. Compared with angiography, it is safer and yields more rapid results. However, the technique is very operator-dependent.

Emergency Department Care and Disposition

1. Before extremity injuries are addressed, immediately life-threatening trauma should be evaluated. Profuse bleeding is initially controlled with **direct pressure.** Clamping or ligation of bleeding vessels should be avoided, when possible, because of the risk of damaging accompanying nerves. Patients with hard signs of arterial injury require either immediate surgical intervention or surgical consultation and angiography. Patients with soft signs rarely require surgery but warrant inpatient observation. The general principles of wound management, including **tetanus prophylaxis,** apply.
2. There is no role for prophylactic antibiotics except for heavily contaminated wounds or in patients who are immunocompromised.
3. **Wound exploration** in the emergency department is reserved for patients with suspected foreign bodies in the wound, for ligamentous involvement, or to control minor venous bleeding. Wound exploration to control arterial or major venous hemorrhage is best reserved for the operating room. Patients with

evidence of joint space involvement require evaluation by an orthopedic surgeon. Often such wounds will be managed by arthroscopic exploration and irrigation. Because of the risk of lead toxicity from retained intraarticular bullet fragments, these should be removed.

Patients with penetrating extremity injury without hard or soft signs, with minimal soft tissue defect, and no signs of compartment syndrome may be discharged with close follow-up after 3 to 12 h of observation and serial examinations.

For further reading in *Emergency Medicine: A Comprehensive Study Guide,* 5th ed., see Chap. 255, "Penetrating Trauma to the Extremities," by Richard D. Zane and Allan Kumar.

FRACTURES AND DISLOCATIONS

164 | Early Management of Fractures and Dislocations

Michael P. Kefer

A delay in diagnosis of several orthopedic emergencies can increase the chance of significant complications or poor functional outcome.

Clinical Features

Knowing the precise mechanism of injury or listening carefully to patients' symptoms is important in diagnosing fracture or dislocation. Pain may be referred to an area distant from the injury (e.g., hip injury presenting as knee pain). If key aspects of the history are not appreciated, specific x-ray views needed may never be ordered.

The physical exam includes (*a*) inspection for deformity, edema, or discoloration; (*b*) assessment of active and passive range of motion of joints proximal and distal to the injury; (*c*) palpation for tenderness or deformity, and (*d*) assessment of neurovascular status distal to the injury. Careful palpation can prevent missing a crucial diagnosis due to referred pain. The neurovascular status should be documented early, before performing reduction maneuvers.

Radiologic evaluation is based on the history and physical exam, not simply on where patients report pain. X-ray of all long bone fractures should include the joints proximal and distal to the fracture to evaluate for coexistent injury. A negative x-ray does not exclude a fracture. This commonly occurs with scaphoid, radial head, or metatarsal shaft fractures. The emergency department (ED) diagnosis is often clinical and is not confirmed until 7 to 10 days after the injury, when enough bone resorption has occurred at the fracture site to detect a lucency on x-ray.

871

An accurate description of the fracture to the consultant is crucial and should include the following details:

Open versus closed.

Location—Mid-shaft, junction of proximal and middle or middle and distal third, or distance from bone end. Intraarticular involvement with disruption of the joint surface may require surgery. Anatomic bony reference points should be used when applicable (e.g., humerus fracture just above the condyles is described as supracondylar, as opposed to distal humerus).

Orientation of fracture line—Transverse, spiral, oblique, comminuted (shattered), and segmental (single large segment of free floating bone).

Displacement—The amount and direction the distal fragment is offset in relation to the proximal fragment should be described.

Separation—Degree the two fragments have been pulled apart. Unlike displacement, alignment is maintained.

Shortening—Reduction in bone length due to impaction or overriding fragments.

Angulation—Angle formed by the fracture segments. Describe the degree and direction of deviation of the distal fragment.

Rotational deformity—Degree the distal fragment is twisted on the axis of the normal bone. It is usually detected by physical exam and not seen on x-ray.

Fractures combined with dislocation or subluxation—Associated disruption of proper joint alignment should be described as fracture-dislocation or fracture-subluxation to clearly communicate the more serious nature of the injury.

Complications resulting from neurovascular deficit may be immediate or delayed. Compartment syndrome that presents with the five classic signs—pain, pallor, paresthesias, pulselessness, and paralysis—is well advanced. This diagnosis should be made presumptively, based on the character of pain, which is the earliest sign. Long-term complications of fracture include malunion, nonunion, avascular necrosis, arthritis, and osteomyelitis.

Emergency Department Care and Disposition

1. Swelling should be controlled with application of cold packs and elevation. **Analgesics** should be administered as necessary. Remove any objects such as rings or watches that may constrict the injury as swelling progresses. Patients should have nothing by mouth if anesthesia will be required.

2. **Prompt reduction of fracture deformity** with steady, longitudinal traction is indicated to (*a*) alleviate pain; (*b*) relieve tension

on associated neurovascular structures; (*c*) minimize the risk of converting a closed fracture to an open fracture when a sharp, bony fragment tents overlying skin; and (*d*) restore circulation to a pulseless distal extremity. Whether the procedure is performed by the emergency physician or the orthopedist depends on practice environment. Of the preceding indications, however, distal vascular compromise is the most time-critical. Postreduction films should be obtained to confirm proper anatomic repositioning.

3. Open fractures as treated immediately with prophylactic antibiotics to prevent osteomyelitis. A common regimen is a **first-generation cephalosporin** and an **aminoglycoside.** Irrigation and debridement in the operating room is indicated.

4. The fracture or relocated joint should be **immobilized.** Fiberglass or plaster splinting material is commonly used. The chemical reaction that causes the material to set is an exothermic reaction that begins upon contact with water. The amount of heat liberated is directly proportional to the setting process, which, in turn, is directly proportional to the temperature of the water. Severe burns, therefore, can result from the splinting material, as the peak temperature to the skin is the sum of the water temperature plus the heat released by the exothermic reaction. The use of water slightly warmer than room temperature is a safe practice. Padding is necessary under the splint to prevent pressure sores and irritation. An adequate length should be used to immobilize the injury. Splints for midshaft fractures should be long enough to immobilize the joint above and below the fracture.

5. **Crutches** are prescribed for patients who have lower extremity injuries that require **non-weight-bearing.** Ideal crutch height is one hand width below the axilla. The pressure of the crutch pads is borne by the sides of the thorax, not the axilla, to avoid injury to the brachial plexus. Walkers and canes are appropriate for partial weight-bearing conditions, and they may be alternatives for patients too weak to use crutches.

6. Patients who are discharged home are instructed to keep the injured extremity elevated above heart level and to seek immediate reevaluation if increased swelling, cyanosis, pain, or decreased sensation develops.

For further reading in *Emergency Medicine: A Comprehensive Study Guide,* 5th ed., see Chap. 259, "Initial Evaluation and Management of Orthopedic Injuries," by Jeffrey S. Menkes.

165 | Wrist and Hand Injuries

Michael P. Kefer

For wrist and hand injuries, the key therapeutic concept is preservation of function by proper splinting, followed by early mobilization.

1. Padded aluminum splints adequately immobilize flexion and extension movement as occurs at the DIP and PIP.
2. Plaster or fiberglass is required to control rotary motion, as occurs at the MCP and wrist.
3. Open fracture or open joint injury is treated in the operating room; immediate intravenous antibiotics are indicated.
4. Fracture or dislocation that compromises neurovascular function or overlying skin requires urgent reduction.
5. Significant crush, artery, or nerve injury requires emergent referral to a hand surgeon.

TENDON INJURIES

Knowing the hand position at the time of injury predicts where, along its course, a tendon is injured. Extensor tendon repair often can be performed by the emergency physician. Flexor tendon repair should be performed by a hand surgeon. Follow-up and rehabilitation of all tendon injuries are necessary.

BOUTONNIERE DEFORMIY

This results from an injury at the dorsal surface of the PIP that disrupts the extensor hood apparatus. Lateral bands of the extensor mechanism become flexors of the PIP and hyperextensors of the DIP. An extensor hood injury is easily missed on emergency department (ED) presentation. Reexamination after 7 days is indicated.

COLLATERAL LIGAMENTS AND VOLAR PLATE

Collateral ligaments form a U-shaped hood around the lateral and volar aspects of the IP and MCP joints. MCP collateral ligaments are taut in flexion and lax in extension. Therefore, to preserve maximum function, the MCP is immobilized at 90° flexion. Abduction and adduction stress is applied to assess collateral ligament stability; hyperextension stress will assess volar plate stability. IP partial sprains are treated by buddy tape splinting. IP complete disruptions are treated by a gutter splint at 20° flexion. MCP partial sprains are treated by an aluminum splint at 90° flexion. MCP complete disruptions are treated by a gutter splint at 90° flexion.

GAMEKEEPER'S THUMB

Gamekeeper's thumb results from forced radial abduction at the MCP with injury to the ulnar collateral ligament of the thumb. This is the most critical of the collateral ligament injuries, since it affects pincer function. A partial tear is diagnosed when abduction stress causes the joint to open up to 20° more, relative to the uninvolved side. A complete tear is diagnosed when abduction stress causes the joint to open >20° more relative to the uninvolved side. Treatment is a thumb spica splint for partial disruption and surgical repair for complete disruption.

DORSAL IP JOINT DISLOCATION

Dorsal IP joint dislocation is relatively common. A radiograph is indicated to distinguish dislocation from fracture-dislocation. Reduction is performed under digital-block anesthesia. The dislocated phalanx should be distracted, slightly hyperextended, then repositioned. Collateral ligament damage should then be assessed and the joint splinted accordingly.

VOLAR IP JOINT DISLOCATION

Volar IP joint dislocation is an uncommon injury. It results in boutonniere deformity from extensor mechanism injury. An x-ray may reveal only dorsal-chip fracture if spontaneously reduced. Early consultation is indicated.

MCP JOINT DISLOCATION

MCP joint dislocation is usually a dorsal dislocation that requires surgical reduction, often due to volar plate entrapment. Closed reduction is attempted with the wrist flexed and pressure applied to the proximal phalanx in a distal and volar direction. The joint should be splinted in flexion.

WRIST FRACTURES

Scaphoid Fracture

Scaphoid fracture is the most common carpal fracture. The patient is tender in the anatomic snuff box. The wrist x-ray is commonly negative, so the diagnosis is based on physical findings. Treatment of the patient with snuff-box tenderness consists of a thumb spica splint and referral. Without proper treatment, there is risk of avascular necrosis of the scaphoid bone.

Triquetrum Fracture

Triquetrum fracture is either a dorsal avulsion or body fracture. There is tenderness dorsally, just distal to the ulnar styloid: The wrist x-ray is often negative, so diagnosis is based on physical findings. Treatment of the patient with tenderness as described consists of a volar splint with 10° wrist extension and referral to a hand surgeon.

Lunate Fracture

Lunate fracture is the most important of the carpal fractures since it occupies two-thirds of the articular surface of the radius. There is risk of avascular necrosis. The patient feels tenderness over the lunate fossa (distal to the rim of the radius at the base of the third metacarpal). Wrist x-ray is commonly negative, so diagnosis is based on physical examination findings. Treatment of the patient with tenderness as described consists of a thumb spica splint and referral.

Trapezium Fracture

Trapezium fracture results in painful thumb movement. Tenderness is present at the apex of the anatomic snuff box and base of the thenar eminence. Treatment consists of a thumb spica splint and referral.

Pisiform Fracture

The pisiform is a sesamoid bone within the flexor carpi ulnaris tendon. There will be tenderness at its bony prominence at the base of the hypothenar eminence. Treatment is a volar splint at 30° flexion with ulnar deviation to relieve tension on the tendon.

Hamate Fracture

Hamate fracture most commonly involves the hook, which is palpable in the soft tissue of the radial aspect of the hypothenar eminence. Treatment consists of a volar splint and referral.

Capitate Fracture

Isolated capitate fracture is rare. It is usually associated with scaphoid fracture. The capitate is also at risk of avascular necrosis. Treatment consists of a thumb spica splint and referral.

Trapezoid Fracture

Trapezoid fracture is extremely rare and difficult to see on x-ray. Treatment consists of a thumb spica splint and referral.

Radial Styloid Fracture

The major carpal ligaments on the radial side of the wrist insert on the radial styloid. Therefore, fracture can produce carpal instability and is associated with scapholunate dissociation. Early consult is indicated.

Ulnar Styloid Fracture

Ulnar styloid fracture may result in radial ulnar joint instability. Treatment consists of splinting the wrist in the neutral position with ulnar deviation.

Colles's and Smith's Fractures

Colles's and Smith's fractures involve the distal radius at the metaphysis. With a Colles's fracture, the distal radius is dorsally displaced, causing a dinner-fork deformity. With a Smith's fracture, the distal radius is volarly displaced causing a garden-spade deformity. Treatment consists of a hematoma block, placement of the hand in a finger trap, and closed reduction.

WRIST DISLOCATIONS

Scapholunate Dissociation

Scapholunate dissociation is a commonly missed diagnosis in the ED. The patient has wrist tenderness that may be localized to the scapholunate joint. The AP view on the wrist x-ray demonstrates a space between the scaphoid and lunate that is >3 mm. Early referral for ligamentous repair is indicated.

Lunate and Perilunate Dislocation

The most common carpal bone dislocations are those of the lunate and perilunate. Lateral, oblique, and AP wrist x-rays reveal the dislocation, as the normal alignment of the radius-lunate-capitate is lost. With a lunate dislocation, the lunate dislocates anterior to the radius, but the remainder of the carpus aligns with the radius. With a perilunate dislocation, the lunate remains aligned with the radius, but the remainder of the carpus is dislocated, usually dorsal to the lunate. Ordinarily, there is concomitant fracture of the scaphoid and the proximal portion of the scaphoid remains with the lunate, while the distal portion dislocates with the carpus. Prompt referral for closed reduction or surgical repair is indicated.

HAND FRACTURES
Distal Phalanx

A tuft fracture is the most common. If associated with subungual hematoma, drainage is recommended. Transverse fractures with displacement are always associated with nail bed laceration, which requires repair. Avulsion fracture of the base results in a mallet finger. If less than one-third of the articular surface is involved, a dorsal extension splint is applied. If greater than one-third of the articular surface is involved, open reduction and internal fixation are recommended.

Middle and Proximal Phalanx Fractures

This diagnosis is often suspected if the fingertips of the closed hand do not point to the same spot on the wrist and the plane of the nail bed of the involved digit is not aligned with the others. Treatment of nondisplaced fractures is a gutter splint in the position of function and referral. Treatment of displaced fractures usually requires surgical intervention. Rotational malalignment is a common problem and requires correction.

Metacarpal Fracture

A fourth or fifth metacarpal neck fracture, the boxer's fracture, is the most common metacarpal fracture. Angulation of 30° in the ring finger and 50° in the fifth finger can be tolerated but, ideally, angulation > 20° should be reduced. Treatment consists of a gutter splint with the wrist extended 20° and the MCP flexed 90° and referral. Second and third metacarpal fractures causing any angulation should be reduced. Treatment consists of a gutter splint and referral. First metacarpal base fracture with intraarticular involvement should be splinted in a thumb spica and referred.

For further reading in *Emergency Medicine: A Comprehensive Study Guide,* 5th ed., see Chap. 260, "Injuries to the Hand and Digits," by Robert L. Muelleman; and Chap. 262, "Wrist Injuries," by Harold W. Chin and Dennis T. Uehara.

166 | Forearm and Elbow Injuries
Stephen W. Meldon

ELBOW DISLOCATION

Clinical Features

Dislocations are predominantly posterior and result from a fall onto an outstretched hand. Clinically, patient has elbows in 45° of flexion. The olecranon is prominent posteriorly; however, this may be obscured by significant swelling. Neurovascular complications occur in 8 to 21 percent of patients, with brachial artery and ulnar nerve injuries most common.

Diagnosis and Differential

While the elbow deformity may resemble a displaced supracondylar fracture, the diagnosis of elbow dislocation is easily confirmed radiographically. On the lateral view, both the ulna and radius are displaced posteriorly. In the anteroposterior view, the ulna and radius have a normal relationship, but may be displaced medially or laterally. Any associated fractures should be noted.

Emergency Department Care and Disposition

Appropriate treatment of elbow dislocations requires adequate reduction and recognition of neurovascular complications, associated fractures, and postreduction instability.

1. Neurovascular compromise must be carefully evaluated by assessing the brachial and radial pulses, along with the ulnar, radial, and median nerves. Any associated fractures should be documented.
2. **Reduction:** After adequate sedation, reduction is accomplished by gentle traction on the wrist and forearm. An assistant applies countertraction on the arm. Distal traction is applied while any medial or lateral displacement is corrected with the other hand. Downward pressure on the proximal forearm will help to disengage the coronoid process from the olecranon fossa. Distal traction is continued and the elbow is flexed. A palpable "clunk" is noted with successful reduction.
3. After reduction, **neurovascular status** should be **reexamined** and postreduction films obtained.
4. **Immobilization** with a long arm posterior splint with the elbow

in 90° of flexion is appropriate. Cylinder casts should not be placed because of the risk of significant subsequent edema.
5. Close orthopedic follow-up should be arranged. Patients with instability in extension require immediate referral.

ELBOW FRACTURES

Radial head fracture is the most common fracture of the elbow and usually results from a fall on an outstretched hand. Intercondylar fractures occur in adults, and any distal humerus fracture in an adult should initially be assumed to be intercondylar. Supracondylar fractures occur most often in children. Of these extraarticular fractures, 95 percent are displaced posteriorly. Fractures of the olecranon are also common and usually result from direct trauma such as a fall.

Clinical Features

Radial hand fractures result in lateral elbow pain and tenderness and inability to fully extend the elbow. Intercondylar and supracondylar elbow fractures typically present with significant swelling, tenderness, and limited mobility. Intercondylar fractures occur from a force directed against the elbow, while most supracondylar fractures result from an extension force. Both can be associated with severe soft tissue injury. Associated neurovascular injuries are common with supracondylar fractures. The anterior interosseus nerve, a motor branch of the median nerve, is particularly prone to injury. Evaluation of this nerve is performed by testing for flexion in the interphalangeal joint of the thumb and the distal interphalangeal joints of the index finger. Acute vascular injuries present with a decreased or absent radial pulse and are most frequently due to transient vasospasm. Clinical findings of olecranon fractures include localized swelling and tenderness and limited range of motion.

Diagnosis and Differential

An anteroposterior and lateral radiograph of the elbow should be obtained. In some undisplaced radial head fractures, the fracture line may not be visible and the posterior fat pad sign may be the only evidence of injury. A careful evaluation for a fracture line separating the condyles from each other and the humerus, which distinguishes intercondylar fractures, should be made. The amount of displacement, rotation, and comminution of the fragments should be noted. In supracondylar fractures, the anteroposterior (AP) radiograph usually reveals a transverse fracture line, while the lateral view shows an oblique fracture line and displacement of the distal fragment proximally and posteriorly. The lateral radiograph may also reveal a posterior and anterior fat pad sign. In olecranon fractures, any displacement (> 2 mm) should be noted.

Emergency Department Care and Disposition

1. Neurovascular compromise should be carefully evaluated.
2. **Splint immobilization** and orthopedic referral are appropriate for nondisplaced fractures. Minimally displaced radial head fractures may be treated with a sling and early range of motion.
3. Displaced fractures and those with neurovascular compromise require immediate **orthopedic consultation**. Supracondylar fractures are often treated with closed reduction followed by pin fixation, while displaced intercondylar and olecranon fractures are usually treated with open reduction and internal fixation. Patients with displaced fractures or severe swelling should be admitted for observation of neurovascular status.

FOREARM FRACTURES

Fractures of both the radius and ulna occur most often from significant trauma, such as a motor vehicle crash or fall from a height. Isolated fractures of the ulna (nightstick fracture) often result from a direct blow to the forearm. Radius fractures are produced by falls on the outstretched hand or by a direct blow.

Clinical Features

Fractures of both bones result in swelling, tenderness, and deformity of the forearm. Open fractures are not uncommon. Isolated fractures of the ulna or radius present with swelling and tenderness over the fracture site. Fracture of the proximal ulnar shaft with radial head dislocation, a Monteggia's fracture-dislocation, causes considerable pain and swelling at the elbow. A distal radial shaft fracture with associated distal radioulnar joint dislocation, referred to as Galeazzi's fracture, will present with localized tenderness and swelling over the distal radius and wrist.

Diagnosis and Differential

Fractures of the radius and ulna are easily diagnosed on an AP anteroposterior and lateral radiograph of the forearm. Displacement, angulation, and longitudinal alignment are easily evaluated. Any rotational malalignment should be noted. Clues to rotational deformity include a sudden change in the bone's width at the fracture site and a change in the normal orientation of the various bony prominences of the radius or ulna. Isolated ulnar fractures are considered displaced if there is greater than 10° of angulation or more than 50 percent displacement. In Monteggia's fracture, the proximal ulnar fracture is clearly visible, but the radial head dislocation may be overlooked. As a rule, the radial head normally aligns with the capitellum in all radiographic views of the elbow. The distal radioulnar joint dislocation seen with Galeazzi's fracture also may be subtle. On the lateral view, the ulna will be displaced dorsally, while the AP view may show only a slightly increased radioulnar joint space.

Emergency Department Care and Disposition

1. Neurovascular complications and evidence of an open fracture should be assessed.
2. **The extremity should be immobilized** and an AP and lateral radiograph should be obtained. The entire forearm including elbow and wrist should be viewed. Evaluate for displacement, alignment, angulation, and associated dislocation.
3. Nondisplaced isolated fractures may be immobilized in a long-arm cast and given orthopedic referral. However, most of these injuries will have significant displacement and require orthopedic consultation and management. Closed reduction is often adequate for both bone fractures in children. Open reduction and internal fixation are usually required for displaced fractures in adults and for Monteggia's and Galeazzi's fracture dislocations.

For further reading in *Emergency Medicine: A Comprehensive Study Guide*, 5th ed., see Chap. 261, "Injuries to the Elbow and Forearm," by Dennis T. Uehara and Harold W. Chin.

---

167 | Shoulder and Humerus Injuries
Stephen W. Meldon

CLAVICLE AND SCAPULA

Clavicle fractures and acromioclavicular (AC) joint injuries are common. Clavicle fractures account for approximately one-half of significant shoulder girdle injuries and are the most common fractures seen in children. While much less common, injuries to the sternoclavicular (SC) joint and scapula are important because of the association with other significant injuries.

Clinical Features

Both clavicle fractures and AC joint injuries result from direct trauma, such as a fall onto the shoulder. Clavicle fractures typically present with swelling, deformity, and localized tenderness. AC joint injuries are usually clinically obvious, with tenderness and deformity of the AC joint. In both cases, the supported arm is slumped inward and downward. Sprains of the SC joint present with localized pain and swelling. Anterior dislocations of this joint result in a prominent medial clavicle that appears anterior to the sternum, while posterior dislocations are less visible and palpable, and may result in impingement of superior mediastinal structures. Scapular fractures present with localized tenderness over the scapula and the affected extremity held in adduction. They usually result from significant trauma, such as motor vehicle collisions or falls.

Diagnosis and Differential

Routine clavicle radiographs usually reveal clavicle fractures in the middle third of the clavicle in 80 percent, distal third in 15 percent, and medial third in 5 percent of cases. AC radiographs help determine the severity of AC injury and any associated fracture. Type I AC injuries have normal radiographs. Type II injuries result in a 25 to 50 percent elevation of the distal clavicle above the acromium, while type III injuries show 100 percent dislocation of the AC joint and coracoclavicular space widening. The diagnosis of SC joint dislocations (which are usually anterior) is suggested clinically. Computed tomography (CT) imaging is indicated, since plain radiographs may not be diagnostic. The differential diagnosis of sternoclavicular sprains should include septic arthritis, especially in intravenous drug users. Fractures of the scapula can be diagnosed with radiographs of the anteroposterior shoulder with axillary and scapular views. Associated injuries to the thoracic cage, lung, and shoulder occur in 80 percent of patients with scapular fractures.

Emergency Department Care and Disposition

1. Carefully **evaluate for neurovascular compromise**. Examine for associated injuries, especially with SC dislocations and scapular

fractures. A chest x-ray is indicated to evaluate for intrathoracic injuries.

2. **Simple immobilization with a sling** is acceptable for most clavicle fractures, scapular fractures, and AC joint injuries. A **figure-of-eight clavicle brace** is acceptable for displaced clavicle fractures and SC dislocations.

3. **Immobilization, ice, analgesics**, and early range-of-motion exercises are appropriate components of conservative treatment. Orthopedic follow-up should be arranged.

4. Orthopedic consultation is indicated for SC dislocations, displaced distal clavicle fractures, articular or complex scapular fractures, and unusual, complicated AC joint injuries.

GLENOHUMERAL JOINT AND ROTATOR CUFF

Dislocation of the glenohumeral joint is the most common major joint dislocation. Anterior dislocations occur in 98 percent of cases. Rotator cuff tears may accompany this injury.

Clinical Features

Glenohumeral joint dislocations are usually suspected clinically. The most common mechanism of injury is a fall onto an extended, abducted arm. The patient typically is in severe discomfort and resists abduction and internal rotation of the affected arm. The shoulder lacks the normal founded contour, and the humeral head can be palpated anteriorly and inferiorly. Associated axillary nerve injuries will present with decreased sensation over the deltoid muscle. The rare inferior dislocation (luxatio erecta) will present with the affected arm fully abducted, elbow flexed, and hand held above the patient's head. Rotator cuff tears will demonstrate tenderness on the greater tuberosity, decreased range of motion, and weakness with abduction and external rotation.

Diagnosis and Differential

Anteroposterior and lateral scapular (Y-view) or axillary radiographs should be obtained before reduction. The Y-view or axillary radiograph will reveal a posterior dislocation, which is rare. Associated bony injuries, such as glenoid rim fractures and compression fractures of the humeral head (Hill-Sachs lesion), should be noted. Associated rotator cuff tears are often missed. Such a tear should be suspected in patients over 40 years old, luxatio erecta dislocations, and patients who are unable to externally rotate or abduct the arm after a glenohumeral dislocation. Diagnosis may require an arthrogram, arthroscopy, or magnetic resonance imaging.

Emergency Department Care and Disposition

Many reduction techniques have been described. The use of conscious sedation is highly recommended, but any technique may be attempted without medication if performed slowly and gradually.

1. Assess and document neurovascular status and any associated bony injury.
2. **Modified Hippocratic technique**. This method uses traction-countertraction. The patient is supine with the arm abducted. A sheet is placed across the thorax of the patient and tied around the waist of the assistant. The physician gradually applies traction while the assistant provides countertraction. Gentle internal and external rotation may aid reduction. A sheet placed around the patient's flexed forearm and the physician's waist may assist with traction.
3. **Milch technique**. With the patient supine, the physician slowly abducts and externally rotates the arm to the overhead position. With the elbow fully extended, traction is applied.
4. **External rotation technique**. With the patient supine and the elbow at 90° flexion, the arm is slowly externally rotated. No traction is applied. This technique must be performed slowly and gently. Reduction is often subtle and occurs prior to reaching the coronal plane.
5. After reduction, **reassess neurovascular status** and obtain **post-reduction radiographs**. A shoulder immobilizer or sling and swathe should be applied and orthopedic follow-up arranged.

HUMERUS FRACTURES

Fractures of the proximal humerus are a relatively common injury and are typically seen in elderly patients with osteoporosis after a fall onto an outstretched hand. In contrast, humerus shaft fractures occur in younger patients following either direct or indirect trauma.

Clinical Features

Patients with proximal humerus fractures usually present with pain, swelling, and tenderness around the shoulder. Crepitus and ecchymoses may be present. Neurovascular injuries may occur and are suggested by paresthesia, pulselessness, or expanding hematoma. Humeral shaft fractures result in localized pain, swelling, and tenderness. Shortening of the upper extremity may occur with displaced fractures. An associated radial nerve injury is common and will be manifested by a wrist drop and decreased sensation over the dorsal first web space. The humerus is also a common site of pathologic fractures.

Diagnosis and Differential

Radiographs consisting of anterioposterior and lateral shoulder and axillary views will diagnose most proximal humerus fractures. The Neer classification is based on the relationship of the proximal humerus segments (greater and lesser tuberosities, anatomic or surgical neck) and the number of fragments significantly displaced (two part, three part, or four part). Over 80 percent of proximal fractures have no significant displacement or angulation and are classified as one-part fractures. The diagnosis of humeral shaft fractures is usually obvious on anteroposterior and lateral radiographs of the humerus.

Emergency Department Care and Disposition

The emergency department management of humerus injuries is relatively straightforward.

1. Assess and document neurovascular status. This is particularly important in complex proximal humerus and humeral shaft fractures.
2. **Immobilize with a sling** and swathe or collar and cuff for simple (one-part) proximal humerus fractures. Humeral shaft fractures can be immobilized by a sugar-tong splint or hanging cast. Alternatively, a simple sling and swathe are often adequate.
3. **Immobilization, ice, analgesia, and orthopedic referral** are indicated for simple fractures. Early range-of-motion exercises are important in simple proximal humerus fractures.
4. Orthopedic consultation is indicated for multipart proximal humerus fractures, significantly displaced or angulated fractures, open fractures, and any fracture with neurovascular complications.

For further reading in *Emergency Medicine: A Comprehensive Study Guide,* 5th ed., see Chap. 263, "Injuries to the Shoulder Complex and Humerus," by Dennis T. Uehara and John P. Rudzinski.

168 | Pelvis, Hip, and Femur Injuries

Judith A. Linden

Although pelvic fractures constitute only 3 percent of all bony fractures, they are associated with high morbidity and mortality rates. Large forces are required to fracture the pelvis, and concomitant abdominal, thoracic, and head injuries are common. The vascularity of the pelvic bones and the proximity of major blood vessels are responsible for large blood loss. Hip fractures are common in elderly patients with osteoporosis and may occur spontaneously or after a fall.

PELVIS FRACTURES

Clinical Features

Pelvic fractures should be suspected whenever there is trauma to the torso or a fall from a height. Pain, crepitus, or instability on palpation of the pelvis suggests a fracture. Hematoma over the inguinal ligament or perineum should increase suspicion. Hypotension may be secondary to abdominal or thoracic injuries or blood loss from disrupted pelvic bones or vessels.

Diagnosis and Differential

Radiographs confirm suspected pelvic fractures. The anteroposterior (AP) pelvic radiograph is the most useful; additional views include oblique hemipelvis, inlet (to evaluate AP displacement), and outlet views (to evaluate superior-inferior displacement). Computed tomography scanning provides more detailed information. Many classifications for pelvic fractures exist; the Young system is helpful because fractures are classified based on mechanism and directional forces (Table 168-1). Four main patterns [suggested by the alignment of pubic rami fractures, pubic symphysis diastasis, and sacroiliac (SI) joint displacement] have been identified: lateral compression (LC), AP compression (APC), vertical shear (VS), and combination (CM). Complications often correlate with, and can be anticipated by, the fracture pattern.

Emergency Department Care and Disposition

1. Standard protocols for evaluation and stabilization of trauma patients should be initiated (see Chap. 151). A careful search for other significant injuries should be made, since there is a strong association with other major injuries.

TABLE 168-1 Injury Classification Keys According to the Young System

Category	Distinguishing characteristics

LC	Transverse fracture of pubic rami, ipsilateral or contralateral to posterior injury:
	  I: Sacral compression on side of impact
	  II: Crescent (iliac wing) fracture on side of impact
	  III: LC-1 or LC-II injury on side of impact; contralateral open-book (APC) injury

APC	Symphyseal diastasis and/or longitudinal rami fractures:
	  I: *Slight* widening of pubic symphysis and/or anterior SI joint; stretched but intact anterior SI, sacrotuberous, and sacrospinous ligaments; intact posterior SI ligaments
	  II: Widened anterior SI joint; disrupted anterior SI, sacrotuberous, and sacrospinous ligaments; intact posterior SI ligaments
	  III: Complete SI joint disruption with lateral displacement; disrupted anterior SI, sacrotuberous, and sacrospinous ligaments; disrupted posterior SI ligaments

VS	Symphyseal diastasis or vertical displacement anteriorly and posteriorly, usually through the S1 joint, occasionally through the iliac wing and/or sacrum
CM	Combination of other injury patterns, LC/VS being the most common

Note: See the text for an explanation of the abbreviations.

2. Administer **100% oxygen**, and secure cardiac monitoring and two IV lines. Blood should be sent for type and cross-matching. Hypotension is treated with early liberal use of **blood products** and pelvic stabilization to prevent further blood loss. Early **external fixation** decreases complications such as acute respiratory distress syndrome and should be considered if there is evidence of continued blood loss with disruption of the posterior elements. **Angiography** for embolization of pelvic vessels is another option for continued major blood losses. Intraabdominal solid organ injuries and other sources of blood loss should be considered. If DPL is performed, a supraumbilical approach should be taken to avoid disruption of pelvic hematoma.

3. If urethral injury is suspected, a Foley catheter should not be placed until a retrograde urethrogram is performed. Rectal examination and, for women, bimanual pelvic examination should be performed for rectal and gynecologic injuries. If blood

is found on pelvic examination, a speculum examination should be performed to evaluate for vaginal lacerations (which may occur with anterior pelvic fractures). Vaginal lacerations mandate operative débridement, irrigation, and intravenous (IV) antibiotics. Rectal injuries are treated with irrigation, diverting colostomy, and antibiotics.

Stable Pelvic Avulsion Fractures

Avulsion fractures involve a single bone that is avulsed during forceful muscular contraction. Avulsion fracture of the anterior superior iliac spine (ASIS) occurs when a forceful contraction of the sartorius muscle causes separation of the ASIS. Symptoms include localized swelling and pain with thigh flexion and abduction. Avulsion fractures of the anterior inferior iliac spine (AIIS) occur after forceful contraction of the rectus femoris muscle. Symptoms include groin pain and inability to flex at the hip. The radiograph reveals downward displacement of the inferior iliac spine. Avulsion of the ischial tuberosity occurs in patients under age 20 to 25 when the hamstring forcefully contracts (jumping). Pain is present on sitting and thigh flexion. There is tenderness on palpation of the tuberosity on rectal examination. Avulsion fractures are stable, heal well, and are treated symptomatically.

Stable Fractures Involving a Single Pelvic Bone

Fracture of a single ischial bone or pubic ramus can occur in the elderly from a fall with direct trauma. A lateral film of the hip is necessary to rule out a hip fracture. The ischial bodies can be injured by a direct fall on the buttocks. Iliac wing (Duverney's) fractures present with pain and swelling over the iliac wing. Intraabdominal injuries may be coexistent. Sacral fractures may occur when large AP forces are applied to the pelvis. They may be difficult to diagnose on radiograph; subtle irregularity, buckling, or malalignment of the sacral foramina is suggestive, and a lateral view may show displacement. A bimanual rectal examination (with one finger in the rectum and a hand on the sacrum) may reveal crepitus. Coccygeal fractures result from a fall in a sitting position. The diagnosis is made clinically by rectal examination, which may reveal tenderness or crepitus. Treatment is symptomatic, with a soft doughnut cushion for sitting, ice, and analgesics.

HIP FRACTURES

Hip fractures are common in elderly patients who present after a fall. The affected leg is classically foreshortened and externally rotated. Morbidity rates are high and are related to premorbid conditions. Complications include infection, venous thromboembolism, avascular necrosis, and nonunion.

The position of the extremity, ecchymoses, deformity, and range of motion should be evaluated. Heel percussion may elicit pain. PA, lateral, and frog-leg views will evaluate the femur and acetabulum. Hip fractures are classified as intracapsular (femoral head and neck) or extracapsular (intertrochanteric and subtrochanteric). Intracapsular fractures may compromise blood supply to the femoral head.

Femoral head fractures are most commonly associated with hip dislocations. Femoral neck fractures are common in elderly patients with osteoporosis. Pain radiates to the groin and inner thigh. The leg is foreshortened and held in external rotation. Nondisplaced neck fractures are treated with pin fixation; displaced fractures are treated with open reduction or prosthesis placement.

Stress fracture of the femur should be suspected if there is significant pain without radiographic abnormality. Radiographs should reveal a fracture, but a bone scan is more sensitive for subtle fractures. Stress fractures are treated conservatively with a bone scan in 1 to 2 days or follow-up radiograph in 10 to 14 days.

Intertrochanteric fractures occur in the elderly after a fall with rotational forces. The leg is foreshortened and externally rotated. Treatment includes nonemergent operative fixation.

Subtrochanteric fractures may be seen in elderly osteoporotic patients and young patients after major trauma. Symptoms include pain, deformity, and swelling. Immobilization with a traction apparatus is recommended, with eventual operative fixation.

Greater trochanter fractures may occur in adults (true fracture) or children (avulsion of the apophysis). Pain is present on abduction and extension. Treatment is controversial and may include conservative treatment or operative fixation (based on the patient's age and displacement of the fragment).

Lesser trochanter avulsions are most common in young athletes after avulsion of the iliopsoas muscle. There is pain during flexion and internal rotation. If there is more than 2 cm of displacement, operative fixation with screws is recommended.

HIP DISLOCATIONS

Hip dislocations are most often the result of massive forces during trauma. Ninety percent are posterior and 10 percent are anterior. Both types are treated with early closed reduction (less than 6 h) in order to decrease the incidence of avascular necrosis. Posterior dislocations, which occur when a posterior force is applied to the flexed knee, may coexist with acetabular fractures. The leg is foreshortened, internally rotated, and adducted. AP, lateral, and oblique views will evaluate the status of the acetabulum and the femoral head. Treatment includes early closed reduction using the Allis maneuver (hip flexion to 90°, then internal and external rotation) or the Stimson maneuver (patient prone, with the leg hanging over the edge of stretcher, and application of gentle traction). Anterior dislocations occur during forced abduction. The leg is held in abduction and external rotation. Treatment includes early closed reduction with strong, in-line traction, and flexing and externally rotating the leg, with abduction, once the femoral head clears the acetabulum.

FEMORAL SHAFT FRACTURES

Femoral shaft fractures typically occur when patients are involved in a motor vehicle crash. Since the femur has a rich vascular supply and is surrounded by soft tissue, it can accommodate 1 L or more of blood, potentially contributing to hypotension and shock after a fracture. Distal neurovascular function should be thoroughly evaluated. Diagnosis is confirmed radiographically. Treatment involves immediate immobilization with Hare or Sager traction or a Thomas splint. Definitive repair is by operative fixation or, in children, traction.

For further reading in *Emergency Medicine: A Comprehensive Study Guide,* 5th ed., see Chap. 265, "Trauma to the Pelvis, Hip, and Femur," by Mark T. Steele.

---

169 | ## Knee and Leg Injuries
| *Judith A. Linden*

Knee injuries are most often the result of ligamentous and cartilage injuries, but may include bony fractures and dislocations. The Ottawa Knee Rules offer guidelines for obtaining radiographs of the knee. Radiographic evaluation is recommended if any of the following criteria are present: (*a*) patient > 55 years old, (*b*) tenderness at the head of the fibula, (*c*) isolated patellar tenderness, (*d*) inability to flex the knee to 90°, or (*e*) inability to transfer weight for four steps both immediately after the injury and in the emergency department (ED).

FRACTURES

Patellar Fractures

Fractures of the patella occur most often from a direct blow or from a fall on a flexed knee but may be caused by forceful contracture of the quadriceps muscle. Symptoms include pain and swelling over the patella. A palpable defect and tenderness are usually found on the patella. The extensor mechanism of the knee should be evaluated. Plain x-rays, including the sunrise view, confirm the diagnosis. Treatment depends on the type of fracture: minimally or nondisplaced fractures, without disruption of the extensor mechanism of the knee, are treated with a knee immobilizer and crutches, followed by 6 weeks in a long-leg cast. Fractures that are displaced > 3 mm, comminuted, or disrupt the extensor mechanism mandate early orthopedic referral for operative repair.

Femoral Condyle Fractures

Femoral condyle fractures often result from a fall from a height or a direct blow. Signs and symptoms include pain, swelling, and deformity, occasionally with shortening and rotation. The integrity of the popliteal artery and the deep peroneal nerve (sensation in the web space between the first and second toe) should be evaluated. The ipsilateral hip and quadriceps apparatus also should be fully evaluated. Orthopedic consultation is indicated. Nondisplaced fractures are treated with immobilization; displaced fractures are treated with *o*pen *r*eduction and *i*nternal *f*ixation (ORIF).

Tibial Spine Fractures

Tibial spine fractures are caused by anterior or posterior forces applied against a flexed knee and are often associated with cruciate ligament avulsions. On exam, the knee is swollen, tender, and cannot be fully extended due to hemorrhagic joint effusion. A positive Lachman's test is present. Nondisplaced fractures are treated with knee immobilization in full extension. Displaced fractures require ORIF.

Tibial Plateau Fractures

Tibial plateau fractures result from a direct blow or axial loading, which forces the femoral condyles onto the tibia. The lateral plateau in most commonly injured. Symptoms include pain and swelling of the knee and decreased range of motion. Radiographs may demonstrate a fracture or joint effusion with a fat/fluid level. Computed tomography (CT) scan is helpful in evaluating the fracture. Treatment for nondepressed fractures is a long-leg cast and non-weight-bearing activity. Depressed fractures are treated operatively with elevation of fragments.

Tibial Shaft Fractures

Tibial shaft fractures present with pain, swelling, and crepitus. A complete neurovascular evaluation is essential. Plain radiographs confirm the diagnosis. Radiographs of the knee and ankle should be included. Treatment depends on the location, amount, and displacement of bony fragments. Most tibial shaft fractures require urgent orthopedic evaluation. Indications for emergent operative repair include open fractures, vascular compromise (not improved with closed reduction), and compartment syndrome.

Fibula Fractures

Fibula fractures most commonly involve the distal fibula at the ankle. Isolated shaft fractures usually occur from direct trauma. Since the fibula is not a large, weight-bearing bone, the majority of fractures are treated with immobilization, crutches, elevation, and analgesics. Stress fractures are most common at the distal third of the fibula. They may be treated with a short-leg walking cast and crutches for patient comfort.

DISLOCATIONS

Patellar Dislocations

Patellar dislocations most commonly present with lateral patellar displacement after a twisting injury. A torn medial knee-joint capsule may be associated with the dislocation. Knee x-rays should be obtained to rule out an associated fracture. Under conscious sedation, reduction is achieved by hyperextending the knee and flexing at the hip while sliding the patella medially back in place. After reduction, the knee should be immobilized in extension. Orthopedic follow-up should be arranged in 1 to 2 weeks.

Knee Dislocation

Posterior knee dislocations are the common form of knee dislocation. On exam, the knee is unstable; occasionally, the dislocation may have reduced spontaneously. A thorough neurovascular exam must be performed since there is a high incidence of associated popliteal artery and peroneal nerve injury associated with this dislocation. Knee x-rays should be obtained to rule out associated fractures. Under conscious sedation, the dislocation should be reduced by applying longitudinal traction. The vascular status should be evaluated before and after reduction with an ankle-brachial index (ABI, see Chap. 163). If there is evidence of vascular insufficiency, an arteriogram should be performed. Some orthopedic surgeons advocate arteriography even if the ABI is normal. Emergent orthopedic consultation and admission are mandated for this injury.

Tendon, Ligamentous, and Meniscal Injuries

Patellar Tendon Rupture

Patellar tendon ruptures are more common in patients < 40 years old who have a history of patellar tendonitis or steroid injections. It occurs after forceful contraction of the quadriceps muscle. The main symptom is pain inferior to the patella. On exam, there is a defect inferior to the patella, with the inability to extend the knee. The patella may be high riding (*patella alta*) or low riding (*patella baja*). Radiographs will rule out patella fracture or avulsion. Treatment requires knee immobilization and orthopedic consultation for operative repair in 7 to 10 days.

Quadriceps Tendon Rupture

Quadriceps tendon rupture is more common in older individuals after sudden contraction of the quadriceps muscle (landing after a jump). Symptoms include sharp pain at the proximal knee on ambulating. If the tear is complete, patients will be unable to extend the leg from knee flexion, although the ability to straight-leg raise may be maintained. There may be a palpable defect, with tenderness and swelling at the suprapatellar region, and the patella may migrate distally (*patella baja*). Radiographs will rule out a patellar of femoral avulsion fracture. Partial tears are treated similarly to quadriceps muscle tears. A complete tear requires orthopedic consultation for operative repair.

Ligamentous Injuries

Patients with ligamentous injuries have pain and swelling at the knee. A hemarthrosis is common but it may be absent if there is complete disruption of the joint capsule. Injury to the anterior cruciate ligament (ACL) is the most common. ACL sprains may be associated with medial meniscal tears. Patients often describe hearing an audible "pop" associated with pain and swelling at the knee. Lachman's and pivot-shift tests are sensitive for diagnosing ACL tears. Posterior cruciate ligament tears are rarer then ACL tears and often involve large posterior forces applied to the lower leg. A posterior drawer sign may be elicited but is not sensitive. Radiographs frequently reveal only a joint effusion. Treatment includes knee immobilization, weight-bearing as tolerated, analgesics, and orthopedic follow-up. Arthrocentesis is beneficial only for symptomatic relief from tense hemarthroses that cause severe pain.

Meniscal Injuries

Symptoms of meniscal injuries include painful locking of the knee, a popping or clicking sensation, or a sensation of the knee giving out. Exam may reveal attophy of the ipsilateral quadriceps muscle. McMurray's test or the grind test may be useful in making the diagnosis. Treatment includes knee immobilization, weight-bearing as tolerated, analgesics, and orthopedic follow-up.

Overuse Injuries

Patellar Tendonitis

Patellar tendonitis, or "jumper's knee," presents with pain over the patellar tendon when running up hills or standing from a sitting position. Treatment includes ice, NSAIDs, and quadriceps-strengthening exercises. Steroid injections play no role in the ED care of patellar tendonitis.

Chondromalacia Patellae

Chondromalacia patellae is caused by patellofemoral malalignment, which places lateral stress on the articular cartilage. It is most common in young active women and presents with anterior knee pain that worsens with climbing stairs or rising from a sitting position. Diagnosis is assisted using the patellar compression test and the apprehension test. Treatment includes nonsteroidal anti-inflammatory drugs, rest, and quadriceps-strengthening exercises.

Shin Splints

Shin splints presents with pain over the anterior or lateral tibia on exertion. Radiographs are helpful for ruling out a stress fracture (but are not sensitive). Treatment includes cessation of the activity for 2 to 3 weeks.

For further reading in *Emergency Medicine: A Comprehensive Study Guide,* 5th ed., see Chap. 266, "Knee Injuries," by Mark T. Steele; and Chap. 267, "Leg Injuries," by Paul R. Haller and Ernest Ruiz.

170 | Ankle and Foot Injuries

Jeffrey D. Dixon

Most ankle and foot injuries are relatively minor and will heal well with conservative therapy. Unrecognized or inadequately treated injuries, however, can result in long-term pain and disability. Thus, prompt and appropriate emergency department (ED) evaluation and treatment are essential.

ANKLE INJURIES

Ankle Sprains

Clinical Features

Most ankle sprains result from a twisting mechanism, with the vast majority due to an inversion mechanism. The ability to bear weight immediately after an injury, with subsequent increase in pain and swelling as the patient continues to ambulate, suggests a sprain rather than a fracture. On physical examination, significant findings include the absence of bony tenderness in the ankle, normal neurovascular examination findings, and tenderness and soft tissue swelling over the involved ankle ligament. The most common sprain involves the anterior talofibular ligament.

Diagnosis and Differential

As with all extremity injuries, the joints above and below the injury should be examined. The patient should be requested to walk four steps: if the patient can transfer weight from one foot to another, and other findings on physical examination are normal, the likelihood of a significant fracture is nil. Both passive and active range of motion should be tested; soft tissue injuries are more likely when there is a significant difference between the passive and active range of motion. Tenderness of the knee, the fibular head, or the proximal fibular shaft suggests a fibulotibial ligament tear or a Maissonneuve fracture. The Achilles tendon also should be examined. Clinically, an Achilles tendon rupture is diagnosed when there is tenderness or a defect over the Achilles tendon, and a positive Thompson's test result (i.e., absence of plantar flexion of the foot when the calf is squeezed).

Classification systems do exist for categorizing sprains of the ankle, but these are of little practical value in the ED. A simpler and more useful approach is to divide the injuries into two groups:

stable and unstable (or potentially unstable). If results of stress testing of the ligaments isare normal, then the patient has a stable ankle sprain and can be appropriately treated. If results of stress testing are clearly unstable or indeterminate because of extensive pain or swelling, then the sprain should be treated as unstable.

The Ottawa Ankle Rules (Fig. 170-1) are simple guidelines that have been extensively validated in numerous clinical trials. When applied properly, they can help the emergency physician identify a subset of patients who can be safely treated without undergoing radiographic studies. Clinical judgment should prevail if the examination is unreliable due to lack of cooperation, intoxication, distracting injury, or diminished sensation in the leg.

Emergency Department Care and Disposition

1. Most studies indicate that patients with ankle sprains who can bear weight easily, whether stable or unstable, should be treated

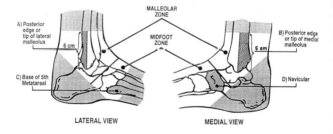

FIG. 170-1   The Ottawa Ankle Rules for ankle and midfoot injuries.

with **rest, ice, compression, and elevation (RICE)** for 24 to 72 h, depending on the amount of swelling and degree of pain. Those who can easily bear weight and have a stable joint should be treated with analgesics and an elastic wrap. They should be instructed to perform near-normal activity as tolerated and to return in 1 week if pain persists. Patients who clearly have an unstable joint should be referred to an orthopedic surgeon, and may benefit from complete immobilization with a **posterior short-leg splint** until follow-up.

2. Most patients may be adequately treated with over-the-counter **acetaminophen** or **nonsteroidal anti-inflammatory drugs**; few will require oral narcotics. A number of types of **ankle braces** (which allow plantar-dorsiflexion but do not allow inversion or eversion of the ankle) are commercially available that provide a degree of comfort and support as patients resume ambulation.

Fractures

Henderson's scheme for classifying ankle fractures is based on their radiographic appearance (unimalleolar, bimalleolar, or trimalleolar) and is adequate for ED treatment purposes.

All fractures of the ankle, with the exception of fibular avulsion fractures, require immobilization, either with casting alone or with surgical reduction and then casting. Isolated avulsion fractures of the distal tip of the fibula may be treated as stable sprains if minimally displaced, small (less than 3 mm), and without evidence of ligamentous instability.

The treatment goals with all other ankle fractures are to restore the anatomic relationship of the ankle, maintain the reduction during the healing process, and institute early mobilization of the ankle. Unimalleolar injuries may be treated with a posterior short leg splint and oral narcotic analgesics. The patient should be kept non-weight-bearing until outpatient orthopedic follow-up in 3 to 5 days.

Bimalleolar and trimalleolar fractures usually require open reduction and internal fixation. Because of this consideration, these patients initially should be given nothing by mouth until definitive management has been discussed with an orthopedist. Parenteral narcotic agents should be administered for pain control.

Dislocations

Dislocations of the ankle joint usually occur with an associated fracture. Patients with fracture-dislocations of the ankle are at significant risk of neurovascular compromise. In cases where there is evidence of such compromise, the emergency physician should proceed with reduction of the injury as expeditiously as possible, without waiting for radiographs, in order to restore vascular integrity. This procedure is best accomplished with the emergency physician grasping the heel and foot with two hands and applying gentle but steady longitudinal traction while an assistant stabilizes the proximal leg. Radiographs may be completed once the reduction has been completed and distal perfusion restored. The patient then should be admitted to the hospital after orthopedic consultation.

Open Fractures

Open fractures should be protected from further contamination by applying a wet, sterile dressing over the wound. Tetanus toxoid should be administered, as necessary, with consideration for tetanus immunoglobulin if the wound is grossly contaminated. The initial antibiotic of choice is a first-generation cephalosporin (usually intravenous **cefazolin** 1 g), or clindamycin (if allergic to cephalosporins). An aminoglycoside (**gentamicin**) also may be added if the wound is grossly contaminated.

Medial Ligament Injuries

Isolated sprains of the deltoid ligament are rare. There is usually an associated fibular fracture or significant tear of the tibiofibular syndesmosis, resulting from an eversion stress. The proximal fibula and fibular shaft should be carefully examined. If radiographs are negative, then a significant syndesmosis tear should be suspected. Treatment is with RICE and early orthopedic referral.

FOOT INJURIES

Although foot injuries are often due to twisting forces, direct blows occur more often than with ankle trauma. Patients with normal findings on examination of the foot and ankle do not need radiographs. Abnormal findings on examination mandate a complete, three-view foot series. If there is tenderness along the heel, an axial view of the calcaneus should be included.

Hindfoot Injuries

Subtalar dislocations and significant fractures of the talus (both rare) often require surgical reduction and merit immediate orthopedic consultation. Fractures of the calcaneus can be caused by any axial load to the heel, such as a fall from a height. Since calcaneal injuries are frequently associated with spinal injuries and other lower extremity fractures, a thorough physical examination is mandatory. Although some fractures of the calcaneus are quite apparent on radiographs, others can be quite subtle. When a radiograph is unremarkable and a calcaneus fracture is still suspected, Boehler's angle—formed by the intersection of a straight line extending along the superior cortex of the body of the os calcis with a line extending from the dome to the anterior tubercle—should be measured on the lateral view of the foot. If the angle is less than 20°, a fracture is likely. Orthopedic consultation should be obtained with all calcaneus fractures.

Midfoot Injuries

Isolated fractures of the tarsal bones are uncommon and usually treated conservatively. When a fracture of the cuboid or cuneiforms is identified, an injury to Lisfranc's joint (tarsometatarsal complex) should be suspected. Injuries to this joint are rare and frequently missed in the ED. A fracture of the base of the second metatarsal may be viewed as pathognomonic of a disruption of the ligamentous complex. This injury should be suspected when there is point tenderness over the midfoot or when there is laxity between the first and second metatarsals. Injuries to the Lisfranc joint may require open reduction or percutaneous pinning, and long-term morbidity may be significant.

Forefoot Injuries

Metatarsal fractures commonly are caused by a crush mechanism. Most non-displaced metatarsal shaft fractures can be treated conservatively. However, any fracture of the first metatarsal shaft must be treated with a period of non-weight-bearing. Displaced fractures of any of the metatarsal shafts are problematic, requiring non-weight-bearing and possibly surgical fixation.

Fifth metatarsal fractures are the most common of the metatarsal fractures. Shaft fractures can usually be treated conservatively, as can the "pseudo-Jones" fracture (i.e., avulsion from the proximal pole). However, the Jones fracture, which is a transverse fracture through the base of the fifth metatarsal, is subject to complications much more frequently, including malunion and non-union. The Jones fracture must be treated with a non-weight-bearing cast and close orthopedic follow-up.

Phalangeal Injuries

Most non-displaced phalangeal fractures can be treated conservatively, with "buddy taping" or a cast shoe. Dislocations and displaced fractures can be reduced by providing a digital block and applying manual traction, followed by buddy taping.

Open Injuries

The special considerations for an open foot fracture are the same as those for an open ankle fracture (see above).

Puncture Wounds

Puncture wounds carry the risk of retained foreign body, deep soft tissue infection, or osteomyelitis. Deep penetration increases the risk of damage to bone and tendons, and penetration through a rubber sole may increase the chance of infection with *Pseudomonas*. Radiographs may be useful in some cases; however, normal x-ray results do not rule out the possibility of bony injury or retained foreign body. The use of prophylactic antibiotics after a puncture wound is controversial and may be best reserved for patients who are immunocompromised, have peripheral vascular disease or diabetes, or have bone or tendon involvement. Patients who present with delayed puncture wounds complicated by infection should have the wound opened and irrigated; any foreign material should be removed, any devitalized tissue excised, and the patient started on antibiotic therapy. The antibiotic of choice is usually a first-generation cephalosporin (e.g., oral **cephalexin** 500 mg qid), although a flouroquinalone (e.g., oral **ciprofloxacin** 500 mg bid) may be added if *Pseudomonas* is suspected. Complicated foot infections, gunshot wounds to the foot, and many lawn mower injuries require consultation for operative débridement.

For further reading in *Emergency Medicine: A Comprehensive Study Guide,* 5th ed., see Chap. 268, "Ankle Injuries," and Chap. 269, "Foot Injuries," by John A. Michael and Ian G. Stiell.

---

171 | Compartment Syndromes

Gary Gaddis

Compartment syndromes may lead to muscle necrosis and are caused by continued elevated pressures within the closed tissue space of one or more anatomic muscle compartments.

Clinical Features

Elevated pressure in a muscle compartment compromises blood flow to that compartment's muscle. This may cause muscle and nerve necrosis if pressures are sufficiently great for a long enough time. Elevated pressure can be caused by decreased or increased compartment size. Constrictive dressings, casts, thermal injury, or frostbite can decrease compartment size. Increased compartment size may be due to edema or hemorrhage within the compartment after blunt or penetrating injuries. Virtually any muscle mass enclosed by fascia can be at risk for the development of a compartment syndrome. Compartment syndromes are more common in anatomic regions where there is relatively less ability to expand, such as the anterior and lateral compartments of the leg.

Conscious patients developing compartment syndromes usually experience severe and constant pain over the involved muscle compartment. Palpation of the affected compartment, active contraction, or passive stretching of muscles in the affected compartments will exacerbate a conscious patient's pain. Muscle weakness and hypoesthesia can appear shortly after the onset of pain when elevated compartment pressures compromise neurologic function. Absent pulses and excessive coolness are unlikely to appear until well after occurrence of pain and neurologic compromise.

Diagnosis and Differential

A high index of suspicion for compartment syndrome should exist in any patient with injury to or compression of an extremity. Missing the diagnosis of compartment syndrome by attributing pain solely to patient's other injuries can lead to morbidity. Suspicion of the diagnosis is even more important in unconscious patients since they cannot express that they are in pain. The mainstay of diagnosis is measurement of compartment pressure. Most muscle compartments normally have pressures of less than 10 mmHg, and such pressures are often normally near 0. The presence of an abnormally elevated pressure confirms the diagnosis.

The differential diagnosis for a compartment syndrome would include other causes of pain, such as fracture or hematoma. Other possible causes of neurologic or vascular compromise must be considered when symptoms advance beyond pain only.

Emergency Department Care and Disposition

Initial stabilization of injuries and measurement of compartment pressures dictate subsequent treatment and disposition. Compartment pressures should be measured by an emergency physician or surgical consultant experienced in the technique.

1. Patients with pressures under 10 mmHg do not require further therapy for their compartment pressures.
2. Pressures of 15 to 20 mmHg require reevaluation in 12 to 24 h, with serial compartment pressure measurements in persistently symptomatic patients. Judgment must be exercised regarding whether to discharge patients based upon their likelihood to follow discharge instructions and return for close follow-up.
3. Pressures greater than 20 mmHg can compromise capillary blood flow and require **hospital admission or surgical consultation**, as persistent pressures in this range can damage nerve and muscle.
4. Pressures over 30 to 40 mmHg place nerve and muscle at risk for necrosis and are grounds for **immediate fasciotomy**. Ice cooling and limb elevation should be avoided since both techniques can decrease perfusion to muscle. Bed rest and serial neurovascular checks are the conservative treatments when immediate fasciotomy is not indicated. The goal of treatment is the avoidance of muscle necrosis, rhabdomyolysis, and nerve damage in the affected area(s).

For further reading in *Emergency Medicine: A Comprehensive Study Guide,* 5th ed., see Chap. 270, "Compartment Syndromes," by Ernest Ruiz.

---

172 | Rhabdomyolysis

Gary Gaddis

Skeletal muscle injury, followed by muscle cell necrosis and release of intracellular contents, underlies the rhabdomyolysis syndromes. Rhabdomyolysis is most strongly associated with alcohol and drug abuse, toxin ingestion, trauma, infection, strenuous physical activity, and heat-related illness.

Clinical Features

Most symptoms are of acute onset, which include myalgias, weakness, muscle stiffness, malaise, low-grade fever, or dark urine. Symptoms directly due to muscular injury, however, may be absent. Other symptoms may include nausea, vomiting, abdominal pain, palpitations, or mental status changes due to uremia.

Risk factors for muscle necrosis should be sought. These factors include physiologic stressors such as unaccustomed muscular exertion (e.g., strenuous exercise, seizures, or delirium tremens), severe heat exposure, altered mental status with prolonged immobility and associated muscular compression, or traumatic crush injury to muscle. Common toxins associated with rhabdomyolysis include drugs of abuse (most notably, cocaine, amphetamines, LSD, heroin, phencyclidine, or ethanol) or medications (e.g., diuretics, narcotics, corticosteroids, benzodiazepines, phenothiazines, and tricyclic antidepressants). Muscular ischemia may result from sickle cell disease, vasculitis, or other toxins.

Involved muscles usually have tenderness, but swelling may not be present until the patient is rehydrated. Muscle involvement may be localized or diffuse. Postural muscles of the lower back, thighs, and calves are most commonly involved. Brownish urine due to myoglobinuria may be absent, especially in mild cases. Highly variable physical findings make history and laboratory clues crucial to diagnosis.

There are numerous complications of rhabdomyolysis. Acute renal failure may be oliguric or nonoliguric and is not correlated with the degree of creatine phosphokinase (CPK) elevation or the degree of myoglobinuria. Common associations include hyperkalemia with renal failure, hyperuricemia with crush injuries, and hyperphosphatemia with hypocalcemia. Disseminated intravascular coagulation, which usually resolves spontaneously, can result in severe hemorrhage. Compartment syndromes can increase the extent of muscle necrosis, which can cause peripheral neuropathy.

Diagnosis and Differential

A fivefold or greater increase in serum CPK level is the hallmark for the diagnosis of rhabdomyolysis. The CPK-MB fraction, originating primarily from cardiac muscle (but which also exists in skeletal muscle), should not exceed 5 percent of the total CPK values. Serum CPK levels rise 2 to 12 h after muscle injury, peak in 24 to 72 h, and then decline about 40 percent daily thereafter. Persistently elevated CPK values suggest ongoing muscle necrosis.

Muscle necrosis releases myoglobin. Myoglobinuria occurs when plasma concentrations exceed 1.5 mg/dL. Reddish-brown urinary discoloration occurs when urine myoglobin exceeds 100 mg/dL. Myoglobin contains heme, which explains why myoglobinuria causes qualitative tests such as the Hemoccult dipstick to be positive when there are no red blood cells evident on the urinalysis. Radioimmunoassays are only slightly more sensitive than dipstick tests for identifying myoglobinuria and are not required for the diagnosis. The absence of myoglobinemia or myoglobinuria does not rule out rhabdomyolysis, as the serum myoglobin level may return to normal within 1 to 6 h after muscle injury.

A serum electrolyte panel; blood urea nitrogen, creatinine, calcium, phosphorus, and uric acid levels; urinalysis; complete blood cell count; and disseminated intravascular coagulation profile should be performed on all patients with suspected rhabdomyolysis to evaluate for the potential complications of this disorder.

The differential diagnosis includes other causes of muscle ischemia or pain, such as sickle cell disease, toxin exposure, inflammatory myopathies, and infectious myalgias.

Emergency Department Care and Disposition

1. Rehydration is the mainstay of therapy. Deficits should be corrected with **IV crystalloid** to maintain a urinary output of at least 2 mL/kg/h, as monitored with a Foley catheter.
2. Cardiac monitoring is required since electrolyte derangement is common. For patients with preexisting cardiac or renal disease, invasive hemodynamic monitoring may be indicated to assist with fluid management.
3. **Sodium bicarbonate** (1 mmol/kg IV bolus) to maintain urinary pH above 6.5 has been recommended to decrease ferrihemate production. However, it can exacerbate the hypocalcemia often observed with rhabdomyolysis.
4. To maintain urinary output, **20% mannitol** (0.5 to 1.0 g/kg over 30 min) or **furosemide** 40 to 200 mg IV has been commonly recommended. Diuretics should be administered only after adequate volume replacement has been instituted.
5. Hyperkalemia often requires ion exchange resins such as **sodium polystyrene sulfonate** (15 to 25 g orally with 50 mL of 20% sorbitol, or 20 g rectally in 200 mL of 20% sorbitol). **Calcium** (10 mL calcium chloride over 10 to 20 min) or **sodium bicarbonate** also should be used when hyperkalemia induces cardiotoxicity. **Glucose** (D50 1 amp) and **insulin** (5 to 10 U regular), though recommended, may not be effective. For patients with acute renal failure, dialysis may be indicated.
6. Use of nonsteroidal anti-inflammatory drugs should be avoided for pain control since they cause renal vasoconstriction.

7. Calcium is seldom required to treat hypocalcemia unless profound signs or symptoms of this disorder occur. Hypercalcemia generally responds to saline infusion and IV furosemide 20 to 40 mg IV.
8. Hyperphosphatemia merits oral phosphate binders, such as sodium polystyrene sulfonate, when serum levels exceed 7 mg/dL. Hypophosphatemia requires treatment if serum levels fall below 1 mg/dL.
9. All patients with rhabdomyolysis require hospital admission to a monitored bed. Nephrology consultation should be obtained in cases with acute renal failure.

For further reading in *Emergency Medicine: A Comprehensive Study Guide,* 5th ed., see Chap. 271, "Rhabdomyolysis," by Francis L. Counselman.

MUSCULAR, LIGAMENTOUS, AND RHEUMATIC DISORDERS

173 | Cervical, Thoracic, and Lumbar Pain Syndromes

Charles J. Havel, Jr.

The list of potential causes of cervical, thoracic, and lumbar pain is long and includes trauma, degenerative disease, infection, neoplasms, congenital malformations, inflammatory processes, and psychic tension. The diagnosis will often be achieved with a thorough history and physical exam accompanied by judicious adjunct testing. Attention in the emergency department (ED) must be paid to identifying causes of permanent disability and life-threatening entities.

Clinical Features

Patients with neck pain will often have associated complaints of stiffness and limited range of motion. They also commonly have an identifiable inciting position or a provocative maneuver that can be reproduced. Localized neck tenderness may or may not be present. Radiation of the pain, particularly in a dermatomal pattern, should suggest a cervical radiculopathy. Pain may be accompanied by a variety of neurogenic symptoms and signs, such as sensory abnormalities, muscle weakness or hypertonicity, reflex changes, sexual or sphincter dysfunction, or incoordination.

Pain from the thoracic spine is less common than either cervical or lumbar pain syndromes. Localized pain and tenderness may or may not be present. Radicular pain is common and may be associated with chest or abdominal pain. If long tract signs are present, (e.g., hyperreflexia, Babinski's sign, or urinary incontinence), then intrinsic or extrinsic spinal cord pathology must be suspected.

Lumbosacral pain carries a long differential diagnosis that includes disease of structures remote from the spine itself. An important goal of evaluation, therefore, is the distinction between musculoskeletal, neurogenic, and more remote causes of pain. Localized bony pain and percussion tenderness points to musculoskeletal disease; radicular pain is common particularly with musculoskeletal and neurologic processes. A neurologic deficit can be associated with either spinal or extraspinal pathology. It is important to note the presence or absence of systemic symptoms and signs; these in association with an abnormal abdominal, neurologic, or rectal examination suggest an extraspinal cause of pain, including potentially life-threatening conditions.

Diagnosis and Differential

The patient's age, medical history, and review of systems can be helpful in prioritizing the differential diagnosis. Other important factors include any history of trauma, mechanism of injury, character and distribution of the pain, identifiable exacerbating or abating positions, and presence or absence of neurogenic or systemic symptoms. In the setting of trauma, the initial physical exam will often be restricted to identifying areas of bony tenderness, crepitus, or step-off and noting any neurologic deficit. Positive findings mandate the need for radiographic imaging before further spinal evaluation and manipulation. For hemodynamically unstable patients, a more focused exam is also done to identify neurologic deficit and other abnormal findings while resuscitation efforts continue. In stable patients with atraumatic pain syndromes, a complete exam can be performed before considering imaging or other testing.

For suspected cervical lesions, range-of-motion testing, spine compression and distraction techniques to reproduce pain and radicular symptoms, assessments of distal upper extremity pulses, and a thorough neurologic exam are important diagnostic procedures. If imaging is required, a three-view cervical spine radiograph should be ordered, with oblique views of flexion-extension views added selectively. A computed tomography (CT) scan or magnetic resonance imaging (MRI) is useful in the work-up for patients with suspected radiculopathy or myelopathy.

The differential diagnosis of neck pain begins with vertebral fracture, especially in the setting of trauma, which can be confirmed by plain films or CT imaging. In the absence of fracture, cervical soft tissue injury, which is an acceleration flexion-extension neck injury (or "whiplash"), is common. These injuries may be accompanied by a host of nonspecific symptoms such as dizziness, dysesthesia, tinnitus, dysphagia, and spacial instability, but without focal neurologic deficits. Patients with a radiculopathy will have neck pain associated with radiation of pain in a dermatomal pattern, with or without demonstrable sensory changes or muscle weakness in the appropriate distribution (Table 173-1). Neck pain with long tract signs signifies a myelopathy, upper extremity hyperreflexia (with Hoffman's reflex indicating a lesion above C5), lower extremity hyperreflexia, up-going great toe, and sphincter changes suggesting cervical stenosis or epidural metastasis. Acute cervical disk herniation may present with a radiculopathy or myelopathy; radicular symptoms in these patients will often be worsened in extension and lateral flexion, and relieved with flexion and distraction. Radiographs may be negative even with large herniations, prompting the need for MRI or myelography to confirm the diagnosis. Chronic degenerative disk disease may continue on to cervical spondylosis and, subsequently, to spinal stenosis, producing a spectrum of symptoms from simple pain and stiffness to myelopathy. Neck pain with reproducible scalp pain when palpated at the occipital notch is diagnostic of occipital neuralgia.

Conditions casuing thoracic pain include fractures resulting from direct trauma and hyperflexion injuries. In the elderly, especially females, pathologic fractures also may occur with minimal or no trauma; those due to osteoporosis are generally stable, while those due to metastatic lesions may present with myelopathy and long tract signs. CT, MRI, or myelography is needed to distinguish between relatively rare thoracic disk herniation and neoplasm. Localized thoracic pain and tenderness are characteristic of acute facet syndrome. Osteoarthritis can cause radicular pain and localized stiffness, and progress to thoracic spinal stenosis. Herpes zoster neuralgia presents with acute thoracic radiculopathy, often before the appearance of the characteristic vesicular skin eruption. Diabetic radiculopathy may have an abdominal pain component as well; electromyography is useful for diagnosis.

The physical exam of patients with lumbar pain must include spinal, neurologic, abdominal, vascular, and lower extremity evaluation. Symptoms and signs of lumbar radiculopathies are listed in Table 173-2. Pelvic and rectal examinations are often valuable as well. Lumbosacral x-rays should be ordered in the setting of trauma and in the elderly, but otherwise are not prerequisite. Additional laboratory testing and imaging studies such as ultrasound and CT scans are indicated in the evaluation of patients with low back pain, other systemic symptoms, and abnormal visceral or vascular physical findings.

Spinal causes of lumbar pain include a spectrum of degenerative spinal processes, inflammatory sacroiliitis, and compression fractures. Acute disk herniation can reveal itself by pain alone or accompanied by radiculopathy or myelopathy; epidural hematoma, abscess, and neoplasm all have a similar neurologic picture. Pain exacerbated by ambulation is typical of both peripheral vascular disease and spinal stenosis and may require arteriography, CT

TABLE 173-1 Symptoms and Signs of Cervical Radiculopathies

Disk space	Nerve root	Pain complaint	Sensory change	Motor weakness	Altered reflex
C1-2	C1-2	Neck, scalp	Scalp	None	None
C4-5	C5	Neck, shoulder, upper arm	Shoulder, thumb	Spinati, deltoid, biceps	Biceps
C5-6	C6	Neck, shoulder, upper scapula, proximal forearm, thumb	Thumb, index finger, lateral forearm	Deltoid, biceps, pronator teres, wrist extensors	Biceps, brachioradialis
C6-7	C7	Neck, posterior arm, dorsal and proximal forearm, chest, medial scapula, middle finger	Middle finger, forearm	Triceps, pronator teres	Triceps
C7-T1	C8	Neck, posterior arm, proximal forearm, medial scapula, medial hand, ring and little fingers	Ring, little fingers	Triceps, flexor carpi ulnaris, hand intrinsic muscles	Triceps

TABLE 173-2 Symptoms and Signs of Lumbar Radiculopathies

Disk space	Nerve root	Pain complaint	Sensory change	Motor weakness	Altered reflex
L2-3	L3	Medial thigh, knee	Medial thigh, knee	Hip flexors	None
L3-4	L4	Medial lower leg	Medial lower leg	Quadriceps	Knee jerk
L4-5	L5	Anterior tibia, great toe	Medial foot	Extensor hallucis longus	Biceps femoris
L5-S1	S1	Calf, little toe	Lateral foot	Foot plantar flexors	Achilles

scan, or MRI for definitive diagnosis. Lumbar pain may be a manifestation of visceral pathology; pyelonephritis and other renal disease, peptic ulcer disease, pancreatic disease, diverticulitis, pelvic disease, abdominal aortic aneurysm, and others fall into this category.

Emergency Department Care and Disposition

1. Patients sustaining significant trauma with or without a neurologic deficit and those with significant life and limb-threatening conditions must be aggressively evaluated and resuscitated. Consultation should be obtained for inpatient care as appropriate. Those with intractable pain, evidence of progression of neurologic deficit, or myelopathy are candidates for initiation of treatment in the ED and hospital admission.

2. The majority of patients, however, can be managed as outpatients; the primary goal being symptomatic relief with nonsteroidal anti-inflammatory drugs (**NSAIDs**). Short-term treatment with an opioid such as **hydrocodone** 5 mg every 4 h for supplemental pain relief may be warranted. Relative rest, cold and heat applications, and other supportive measures may provide additional seymptomatic relief. Close follow-up is advisable to monitor for the appearance or progression of neurologic deficits.

For further reading in *Emergency Medicine: A Comprehensive Study Guide,* 5th ed., see Chap. 273, "Neck Pain," by Myron M. LaBan; and Chap. 274, "Thoracic and Lumbar Pain Syndromes," by Paul J. W. Tawney, Cara B. Siegel, and Myron M. LaBan.

174 Shoulder Pain

Charles J. Havel, Jr.

Shoulder pain is a common musculoskeletal complaint, especially in patients over 40 years of age. Occupational, recreational, and normal daily activities all stress the shoulder joint and may result in pain from either acute injury or, more commonly, chronic overuse conditions. Complicating the evaluation of this complaint is that the origin of pain may be either pathology intrinsic to the shoulder joint or that to extrinsic disorders causing referred pain.

Clinical Features

The pain of musculoskeletal shoulder pathology is often described by patients as an aching sensation, particularly in the setting of a more chronic process. Specific motions may exacerbate it, and this history is helpful in making a specific diagnosis. Decreased range of motion, crepitus, weakness, or muscular atrophy may be associated with certain conditions. Any systemic symptoms (e.g., shortness of breath, fever, or radiation of pain from the chest or abdomen) should raise suspicion for extrinsic and potentially life-threatening problems.

Diagnosis and Differential

The primary diagnostic maneuver is a thorough history and physical exam. Examination of the shoulder joint should include range of motion and muscle strength testing, palpation for local tenderness or other abnormality, and identification of any neurovascular deficit. Specific tests for impingement and rotator cuff muscle function are often helpful in intrinsic disease. Plain radiographic studies of the shoulder joint are rarely diagnostic but may be helpful to rule out bony abnormalities in selected patients or to evaluate for abnormal calcifications. In patients in whom extrinsic causes of shoulder pain are suspected, further diagnostic testing may be indicated such as laboratory studies, additional x-rays, and electrocardiograms.

The differential diagnosis includes a variety of intrinsic musculoskeletal disorders, and individual patients may exhibit considerable overlap in their symptoms manifesting a combination of specific conditions. *Impingement syndrome* is a painful overuse condition characterized by positive findings with impingement testing and relief of pain with anesthetic injection of the subacromial space. Both *subacromial bursitis* and *rotator cuff tendinitis* are associated with impingement. Subacromial bursitis is generally seen in patients < 25 years of age and will present with positive impingement tests with varying degrees of tenderness at the lateral proximal humerus or in the subacromial space. Rotator cuff tendinitis is distinguished by an incidence primarily in the 25- to 40-year-old age group and findings of tenderness of the rotator cuff with mild-to-moderate muscular weakness. Signs of impingement are commonly found. In more chronic disease, crepitus, decreased range of motion, and osteophyte formation visible on x-ray may also be apparent. *Rotator cuff tears* occur primarily in patients older than 40 years and are associated with muscular weakness (especially with abduction and external rotation) and cuff tenderness. Ninety percent will be chronic tears with a history of minimal or no trauma; in severe disease, muscular atrophy may be present. Acute tears may occur in patients of any age and result from significant force, producing a tearing sensation with immediate pain and disability. In patients between the ages of 30 and 50, abnormal calcifications on x-ray in the clinical setting of a painful shoulder with rotator cuff tenderness and, often, crepitus suggest the diagnosis of calcific tendinitis. *Osteoarthritis* is characteristically associated with degenerative disease in other joints (primary), previous fracture, or other underlying disorder (secondary). The hallmark of *adhesive capsulitis* is significantly painful and limited range of motion, often but not always associated with a period of immobilization. X-rays should be done to rule out posterior glenohumeral dislocation.

Also to be considered as a cause of shoulder pain are a number of extrinsic conditions. *Pancoast's tumor* may compress the brachial plexus and thus manifest itself as shoulder pain. *Degenerative disease of the cervical spine, brachial plexus disorders, and suprascapular nerve compression* are all neurologic processes that should be sought in patient evaluation. Vascular pathology, notably *axillary artery thrombosis,* also may cause shoulder pain. Last, acute cardiac, aortic, pulmonary, and abdominal pathology may cause pain referred to the shoulder, and the clinician must remain alert to this possibility.

Emergency Department Care and Disposition

1. For intrinsic disease, the primary goals of emergency department care are to reduce pain and inflammation and prevent progression of disease. For most conditions, this translates to

relative rest of the joint assisted by use of a sling (full immobilization is not suggested), **nonsteroidal anti-inflammatory drugs (NSAIDs)**, further analgesics as needed, and the application of **cold packs.**

2. **Joint space injection** with glucocorticoids (e.g., triamcinolone 20 to 40 mg) with or without a local anesthetic such as lidocaine should be used judiciously in view of the potential deleterious effects on soft tissues, tendon rupture with direct injection, and a recommended limitation of three injections into a single area. **Needling of calcifications** with an 18-gauge needle can be performed in calcific tendinitis when calcifications can be localized. For all intrinsic disorders, follow-up with a primary care physician with expertise in joint disease or orthopedic referral is suggested within 7 to 14 days. Physical therapy referral may also be valuable and can be accomplished in consultation with the primary care or orthopedic physician.

3. In extrinsic disease, the treatment and referral pattern will be diagnosis-dependent. Neurologic problems will require analgesia and anti-inflammatory medications and may require neurology or neurosurgical follow-up. Vascular causes of shoulder pain must be carefully evaluated and, with axillary artery thrombosis, immediate consultation made to initiate thrombolysis. Treatment of other extrinsic conditions depends on the specific diagnosis and may entail consultation with other specialists.

For further reading in *Emergency Medicine: A Comprehensive Study Guide,* 5th ed., see Chap. 275, "Shoulder Pain," by D. Monte Hunter.

---

175 | Acute Disorders of the Joints

David A. Peak

Acute disorders of the joints and bursae are common emergency conditions that involve a wide spectrum of age, acuity, and causes.

Mismanagement of certain causes can lead to significant disease and even death.

Clinical Features

Multiple pathways can cause disruption of the normal joint milieu, leading to acute joint complaints. These changes invariably lead to pain, the most common complaint of patients with a joint problem. It is important to elicit whether a diagnosis already has been established and whether the pain is acute, chronic, or acute on chronic. The number and distribution of joints affected narrows the differential diagnosis (Table 175-1).

On physical examination, arthritis should be distinguished from more focal periarticular inflammation, such as cellulitis, bursitis, and tendinitis. True arthritis produces joint pain exacerbated by both active and passive motion.

Diagnosis and Differential

Synovial fluid should be sent for culture, Gram's stain, cell count, and crystal evaluation (Table 175-2). The white blood cell count and erythrocyte sedimentation rate lack the sensitivity and specificity to be reliable discriminators.

Radiographs should be obtained when the differential diagnosis

TABLE 175-1 Classification of Arthritis by Number of Affected Joints

No. affected joints	Differential considerations
1 = Monarthritis	Trauma-induced arthritis Infection/septic arthritis Crystal-induced (gout, pseudogout) Osteoarthritis (acute) Lyme disease Avascular necrosis Tumor
2–3 = Oligoarthritis	Lyme disease Reiter's syndrome Ankylosing spondylitis Gonococcal arthritis Rheumatic fever
> 3 = Polyarthritis	Rheumatoid arthritis Systemic lupus erythematosus Viral arthritis Osteoarthritis (chronic)

TABLE 175-2 Examination of Synovial Fluid

	Normal	Noninflammatory	Inflammatory	Septic
Clarity	Transparent	Transparent	Cloudy	Cloudy
Color	Clear	Yellow	Yellow	Yellow
WBC/mL	< 200	< 200–2000	200–50,000	> 50,000
PMNs, %	< 25	< 25	> 50	> 50
Culture	Negative	Negative	Negative	> 50% positive
Crystals	None	None	Multiple or none	None
Associated conditions		Osteoarthritis, trauma, rheumatic fever	Gout, pseudogout, spondyloarthropathies, rheumatoid, Lyme disease, SLE	Nongonococcal or gonococcal septic arthritis

Note: The white blood cell count (WBC) and percent polymorphonuclear leucocytes (%PMNs) are affected by a number of factors, including disease progression, affecting organism, and host immune status. The joint aspirate WBC and %PMNs should be considered part of a continuum for each disease, particularly septic arthritis, and should be correlated with other clinical information. SLE, systemic lupus erythematosus.

includes trauma, osteomyelitis, neoplasm, avascular necrosis, slipped capital femoral epiphysis, or Legg Calvé Perthes disease. More sophisticated modalities, such as computed tomography or magnetic resonance imaging (for sternoclavicular or sacroiliac joint disease and transient synovitis), and radioisotope scanning (for avascular necrosis, occult fracture, and osteomyelitis) are employed in rare cases.

Emergency Department Care and Disposition

Septic Arthritis

Septic arthritis is a condition that can rapidly lead to irreversible joint destruction if inadequately treated. It typically presents as a monarticular arthritis and may be associated with fever, chills, or malaise. The synovial fluid confirms the diagnosis. Therapy requires admission for parenteral antibiotics and repeated needle aspiration, arthroscopy, or open surgical drainage.

Traumatic Hemarthrosis

Traumatic hemarthrosis is associated with intra-articular fracture or ligamentous injury. Aspiration of large effusions may decrease pain and increase range of motion. Treatment is supportive. Spontaneous hemarthrosis may be associated with coagulopathies requiring specific clotting factor replacement.

Crystal-Induced Synovitis

Crystal-induced synovitis generally affects middle-aged to elderly patients. Gout (uric acid crystals) typically affects the great toe, tarsal joints, and knee, while pseudogout (calcium pyrophosphate crystals) typically affects the knee, wrist, ankle, and elbow. Pain evolves over hours to days and may be precipitated by trauma, surgery, significant illness, dietary or alcohol indiscretions, or certain medications. The synovial fluid is inflammatory with negative birefringent needle-shaped (gout) or weakly positive birefringent rhomboid (pseudogout) crystals. Treatment is with nonsteroidal anti-inflammatory drugs [NSAIDs; e.g., oral (PO) indomethacin 50 mg tid for 3 to 5 d], corticosteroids (e.g., intramuscular ACTH 40 U), or colchicine (0.6 mg/h PO until resolution of symptoms or intolerable gastrointestinal side effects).

Osteoarthritis

Osteoarthritis is a chronic, symmetric, polyarticular destruction of joints (including the distal interphalangeal DIP correctly expanded joints) distinguished by a lack of constitutional symptoms. Patients may present with acute monarticular exacerbations with a small, amount of non-inflammatory synovial aspirate and characteristic joint space narrowing on radiographs. Treatment involves rest and analgesics.

Lyme Arthritis

Lyme arthritis is a monarticular or symmetric oligoarticular arthritis (especially of the large joints) with brief exacerbations followed by complete remission occuring weeks to years after the primary infection. Synovial fluid is inflammatory and cultures are usually positive. Treatment with appropriate antibiotics (e.g., doxycycline, penicillin, erythromycin, and amoxicillin) is effective.

Gonococcal Arthritis

Gonococcal arthritis is an immune-mediated infectious arthritis that typically affects adolescents and young adults. Fever, chills, and migratory tenosynovitis or arthralgias typically precede mon- or oligoarthritis. Vasiculopustular lesions on the distal extremities are characteristic. Synovial fluid is usually inflammatory and often culture negative; cultures of the pharynx, urethra, cervix, and rectum increase the culture yield. The patient should be admitted for pain control and parenteral antibiotic therapy. Orthopedic consultation is advised.

Acute Rheumatic Fever

Acute rheumatic fever is a non-infectious immune disease featuring migratory or additive symmetric oligoarthritis (primarily in larger joints) appearing 3 to 4 weeks after an untreated group A beta-hemolytic streptococcus infection. Diagnosis consists of two major criteria (carditis, migratory polyarthritis, chorea, erythema marginatum, and subcutaneous nodules) or one major and two minor criteria (fever, arthralgia, prior history or rheumatic fever, and elevated acute-phase reactants). Synovial fluid is inflammatory. Treatment consists of penicillin or erythromycin and analgesics.

Reiter's Syndrome

Reiter's syndrome is a seronegative reactive spondyloarthropathy characterized by acute asymmetric oligoarthritis (especially the lower extremities) preceded by an infectious illness, such as urethritis or enteric infection, 2 to 6 weeks earlier. The classic triad of arthritis, conjunctivitis, and urethritis is not required for diagnosis. Synovial fluid is inflammatory. Treatment is symptomatic.

Ankylosing Spondylitis

Ankylosing spondylitis is a seronegative spondyloarthropathy that primarily affects the spine and pelvis and may be associated with morning stiffness, fatigue, and weakness. Hereditary predeliction (characterized by HLA-B27 antigen and absence of rheumatoid factor) is significant. Radiographic findings include sacroiliitis and squaring of the vertebral bodies (bamboo spine). Treatment is symptomatic.

Rheumatoid Arthritis

Rheumatoid arthritis is a chronic, symmetric, polyarticular joint disease (with sparing of the distal interphalangeal DIP expanded correctly joints) associated with morning stiffness, depression, fatigue, and generalized myalgias. Pericarditis, myocarditis, pleural effusion, pneumonitis, and mononeuritis multiplex may occur. Synovial fluid is inflammatory. Treatment of an acute exacerbation involves immobilization, NSAIDs and, occasionally, corticosteroids. Antimalarials, gold, and methotrexate are used for long-term therapy.

Viral Arthritis

Viral arthritis is an acute, symmetric, usually polyarticular immune-mediated arthritis associated with the prodromal features of the common viral causes (rubella, hepatitis B, entero- and adenoviruses, mumps, and Epstein-Barr virus). Synovial fluid is noninflammatory to inflammatory. Treatment is supportive.

Bursitis

Bursitis is an inflammatory process involving any of the more than 150 bursae throughout the human body and may be caused by infection, trauma, rheumatologic diseases, or crystal deposition. Certain repetitive activities also may precipitate bursitis: "carpet layer's knee" (prepatellar bursitis) or "student's elbow" (olecranon bursitis). A suspicion for septic bursitis, especially in olecranon bursitis, necessitates aspiration of bursitis fluid. Septic bursal fluid characteristically is purulent in appearance, with greater than 15,000 leukocytes/mL, and culture positive. Treatment includes rest, compressive dressing, analgesics, and antibiotics (amoxicillin clavulanate 500 mg PO tid for 10 d) for septic bursitis.

For further reading in *Emergency Medicine: A Comprehensive Study Guide*, 5th ed., see Chap. 278, "Acute Disorders of the Joint and Bursae," by John H. Burton.

176 | Musculoskeletal Disorders in Adults

Michael P. Kefer

RHEUMATIC EMERGENCIES ASSOCIATED WITH RISK OF DEATH

Respiratory System

Death may result from airway obstruction, respiratory muscle failure, or pulmonary tissue involvement.

Airway Obstruction

Relapsing polychondritis begins with abrupt onset of pain, redness, and swelling of the ears or nose. The tracheobronchial cartilage is involved in approximately 50 percent of cases. Hoarseness and throat tenderness over cartilage is noted. Repeated attacks can lead to airway collapse. Treatment of an exacerbation is with high-dose steroids and admission for observation.

Rheumatoid arthritis may involve the cricoarytenoid joints, causing pain with speaking, hoarseness, or stridor. The joints may fix in a closed position, mandating emergency tracheostomy.

Respiratory Muscle Failure

Dermatomyositis and polymyositis may lead to respiratory failure from respiratory muscle involvement in poorly controlled disease.

Pulmonary Tissue Involvement

Pulmonary hemorrhage complicates Goodpasture's disease, systemic lupus erythematosus, Wegener's granulomatosis, and other vasculitic conditions.

Pulmonary fibrosis complicates ankylosing spondylitis, scleroderma, and other conditions.

Pleural effusion complicates rheumatoid arthritis and systemic lupus erythematosus.

The Heart

Many rheumatologic conditions involve the heart.

Pericarditis occurs in rheumatoid arthritis and systemic lupus erythematosus. Myocardial infarction may occur from coronary artery involvement in Kawaski's disease or polyarteritis nodosa.

Pancarditis is noted in acute rheumatic fever.

Valvular heart disease is noted in ankylosing spondylitis, relapsing polychondritis, and rheumatic fever. Further involvement may extend into the conduction system.

Adrenal Glands

Glucocorticoids are used often in the treatment of many rheumatic conditions. Any acute condition that prevents the patient's steroid requirement from being met, such as vomiting or acute illness or injury that increases the physiologic requirements, may result in adrenal insufficiency. The patient should receive stress-dose steroid therapy. Other medications used to treat rheumatic conditions, such as nonsteroidal anti-inflammatory drugs (NSAIDs), cyclophosphamide, chlorambucil, methotrexate, and hydroxychloroquine, can be safely held during brief periods of vomiting .

RHEUMATIC PRESENTATIONS ASSOCIATED WITH RISK OF MORBIDITY

Cervical Spine and Spinal Cord

Patients with rheumatologic involvement of the cervical spine may be at high risk for serious cervical spine or spinal cord injury from otherwise trivial trauma, including manipulation during endotracheal intubation if extreme caution is not exercised. Ligamentous destruction of the transverse ligament of C2, with resultant symptoms of cord compression, may complicate rheumatoid arthritis. Cervical spine inflexibility from ankylosing spondylitis predisposes to injury out of proportion to the mechanism. Anterior spinal artery syndrome may result from rheumatologic conditions causing vasculitis, aortic dissection, or embolism.

The Eye

Rheumatologic involvement of the eye ranges from mild irritation to complete blindness.

Temporal arteritis is a cause of sudden blindness and should be considered in any patient older than 50 who presents with new-onset headache, visual changes, or jaw or tongue claudication. Laboratory investigation reveals an elevated erythrocyte sedimentation rate (greater than 50 mm/h), anemia, and elevated alkaline phosphatase levels. Treatment consists of **prednisone** 60 mg/day and is initiated immediately, based on clinical and laboratory findings. Treatment is not delayed for definitive diagnosis, which requires temporal artery biopsy. Biopsy, however, must be obtained within the first week of treatment to be accurate.

Dry eyes and dry mouth from Sjögren's syndrome may occur alone or coexist with many rheumatologic conditions.

Episcleritis is a self-limiting, painless injection of the episcleral vessels. It is in the differential diagnosis of the red eye in patients with rheumatoid arthritis.

Scleritis, also seen in patients with rheumatoid arthritis, presents with marked ocular tenderness. The eye has a purple discoloration. The potential for visual impairment and scleral rupture mandates emergent ophthalmologic consult and high-dose steroids.

Hypertension

Hypertension can complicate any rheumatologic condition that affects the kidneys either directly, as in polyarteritis nodosa or systemic lupus erythematosus, or indirectly, as from nephrotoxic drugs used to treat the underlying disorder.

The Kidney

Renal insult is common in rheumatologic conditions and is due either to the primary disease process, the drugs used to treat the disease, or both.

Nephritis is a common complication of systemic lupus erythematosus and systemic vasculitis. Renal dysfunction from malignant hypertension occurs with scleroderma.

Nephrotic syndrome in patients with systemic lupus erythematosus predisposes to renal vein thrombosis.

Renal insufficiency from prostaglandin inhibition by NSAIDs is more frequent in the elderly. It also may result from rhabdomyolysis in the patient with florid myositis.

For further reading in *Emergency Medicine: A Comprehensive Study Guide,* 5th ed., see Chap. 276, "Emergency in Systemic Rheumatic Diseases," by Mary Chester Morgan Wasko.

177 | Infectious and Noninfectious Inflammatory Conditions of the Hand

Michael P. Kefer

Rest and elevation are the mainstay of treatment of nontraumatic conditions to decrease inflammation, avoid secondary injury, and prevent spread of any existing infection. The optimal position of the hand for splinting is the position of function: wrist in 15° extension, MCP in 50 to 90° flexion, PIP in 10 to 15° flexion, and DIP in 10 to 15° flexion.

INFECTIOUS CONDITIONS

Infections of the hand are often polymicrobial. Skin organisms are frequently involved. Infections from animal bite wounds may be infected with *Pasteurella multocida,* and human bite wounds with *Eikenella corrodens.* Abscesses always require surgical drainage. Table 177-1 summarizes the common infections of the hand, the likely organisms involved, and recommended antibiotic therapy.

Cellulitis

Cellulitis is a superficial infection presenting with localized warmth, erythema, and edema. The examiner must exclude the involvement of deeper structures by demonstrating absence of tenderness on deep palpation and range of motion of the hand. Emergency department (ED) care consists of antibiotics, splinting in the position of function, elevation, and close follow-up.

Pyogenic Flexor Tenosynovitis

Pyogenic flexor tenosynovitis is diagnosed on exam by the presence of the four cardinal signs: (*a*) tenderness over the flexor tendon sheath; (*b*) symmetric swelling of the finger; (*c*) pain with passive extension; and (*d*) flexed position of the involved digit. ED care consists of splinting, elevation, intravenous antibiotics, and orthopedic consult.

TABLE 177-1 Initial Antibiotic Coverage for Common Hand Infections

Infection	Initial antibiotic	Likely organisms	Comments
Cellulitis	First-generation cephalosporin (cephalexin) *or* antistaphylococcal penicillin (amoxicillin-clavulanate, dicloxacillin)	*Staphylococcus pyogenes, S. aureus*	Consider vancomycin for intravenous drug abusers
Felon/paronychia	First-generation cephalosporin (cephalexin) *or* antistaphylococcal penicillin (amoxicillin-clavulanate, dicloxacillin)	Polymicrobial, *S. aureus*, anaerobes	Antibiotics indicated for infections with associated localized cellulitis
Flexor tenosynovitis	β-Lactamase inhibitor (ampicillin/sulbactam) *or* first-generation cephalosporin (cefazolin) and penicillin	*S. aureus*, streptococci, anaerobes, gram-negatives	Parenteral antibiotics are indicated; consider ceftriaxone for *N. gonorrhoeae*
Deep space infection	β-Lactamase inhibitor (ampicillin/sulbactam) *or* first-generation cephalosporin (cefazolin) and penicillin	*S. aureus*, streptococci, anaerobes, gram-negatives	Inpatient management
Animal bites (including human)	β-Lactamase inhibitor *or* first-generation cephalosporin and penicillin	*S. aureus*, streptococci, *Eikenella corrodens* (human), *Pasteurella multocida* (cat), anaerobes and gram negatives	All animal bite wounds should receive prophylactic oral antibiotics
Herpetic whitlow	None, unless secondary bacterial contamination is present	Herpes simplex	Consider acyclovir; no surgical drainage is indicated

Deep Space Infections

Web space infection occurs after penetrating injury to the web space. Clinically, dorsal and volar swelling of the web space with separation of the digits is noted. Midpalmar space infection occurs from spread of a flexor tenosynovitis or penetrating wound to the palm causing infection of the radial or ulnar bursa of the hand. ED care consists of splinting, elevation, intravenous antibiotics, and orthopedic consult.

Closed Fist Injury

Closed fist injury is essentially a human bite wound to the MCP that results from punching an individual in the teeth. Risk of infection spreading along the extensor tendons is high. Wounds penetrating the skin should be explored, irrigated, and allowed to heal by secondary intention. When inspecting for extensor tendon injury, physicians should remember to consider the position of the hand at the time of injury. ED care consists of intravenous antibiotics, splinting, and orthopedic consult for admission. Extensor tendon repair is delayed until the risk of infection has passed.

Paronychia

Paronychia is an infection of the lateral nail fold. ED care of a small paronychia consists of inserting a number 11 blade into the nail fold parallel to the nail to drain the abscess. In an advanced infection or that where pus is seen beneath the nail, the corner of the paronychium should be incised and the nail fold lifted. A portion of the nail may have to be removed and packing placed for adequate drainage. Injury to the nail bed should be avoided. The wound should be checked in 24 to 48 h, the packing pulled, and warm soaks begun.

Felon

Felon is an infection of the pulp space of the fingertip. Pain results from buildup of pus in the fibrous septae of the finger pad. ED care consists of drainage by the lateral approach to protect the neurovascular bundle. An incision should begin 5 mm distal to the DIP crease and continue just palmar to, and parallel with, the paronychium, stopping distally at the phalangeal tuft. The incision should be deep enough to extend across the entire finger pad to divide the septae at the bony insertions. Unless there is a pointing abscess, the radial aspect of the index and long finger, and the ulnar aspect of the thumb and small finger, should be avoided. The wound should be packed loosely, and the hand splinted in the position of function. The wound should be checked in 24 to 48 h, the packing pulled, and warm soaks begun.

Herpetic Whitlow

Herpetic Whitlow is a viral infection of the fingertip involving intracutaneous vesicles. Clinically, it may present similar to a felon. ED care consists of protection with a dry dressing to prevent autoinoculation and transmission, immobilization, and elevation. Antiviral agents may shorten the duration.

Noninfectious Conditions

Tendonitis and Tenosynovitis

Tendonitis and tenosynovitis are usually due to overuse. ED care consists of immobilization and nonsteroidal anti-inflammatory drugs. Noninfectious synovitis may also be treated by injection of deposteroids. Triamcinolone 40 mg/mL mixed with 0.5% bupivicaine is injected into the synovial sheath.

Trigger Finger

Trigger finger is a tenosynovitis of the flexor sheaths of the digits and may result in stenosing of the tendon sheath. Impingement and snap release of the tendon occur as the finger is extended from a flexed position. Steroid injection may be effective treatment for early stages. Definitive treatment is surgery.

DeQuervain's Tenosynovitis

DeQuervain's tenosynovitis is a tenosynovitis of the extensor pollicis brevis and abductor pollicis tendons. Pain occurs at the radial aspect of the wrist and radiates into the forearm. Finkelstein's test is diagnostic: with the involved hand, patients grasp the thumb in the fist and deviate the hand ulnarly reproducing pain along the tendons. ED care consists of a thumb spica splint and NSAIDs. Steroid injection may be useful.

Carpal Tunnel Syndrome

Carpal tunnel syndrome results from compression of the median nerve by the transverse carpal ligament. The cause is usually edema secondary to overuse, pregnancy, or congestive heart failure. Pain in the median nerve distribution of the hand tends to be worse at night. Tinel's sign (reproducing symptoms by tapping over the median nerve at the wrist) and Phelan's sign (holding the wrist flexed maximally for > 1 min) support the diagnosis when pain is elicited distally in the median nerve distribution. ED care consists of a wrist splint and NSAIDs. Steroid injection may be useful.

Advanced cases will require referral for elective surgical decompression.

Dupuytren's Contracture

Dupuytren's contracture results from fibrous changes in the subcutaneous tissues of the palm, which may lead to tethering and joint contractures. Referral to a hand surgeon is indicated.

For further reading in *Emergency Medicine: A Comprehensive Study Guide,* 5th ed., see Chap. 277, "Hand Infections," by Mark W. Fourre.

---

178 | Soft Tissue Problems of the Foot

Mark B. Rogers

TINEA PEDIS

Clinical Features

The most common form of tinea pedis is interdigital, usually a fissure between the fourth and fifth digit. The webspace is often white, macerated, and soggy and is caused by polymicrobial organisms (dermatophytes and bacteria). The lesions can be pruritic and painful. Other forms can affect the entire plantar surface with scaling, erythema, and fissures or with vesicles.

Emergency Department Care and Disposition

Due to the polymicrobial nature of tinea pedis, the ideal medication must be antifungal and antibacterial, as well as have local drying and anti-inflammatory properties. The **topical imidazole antifungals** (e.g., miconazole, econazole, ketoconazole, oxiconazole, sulconazole, and tioconazole) are the agents of choice and should be applied for 2 to 3 weeks. Creams and solutions are preferred, but sprays are also effective. Ointments should not be used on moist and oozing lesions. Alternatively, topical terbinafine and butenafine can be applied for 1 to 2 weeks. One week of **oral antifungal therapy** has been advocated (e.g., itraconazole, fluconazole, and terbinafine). Other aspects of therapy include better **foot hygiene** with daily foot cleaning, drying, and changes in socks and footwear.

ONYCHOMYCOSIS

Clinical Features

Nail plate invasion by dermatophyte fungi lead to severe disturbances in nail growth. Infection spreads from surrounding skin causing the nail to appear opaque, discolored, and hyperkeratotic. Patients at high risk include the elderly, those with diabetes, and those who are immunocompromised.

Emergency Department Care and Disposition

Newer **oral antifungals** (itraconazole, terbinafine, and fluconazole) are preferred first-line agents because topical medications are poorly absorbed. Treatment may be continuous (daily for 12 weeks) or, more preferably, "pulse dosing" (daily for one week per month for 3 to 4 months). Pulse therapy with terbinafine (500 mg orally once daily) appears to be most cost-effective. Adjunctive therapy may include surgical or chemical debridement of the nail matrix prior to oral antifungals. Since the recurrence rate is very high, referral to a podiatrist is needed for long-term care.

ONYCHOCRYPTOSIS (INGROWN TOENAIL)

Clinical Features

Ingrown toenails occur when part of the nail plate penetrates the nail sulcus and subcutaneous tissue. This is most commonly due to the curvature of the nail and is often associated with external trauma or self-treatment. Inflammation, swelling, and infection of the medial or lateral toenail are present, usually involving the great toe. Patients with underlying diabetes, arterial insufficiency, cellulitis, ulceration, or necrosis are at risk for amputation if treatment is delayed.

Emergency Department Care and Disposition

If infection is not present, elevation of the nail with a wisp of cotton between the nail plate and skin, daily foot soaks, and avoiding pressure on the area is often sufficient. After a digital block, a spicule of the offending nail can also be removed and the nail groove debrided. If granulation tissue or infection is present,

partial removal of the nail is indicated. After a digital block, one quarter or less of the nail should be cut longitudinally, including the nail beneath the cuticle, using a nail splitter or scissors. The cut portion should then be grasped by hemostats and removed using a rocking motion. The nail groove should be debrided and nonadherent gauze with antibiotic ointment applied. A bulky dressing should be placed, and the wound checked in 24 to 48 h.

BURSITIS

There are many bursae in the foot, any of which may become painful due to various causes. Noninflammatory bursae are pressure-induced over the bony prominences. Inflammatory bursae are due to gout, syphilis, or rheumatoid arthritis. Suppurative bursae are due to pyogenic organisms, usually from adjacent wounds. Complications include a hygroma, calcified bursae, fistula, and ulcer formation. Diagnosis is dependent on aspirated bursal fluid. Fluid should be sent for cell count, crystal analysis, gram stain, culture, and protein, glucose, and lactate levels. Treatment depends on the cause. Patients should be instructed to **avoid pressure to the area** and be **non-weight-bearing.** Septic bursitis should be treated with nafcillin or oxacillin. Repeated aspiration or incision and drainage may become necessary.

PLANTAR FASCIITIS

The plantar fascia is connective tissue that anchors the plantar skin to the bone protecting the arch of the foot. Inflammation of the plantar aponeurosis usually is caused by overuse or in those unaccustomed to activity. Patients have point tenderness over the anterior-medial calcaneus that is worse on arising and after activity. Plantar fasciitis is usually self-limited. Treatment includes **rest, ice, and nonsteroidal anti-inflammatory agents (NSAIDs).** Glucocorticoid injections are not recommended in the emergency department. Severe cases may need a short-leg walking cast and should be referred to a podiatrist.

GANGLIONS

A ganglion is a benign synovial cyst attached to a joint capsule or tendon sheath. The anterolateral ankle is a typical site. Ganglions may appear suddenly or gradually, enlarge or diminish in size, and may be painful or asymptomatic. A firm, usually nontender, cystic lesion is seen on examination. The diagnosis is clinical, but magnetic resonance imaging or ultrasound can be used if in doubt. Treatment includes **aspiration and injection of glucocorticoids,** but most require surgical excision.

TENDON LESIONS

Tendon lesions usually require consultation with an orthopedist. Tenosynovitis or tendonitis usually occurs due to overuse and presents with pain over the involved tendon. Treatment includes ice, rest, and NSAIDs.

Tendon lacerations should be explored and repaired if the ends are visible in the wound; however, due to the high complication rate, specialty consultation is recommended. After repair, extensor tendons are immobilized in dorsiflexion and flexor tendons in equinus.

Rupture of the Achilles' tendon presents with pain, a palpable defect in the area of tendon, inability to stand on tiptoes, and absence of plantar flexion with squeezing of the calf (Thompson's sign). Treatment is generally surgical in younger patients and conservative (casting in equinus) in the elderly. Rupture of the anterior tibialis tendon results in a palpable defect and mild foot drop. Surgery is usually not necessary. Rupture of the posterior tibialis tendon is usually chronic and insidious and presents with a flattened arch and swelling over the medial ankle. Examination may show weakness on inversion, a palpable defect, and inability to stand on tiptoes. Treatment may be conservative or surgical. Rupture of the flexor hallucis longus presents with loss of plantar flexion of the great toe and, in athletes, must be surgically repaired. Disruption of the peroneal retinaculum occurs with a direct blow during dorsiflexion, causing localized pain behind the lateral malleolus and clicking while walking as the tendon subluxes. The treatment is surgery.

IMMERSION FOOT (TRENCH FOOT)

Immersion foot results from prolonged exposure to moist, nonfreezing (<65°F or <15°C), and occlusive environment. It is classically seen in military recruits and in the homeless. At first, the involved area is pale, anesthetic, pulseless, and immobile, but not frozen. With rewarming, one sees hyperemia (lasting up to weeks) with severe burning pain and return of sensation. Edema, bullae, and hyperhidrosis may develop. The differential includes cellulitis and fungal infections. Treatment includes **admission for bed rest, leg elevation, and air drying at room temperature**.

FOOT ULCERS

Clinical Features

Foot ulcers are classified as ischemic or neuropathic. Diabetics are most prone to both types and are more apt to develop infections.

Ischemic ulcers are due to vascular compromise of the larger vessels. The examination shows a cool foot, dependent rubor, pallor on elevation, atrophic shiny skin, and diminished pulses. Neuropathic ulcers are pressure ulcers due to poor sensation. The ulcers appear well-demarcated with surrounding white callus-like material. The foot (in the absence of severe vascular disease) has normal temperature, color, and pulses. Decreased touch, pressure, and proprioception are common.

Emergency Department Care and Disposition

The treatment of an ischemic ulcer requires vascular surgery. Non-infected neuropathic ulcers require relief of pressure and referral to an appropriate foot care specialist. Treatment of an infected ulcer initially consists of **debridement, pressure relief via bed rest or total contact casting, and broad spectrum antibiotics** (e.g., ampicillin/sulbactam 3 g IV every 6 h). Cultures of purulent drainage should be obtained. X-rays should be obtained to rule out gas in the soft tissue, foreign body, osteomyelitis, or Charcot foot. Palpation of bone in an infected ulcer strongly correlates with osteomyelitis. Serum glucose levels should be checked. Consultation with a vascular surgeon and admission are often warranted.

For further reading in *Emergency Medicine: A Comprehensive Study Guide,* 5th ed., see Chap. 279, "Soft Tissue Problems of the Foot," by Frantz R. Melio.

PSYCHOSOCIAL DISORDERS

179 | Clinical Features of
Behavioral Disorders

John Sverha

Psychiatric disorders are common in emergency department (ED) patients. Sometimes, the psychiatric disorder is clearly the primary reason for a patient's visit. In other cases, a patient's psychiatric disorder leads to injury or illness. It is essential for the emergency physician to recognize and understand the clinical features of major psychiatric disorders.

CLINICAL PSYCHIATRIC SYNDROMES

Cognitive Disorders

Dementia

The hallmark of dementia is a pervasive disturbance in cognitive function that affects memory, abstract thinking, judgment, and personality. The onset of dementia is typically gradual, with memory disturbances being the first signs to appear. An acute worsening in the mental status of a patient with dementia can be caused by a superimposed medical illness, an adverse drug effect, or an environmental change. The most common cause of dementia is Alzheimer's disease, followed by multi-infarct dementia. Reversible causes of dementia include endocrine disorders, polypharmacy, and depression.

Delirium

Delirium is similar to dementia in that it is also characterized by a global impairment of cognitive function. It differs from dementia in that there is a "clouding of consciousness" manifested in a decreased ability to sustain attention to external stimuli. Delirium also differs from dementia in that it is rapid in onset and usually reversible. Common causes of delirium include infection, electrolyte imbalance, toxic ingestions, and head injury.

Substance-Induced Disorders

Intoxication can be defined as impairment of judgment, perception, attention, emotional control, or psychomotor activity following the ingestion of an exogenous substance. Repeated episodes result in the diagnosis of substance abuse disorder. Withdrawal is a syndrome that occurs following the reduction or cessation in the use of substance of abuse. Symptoms vary and depend on the substance whose use is being curtailed. *Withdrawal* should generally be used to describe mild symptoms (i.e., not delirium) in patients abstaining from a drug of abuse.

Schizophrenia and Other Psychotic Disorders

The primary features of psychotic disorders are delusions and hallucinations. Delusions are fixed false beliefs that are not amenable to arguments or facts to the contrary and that are not shared by others of similar cultural background. Hallucinations are false perceptions experienced in a sensory modality and occurring in clear consciousness.

Schizophrenia

Schizophrenia is the most common of the psychotic disorders. Onset of symptoms is usually in late adolescence or early adulthood. The features of schizophrenia are (1) deterioration in functioning; (2) the presence of hallucinations, delusions, disorganized speech, or catatonic behavior for at least 1 month; and (3) the absence of a mood disorder. Antipsychotic medications reduce the severity of delusions and hallucinations but are less effective in treating symptoms such as lack of volition, anhedonia, and inattention.

Brief Psychotic Disorder

A brief psychotic disorder is a psychosis lasting less than 4 weeks that occurs following a traumatic life experience, such as death of a loved one or a life-threatening situation.

Delusional Disorder

Persistent nonbizarre delusions are the hallmark of this disorder. Unlike schizophrenia, delusional disorder is rarely characterized by impairment in daily functioning. Onset of symptoms is in middle or late adulthood, with delusions typically developing over the course of months or years.

Mood Disorders

Mood or affective disorders are the most common psychiatric disorders and affect 10 to 15 percent of the general population during their lifetimes. Symptoms tend to be episodic with periods of remission and normal function.

Major Depression

The features of major depression include a persistent dysphoric mood and loss of interest in usual activities lasting for at least 2 weeks. Feelings of self-reproach, worthlessness, and anhedonia and recurrent thoughts of death or suicide are common. Vegetative symptoms are also present and include loss of appetite, sleep disturbances, fatigue, and inability to concentrate. The illness is more common in women, persons with a family history of depression, and people with preexisting medical or psychiatric illnesses.

Bipolar Disorder

Mania is the main characteristic of this disorder, formerly termed manic-depressive illness. Manics are expansive, energetic, and elated but quickly become argumentative, hostile, or sarcastic if their plans are thwarted. Other signs include decreased need for sleep, rapid speech, and racing thoughts. Poor judgment in monetary or sexual matters may lead to problems that prompt treatment. Manics often have grandiose ideas and lack insight into their surroundings; thus, consultation with family or friends is important. Patients also have periods of depression. The disorder has no sex preference and has onset in the third or fourth decades. Depressive episodes are more common than manic ones, and suicide and drug abuse are common.

Dysthymic Disorder

Dysthymic disorder is a chronic and less severe form of depression. A depressed mood must be present more days than not for at least 2 years. Patients have a lifelong gloomy outlook but remain functional.

Anxiety Disorders

Panic Disorder

Recurrent episodes of severe anxiety are the hallmark of this disorder. Attacks consist of a sudden surge of anxiety, along with autonomic signs, including palpitations, tachycardia, shortness of breath, chest tightness, dizziness, and sweating. Patients often present to the ED with these symptoms. Presenting complaints mimic a variety of medical emergencies, and careful exclusion of an organic cause is mandatory.

Generalized Anxiety Disorders

Patients with generalized anxiety disorder have chronic anxiety instead of discrete panic attacks. Symptoms must persist at least 6 months for this diagnosis.

Phobic Disorders

Phobic disorders are anxiety disorders associated with specific exposures, such as height, social occasions, and so on. The symptoms are similar to those of panic disorder.

Somatoform Disorders

In somatoform disorders, patients have symptoms for which no medical explanation can be identified. When the complaint is an acute loss of physical functioning, such as paralysis, the diagnosis of conversion disorder can be made (see Chap. 181). Less specific complaints, which are typically chronic in nature, are diagnosed as somatization disorder. Patients with somatization disorder typically have the onset of their symptoms in their teens or twenties and often undergo considerable unnecessary medical and surgical intervention. Making a new diagnosis of somatoform disorder in the ED is difficult. As always, a careful search for a treatable medical disorder is necessary and, if none is found, the patient should be reassured. Follow-up with a general internist or family practitioner is strongly encouraged.

Dissociative Disorders

Dissociative disorders share as a central feature a sudden disruption of the normal integrity of identity and consciousness. The dissociation often occurs under severe stress and is usually temporary. Examples include psychogenic amnesia, in which there is a sudden loss of memory for personal details, and psychogenic fugue, in which a similar loss of personal memory occurs accompanied by travel away from home.

Personality Disorders

A personality disorder is present when a person exhibits a lifelong pattern of difficulty in interpersonal relationships that results in significant impairment in social and occupational functioning. The most common personality disorder seen in the ED is the antisocial personality disorder. These patients show a consistent disregard for the rights of others and often have a history of criminal behavior, violence, financial irresponsibility, and an inability to sustain enduring attachments to others. These patients are often manipulative and can be difficult to treat in the ED. It is important to establish firm limits on their behavior and focus on the chief complaint.

For further reading in *Emergency Medicine: A Comprehensive Study Guide,* 5th ed., see Chap. 280, "Behavioral Disorders: Clinical Features," by Douglas A. Rund.

---

180 | Behavioral Disorders: Emergency Assessment and Stabilization

Burton Bentley II

Patients with behavioral disorders frequently go to the emergency department (ED). Their abnormal behavior may be either a presenting complaint or a secondary finding. The care of these patients must be approached in a systematic fashion in order to distinguish functional from organic etiologies. Specific techniques may be required in the management of violent, suicidal, or otherwise distraught patients.

ACUTE BEHAVIORAL DISORDERS

Diagnosis and Differential

A thorough medical-psychiatric history and physical examination are the most effective tools for the emergency evaluation of behavioral disorders. An immediate goal is to attempt to distinguish *organic* from *functional* disorders. Since few functional disturbances begin abruptly, the sudden onset of a major change in behavior, mood, or thought is most likely to result from an organic cause. The following life-threatening conditions may result in abrupt behavior disturbances and must be systematically ruled out:

1. Central nervous system (CNS) infection (meningitis or encephalitis)
2. Intoxication
3. Alcohol or drug withdrawal
4. Hypoglycemia
5. Hypertensive encephalopathy
6. Hypoxia
7. Intracranial hemorrhage
8. Poisoning
9. Head trauma
10. Seizure
11. Acute organ system failure

For the severely impaired patient, third-party accounts may be the only reliable source of historical information. The change in behavior is an excellent starting point for inquiry, and it should always be evaluated relative to the patient's previous level of functioning. In addition to the standard questions asked during the history of a present illness, the evaluation of the behaviorally disturbed patient should include the following data:

1. Thorough review of systems focusing on neurologic symptoms (e.g., confusion, recently impaired speech, and headaches).
2. Description of previous and recent highest level of functioning.
3. Previous psychiatric illness and treatment.
4. History of substance abuse, prescription drugs, and over-the-counter medications.
5. Exposure to occupational hazards or toxins (e.g., heavy metals and organic solvents).
6. Identity of stressors in the patient's environment that may provoke or accentuate disturbed behavior.

Mental Status Examination

Important components of the mental status examination include assessment of affect, orientation, language, memory, thought content, perceptual abnormalities, and judgment. Impaired language performance, including difficulty with speech, reading, writing, and word finding, may indicate a neurologic disorder. The patient's affect should be evaluated for sadness, euphoria, or anxiety. This observation may help to distinguish between psychiatric illness induced by affective disorders versus true organic dementia. The experience of hallucinations should also be reviewed; visual hallucinations favor organic etiologies whereas auditory hallucinations are often functional. Last, the "clock face test" may be useful. To perform this test, the physician draws a circle and asks the patient to fill in the numbers and hands to form the face of a clock. The inability to perform this task suggests organic disease.

Physical and Laboratory Evaluations

The physical examination should identify problems that may have caused or impacted upon the behavioral disorder being evaluated. Additionally, it should uncover medical problems that require special care or that may be inappropriate for management in a psychiatric hospital setting. All patients must be thoroughly examined for signs of trauma, since it is frequently both unsuspected and underreported. Last, the neurologic examination should include a search for focal neurologic deficits such as apraxia, aphasia, asymmetric reflexes, and paresis.

Many medical illnesses cause both acute behavioral disturbances and a change in vital signs. Abnormal vital signs must therefore never be dismissed as being secondary only to the behavioral disturbance itself. Examples of *specific signs* and their potential causes include the following:

1. *Bradycardia*: hypothyroidism, Stokes-Adams syndrome, elevated intracranial pressure, and cholinergic poisoning.
2. *Tachycardia*: hyperthyroidism, infection, heart failure, pulmonary embolism, alcohol withdrawal, and anticholinergic or sympathomimetic poisoning.
3. *Fever*: thyroid storm, vasculitis, alcohol withdrawal, sedative-hypnotic withdrawal, and infection.
4. *Hypothermia*: sepsis, hypoendocrine status, CNS dysfunction, and alcohol intoxication.
5. *Hypotension*: shock, Addison's disease, hypothyroidism, and medication side effect.
6. *Hypertension*: hypertensive encephalopathy and stimulant abuse.
7. *Tachypnea*: metabolic acidosis, pulmonary embolism, cardiac failure, and fever.

The selection of appropriate laboratory tests must be guided by clinical history and presentation. Bedside glucose determination should be the first test performed on any patient with an altered level of consciousness or agitation. Urine and serum drug screens, as well as specific toxicologic assays, may be performed when appropriate. Electrocardiograms are useful in elderly patients who may sometimes have behavioral changes as a manifestation of myocardial ischemia. A qualitative B-HCG test should be obtained on all women of child-bearing age since a positive pregnancy test may impact further treatment plans. Additional tests may be ordered as indicated. These include serum electrolyte levels, renal and liver function tests, arterial blood gas analysis, cerebrospinal fluid analysis, electroencephalography, computerized tomographic studies, and magnetic resonance imaging.

Emergency Department Care and Disposition

1. In order to protect patients from harming themselves and others, *violent behavior demands immediate physical restraint.* This action should only be undertaken by trained personnel such as the hospital security teams or local police. An initial show of force may be sufficient to induce the patient to accept physical or chemical restraint without further resistance. This approach usually requires five team members with each one assigned to a limb and the leader controlling the head. When approached from different directions and grabbed simultaneously, the violent person can usually be immobilized. All restrained patients should be disrobed, gowned, and searched for weapons.

2. Chemical restraint is indicated for those patients whose behavior remains dangerously uncontrolled despite adequate physical restraint. **Lorazepam** (Ativan) is often considered to be the agent of choice for control of the agitated patient. It has a rapid onset of action, a wide therapeutic index, and may be given orally, IV, or IM. Typical starting doses of lorazepam are 1 to 2 mg IM or 1 mg IV repeated every 30 min as necessary. Respiratory depression may occur and can be treated with **flumazenil** (Romazicon), 0.2 mg IV with subsequent doses of 0.3 mg and 0.5 mg if necessary. **Haloperidol** (Haldol) and **droperidol** (Inapsine) are neuroleptic tranquilizers that may be used as single-line agents or to augment the effect of lorazepam. They are particularly good for patients whose agitation has psychotic features. The dose of haloperidol may be titrated, starting at 2.5 to 5 mg IM. Droperidol's onset of action is rapid by both the IV and IM routes and is usually started at 2.5 to 5 mg via either route. Hypotension from either agent usually responds to crystalloid infusion.

3. Potentially violent behavior requires a nonthreatening attitude by the physician and staff while an adequate back-up force is summoned. This force should be clearly visible, and the patient must be informed that certain types of unacceptable behavior will result in restraint. The physician should avoid excessive eye contact, maintain a somewhat submissive posture, and stand in a location that neither threatens the patient nor blocks his

own retreat from the room. Potentially violent situations may be defused by allowing the patient to ventilate feelings verbally while the physician makes neutral comments and sets limits on behavior.

4. The decision to release a patient from restraints should be made jointly by medical and nursing personnel on the basis of the patient's behavior and not as a result of bargains or threats. Restraints are then released in a stepwise fashion, limb by limb, over time.

SUICIDE

Suicide attempts are made by roughly 1 percent of the population and regardless of how trivial the attempt may seem, the action must be taken seriously. All staff members should be empathetic while protecting the patient from further attempts at injury. Medical problems must be addressed efficiently, and the suicide risk should be assessed.

Clinical Features

Schizophrenia, substance abuse, and depression are psychiatric diagnoses that place patients at a relatively high suicide risk. Personality or adjustment disorders are frequent diagnoses in people who attempt suicide, though they have a lower risk of completion. Violent suicide actions (e.g., shooting and hanging) place patients at a high risk for future attempts. In general, the risk of a successful suicide increases with advancing age. Other factors that contribute to suicide risk include male gender, divorced/widowed marital status, unemployment, poor health, prior suicide attempts, history of poor achievement, and social isolation.

Emergency Department Care and Disposition

1. During the clinical interview, patients who display hopelessness, helplessness, exhaustion, overwhelming depression, or clear suicidal intent obviously remain at high risk; immediate psychiatric consultation and hospitalization is required. Patients at lower suicide risk often show remorse or embarrassment about the attempt, and the action may have been taken during a period of transient anger. Patients who refuse to provide any information about the event must be considered to be at high risk. Patient disposition can also be aided by considering the lethality of the attempt and the likelihood of rescue. For example, the patient who attempts to hang himself while alone at home is at much

greater risk than the patient who takes a few pills in front of friends.

High-risk patients with strong suicidal intent require immediate psychiatric hospitalization. *Moderate-risk patients* are those who have a positive response to initial intervention and favorable social support. They are judged not to be in immediate danger and may often be treated right away in the outpatient setting. This determination is made in concert with a psychiatric consultant and requires the support of family or friends. *Low-risk patients* often present following suicide threats or minor attempts that occur in the context of a clearly definable external crisis. Provided that they have a responsive and available social support system, they may be managed as outpatients once immediate follow-up has been arranged.

2. Consideration of the following criteria is suggested before discharging a potentially suicidal child, adolescent, or adult from the ED:
   a. The patient must not be imminently suicidal.
   b. The patient must be medically stable.
   c. The patient agrees to return to the emergency department if suicidal intent returns.
   d. The patient must not be intoxicated, delirious, or demented.
   e. Potentially lethal forms of self-harm have been removed.
   f. Treatment of underlying psychiatric diagnoses has been arranged.
   g. Acute precipitants to the crisis have been addressed, and attempts have been made to resolve them.
   h. The physician believes that the patient and family will follow through on treatment recommendations.
   i. The patient's caregivers and social supports are in agreement with the discharge plans.

Any patient whose suicide risk cannot be determined must be evaluated by a psychiatric consultant and considered for hospitalization.

For further reading in *Emergency Medicine: A Comprehensive Study Guide,* 5th ed., see Chap. 281, "Behavioral Disorders: Emergency Assessment and Stabilization," by Jeffrey C. Hutzler and Douglas A. Rund.

181 | Conversion Disorder

John Sverha

Conversion disorder (or conversion reaction) is a psychologically produced acute loss of physical functioning.

Clinical Features

Most patients with conversion disorder have neurologic symptoms. Motor disorders (e.g., pseudoseizures, localized paralysis, and difficulty swallowing) are more common than are alterations in sensation (e.g., blindness, numbness, and paresthesias). Rarely, autonomic or endocrine symptoms are described. The symptoms of conversion disorder typically have an acute onset and are often related to a severe stress. Although psychologic in origin, the patient is not conscious of purposely producing the symptom. Some patients describe their symptoms with a surprising lack of concern (*la belle indifference*), although this is not universal or diagnostic.

Diagnosis and Differential

Conversion disorder is a diagnosis of exclusion. A careful history and physical exam is essential. Often, the neurologic exam in patients with conversion disorder is not consistent with known anatomic or pathophysiologic states. Physical examination techniques that can help detect pseudoparalysis include the hand drop test (an extremity dropped above the face will miss it) and the Hoover test (the patient will press downward with the affected leg when elevating the normal leg). Sensory deficits can be tested with the "strength" test. The patient is asked to close his eyes, and "strength" is tested by lightly touching the finger to be moved. True lack of sensation would not allow the patient to ascertain which finger should be moved. In cases of hysterical blindness, testing with an optokinetic drum will produce nystagmus.

If the history and physical exam are not definitive, appropriate laboratory and radiologic studies should be performed. Central nervous system masses, infections, or atypical seizure disorders must be considered. A high index of suspicion should also be maintained for physical disorders that have a vague onset of non-specific symptoms (e.g., systemic lupus erythematosus, multiple sclerosis, polymyositis, Lyme disease, and drug toxicity). Neurologic and/or psychiatric consultation may be necessary if the diagnosis is unclear.

Emergency Department Care and Disposition

Several psychologic strategies are recommended for managing patients with conversion disorder. Do not confront the patient or trivialize their symptoms. Instead, review test results with the patient and offer reassurance. Suggesting that their symptoms will improve is helpful and creates an expectation for recovery. The patient should also be educated as to the cause of their symptoms, although this often must be done gradually in order to be accepted by the patient. Referral to appropriate psychiatric and medical resources is highly recommended.

For further reading in *Emergency Medicine: A Comprehensive Study Guide,* 5th ed., see Chap. 285, "Conversion Disorder" by Gregory P. Moore and Kenneth C. Jackimczyk.

182 | ## Child and Elderly Abuse

Stephen W. Meldon

PEDIATRIC ABUSE

The spectrum of pediatric abuse includes child neglect, physical abuse, sexual abuse, and Munchausen's syndrome by proxy (MSBP). The physical stigmata of such abuse may be characteristic or subtle. Recognition of abuse is aided by knowledge of normal child development.

Clinical Features

Child neglect in early infancy results in the syndrome of failure to thrive (FTT). Overall physical care and hygiene are frequently poor. FTT infants have very little subcutaneous tissue, prominent-appearing ribs, and loose skin over the buttocks. Muscle tone is usually increased. Distinct behavioral characteristics include wariness, poor eye contact, difficult consolability, and even irritability with interpersonal interaction. Children over the age of 2 to 3 years with emotional neglect are termed psychosocial dwarfs. These children manifest the classic triad of short stature; bizarre, voracious appetite; and a disturbed home environment. They are frequently hyperactive and have delayed speech.

While the spectrum of injuries in physical abuse is wide, certain clinical features should be suggestive. Suspicion should be raised when observing multiple areas of ecchymoses, especially over the lower back, buttocks, thighs, cheeks, ear pinnae, ankles, or wrists, and bruises that are uniform but well-demarcated (caused by belts or cords). Scald burns caused by immersion in hot water do not show a splash configuration but, rather, involve an entire hand or foot ("glove-and-stocking" pattern) or the buttocks and genitalia. Skeletal injuries often present with unexplained swelling of an extremity or the refusal to walk or use an affected extremity. Head injuries may be manifested by subgaleal hematomas, bruising around the eyes or ears, or mental status changes. Intracranial hemorrhage with associated retinal hemorrhages may result from vigorous shaking of an infant. Injuries to the abdomen are equally

945

serious. Signs and symptoms include recurrent vomiting and abdominal pain, with abdominal tenderness and distention on examination. Finally, abused children are often submissive and compliant, do not resist painful medical procedures, and may be overly affectionate to the medical staff.

The clinical features of sexual abuse are also varied. Genitourinary symptoms, including vaginal discharge or bleeding and urinary tract infections, and behavioral disorders, such as sexually oriented behavior, encopresis, regression, and nightmares, are common. Genital and perianal injury may result in abrasions, hematomas, fissures, or scarring. Erythema, however, may be secondary to irritation or inflammation and is not specific for abuse.

MSBP is a relatively uncommon form of child abuse in which a parent induces or fabricates an illness in a child. Typically, reported symptoms include bleeding, seizures, apnea, diarrhea, vomiting, and fever.

Diagnosis and Differential

The diagnosis of child abuse should be suggested by an inconsistent history and the previously mentioned clinical features. A high index of suspicion must be maintained when evaluating children for genitourinary complaints or serious trauma. Weight, length, and head circumference should be measured in FTT infants. The body mass index [BMI = weight (kg)/height (m^2)] may be less than 5 percent. Weight gain after hospital admission is considered to be the sine qua non of environmental FTT. Children with suspected physical abuse should be evaluated with a complete blood cell count, including platelets, coagulation studies, and a skeletal survey. Inflicted injuries are suggested by spiral fractures of a long bone, metaphyseal chip fractures, multiple fractures at different stages of healing, and unusual fracture sites, such as ribs, lateral clavicle, and scapula. Infants and children with suspected intracranial or intraabdominal trauma should be evaluated with computed tomography scan. Rarely, pathologic conditions such as leukemia, aplastic anemia, and osteogenesis imperfecta can mimic physical abuse.

The diagnosis of sexual abuse can often be confirmed by careful inspection of the genital and perianal areas. The hymeneal orifice should be measured and any hymeneal notches (concavities) noted. Anal tone should be assessed. Children seen immediately after an assault should be evaluated for the presence of forensic evidence, such as semen. Swabs of the vagina, rectum, and oral cavity should be performed. These areas should also be cultured for gonorrhea. A vaginal culture for chlamydia should be included. Rapid antigen assays for chlamydia are unreliable in prepubescent children. It is important to remember that the absence of physical findings does not exclude abuse.

Emergency Department Care and Disposition

The medical management of pediatric abuse should be guided by the physical findings and nature of injury. A full **social service assessment** should be obtained. Infants with significant environmental FTT and MSBP should be admitted. Victims of physical abuse frequently require admission. **Reporting of suspected cases** of abuse is mandatory, and a verbal report should be made to the police department or child protection agency. A suspicion of child sexual abuse also mandates such reporting. Although there is the likelihood that the child may be removed from the home, a follow-up appointment for culture results and a referral for psychological counseling should be arranged.

ELDER ABUSE

Elder abuse continues to be underrecognized and underreported. Research suggests that elder abuse affects 3 to 4 percent of the elderly population.

Clinical Features

Most elderly victims of abuse live with the perpetrator. The abuser is often dependent on the victim for housing and financial or emotional support. Functional disability and worsening cognitive impairment are significantly associated with elder mistreatment. Other important historical features include presence of caretaker mental illness or drug or alcohol abuse, family history of violence, patient isolation, and recent stressful life events for the caretaker. The physical examination should note signs or symptoms of poor personal hygiene; inappropriate, soiled clothing; dehydration; malnutrition; and decubiti. Specific injuries suggestive of abuse include unexplained fractures, lacerations, or ecchymoses; injuries to the head or face; and unusual burns. In addition, certain interactions between the patient and caretaker are suggestive of abuse. These include patient fear; conflicting accounts of the injury or illness; an indifferent or angry attitude; inordinate concern with the cost of treatment; and denial by the caretaker of opportunity for the patient to interact privately with the medical staff.

Diagnosis and Differential

A high index of suspicion is necessary for diagnosis of elder abuse. It should be considered in the differential diagnosis when evaluating the patient with frequent falls, failure to thrive, dementia, and dehydration or malnutrition. The diagnosis can be made in most cases by simple direct questioning regarding abusive relationships and careful physical examination.

Emergency Department Care and Disposition

Management of elder abuse involves both specific treatment for the injuries or illnesses detected, and immediate intervention. **Social services consultation** and **adult protective services** involvement should be obtained in cases of proven or strongly suspected elder abuse. Elderly patients with medical problems requiring hospital admission should be admitted to the appropriate medical service. Patients who do not medically require admission may need to be admitted for protective placement if they cannot be safely discharged. If indicated, caregivers should be provided with intervention options such as home health services, Meals on Wheels, transportation, and medical and mental health services. The majority of states have mandatory reporting laws that require disclosure of suspected elder mistreatment despite the victim's wishes.

For further reading in *Emergency Medicine: A Comprehensive Study Guide,* 5th ed., see Chap. 289, "Child Abuse and Neglect," by Carol D. Berkowitz; and Chap. 292, "Abuse in the Elderly and Impaired," by Ellen H. Taliaferro and Patricia R. Salber.

---

183 | Sexual Assault

Stephen W. Meldon

Sexual assault accounts for 5 percent of reported violent crimes. Prevalence studies suggest that one in five women have been victims of rape, although it is estimated that only one in three cases are reported. Male sexual assault is similarly underrecognized and underreported, and has an estimated incidence of 2 to 4 percent of reported rapes.

Clinical Features

A brief, tactfully obtained history should include the following components: (1) who (whether the assailant was known and the number of attackers), (2) what happened (including other physical assaults and injuries), (3) when (time since assault), (4) where (vaginal, oral, or rectal penetration), and (5) whether the patient has douched, showered, or changed clothes since the attack. All of these activities should be documented. Important past medical history includes date of last menstrual period, birth control method, time of last intercourse, and drug allergies. The physical examination should document bruises, lacerations, and other trauma. As many as 50 percent of rape survivors have injuries outside the genital region. The victim's face, oral cavity, neck, breasts, wrists, thighs, and buttocks should be inspected. A pelvic examination may reveal vaginal discharge or genital lacerations or abrasions. Application of toluidine blue stain to the posterior fourchette may reveal small, subtle vulva lacerations, which will appear as a linear blue stain. When oral or rectal penetration has occurred, a careful examination should be performed, with attention to ecchymoses, lacerations, or fissures. The male rape examination should entail the same history taking as noted above. The physical examination should search for abrasions to the abdomen or anterior chest. The anal area should be inspected for signs of trauma. Approximately half of victims have minor genital injuries, such as perineal contusions, anal fissures, or rectal mucosal tears.

Diagnosis and Differential

Rape is a legal determination, not a medical diagnosis. The legal definition contains three elements: carnal knowledge, nonconsent, and compulsion or fear of harm. Because of the legal considerations, careful documentation and sample collection are important. Informed consent should be obtained and a system to maintain "chain of evidence" established. Preprinted diagrams can aid in accurate representation of injuries. A prepackaged rape kit with equipment and directions on sample collection should be used. If no kit is available, smears from the vagina and cervix are made, labeled, and air dried. A wet mount from the same areas should be microscopically inspected for sperm. A vaginal aspirate using 5 to 10 mL of normal saline solution should be tested for acid phosphatase. Premoistened rectal or buccal swabs for sperm should be collected. A Wood's lamp will cause semen to fluoresce and may aid in sperm collection. If sodomy has occurred, rectal swabs should be taken and slides made, labeled, and air dried. A rectal aspirate using 10 mL of normal saline solution should be examined for sperm. Additional forensic laboratory evaluation may include glycoprotein p30 testing and genetic (i.e., DNA) typing.

Emergency Department Care and Treatment

Care of the rape victim includes management of any injuries, such as laceration repair, and tetanus prophylaxis, counseling, and pregnancy and sexually transmitted disease (STD) prophylaxis.

1. Although the risk of pregnancy is very low, women rape victims should be offered **pregnancy prophylaxis**. Currently accepted therapy is **Ovral** (norgestrel and ethinyl estradiol) 2 tablets initially and 2 tablets in 12 h later. A negative pregnancy test result should be documented prior to providing this regimen. Prophylaxis must be initiated within 72 h of the sexual assault to be effective.
2. STD prophylaxis for gonorrhea and chlamydia should also be given. Current recommendations include **ceftriaxone** 125 mg IM or **ciprofloxacin** 500 mg orally once, followed by **doxycycline** 100 mg orally twice a day for 7 d or **azithromycin** 1 g orally once. In addition, a baseline VDRL should be obtained. HIV testing and counseling should be discussed with the patient, emphasizing the need for repeat testing and that the risk of transmission is very low. Physicians who consider offering post-exposure therapy with antiretroviral agents should consider the likelihood of HIV exposure and the risks versus the benefits of such therapy.
3. Indications for admission are related to the nature of injuries sustained. Only 1 to 2 percent of patients require hospitalization. Counseling, ideally, should be available 24 h a day. Often the rape counselor can assess and prepare the patient for examination prior to physician assessment. If counseling is not immediately available, follow-up with a local mental health or rape counseling center should be provided. A follow-up medical appointment in 7 to 14 days is appropriate.

For further reading in *Emergency Medicine: A Comprehensive Study Guide,* 5th ed., see Chap. 290, "Female and Male Sexual Assault," by Kim M. Feldhaus.

INDEX

Note: Page numbers followed by the letters *f* and *t* indicate figures and tables, respectively.

Notes

Notes

Notes

Notes

Notes

Notes

Notes

Notes

Notes

PHYSICAL AIDS TO THE ORGANIC CHEMIST

ELSEVIER MONOGRAPHS

CHEMISTRY SECTION

ELSEVIER PUBLISHING COMPANY

AMSTERDAM–NEW YORK

PHYSICAL AIDS
TO
THE ORGANIC CHEMIST

by

M. ST. C. FLETT

Research Chemist,
I.C.I. (Dyestuffs Division) Ltd.,
Blackley, Manchester
(Great Britain)

ELSEVIER PUBLISHING COMPANY

AMSTERDAM—NEW YORK

1962

SOLE DISTRIBUTORS FOR THE UNITED STATES AND CANADA
AMERICAN ELSEVIER PUBLISHING COMPANY, INC.
52 Vanderbilt Avenue, New York 17, N.Y.

Library of Congress Catalog Card Number 62–10358

With 109 figures and 38 tables

PRINTED IN THE NETHERLANDS BY
NEDERLANDSE BOEKDRUK INRICHTING N.V., 'S-HERTOGENBOSCH

PREFACE

In view of the increasing extent to which physical methods are being applied to problems of separation, structural determination, and analysis in organic chemistry, this book is offered to students and practising organic chemists who wish to expand their knowledge of such methods. Although the topics considered have already been the subjects of monographs and large volumes written by groups of experts, it is thought that there is a need for a small, fairly cheap book, which anyone who so desires may purchase for day-to-day use.

Each chapter begins with a short description of the theoretical principles and experimental methods of the technique under discussion. The main emphasis throughout is, however, on the applicability of the various methods to organic chemistry, and most of the book is therefore devoted to examples of chemical applications.

Since the field to be covered is rather wide, I have been very fortunate in that colleagues with expert knowledge of particular topics have read sections of the manuscript. In this connection I am particularly grateful to Dr. J. H. Beynon (who read the whole manuscript), Dr. J. K. Becconsall, Mr. R. A. Saunders, and Dr. A. F. Wells. I wish also to thank the editors of various journals for permission to reproduce figures, my wife for assistance with the diagrams, and I.C.I. (Dyestuffs Division) Ltd., for typing facilities.

I.C.I. (Dyestuffs Division) Ltd.,   M. St. C. Flett
Blackley, Manchester,
May, 1961

ACKNOWLEDGEMENTS

Thanks are due to the copyright holders and authors who kindly permitted the reproduction of published diagrams: to Interscience Publishers, Inc., for Figs. 5 and 62: to Butterworths Scientific Publications for Figs. 6 and 44: to Analytical Chemistry for Figs. 7(a), 15, 19(a) and (b), and 106: to the Society for Analytical Chemistry for Figs. 7(b) and 21: to the Society of Chemical Industry for Figs. 7(c), 19(c) and (d), and 39: to Nature for Fig. 19(e): to the Institute of Petroleum for Figs. 22 and 97: to John Wiley and Sons for Fig. 26, from Zone-Melting, by Pfann, and Fig. 30 from Ultra-Violet Spectra of Organic Compounds, by Friedel and Orchin: to the Clarendon Press for Figs. 32 and 36, from Bowen, Chemical Aspects of Light: to the American Chemical Society for Figs. 41, 42 and 82: to the Faraday Society for Figs. 52(a) and (b), 70, 71 and 77: to the Royal Society for Fig. 55: to the American Institute of Physics for Figs. 78 and 80: and to the McGraw-Hill Book Co., Inc., for Figs. 87(a), (b) and (c), 89(a) and 91, which are from High-Resolution Nuclear Magnetic Resonance by Pople, Schneider and Bernstein. Figs. 87(d) and (e), and 88(b), (c) and (d) are based on curves which originally appeared in the "NMR at Work" series of advertisements by Varian Associates.

CONTENTS

INTRODUCTION

In some ways the task of the organic chemist is becoming more and more difficult. For example, workers in the field of natural products are trying to elucidate the chemistry of such compounds as alkaloids, nucleic acids, vitamins and proteins of increasing complexity. The demands by industry for specialised products to perform specific tasks, for example, as dyes, wetting agents, rubber chemicals and pharmaceuticals place an increasing burden on the industrial research chemist. To satisfy these needs, he may have to synthesise new molecules, probably based on a ring system which a generation ago was an academic curiosity, and carrying several functional groups. The rapid development of synthetic polymers for the plastics and fibre industries has opened up a new and difficult field.

When the synthetic and degradative reactions of classical organic chemistry are applied to complicated molecules, the chances of their following unsuspected courses or giving large amounts of by-products are greatly increased. It therefore frequently happens that the chemist is uncertain of the composition and structure of his reaction products. For investigating these products he has on the one hand the tools of classical organic chemistry. These comprise distillation and recrystallisation as means of separation and purification of the products, followed by elementary analysis, molecular weight determination, and the formation of derivatives as means of elucidating structure. Unfortunately, particularly in polymer chemistry, these tools are much less effective than in simple systems. High molecular weight substances are frequently difficult to purify by normal methods, and the accuracy of elementary analyses may be insufficient to reveal small structural differences. Similarly, because of insolubility in suitable solvents, molecular weight determination and the formation of derivatives may be difficult.

During the last twenty years several new and valuable methods have emerged from the field of pure physics to assist the organic chemist. Techniques such as infra-red and mass spectroscopy which before the war were practised only in academic physics laboratories are now being applied daily to chemical problems throughout the world. This transformation began when, under the pressure of wartime conditions, chemists particularly in the petroleum industry had to find rapid methods of analysis and turned to the physicist for help. The extent of this co-operation has increased steadily and has been aided by instrument manufacturers who have developed equipment of greatly improved sensitivity, speed and above all, reliability, thereby making possible the application of physical techniques for day-to-day problems in chemical laboratories.

From what has been said, it is clear that if an organic chemist is to work at full efficiency, he must make full use of physical aids. This is not entirely easy to achieve. Since fairly complicated apparatus is often involved, the operation of these techniques is often under the supervision of physicists, who may also be responsible for interpretation of the records. The physicist, no matter how willing, cannot help the chemist until the latter approaches him and tells him of his problems. Unfortunately, by no means all organic chemists can recognise when a physical technique is applicable, and if so, which one is most suitable in a given case. Although the teaching of chemistry at most universities now includes some indication of how physical methods are applied, an undergraduate whose main interest is organic chemistry may well fail to find time properly to study the application of physics to his art. The situation of the practising chemist who graduated before such methods became popular is also difficult. There are available excellent monographs dealing with the subjects described in this book, and also collective volumes, written by several authors, each an expert on some topic. However, such books often deal with the subject from too physical an aspect, considerable space being devoted to underlying theory and experimental methods, at the expense of examples of chemical applications. This gives a chemist reading such a book the impression that the subject is difficult and remote from his own work.

This book attempts to meet these difficulties by describing a number of well-established physical aids, in sufficient detail to enable an organic chemist to form his own judgment, as to whether they are applicable to his problems. Discussions of theory and instrumental methods have been kept to a minimum, since it is felt that no profound knowledge of either is required in many chemical applications. What the chemist must know is what type of problem each technique can tackle, the form in which his samples must be presented, and the expenditure of time and effort involved in obtaining the results. The book attempts to answer these questions, largely by the use of illustrative examples.

The choice of topics is based on the author's experience during several years in a group whose main function is to supply a service of physical aids to a large research organisation, staffed mainly by organic chemists engaged in the invention and development of new products. All the methods described have been in continuous use in these laboratories for several years, and have been found consistently useful. Although several techniques have not been discussed, it is thought that the solution of the vast majority of organic chemical problems will be speeded by one or other of the methods described here.

The next three chapters deal with techniques which are primarily means of separating the components of mixtures, so that they can more readily be identified. Chapter 2 describes various aspects of chromatography, whilst gas chromatography which, since its discovery in 1952, has been developed extremely rapidly as a method of separating volatile mixtures, is the subject of Chapter 3. Purification by zone-melting provided the key to the preparation of germanium and silicon in the very high state of purity demanded by transistor applications. The method is now being applied increasingly in organic chemistry, both for the preparation of ultra-pure samples, and to concentrate impurities to facilitate their identification. Most applications of physical methods to mixtures are assisted by the preliminary use of one of these methods.

Four chapters follow which deal with the absorption of electromagnetic radiations at various wavelengths. Chapter 5 treats absorption spectroscopy in the visible and ultra-violet regions, one of the earliest physical techniques to be applied to organic problems. In addition to well-established uses in impurity detection and structural diagnosis, the recent applications of electronic spectra to the study of steric effects within molecules, and the properties of metastable radicals and triplet state molecules are described. The next chapter covers infra-red spectroscopy. Of all the physical techniques described here, this is perhaps the most widely applicable. Recent instrumental developments enable the infra-red spectrum of any sample, solid, liquid or gas to be obtained rapidly, thus providing the best available means of fingerprinting organic compounds. Not only is the infra-red spectrum a powerful means of identifying an unknown whose spectrum is in any of the available collections, but the possibility of associating bands at certain wavelengths with particular chemical groups is invaluable in determining the structures of compounds which have not previously been examined.

Absorption of radiation of much longer wavelengths, in the microwave and radio-frequency regions, form the subject of Chapters 7 and 8. Since the electron spins about its axis, it has associated with it a magnetic moment, so that free radicals, which contain unpaired electrons, absorb energy in a magnetic field. Electron Spin Resonance Spectroscopy utilises this effect, and is the most powerful method available for determining the concentrations and structures of free radicals. Similarly the spin properties of atomic nuclei lead to Nuclear Spin Resonance Spectroscopy, which can be applied in much the same way as infra-red spectroscopy, since signals are obtained at positions in the spectrum, which are characteristic of the chemical binding of the proton or other nucleus, satisfying the conditions for resonance.

Mass spectroscopy has also become of great importance during the last fifteen years. It first provided a method for the quantitative analysis of multicomponent hydrocarbon mixtures, but more recently its power in impurity detection and in the determination of the molecular weights and structures of unknowns has become apparent. The ability of mass spectroscopy to reveal impurities at a level far below the detection limit of most physical methods is a valuable feature. Its applicability is limited only by the need for the sample to show appreciable vapour pressure below its decomposition temperature.

In the final chapter, the uses of X-ray crystallography are summarised. This method may become even more valuable as a result of improvements in computer methods, which speed up the rather laborious calculations sometimes required.

CHAPTER 2

CHROMATOGRAPHIC SEPARATION

Many of the products handled by organic chemists are mixtures of several components, or may contain small amounts of impurity which affect their properties. All the methods described in the later chapters can be applied more effectively in identifications and structural determinations, to pure compounds than to mixtures. The book therefore begins with three chapters dealing with methods which, though sometimes themselves capable of identifying unknowns are primarily methods of separation and purification.

A. METHODS OF CHROMATOGRAPHY

All chromatographic methods depend basically on the distribution of the substances to be separated between two phases, one fixed and the other moving. The fixed phase takes the form of a column or strip, through which flows the moving phase, in which the substances to be separated are dissolved. Either a liquid or, in the case of volatile materials, a gas may be used as solvent. The molecules of those solutes which interact strongly with the fixed phase will spend a high proportion of their time stationary, so such solutes will move only slowly through the column. On the contrary, substances which are only weakly attached will be washed through more rapidly. If as in Fig. 2a a mixture is introduced on the top of the column, in the form of a concentrated solution, followed by a flow of solvent, the various solutes move at different rates, and a separation is effected. There are many variants of the process, as set out in Fig. 1.

Chromatographic methods are of three types, according to the nature of the fixed phase. This may be a solid which is quite insoluble in the solvents used. The essential step is then adsorption from solution on to the solid, the process being called adsorption chromatography. Again the stationary phase may be a solid on to which a liquid is so firmly adsorbed as to be

Fig. 1. Types of chromatography.

virtually stationary. Distribution of solutes then occurs between this first liquid and the flowing solvent, with which it is immiscible, the process being termed partition chromatography.

Paper chromatography, in which the "column" takes the form of a paper strip, through which flows the mixture in an organic solvent, is usually regarded as a branch of partition chromatography, the layer of adsorbed water which is always carried by paper acting as the fixed liquid.

In the third form, known as ion-exchange chromatography the separation depends on the differing attractions of, for example, a column material containing basic centres for the components of a mixture of acids of various strengths. Further sub-divisions of these three types are possible according to whether the moving solvent is liquid or gaseous.

With a given fixed phase, there are various possible ways of operating the column. By far the commonest is elution analysis. Here the mixture is introduced at the top of the column (Fig. 2a) in the form of a concentrated solution, and the separation is "developed" by flow of pure solvent. The process may either be stopped at the stage of Fig. 2b with the separated constituents

Fig. 2. Basic experiment of chromatography.

on the column, or continued till each solute in turn reaches the foot of the column and is collected. With colourless substances the latter method is usually adopted. It is sometimes possible to measure continuously some physical property of the effluent solution in order to monitor the components of the solution. If this property is plotted against the volume of liquid which has passed through, a curve of the form shown in Fig. 3a is obtained, with a peak corresponding to each separated component.

Elution analysis suffers from the defect that so-called "tailing" of the bands may occur. In this event, if concentration of solute in the effluent is plotted against volume of solvent passed through

Fig. 3. (a) Complete separation of A, B and C; (b) Incomplete separation because of "tailing".

Fig. 4. Development by displacement.

the column, a curve such as is shown in Fig. 3b, rather than 3a is obtained. Separation is thus incomplete so it may pay to try another method of operation, called displacement analysis. Here the separation is effected not by pure solvent, but by a developing solution containing a solute which is more strongly adsorbed than any of the solutes to be separated. This solution acts as a

piston pushing the solutes down the column at a rate dependent
on how strongly they are adsorbed. The result may be a very
sharp separation. If some suitable property of the issuing
solution is now plotted against volume of solvent, a diagram
similar to Fig. 4 is obtained, each step corresponding to a
different solute.

A third method called frontal analysis in which a solution
flows continuously through the column was introduced by
Tiselius and Claesson[1,6], and has advantages in certain difficult
cases.

The theory of chromatographic separations has been considered in terms of partition coefficients, adsorption isotherms,
and rates of adsorption and has been treated by several authors.
Since a simple theory which is universally accepted has not yet
emerged, the subject will not be dealt with here. For a simple
account the reader is referred to Martin[41], and many of the
texts listed in the selected bibliography give fuller treatments.

B. SELECTION OF A CHROMATOGRAPHIC METHOD

Before describing the various branches of chromatography
summarised in Fig. 1, it may be helpful to discuss the factors
governing the selection of a method in a given case. There is
little doubt that, provided the system is sufficiently volatile,
gas–liquid partition chromatography will normally be the most
convenient method. Since modern columns can be operated up
to 300°C, it is sufficient that the mixture should have a vapour
pressure of a few centimetres at this temperature. The danger
of decomposition on the column at high temperatures must, of
course, be considered. Gas chromatography has the great
advantage that no problems of removing the separated components from the column or the solvent arise. They emerge in a
form ideally suited to subsequent study by some other physical
technique. As shown in the next chapter the technique is fairly
simple, and may be operated by the organic chemist himself if
he wishes.

It must, of course, be admitted that volatility limits the

application of gas–liquid chromatography. A very convenient method of separation, which does not depend on volatility is afforded by liquid chromatography with paper strips or cellulose columns. The limitation here is that, since the separation depends on distribution between an organic solvent, and water adsorbed on to the paper, appreciable water solubility is required. Although the method is thus singularly well suited to the separations of many natural products, which normally occur in aqueous media, many classes of organic compound are ruled out.

For substances which are involatile and quite insoluble in water, there remains adsorption and partition column chromatography.

C. ADSORPTION CHROMATOGRAPHY

The basic experiment of adsorption chromatography is illustrated in Figs. 2a, b and c. As already mentioned, the process may either be stopped at stage (b) or continued till each solute in turn is washed from the bottom of the column.

1. Technique and materials

As seen from the figure very simple apparatus may be used, to which minor modifications may be made if, for example, one wishes to speed the process by suction or to work in an inert atmosphere. Columns from a few millimetres to several centimetres in diameter may be used, according to the scale of the experiment. Generally speaking a long thin column gives the best separation in difficult cases, but large quantities of readily separable substances can be treated more rapidly in a wide column. Great care must be taken in filling the column, since any irregularities may lead to mixing of the separated zones, and channels through which the solution can flow unchanged. The methods commonly used are either to add the adsorbent in small amounts, pressing it down after each addition, or to make a slurry with solvent which is poured in and allowed to settle. In the former case the column should be wetted with solvent before use. A good account of these methods is given by Williams[3].

References p. 34

Successful separations depend on proper selection of both solvent and column material. This is partly a matter of trial and error, but there are certain guiding principles. The rate at which a solute is carried through a column is difficult to predict since it depends both on specific effects such as hydrogen bonding between solute and column material, and on the general affinity of the solute for solvent and solid. Some classes of compound are adsorbed much more strongly than others. Roughly speaking acids and strong bases are most strongly adsorbed, followed by alcohols and amines, then by aldehydes, ketones and esters. Lower in the list come unsaturated and aromatic hydrocarbons, and finally saturated hydrocarbons. For strongly adsorbed compounds it is usually best to use a polar solvent such as an alcohol, pyridine, or an ester, whereas with weakly adsorbed solutes the solvent is normally petroleum ether, carbon tetrachloride or cyclohexane, from which adsorption takes place more readily.

Alumina is by far the most commonly used adsorbent, and can be purchased in suitable quality. If necessary its activity can be controlled by additions of small amounts of water before use[4]. Alumina may, however, sometimes adsorb too strongly for rapid separation. A few other possible materials, listed below in order of decreasing adsorption strength are: dry alumina, charcoal > calcium carbonate, magnesia > sucrose, starch, talc.

2. Isolation and identification of the separated components

When the separation has been carried out there remains the problem of isolating and identifying the components. This is much simpler in the case of coloured substances. The separation can then be followed visually, and stopped at the right point (Fig. 2b). The contents are then pushed out bodily (which is not always entirely easy) and cut into the various coloured zones, from which the components may be dissolved and recovered.

With colourless materials, the possibility of forming coloured derivatives should first be considered. Mixed aldehydes and ketones could, for example, be converted to dinitrophenyl hydrazones. Where this is impossible, colourless samples may sometimes be rendered visible on the column by fluorescence, excited by an ultra-violet lamp. Alternatively the column material may be rendered fluorescent by admixture of luminous paint or morin[5], whereupon zones of adsorbed solute show up as dark areas upon illumination.

Usually with colourless materials it is, however, best to continue the elution till all the sample has been washed through the column, collecting a large number of fractions. This is greatly simplified by an automatic fraction collector. These collectors automatically change the receiver after a given weight of solution has collected, or after a given time, and are available commercially. Chemical or physical methods of analysis can then be applied to the fractions.

Another method of deciding when the various fractions emerge involves passing the effluent before collection through a cell, for measurement of a physical property such as conductivity, refractive index or ultra-violet spectrum. The successive appearance of the components is then signalled and the receiver can be changed accordingly. A very elegant variant of this method, in which refractive indices are measured by an interferometer, has been described by Claesson[6].

3. Applications of column adsorption chromatography

The simplest application is the removal of small amounts of impurities whose structures differ widely from that of the major component. It is usually possible to select a column material through which the latter passes readily, whilst the impurities are strongly adsorbed, and may be recovered if required. Many solvents may be purified for spectroscopy by this means[7]. For example, it has been reported that commercial samples of aliphatic hydrocarbons may be sufficiently freed from aromatic and unsaturated impurities by a single passage through silica gel columns, for use in ultra-violet spectroscopy. Activated alumina has also given good results.

Adsorption chromatography provides a good method of

testing the homogeneity of coloured components. It must, however, be stressed that formation of a single band does not necessarily imply purity. To be certain of this one should try more than one solvent.

The commonest application is separation of structurally similar compounds. Table 1 lists some classes of compound which are well suited to this type of chromatography.

TABLE 1

APPLICATION OF ADSORPTION CHROMATOGRAPHY

Class of compound	Column material	Solvent	References
Long-chain fatty acids	Alumina	Benzene, petroleum ether	8, 9
Terpene hydrocarbons and alcohols	Alumina	Petroleum ether	8
Phenols	Alumina or magnesia	Methanol	8
Condensed polycyclic hydrocarbons	Alumina	Petroleum ether and benzene	8
Alkaloids	Various	Benzene, alcohol, ether, chloroform	8
Anthocyanines	Alumina	Water	8, 10
Chlorophylls	Sucrose	Petroleum ether, benzene	11
Carotenoids	Various	Various	8
Azobenzenes	Alumina, silica, calcium sulphate	Various	5
Anthraquinones	Alumina	Toluene	4

The method has been applied to the purification of many natural products, including sugars, amino acids, sterols and vitamins. Many examples are given in Ref.[9] and by Strain[8], including a most striking case where a mixture of xanthophylls extracted from leaves, was separated into thirteen components (Fig. 5). Another typical separation concerns the estimation of anthracene in tar oils. A preliminary separation is required because the ultra-violet bands which are used to measure the

anthracene content are overlaid by bands of related hydrocarbons also present. When the tar, dissolved in a mixture of
chlorobenzene and petroleum ether is passed down an alumina

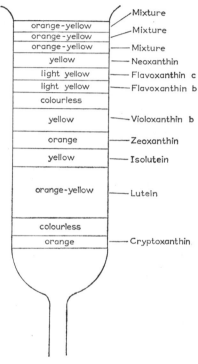

Fig. 5. Separation of leaf xanthophylls on a magnesia column[8].

column, little separation is apparent in ordinary light, but on
illumination with an ultra-violet lamp, a zone showing the
typical anthracene fluorescence can be picked out. This portion
of the column may be separated mechanically, and the anthracene
dissolved and estimated.

References p. 34

An interesting technique, described as "continuous gradient elution chromatography", has recently been developed for the separation of polymer mixtures. For example Hartley[13] has applied it to the separation of graft co-polymers formed during the polymerisation of vinyl acetate in the presence of polyvinyl alcohol. A sample containing the graft co-polymer with a large excess of polyvinyl acetate and polyvinyl alcohol was introduced in suitable form at the top of a column filled with glass beads. The column was then eluted, not as normally with a solvent of fixed composition, but with a mixture of ethyl alcohol and water whose composition varied continuously with time from pure water to pure ethanol. Fractions were collected automatically at the foot of the column for further analysis. By this means good separations were obtained, because polymers such as polyvinyl alcohol with a high water solubility were washed through first, whilst those like polyvinyl acetate which were not soluble in water passed through only towards the end of the experiment.

4. Gas adsorption chromatography

As indicated by the title, the solvent is replaced in this technique by a "carrier" gas, such as nitrogen. The column is usually of charcoal, alumina, or silica, and the method is normally applied to the separation of mixtures of permanent gases or low boiling hydrocarbons. With more polar or less volatile materials, attachment to the column is usually too strong, causing inconveniently long separation times. In this event gas–liquid partition chromatography is more suitable.

The experimental methods are very similar to those of gas–liquid chromatography (p. 37). The mixture to be separated, if liquid, is introduced at one end of the column from a hypodermic syringe, through a serum bottle cap, or, if gaseous, by some such device as that described by Phillips[14], and shown in Fig. 6. The taps are initially set so that carrier gas flows via A and B. The separation is begun by turning them so that the new passage via C and D carries the mixture on to the column, and flow continues till each component in turn reaches the end of the column and is carried to the detector (p. 40) where its presence, and if required, its concentration are recorded.

Both elution and displacement methods have been used. For

Fig. 6. Introduction of gaseous samples[14].

example Ray[15] separated a mixture of hydrogen, methane, carbon dioxide, ethylene and ethane by elution on a charcoal column, with nitrogen as carrier gas. Fig. 7a, where the detector signal is plotted against time, illustrates this separation. Similarly Patton *et al.*[16] separated hydrogen, oxygen and methane on charcoal, but found that columns of activated alumina or silica, at temperatures between 25° and 100°C were better for hydrocarbon separations (Fig. 7b).

The peaks of Fig. 7 are seen to be asymmetrical, showing marked "tailing". This is an inherent fault of the elution method in gas adsorption work, and introduces difficulties in quantitative analysis, which depends on the peak heights. Displacement methods were applied by Phillips[17], who analysed hydrocarbon mixtures by adsorption on charcoal, followed by displacement by carrier gas incorporating ethyl acetate, which progressively displaced the hydrocarbons. Accurate quantitative analyses are possible, but the method is rather slow.

Excellent results in the analysis of permanent gas mixtures

have been reported by Timms, Konrath and Chirnside[18]. They avoid the above difficulties by the use of "molecular sieves" as adsorbents. These are zeolites from which the water is removed

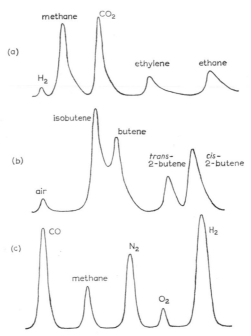

Fig. 7. Separations by adsorption chromatography. (a) Permanent gases on charcoal[15]; (b) Vapours on silica[16]; (c) Permanent gases on zeolite[18].

by heating, leaving holes of molecular dimensions. Their specific problem was the analysis of impurities in carbon dioxide for nuclear reactor coolants. After removal of the carbon dioxide, the gas was carried by argon through a 6 foot column. As shown by Fig. 7c, rapid and complete separation was achieved, with peaks eminently suitable for quantitative analysis.

D. PARTITION CHROMATOGRAPHY

As explained above this technique depends on distribution of solutes between a moving solvent, and a second liquid firmly attached to the solid. It has the following inherent advantages over the adsorption method.

(a) Recovery of the separated material from the column is easier, and can be done quantitatively.

(b) Conditions can be more easily reproduced, since the properties of dry adsorbents are rather variable.

(c) The phenomenon of "coning", that is the tendency of material at the centre of the column to move more quickly than at the edges, is less troublesome.

1. Column partition chromatography

The earliest practical application was by Martin and Synge[19], who used a column of silica gel with adsorbed water to separate amino acids in a chloroform–butanol solvent. The separation was followed by incorporating methyl orange in to the column, which serves to locate the separated acids. Such a method is only applicable where the solutes have some water solubility. It has subsequently been found that in such cases the separation can usually be carried out more conveniently on paper, a much more reproducible material than silica gel. Column partition chromatography is not therefore widely practiced, though it is worth considering where a suitable pair of solvents is available. For example the stereoisomeric hexa-chloro cyclohexanes were separated using nitromethane as stationary liquid and hexane as solvent[20]. Fatty acids have been separated from a paraffin solution, with methanol as stationary liquid. A good account of methods by which the limitation imposed by water solubility can be overcome is given by Levi[21]. Applications of column partition chromatography are fully discussed in Refs.[2,9].

2. Paper chromatography

Paper chromatography is usually regarded as a partition process, in which the stationary phase is paper, carrying in its natural state enough adsorbed water to serve as the fixed liquid, whilst an organic solvent carries the solute. There is, however, no doubt that in such cases as the separation of water soluble dyes, the adsorption properties of the paper itself play a part.

Apparatus and materials

The simplest form of separation on paper is illustrated in Fig. 8. About a milligram of the mixture in solution is spotted from a micro burette on to the paper, which is then dipped into

Fig. 8. Separation by paper chromatography.

the developing solvent. This rises by capillary attraction, and the components are carried through the paper at different rates. After a few hours the paper is removed and dried, and the separated spots, if colourless, rendered visible by treatment with a reagent. The only basic limitation to this simple method is that capillary attraction will not lift the solvent front more than about 30 cm. Therefore in difficult separations where rates of travel are not very different, a descending method is preferable in which the solvent is siphoned from a trough through the paper[2]. As one often wishes to attempt several separations simultaneously, or to run reference substances under the same conditions, rather more elaborate equipment is sometimes used. The basic requirements are:

(a) An airtight vessel into which the assembly of paper, solvent trough, etc., will fit, to prevent evaporation of solvent from the paper. A reservoir of solvent may be placed in this vessel to saturate its atmosphere.

(b) A glass or plastic trough holding the solvent, and some arrangement of supports (usually glass rods) to enable the paper strip or sheet to dip in the solvent.

TABLE 2

TYPICAL WHATMAN PAPERS FOR CHROMATOGRAPHY

Fast running	No. 15 (a thick paper)
	No. 4
Medium	No. 1
	No. 3 mm (a thick paper)
Medium slow	No. 11 (a thin paper)
	No. 2
Slow	No. 20

(c) An oven for drying the paper after the separation.

(d) An atomiser with which to spray the paper after drying, with a reagent capable of rendering colourless substances visible.

Good descriptions of the apparatus are given by Cramer[22], and Brimley and Barrett[2]. The equipment is available commercially, or can be made up in any laboratory with elementary workshop facilities.

Methods of handling several sheets simultaneously have been described by Datta *et al.*[23].

A variety of Whatman papers are available, as described by Balston and Talbot[24], and in the manufacturers' literature. Typical papers for qualitative work are listed in Table 2 (from Ref.[24]).

Two factors govern the choice of a paper. If the solutes are strongly adsorbed and slow moving, a fast running paper is required and vice versa. Secondly, it is clearly possible to handle larger quantities on a thick than a thin paper.

Experimental techniques

The best separations are attained by spotting about a milligram of mixture on to the paper. Generally speaking the less there is of a component, the sharper will be the corresponding spot, but clearly a limit is set by the sensitivity of detection. There are three main experimental methods in paper chromatography.

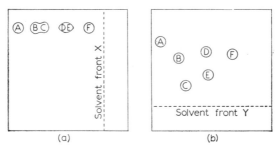

Fig. 9. Two-dimensional paper chromatography.

(a) Straightforward one-dimensional separation has already been described. This has the disadvantage that with any one eluting solvent separation may be incomplete as in Fig. 9a, where D and E are not separated.

(b) Two-dimensional method. In this variation the initial spot is placed near one corner of a square sheet, and eluted in the usual way with solvent X (Fig. 9a). X is then dried off, the paper turned through 90°, and eluted with another solvent Y. By suitable choice of X and Y, a complete two-dimensional separation may be obtained, as in Fig. 9b. An outstanding example of this is given by Dent[25], in which a mixture of no fewer than sixty-two amino acids was separated.

(c) Chromatography on circular papers. This method has proved particularly useful in separating mixtures of dyestuffs. A circular paper is held between two discs of glass or plastic, the upper of which has a hole at its centre (Fig. 10). The mixture

Fig. 10. Circular paper chromatography. B is the major component, A and C minor components.

TABLE 3

SEPARATION BY PAPER CHROMATOGRAPHY

Class of compound	Solvents	Detecting agents	References
Amino acids	Phenol, collidine, butanol–acetic acid	Ninhydrin	26
Sugars	Water-saturated phenol or collidine. Upper layer of *n*-butanol, acetic acid, water (4:1:5)	Ammoniacal silver nitrate	27
Carboxylic acids (as sodium or ammonium salts)	*n*-Butanol–aqueous ammonia	Bromo-thymol blue	28
Aldehydes and ketones (as dinitro phenyl hydrazones)	Diethyl ether-light petroleum. Aqueous acetone–petroleum	None required	29
Alcohols (as 3,5-dinitrobenzoates)	20% aqueous dioxane	0.5% 1-naphthyl-amine in ethanol	29
Flavonoid pigments	*n*-Butanol–acetic acid–water (4:1:5)	None required	30
Porphyrins	Water-saturated lutidine	Natural colours or fluorescence	31
Aromatic amines	Mixtures of benzene, amyl alcohol, methanol and water	By diazotisation	32
Penicillins	Water-saturated ether	Inhibition of spore growth	33
Steroids (as Girard T derivatives)	Water-saturated *n*-butanol	An iodoplatinate solution	24
Dyestuffs	Aqueous acetic acid, aqueous ammonia, aqueous caustic soda, aqueous cellosolve	None required	34

(in solution) is placed in the centre hole followed dropwise by solvent, which spreads as before by capillary attraction carrying the components into concentric rings as in Fig. 10. With coloured substances a circular trough may be cut in the lower disc, and elution continued until each ring is washed to the edge, collected, and drained off for subsequent recovery. The circular method has the following advantages over the others:

(1) The apparatus is even simpler, no airtight container being needed. (2) The run out is very rapid (32 cm in 4–5 h). (3) Separations are usually sharper, probably as a result of progressive dilution as the components spread out. (4) The effectiveness of various possible developers on colourless systems can be tried by cutting sectors from the paper. (5) Much larger quantities, up to 100 mg of mixture can be handled.

Typical separations on paper

The use of paper chromatography is so widespread that it is difficult to choose specific examples. Table 3 lists classes of compound to which the method has been applied, with the appropriate solvents and detecting agents. The data is largely taken from Balston and Talbot[24] where much more detailed descriptions with many examples will be found.

Paper chromatography as a means of identification (${R_F}$ values)

The use of paper chromatography in identification of unknowns depends on the high reproducibility of modern papers. Provided that the same paper, solvent, and conditions are used, the rate of movement of the spot corresponding to a pure substance is constant. If then a mixture is separated alongside spots of the likely components, identification by direct comparison is possible. Moreover the principle can be applied in the absence of reference compounds, since much data on rates is available in the literature. This is usually given in the form of R_F values, R_F being the ratio of distance moved by the spot to distance moved by the solvent front. In Fig. 11, for substance C, $R_F = b/a$. One of the objects of the recently introduced *Journal of Chromatography* is to collect together R_F values. "*Chromatography*" by Lederer and Lederer[9] also contains many R_F values. The disadvantage of R_F values is that, unlike for example melting points or infra-red spectra, they are significant only in conjunction with a particular solvent, paper and temperature.

References p. 34

The above method inevitably fails frequently because of lack of reference data. Identification then usually depends on isolation of the separated materials from the paper, for examination by

Fig. 11. Determination of the R_F value of C.

another method. The quantities normally used (as little as 50 μg of each component) are often insufficient for this. This difficulty may be overcome by using the circular method, with two or three layers of a fairly thick paper. Five or ten milligram quantities may thus be handled. Care must be exercised in removing separated materials from filter paper, since even special grades of paper yield, when extracted with certain solvents, sufficient impurity to affect the physical properties of the extract. A method of concentrating the product in preparation scale paper chromatography has been described[35] in which, by selective evaporation, a relatively large concentration of separated components build up on the paper.

The direct measurement of infra-red spectra of samples while still on the paper has been described by Bellamy[36]. Only very thin paper can be used because of the strong infra-red absorption of cellulose. This limits the quantities which can be handled.

Quantitative analysis

Micro-analytical techniques have been evolved which make possible quantitative analysis of microgram quantities by paper chromatography. Two principles are used. It has been found empirically that the area of a spot is roughly proportional to the quantity of the substance giving rise to it. By suitable comparison of the chromatogram of a mixture with those of its pure components, rough quantitative analyses can be performed.

More satisfactory results are usually obtained by comparison of the colour intensity of the spots of separated component and pure substances, after treatment where necessary with the appropriate reagent. This is best done with a photoelectric colorimeter after light scattering by the paper has been minimised by immersing it in a medium whose refractive index is similar to that of paper.

3. Cellulose powder column chromatography

This branch is the logical extension of paper chromatography, if larger quantities must be handled. As in adsorption column work care must be taken to avoid trapped air in packing the column, which will cause channelling. An improvement may be effected by treating the glass of the column with a silicone preparation to render it water repellent. The column should be well washed with solvent before the separation is begun, and the operation of the column is very similar to that of column adsorption work.

4. Paper electrophoresis

Paper chromatography has the disadvantage, particularly when applied to substances of high molecular weight such as proteins or peptides, that separations may be unduly slow, with resulting enlargement of the spots by general diffusion. One method of overcoming this is by mounting the strips in a centrifuge, thus adding a radial force to the normal flow under gravity. A more commonly used alternative is paper electrophoresis. Although not strictly a branch of chromatography, the technique will be described briefly at this point, since its applicability is very similar to that of paper chromatography.

In the simplest form a solution of the materials to be separated is placed on a paper moistened with suitable buffer solution, the ends of which dip into electrode vessels. The paper acts merely as a porous supporting material which prevents remixing by

Fig. 12. Apparatus for paper electrophoresis.

diffusion of the components, which separate by virtue of moving at different speeds in the applied electric field. Clearly the method applies only to such substances as acids, bases, amino acids and proteins which carry charge in a buffer of suitable pH. Provided fairly low voltages (5–10 V/cm) are used, very simple apparatus will suffice. However, with low voltages separation times remain long, and the separations are not very sharp owing to diffusion.

It is therefore much better to work with higher voltages, 50 V/cm and upwards. This, however, introduces a serious experimental difficulty, since the heat generated in the strip increases with the square of the voltage, with resultant risks of evaporating the solvent. The difficulty is best overcome by enclosing the strip between two glass plates, one of which is cooled. The usual experimental arrangement is shown in Fig. 12. The strip should be just moist enough to conduct, so as to avoid diffusion. Cellophane membranes prevent its becoming too moist through adsorption from the buffer vessels, which are connected by bridges to reversible electrodes. Good accounts of the experimental arrangements are given by Michl[37], and by Grassmann[38]. After the experiment, the separated zones must be rendered visible by drying the paper, and spraying as in chromatography. Fig. 13 shows the nature of the final paper. If the paper is mounted in oil so as to make it transparent, the intensities of the zone colours can be used to estimate quantitatively the amounts of the corresponding components.

Fig. 13. Amino acid separation by paper electrophoresis (after treatment to render the strips visible).

Careful choice of buffer is required for the best results. In general the pH of the buffer should be roughly in the middle of the pK range of the substances to be separated. Anomalous results are, however, sometimes found as a result of adsorption on to the paper. In some cases[38] it proves advantageous to replace conventional aqueous buffers by such mixtures as pyridine-acetic acid, ammonia–formic acid, and trimethylamine–formic acid. These organic solvents extend the applicability of the method to water-insoluble substances, but have the disadvantage of lower conductivity than aqueous media.

Fig. 14. Continuous paper electrophoresis.

Paper electrophoresis has been applied widely for separations of amino acids, peptides, proteins, carbohydrates (as their boric acid complexes), purines, biological acids, alkaloids, and inorganic ions. Valuable medical diagnostic techniques have also been devised.

A particularly valuable development is paper electrophoresis on a continuous basis[38], which may be used for quite large scale separations. Fig. 14 illustrates the principle. A sheet of paper is clamped vertically between two strips which serve as electrodes. The mixture flows continuously on to the paper at P, and each component then moves under the joint influence of gravity and the electric field, at an angle α given by

$$\tan \alpha = \frac{\text{electrophoretic rate}}{\text{flow rate}}$$

On reaching the bottom of the paper, the components have fanned out and are collected separately.

Electrophoresis and paper chromatography can sometimes be profitably combined. For example, a protein hydrolysate was separated by continuous paper electrophoresis into glutamic acid, aspartic acid, cysteic acid, a group of neutral amino acids, and a group of basic amino acids. Each of the groups was then resolved by normal paper chromatography.

5. Gas–liquid partition chromatography

This is discussed separately in Chapter 3.

E. ION-EXCHANGE CHROMATOGRAPHY

The ion-exchanging ability of minerals such as the zeolites has long been realised. An important method of softening hard water depends on the ability of these materials to exchange sodium ions for the magnesium and calcium ions of water which flows through them. The application of such materials to analytical chemistry had, however, to await the discovery during the thirties of organic resins which exchange groups of a specific kind. For example, cross-linked sulphonated polystyrene provides in effect a porous network studded with sulphonic acid groups, where hydrogen ions may be exchanged for those of inorganic or organic cations.

Ion-exchange chromatography found its first major application in the separation and isolation of certain rare earth metals and their salts, the physical and chemical properties of which are so similar, that their separation has long been one of the most difficult tasks of analytical chemistry[39]. In this experiment a column of strongly acid resin was first treated with hydrochloric acid to ensure that all the exchange points were initially occupied by hydrogen ions. The mixed rare earths were then applied in the form of their chlorides, whereupon the cations displaced hydrogen ions, forming a compact band at the top of the column. Elution by water being unduly slow, development of the chromatogram depended on the formation by the cations of complexes of differing stabilities with citric acid. When the column was eluted with citric acid solution, the cations moved down the column at rates depending on the stability of the corresponding complex, and were identified as they emerged, by following the absorption spectrum of the liquid.

More recently several organic resins have become available, whose exchange centres vary from strongly acid, as in sulphonated polystyrene, through weakly acid as in cross-linked polymethacrylic acid, to strongly basic, as in polystyrene incorporating quaternary ammonium groups. This has opened up the possibility of separating organic mixtures of amino acids, purine and pyrimidine bases, nucleotides, alkaloids and even proteins. The choice of resin is governed by the acid and base strengths of the mixture, but generally the strongly acidic and basic resins are most effective.

In some cases ion-exchange methods have marked advantages over the adsorption and partition techniques. The capacity of these resins is quite large, so that 0.1 g or more can readily be handled. Also recovery from the column is virtually complete, which is, of course very important in quantitative work.

Experimental technique

Since as in the inorganic case cited above, elution of organic mixtures from an ion-exchange column is usually too slow, displacement is used. In order to increase the sharpness of separation, two or three columns of decreasing diameter may be used in conjunction. The separation commences in the largest of these columns. By the time the front of a solute band has reached the bottom of this, its initial planeness will have been partly destroyed. However, if the effluent is now led to a second narrower column, a small part from the centre of the curved front is in effect selected, so much of the planeness is restored. The process may be repeated with a third column, which again acts as a "front straightener". Linstead *et al.*[40] show a simple arrangement of three columns, giving very sharp separations.

Fig. 15. Amino acid separation on an ion-exchange column, with automatic recording of the effluent composition[12].

In carrying out a typical amino acid separation the columns are first filled with sulphonated polystyrene, which has been slurried with $2N$ hydrochloric acid, to ensure that all the active centres are in the acid form. The assembly is next washed free from excess HCl by distilled water. An aqueous solution of the amino acid mixture, which may contain as much as 0.1 g of each component is then placed in the top column, where insoluble salts with the sulphonic acid groups are formed

$$RSO_3H + B \rightarrow RSO_3^- \cdot BH^+$$

Dilute caustic soda solution now flows through the column, where, being a strong base it displaces the amino acids from their salts,

$$RSO_3^-BH^+ + OH^- \rightarrow B + H_2O + RSO_3^-$$

with a facility depending on the base strengths of the components. Accordingly they are carried to the bottom at differing speeds, where fractions are collected, and their contents identified by paper chromatography or otherwise. Fig. 15 illustrates an amino acid separation by this method[12], with automatic recording.

REFERENCES

1 A. Tiselius, *Advances in Colloid Science*, Vol. III, Academic Press, New York, 1947, p. 67.
2 R. C. Brimley and F. C. Barrett, *Practical Chromatography*, Chapman and Hall, London, 1954, p. 52.
3 T. I. Williams, *The Elements of Chromatography*, Blackie and Son, London, 1954, Chapter II.
4 A. Stewart, *Discussions Faraday Soc.*, 7 (1949) 65.
5 H. Brackmann, *Discussions Faraday Soc.*, 7 (1949) 58.
6 S. Claesson, *Arkiv Kemi, Mineral., Geol.*, 23A, No. 1, 1946.
7 C. R. N. Strouts, J. H. Gilfillan and H. N. Wilson, *Analytical Chemistry*, Vol. II, Clarendon Press, Oxford, 1955, p. 731.
8 H. H. Strain, *Chromatographic Adsorption Analysis*, Interscience, New York, 1945.
9 E. Lederer and M. Lederer, *Chromatography*, Elsevier, Amsterdam, 1957.
10 J. R. Price and R. Robinson, *J. Chem. Soc.*, (1937) 449.
11 A. Winterstein and G. Stein, *Z. Physiol. Chem.*, 220 (1933) 263.
12 D. H. Spackman, W. H. Stein and S. Moore, *Anal. Chem.*, 30 (1958) 1190.
13 F. D. Hartley, *J. Polymer Sci.*, 34 (1959) 397.
14 C. Phillips, *Gas Chromatography*, Butterworths, London, 1956.
15 N. H. Ray, *J. Appl. Chem.*, 4 (1954) 82.
16 H. W. Patton, J. S. Lewis and W. I. Kaye, *Anal. Chem.*, 27 (1955) 170.
17 C. S. G. Phillips, *Discussions Faraday Soc.*, 7 (1959) 241.
18 D. G. Timms, H. J. Konrath and R. C. Chirnside, *Analyst*, 83 (1958) 600.
19 A. J. P. Martin and R. M. L. Synge, *Biochem. J.*, 35 (1941) 1358.
20 L. L. Ramsey and W. I. Patterson, *J. Assoc. Offic. Agr. Chem.*, 29 (1946) 337.
21 A. A. Levi, *Discussions Faraday Soc.*, 7 (1949) 124.
22 F. Cramer, *Paper Chromatography*, Macmillan, London, 1959.
23 S. P. Datta, C. E. Dent and H. Harris, *Biochem. J.*, 46 (1950) xlii.
24 J. N. Balston and B. E. Talbot, *A Guide to Filter Paper and Cellulose Powder Chromatography*, Reeve Angel, London, 1952.
25 C. E. Dent, *Biochem. J.*, 43 (1948) 169.

[26] R. Consden, A. H. Gordon and A. J. P. Martin, *Biochem. J.*, 38 (1944) 224.

[27] S. M. Partridge, *Nature*, 158 (1946) 270.

[28] F. Brown and L. P. Hall, *Nature*, 166 (1950) 66.

[29] R. G. Rice, G. J. Keller and J. G. Kirchner, *Anal. Chem.*, 23 (1951) 194.

[30] E. C. Bate-Smith, *Nature*, 161 (1948) 835.

[31] R. E. H. Nicholas and C. Rimington, *Biochem. J.*, 48 (1951) 306.

[32] P. Edman, *Acta. Chem. Scand.*, 2 (1948) 592.

[33] R. R. Goodall and A. A. Levi, *Nature*, 158 (1946) 675.

[34] H. Midgelow, *Hexagon Digest (I.C.I. Ltd., Dyestuffs' Div.), No. 3* (1948).

[35] E. Kawerau, *Biochem. J.*, 48 (1951) 281.

[36] L. J. Bellamy, *J. Appl. Chem.*, 3 (1953) 421.

[37] H. Michl, *Chromatographic Reviews*, Vol. I, Elsevier, Amsterdam, 1959, p. 11.

[38] W. Grassmann in *Paper Electrophoresis*, Churchill, London, 1956.

[39] F. H. Spedding, *Discussions Faraday Soc.*, 7 (1949) 214.

[40] R. P. Linstead, J. A. Elvidge and M. Whalley, *Techniques of Organic Chemistry*, Butterworths, London, 1955, p. 23.

[41] A. J. P. Martin, *Endeavour*, 6 (1947) 21.

SELECTED BIBLIOGRAPHY TO CHAPTER 2

Balston, J. N. and B. E. Talbot, *A Guide to Filter Paper and Cellulose Powder Chromatography*, Reeve Angel, London, 1952, 145 pp. Many separations of mixtures of members of various classes of organic compounds are described.

Brimley, R. C. and F. C. Barrett, *Practical Chromatography*, Chapman and Hall, London, 1953, 128 pp. The theory and practice of adsorption, partition and ion-exchange methods are clearly discussed.

Cassidy, H. G., *Fundamentals of Chromatography*, Interscience, New York, 1957, 465 pp. This work deals mainly with the underlying theory of chromatographic separations.

Cramer, F., *Paper Chromatography*, Macmillan, London, 1959, 124 pp. This book includes very clear descriptions of experimental techniques, and lists many applications to organic chemistry. Paper electrophoresis is also dealt with.

Journal of Chromatography, Elsevier, Amsterdam. The journal consists of review articles and original papers on chromatographic subjects, and assembles published R_F values.

Lederer, E. and M. Lederer, *Chromatography*, Elsevier, Amsterdam, 1957, 712 pp. The treatment of both practical methods and applications is comprehensive, with numerous literature references, and R_F values.

Lederer, M., *Introduction to Paper Electrophoresis and Related Methods*, Elsevier, Amsterdam, 1957, 214 pp.

STRAIN, H. H., *Chromatographic Adsorption Analysis*, Interscience, New York, 1945, 222 pp.

WILLIAMS, T. I., *The Elements of Chromatography*, Blackie and Son, London, 1954, 90 pp. This book is perhaps the best available introduction to chromatography.

WUNDERLY, CH., *Principles and Applications of Paper Electrophoresis*, Elsevier, Amsterdam, 1961, 223 pp. An up-to-date treatment of principles and results is given, including many references.

CHAPTER 3

GAS–LIQUID CHROMATOGRAPHY

In accordance with the recommendation of the Hydrocarbon Research Group of the Institute of Petroleum, gas–liquid partition chromatography will be referred to as "gas–liquid" chromatography. Since the discovery of gas–liquid chromatography in 1952, the growth of its applications in the separation of mixtures, and qualitative and quantitative analysis has been phenomenally rapid. Consequently the technique is now an essential in any well equipped organic or analytical laboratory. The applications of gas–liquid chromatography are broadly of four kinds.

(1) Separation of mixtures and identification of the components from their behaviour on the column. Accurate control of the column conditions are required for such applications.

(2) Separation with a view to identification of the components by another method. A much less refined column technique may be used for this.

(3) Quantitative analysis of mixtures. Again accurate column control is required.

(4) The use of gas–liquid chromatography on a preparative scale (up to 10 g or more) as an alternative to purification by distillation.

A. EXPERIMENTAL METHODS

Before these applications are discussed a brief description will be given of the experimental methods involved.

Fig. 16 shows a block diagram of a typical set-up. The components will be briefly described in turn.

1. Carrier gas

As will be seen later, the choice of carrier gas is governed to some extent by the detector used. The first detector to come into universal use, the katherometer, depends on conduction of heat from a hot wire by the effluent gas. The relative merits of gases

Fig. 16. Arrangement of apparatus for gas–liquid chromatography.

of low thermal conductivity such as carbon dioxide or nitrogen, against those of high conductivity, such as helium and hydrogen have been argued at length[1], with the general conclusion that the latter type give greater sensitivity. Against this, however, hydrogen introduces an explosion hazard and helium is not readily obtainable in all countries. Accordingly cylinder nitrogen is perhaps the most commonly used carrier gas, and is usually quite satisfactory.

2. Control valve and flowmeter

Accurate control of the pressure and flow rate is essential for applications of types (1) and (3). For (2) and (4) ordinary cylinder control valves and a simple flowmeter are adequate.

3. Sample introduction system

Normally 10–50 mg of sample is injected in liquid form, or in solution from a hypodermic needle, pushed through a serum bottle cap. If the highest resolution is sought, a small heater in the vicinity helps to ensure immediate vaporisation of the sample. Even in quantitative analysis the necessity to measure accurately the small quantity of sample injected is usually avoided by the "normalisation" method described below.

4. Columns

The column may be straight, U-shaped, W-shaped or coiled if compactness is essential, though it is more difficult to pack a coiled column uniformly. It may vary in diameter from a few thousandths of an inch (capillary columns see p. 54), if the highest possible resolution is sought on a micro scale, up to 3 inches for large scale preparative work. For most purposes a convenient size is about 4 feet in length by 0.5–1 cm in diameter.

By far the most commonly used fixed solid is kieselguhr, which is sold commercially in a suitable form as "Celite". Firebrick has also been used, and it has recently been claimed that a purified form of the detergent "Tide" has advantages in certain cases[2,40]. The choice of a fixed liquid presents more difficulty, since its polarity markedly affects the relative rates at which different classes of compound pass through. Thus a separation which is difficult, or impossible, with one partitioning liquid may be easy with a more suitable one. Several liquids should therefore be tried before any separation is abandoned as impossible. Volatility is the other factor governing choice of liquid, since one which is too volatile may contaminate the detector, or, in cases where for example infra-red analysis of the products is envisaged, may swamp the analytical device.

Table 4 lists some liquids commonly used for separations in the boiling ranges and chemical fields indicated.

TABLE 4

FIXED LIQUIDS IN GAS–LIQUID CHROMATOGRAPHY

Liquid	Boiling range (°C)	Type of compound
Dinonylphthalate	20–100	Hydrocarbons, esters, ketones, halogenated hydrocarbons
Benzyldiphenyl	80–150	Aromatic compounds, fatty acids, halogen compounds, hydrocarbons
Dimethylformamide	—20–+20	Light hydrocarbons
Silicone oil	High temperatures	General purposes
Diglycerol	20–150	Oxygenated compounds, aliphatic amines
Squalene	20–150	Hydrocarbons (e.g. branched chain and cyclic alkanes)
Triethanolamine	Approx. 20–60	Amines, pyridine bases
Tritolylphosphate	20–170	Alcohols, aromatic hydrocarbons, halogenated hydrocarbons

To obtain the best separations, the column should be held at as low a temperature as is consistent with reasonably rapid elution of the sample. In practice this normally means that the column temperature will be about 50°C below the mean boiling point of the sample.

Early workers used jackets of vapour in equilibrium with a boiling liquid, but thermostatically controlled wound heaters or air thermostats are now normally used. Control to about 0.1°C is advisable for application of types (1) and (3), but problems (2) and (4) allow much more latitude. The special problems associated with work at high temperatures, to handle relatively involatile substances, have been discussed by several workers[3,5a].

5. Detectors

The method of detection originally used by James and Martin[24] involved automatically titrating separated mixtures of acids or bases. This is of rather limited applicability, and was superseded by the katherometer, which consists of an electrically heated wire which forms one arm of a Wheatstone bridge. When pure carrier gas flows over the wire it assumes a steady temperature and resistance. However, as the separated components reach the wire its temperature increases as a result of the decreased thermal conductivity of its surroundings, and the resulting change in its resistance is measured. This change is proportional to the concentration of component. To eliminate zero drift two hot wires are commonly used, over one of which flows the carrier gas before reaching the column. Because of the danger of vapour condensation in the detector, it should be maintained at about the same temperature as the column. An improved version of this detector has been developed by the Perkin-Elmer Corporation in their vapour fractometer (Fig. 17a). The hot wires are replaced by thermistors which not only eliminates danger of decomposition on the hot wire, but also increases sensitivity.

Fig. 17. Detectors: (a) Thermal conductivity detector (Perkin-Elmer); (b) Flame ionisation detector.

In the quest for even more sensitive detectors, particularly for use with involatile substances and micro quantities, various other devices have been developed. A fundamentally different principle was developed by Scott[6]. Using hydrogen as carrier gas, he burnt the effluent in a small flame just above which was suspended a thermocouple. When an organic compound emerges from the column, the flame temperature increases somewhat, causing a change in the thermocouple signal, proportional to the vapour concentration. The device is very simple to construct, gives a linear relation between concentration and signal, and is very sensitive. Even greater sensitivity is obtained by a development due to McWilliam and Dewar[9]. Again a hydrogen flame is used, in which is placed an electrode at a potential about 200 V above that of the jet, which serves as the other electrode (Fig. 17b). Under these conditions an ionisation current flows, the magnitude of which is extremely sensitive to organic compounds in the gas stream. Whereas in the absence of organic vapours the resistance is about 10^{12} ohms, this value may fall to 10^6 ohms when organic material is being eluted. Because of its great sensitivity, simplicity and stability, this device is likely to be widely used. It has the advantage that its large output reduces subsequent recording problems; if necessary it can be coupled directly to a recording galvanometer, eliminating the normal costly amplifier and recorder. Destruction of the effluent components, if it is desired to collect and identify them, may be avoided with this type of detector, by by-passing a fraction only of the gas-stream to be burnt. The only difficulty associated with this and other ultra-sensitive detectors is the frequent necessity to dilute the sample with a material such as CS_2, to which the device is insensitive, so as to avoid signals too large to be accurately measurable.

Finally mention must be made of another ultra-sensitive device, the argon detector, which was invented by Lovelock[10], and is used commercially in the Pye Argon Chromatograph. The carrier gas (argon) flows through an ionisation chamber, with a radioactive source. Electrons are ejected which are accelerated by an electric field, and by collisions produce large numbers of metastable argon atoms. When an organic vapour reaches the detector its molecules collide with these atoms, producing many more electrons, and causing the ionisation current to increase. The device is sensitive enough to detect 10^{-13} mol of most organic compounds, but has the disadvantage of being insensitive to halogens and other materials of high ionisation potential.

6. Recorders

All the above detectors are normally coupled to a pen recorder, so that a record of time against concentration of organic vapour in the carrier gas is obtained (Fig. 18). This usually starts with

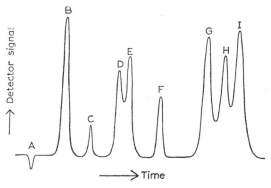

Fig. 18. Typical gas–liquid chromatogram.

a false peak, A, due to air injected with the sample reaching the detector. There follow several peaks, some, such as B, C and F being single and symmetrical, and corresponding to perfectly separated components. There may also be groups such as DE and GHJ, indicating components which are only partially separated under the conditions used. With a satisfactory detector the peak height gives a fair measure of the amount of component.

However, some peak distortion may occur, so in quantitative work it is better to use the areas under the peaks.

7. Fraction collectors

If the separated components are to be collected for subsequent identification or chemical experiments, provision must be made for their efficient condensation from the gas stream. Basically fraction collectors consist of U-tubes immersed in ice, acetone-Drikold, or liquid nitrogen*, according to the volatility involved. In practice the last mentioned coolant is usually by far the most effective, but traps must be carefully designed to ensure that a large cold surface is presented to the gas. This may be done by packing the tube with glass beads, or a spiral of metal foil. Fog-formation rather than liquefaction must be guarded against. With well-designed traps 85–95% recovery of components from the carrier gas is possible.

B. APPLICATIONS OF GAS–LIQUID CHROMATOGRAPHY

The technique has been applied to the separation of a very wide variety of mixtures and is in fact applicable in any case where the components are appreciably volatile, and stable, at temperatures not exceeding about 250°C. Fig. 19 shows a few typical separations. In the majority of cases clean separations of multicomponent mixtures of structurally similar compounds are possible. The applications will now be considered under the four headings suggested on p. 37.

1. Use of gas–liquid chromatography to identify components of mixtures solely by their behaviour on the column

This application depends on reproducing column conditions accurately enough for precise values to be measured of the rates at which compounds move along it. In paper chromatography the quantity R_F, the ratio of the distance moved by a spot over the simultaneous distance moved by the solvent front, serves as

---

* Condensation of liquid oxygen in the trap is a possible hazard in this case.

a means of identification. Although the corresponding quantity in gas chromatography, that is, the relative movements of component and carrier gas, is inconveniently small, a related

Fig. 19. Typical separations: (a) aliphatic hydrocarbons[36]; (b) anilines[19]; (c) pyridines[37]; (d) aromatic hydrocarbons[38]; (e) esters[39].

References p. 56

quantity can be used. Suppose that while passing through the column, a component R distributes itself between carrier gas and fixed liquid so that there are f molecules in the liquid for each one in the gas. Then if a carrier gas molecule takes time t_0 to flow through the column, a molecule of R will take

$$t_R = t_0(1 + f)$$

Since f depends only on the solubility of R in the fixed liquid at the column temperature, then for a given liquid and temperature, t_R is a constant, known as the retention time of R. More often a related quantity *the retention volume* given by

$$V_R = t_R \times \text{rate of flow of carrier gas, at the exit pressure}$$

is used. V_R provides, like R_F, a convenient means of recording the behaviour of a compound on a column. In accurate work V_R should be corrected for the inevitable pressure difference between the ends of the column. The formulae

$$\frac{V_R}{V_R(\text{corrected})} = \frac{2}{3} \frac{(p_1/p_0)^3 - 1}{(p_1/p_0)^2 - 1}$$

may be applied, where p_1 and p_0 are the pressures at the inlet and outlet. It must be stressed that the usefulness of V_R is limited, in that it applies only to a particular column material at a given temperature. V_R values are very sensitive to temperature, a temperature change of 1°C frequently causing a 5% change in V_R. For this reason it is now usual to deal with retention volumes measured relative to some given pure substance. This substance is then added to a mixture in which it is desired to study unknowns, and their retention volumes are measured relative to it. This eliminates the need for accurate control of column temperature and flow rate.

The procedure for identifying an unknown may now be outlined. Suppose in the first case that one has, from chemical evidence, a fair idea of what its structure may be. The problem then is to find which member of its class has the same retention volume as the unknown, within the experimental error. If samples of likely compounds are available, it is best to put these through the same column and perform the identification directly. In the absence of such samples, recorded values of V_R must be sought. Unfortunately these are scattered through the literature and books on gas chromatography, but an attempt is being made by the Journal of Chromatography to collect together V_R values. Compounds which have been studied include hydrocarbons[8,11,12,14], halogenated compounds[5b], amines [15,18], anilines[19], pyridines[13], acids[16,17], esters[17], phenols[20,21], and others[22,23].

If the homologous class of the unknown is known, its identification may be possible even if its V_R value cannot be matched. This depends on the simple relationship usually found between V_R and number of carbon atoms, in such a series. Fig. 20

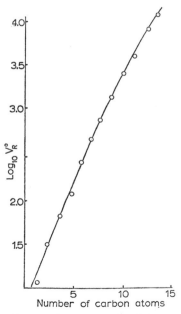

Fig. 20. Retention volume and number of carbon atoms in fatty acids[25].

References p. 56

illustrates the case of fatty acids[24], where a higher member could be identified by extrapolation.

An even more difficult problem, which arises if even the chemical class of the component is unknown, is considered in some detail in Ref.[26]. The best approach is to study the unknown on two columns, of materials with different polarities. Fig. 21 shows how, for example, the study of an unknown amine on columns of Lubrol MO and liquid paraffin would yield a point, which should fall on one or other of the three lines corresponding to primary, secondary and tertiary amines[25]. Its type might thus be found, and the identification possibly completed by the methods of the last paragraph. The striking

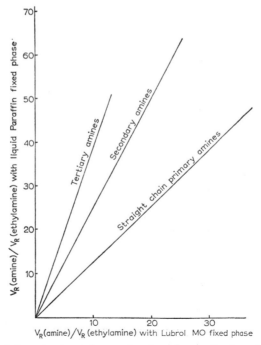

Fig. 21. Relative retention volumes of various classes of amine with paraffin and Lubrol MO, as fixed liquids[25].

difference of behaviour of tertiary amines from the others in Fig. 21 arises because, whereas the three types have roughly equal affinities for paraffin, primary and secondary amines have much the stronger affinity for Lubrol MO (a polyether), since they can form hydrogen bonds.

2. Identification of components by use of gas–liquid chromatography in conjunction with another physical method

From what has been said above, identification by gas–liquid chromatography is clearly limited, basically because only a single datum is measured, so the use of columns for separation, followed by identification by another method must be considered.

The first possibility is to collect each component as it emerges in a cooled trap (see p. 44). The difficulty here is that, since gas chromatography is usually operated with milligram or even microgram quantities, the fractions so obtained are very small. This often precludes identification chemically, and by many physical methods, but it is possible to use mass and infra-red spectroscopy for the purpose. The main objection to the mass spectrometer method is the time consumed, since each fraction must be introduced, measured, and pumped out again before the next can be examined. Identification of all the components of a complex mixture might then take several days. Beynon et al.[27] have described the collection of the separated components by direct condensation of the vapour into the sample system of a mass spectrometer.

Following the initial condensation of a component, there are two possible methods of obtaining its infra-red spectrum[41]. If volatile, the material may be re-evaporated into a suitable gas cell, and measured in this state. If it is high boiling the vapour pressure will be insufficient to yield a good gas spectrum, and it is preferable to redistil into a capillary tube, from which transfer to an infra-red micro cell is possible. Although these methods can be applied to well under a milligram of sample, grave difficulties are presented by components present only in impurity amounts.

References p. 56

Another possibility is to lead the effluent gas directly through an instrument which performs the identification, without the intermediate fraction collecting and transfer. In the mass spectroscopy case this has been achieved by Gohlke[28]. This method depends on the use of a special type of mass spectrometer known as "time of flight", (see p. 314) in which the mass spectrum can be scanned several times per second and displayed on a cathode-ray oscillograph screen. Ideally it is necessary only to watch the screen as the elution proceeds, photograph it as the pattern changes, and subsequently identify the components from their mass spectra. This combination is clearly a most powerful tool for identification of volatile mixtures, but has the disadvantage that the sensitivity is limited by the fact that a large amount of carrier gas dilutes the sample.

Similar arrangements using infra-red spectra have been reported[29]. If the effluent were passed through a normal infra-red gas cell, the bands would be too weak because of the small vapour concentration. However, this can be overcome by a multiple reflection cell, giving a very large effective cell length. Unfortunately these cells require a fairly large volume of gas. The use of such a cell in conjunction with an infra-red spectrometer, adapted so that the spectrum is displayed continuously on an oscillograph, is an attractive possibility, which appears not yet to have been realised in practice.

3. Quantitative analysis

Gas–liquid chromatography provides a convenient and, in suitable cases, highly accurate method for quantitative analysis of small quantities, provided all the components are known. This application uses the strength of the bands. As previously mentioned this is given by their peak height, or, if high accuracy is required, by the area under the peak, which in turn is given fairly closely by the product of the height times the width at half height. With the commonly used detectors the strength of a peak is proportional to the quantity of the corresponding component. Thus it is possible in principle to perform analyses by direct comparison of the strengths observed in a mixture, with those obtained when known amounts of each component are passed separately through the column. In practice there are two difficulties. Firstly such a procedure involves accurate measurement of the very small quantities used (about 1 milligram). Secondly very accurate reproduction of the column conditions between measuring the samples and the pure components is required. Of two methods used to overcome these difficulties, the most accurate involves use of an internal standard. Known mixtures are first made up of each component with the standard, which should be of similar volatility. For example, in analysing mixtures of benzene, toluene and higher homologues Bradford et al.[30] used acetone. A calibration is then set up, in which percentage of component is plotted against the relative height (or area) of its peak over that of the standard (Fig. 22). When unknown mixtures are then analysed, the proportions of each component can be read directly from the calibration chart.

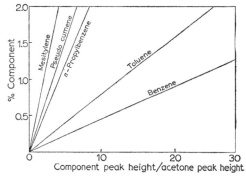

Fig. 22. Calibration chart for quantitative analysis[30].

A second method depends on a special property of certain detectors, such as the katherometer with helium or hydrogen as carrier gas. In this case the strength of a peak is independent of the substance causing it, depending only on the concentration. A normalisation method may then be used. The band heights (or areas) of all the peaks are added up and the proportion, x, of component A may be obtained from the equation

$$x = \frac{\text{Height (or area) of peak A}}{\text{Total height (or area) of all peaks}}$$

Phillips[26] quotes figures which illustrate the accuracy obtainable.

4. *Preparative scale gas chromatography*

The applications described hitherto are usually performed with an analytical scale column, of diameter about 5 mm and length not greater than 6 feet, capable of handling quantities up to about 50 milligrams. One often wishes to isolate the components in quantities of a gram or more, to perform further physical or chemical experiments on them. In this event, preparative scale gas–liquid chromatography may have distinct advantages over fractional distillation. It is fundamentally a more efficient separation process. Whereas the best fractionating columns attain efficiencies only of a few hundred theoretical plates, both analytical and preparation scale columns may give the effect of many thousands of plates. Also azeotrope formation, which presents insoluble problems in distillation, has no counterpart in chromatography. Whereas only one set of conditions is possible in distillation, a variety of stationary liquids may be tried, to obtain the best chromatographic separation. Distillation also suffers from the disadvantage that the whole column must be filled with the vapour–liquid mixture. This means in practice that at least one hundred cm^3 is usually required for an efficient separation.

There is no fundamental difficulty about scaling up separations. Roughly speaking, the amount of sample which can be handled with a given efficiency, increases as the cross sectional area of the column and is proportional to the square root of its length. Thus, for example, a four-fold increase of length and a ten-fold increase of diameter would permit the use of two hundred times as much sample. In practice this ratio may be greatly exceeded in the case of easy separations, where the column is deliberately overloaded and some loss of resolution can be tolerated. For example, Tatlow and Evans[31], using a column 16 feet long and 30 mm in diameter find that whereas only 0.5 g of a mixture of chemically similar components boiling 1°C apart can be handled, as much as 10 g of a more easily separable mixture can be treated. Kirkland[4], using a column of similar dimensions, separates between 2 and 15 gram quantities, according to the difficulty involved.

Particular attention must be paid to certain experimental points in scaling up. Steps must be taken, by use of a preheater, to ensure very rapid volatilisation of the sample, so that it all enters the column at once. A motor driven plunger to speed the process is described in Ref.[4]. Effective collection of the issuing components is also essential. Especial care must also be taken with large columns that contamination does not arise from volatility or decomposition of the stationary liquid.

Examples of purifications by preparative gas chromatography include *n*-butanol, where trouble is caused in distillation by azeotrope formation with water and organic impurities. *p*-Methoxy acetophenone, which normally contains three close boiling impurities which are difficult to eliminate by distillation or recrystallisation, has been purified by gas–liquid chromatography.

The method has been widely used by Tatlow and others[7,31] in fluorine chemistry. For example, the fluorination of benzene with cobaltic fluoride gives a mixture of polyfluoro cyclohexanes, which cannot be separated by distillation. Analytical gas chromatography showed five components, only two of which could be identified from their retention times. Using the experience gained with the analytical column, larger quantities were chromatographed and sufficient of the unknowns isolated to react them with aqueous alkali. Finally the products of the hydrolyses were identified chromatographically, and from this

References p. 56

the structures of the products were shown to be:

and

Another approach to large scale separation has been pioneered by Atkinson and Tuey[32]. Instead of attempting to separate a single very large amount of mixture, they arranged their apparatus so that at twenty-seven minute intervals a cycle of automatic operations began, from introduction of the sample to final collection of the separated components. By this means 50–100 cm^3 of an ethanol–toluene mixture could be separated in twenty-four hours.

C. RECENT ADVANCES IN GAS–LIQUID CHROMATOGRAPHY

Mention must be made of two recent improvements in the technique. The first concerns the use of capillary columns. Only columns of diameter about 0.5 cm and upwards were used, until it was recently suggested by Golay[33], that great improvements in resolution might result from using long (100–200 ft) capillary columns of internal diameter about 0.01 inches. The idea was developed in practice by Desty. Such a column cannot be packed normally, and in fact requires no supporting solid. A dilute solution of the stationary liquid in a volatile solvent is forced into the tube, and the solvent carefully pumped out, leaving a thin layer of liquid on the capillary walls.

The enormous resolution obtainable with such columns, is illustrated by the ease with which they resolve *meta*- and *para*-xylenes, an extremely difficult separation with conventional columns. Examples of their efficiency in the field of natural products are given by Lipsky *et al.*[34]. Various mixtures of fatty acids and esters were resolved chromatographically for the first time, including the separation of the cis-trans isomers methyl elaidate and methyl oleate.

A somewhat different way of using capillary columns has been suggested by Scott[35]. By sacrificing some efficiency they can be made to carry out separations in seconds, rather than minutes or hours with normal columns. With suitable detection and amplification it is possible to display an entire chromatogram on the screen of a long-persistence oscilloscope. Possible applications include the chromatography of reacting systems, and plant control, where immediate action is required following a variation in the composition of a gas stream.

Fig. 23. Three-stage separation of a mixture.

References p. 56

Capillary columns can, of course, handle only extremely small (microgram) quantities, and require very sensitive detectors such as the argon and hydrogen flame devices.

The other development concerns the use of multiple column apparatus. In a mixture of many components it may be impossible to separate them all with any one stationary liquid and temperature. Suppose that on passing a hypothetical mixture of twenty components through column A (Fig. 23a), only partial separation is achieved, many of the components passing too rapidly for resolution. The unresolved portion (1–12) is now fed to a second column, with a different stationary liquid, leading to some further separation (Fig. 23b), followed finally by a third column which completes the separation. This principle is applied in the Perkin-Elmer Corporation's Model 188 Vapour Fractometer.

REFERENCES

1 L. J. SCHMAUCH AND R. A. DINERSTEIN, *Nature*, 183 (1959) 673.
2 A. W. DECORA AND G. U. DINNEEN, *Anal. Chem.*, 32 (1960) 164.
3 V. T. COATES et al., (Eds.): *Gas Chromatography*, Academic Press, New York, 1958, pp. 131 and 155.
4 J. J. KIRKLAND, *Ibid.*, p. 203.
5 D. H. DESTY AND C. L. A. HARBOURN, (Eds.): *Vapour Phase Chromatography*, Butterworths, London, 1957. (a) pp. 222, 266 and 316; (b) pp. 117 and 336.
6 R. P. W. SCOTT, *Ibid.*, p. 131.
7 J. C. TATLOW AND D. E. M. EVANS, *Ibid.*, p. 256.
8 M. M. WIRTH, *Ibid.*, p. 162.
9 I. G. MCWILLIAM AND R. A. DEWAR, *Nature*, 181 (1958) 760.
10 J. E. LOVELOCK, *J. Chromatog.*, 1 (1958) 35.
11 L. J. SULLIVAN, J. R. LOTZ AND C. B. WILLINGHAM, *Anal. Chem.*, 28 (1956) 495.
12 V. T. BROOKS AND G. A. COLLINS, *Chem. & Ind. (London)*, (1956) 921.
13 V. T. BROOKS AND G. A. COLLINS, *Ibid*, p. 1021.
14 D. H. DESTY AND B. H. F. WHYMAN, *Anal. Chem.*, 29 (1957) 320.
15 A. T. JAMES AND A. J. P. MARTIN, *Biochem. J.*, 51 (1952) 323.
16 A. T. JAMES AND A. J. P. MARTIN, *Ibid.*, 50 (1952) 679.
17 A. T. JAMES AND A. J. P. MARTIN, *Ibid.*, 63 (1956) 144.
18 A. T. JAMES, *Biochem. J.*, 52 (1952) 242.
19 A. T. JAMES, *Anal. Chem.*, 28 (1956) 1564.
20 J. JANÁK AND R. KOMERS, *Z. anal. Chem.*, 164 (1958) 69.

[21] G. BERGMANN AND D. JENTZSCH, *Ibid.*, 164 (1958) 10.

[22] G. RAUFF, *Ibid.*, 164 (1958) 135.

[23] H. KIEBER, *Angew. Chem.*, 71 (1959) 218.

[24] A. T. JAMES AND A. J. P. MARTIN, *Biochem. J.*, 50 (1952) 238.

[25] A. T. JAMES AND A. J. P. MARTIN, *Analyst*, 77 (1952) 915.

[26] C. PHILLIPS, *Gas Chromatography*, Butterworths, London, 1956.

[27] J. H. BEYNON, R. A. SAUNDERS AND A. E. WILLIAMS, *J. Sci. Inst.*, 36 (1959) 375.

[28] R. S. GOHLKE, *Anal. Chem.*, 31 (1959) 539.

[29] J. U. WHITE, N. L. ALPERT, W. M. WARD AND W. S. GALLAWAY, *Anal. Chem.*, 31 (1959) 1267.

[30] B. W. BRADFORD, D. HARVEY AND D. E. CHALKLEY, *J. Inst. Petrol.*, 41 (1955) 80.

[31] D. E. M. EVANS, W. E. MASSINGHAM, M. STACEY AND J. C. TATLOW, *Nature*, 182 (1958) 591.

[32] A. P. ATKINSON AND G. A. P. TUEY, in *Gas Chromatography*, Ed. D. H. DESTY, Butterworths, London, 1958, p. 270.

[33] M. J. E. GOLAY, *Ibid.*, p. 36.

[34] S. R. LIPSKY, R. A. LANDSDOWNE AND J. E. LOVELOCK, *Anal. Chem.*, 31 (1959) 852.

[35] R. P. W. SCOTT, *Nature*, 185 (1960) 312.

[36] E. M. FREDERICKS AND F. R. BROOKS, *Anal. Chem.*, 28 (1956) 297.

[37] W. J. MURRAY AND A. F. WILLIAMS, *Chem. & Ind. London*, (1956) 1020.

[38] A. T. JAMES AND A. J. P. MARTIN, *J. Appl. Chem.*, 6 (1955) 114.

[39] M. L. VOSBECK, L. R. MATTICK, F. A. LEE AND C. S. PEDERSEN, *Nature*, 187 (1960) 689.

[40] E. M. BENS, *Anal. Chem.*, 33 (1961) 178.

[41] J. HASLAM, A. R. JEFFS AND H. A. WILLIS, *Analyst*, 86 (1961) 44.

SELECTED BIBLIOGRAPHY TO CHAPTER 3

BAYER, E., *Gas Chromatography*, Elsevier, Amsterdam, 1961, 240 pp. This book stresses practical applications of the subject, and includes large numbers of literature references and tables of retention volumes.

COATES, V. J., H. J. NOEBELS AND I. S. FAGERSON (Eds.), *Gas Chromatography*, Academic Press, New York, 1958, 323 pp. This volume consists of papers on all aspects of gas chromatography.

DESTY, D. H. (Ed.), *Gas Chromatography*, Butterworths, London, 1958, 383 pp.

DESTY, D. H., AND C. L. A. HARBOURN (Eds.), *Vapour Phase Chromatography*, Butterworths, London, 1957, 436 pp. This book, the previous one and that of R.P.W. Scott, report the proceedings of meetings of the Gas Chromatography Group of the Institute of Petroleum and provide up-to-date accounts of the theory, practice, and applications of gas chromatography.

Journal of Chromatography, Elsevier, Amsterdam. This journal contains review articles, original papers, and retention volume data.

KNAPMAN, C. E. H. (Ed.), *Gas Chromatography Abstracts 1958*, Butterworths, London, 1960, Vol. 1, 262 pp. This book and similar volumes to appear annually, provide a convenient coverage of the rapidly growing literature of this subject.

KEULEMANS, A. I. M., *Gas Chromatography*, Reinhold, New York, 1959, 234 pp. This book includes a thorough treatment of the theoretical side of the subject.

PESCOK, R. L., *Principles and Practice of Gas Chromatography*, Wiley, New York, 1959, 226 pp.

PHILLIPS, C. G. C., *Gas Chromatography*, Butterworths, London, 1956, 105 pp. This is an excellent concise, but comprehensive introduction to the subject.

SCOTT, R. P. W. (Ed.), *Gas Chromatography 1960*, Butterworths, London, 1960, 466 pp.

Chapter 4

ZONE REFINING

One of the most frequent problems in organic chemistry is the purification of a crude solid. This is traditionally performed by fractional crystallisation, by which satisfactory material can often be obtained. Indeed extremely difficult separations, such as that of radium by the Curies, and of the rare earths, have been made in this way by careful workers. High purity however usually calls for many recrystallisations, which are inevitably time-consuming, and may lead to serious reduction of yield. Should it be necessary also to isolate or concentrate the impurities of the crude for their identification, crystallisation has the disadvantage that these substances end up in a solvent in which they are very soluble, and from which their isolation is difficult. For these reasons, an alternative to fractional crystallisation must sometimes be sought. Chromatographic techniques immediately come to mind, but, with the possible exception of gas–liquid chromatography of fairly volatile samples, they cannot readily handle large quantities.

Provided that a solid satisfies the basic requirement that it is completely stable at its melting point, zone refining is frequently the most convenient way of obtaining a very pure sample, and of concentrating impurities prior to their identification by some other method. This technique, which consists basically of passing a narrow molten zone along a sample in the form of a long bar, was discovered by W. G. Pfann, a metallurgist of the Bell Telephone Company, in 1952[1,2]. It was applied with striking success to various problems in the semi-conductor field, providing the only satisfactory method of obtaining germanium and silicon of the extreme purity required for transistors. Also modifications of the method enabled a necessary impurity to be distributed very uniformly through samples of these materials

and made possible the formation of precisely controlled discontinuities in impurity concentration, as required in the
transistor analogues of certain thermionic valves.

By 1956 applications to organic chemistry were being made[3],
the extent of which have increased steadily since that date[4]. One
valuable feature from a chemical viewpoint is that relatively
simple, cheap apparatus is used, which does not necessarily
require the supervision of a trained physicist. Moreover, although
the separations are not always rapid, the process requires little
attention, so that the cost in man-hours is small.

A. THEORETICAL CONSIDERATIONS

Consider first the common situation where a solid A contains a
small amount of impurity B, which depresses the melting point.
The phase diagram for such a system usually resembles Fig. 24.
Here the two curves are known as the solidus and liquidus of the
system, and the diagram has the property that at temperature
T_0, solid of composition C_1 is in equilibrium with liquid of
composition C_0. Suppose that a sample of composition C_0 is
melted, and then slowly cooled. The system will remain liquid
above T_0, at which temperature the liquid is in equilibrium with
solid of composition C_1. In other words the solid which begins
to separate on further cooling has a much lower impurity content
than the original solid. The ratio C_1/C_0 is defined as the partition
coefficient k, and is the vital factor governing the success or
otherwise of a purification by zone refining. It is approximately
constant for low concentrations of impurity.

Zone refining will now be considered in the light of Fig. 24.
Suppose that a sample is contained in a long cylindrical tube,
and that a heater capable of melting a length 1 of it, moves
slowly along the tube. When the melting front has covered a
distance 1, separation of solid at the freezing front will commence,
the composition of which will be C_1. This will leave the advancing molten zone richer in impurity, so that as it advances,
the impurity contents of both liquid and separating solid will
increase, in accordance with Fig. 24. The composition of the

re-solidified bar along its length therefore follows curve b, Fig. 25, assuming diffusion in the solid to be very slow. By the time point A is reached, the impurity content of the freezing solid has risen to the level of the original sample, so that no

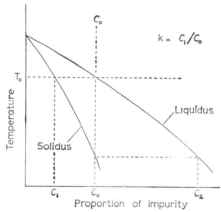

Fig. 24. Typical solid–liquid equilibrium diagram.

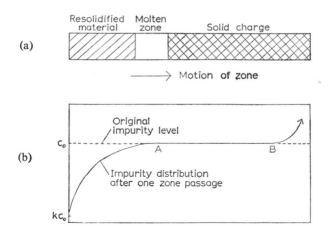

Fig. 25. Purification by zone-refining. (a) Motion of zone; (b) Resulting change of composition.

change in composition between A and B takes place. When finally the melting front reaches the end of the bar, the final length 1 of liquid, being in equilibrium with solid C_0, will have an impurity concentration C_2. As it freezes the purity of the separating solid decreases steadily, as in the figure.

Inspection of curve b, Fig. 25 shows the net effect of one zone passage to be the transfer of impurity from one end to the other. The magnitude of the concentration changes depends on the distribution coefficient k, which varies widely from case to case. If the passage of one zone does not produce useful results, it is an easy matter to repeat the process with suitable automatic equipment, so that twenty or fifty passes can be made quite readily. This ease of repetition is perhaps the greatest advantage of zone refining over fractional crystallisation. Fig. 26 shows the theoretical effect of repeated passages in a typical case, where

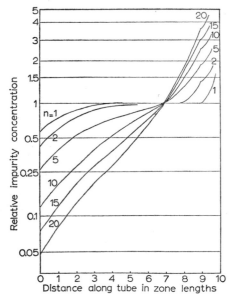

Fig. 26. Effect of increasing the number of passes (n). $k = 0.7$. Zone length $= 1/10$ sample length.

$k = 0.7$, and the length of the molten zone is one tenth that of the sample. Precise calculations in the region where the final zone is freezing are not possible. By the definition of k, a single passage yields at one end solid with 70% of its original impurity content, whilst at the far end a two or three fold concentration has taken place. After twenty passes only about 6% of the original amount of impurity remains at the end first melted, and there is ten times as much impurity at the other end as there was initially. As would be expected on common sense grounds, small values of k lead to easy separations, and vice-versa. Where $k = 0.2$ for example, ten passes cause a relative impurity concentration of only 2.10^{-5} at one end, and an over ten-fold increase at the other. A large number of computed cases are given in Pfann's book[1], from which the efficiency of a proposed separation can be estimated, if k is known.

It must be stressed that the above account is very much over-simplified. Only one type of phase-rule diagram has been considered. Cases are known both in alloy systems, and among organic compounds, where an impurity elevates the melting point. Similar arguments show that in this case the impurities concentrate in the end from which melting starts. Should a compound contain several impurities, neither end of the refined sample need necessarily be pure. It has also been assumed throughout that true equilibrium is maintained between the liquid zone and the freezing solid. This implies that the liquid is sufficiently turbulent for its composition to be uniform, and that the freezing surface grows perfectly smoothly with no occlusion of liquid. Since neither of these conditions is normally realised in practice, actual purifications are often less efficient than those predicted by theory. Finally it must be pointed out that complications arise where the components form eutectic mixtures, or addition compounds, a topic fully discussed by Goodman[5]. Such phenomena normally interfere only when large amounts (say over 5%) of impurity are present. Zone refining is therefore on the whole most effective when the starting material is already reasonably pure.

References p. 72

B. EXPERIMENTAL METHODS

The design of practical zone refiners for organic compounds is governed by many factors. Since, unlike liquid metals, organic liquids have low surface tensions, the sample must be surrounded by a container such as a glass tube. Most compounds expand on melting, so that the molten zone must be started at a free surface, to avoid tube breakage. Experiments having shown that in a horizontal tube the liquid zone tends to diffuse into the solid, a vertical position is normally used. The normal practice is thus to pass the heater down from the top of a vertical tube, or, conversely to pass the tube upwards through a fixed heater. One other advantage accrues from this arrangement. The need for thorough mixing of the molten zone if good separations are to be obtained has already been referred to. With a vertical tube the lower end of the molten zone becomes somewhat hotter than its top, so that convection currents effectively stir the liquid.

Steps must be taken to stabilise the heater current to avoid the danger that the liquid zone, whilst passing along the tube, may become overheated and expand, breaking the tube. For the same reason zone refiners should be shielded from draughts. With very impure samples one may even have to reduce the heat input as the zone moves down the tube, since, as impurities move downwards, the melting point will decrease.

The rate at which a zone may be passed through a sample is limited by the need for a close approximation to equilibrium between the liquid and freezing surface, if the separation efficiency is to approach the theoretical. Too rapid a motion causes the solid to deposit as a mass of fine crystals, in which pockets of liquid are trapped. In practice speeds of about one inch per hour are commonly used, though the loss of efficiency resulting from a two or three-fold increase may be offset by ability to make more passes in a given time. Since sample lengths are usually between one and four feet, and several passages are usually necessary, it will be seen that days or weeks, rather than hours, are usually required for the purification. However, as explained later, the apparatus does not normally require attention, and several samples can be handled simultaneously.

Practical considerations lay fairly rigid upper and lower limits to the quantities that can be treated. The maximum usable tube diameter is about $1\frac{1}{2}''$, for two main reasons. As most organic compounds are poor thermal conductors, heat from normal radiant heaters will not penetrate to the centre of a thick tube, without excessive spreading of the zone near the walls. This can be overcome by using dielectric heating, but there is no known means of abstracting heat from the centre of a wide tube, enabling the freezing surface to grow smoothly. The maximum charge is thus about 1500 g, assuming a four foot tube. At the other end of the scale, tube diameters below about 2 mm are unsatisfactory, partly because convection in the molten zone becomes inadequate. Also, unless the sample is carefully degassed, bubbles become trapped at the freezing surface, destroying the efficiency of the process. For these reasons at least 0.5 g of sample is required.

The relative lengths of molten zone and sample have an important effect on the separation. Generally speaking a long zone leads to rapid transport of impurities, but a narrow one gives a better ultimate distribution, provided time permits a sufficient number of passes. In practice these advantages can be combined, by using for the first two or three passes a wide zone, which is subsequently narrowed to about one twentieth (or less) of the sample length.

In principle zone refining can readily be speeded up by passing several zones simultaneously along the sample. They must however be well separated, as organic liquids in a cylindrical tube tend to resolidify with a hollow central core, which might connect two closely spaced molten zones.

Unlike many of the techniques discussed in this book, zone refining uses apparatus simple enough to be constructed in any laboratory with workshop facilities. Equipment is also available commercially. Typical modern apparatus has recently been described by Beynon and Saunders[4]. Fig. 27 shows diagram-

References p. 72

matically their apparatus for handling large and small samples, and for those with low melting points. More detailed drawings are given in the original paper. The large scale refiner (Fig. 27a) utilizes a framework of three stout brass rods, clamped to a wall at the top, for additional rigidity. Along these bars slides a platform carrying six electrical heaters (of which only two are shown for simplicity) with adaptors enabling them to fit closely

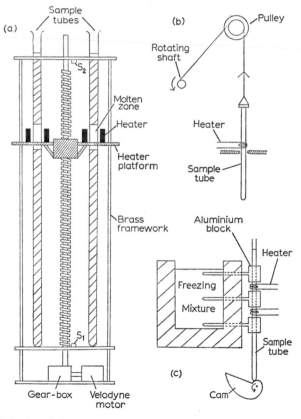

Fig. 27. Zone-refining apparatus. (a) Large-scale; (b) Micro-scale; (c) For use at low temperatures.

over any tube between $\frac{1}{4}$ and $1\frac{1}{2}$ inches in diameter. Six tubes can thus be handled simultaneously. The heater platform is fixed to a nut, running in a screw thread, which is turned, via a gear-box by a "velodyne" motor. During normal operation this causes the heater assembly to move steadily downwards at about one inch per hour. At the bottom a microswitch S_1 is activated which affects the velodyne circuit in such a way as to reverse the motor and greatly to increase its speed, thus returning the heaters to the top, where a second microswitch restores the downward motion. This refiner thus performs any required number of passes automatically. Fig. 27b demonstrates the principle of a very simple micro zone-refiner. Upward motion of the tube is achieved simply by winding a thread on to a slowly rotating shaft such as that driving the hour hand of a clock, and the heater, which in this case is fixed, is a single coil of nichrome wire.

Substances with melting points within 30°C of room temperature solidify too slowly for the above types of apparatus to be suitable. To overcome this difficulty, alternate regions of heating and cooling must be provided. Beynon and Saunders obtain cold zones from a series of cooled aluminium blocks, which are connected by thermally conducting bars to the inside of an insulated vessel containing freezing mixture. The refining tube passes through these blocks, an intermediate glass tube being used to prevent freezing of the sample tube to the aluminium. An eccentric cam, driven continuously, moves the sample slowly up and rapidly down through the succession of cold zones and heaters. The pitch of the motion equals the distance between adjacent heaters so that effectively continuous movement of the zones is achieved. Satisfactory results have been obtained with substances which melt between —30 and 50°C.

Experience is needed to know how long a zone-refining experiment should be continued to obtain the optimum result. Frequently the process can be followed by colour changes along the tube. The impure end usually becomes steadily darker, whilst the colour (if any) at the pure end brightens. A fair idea of the degree of purification can thus be obtained visually. It has also been noticed that, whereas impure materials resolidify in a polycrystalline mass, very pure samples tend to form large single crystals. This phenomenon may also be taken as a sign that high purity is being approached.

C. APPLICATIONS TO ORGANIC CHEMISTRY

There are two main uses of zone-refining in organic chemistry. Very pure samples are sometimes required, for example for use as intermediates in the polymer field, where small amounts of impurity may have large effects on the physical properties of the resulting polymer. Such techniques as mass spectrometry which can detect impurities down to a few parts per million also demand exceptionally pure reference standards. In such cases zone-refining may have advantages over fractional crystallisation. The technique may also help to solve the very common industrial problem, where the quality of a compound varies from batch to batch because of impurities. It may be essential to identify these impurities before the necessary alterations to the process can be made. If, as often happens, the impurity level is too low for the usual methods of identification, such as infra-red spectroscopy to be usable, a concentration of up to 10^4 times can sometimes be effected by zone-refining, whereupon another method may be used to complete the identification. The applicability of zone-refining is very wide, being limited only by the necessity for absolute stability just above the melting point. It will be appreciated that, since during purification the material may be molten for several hours, the slightest tendency to decomposition may invalidate the procedure. Subject to this condition, the authors of reference[4] report that almost every sample they examined responded to zone-refining. Substances melting up to 300°C have been successfully treated, but, as previously mentioned, special apparatus is needed with melting points within 30°C of ambient. Purifications may sometimes be speeded up by starting with a large tube, and, after a few passes transferring the material of the pure end to a much smaller tube. By thus proceeding in stages the number of passes required may be minimised. In selecting samples care must be taken to avoid concentrating explosives, for example from a nitration where poly-nitro impurities may be concentrated to a point where an explosion might occur.

Several examples follow of typical purifications. The best available collection of such examples is due to Beynon and Saunders[4]. Among other compounds, they have successfully treated amides, amines, acids, alcohols, anthraquinones, azo compounds, esters, hydrocarbons, indoles, ketones, phenols and pyrazolones.

(a) Benzene: An example of the purification of a liquid is given by Rock[6]. Zone-refining of benzene, the whole apparatus being immersed in an ice bath, reduced the mole fraction of impurity, as indicated by the melting point, from $6.3 \cdot 10^{-3}$ to less than $8 \cdot 10^{-5}$ molar.

(b) Naphthalene[3,4]: Zone-refining proved a very efficient means of reducing the anthracene content of naphthalene. According to Herington et al.[3], seven passes were sufficient to reduce the concentration of anthracene, judged by comparing the fluorescence of the sample with those of standards, from 0.2% to less than 0.00002%. Crude naphthalene also responded[4], nine passes raising the melting point of the pure end from 73.5 to 80.2°C, and concentrating the impurities sufficiently for no fewer than seventeen of them to be identified by mass spectroscopy.

(c) Anthracene[4]: The effect of zone refining on the concentrations of three impurities in anthracene as measured by mass

TABLE 5

IMPURITIES IN ANTHRACENE

	% Carbazole	% Hexahydro-anthracene	% Methylanthracene
Initial	0.80	0.64	0.19
After 18 passes	0.38	0.05	<0.005
After 32 passes	0.11	<0.005	<0.005

References p. 72

spectrometry is shown in Table 5. Of the three, carbazole is clearly much the most difficult to remove. By starting with six tubes, and transferring the partially refined materials from them to a new tube, a carbazole content of less than one part in twenty thousand was ultimately attained.

TABLE 6

DISTRIBUTION OF IMPURITIES ALONG A TUBE OF 1-AMINO-2-METHYL
ANTHRAQUINONE, AFTER THIRTY-THREE PASSES

	% Diaminomethyl anthraquinone	% Aminodimethyl anthraquinone
Initial concentration	0.31	0.31
Top layer	0.20	0.05
3 in. from top	0.20	0.05
6 in. from top	0.20	0.07
9 in. from top	0.25	0.14

TABLE 7

DISTRIBUTION OF IMPURITIES ALONG A TWENTY-FOUR INCH TUBE
OF 3-METHOXYBENZANTHRONE, AFTER FORTY-EIGHT PASSES

	% Chloromethoxy-benzanthrone	% Dimethoxy-benzanthrone	% Chloro-benzanthrone
Initial concentration	2.0	0.12	0.66
Top layer	3.4	0.04	0.12
8 in. from top	2.1	0.06	0.19
16 in. from top	1.07	0.11	0.78
bottom layer	0.70	0.17	0.78

(d) Benzoic acid[4]: A $1\frac{1}{2}$ kg sample of A.R. material was purified by seven passes in a $1\frac{1}{2}$ inch tube. During the process the purity at the top, judging from the melting point, rose from 99.3 to 99.97%. After a few passes, the top of the sample began to grow in a single crystal, which however cracked on cooling.

(e) 1,4,5-Trichloro-anthraquinone: During thirty zone passages, this compound developed marked colour variations along the tube. The top few inches developed a green shade, which was shown by infra-red spectroscopy to arise from the 1,4,5,8-tetrachloro compound. This impurity elevates the melting point, and therefore moves in a direction counter to that of the molten zone. The centre of the tube contained 1,4,5-trichloro-anthraquinone, which, from the brightness of its yellow colour seemed much purer than the starting material, whilst the bottom section, containing most of the other impurities was much darker.

(f) 1-Amino-2-methylanthraquinone: Table 6 shows the distribution of the two main impurities along a tube after thirty-three passes. These figures emphasise the wide variations in efficiency from one impurity to another.

(g) 2-Methoxybenzanthrone: Table 7 shows the concentrations of three impurities along a twenty-four inch tube, after forty-eight passes. Chloromethoxybenzanthrone is another example of a compound which elevates the melting point. As borne out by the figures, such compounds usually move abnormally slowly, being unable to move more than a single zone length per pass.

(h) Purification of waxes and polymers: A modification of zone-refining has recently been reported[7], which extends the technique to non-crystalline materials. A small amount of a solvent such as chloroform or butyl alcohol is incorporated into a tube filled with the sample. When a heater is passed along the tube, the solid dissolves in the hot region, and reprecipitates as the heater moves on. The separation thus depends on the different solubilities of the components of a mixture, those of greatest solubility being concentrated behind the moving zone. Mechanically, the process is identical with zone melting. Problems which have been tackled include purification of waxes, fats and rubbers, and separation of polymers such as polystyrene into molecular weight fractions.

REFERENCES

1 W. G. PFANN, *Zone Melting*, John Wiley & Sons, New York, 1958.
2 W. G. PFANN, *J. Metals*, 4 (1952) 747.
3 E. F. G. HERINGTON, R. HANDLEY AND A. J. COOK, *Chem. & Ind. (London)*, (1956) 292, 304.
4 J. H. BEYNON AND R. A. SAUNDERS, *J. Appl. Phys.*, 11 (1960) 128.
5 C. H. L. GOODMAN, *Research*, 7 (1954) 168.
6 H. ROCK, *Naturwiss.*, 41 (1954) 425.
7 Esso Research, *Chem. Eng. News*, 39 (1961) 74.

CHAPTER 5

ELECTRONIC ABSORPTION SPECTROSCOPY

A. INTRODUCTION, UNITS, DEFINITIONS

This chapter and the next three deal with the absorption of radiation in various parts of the electromagnetic spectrum. Inspection of Fig. 28 shows how X-rays, ultra-violet and visible light, infra-red radiation, and radio waves, which are all similar in nature, differ greatly in wavelength, so much so that it is inconvenient to use the same units throughout to specify a position in a spectrum. Since a wave has associated with it both a wavelength (λ) and a frequency (ν) connected by the equation

$$c = \nu\lambda$$

where c is the velocity of light, it is possible to determine spectral positions either on a frequency or a wavelength basis.

At one end of the scale, radio waves have wavelengths of the order of tens and hundreds of metres, and frequencies of megacycles/sec. Passing to the infra-red region, the wavelength becomes too short to be conveniently described in metres or centimetres, the normal unit being the micron (μ) where

$$1\ \mu \equiv 10^{-4}\ \text{cm}$$

The infra-red region most useful in chemical applications then extends from about 2 to 20 μ. In the visible and ultra-violet regions, the micron is inconveniently large, and is usually replaced either by the millimicron or the Ångstrom unit, where

$$1\ \text{m}\mu \equiv 10\ \mathring{A} \equiv 10^{-7}\ \text{cm}$$

In these units, the visible region and that part of the ultra-violet where measurements can readily be made, stretch from 185 to 800 mμ or 1,850–8,000 $\mathring{A}$.

References p. 134

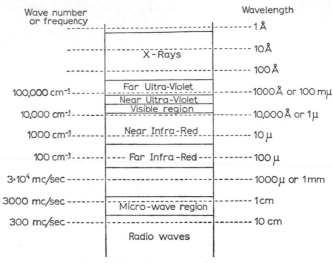

Fig. 28. The electromagnetic spectrum.

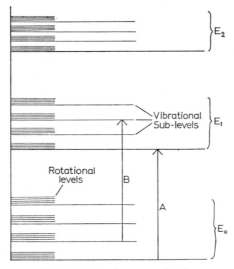

Fig. 29. Molecular energy levels.

Except with radio waves, frequencies are too great to be a useful unit. However, the wave-number, or number of waves which fit into one centimetre, is often used to locate bands in the infra-red, and less commonly in the ultra-violet region. This unit, which is written cm^{-1}, equals $1/\lambda$ if the latter is expressed in centimetres, or $10^4/\lambda$ if the wavelength is in units of μ. It follows that the useful infra-red region stretches from about 500 to 5,000 cm^{-1}, whilst the near ultra-violet and visible extend from 12,500 to 55,000 cm^{-1}. Interconversion from wavelength to wave-number units can readily be made with a slide-rule or reciprocal tables.

Absorption spectroscopy depends on the fact that most forms of molecular energy are quantised, including the potential energy of the electrons around their nuclei, the vibrational energy of the atoms against one another, and the rotational energy of the molecule as a whole. That is to say, a molecule has associated with it a series of energy levels (Fig. 29), and can take up or lose energy only in steps corresponding to the differences between these levels. As seen from the figure, the electronic energy levels are relatively far apart, and the vibrational levels much closer. Each vibrational energy level is further subdivided into rotational levels.

Although in order to explain such phenomena as diffraction and interference, light must be regarded as a wave motion, it is also clear from the photoelectric effect, that a light beam may also behave as a stream of particles. For the present purpose one may regard a monochromatic light beam of frequency ν_1, as a stream of particles, called photons, each with an energy given by

$$E = h\nu_1$$

where h is Planck's constant. Similarly a beam of white light consists of a mixture of photons of various energies.

If, then, light from a source which emits continuously over the frequency range to be studied is passed through a sample, and if the molecules have energy levels E_0, E_1, E_2, etc., light

References p. 134

may be absorbed at frequencies given by

$$E_1 - E_0 = h\nu_1$$
$$E_2 - E_0 = h\nu_2$$

and so on. If the emergent beam is analysed in a spectrometer, absorption bands will be found at ν_1, ν_2 etc.

Since electronic energy levels are fairly well separated, the corresponding absorption bands are at rather high frequencies, or short wavelengths, in the ultra-violet and visible regions. The vibrational energy levels being much closer, transitions between them cause bands of longer wavelengths in the near infra-red, whilst still further into the infra-red come bands corresponding to the closely spaced rotational levels.

Absorptions in both the visible and near ultra-violet being due to electronic transitions, they are dealt with together in the present chapter. Suppose that light from a source which emits continuously between 200 and 400 mμ is passed through a sample, diluted if necessary with a transparent solvent, and then to a spectrophotometer (p. 97). A spectrum may then be obtained (Fig. 30a) of wavelength against percentage absorption, which will usually have several bands, corresponding to various electronic transitions. Such a spectrum may, however, suffer from the disadvantage that the bands differ so much in intensity that measurements at several dilutions will be required to show each band at a satisfactory level. Rather than present a series of curves, the band strengths are often converted to a logarithmic scale. If at any wavelength, I_0 is the incident light intensity, and I its value after passing through the sample, then the optical density, or absorbance, is defined as

$$d = \log_{10} I_0/I$$

As expressed in the laws of Beer and Lambert, it is found experimentally that

$$d = kcl$$

where c is the concentration of solute, l is the cell length, and k

the extinction coefficient, which is a constant at any wavelength. For pure substances, if c is expressed in moles/l, and l in centimetres, the equation may be written

$$d = \varepsilon c l$$

where ε is the molecular extinction coefficient. Since a series of measurements on solutions of different strengths can be combined in a single graph of ε against wavelength, this is the method normally used in the literature for showing spectra. Of particular importance are the values ε_{max} of ε at the band peaks, which are often quoted together with the wavelength. If, as sometimes happens, intensity variations from band to band are too great even for ε to be satisfactory, $\log_{10}\varepsilon$ is used for the ordinate (Fig. 30d).

Two general points about the phenanthrene spectrum of Fig. 30 may be noted. Whereas it might be expected that all bands would have equal intensity, in practice they differ greatly,

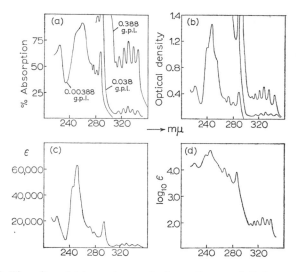

Fig. 30. The ultra-violet spectrum of phenanthrene, plotted on various intensity scales.

for reasons to be discussed later (p. 83). Also they are comparatively wide, showing that in fact absorption over a range of
wavelengths takes place. This arises mainly from the changes of
vibrational energy which accompany electronic transitions.
Returning to Fig. 29, the lines A and B which represent the
same electronic energy change clearly differ. Whereas A involves
the zero vibrational level of both electronic states, B is accompanied by a vibrational change. The band near 270 mμ in the
phenanthrene spectrum shows several sub-peaks, due to
vibrational changes. Frequently these sub-peaks are not
resolved, but nevertheless broaden the band.

B. ELECTRONIC ENERGY LEVELS AND SPECTRA OF SIMPLE MOLECULES

Before attempting a description of the electronic spectra of
organic molecules, it may be helpful to discuss briefly the nature
of the electronic energy levels. A thorough discussion of this
subject by quantum theory is clearly beyond the scope of this
book. However, various simple treatments have been attempted[1-3], of which that in terms of molecular orbitals is
perhaps the best.

In Bohr's original quantum theory picture of an atom, the
electrons were thought of as revolving in circular or elliptical
orbits around the nucleus, like planets in a solar system. The
energies of the electrons increased with the diameter of the
orbit, and an electron could pass from one orbit to another of
higher energy by absorption of light, of frequency v, according
to the equation

$$E_1 - E_2 = hv$$

This simple model has now been rejected for two main reasons.
Firstly it fails to account for many more recent observations on
atomic spectra. Also, there is now overwhelming evidence that
it is fundamentally unsound to attempt to treat a particle of the
nature of an electron by the laws of classical mechanics, as Bohr
did. Modern quantum mechanics uses the discovery that in
many ways moving electrons behave rather as waves than as

particles. As a result of its wave character, an electron bound to an atomic nucleus has associated with it a wave function ψ, which in simple cases can be obtained by solving Shroedinger's equation, the fundamental equation of quantum mechanics. It is found that this equation can only be solved for certain discrete values of the energy of the electron. Thus modern quantum mechanics predicts, as did the old theory, a set of discrete energy levels which electrons may occupy. These are called orbitals, by analogy with the orbits of Bohr's theory. By means of the Shroedinger equation, ψ may be calculated at various points in space around the nucleus, for each of the possible orbitals. One can then, as represented in Fig. 31, construct three-dimensional figures illustrating the distribution of ψ in space, for the various energy levels. Outside the surfaces drawn, ψ falls rapidly to a negligible value. It is important to note that ψ may be either positive or negative. Although the physical significance of ψ itself is not easy to see, ψ^2 at any point represents the probability that the electron will be there at a given instant. Alternatively, one may regard the electron as a "smeared out" charge distributed through its orbital, the charge at any point being proportional to ψ^2.

An atom has therefore associated with it a family of orbitals of various shapes and energies. By the Pauli Exclusion Principle, only two electrons may occupy any orbital, and then only provided their spins are in opposite directions. Hence, if an atom has $2N + 1$ electrons, they will tend to occupy the N orbitals of lowest energy, leaving one which will be accommodated in a higher energy orbital, and will therefore be more liable to be involved in chemical reactions. Above the occupied orbitals is a manifold of empty levels. Light absorption may therefore take place, in which an electron from the highest occupied level is raised to an empty one. Emission is the result of the reverse process.

Many properties of orbitals can be understood by considering their shapes. Of particular importance in the fairly small atoms of organic chemistry are s and p type orbitals. The lowest energy level is designated 1*s*, and is spherical and symmetrical about the nucleus (Fig. 31). Above this come the 2*s* and 2*p* orbitals which have the same energy, but differ in shape. Whereas 2*s* is again spherically symmetrical, the 2*p* orbitals are dumb-bell shaped, and may have their axes in one of three possible directions. Because the sign of ψ is different in its two halves, a 2*p* orbital is said to be antisymmetrical about a plane through the nucleus.

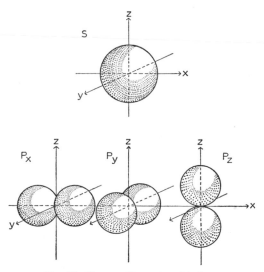

Fig. 31. Shapes of atomic orbitals.

In the same way as the electrons in atoms occupy atomic orbitals, those of molecules exist in pairs in molecular orbitals, which again may be specified in terms of energy and shape. Consider first, for simplicity, a diatomic molecule. The inner electrons will be little affected by bond formation, so, in the molecule, will continue to occupy orbitals very similar in shape and energy to those of the isolated atoms. This applies also to "lone pair" electrons of, for example, oxygen and nitrogen, which are not involved in chemical bonding. However, the outer occupied orbitals, which hold the valency electrons of the atom, will be considerably altered. For the hydrogen molecule, Fig. 32 shows on the left some combinations of two isolated atoms, in which the electrons are located in various orbitals. If in each

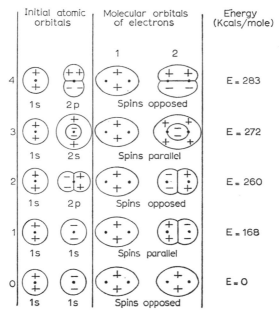

Fig. 32. Molecular orbitals of hydrogen.

case a hypothetical combination of the atoms is carried out, the centre of the figure shows the molecular orbitals occupied by the two electrons in the resulting molecule. Although they are enlarged, since they must now enclose two nuclei, their shapes are similar to those of the corresponding atomic orbitals.

At the bottom of the figure, two hydrogen atoms, each with its electron in the lowest (1s) orbital, combine to give a normal, stable hydrogen molecule. The letter σ is used to describe

References p. 134

molecular orbitals (or electrons) of the lowest, most symmetrical kind. All the other combinations yield electronically excited molecules, the energies of which, relative to the stable ground state, are given on the right of the figure. It will be noticed that, in some of these states, including the ground state, the electron spins are in opposite directions or opposed. Such states are described as "singlet", whereas others such as 1 and 3, in which the electron spins are parallel, are "triplet" states.

Light absorption by molecular hydrogen will now be considered in terms of Fig. 32. Since the energy gap from the ground state even to the lowest excited level is large, the bands fall at very high frequencies (since $\Delta E = h\nu$) or short wavelengths, in the far ultra-violet. At first sight one might expect four absorption bands, corresponding to transitions from the ground state to 1, 2, 3 and 4. In practice, only transitions $0 \rightarrow 2$ and $0 \rightarrow 4$ cause absorption, for reasons which are of fundamental importance in spectroscopy.

The absence of a band corresponding to $0 \rightarrow 1$ provides an example of a general rule, which forbids absorption arising from transitions between singlet and triplet states, involving reversal of an electron spin. Transition $0 \rightarrow 1$ is described as "spin forbidden".

There is another important restriction on light absorption. An electronic transition can be induced by light absorption only if it is accompanied by a so-called dipole moment of transition, or transition moment. This does not imply that there need be a change in the permanent dipole moment of the molecule. However, in a transition such as $0 \rightarrow 2$, examination of the plus and minus signs associated with the wave function in the upper and lower states, reveals a change of symmetry which causes the molecule to acquire an instantaneous dipole moment. Quite generally, unless a transition is accompanied by a change of symmetry in the wave function (or orbital), it is described as "forbidden" and no strong band will result.

Reconsidering the hydrogen molecule in the light of these two selection rules, one sees that although transition $0 \rightarrow 1$ is "permitted" on symmetry grounds, it is spin forbidden. Since $0 \rightarrow 2$ involves a symmetry change, but no spin reversal, it gives rise to a strong absorption band. $0 \rightarrow 3$ is forbidden on both symmetry and spin grounds, but there are no such restrictions on $0 \rightarrow 4$, and a band results.

The concept of transitions which are permitted or forbidden explains most of the intensity variations of bands in ultra-violet and visible spectra. For example, in the phenanthrene spectrum (Fig. 30), band A corresponds to a permitted transition, and B to a forbidden one.

Similar arguments can be applied to the bonds of saturated aliphatic compounds, such as paraffins, naphthenes, alcohols and ethers. As with the hydrogen molecule, the electrons of each bond fall into the lowest σ orbitals, and there is a large energy gap between the highest occupied and lowest unoccupied levels. Consequently these compounds have no strong ultra-violet bands at wavelengths longer than about 160 mμ, so that ultra-violet spectroscopy cannot readily be applied to problems involving them.

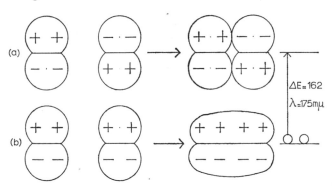

Fig. 33. π-orbitals of ethylene.

Compounds containing unconjugated double bonds will next be considered. Double bond formation between two carbon atoms involves both s and p type electrons. Since the latter are of much higher energy, the formation of the double bond may be regarded crudely as two distinct processes. In the first, two $2s$ orbitals, one from each atom, combine forming a σ type molecular orbital. Simultaneously the two $2p$ orbitals, whose axes become aligned, may combine in one of two possible ways, according to whether the signs of ψ are "head to head" or "head to tail". Two π orbitals result (Fig. 33), of which the more symmetrical one (b), has the lower energy. Accordingly, two of the four double bond electrons occupy the orbital, and, in the ground state, the other two fill the lower π orbital. The important point, however, is that the energy difference between the two π orbitals is less than between the occupied and unoccupied levels of the molecules previously considered.

Consequently, ethylene has a strong band at 175 mμ, just beyond the range of most ultra-violet spectrophotometers, its strength arising from the permitted nature of the transition. Alkyl substituents, by secondary effects, move the band to rather longer wavelengths where it can be conveniently studied. The terms $N \rightarrow V$ and $\pi \rightarrow \pi^*$ are used in describing transitions of this kind between two molecular orbitals formed from the same atomic orbitals.

Similar ideas apply to other isolated double bonds, including $C{=}O$, $C{=}S$, $C{=}N$, $N{=}N$ and $N{=}O$. As these, and more complicated unsaturated groups are the cause of absorption in the ultra-violet and visible regions, the term chromophore is applied to them.

Another type of transition is possible with double bonds involving nitrogen and oxygen atoms, in which a lone pair electron, from a non-bonding orbital, is raised to the excited π^* orbital. Fig. 34 illustrates the situation with the carbonyl group. In contrast to $N \rightarrow V$, these $n \rightarrow \pi^*$ (or $N \rightarrow Q$) transitions are symmetry forbidden, so the band is weak. Aliphatic aldehydes and ketones show a weak $n \rightarrow \pi^*$ band at 280 mμ. Similarly, in addition to strong absorption near 210 mμ, aliphatic nitro compounds show a weak band near 270 mμ. Since the lone pair electrons in the sulphur atom are at a higher level, thioketones show the corresponding band at a longer wavelength, near 460 mμ. Aliphatic azo compounds provide a final example of $n \to \pi^*$ transitions, azomethane, for example, absorbing weakly at 347 mμ, and diazo methane at 410 mμ.

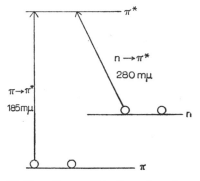

Fig. 34. Transitions within the carbonyl group.

TABLE 8

ELECTRONIC ABSORPTION BANDS OF SOME ALIPHATIC COMPOUNDS

Compound	Band 1		Band 2*	
	λ_{max}	ε_{max}	λ_{max}	ε_{max}
Ethylene	175	c. 5,000	—	—
Mono alkyl ethylenes	173–188	c. 5,000	—	—
Dialkyl ethylenes	185–205	c. 5,000	—	—
Trialkyl ethylenes	190–216	c. 5,000	—	—
Tetra alkyl ethylenes	215–232	c. 5,000	—	—
Aldehydes	c. 210	strong	285–295	10–30
Ketones	c. 195	c. 1,000	270–285	10–30
Carboxylic acids	207–210	50–70	—	—
Esters	c. 205	c. 50	—	—
Thioketones	c. 200	strong	c. 400	weak
Oximes	190	c. 5,000	—	—
Nitro compounds	210	strong	270	10–20
Acetylenes	c. 180	c. 6,000	—	—

* $n \to \pi^*$ transition.

References p. 134

Table 8 lists the approximate λ_{max} and ε_{max} values of compounds with unconjugated double bonds. As previously mentioned, many aliphatic compounds are virtually transparent in this region, including paraffins, alicyclic hydrocarbons, ethers, alcohols, thiols and amines. Those with an isolated double bond usually absorb strongly near 200 mμ, and sometimes weakly at longer wavelengths.

C. ELECTRONIC LEVELS AND SPECTRA OF CONJUGATED SYSTEMS

It has so far been seen that single bonds and isolated double bonds cause strong absorption only towards the short wavelength end of the accessible region. Absorption of longer wavelength ultra-violet and visible light occurs only with molecules containing two or more conjugated double bonds. Such groups as —OH, —NH$_2$, and —NMe$_2$, known as auxochromes, also move the absorption of a given chromophore to longer wavelengths, and intensify it.

1. Polyenes and related compounds

The principles governing the spectra of conjugated systems may well be illustrated by the polyene case. As previously explained for ethylene, the $2p$ orbitals of the two carbon atoms combine, forming two π orbitals, of which the lower is occupied by the two π electrons of ethylene in its ground state, whilst the absorption near 175 mμ arises from a transition to the upper π^* orbital. In the next simplest case, that of butadiene, there are four carbon atoms. As with ethylene, three σ type orbitals are formed, leaving four valence electrons to occupy higher levels. Each carbon atom contributes one $2p$ orbital to the molecular orbitals of butadiene. According to the signs of their wave functions, four distinct orbitals may be formed, as shown in Fig. 35. In the ground state of the molecule, the four electrons occupy the lowest two levels, and light absorption is caused by transitions to the upper ones. Butadiene absorbs near 210 mμ, in good agreement with theory.

When the theory is applied to the general case of a polyene

with n carbon atoms, each contributing one atomic orbital, it transpires that, if n is large, the energy difference between the highest occupied and lowest unoccupied levels is

$$\Delta E = K/(n-1)$$

K being a constant, so that the longest wavelength of absorption is

$$\lambda = hc/\Delta E = (n+1)hc/K$$

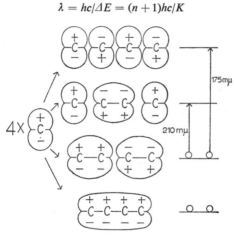

Fig. 35. π-orbitals of butadiene.

TABLE 9

ELECTRONIC ABSORPTION BANDS OF POLYENE SYSTEMS[4]

Compound	Number of double bonds	λ_{max}	ε_{max}	Colour
Ethylene	1	175	c. 5,000	colourless
Butadiene	2	217	21,000	colourless
Hexatriene	3	258	35,000	colourless
Dimethyloctatetraene	4	296	52,000	pale yellow
Decapentaene	5	335	118,000	pale yellow
Dimethyl dodecahexaene	6	360	70,000	yellow
Dihydro-β-carotene	8	415	210,000	orange
Lycopene	11	470	185,000	red
Dehydrolycopene	15	504	150,000	violet

Hence the absorption moves steadily to longer wavelengths, as the number of double bonds increases. This is one of the most important principles governing electronic spectra. The value of ε_{max} also increases, as shown in Table 9, which also shows how colour develops with increasing chain length. Similar effects are found when other double and triple bonds are conjugated, as shown in Table 10.

TABLE 10

ABSORPTION BANDS OF CONJUGATED SYSTEMS[4]

System	Example	λ_{max}	ε_{max}
C=C—C≡C	vinyl acetylene	219	6,500
C=C—C=N	n-butyl crotonaldimine	220	23,000
C=C—C=O	crotonaldehyde	217	16,000
		321*	20
O=C—C=O	diacetyl	435*	18
C=C—NO₂	1-nitro-2-propene	229	9,500
C=C—C=C—C=O	sorbaldehyde	263	27,000
O=C—C=C—C=O	diacetylethylene	226	14,500
		338*	70
C—(C=C)₂—NO₂	5-nitro-2,4-pentadiene	298	12,500

* $n \rightarrow \pi^*$ transition.

2. The Benzene Chromophore – substituent effects

The electronic absorption of benzene and its derivative differs markedly from that of the corresponding open chain compound, hexatriene. As with olefines the bonding in the benzene hexagon may be thought of as in two parts. Six electrons occupy σ type C–C orbitals, whilst π orbitals are formed by overlap of the six $2p$ orbitals of the carbon atoms, arranged with their axes perpendicular to the plane of the ring, which may combine in six possible ways, according to the signs of the wave functions. Long wavelength absorption results from transitions between these π levels. In benzene however, the longest wavelength band, near 260 mμ, corresponds to a forbidden transition which is not accompanied by a change of symmetry. However the carbon-carbon distances are slightly different in the upper and lower electronic states, so the transition readily induces a molecular vibration, which slightly distorts the hexagon, partially removing the symmetry restriction. A weak band near 260 mμ (ε about 200) results. The effect of the vibration shows clearly in the band (Fig. 36), which has five well defined sub-peaks, whose spacing corresponds to the vibrational frequency.

Fig. 36. Spectra of solutions of polyacenes[2].

Benzene also absorbs more strongly near 185 and 202 mμ. The terms K band and B band are sometimes used respectively to describe the benzenoid absorptions near 200 and 260 mμ.

Substituent effects may conveniently be discussed here, since the behaviour of the benzene band at 260 mμ shows these effects very clearly, lying at a convenient wavelength near the middle of the near ultra-violet, and being weak enough for intensity variations to be accurately measurable. Moreover many substituents have rather similar effects on other aromatic systems.

Roughly speaking, substituents in benzene are of three kinds. Such groups as alkyl and halogen influence the ring mainly by an inductive, rather than a mesomeric effect. This affects the upper and lower energy states to about the same extent, so that

the band position is not much changed. Slight band intensification, however results since substituents reduce the symmetry of
the ring, making the transition less forbidden. Alkyl groups
move the band to slightly longer wavelengths, through hyper-
conjugation in which methyl groups show some tendency to
donate electrons to the ring mesomerically.

Much more striking effects are produced by —NH_2, —NMe_2,
—OH, —OMe and similar groups, whose electrons interact
strongly with the π electrons of the ring. The term auxochrome
is used in describing such groups, which, though not themselves
capable of absorption in the visible or near ultra-violet, profoundly affect other chromophores. In molecular orbital
language the interaction is attributed to the ability of the lone
pair orbitals of the nitrogen and oxygen atoms, partially to mix
with the ring carbon $2p$ orbitals, leading to a modified set of
energy levels. Alternatively on valence-bond theory, the effect is
ascribed to resonance forms such as

where the lone-pair electrons are transferred to the ring. The
net effect is that these substituents, as shown by Table 11 greatly
intensify the band, and move it to longer wavelengths. A striking
comparison may be made between the spectrum of aniline, and
that of the anilinium ion, which, as a result of immobilisation
of the lone-pair electrons, is very similar to that of benzene.

Finally substituents with a double bond adjacent to the ring
must be considered. Groups such as —$CH{=}CH_2$, —CHO, and
NO_2 have an effect analagous to the addition of another $C{=}C$
unit in polyenes. Their double bond orbitals mix completely
with those of the ring, giving a new set of molecular orbitals.
Table 11 shows the effect on the spectrum, which is again
intensified and moved to longer wavelengths. This effect is
confined to the case where the double bond adjoins the ring.
Should they be separated, for example, by a —CH_2— group, the

TABLE 11

EFFECT OF SUBSTITUENTS ON THE SPECTRUM OF BENZENE[10]

Compound	K band		B band	
	λ_{max}	ε_{max}	λ_{max}	ε_{max}
Benzene	198	8,000	255	230
Toluene	—	—	263	270
p-Xylene	—	—	269	750
Chlorobenzene	210	7,400	264	205
Aniline	230	7,000	290	1,470
Phenol	—	—	273	2,050
Thiophenol	236	10,000	269	700
Anisole	—	—	265	2,300
Nitrobenzene	252	10,000	280	1,000
Styrene	244	13,000	282	2.7
Acetophenone	244	16,000	278	1,000
Benzophenone	252	20,000	*	*
Diphenyl	246	20,000	*	*
Trans-stilbene	295	27,000	*	*
$C_6H_5 \cdot N = N \cdot Me$	261	8,000	*	*
Azobenzene	319	20,000	*	*

* Obscured by the strong K band.

spectrum is simply that of benzene plus that of a double bond. The third type of substituent also moves the strong 200 mμ absorption of benzene to longer wavelengths, as shown in the table. In extreme cases the weaker 260 mμ band is completely overlaid by the shifted K band.

3. Polyphenyls and condensed ring hydrocarbons

Table 12 summarises data on some such compounds. Since the two benzene rings of diphenyl are roughly co-planar, large molecular orbitals can be formed, covering both rings. These cause new transitions and the weak 260 mμ band is obscured by a strong band analogous to the 202 mμ band of benzene. As only two of the three rings of m-terphenyl can lie in the same plane for steric reasons, its spectrum is very similar to that of diphenyl. p-Terphenyl and tetraphenyl, on the contrary, form larger

References p. 134

TABLE 12

SPECTRA OF POLYPHENYLS AND POLYACENES[4]

Compound	Band 1		Band 2		Band 3	
	λ_{max}	ε_{max}	λ_{max}	ε_{max}	λ_{max}	ε_{max}
Benzene	184	46,700	202	6,920	255	170
Diphenyl	—	—	246	20,000	—	—
m-Terphenyl	—	—	252	44,700	—	—
p-Terphenyl	—	—	280	27,500	—	—
p-Tetraphenyl	—	—	300	38,900	—	—
Naphthalene	220	112,000	275	5,620	312	175
Anthracene	252	199,000	375	7,940	—	—
Naphthacene	278	126,000	473	11,200	—	—
Pentacene	310	282,000	580	15,800	—	—

conjugated systems, and the bands move to longer wavelengths and become stronger.

The polyacene series, benzene to pentacene, provide an excellent example of the effect of increasing length of a conjugated system on wavelength of absorption. As seen from Fig. 36, the similar fine structure of the longest wavelength band in each spectrum shows them to be analogous to the 255 mμ band of benzene, though increased in strength. Bands at 184 and 202 mμ in the benzene spectrum show similar effects.

Generally speaking, as the number of rings in a condensed ring hydrocarbon goes up, it absorbs increasingly in the visible range. The limit is reached with graphite, which absorbs throughout the visible region.

4. Heterocyclic systems

As seen in Table 13, the five-membered ring heterocyclics furan, thiophene and pyrrole absorb at shorter wavelengths than benzene. This may possibly be correlated with the fact that chemically they are more reactive, and less aromatic in character than benzene.

Turning to heterocyclic analogues of aromatic hydrocarbons, the most striking feature is that replacement of —CH= by

TABLE 13

SPECTRA OF HETEROCYCLIC SYSTEMS[4,52] AND SOME RELATED COMPOUNDS

Compound	λ_{max}	ε_{max}	λ_{max}	ε_{max}
Furan	205	6,000	—	—
Thiophene	235	4,500	—	—
Pyrrole	210	10,000	—	—
Benzene	255	230	—	—
Pyridine	250	2,000	—	—
Pyrimidine	243	3,000	275	300
Pyrazine	260	5,200	311	580
Stilbene (*trans*)	295	27,000	—	—
Benzalaniline	263	12,000	—	—
Azobenzene	319	20,000	445	300
Naphthalene	276	5,600	312	250
Quinoline	275	4,500	311	6,300
Isoquinoline	262	3,700	318	3,600
Anthracene	252	200,000	375	8,000
Acridine	252	170,000	347	7,900
Phenazine	250	120,000	370	1,600

—N=, or of —CH₂— by —NH— or —S— produces little change in wavelengths, though some intensification may result from reduction of the symmetry. Some examples are given in the table. The absorption of nitrogen compounds extends to rather longer wavelengths, partly because of additional weak $n \rightarrow \pi^*$ bands.

5. Systems with several chromophores

This brief survey of the spectra of organic compounds concludes with an indication of how several chromophores in the same molecule interact. Provided they are not insulated by such groups as —CH₂—, their individual bands are usually lost, and replaced by stronger bands at longer wavelengths. Even in cases where, formally, conjugation between two chromophores is possible, a further condition must be satisfied. It will be recalled that the formation of larger molecular orbitals depends on alignment of the axes of all the 2p orbitals perpendicular to the plane of the σ bond skeleton. This cannot happen if, for steric reasons, co-planarity is impossible. For example bulky ortho substituents in diphenyl cause its spectrum to revert to that of two isolated benzene rings. *Cis* and *trans* stilbene show the same effect. In the latter molecule, the rings are co-planar, whereas in the former co-planarity is prevented by the relatively close approach of two ortho hydrogen atoms. This causes *cis*-stilbene to absorb at 280 mμ ($\varepsilon = 13,500$) compared to 295 mμ ($\varepsilon = 27,000$) for the other isomer.

Dyestuff molecules often contain several conjugated chromophores. Owing to their complexity, no comprehensive quantum mechanical method has yet been evolved, by which their spectra can be calculated. Nevertheless considerable success has been achieved within certain classes of dye. For example, Brooker[5], using a form of the valence-bond theory, has explained many features of the spectra of cyanine dyes. Dewar[3] has used a modified molecular orbital method to account for the longest wavelength absorptions of many triphenyl methane dyes. In a comprehensive article on the relation between constitution and colour, Lewis and Calvin[6], regarding the electron cloud of a molecule as a two dimensional oscillator, made several valuable generalisations.

D. DETERMINATION OF ABSORPTION SPECTRA

Before applications to problems are discussed, a brief description of experimental methods will be given. Until about 1950, photographic methods of recording spectra were often used. However the conversion of a photographed spectrum to a curve of optical density against wavelength, which is usually required, is at best a laborious and inaccurate process. Accordingly, following recent great improvements in ultra-violet sensitive photocells, and electron multipliers, photographic techniques have been largely superseded by photoelectric methods of recording absorption spectra. Basically a photoelectric spectrophotometer consists of a light source, emitting continuously over the required range, a monochromator by which light of any given wavelength may be selected, a suitable cell containing the sample, and a detector to determine the proportion of light transmitted. The current from this detector is used in single-beam operation to indicate the percent transmission or optical density on a scale, and in double-beam instruments to operate a recorder. Spectra are obtained by selecting each wavelength in turn with the monochromator, and measuring the corresponding transmission or density.

1. Sources, detectors, cells and solvents

Since these matters are common to single and double beam spectrophotometers, they will be discussed first.

By far the commonest continuous source of ultra-violet light is the hydrogen discharge tube. Several designs of this lamp, which must of course be enclosed in a quartz envelope, have been marketed. The intensity is adequate from about 350 mμ, down to about 185 mμ, where atmospheric absorption curtails the range of most spectrophotometers. In the visible region a tungsten filament lamp is normally used. Spectrophotometers are usually fitted with both these sources, and provision is made for their interchange at about 360 mμ.

Many photoelectric instruments use, as detectors, photocells of the photoemissive (potassium and caesium oxide) types. Two such tubes cover the range from 200 to 800 mμ with good sensitivity. Recently, in recording instruments where a large detector output is desirable, electron multipliers have often replaced photocells. Multipliers are available which cover the near ultra-violet and visible regions, but if one wishes to extend the range of an instrument into the near infra-red, a second detector must be added, normally a lead sulphide photoconductive cell.

Sample cells present no major problems in electronic spectroscopy. They are often used in matched pairs, so that, if a solvent is used, its absorption, if any, will cancel out between sample and blank cells. Cell windows for the ultra-violet regions must be of optical quality quartz or silica, glass being opaque below

References p. 134

about 300 mμ. Thicknesses between 0.1 and 3 cm are normally used. Vertical cells of rectangular cross-section, with the windows fused to a glass body are easy to clean and suitable for most purposes. In quantitative work special precautions must be taken to prevent the evaporation of volatile solvent from the cell. Variable thickness micrometer cells, where the windows are held at an adjustable distance apart in a former of steel or other inert material, also have advantages, but are expensive.

Except in problems of impurity detection, it is usually essential greatly to dilute the sample with a transparent solvent to obtain bands of convenient intensity. Fortunately a wide range of solvents are transparent through the visible and much of the near ultra-violet range. The lower limits to which some common solvents can be used in a 1-cm cell are given in Table 14. Since unsaturated and aromatic impurities absorb strongly, it is vital that solvents be very pure.

TABLE 14

SOLVENTS FOR ELECTRONIC SPECTROSCOPY

Solvent	Quality	Useful limit (mμ)	Solvent	Quality	Useful limit (mμ)
Water	distilled	200	dioxan	purified	220
iso-Octane	S.P.*	200	ethyl acetate	S.P.	250
n-Hexane	S.P.	200	chloroform	B.P.	250
Cyclohexane	S.P.	200	carbon tetrachloride	A.R.	250
Methanol	A.R.	210	dimethyl formamide	distilled	270
Ether	—	220	benzene	A.R.	275

* S.P. = Spectroscopically pure.

Specially purified grades for spectroscopy may be bought, but for many purposes the cheaper A.R. or B.P. materials will suffice. Whilst it is uneconomical to purify crude solvent for spectroscopy, either chromatographic (p. 13) or chemical methods may be used to remove small amounts of impurity.

During purification the solvent should be checked at each stage by running the spectrum of a thick layer (about 3 cm). A good account of solvent purification is given in Ref.[7], p. 731.

It is noteworthy that water and the alcohols are possible ultra-violet solvents, whilst their use in the infra-red is very limited. For the reasons outlined in section B, most saturated aliphatics are reasonably suitable as ultra-violet solvents. If however a choice is available on solubility grounds, a non-polar rather than a polar solvent should be chosen, since sharper bands are usually found with the former type, and there is no danger of modification of the solute absorption by hydrogen bonding.

2. Single-beam manual photoelectric spectrophotometers

The first commercially available instrument of this type was the Beckman DU, which has been followed in Great Britain by the

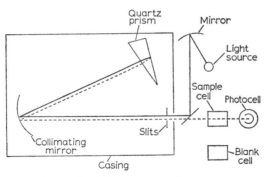

Fig. 37. Single-beam spectrophotometer.

Hilger Uvispek and the Unicam S.P. 600 spectrophotometers. All these use quartz prism monochromators, and are basically rather similar. More recently the Optica CF. 4 has been marketed, with a diffraction grating rather than a prism as its dispersing element.

Fig. 37 illustrates the optical layout of several prism spectro-photometers. Light from one of the sources is focussed by mirrors on to the entrance slit. A diverging beam from this is rendered parallel by the collimating mirror, and directed to the prism, which is of pure quartz. After reflection from the back of the prism, the light beam, now split up into a spectrum returns to the collimating mirror at a slightly different vertical angle. It is again focussed, giving a spectrum in the plane of the exit slit, which is vertically below the entrance slit. By turning the prism, light of any required wavelength in this spectrum can be made to fall on the exit slit and pass through it to the absorp-tion cell and detector.

In operating this type of instrument, the required wavelength is first selected by the appropriate knob. A cell full of solvent is then placed in the beam, causing a certain current from the photocell, which is balanced by adjusting a potentiometer till the indicating galvanometer reads zero. The solvent cell is now replaced by that containing the solution and the photocell current again balanced. By suitable arrangement of the electrical circuits, a scale to which the potentiometer is attached is made to read directly the transmission or optical density of the sample at the wavelength in question.

For quantitative analysis and routine checks on purity, where measurements at only a few wavelengths are required this type of instrument is eminently suitable. If however identifications or structural diagnoses are to be undertaken, the spectrum must be measured over a wide range of wavelengths. In this event the density may have to be measured at a hundred points or more, a laborious and time-consuming process. The answer to this difficulty is provided by automatic recording double-beam spectrophotometers.

3. Double-beam recording spectrophotometers

Whilst it is quite possible to adapt a single-beam instrument so as to obtain an automatic record of photocell output against wavelength, the result is not very satisfactory, since the output of the source varies with wavelength, and the spectrum is therefore superimposed on its wavelength–emission curve. Moreover cancellation of solvent absorption is no longer possible. Double-beam instruments have therefore been developed, in which light, after passing through the monochromator is split into two equivalent beams, of which one passes through the sample and the other through the solvent, before they are recombined on the detector.

The Cary Spectrophotometer (Applied Physics Corporation) is of this type, and has been available for several years. This instrument is built to a very searching specification and is therefore rather expensive. More recently several manufacturers including Beckman and Perkin-Elmer in America and Optica

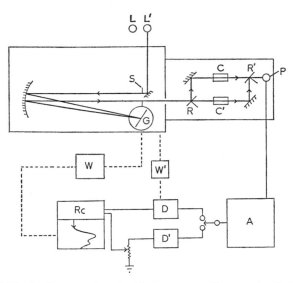

Fig. 38. Block diagram of a double-beam recording spectrophotometer (Optica CF4DR). L and L′ represent the light sources, S the slits, G the diffraction grating, R and R′ rotating mirrors, C and C′ the blank and sample cells, P the electronmultiplier, A the amplifier, D and D′ the reference and sample signal demodulators, Rc the recorder, and W and W′ the wavelength and slit drives.

United Kingdom, Unicam and Hilger in Great Britain have marketed cheaper instruments. Fig. 38 illustrates the optical and electronic arrangements of the Optica CF4DR, which, though using a grating rather than a prism is similar in principle to the others mentioned.

Light from one of the alternative sources passes first through a monochromator identical to that used in the corresponding single-beam instrument. On leaving the exit slit it enters the double-beam unit, where two rapidly rotating mirrors (R and R') pass the light alternately through the sample and blank cells several times per second. The electron multiplier output therefore carries two distinct alternating signals, which differ in phase and amplitude, corresponding to the light intensity transmitted by solvent and sample. These are amplified together, and then separated by an electronic switching circuit which operates in step with the rotating mirrors. Finally the two separated signals reach demodulators, where they are converted to two direct current voltages the ratio of which is indicated by the recorder. In operation the grating is rotated and the recorder chart is driven continuously by synchronous motors, so that a record is drawn of wavelength against percent transmission, or optical density if a special recorder is used. To ensure optimum performance throughout the spectrum, the slit width is varied continuously to maintain constant energy in the reference beam.

The outstanding merit of automatic recording instruments is their speed, which enables a spectrum with several peaks to be obtained in about ten minutes. It must however be stressed that for measuring optical densities to the highest possible accuracy in quantitative analysis, single-beam instruments remain superior.

E. APPLICATIONS OF ELECTRONIC SPECTROSCOPY

This section describes some straightforward applications which depend basically on direct comparison of spectra under investigation with those of known substances. In the absence of suitable comparison data, deduction of the chromophores present must be attempted by the methods of section F.

1. Identification by comparison

Two identical substances in the same solvent must of course yield the same spectrum. However the usefulness of this is limited, since the spectra of large molecules which differ only slightly in structure, may be very similar. Moreover electronic spectra sometimes consist of only two or three fairly wide, overlapping bands, and are therefore less useful for "finger-printing" molecules than infra-red spectra. This is illustrated by many of the spectra of Ref.[8].

Ultra-violet methods are however sometimes effective where infra-red techniques cannot be applied. For example, a substance available only as a dilute aqueous solution could readily be examined in the ultra-violet, but not in the infra-red region. Whereas dilute solutions are adequate for electronic spectroscopy, only undiluted samples or rather strong solutions are usable in the infra-red. Chromatographically separated fractions provide another case where electronic spectral measurements are straightforward, but infra-red work requires preliminary concentration.

The other limiting factor in spectroscopic identification is availability of reference spectra. Many hydrocarbon spectra have been published by the American Petroleum Institute, whilst a book by Friedel and Orchin[8] offers a valuable collection of organic spectra of all classes. Recently the well known Sadtler Collection[9] has been extended to the ultra-violet region. The essential features of these spectra have been coded on punched cards in such a way that an unknown may be identified by sorting the cards with regard to its peak wavelengths, provided its spectrum is in the Sadtler collection.

Generally speaking the chances of identifying an unknown from its electronic spectrum are greatly improved, if full use is made of other physical and chemical information. In restricted fields, where the chemical class of the unknown is already established, there is a much better prospect of success. This applies for example to carotenoids[10], and to polynuclear aromatic hydrocarbons, where Karr[11] has arranged many such compounds in order of their longest wavelength peak.

In conclusion it may be pointed out that, as with many other physical methods, identification is usually successful only when dealing with a fairly pure substance. Preliminary purification, for example by chromatography may therefore be essential.

2. Impurity detection

Electronic spectroscopy is a powerful method of impurity detection for two main reasons. Firstly the bands are often very intense, so that for example 0.005% of an impurity, the ε value of whose band is 2000 can readily be detected in a transparent major component. Also organic compounds can be divided fairly sharply into saturated compounds, with little absorption, and those with conjugated groups and hence strong bands. For example, from its normal method of preparation, the most likely impurity in cyclohexane is benzene, which can readily be detected by its absorption near 255 mμ. The successful manufacture of nylon depends on rigorous purification of the starting materials, hexamethylenediamine and adiponitrile. Traces of unsaturated and aromatic impurities in these interfere with the formation of long, unbranched chains which are vital to good quality polymer. Since the monomers are themselves transparent in the near ultra-violet, spectra provide an excellent method of detecting the undesirable impurities.

In suitable cases traces of unreacted monomer can be detected in a polymer. Since the styrene chromophore has one double bond more than that of polystyrene, the monomer absorbs more intensely and at longer wavelengths, and can therefore be detected.

By the same principle small numbers of unsaturated groups in the chains of polyvinyl alcohol and polyvinyl chloride can be seen. Campbell et al. for example[12], on the basis of the ultra-violet spectrum of thermally degraded polyvinyl chloride, deduced the presence of polyene units, formed by removal of hydrogen chloride from the polymer. Whilst pure polyvinyl alcohol, ($-CH_2 \cdot CHOH)_n$, would not be expected to show any near ultra-violet absorption, the product of polyvinyl acetate hydrolysis under certain conditions shows bands at 225, 280 and 330 mμ[13]. These can plausibly be attributed to oxidation of —CHOH— units to carbonyl, followed by elimination of water between the resulting activated methylene group and an adjoining hydroxyl group, giving units such as —CO·CH=CH—, —CO(CH=CH)$_2$—, and —CO(CH=CH)$_3$—.

Plasticisers, including dibutyl and other phthalates can be detected in poly(methyl methacrylate) by their benzenoid absorption, either by dissolving the polymer in chloroform, or by direct measurements on polymer sheet. Ultra-violet absorbers are often added to polythene and polystyrene to prevent degradation caused by the ultra-violet radiation in sunlight. These substances absorb near 300 mμ, and show readily in an ultra-violet spectrum.

3. Quantitative analysis

Whenever the electronic spectra of the components differ considerably, they offer a method for the quantitative analysis of mixtures. Because of band overlap the method is however often inferior to infra-red spectroscopy or gas chromatography. The simplest case arises when only one of the components, X, absorbs at some wavelength. Suppose the sample is diluted with a transparent solvent to a concentration w. Again the fundamental equation (p. 76)

$$d = \log_{10} I_0/I = kcl$$

is used. Since d may be measured, l is known, and k may be determined in a separate experiment using a pure specimen of X, its concentration, c, in the solution may be obtained, and divided by w to yield the proportion of X in the original sample.

In practice band overlap must normally be allowed for. Consider a mixture of two components in the proportion x/y. Two wavelengths, λ_1 and λ_2 are chosen, where the difference between the extinction coefficient of the two components is as

References p. 134

great as possible. If d_1 and d_2 are the corresponding optical densities of a solution, then

$$d_1 = k_1{}^1 xl + k_2{}^1 yl$$
$$d_2 = k_1{}^2 xl + k_2{}^2 yl$$

As before the four coefficients $k_1{}^1$ etc. may be measured in separate experiments on solutions of the pure components. There remain two unknown concentrations x and y, which may be obtained by solving the two simultaneous equations.

This procedure may in principle be applied to any number of components (n), measuring the density at n wavelengths, and solving a set of n simultaneous equations of the type

$$d_i = k_1{}^1 xl + k_2{}^1 yl + k_3{}^1 zl + \dots.$$

In practice this is usually satisfactory only with binary or ternary mixtures, for two main reasons. Intermolecular interactions may cause failure of Beer's Law, causing the k's no longer to be true constants. Also small instrumental errors in the densities tend to be multiplied during solution of the equations, causing large errors. Attempts have recently been made[14,15] to avoid this difficulty by a more complicated method of calculation in which optical density measurements at a number of wavelengths much greater than n are used, and the best solution of the resulting equation is obtained with a computer.

Systems which have been analysed include mixtures of the three xylenes and ethyl benzene[16], anthracene in tar and tar oil fractions, naphthalene and methyl naphthalenes in oils, and small amounts of crotonaldehyde and acetaldehyde in vinyl acetate[17]. Several examples are described fully in Ref.[7], where the experimental details and difficulties are discussed.

4. Molecular weight determination

Electronic spectroscopy sometimes provides a convenient method of molecular weight determination. For example, many aromatic hydrocarbons and amines form picrates, which are stable enough to be purified by recrystallisation. Because of the loose chemical binding between the molecules, the absorption spectrum of picric acid is little affected by complex formation. In particular there is no change in the molecular extinction coefficient of the strong band near 380 mμ, which is not appreciably overlapped by the bands of hydrocarbons and amines. If then solutions of equal concentrations of picric acid (M.W. 229) and of a complex with a compound of molecular weight m, have optical densities d and d', with the same cell and solvent,

$$(229 + m)/229 = d/d'$$

or $$m = 229(d/d' - 1)$$

In the same way the molecular weights of aliphatic alcohols may be found by measurements on their solid esters with an aromatic acid such as β-(2,4-dinitrophenyl)propionic acid, which has a strong band at 242 mμ, well clear of any alcohol absorption. The 2,4-dinitrophenyl hydrazones can be used similarly with aliphatic aldehydes and ketones, although in this case the accuracy is less, because the extinction coefficient of the hydrazone is somewhat dependent on the particular carbonyl compound.

F. STRUCTURAL DIAGNOSIS BY ELECTRONIC SPECTROSCOPY

Where identification by the method E1 is impracticable, much information about an unknown structure may nevertheless be obtainable from the spectrum. Even in the extreme case where nothing is known on chemical grounds about the structure, certain inferences can be drawn, by using the extensive data which has been accumulated about the band positions and intensities of chromophores. If, for example, the unknown has no appreciable absorption between 200 and 800 mμ, it may be an aliphatic or alicyclic hydrocarbon, alcohol, ether, acid or ester. A weak structureless band near 280 mμ suggests an aldehyde or ketone, but care must be taken in drawing such inferences, since the band could also be caused by a small amount of an intensely absorbing impurity. Similarly a strong band between 220 and 300 mμ might be due to a two, three or

References p. 134

four unit conjugated system, whilst a medium intensity band with fine structure near 260 mμ indicates a benzene ring.

It is however only rarely that much progress is made with the elucidation of an unknown structure by these methods. Spectra are normally valuable only when sufficient chemical and other physical work has been done for possible structures to be suggested. It may happen that the structures have fairly large chromophoric units whose spectra are not much affected by their molecular surroundings. The presence or absence of such units can then be decided by comparison with simpler compounds containing the same chromophores.

When there are several possibilities, the positions and intensities of their bands can sometimes be predicted, and compared with the observed spectrum. This procedure has been particularly valuable with alkaloids, terpenes, steroids and other natural products, where the proposed structures contain double bonds which may or may not be conjugated. The examples below illustrate these methods. Many other examples have been collected in Ref.[10] (Chapter 14) and in Ref.[4] (Chapter 4).

1. Structures with one double bond

Occasionally problems can be settled by observing the absorption of an unconjugated double bond. Some light is thrown on the structure of chloral hydrate by its spectrum. Anhydrous chloral in hexane shows the expected carbonyl band at 290 mμ ($\varepsilon = 33$), but in aqueous solution no such band is found. The inference is that chloral hydrate has structure II rather than I

$$CCl_3 \cdot CHO \cdot H_2O$$

$$CCl_3 \cdot \overset{\displaystyle H}{\underset{\displaystyle OH}{C{-}OH}}$$

I   II

2. Structures with two double bonds

It is easy to say from the spectrum whether or not two double bonds are conjugated. For example there are two isomers, III and IV, of mesityl oxide, the self-condensation product of acetone.

$$CH_3-C=CH\cdot COMe \qquad\qquad CH_2=C-CH_2\cdot COMe$$
$$| \qquad\qquad\qquad\qquad\qquad\qquad |$$
$$CH_3 \qquad\qquad\qquad\qquad\qquad CH_3$$
$$III \qquad\qquad\qquad\qquad\qquad IV$$

Structure III is assigned to the compound with a maximum at 235 ($\varepsilon = 12{,}000$) and IV to the one with no strong absorption above 220 mμ.

As already mentioned (p. 93), the degree of interaction even in cases where formally two double bonds are conjugated, may vary. For example there is a marked difference between the band maxima of alicyclic dienes (λ_{max} about 250 mμ, ε about 5000) compared to straight chain and exocyclic dienes (λ_{max} about 225, ε about 10,000)[10]. This has found important applications in the terpene field. For example the correct formulae can be assigned to the isomers α- and β-phellandrene on this basis:

α-Phellandrene
$\lambda_{max} = 263$ mμ, $\varepsilon = 2500$

β-Phellandrene
$\lambda_{max} = 231$ mμ, $\varepsilon = 9000$

Abietic and laevopimaric acids are isomers, where chemical methods have elucidated the ring system, and shown that both molecules have two double bonds. Their absorption spectra show the probable locations of these bonds.

Abietic acid
$\lambda_{max} = 238$ mμ, $\varepsilon = 16000$

Laevopimaric acid
$\lambda_{max} = 273$ mμ, $\varepsilon = 7000$

References p. 134

3. Structural diagnosis by finding the length of a conjugated system

The structures of α- and β-ionone may be assigned on the grounds that the α-isomer shows a peak at 228 mμ ($\varepsilon = 14{,}000$) indicating two conjugated bonds, whilst β-ionone has a band at 296 mμ ($\varepsilon = 11{,}000$) showing a longer conjugated system.

α-Ionone   β-Ionone

A rather similar situation arose with the mould product patulin. Formula V was originally suggested on chemical grounds. Having only a two unit chromophore, this would not be expected to absorb above 260 mμ. Partly in view of a band at 276 mμ ($\varepsilon = 16{,}000$), Woodward and Singh[18] suggested the alternative formula VI, which was subsequently confirmed by synthesis.

V   VI

4. Structural diagnosis by analogy

When carbon disulphide reacts with acetaldehyde ammonia, the most likely structures for the product, carbothialdine, are VII and VIII

VII	VIII	IX	X
$\lambda_{max} = 288$,	$\varepsilon = 12{,}800$	$\lambda_{max} = 217$	$\lambda_{max} = 276$, $\varepsilon = 1($
and $\lambda_{max} = 243$,	$\varepsilon = 5{,}000$	$\varepsilon = 8000$	and $\lambda_{max} = 246$, $\varepsilon = 8$

No decision on chemical grounds is possible. However comparison with the spectra of the simple compounds IX and X, which carry the same chromophores as VII and VIII leaves little doubt that VII is the correct structure. Interaction of the nitrogen lone-pair electrons with the C=S unit no doubt accounts for the long-wavelength absorption.

Degradation of the antibiotic terramycin yields an acid, decarboxyterracinoic acid for which probable structures are

The point was settled by its ultra-violet spectrum, which was very similar to that of 5-hydroxy indanone, but quite different from that of the 7 compound, favouring structure XII.

As a final example, the contribution of ultra-violet spectroscopy in elucidating the structure of Vitamin K may be mentioned. Bands near 250 and 330 mμ suggested a naphthaquinone nucleus, the presence of which was confirmed by the replacement of these bands by one near 230 mμ on reductive acetylation. Comparison with the spectra of several alkyl naphthaquinones showed the compound to be a 2:3-dialkyl derivative. Its structure was finally shown to be 2-methyl-3-phytyl-1:4-naphthaquinone.

G. STUDY OF EQUILIBRIA IN SOLUTION

Since the majority of solvents are transparent in the visible, and part of the ultra-violet region, electronic spectroscopy provides an excellent method of studying equilibria, whenever the components absorb at reasonably long wavelengths. This section describes applications to acid-base equilibria, tautomeric systems, molecular complexes, and cis-trans isomerism.

1. Acid–base equilibria

With most aromatic acids and bases, the spectrum is appreciably changed by addition of a proton to the basic form. Spectrophotometric methods compare favourably with the conventional conductivity and electromeric techniques for accurate determination of acid–base equilibrium constants, particularly with very weak acids and bases. Consider the equilibrium

$$B + H^+ \rightleftharpoons BH^+$$

and suppose that at some wavelength where the spectra of B and BH^+ differ considerably, one measures the optical density of the compound at the same concentration, C_0, and cell thickness, in a strongly acid medium where only BH^+ is present, in alkali with B only, and in some buffer of intermediate known pH. Then if ε_A and ε_B are the extinction coefficients of BH^+ and B, one has in the acid, alkaline and intermediate solutions,

$$d_{acid} = \varepsilon_A \cdot C_0 \cdot l,$$

$$d_{alk.} = \varepsilon_B \cdot C_0 \cdot l$$

and $d_{buffer} = \varepsilon_B \cdot C_B \cdot l + \varepsilon_A \cdot C_{BH^+} \cdot l$, with $C_0 = C_B + C_{BH^+}$

Algebraic combination of these with the definitions

$$pK_A = -\log K_A = -\log \frac{[B][H^+]}{[BH^+]} \text{ and } pH = -\log[H^+],$$

leads readily to the condition that

$$pK_A = pH + \log \frac{(d_{buffer} - d_{alk.})}{(d_{acid} - d_{buffer})}$$

A careful application of this method is described by Brown et al.[19], who wished to measure accurately the fairly small changes of base strength caused by adding alkyl groups to the pyridine nucleus. Each base was measured in $N/10$ HCl, $N/10$ NaOH and in two buffer solutions, at four different wavelengths. Accordingly eight equations of the above type were available in each case, and, by averaging, high accuracy was assured. A correction was also applied for the small errors due to neglect of activity coefficients in the above treatment.

The method was also chosen by Gage[20] in an attempt to correlate the basicities of several alkyl-aryl diguanidines based on the structure

$$
\begin{array}{ccc}
NH & & NH \\
\| & & \| \\
C_6H_5 - NH - C - NH - C - NH_2,
\end{array}
$$

with their antimalarial activities. His results showed that these compounds are diacid bases, and that at physiological pH values, they are normally present as singly charged cations. A recent paper by Biggs *et al.* reports data on many substituted phenols and anilines[53].

One of the most important applications of light absorption in this connection was the determination by Hammett *et al.*[21] of the pK values of very weak bases. Many substances, including mono-, di- and tri-nitro-anilines, chloronitroanilines, benzal acetophenone, benzoic acid, acetophenone and anthraquinone, though too weak to behave as bases in water, have been shown by freezing point measurements in sulphuric acid to be strong bases in this solvent, ionising according to the equation

$$ B + H_2SO_4 \rightleftharpoons BH^+ + HSO_4^- $$

With carbonyl compounds the proton adds on to the carbonyl oxygen atom. This raises the possibility of measuring their pK values in some mixture of water and sulphuric acid, where they are partially ionised. Conductiometric and electrometric methods being clearly inapplicable in such media, Hammett used the changes in light absorption which accompany conversion of a base to its conjugate acid. Where the basic form is coloured and the acid colourless, colorimetric methods were used, but otherwise ultra-violet absorption spectra were measured to obtain the equilibrium constants.

2. Tautomeric equilibria

In many tautomeric systems, one form has a more highly conjugated chromophore, and hence stronger ultra-violet absorption than the other. The classical example is ethyl acetoacetate, where the equilibrium is

$$CH_3 \cdot CO \cdot CH_2 \cdot COOEt \rightleftharpoons CH_3 \cdot C(OH) = CH \cdot COOEt$$

$$\lambda = 275 \text{ m}\mu, \ \varepsilon = 16 \qquad \lambda = 244 \text{ m}\mu, \ \varepsilon = 16{,}000$$

and the keto form has only the weak $n \rightarrow \pi^*$ band of an isolated carbonyl group, whilst the $-CH=CH-C=O$ unit of the enol absorbs strongly. Consequently a measure of the proportion of the tautomers at equilibrium in various solvents can be obtained from the strength of the 244 mμ band. In hexane, ether and alcohol for example the percentages of enol are respectively 51, 32 and 12. Similar methods can be applied to other aceto-esters and to enolisable diketones.

An interesting related example arises from the controversy as to whether sugars in solution have an open chain (XIII) or a cyclic structure (XIV):

$$HO \cdot CH_2 \cdot (CHOH)_4 \cdot CHO \qquad \overset{\displaystyle O}{\overline{HO \cdot CH_2 \cdot CH \cdot (CHOH)_4}}$$

$$\text{XIII} \qquad\qquad\qquad \text{XIV}$$

From studies of the carbonyl band near 280 mμ[22], it has been shown that with d-glucose in neutral aqueous solution there is less than 0.01% of open chain form, but that in strong acid this may rise to 0.1%.

Passing to aromatic compounds, the tautomeric properties of the rubber accelerator 2-mercaptobenzthiazole have been studied[23]:

Here it is impossible to associate specific bands with the $C=S$ and $C=N$ groups, but, as reference compounds, the corre-

sponding N-methyl and S-methyl derivatives can be synthesised
by unambiguous routes. Comparison of their spectra with that
of mercaptobenzthiazole in alcohol, benzene and chloroform
leaves no doubt that in these solvents almost exclusively the
thione form is present. Only in alkaline solution does the
equilibrium pass to the left, presumably because of the acidity
of the thiol group.

Fig. 39. The effect of solvent on the tautomerism of benzene-azo-β-naphthol[24].

Burawoy and his co-workers[24] have studied azo-hydrazo
tautomerism in benzene-azo-naphthol derivatives. Fig. 39 shows
the spectrum of benzene-azo-β-naphthol in four solvents, the
equilibrium being

Clearly there are wide differences in the positions of equilibrium. Since both OH and NH groups are involved in internal hydrogen bonding, external bonds to solvent molecules do not play an important role, and the equilibrium position is determined mainly by the dielectric constant of the solvent, increase of which favours the more polar hydrazo form. In agreement with this, the proportions of hydrazone increase in the order hexane < benzene and ethanol < chloroform < acetic acid < water.

An interesting comparison was made between these equilibrium positions, and those of the corresponding 4-arylazo-1-naphthols. Here, in the absence of internal bonding, an important factor is the greater tendency of an OH than a NH group to form external hydrogen bonds. Consequently the proportion of azo form is anomalously high in, for example, ethanol. The effect is even more marked on introducing an *ortho* substituent which prevents sterically external bonding of the NH group of the hydrazone. Thus, although 4-(*o*-chlorophenylazo)-1-naphthol is mainly hydrazone in hexane and benzene, a considerable amount of azo form can be detected in the more polar ethanol, as a result of preferential hydrogen bonding to solvent molecules.

3. Molecular complex formation

Since comparatively weak intermolecular forces considerably affect the energies of the electrons mainly responsible for electronic absorption, spectra provide a sensitive method for the study of complex formation. When two substances are mixed in solution, their spectra are normally additive and any marked deviation from this indicates complex formation.

A good example is afforded by the work of Derbyshire and Peters[25] on mixed solutions of the dyes Chlorazol Sky Blue FF and Chrysophenine G. As shown in Fig. 40, the observed spectrum of a fifty-fifty mixture differs considerably from half the sum of the two individual spectra. Measurements on solutions with an excess of Sky Blue FF gave curves which could plausibly be ascribed to a 1:1 complex plus excess free dye.

With Chrysophenine G in excess however, the authors concluded that other complexes, with two or more moles of this dye to one of the other, were also present. Clearly complex formation is a possible source of error in analyses of dyestuff mixtures in solution by spectroscopy.

Fig. 40. Spectra of aqueous solutions of Chrysophenine G and Chlorazol Sky Blue FF.
  (i) Chlorazol Sky Blue FF (0.02 g/l)
 (ii) Chrysophenine G (0.02 g/l)
(iii) Sum of (i) and (ii)
(iv) Mixture of (i) and (ii) (total concentration 0.04 g/l).

It has long been known that the colours of solutions of iodine in various solvents differ. One suggested explanation is in terms of solvent-iodine complexes. This was first investigated systematically by Benesi and Hildebrand[26]. They found that, not only did the peak absorption position in the visible vary, but, in aromatic solvents, an intense band between 280 and 350 mμ appeared, which had no analogue in aliphatic solvents. They attributed this to iodine-aromatic ring complexes, and made precise studies with various concentrations of iodine and benzene derivatives, in the inert solvent carbon tetrachloride. Deducing from the direct proportionality of the intensity of the new band in pure benzene to the iodine concentration, that the equilibrium is of the type

$$I_2 + B \rightleftharpoons I_2B$$

they derived the equation

$$[I_2]l/\log I_0/I = 1/K[A] + 1/\varepsilon_c$$

where $[I_2]$ and $[A]$ are the initial concentrations of iodine and hydrocarbon, K the equilibrium constant, l the cell length and ε_c the extinction coefficient of the complex. On plotting $[A]$ against $[I_2]/\log I_0/I$, ε_c and K could be obtained from the slope and intercept of the line. A more rigorous derivation of equilibrium constants from data of this kind[27] has provided substantial confirmation of the work. Much data has now been collected on the equilibrium constants of complexes of halogens with aromatic hydrocarbons. This has a bearing on the mechanism of halogenations, and has provided theoretical chemists with valuable data to test their theories about the bonds holding complexes together.

Self association of dyes in concentrated solution sometimes causes spectral changes. For example an alcoholic solution of pseudocyanine

where the dye is monomeric, absorbs at 525 mμ. In dilute aqueous solution, this band and another at 485 mμ indicate a monomer-dimer equilibrium, but in concentrated solution a new sharp band at 573 mμ is found. The last band has been attributed to polymers, in which the molecules are held together, as in a stack of coins, by Van der Waals forces. In the biological field complexes of dyes with proteins have been studied spectroscopically, in connection with photosynthesis[28].

Absorption spectra have been used extensively to study metal chelation in solution (Ref.[29], Chapter 2). In favourable cases not only can the proportions of metal ion and chelate in the complex be determined, but the stability constant may be calculated. Where the chelate gives a new band little overlapped by those of the parent ion, it has been shown by Job[30], that, for a constant total concentration of metal plus chelating agent, the concentration of complex, (and hence the band intensity), reaches a maximum when the components are brought together in the ratio in which they exist in the complex. For example it was shown by this method[31] that in the complex of uranyl ion and sulphosalicylic acid, metal and chelating agent are in the ratio 1:1. The derivation of stability constants from spectra is described in Ref.[29] (Chapter 3).

4. Cis-trans isomerism

In simple compounds with one double bond, where the barrier to rotation about the bond is high, *cis* and *trans* isomers are usually well defined compounds, which can be isolated and purified, and show different melting points and other physical properties. On the contrary, in conjugated systems such as carotenoids, stilbenes, and aromatic azo compounds, the carbon-carbon or nitrogen-nitrogen double bonds have a fair amount of single bond character, rendering *cis-trans* interconversion much easier. Other isomers therefore revert to the most stable one, usually the all-trans form. These unstable isomers are nevertheless of great importance in photochemical reactions, and occasionally cause problems with commercial azo dyes, where the *cis* and *trans* forms may have different shades.

Unstable isomers of conjugated systems are usually made by intense illumination of a solution of the stable form. By a mechanism which has been discussed by Wyman[32] a meta-stable equilibrium may then be set up, containing a relatively high proportion of the unstable form. On removal of the illumination, the *cis* isomer reverts to *trans* at a rate which is often slow enough for its spectrum to be measured normally. Alternatively the spectrum of the unstable species may be measured[33] with a rotating shutter so arranged that the sample is irradiated and measured simultaneously. The spectra of *cis* and *trans* forms often differ sufficiently to provide a good method of characterisation.

Having observed striking changes in the spectrum of a solution of benzalacetophenone ($C_6H_5 \cdot CH = CH \cdot CO \cdot C_6H_5$) on irradiation, Lutz and Jordan[34] inferred that a cis isomer was being formed, and eventually managed to isolate it by low temperature crystallisation. Fig. 41 shows the great difference

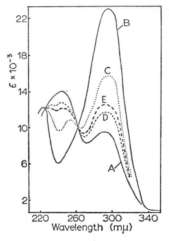

Fig. 41. Spectra of benzalacetophenone solutions[34]: (A) cis isomer; (B) trans isomer; (C) trans isomer exposed to sunlight for two minutes; (D) cis isomer exposed to sunlight for two minutes; (E) either isomer exposed to sunlight for twelve minutes.

between the *cis* and *trans* spectra, and illustrates the value of spectroscopy in following the effect of light on the pure isomers. Clearly in sunlight an equilibrium is set up in which the rate at which *cis* molecules are formed by light absorption equals their rate of thermal decay.

In the dyestuffs field thioindigo and its derivatives show *cis-*

trans phenomena. Solutions of the dyes were irradiated for five to ten minutes with light of various colours[35], and their absorption spectra measured immediately afterwards. These spectra showed marked differences which were explained by postulating varying degrees of *trans* to *cis* conversion. Since in these dyes reversion to the stable form was rather slow, it proved possible to isolate the cis form by chromatography of an irradiated solution. Fig. 42 shows the spectra of the pure *cis* and *trans* isomers of thioindigo, and of the trans after illumination with blue, green and yellow light. Clearly the degree of conversion to cis depends on the wavelength. The different proportions of

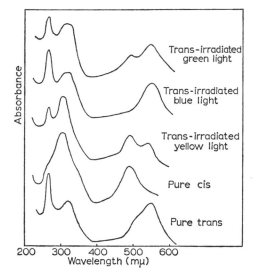

Fig. 42. Effect of irradiation on thioindigo in chloroform[32].

isomers in the three cases were explained by supposing that the maximum conversion is achieved with light rich in the wavelength of the longest wavelength band of the stable isomer.

References p. 134

Most indigo derivatives on the contrary exhibit no *cis-trans* effects, probably because of internal hydrogen bonding,

which greatly stabilises the trans form. In support of this explanation, N,N'-dimethyl and N,N'-diacetyl indigo behave much as thioindigo.

Cis-trans isomerism about the $N=N$ bond has been observed in many azo compounds and dyes. The cis forms of azobenzene and many of its alkyl, halogen and nitro derivatives are stable enough to be separated from irradiated solutions by chromatography. Solutions of 2-hydroxy azobenzene and similar compounds show no change of spectrum on illumination, no doubt because the trans form is again stabilised by internal hydrogen bonding.

Atherton and Peters[36] measured the rates and energies of activation of the *cis* → *trans* dark reaction for several substituted benzene-azo-β-naphthols. Activation energies of about 20 kcals. per mole were found. They also investigated the phototropic behaviour of the azo dye Chrysophenine G,

in which isomerism about the $N=N$ bond takes place in light. It has been found that the spectrum of this and several other azo dyes in solution, or dyed on to cellulose acetate (where they probably go in to solid solution) change appreciably on irradiation. This has obvious practical consequences. Cellulose dyed with Chrysophenine G shows on the contrary no change of spectrum under illumination, probably because the trans form is too firmly anchored to the cellulose chains by hydrogen bonds between azo and hydroxyl groups, for a *trans* → *cis* change to be possible.

H. SPECTROSCOPIC DETERMINATION OF REACTION RATES

If the spectra of the products of a reaction differ significantly from those of the starting materials, spectroscopy is often the best method of following the reaction. In this connection the visible and ultra-violet regions have advantages over the infrared, in that those solvents in which reactions are normally studied are transparent.

1. Experimental methods

Broadly speaking there are two possible approaches, the first by removing samples periodically from a reaction vessel, treating them so as to stop the reaction, and then measuring their spectra. This procedure requires no modification of a standard spectrophotometer, and is normally to be preferred if the reaction is fairly slow, and a reagent is available to stop further reaction in the withdrawn samples.

With fast reactions it is obviously better to place the reacting mixture directly in the spectrophotometer beam. Should the reaction be very rapid, or if a single beam instrument is to be used, one wavelength should be selected, preferably the peak of a band due to one of the products, where the reactants do not absorb, or a band which disappears during the reaction. By frequent optical density measurements at this wavelength, or in the case of a recording instrument, by allowing the chart to run with the wavelength fixed, the change in concentration of one of the compounds can be followed continuously. When automatic equipment is available, the spectrum can be scanned in ten minutes or less. It may then be advisable to run through the spectrum as frequently as possible, so that bands due to more than one component may be followed, and cross-checks obtained on the concentration variations.

Direct spectroscopic studies create certain practical difficulties.

For accurate work one must fit into the very limited space of the instrument's cell compartment a small thermostat, and a cell with provision for stirring and introduction of the reagents. Suitable thermostats consisting essentially of a metal block, which can be heated electrically to a thermostatically controlled temperature, have been described. A good example of the type of cell required is given in Ref.[38].

In view of these difficulties another possibility merits consideration. The reaction may be carried out in a large well-stirred, thermostatted vessel, from which a small volume of liquid is circulated through a cell in the spectrometer beam.

2. Typical applications

A simple reaction which can very conveniently be followed spectroscopically is the isomerisation of α-phenyl allyl alcohol,

$$C_6H_5 \cdot CH(OH) \cdot CH = CH_2 \rightarrow C_6H_5 \cdot CH = CH \cdot CH_2OH$$

in an acidified dioxane–water mixture[39]. At 50°C with $N/10$ HCl, the reaction is slow enough for samples to be withdrawn at twenty minute intervals, quenched in buffer solution, and their optical density at 251 mμ measured. As the product, having a double bond conjugated with a benzene ring absorbs much more strongly at this wavelength than the other isomer, the density increase enables the reaction to be followed. The equation for a first order reaction may be written

$$k = \frac{2.303}{t} \log_{10} \frac{a}{(a - x)}$$

a being the initial concentration, and x the amount of product found after time t. If d_0 and d_∞ are the initial and final optical densities in a cell of suitable thickness, $(d_\infty - d_0)$ is proportional to a, and $(d_\infty - d_t)$ proportional to $(a - x)$, so the equation may be written

$$k = \frac{2.303}{t} \log_{10} \frac{(d_\infty - d_0)}{(d_\infty - d_t)},$$

and values of the rate constant obtained at various times and averaged.

Vat dyeing is usually carried out by reducing the quinone form of the dye to its leuco (hydroquinone) form by stirring a suspension of the insoluble quinone with aqueous hydrosulphite solution. Marshall and Peters[38] measured the rates of reduction

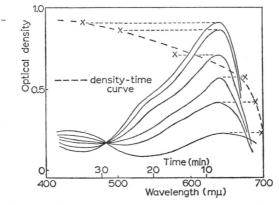

Fig. 43. The use of spectrophotometry to follow the reduction of Caledon Jade Green. The strong peak near 640 mμ which grows with increasing time is due to the leuco derivative[38].

of several vat dyes under these conditions, since the process is by no means instantaneous, and its rate is clearly of commercial importance. Since the bands, in the visible region, of soluble leuco compounds were much stronger than those of the initial suspension, they used spectrophotometry to follow the reaction. Fig. 43 shows typical curves obtained with Caledon Jade Green, on a Hardy Recording Spectrophotometer. The band near 650 mμ due to the leuco form increases with time, and, as shown in the figure, a curve connecting degree of reduction with time can readily be obtained.

Other examples are quoted by Gillam and Stern[10]. Autoxidation of fatty acids has been shown to proceed via an intermediate conjugated system, and the acid catalysed isomerisation of various vinylethynyl carbinols.

$$CH_2=CH \cdot CHOH - CH=CH_2 \rightarrow CH_2=CH - CH=CH \cdot CH_2OH$$

References p. 134

4-Nitroanilines (in 96% ethanol)	λ_{max}	ε_{max}	Anilines (in iso-octane)
H	376	15,500	H
3-Me	374	13,200	2-Me
2,3-di-Me	382	9,750	2,4,6-tri-Me
3,5-di-Me	385	4,840	2-t-butyl
2,3,5,6-tetra-Me	396	1,560	2,4,6-tri-t-butyl
3,5-di-t-butyl	401	540	2,6-di-t-butyl

has been followed. Kinetic studies of the very rapid decomposition of oxyhaemoglobin by reducing agents have been carried out with special apparatus.

I. DETECTION OF STERIC HINDRANCE

It has already been pointed out (p. 94) that complete conjugation of two or more chromophores or auxochromes is possible only in planar structures. Prevention of coplanarity by steric factors is reflected in the spectrum. Spectroscopic methods are therefore sometimes useful in deciding whether anomalous reaction rates and base strengths can be attributed to steric hindrance.

Two kinds of behaviour have been observed[40], and referred to as type 1 and type 2. Type 1 is exemplified by alkyl derivatives of *p*-nitroaniline. This compound shows a band near 390 mμ, which has no counterpart in the spectra of aniline or nitrobenzene. It is therefore associated with strong interaction between the ring π electrons, the nitrogen lone-pair electrons, and those of the nitro group. On valence-bond theory the band occurs because of a large resonance contribution from the form

$$\overset{+}{H_2}N=\!\!\!=\!\!\!=\!\!\!=\!\!\!=NO_2^-$$

Because of the resulting double bond character of the C—N

λ_{max}	ε_{max}	N,N-dimethyl anilines (in iso-octane)	λ_{max}	ε_{max}
234	9,130	H	251	15,500
234	8,800	2-Me	248	6,360
236	8,600	2,4,6-tri-Me	257	2,500
237	7,850	2-t-butyl	250	630
242	8,750			
240	6,900			

links, rotation about them is restricted, and both the amino and nitro groups, though not rigidly held in the plane of the ring, will oscillate about the plane. At a given instant therefore a large proportion of the molecules will be uniplanar, so that the 390 mμ band, corresponding to a high degree of conjugation, is strong.

Consider now the effect of alkyl substituents on the band, as set out in Table 15[41]. Clearly methyl and t-butyl groups, particularly when *ortho* to the nitro group, weaken the band but do not greatly affect its wavelength. In the extreme case, that of the 3,5-di-t-butyl compound, the strength falls to 3% of its initial value. The explanation lies in a reduction of the number of planar molecules at a given moment, through steric interaction between the nitro group and the substituent. With for example a t-butyl group, the nitro group will now oscillate about a plane far removed from that of the ring, so that the chance of absorption by a planar molecule, contributing to the 390 mμ band, is small, and the band weak.

Similar effects have been found with nuclear alkylated anilines, and N,N-dimethylanilines. From the data in the table, it appears that bulky ortho alkyl groups do not interfere with an amino group. Even a single ortho methyl however pushes a dimethylamino group from the plane of the ring, an effect which is even more pronounced with the t-butyl derivatives. An interesting comparison of these spectroscopic changes with base strength variations is given by Wepster[41].

In cases of more severe hindrance (type 2 behaviour), the band is not only weakened, but is also shifted to shorter wavelengths. The diphenyls provide an example of this. Beavan[42] has reported the spectra of many methyl and *t*-butyl substituted diphenyls. In the absence of substituents *ortho* to the ring junction, the spectra differ little from that of diphenyl itself, the main feature of which is an intense band near 260 mμ, associated with a measure of ring co-planarity. As shown by Fig. 44, one *ortho* methyl group slightly shifts and weakens the band, two profoundly affect it, and four methyl or two *t*-butyl groups completely remove the conjugation band, the spectrum becoming similar to twice that of hexamethyl benzene. Clearly in the last case co-planarity has become quite impossible, the rings being forced to lie in perpendicular planes.

Another example, from the field of azo dyes, has been described by Brode[37]. This concerns a series of benzidine dyes,

Fig. 44. Spectra of diphenyls[42]: (1) unsubstituted; (2) 2,2′-dimethyl; (3) decamethyl; (4) 2 × hexamethylbenzene; (5) 2-methyl.

where the strong band near 450 mμ (Fig. 45) results from conjugation through the four benzene rings and two azo groups. Methyl groups in the central rings destroy the co-planarity necessary for this, causing disappearance of the band, and its replacement by a spectrum at shorter wavelengths, almost equal to twice that of an isolated half of the molecule.

Fig. 45. Steric effects on spectra of azo dyes[37].

J. SPECTRA OF TRANSIENT SPECIES

The molecules of the majority of stable organic compounds are uncharged species, whose electrons occupy energy levels in pairs, the spins of which are in opposite directions (anti-parallel). Under the influence of intense illumination, a rearrangement of the electrons sometimes takes place, yielding excited molecules of high energy. Although the life-times of these unstable species are seldom more than a few milliseconds, and high concentrations of them cannot normally be built up, their greatly enhanced reactivity nevertheless endows them with considerable importance as intermediates, particularly in photochemical reactions. Methods of detecting and characterising them are therefore required.

Possible effects of light on a molecule include the following:

(a) A covalent bond may break, giving two fragments called free radicals, each with one unpaired electron:

$$A : B \rightarrow A\cdot + B\cdot$$

Although electronic spectroscopy has been applied to their study, electron spin resonance spectroscopy is a more powerful tool for the purpose, and free radicals are further discussed in Chapter 7, where examples of their importance in chemistry are quoted. The latter technique however suffers from the disadvantage that a period of minutes is required to measure the spectrum. Where radical lifetimes are very short the electronic absorption method is therefore the only one available, since the spectrum in this region can be determined in a few milliseconds.

(b) The molecule may pass to an upper electronic state in which the spin of an outer electron becomes reversed, leading to a molecule with two unpaired electrons. This is in effect internal radical formation, and may crudely be written, for ethylene, as follows:

$$H_2C : : CH_2 \rightarrow H_2\dot{C} : \dot{C}H_2$$

Such molecules are said to be in the triplet state, the multiplicity of any state being defined as $2S + 1$, where S is the net spin of the electrons. Information about triplet molecules has been obtained almost exclusively from electronic spectra, as they are not normally amenable to electron resonance methods.

(c) Photoionisation may take place, yielding either a positive or a negative ion, or a free electron plus a positive ion:

$$A : B \rightarrow A^+ + :B^-$$

$$AB \rightarrow AB^+ + e$$

1. Experimental techniques with unstable molecules

Two distinct methods have been used. When radical or triplet molecules are formed by the action of light on solutions at room temperature, they survive only a few milliseconds before recombining or losing their excess energy to the solvent. One method of avoiding this is to replace conventional solvents by a rigid solvent or glass. Boric acid glasses have been used at ordinary temperatures for the purpose, but suffer from the disadvantage of being translucent, and therefore not very suitable spectroscopically. Most recent work has therefore been done in glasses formed by cooling suitable solvent mixtures in liquid nitrogen, whereupon they set to rigid glasses. It is of course essential to use a mixture which does not crystallise on cooling. Commonly used mixtures include EPA (five parts ether, five parts pentane and two parts alcohol), and isopentane

Fig. 46. Apparatus for flash photolysis.

plus methyl cyclohexane in the proportion of three to two. A great many organic compounds, when irradiated in rigid media, yield radicals and triplets which persist for long periods, and can be studied spectroscopically. Typical apparatus has been described by Norman and Porter[43]. Light from a mercury lamp is first admitted through the quartz windows of a Dewar, causing photolysis, after which the cell is turned through 90°, and the spectrum measured by passing light from a hydrogen discharge lamp through the cell and in to the spectrometer.

A more direct approach is the flash photolysis method, which can be applied to solutions at room temperature. Here a high concentration of transient species is formed instantaneously by subjecting the sample to an intense flash of light. The difficulty is to measure the spectrum during the few milliseconds between the conclusion of the photolysing flash, and the decay of the transients formed. This is accomplished (Fig. 46) by using two intense light flashes, of which the first, from a discharge tube lying parallel to the tube containing the substance under investigation in a carefully degassed solvent, causes photolysis. Electronic circuits cause a second flash tube to operate a few milliseconds later, light from which passes lengthwise through the tube into a spectrometer, where the spectrum is photographed. By taking a series of photographs, with increasing small intervals between the two flashes, the progressive weakening of the bands due to the transients may be followed, and their lifetimes deduced. This opens up the possibility of studying the kinetics of decay of a transient in various environments, and thus discovering its chemical properties.

2. Triplet state molecules

Since almost all chemical reactions involve unpairing of electrons, it seems likely that triplet formation, where unpairing takes place without actual breaking of bonds, may not infrequently be the first step in a reaction. It may also be significant that the lowest electronically excited state of a molecule is normally the lowest triplet level. This may be particularly important in biological processes, where the energy quanta are small. Another factor contributing to the importance of triplet molecules in kinetics is their lifetime, which, though short, is about a million times that of the excited singlet. Much higher concentrations may therefore be built up, increasing the chances of triplet reactions.

Many substances, particularly aromatic hydrocarbons and dyestuffs, exhibit phosphorescence with lifetimes of several seconds, when illuminated in a boric acid glass or rigid solvent. Largely as a result of the work of the school of Lewis[44], phosphorescence is now well understood. Light absorption first raises the molecule to an excited singlet state. Although many of these excited molecules lose their excess energy by thermal degradation, a certain number pass to the lowest triplet level, which is responsible for phosphorescence. Since the light emission accompanying the return from the triplet to the ground state is a forbidden process, the molecule spends a relatively long time in the triplet state. Emission of phosphorescent light may therefore continue for several seconds after removal of the illumination, in a rigid medium. Fig. 47 shows the relationship between these energy levels, and the emission of phosphorescence and fluorescence.

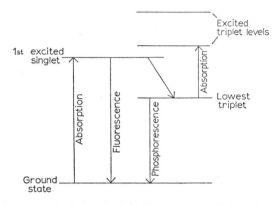

Fig. 47. Energy levels involved in fluorescence and phosphorescence.

The phosphorescent emission method is of limited scope in studying triplets, and has been largely replaced by flash photolysis. This has the advantage that the triplets may be formed in any required solvent at ordinary temperatures, and their reactivities toward various reagents obtained from the effects of the latter, on the lifetimes of the triplet molecules. A typical study is that of Porter and Windsor[45] on naphthalene, anthracene, phenanthrene, and many other condensed ring hydrocarbons in hexane. Provided the solvent was carefully freed from oxygen, excitation to the triplet level was observed in every case, and by taking a series of photographs at various times after the initial flash, the lifetimes of the excited molecules could be found. The decay of triplet anthracene under various conditions was studied, and was found to follow first-order kinetics. Dissolved oxygen had a profound effect on the lifetime, indicating a rapid reaction between molecular oxygen and triplet anthracene. Experiments in various solvents revealed a steady decrease of decay rate with increasing viscosity.

Many reactions in which triplet state intermediates have been postulated are described in Chapter 5 of Reid's book[46]. It is well established that certain *cis → trans* isomerisations, including those of maleic acid and diethyl maleate, proceed via a triplet mechanism. Other examples include the photoreduction of eosin Y with alkyl thiourea[47] and the photo-oxidation of zinc chlorin to the corresponding porphyrin by naphthoquinone. Chlorophyll has been shown readily to pass to a triplet level on irradiation. In connection with the photosynthesis of green plants the stability of triplet chlorophyll has been measured in the presence and absence of oxygen, quinone, carotene, and other reducing agents[48].

3. *Spectra of free radicals*

Both the rigid solvent and the flash photolysis methods have been used to obtain free radical spectra. Typical of the former approach is the work of Norman and Porter[43]. Using solutions in rigid solvents at the temperature of liquid nitrogen, they found that many compounds could be photolysed to yield radicals, stable enough under these conditions for their spectra to be recorded. Ethyl iodide split into ethyl radicals and iodine atoms. The colour of an iodine solution completely disappeared and returned on warming, showing the molecules to have been dissociated into atoms. Although benzene showed no evidence of radical formation, toluene, benzyl chloride and benzylamine all gave a spectrum with sharp bands at 318.7, 305.2, and 308.9 mμ, which was attributed to the benzyl radical. By irradiation of the corresponding compounds, spectra were used to characterise the radicals $p-CH_3 \cdot C_6H_4 \cdot CH_2^{\cdot}$, $(C_6H_5)_2CH^{\cdot}$ and $(C_6H_5)_3\dot{C}$. In the case of aniline, bands were found arising from both the radical $C_6H_5NH^{\cdot}$ and the ion $C_6H_2 \cdot \overset{+}{N}H_2$, whilst o-toluidine yielded both

Phenol and anisole gave identical spectra, probably due to the $C_6H_5 \cdot O^{\cdot}$ radical.

A recent application of flash photolysis in elucidating the mechanism of a photochemical reaction has been described by Porter and Bridge[49]. It has long been known that certain anthraquinone vat dyestuffs, on cellulosic fibres, catalyse oxidation of the fibre in sunlight, whilst themselves remaining unchanged. Clearly reactive transients are responsible, but their identification by chemical means has not proved possible. To simulate phototendering these authors flashed solutions of duroquinone in various solvents, and succeeded in identifying the transients formed. In liquid paraffin two new bands appeared, one of which, with a very short lifetime, was associated with triplet quinone molecules, and the other, of longer life, was attributed to a radical or radical ion formed by abstraction of a hydrogen atom from the solvent. The transient spectra found in ethanol depended on the pH of the solution. On the alkaline side, peaks at 415 and 438 mμ, decaying at the same rate, were assigned to the semi-quinone radical ion, by comparison with known spectra. Spectra from solutions in pure ethanol and acidified aqueous ethanol led to the conclusion that an equilibrium is set up between the semi-quinone radical and radical ion, following initial removal of a hydrogen atom from the solvent by an activated quinone molecule.

References p. 134

This work established clearly that the initial step in photo-tendering is removal of a hydrogen atom from cellulose by an excited dye molecule. Kinetic studies in liquid paraffin revealed no parallelism between the rates of decay of triplet molecules, and formation of radicals. Hence it seems likely that the latter arise from reactions between excited singlet molecules and the solvent.

4. Photo-ionisation

Mention must finally be made of the dissociation of organic molecules into ions by the action of light. An early example was observed by Lewis and Lipkin[50]. They irradiated tetra-phenylhydrazine at low temperatures in a rigid solvent. The solution developed colour, and gave a spectrum with three peaks, which were shown to correspond to three distinct species. By comparison with the spectra obtained by irradiating several molecules including $(C_6H_5)_3C \cdot N(C_6H_5)_2$, $(C_6H_5)_2N \cdot NO$, $(C_6H_5)_2N \cdot NH_2$ and $(C_6H_5)_2N \cdot Li$, it was shown that the three bands from tetraphenylhydrazine correspond to $(C_6H_5)_2N \cdot$, $(C_6H_5)_2N^+$ and $(C_6H_5)_2N \cdot N(C_6H_5)^+$.

It has recently been reported[51] that perylene, 3:4-benzpyrene, triphenyl, quaterphenyl and coronene, when irradiated in boric acid glass at room temperature become coloured, as a result of the formation of positive ions. On slowly heating the glasses, the colour disappears, with emission of phosphorescence.

REFERENCES

[1] C. A. COULSON, *Valence*, Oxford University Press, London, 1951.
[2] E. J. BOWEN, *Chemical Aspects of Light*, 2nd ed., Oxford University Press, London, 1946.

3 M. J. S. DEWAR in: *Recent Advances in the Chemistry of Colouring Matters*, Special Publication No. 4, The Chemical Society, London, 1956, p. 64.

4 E. A. BRAUDE in: *Determination of Organic Structures by Physical Methods*, Academic Press, New York, 1955, p. 147.

5 L. G. S. BROOKER, *Revs. Modern Phys.*, 14 (1942) 275; *Chem. Revs.*, 41 (1947) 325.

6 G. N. LEWIS AND M. CALVIN, *Chem. Revs.*, 25 (1939) 273.

7 C. R. N. STROUTS, J. H. GILFILLAN AND H. N. WILSON, *Analytical Chemistry*, Vol. II, Oxford University Press, London, 1955.

8 R. A. FRIEDEL AND M. ORCHIN, *Ultra-violet Spectra of Aromatic Compounds*, Wiley, New York, 1951.

9 Sadtler Research Laboratories, 1517 Vine St., Philadelphia 2, Penna, U.S.A.

10 A. E. GILLAM AND E. S. STERN, *Electronic Absorption Spectroscopy*, Arnold, London, 1954, p. 152.

11 C. KARR, *Appl. Spectroscopy*, 13 (1959) 15.

12 J. E. CAMPBELL AND W. H. RAUSCHER, *J. Polymer Sci.*, 18 (1955) 461.

13 M. MATSUMOTO, K. IMAI AND Y. KAZUSA, *J. Polymer Sci.*, 28 (1958) 426.

14 J. C. STERNBERG, H. S. STILLO AND R. H. SCHWENDEMAN, *Anal. Chem.* 32 (1960) 84.

15 R. P. BAUMAN, *Appl. Spectroscopy*, 13 (1959) 156.

16 R. R. GORDON AND H. POWELL, *J. Inst. Petrol.*, 31 (1945) 428.

17 C. CAPITANI AND E. MILANI, *Chim. e ind. Milan*, 37 (1955) 177.

18 R. B. WOODWARD AND G. SINGH, *Experientia*, 6 (1950) 238.

19 H. C. BROWN AND X. R. MIHM, *J. Am. Chem. Soc.*, 77 (1955) 1723.

20 J. C. GAGE, *J. Chem. Soc.*, (1949), 221.

21 L. P. HAMMETT, *Physical Organic Chemistry*, McGraw-Hill, New York, 1940.

22 E. PACSU AND L. A. HILLER, Jr., *J. Am. Chem. Soc.*, 70 (1948) 523.

23 H. P. KOCH AND J. FABIAN, *J. Chem. Soc.*, (1949), 405.

24 A. BURAWOY, A. G. SALEM AND A. R. THOMPSON, *Chem. & Ind. London*, (1952) 668; A. BURAWOY AND A. R. THOMPSON, *J. Chem. Soc.*, (1953) 1443.

25 A. N. DERBYSHIRE AND R. H. PETERS, *J. Soc. Dyers Colourists*, 72 (1956) 268.

26 H. A. BENESI AND J. H. HILDEBRAND, *J. Am. Chem. Soc.*, 71 (1949) 2703.

27 N. J. ROSE AND R. S. DRAGO, *J. Am. Chem. Soc.*, 81 (1959) 6138.

28 E. I. RABINOWITCH, *Photosynthesis*, Vol. II, Chapter 22, Interscience, New York, 1951.

29 A. E. MARTELL AND M. CALVIN, *Chemistry of Metal Chelate Compounds*, Prentice-Hall, New York, 1952.

30 P. JOB, *Ann. chim.*, (10) 9 (1928) 113; (11) 6 (1936) 97.

31 R. T. FOLEY AND R. C. ANDERSON, *J. Am. Chem. Soc.*, 71 (1949) 909.

[32] G. M. Wyman, *Chem. Revs.*, 55 (1955) 625.

[33] W. R. Brode, J. H. Gould and G. M. Wyman, *J. Am. Chem. Soc.*, 74 (1952) 4641.

[34] R. E. Lutz and R. H. Jordan, *J. Am. Chem. Soc.*, 72 (1950) 4300.

[35] G. M. Wyman and W. R. Brode, *J. Am. Chem. Soc.*, 73 (1951) 1487.

[36] E. Atherton and R. H. Peters in: *Recent Advances in the Chemistry of Colouring Matters*, Special Publication No. 4, The Chemical Society, London, 1956, p. 17.

[37] W. R. Brode, *ibid*, p. 1.

[38] W. J. Marshall and R. H. Peters, *J. Soc. Dyers Colourists*, 68 (1952) 289.

[39] R. P. Linstead, J. A. Elvidge and M. Whalley, *Modern Techniques of Organic Chemistry*, Butterworths, London, 1955, p. 29.

[40] E. S. Waight and R. L. Erskine in: *Steric Effects in Conjugated Systems*, (Ed. G. W. Gray), Butterworths, London, 1958, p. 73.

[41] B. M. Wepster, *ibid*, p. 82.

[42] G. H. Beavan, *ibid*, p. 22.

[43] I. Norman and G. Porter, *Proc. Roy. Soc. London*, A 230 (1955) 399.

[44] M. Kasha, *Chem. Revs.*, 41 (1947) 401.

[45] G. Porter and M. W. Windsor, *Discussions Faraday Soc.*, 17 (1954) 178.

[46] C. Reid, *Excited States in Chemistry and Biology*, Butterworths, London, 1957.

[47] G. Oster and A. H. Adelman, *J. Am. Chem. Soc.*, 78 (1956) 913.

[48] E. Fujimori and R. Livingstone, *Nature*, 180 (1957) 1036.

[49] G. Porter and N. K. Bridge, *Proc. Roy. Soc. London*, A, 244 (1958) 259.

[50] G. N. Lewis and D. Lipkin, *J. Am. Chem. Soc.*, 64 (1942) 2801.

[51] P. Bennema, G. J. Hoijtink, J. H. Lupinski, L. J. Oosterhoff, P. Selier and J. D. W. van Voorst, *Mol. Phys.*, 2 (1959) 431.

[52] F. A. Matsen in: *Chemical Applications of Spectroscopy*, (Ed. W. West) Interscience, New York, 1956.

[53] A. I. Biggs and R. A. Robinson, *J. Chem. Soc.*, (1961) 388.

SELECTED BIBLIOGRAPHY TO CHAPTER 5

Bowen, E. J., *Chemical Aspects of Light*, 2nd ed., Oxford University Press, London, 1946, 300 pp. This is an excellent non-mathematical account, in terms of wave mechanics, of light absorption, fluorescence, phosphorescence, and photochemistry.

Braude, E. A., in: *Determination of Organic Structures by Physical Methods*, (Eds. E. A. Braude and F. C. Nachod), Academic Press, New York, 1955. Chapter 4 of this book (pp. 131–186) contains a valuable summary of the main features of the ultra-violet spectra of organic compounds, together with many examples illustrating the use of spectra in structural diagnosis, reaction velocity studies, tautomerism, etc.

COULSON, C. A., *Valence*, Oxford University Press, London, 1952, 338 pp. The book discusses at a fairly elementary level the quantum mechanics required for a full understanding of electronic absorption spectroscopy.

The Chemical Society, Special Publication No. 4, *Recent Advances in the Chemistry of Colouring Matters*, London 1956.

FRIEDEL, R. A., AND M. ORCHIN, *Ultra-violet Spectra of Aromatic Compounds*, Wiley, New York, 1951, 618 pp. Following a brief description of the practical side of ultra-violet spectroscopy, the work reproduces the spectra of several hundred compounds, covering a wide range of structures.

GRAY, G. W. (Ed.), *Steric Effects in Conjugated Systems*, Butterworths, London, 1958, 181 pp. This is a collection of papers presented at a symposium, many of which deal with electronic spectra.

GILLAM, A. E. AND E. S. STERN, *Electronic Absorption Spectroscopy*, Arnold, London, 1954, 283 pp. This book, written specifically as a guide to the interpretation of the spectra of organic molecules, is an essential handbook in any laboratory where such work is undertaken.

HERSHENSON, H. M., *Ultra-violet and Visible Absorption Spectra*, Academic Press, New York, 1956. In this book compounds whose electronic spectra appeared in the literature between 1930 and 1954 are arranged alphabetically, with the appropriate references.

LOTHIAN, G. F., *Absorption Spectrophotometry*, Hilger & Watts, London, 1958. 246 pp. The book is in three parts, dealing with principles and laws, applications and techniques of spectrophotometry in the ultra-violet, visible and infra-red regions.

MATSEN, F. A., in: *Chemical Applications of Spectroscopy*, (Ed. W. WEST) Interscience, New York, 1956. Chapter 5, Part 2 of the book (pp. 629–705) describes very clearly the electronic transitions responsible for absorption by simple organic molecules.

RAO, C. N. R., *Ultraviolet and Visible Spectroscopy*, Butterworths, London, 1961, 164 pp.

STROUTS, C. R. N., J. H. GILFILLAN AND H. N. WILSON, *Analytical Chemistry*, Oxford University Press, London, 1955. Chapter 22 of Volume II of the book deals with both qualitative and quantitative applications to analysis.

Organic Electronic Spectral Data, Vol. I (1946–1952, Ed. M. J. KAMLET) and Vol. II (1953–55, Ed. H. E. UNGNADE), Interscience, New York, 1960. The volumes provide comprehensive coverage of literature spectra.

CHAPTER 6

INFRA-RED SPECTROSCOPY

Of all the methods considered in this book, infra-red spectroscopy is perhaps the most widely used at the present time. Although it may be applied to organic chemical problems, in a purely empirical fashion, some knowledge of the underlying principles is desirable. For this reason, the next section describes the information which can be obtained from a detailed consideration of the infra-red spectrum of a simple molecule, of not more than about ten atoms. Apart from its intrinsic interest, an acquaintance with this subject should lead to a more intelligent application of the information on the spectra of complex organic molecules contained in section B.

A. SPECTRA OF SIMPLE MOLECULES

Both infra-red and Raman spectroscopy depend on interatomic vibrations in molecules. Whereas infra-red spectra are obtained by direct absorption of radiation, Raman spectra arise when a sample is irradiated with monochromatic visible light (usually the blue mercury line). When the light scattered at right-angles to the incident beam is examined carefully in a spectrometer, it is found to contain not only light of the frequency of the exciting line, but also weak lines separated from this line by amounts equal to the molecular vibration frequencies.

The applications of the two methods are complementary. Raman spectroscopy is not, however, very much used in day-to-day problems, mainly because of difficulties in sample preparation. It is not easy to obtain a satisfactory Raman spectrum except from a colourless liquid or concentrated solution.

1. Vibrations of simple molecules

Molecules may be thought of as approximating to point masses connected by small springs representing the bonds. It is well established mathematically that such a system has associated with it a number of vibrational motions of the atoms against one another. If the natural frequency of one of these is ν, the molecule may absorb a light quantum of energy $h\nu$, the energy of which is converted to vibrational motion of the atoms.

A diatomic molecule presents the simplest case. Here only one type of vibration is possible, and it can easily be shown that the atoms execute a simple harmonic motion of frequency

$$\nu = 4 \cdot 125 \, (k/\mu)^{1/2}$$

where ν is in cm^{-1} (p. 75), k is the force constant in dynes/cm, and μ the reduced mass of the system, given by $m_1 m_2/(m_1 + m_2)$.

With polyatomic molecules, complications immediately arise, since there are several ways in which the molecule may vibrate. It can, however, be shown that there is a fixed number of so-called normal or fundamental modes of vibration, by superimposition of which any vibratory motion of the molecule can be built up. These normal modes have the property that, as the molecule vibrates, each atom oscillates about its equilibrium position with the frequency of the mode in question. Any molecule has therefore associated with it a definite set of frequencies, each of which may cause light absorption, provided that the selection rules are satisfied.

The number of normal modes of a molecule can readily be deduced from the number of its atoms. With N atoms, a total of $3N$ data are required completely to specify the positions of every atom in space, so that the system has $3N$ degrees of freedom. In considering the interatomic vibrations, one must first express the condition that the molecule as a whole is neither moving nor rotating in space. Three data are required to specify the position of the centre of gravity, and a further three to forbid rotation about any axis. $3N - 6$ internal degrees of freedom therefore remain, corresponding to the normal modes of vibration, except in the case of a linear molecule where, since there are only two rotational degrees of freedom, the number is $3N - 5$.

This expression confirms that a diatomic molecule has only one mode of vibration, whilst tri- and tetra-atomic ones have respectively three and six. In these very simple cases one can intuitively decide the form of the normal vibrations. Fig. 48 shows their form for linear and bent triatomic molecules, and for a planar molecule of four atoms, such as formaldehyde.

Fig. 48. Normal vibrations of simple molecules: (a) H_2O; (b) CO_2; (c) formaldehyde.

Motions perpendicular to the plane of the paper are indicated by $+$ and $-$ signs. Two points of general interest may be noted. Certain vibrations, such as ν_1 and ν_3 of (a) and (b), and ν_1 and ν_4 of (c), involve essentially stretching rather than bending of the bonds, because of the large amplitudes of the light hydrogen atoms. These are described as stretching vibrations, and are sometimes indicated by the symbol ν_{X-Y}, if $X - Y$ is the bond in question. Others, including ν_2 of (a) and (b), are bending vibrations, to which the letter δ is sometimes applied.

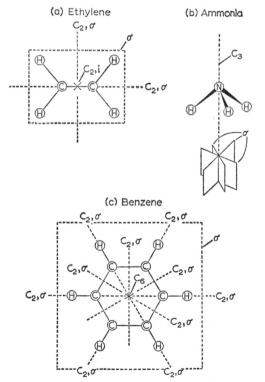

Fig. 49. Symmetry elements in molecules: (a) ethylene; (b) ammonia; (c) benzene. C_n indicates an n-fold symmetry axis, σ a plane, and i a centre of symmetry.

It may happen in molecules with a more than twofold axis of symmetry (below), that two of the normal modes are identical in frequency, differing only in their orientation in space. An example is provided by v_2 of carbon dioxide, which occurs with equal frequency in the plane of the paper and perpendicular to it. Such vibrations are said to be doubly degenerate.

Before the discussion of normal modes is continued, a brief account of molecular symmetry properties must be given. Three kinds of symmetry element may be shown by simple molecules. These include symmetry planes (often denoted by σ), which have the property that reflection in such a plane produces an identical atomic arrangement. The water molecule, for example, has two mutually perpendicular symmetry planes. Secondly, if by rotation through half a revolution an identical configuration is obtained, the molecule is said to have a two-fold symmetry axis (C_2). The water molecule has such an axis, whilst ammonia, being unchanged by rotation through one-third of a revolution about its central axis, is said to have a three-fold symmetry axis (C_3). More highly symmetrical molecules may also have centres of symmetry, with the property that reflection of every atom in a straight line through the centre produces no change.

Fig. 49 illustrates the symmetry elements of typical molecules. Ethylene has three symmetry planes, three two-fold axes, and a centre. Ammonia, whose molecule is a symmetrical pyramid, shows three planes and a three-fold axis, whilst the highly symmetrical benzene molecule has a centre, a six-fold axis, a three-fold axis, seven two-fold axes, and seven symmetry planes.

It can be shown, either by trial and error or mathematically, that only certain combinations of symmetry elements are possible. For example, one cannot have three mutually perpendicular planes without a centre of symmetry. The term "point group" is used to describe these permitted combinations, and any molecule must belong to one particular point group. Table 16 lists the symmetry elements of a few common point groups, together with examples of molecules belonging to some of them.

The presence of symmetry elements enables the normal

TABLE 16

POINT GROUPS OF MOLECULES

Point group	No. of planes	Axis of symmetry 2-fold	3-fold	6-fold	Centre of symmetry	Examples
C_1	0	0	0	0	0	CHFClBr
C_2	0	1	0	0	0	
C_{2v}	2	1	0	0	0	H_2O, HCHO
C_{3v}	3	0	1	0	0	NH_3
C_{2h}	1	1	0	0	1	trans planar $Cl — CH = CHCl$
C_{3h}	1	0	1	0	0	
D_{2d}	2	3	0	0	0	$CH_2 = C = CH_2$
D_{3d}	3	3	1	0	1	cyclohexane (chair form)
D_{2h}	3	3	0	0	1	$CH_2 = CH_2$ (planar)
D_{3h}	4	3	1	0	1	BCl_3 (planar)
D_{6h}	7	7	1	1	1	benzene
T_d	6	3	4	0	0	methane

TABLE 17

VIBRATION CLASSES OF FORMALDEHYDE

Class	σ_{xz}	σ_{yz}	Vibrations
A_1	+	+	ν_1, ν_2, ν_3
A_2	—	—	None
B_1	+	—	ν_4, ν_5
B_2	—	+	ν_6

vibrations of a molecule to be divided into classes, according to whether they are symmetric or anti-symmetric with respect to the elements. In the former case, application of the symmetry operation leads to an identical configuration of the vibrating molecule, whereas in the latter case a mirror image results. Of the three vibrations of the water molecule, ν_1 and ν_3 are symmetric with respect to the symmetry plane perpendicular to the paper through the oxygen atom, whereas ν_3 is anti-symmetric. ν_1 may therefore be described as the symmetric O – H stretching mode, and ν_3 as the anti-symmetric stretching mode. Since formaldehyde (Fig. 48c) has symmetry planes co-incident with that of the paper (σ_{xz}) and perpendicular to it (σ_{yz}), its vibrations are of four symmetry types, as shown in Table 17, where $+$ and $-$ signs indicate symmetric and anti-symmetric. Each vibration belongs to one class. Increasing the number of symmetry elements leads to larger numbers of symmetry classes. For example, the twelve vibrations of ethylene are distributed among eight classes (Table 18), and those of benzene among twelve.

It is relatively easy, for each of the point groups, to determine the number of symmetry classes. As described in Herzberg's book (Ref.[1], pp. 131 *et seq.*), rather more detailed symmetry considerations enable one also to predict, from the number of atoms in a molecule, the number of vibrations in each class. The importance of this in deducing the shapes of simple molecules will become apparent in the next section.

2. *The Infra-red and Raman spectra of simple molecules – molecular shapes*

Although a molecule of N atoms normally has $3N - 6$ normal modes, it does not follow that they all cause infra-red absorption bands and Raman lines. The intensity of an infra-red band is proportional to the square of $\delta\mu/\delta\eta$ where μ is the dipole moment of the molecule, and η a co-ordinate related to the displacements of the atoms. In other words, the band has appreciable intensity only if the corresponding vibration is accompanied by a change of dipole moment. For such simple molecules as water and carbon dioxide, it is obvious whether or not a particular vibration is "infra-red active". All three vibrations of the former clearly change the moment and are active. During ν_1 of carbon dioxide, on the contrary, the dipole moment of the system remains zero. The spectrum therefore shows only two strong bands. Selection rules also govern the production of Raman lines. A vibration is active only if it involves a change of polarisability. For example, whilst a molecule of carbon dioxide executes ν_1, the polarisability varies from a small value in the compressed form, through its normal value at the equilibrium position, to a larger value in the extended molecule. The polarisability thus changes continuously during the vibration, which is therefore Raman active, whilst v_2 and v_3 are inactive.

With larger molecules it becomes increasingly difficult to predict on commonsense grounds whether a vibration will be active in the infra-red spectrum, the Raman spectrum, both, or neither. This problem has, however, been solved quite generally,

TABLE 18

NORMAL VIBRATIONS OF ETHYLENE

Symmetry class	σ_{xy}	σ_{xz}	σ_{yz}	No. of vibrations	Activity
A_g	+	+	+	3	R
A_u	—	—	—	1	inactive
B_{1g}	+	—	—	2	R
B_{1u}	—	+	+	1	I.R
B_{2g}	—	+	—	1	R
B_{2u}	+	—	+	2	I.R
B_{3g}	—	—	+	0	R
B_{3u}	+	+	—	2	I.R

and the results tabulated, for example in Ref.[1] (p. 252). By referring to such tables, one can discover for any given point group which classes of vibration are active in the two types of spectrum. Table 18 illustrates the case of ethylene. This planar molecule belongs to the point group D_{2h}, and, as can readily be found from Herzberg's book, its vibrations have the properties listed in the table. Of the twelve, five would be expected to give strong infra-red bands, and six to give Raman lines, whilst the final vibration (the twisting motion) is active in neither spectrum. In practice, the spectrum of ethylene agrees substantially with this. None of the vibrations of ethylene are active in both the infra-red and Raman spectrum. This is true of any molecule with a centre of symmetry, and, conversely, if there are no coincidences between the infra-red and Raman frequencies of an unknown structure, it cannot have a centre of symmetry.

Considerations of this kind can be applied in deciding the shapes of simple molecules. Suppose, for example, that it is not known whether a molecule XY_3 is pyramidal or planar. In the former case, since the point group is D_{3h}, one would predict four fundamentals (two of them doubly degenerate), all of which would be active in both the infra-red and Raman spectrum. If the molecule were planar, however, one frequency would be missing from each spectrum. By this means BF_3, BCl_3 and BBr_3 have been shown to be planar, whilst the trihalides of phosphorus, arsenic, antimony and bismuth, all of which show four strong Raman lines, are probably pyramidal.

There are several possible shapes for the hydrogen peroxide molecule, including those given below, of which IV is non-planar.

$$H-O-O-H \qquad \begin{matrix} H \\ / \\ O-O \\ / \\ H \end{matrix} \qquad \begin{matrix} H \quad H \\ \searrow \quad / \\ O-O \end{matrix} \qquad \begin{matrix} H \quad H \\ / \quad \searrow \\ O-O \\ / \\ H \end{matrix}$$

$$\text{I} \qquad\qquad \text{II} \qquad\qquad \text{III} \qquad\qquad \text{IV}$$

Since the two strongest bands in the infra-red and Raman spectra coincide, the molecule cannot have a centre of symmetry, which rules out I and II. On the whole, the data fits IV fairly well.

Extensive studies of the Raman and infra-red spectra of benzene and deuterated benzenes by Ingold et al.[2], proved the molecule to be a plane, symmetrical hexagon, thus settling a long-standing controversy in organic chemistry. Again, the lack of coincidences between infra-red and Raman frequencies proved the presence of a centre of symmetry. A great many cases where studies of this kind have contributed to problems of molecular structure are described by Herzberg[1].

3. Determination of force constants

It is usually possible by measuring both the infra-red and Raman spectra of a simple molecule to obtain the frequencies of all the $3N - 6$ normal modes. Armed with this information, one may attempt the calculation of the force constants associated with bond stretching and bending, provided the interatomic distances and angles are known. For diatomic molecules this is a simple matter (p. 139), but even with three atoms, the equations connecting the frequencies, the molecular dimensions, and the force constants become much more complicated. Since the number of frequencies is usually smaller than the number of force constants required to specify the resistance of every bond to stretching and bending, simplifying assumptions must be made. A valence force field is often assumed, in which one postulates a strong restoring force in the line of every valence bond, and a force opposing bending of each bond, other interatomic forces being neglected.

TABLE 19

FORCE CONSTANTS OF BONDS

Bond	Molecule	$k \cdot 10^{-5}$ (dynes/cm)	Bond	Molecule	$k \cdot 10^{-5}$ (dynes/cm)
C — H	C_2H_6	5.1	C — N	oximes	c. 10.4
C — H	C_2H_4	5.1	C — N	CH_3CN	17.5
C — H	C_2H_2	5.9	C — O	CH_3OH	5.0
C — H	HCN	5.9	C — O	CO_2	15.5
C — C	C_2H_6	4.5	C — O	CH_2O	12.3
C — C	C_2H_4	9.8	C — O	CO	18.9
C — C	C_2H_2	15.6	C — Cl	CH_3Cl	3.4
C — C	$CH_2=C=CH_2$	9.7	N — H	NH_3	6.5
C — C	C_6H_6	7.6	O — H	CH_3OH	7.6
C — N	Single	c. 4.8	S — S	S_2	5.0

Table 19 lists the force constants of a few typical bonds. They show interesting parallels with several other bond properties[3]. For example, as one proceeds up the periodic table in the series B—H, C—H, N—H, O—H and F—H, the force constant increases steadily from 3.6 to 9.0 units. All single bonds involving carbon have constants near 5 units, whilst carbon double bonds show values around 10 units, and triple bonds fall near 15. Variations within one of these classes can often be explained in terms of bond order. For example, the figures for carbon monoxide, carbon dioxide and formaldehyde are respectively 18.5, 15.5 and 12.3, showing the bonds of the dioxide to be intermediate between double and triple. Similarly, the value for the C—C bond of benzene falls between those of ethylene and ethane. The C—Cl bond force constant has the much higher value of 5.3 in cyanogen chloride, than in methyl chloride (3.4), probably because of a large resonance contribution from an ionic form:

$$Cl — C \equiv N \longleftrightarrow Cl^+ = C = N^-$$

Various formulae have been suggested, connecting bond lengths with force constants. One of the most successful, due to Gordy[4], is of the form

$$k = 1.67N(x_A x_B / d^2)^{3/4} + 0.30$$

where x_A and x_B are the Pauling electronegativities of the atoms, d the bond length, and N its order.

4. Determination of thermodynamic quantities

It sometimes happens that the heat capacity or entropy of a gas may be required at temperatures where it cannot be measured directly. Also, discrepancies between measured and calculated heat capacities sometimes serve to determine the height of a barrier to internal rotation. The calculation of heat capacities and entropies involves computing separately the contributions from molecular translation, rotation, and internal vibrations. Of these, the first can be obtained approximately from kinetic theory, the second from the moments of inertia of the molecule, and the third from a knowledge of the frequency of every fundamental mode of vibration. The vibrational contributions to the heat capacity and entropy are given by the equations

$$C_p{}^0 = R(hc/kT)^2 \sum_i (d_i\nu_i{}^2 e^{-\nu_i hc/kT})/(1 - e^{-\nu_i hc/kT})^2$$

$$S_0 = -R \sum_i d_i \log_e (1 - e^{\nu_i hc/kT})$$

where d_i is the degeneracy of the ith vibration. Arithmetical substitution in these formulae is laborious, but can be avoided by the use of tables compiled by Aston (Ref. [5], p. 655), from which the contribution in calories or cals/degree of a given frequency to the heat capacity or entropy can be read directly. Even in complex molecules where not all the fundamentals have been assigned, it is often possible to devise a set which enables the vibrational contributions to be estimated with useful accuracy[6].

5. Interactions of molecular vibration and rotation

As shown in Fig. 29, each vibrational energy level of an isolated molecule is subdivided into much more closely spaced rotational levels. Since quantised rotation of molecules does not take place in the solid or liquid states, or in liquid solutions, rotational effects do not influence infra-red spectra as normally measured. Spectra of molecules in these states consist of relatively wide bands, symmetrical in shape (Fig. 50a). In gases, however, where vibrational transitions are accompanied by changes in the rotational sub-levels, the bands may present a much more complex pattern. Fig. 50b is typical of the results obtained with good instrumental resolution for light molecules of not more than about six atoms, where the rotational fine structure is well resolved. With heavier molecules, even as gases, the rotational lines become so close that they cannot be resolved, since the spacing decreases with increasing moment of inertia. There remains, however, an envelope indicating the shape of the band (Fig. 50c). The HCN band shows two sub-groups of lines, called the P and R branches, with a single central peak, the Q branch. The other resolved band shows no Q branch.

Valuable information about the structures of simple molecules can be obtained from the rotational structure. In the first place, from the intensity pattern of the lines, it is often possible to say whether the band corresponds to a vibration in which the dipole moment change is perpendicular or parallel to a symmetry axis

Fig. 50. Effect of molecular rotation on infra-red bands: (a) typical bands in solids and liquids; (b) rotational fine structure in bands of simple gases; (c) rotational contours of gases of higher molecular weight.

in the molecule. This helps in assigning frequencies to modes of vibration, and is applicable even to molecules too large for the individual lines to be resolved. From the spacing of the rotational lines, molecular moments of inertia may sometimes be deduced. Formulae have been derived relating this spacing to the moments for linear and spherical molecules which have only one moment of inertia, and for symmetrical tops with two. For a band of a linear molecule where the dipole moment change is perpendicular to the axis, the lines of the P, R and Q branches are given respectively by:

$$\nu = \nu_0 + h(J+1)/4\pi^2 I \ldots\ldots J = 0,1,2\ldots$$
$$\nu = \nu_0 - hJ/4\pi^2 I \qquad \ldots\ldots J = 1,2,3\ldots$$
$$\nu = \nu_0$$

where I is the moment of inertia, and J takes the values indicated. From the formulae, I can readily be calculated, and from it values of interatomic distances. The formulae for other types of molecule are more complicated, and the reader is referred to Ref. [1].

B. SPECTRA OF COMPLEX ORGANIC MOLECULES

As has already been stressed, the calculation of force constants, bond lengths, etc., is possible only for simple molecules of not more than about ten atoms. Nevertheless many types of information are obtainable from the spectra of larger molecules, although a detailed assignment of each band to a particular mode of vibration is no longer possible.

1. General considerations

On the basis of the $3N - 6$ rule, organic molecules are expected to have very large numbers of vibration frequencies. Typical numbers are fifty-seven for hexane, thirty-three for benzene and fifty-one for naphthalene. Although the number may be somewhat reduced by symmetry, an infra-red spectrum therefore comprises very many bands. Since their frequencies are determined by molecular geometry and force constants rather than by the physical properties of the substance, every compound has a unique infra-red spectrum, which provides perhaps the best available method of "finger-printing" an organic compound, so that it may be identified or detected in mixtures. In this respect there is a great advantage over ultra-violet spectra, where only a few bands are normally found.

From what has just been said, it might appear that the spectra of organic molecules are too complicated for any interpretation to be possible. There are however a number of simplifying factors. The bands may first be divided into those due to fundamental modes of vibration, and those arising from overtones and combinations of these. Most fundamental frequencies of organic molecules fall between 2.7 and 20 μ (500 and 3,700 cm^{-1})*, but weak overtones are found at shorter wavelengths.

Fundamental frequencies of molecules are of two types. In the first kind, the vibrations involve the whole, or a large part of the molecular framework, and are described as "skeletal". Of much greater importance to the organic chemist, are the so-called characteristic or group frequencies. Whenever a molecule contains atoms such as hydrogen and deuterium, which are much lighter than its other atoms, it can be shown mathematically that there will be a mode, or modes of vibration, in which the motion is largely localised in the light atom, the other atoms being essentially at rest. In such a vibration, since the molecule behaves largely as a diatomic molecule, the frequency is determined mainly by the force constant of the X–H link, and depends little on the rest of the molecule. It follows that such groups as C—H, O—H, N—H and S—H have characteristic frequencies, which vary only slightly from molecule to molecule. Similarly molecules containing —CH$_2$—, —NH$_2$ and similar groups have vibrations in which the motion is confined to these groups, behaving as triatomic molecules. Such groups thus have three characteristic frequencies, similar in form to those of the water molecules (Fig. 47), a symmetrical and an anti-symmetrical stretching mode, and a scissors-like deformation mode.

Calculations and experiment agree that characteristic frequencies also result when one bond of a molecule is much stronger than the others. For this reason such groups as C $\equiv$ N, C$\equiv$C, C$=$O, C$=$N and C$=$C give group frequencies, whilst —NO$_2$ and —SO$_2$— behave as triatomic molecules, having two characteristic stretching vibrations. Frequencies connected

---

* See p. 73 for definitions.

with the single bonds C—C, C—O, C—N, C—S, etc. are much more dependent on the masses of other atoms in the molecule.

Characteristic frequencies may greatly simplify a spectrum. For example, of the large number of vibrations of a long chain hydrocarbon such as polythene, many, being C—H stretching modes, fall together near 2940 cm^{-1}. Similarly all the C—H bending frequencies fall together, with the net effect that the spectrum of polythene is much simpler than those of many smaller molecules.

Enough has been said for a rough idea to be formed of the infra-red spectrum to be expected from an organic molecule (see Fig. 51). Proceeding from the end of the visible region, only

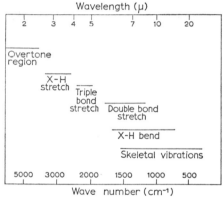

Fig. 51. Absorption regions and types of vibration.

weak overtones are to be expected down to about 3,600 cm^{-1} (2.8 μ). From this point to about 1,300 cm^{-1}, most of the bands are characteristic frequencies of X–H groups and multiple bonds. This region of the spectrum is therefore useful rather for the detection of these groups in unknowns, than for finger-printing molecules. For the latter purpose the most useful range is that from 1300 to about 500 cm^{-1}, which comprises most of the skeletal vibrations, together with some characteristic bending

References p. 218

frequencies of X–H links. At still longer wavelengths there are fewer bands, usually arising from motions involving heavy atoms, and from bending vibrations of such groups as C—O—C and C—C—C.

As with simple molecules, the intensity of each band is determined by the rate of change of dipole moment. Wide variations from band to band in a spectrum are to be expected. Motions localised in relatively nonpolar groups such as C=C

Fig. 52. Effect of state on spectra: (a) liquid *n*-propyl bromide; (b) solid *n*-propyl bromide[125]; (c) copper phthalocyanin, α-form; (d) β-form.

and C=N give weak bands, in contrast for example to the C=O group, which, being partially ionic, causes strong bands. Very roughly one may say that the less polar compounds, such as aliphatic hydrocarbons, give rather weak bands, compared to such polar compounds as ethers, esters and sulphonic acids.

One other general feature must be mentioned. Although a spectrum is determined mainly by the forces within the molecule, it is modified by intermolecular forces. For this reason the spectrum of a given compound is by no means identical in the solid, liquid and gas states. The effect of rotation on gas spectra has already been mentioned. Solid–liquid transitions, and even polymorphic changes in the solid state can produce minor changes. On freezing a liquid the bands usually sharpen, and doubling of peaks may occur. The magnitude of such effects is illustrated by the spectra of Fig. 52. For similar reasons, spectra of solutions depend slightly on the solvent, and differ from those of the solid or liquid solute. This is particularly marked where solvent-solute hydrogen bonding occurs.

2. The overtone and combination region (1–2.5 μ)

Although this region is applied much less to chemical problems than longer wavelengths, it sometimes has distinct advantages[7,8]. Most of the bands between 1 and 2.5 μ are overtones or combination frequencies based on the C—H, OH and NH stretching fundamentals near 3 μ. Only the first overtone (at twice the fundamental frequency), which has about one hundredth its intensity, is normally strong enough to be useful. Combinations of the stretching and bending frequencies of a group such as —CH_2— give bands of similar intensity. Table 20 lists such bands.

TABLE 20

OVERTONE AND COMBINATION BANDS

Bond or group	Type of compound	Type of vibration	Wave-number	Wavelength in μ
O—H	alcohols and phenols	1st overtone	7,150–6,850	1.40–1.45
	alcohols and phenols	combination	5,130–4,650	1.95–2.15
	water	combination	5,350–5,260	1.87–1.90
N—H and NH_2	amines and amides	1st overtone	6,900–6,200	1.4 –1.6
C—H	aliphatic and aromatic	1st overtone	6,100–5,700	1.61–1.75
	aliphatic	combination	4,550–4,200	2.2 –2.4
	aromatic	combination	4,250–4,000	2.35–2.5

The overtone region has the advantage of being available to instruments with quartz optics, designed primarily for use in the ultra-violet and visible regions, and to simple, cheap grating spectrometers with lead sulphide detectors. Where the nature of the sample precludes the preparation of the very thin layers normally required for infra-red spectroscopy, the weakness of overtone bands may be turned to advantage. Layers between 0.5 and 10 mm thick are normally used.

Since most bands in this region are connected with X–H links, its use in structural diagnosis is very limited. However many examples have been reported, where analytical problems are best tackled in the region, since the overtone spectra of the components are better separated than their fundamental frequencies. Examples include the detection of residual monomer by means of its $>C=CH_2$ units in acrylic polymers[8], the estimation of water in alcohols and various applications in hydrocarbon analysis[9].

3. Characteristic frequencies

During the last fifteen years, infra-red spectroscopy has been applied extensively to all kinds of organic compounds. A very large volume of data has been accumulated concerning the characteristic frequencies of functional groups and chemical classes. This information has been admirably collated in books by Bellamy[10] and by Jones and Sandorfy, writing in *Chemical Applications of Spectroscopy*[11]. A selection of such data is presented in the next few pages. The best form of presentation depends on the use to which the material is to be put. Some information can be obtained from the spectrum of a completely unknown sample, by observing bands at characteristic frequencies, and deducing the presence of the corresponding groups. Fig. 53 consists of charts from which the presence of groups in unknowns can often be inferred from their bands. Similar charts have been published by various authors[12,13,124], but there is a definite limit to the amount of information which can be included without making the chart unduly large or confused.

For this reason data on the I.R. spectra of the commoner classes of organic compound are also presented in tabular form, in Table 22 (pp. 162 ff.). Band positions are given for convenience in both wavelength and wavenumber units, since unfortunately both are still used freely in the literature. Although, as described in the next section quantitative data on group intensities is accumulating, only qualitative band intensity estimates are given.

Fig. 53. Correlation charts (pp. 157–160).

Bands in the spectral region 2700–3700 cm⁻¹ are almost invariably due to stretching of X–H links, which are thus readily detectable in unknowns. Although all C—H bonds absorb between 2800 and 3100 cm⁻¹, the number of sub-peaks and their precise location depends on the nature of the C—H link. A —CH₂— group for example has two bands near 2950 and 2850 cm⁻¹, due to its symmetrical and anti-symmetrical

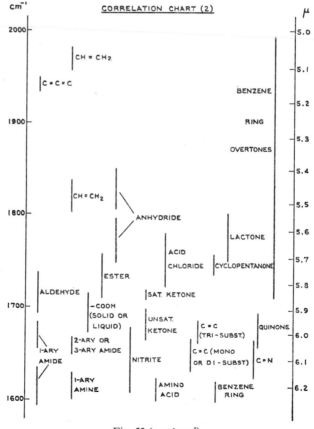

Fig. 53 (*continued*).

stretching modes, a methyl group gives three bands in the same region, and benzene rings, with several adjacent C—H links give three or more peaks between 3000 and 3100 cm^{-1}. Likewise, as can be seen from the table, an —NH$_2$ unit gives two bands near 3300 cm^{-1}, the exact positions of which enable amines and amides to be distinguished. Primary amines can be distinguished

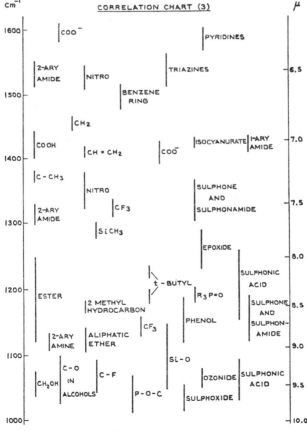

Fig. 53 (*continued*).

References p. 218

from secondary ones, which normally give only a single N—H peak. Fig. 54 illustrates various absorption patterns arising from X—H groups.

Table 21 lists the hydroxyl frequencies of several compounds, measured in dilute carbon tetrachloride solution to avoid complications from association. There is invariably a band near

Fig. 53 (*continued*)

TABLE 21

HYDROXYL STRETCHING FREQUENCIES IN DILUTE CCl_4 SOLUTION

Compound	Wave number	Compound	Wave number	Sigma factor
Ethyl alcohol	3,632	p-Methoxyphenol	3,614	—0.27
n-Propyl alcohol	3,634	p-Methylphenol	3,612	—0.17
n-Butyl alcohol	3,636	Phenol	3,609	0.00
sec.-Butyl alcohol	3,626	p-Chlorophenol	3,606	0.23
iso-Propyl alcohol	3,620	m-Nitrophenol	3,600	0.71
tert.-Butyl alcohol	3,616	p-Nitrophenol	3,592	1.27

Fig. 54. Typical spectra in the X—H stretching region.

3600 cm^{-1}, and by careful wavelength measurements one can differentiate between primary, secondary and tertiary alcohols, phenols, acids, and oximes. Structural inferences of this kind can often be further substantiated by considering intensities as in the next section.

References p. 218   *(Text continued on p. 184)*

Class of compound	Type of vibration	Wave-number range	Wavelength range
Acetylenes	$\equiv$C—H stretch	c. 3,250	c. 2.98
H—C$\equiv$C—R	C$\equiv$C stretch	2,100–2,140	4.762–4.673
R—C$\equiv$C—R	C$\equiv$C stretch	2,190–2,260	4.566–4.425
—C$\equiv$C—C$=$C—	C$\equiv$C stretch	2,220–2,270	4.505–4.405
—C$\equiv$C—C$=$O	C$\equiv$C stretch	c. 2,250	c. 4.425
Acid chlorides			
aliphatic	C$=$O stretch	1,770–1,785	5.65–5.60
aromatic	C$=$O stretch	1,740–1,770	5.75–5.65
	C$=$O stretch	1,775–1,785 and 1,745–1,765	5.634–5.602 an 5.760–5.670
Alcohols	O—H stretch	c. 3,300	c. 3.03
primary	O—H stretch	3,630–3,636	2.755–2.751
secondary	O—H stretch	c. 3,620	c. 2.762
tertiary	O—H stretch	3,612–3,620	2.768–2.762
With internal O—H $\cdots$ O or O—H $\cdots$ N bonds	O—H stretch	3,300–3,450	3.03–2.90
primary	C—O stretch	1,030–1,060	9.71–9.43
secondary	C—O stretch	c. 1,100	c. 9.09
tertiary	C—O stretch	c. 1,140	c. 8.77
Aldehydes	C—H stretch	2,720–2,740 and c. 2,820	3.671–3.650 an c. 3.546
sat. aliphatic	C$=$O stretch	1,740–1,720	5.841–5.747
	C$=$O stretch	c. 1,735	c. 5.764
α-β unsaturated	C$=$O stretch	1,685–1,690	5.934–5.917
	C$=$O stretch	c. 1,705	c. 5.866
aromatic	C$=$O stretch	1,700–1,710	5.882–5.848
Allenes	C$=$C$=$C antisym. stretch	1,940–1,950	5.155–5.128
	—CH$_2$ deformation	c. 850	c. 11.76
Amides			
primary	N—H stretch	3,390–3,400 and 3,520–3,530	2.950–2.940 an 2.841–2.832

RISTIC FREQUENCIES

Intensity	Remarks	References
edium-strong	Very useful diagnostically	14, 15, 16
very weak	May be missed in unknowns	
very weak		
medium		
strong		
strong		17
strong	Liquid or solid states	
variable	In dilute CCl_4 solution	
strong	Solid or liquid state, broad band	18, 19
strong	In dilute CCl_4 solution, in absence of intermolecular	
strong	hydrogen bonding	
strong		
strong		
strong		
strong	Lower wave-number with branching	
strong		
medium	Well separated from other C—H bands	20, 21
strong	Solid or liquid state	
strong	Dilute solution	
strong	Solid or liquid state	
strong	Solid, liquid or dilute solution	
strong		
v. strong	Doublet in $CH_2=C=CHR$ if R = —COOH, —COOR,	22
	or similar group	
strong		
strong	In dilute solution. Very sharp bands	23, 24
strong		

TABLE 2

Class of compound	Type of vibration	Wave-number range	Wavelength range
primary	N—H stretch	c. 3,180 and c. 3,350	c. 3.145 c. 2.985
primary	C=O stretch and N—H def.	c. 1,620 and 1,670–1,690	c. 6.17 5.99–5.92
primary	as above	1,620–1,670	6.17–5.92
secondary	N—H stretch	c. 3,430	c. 2.915
secondary	N—H stretch	c. 3,270	c. 3.06
secondary	origin uncertain	c. 3,070	c. 3.28
secondary	C=O stretch	1,660–1,680	6.02–5.98
secondary	C=O stretch	1,640–1,670	6.098–5.988
secondary	N—H def. + C—N stretch	1,530–1,570	6.53–6.37
secondary	origin uncertain	c. 1,300	c. 7.69
tertiary	C=O stretch	1,640–1,670	6.10–5.99
Amines			
primary aliphatic	N—H stretch	c. 3,300	c. 3.03
primary aliphatic	N—H def. in-plane	1,600–1,610	6.25–6.21
primary aliphatic	N—C stretch	1,030–1,080	9.71–9.27
primary aliphatic	N—H def. out-of-plane	776–794 and 825–840	12.88–12.59 12.12–11.9
primary aromatic	N—H antisym. and sym. stretch	3,380–3,420 and 3,450–3,510	2.958–2.925 2.902–2.855
primary aromatic	N—H def. in-plane	1,600–1,630	6.25–6.135
secondary aliphatic	N—H stretch	c. 3,400	c. 2.95
secondary aliphatic	C—N stretch	1,139–1,181	8.78–8.47
secondary aliphatic	? N—H def.	768–739	13.9–13.5
secondary aromatic	N—H stretch	3,430–3,450	2.915–2.898
secondary aromatic	N—H stretch	3,300–3,400	3.03–2.94
Amine hydrochlorides	N—H stretch	2,800–2,300	3.570–4.35
	?	c. 2,000	c. 5.0
	? N—H def.	1,600–1,500	6.25–6.67
Amino acids	N—H stretch	3,000–3,200	3.333–3.125
	?	c. 2,100	c. 4.76
	C—O sym. stretch	1,590–1,600	6.29–6.25
	C—O antisym. stretch	c. 1,400	c. 7.14
	? N—H def.	1,550–1,485	6.45–6.73

Continued)

Intensity	Remarks	References
strong	Solid state	
strong		
v. strong	In dilute solution	
v. strong	Solid state. Doublet in the range	
strong	Dilute solution. May be doublet	
strong	Solid or liquid state	
weak	Solid or liquid state	
strong	In dilute solution	
strong	Solid or liquid state	
strong	Very useful diagnostically	
strong		
strong		
medium-weak	Broad band	17, 25, 26
strong	Very useful diagnostically	
medium	Less useful	
strong	Less useful	
strong-medium	Dilute solution. c.100 wave-numbers lower in the solid state	
strong		
weak		
medium	Very useful	
variable		
strong	Dilute solution	
strong	Solid or liquid state	
strong	Very useful diagnostically	27
medium		
medium		
strong	Unsubstituted amino acids only	28
weak		
strong		
weaker than sym.		
fairly strong		

        (*continued*)

TABLE 2

Class of compound	Type of vibration	Wave-number range	Wavelength range
Anhydrides	C=O stretch	1,780–1,865 and	5.62–5.36
		1,720–1,810	5.81–5.52
	C—O—C stretch	1,175–1,210	8.51–8.26
	C—O—C stretch	1,210–1,310	8.26–7.63
Benzene derivatives	C—H stretch	3,010–3,110	3.332–3.215
	Overtone and combination bands	2,000–1,660	5.00–6.02
	C=C stretch	1,480–1,520 and	6.76–6.58
		1,590–1,630	6.29–6.13
	C—H in-plane def.	950–1,225	10.5–8.17
	C—H def. out- of- plane	650–900	15.4–11.1
mono-substituted	— do. —	694–701 and	14.4–14.3
		750–760	13.4–13.2
1,2-disubstituted	— do. —	740–760	13.5–13.2
1,3-disubstituted	— do. —	690–710 and	14.5–14.1
		778–800	12.8–12.5
1,4-disubstituted	— do. —	810–833	12.4–12.0
1,2,3-trisubstituted	— do. —	705–745	14.2–13.4
1,2,4-trisubstituted	— do. —	805–825 and	12.4–12.1
		870–885	11.5–11.3
1,3,5-trisubstituted	— do. —	830–850	12.1–11.7
Carboxylic acids	O—H stretch	c.3,550	c.2.82
	C=O stretch	c.1,760	c.5.68
	O—H stretch	2,400–3,000	4.17–3.33
aliphatic and unsat. acids only	C=O stretch	1,700–1,720	5.88–5.81
aromatics only	C=O stretch	1,680–1,700	5.95–5.88
	C—O stretch + O—H def.	1,400–1,440	7.14–6.94
	—CH₂-wagging	1,345–1,180	7.43–8.47
	O—H def.	915–955	10.9–10.5
salts of carboxylic acids	C=O stretch (anti.)	1,650–1,610	6.45–6.21
	C=O stretch (sym.)	1,300–1,400	7.69–7.14
Carbodiimides	N=C=N stretch	2,100–2,150	4.762–4.651

(Continued)

Intensity	Remarks	References
strong	5-rings cause high frequencies and unsaturation low ones	
strong	Open chain compounds	
strong	Anhydrides with ring strain	
medium	Usually 3 or 4 peaks	10, 29
weak	Band pattern is characteristic of the substitution type	
strong or medium		
medium	Not very useful	
strong	These provide the best method of determining substitution type. The correlations do not, however, always hold	
strong	with highly polar substituents	
strong		
strong		
strong		
strong		
strong		
strong		
strong	Monomers in dilute solution	30, 31, 32
strong	Monomers in dilute solution	
strong	Solids and liquids. Very broad band	
strong	This and the other correlations apply to solids and liquids	
strong		
medium	Less useful diagnostically	
medium	Long chain acids and salts show band progressions, the spacing of which depends on the chain length	
very strong	Very useful in diagnosis	
weaker than anti.		
very strong		33

TABLE 22

Class of compound	Type of vibration	Wave-number range	Wavelength range
Epoxides	C—H stretch	3,000–3,050	3.333–3.279
	origin unknown	1,279–1,244	7.82–8.04
	origin unknown	951–863	10.52–11.58
	origin unknown	864–786	11.57–12.72
Esters	overtone	c.3,450	c.2.90
saturated esters	C=O stretch	1,735–1,740	5.76–5.75
	C=O stretch	1,740–1,750	5.75–5.71
unsat. esters and benzoates	C=O stretch	1,705–1,720	5.87–5.81
R·CO·O·C=C—	C=O stretch	c.1,770	c.5.65
enolised keto-esters and salicylates	C=O stretch	c.1,670	c.5.99
formates	C—O—C stretch	c.1,158	c.8.44
acetates	C—O—C stretch	c.1,245	c.8.03
propionates	C—O—C stretch	c.1,190	c.8.40
n-butyrates	C—O—C stretch	c.1,190	c.8.40
benzoates	C—O—C stretch	c.1,290 and c.1,110	c.7.75 and c.9.00
Ethers			
dialkyl	C—O—C stretch	1,110–1,140	9.01–8.89
benzyl ethers	C—O—C stretch	c.1,090	c.9.17
alkyl-aryl ethers	C—O—C stretch	1,240–1,270 and 1,020–1,050	8.07–7.87 and 9.80–9.52
vinyl ethers	C=C stretch	1,610 and 1,620–1,650	6.21 and 6.17–6.06
	C—H def.	810 and 960	9.09 and 10.4
	C—O—C stretch	1,020–1,075 and 1,200–1,275	9.80–9.30 and 8.33–7.84
—C—O—C— in ring	stretch	1,170–1,250	8.55–8.00
Halogenated compounds			
fluorine compounds	| —C—F stretch |	1,000–1,100	10.0–9.09
	—CF₂— stretch	1,100–1,300	9.09–7.69
	CF—CF₃	745–730	13.4–13.7
	—CF₃, aromatic	c.1,140 and c.1,320	c.8.8 and c.7.6
chlorine compounds	C—Cl stretch	600–800	16.7–12.5

(Continued)

Intensity	Remarks	References
weak fairly strong variable variable	None of these bands are very satisfactory for diagnosis	34, 35
weak strong strong strong strong very strong	 Liquid state In carbon tetrachloride solution	36, 37, 21
strong strong strong strong strong	All refer to liquids	
very strong strong strong weaker very strong	Solids, liquids and solutions	38, 39
very strong strong		
strong		
strong		
very strong very strong very strong	 Useful in diagnosis	
medium	Of limited use in diagnosis	

TABLE 22

Class of compound	Type of vibration	Wave-number range	Wavelength range
bromine compounds	C—Br stretch	500–600	20.0–16.7
iodine compounds	C—I stretch	c.500	c.20
Hetero aromatics	C—H stretch	3,100–3,000	3.23–3.33
six-rings	C=C stretch	1,430–1,605	6.99–6.22
five-rings	C=C stretch	1,400–1,590	7.14–6.29
	C—H def.	750–900	13.3–11.1
Hydrocarbons, alicyclic			
cyclopropanes	origin unknown	1,020–1,000 and	9.8–10.0 a
		870–855	11.5–11.7
cyclobutanes	origin unknown	900–920	11.1–10.9
cyclohexanes	origin unknown	1,000–1,050 and	10.0–9.52 a
		950–1,000	10.5–10.0
Hydrocarbons, paraffinic			
$CH_3 \cdot (CH_2)_n$, $n = 2$	—CH₂— rocking	734–743	13.62–13.46
$n = 3–5$	—CH₂— rocking	723–730	13.8–13.7
$n = 6$, or greater	—CH₂— rocking	722–724	13.85–13.81
2,3-dimethyl group	origin unknown	1,116–1,130	8.96–8.85
2-methyl group	origin unknown	1,168–1,171	8.56–8.54
	—CH₃ def.	1,368–1,372 and	7.309–7.272 a
		1,381–1,389	7.241–7.197
2,2-dimethyl group	—CH₃ def.	1,366–1,374	7.320–7.277
	origin unknown	1,235–1,253	8.098–7.981
	origin unknown	1,163–1,208	8.598–8.282
Hydrocarbons, polynuclear aromatic			
napthalenes	C=C stretch	1,580–1,620	6.33–6.17
	C=C stretch	1,505–1,550	6.65–6.45
	origin unknown	1,390–1,400	7.19–7.14
	C—H def.	c.777 and	c.12.9 a
		c.792	c.12.6
	C—H def.	c.750 and	c.13.3
		c.815	c.12.3
anthracenes	C=C stretch	1,620–1,640	6.17–6.10
	C=C stretch	c.1,510	c.6.45
	C—H def.	700–900	14.3–11.1

Intensity	Remarks	References
medium		
—		
medium	Similar to benzene derivatives	40
variable	Usually four bands	
variable	Usually three bands	
strong	Often several bands	
variable	Neither is very strong or reliable	41, 42
variable	May be rather weak	
medium	Cyclohexane itself is an exception	
medium	The band splits into two components in the solid state	29, 43
medium		
medium		
medium		
medium	*i.e.* isopropyl compounds	
strong		
strong	*i.e.* *t*-butyl compounds	
variable	Useful diagnostically	
variable	Useful diagnostically	
medium	One or two bands	44, 45, 46
medium		
medium		
strong	α-Mono-substituted compounds	
strong	β-Mono-substituted compounds	
medium		
variable		
strong	Position and number of peaks indicates type of substitution	

TABLE 2

Class of compound	Type of vibration	Wave-number range	Wavelength range
phenanthrenes	C=C stretch	c. 1,600	c. 6.25
	origin unknown	c. 1.500	c. 6.67
	C—H def.	650–900	15.4–11.1
Hydroperoxides			
	—OH stretch	c. 3,560	c. 2.81
	—OH stretch	c. 3,400	c. 2.94
	—O—O— stretch	877–848 and	11.4–11.8
		833–800	12.0–12.5
	origin unknown	830–845	12.1–11.8
Isocyanates	N=C=O stretch (antisym.)	2,265–2,280	4.415–4.386
Isocyanurates	C=O stretch	c. 1,710	c. 5.85
	origin unknown	c. 1,420	c. 7.05
Isonitriles			
alkyl	N⇒C stretch	2,150–2,170	4.651–4.608
aromatic	N⇒C stretch	2,110–2,130	4.739–4.695
Isothiocyanates			
aliphatic	C=N=S stretch (antisym.)	2,080–2,140	4.81–4.67
aromatic	C=N=S stretch (antisym.)	2,040–2,090	4.96–4.78
Ketones			
dialkyl	C=O stretch	1,705–1,715	5.866–5.832
	C=O stretch	c. 1,720	c. 5.814
methyl ketones	uncertain	near 1,170, 1,370 and 1,420	near 8.55, 7.? and 7.04
unsat. ketones and acetophenones	C=O stretch	1,670–1,700	5.988–5.882
benzophenones	C=O stretch	1,650–1,670	6.061–5.988
enolised β-diketones	C=O stretch	c. 1,610	c. 6.2
cyclopentanones	C=O stretch	1,740–1,750	5.747–5.714
	unknown	c. 1,150	c. 8.7

(Continued)

Intensity	Remarks	References
fairly strong		
variable		
strong	About four bands	
strong	Dilute solution, unbonded	47, 48
strong	Hydrogen bonded	
weak	Of limited usefulness	
weak		
medium	Tertiary hydroperoxides only	
very strong	Range covers solids, liquids and solutions	49, 50
strong		
very strong		
		51
weak	Rather stronger band than in nitriles	
variable		
		50
strong	Usually several sub-peaks	
very strong		
		21, 36
strong	Liquid or solid	
strong	Dilute carbon tetrachloride solution	
strong		
strong		
strong		
very strong		
strong		
strong		

TABLE 22

Class of compound	Type of vibration	Wave-number range	Wavelength range
Lactones			
saturated 7-rings	C=O stretch	c.1,727	c.5.791
saturated 6-rings	C=O stretch	c.1,740	c.5.747
saturated 5-rings	C=O stretch	c.1,770	c.5.650
$\Delta_{\alpha\beta}$ 5-rings	C=O stretch	c.1,750	c.5.714
$\Delta_{\beta\gamma}$ 5-rings	C=O stretch	c.1,800	c.5.556
Mercaptans	S—H stretch	c.2,580	c.3.88
	C—S stretch	550–700	18.2–14.3
Methyl			
hydrocarbons	C—H stretch	2,850–2,970	3.509–3.367
—O—CH₃	C—H stretch	2,832–2,815	3.532–3.553
$\diagdown$ N—CH₃ $\diagup$	C—H stretch	2,780–2,820	3.597–3.546
$\begin{array}{c} \text{Me} \\ \diagup \\ -\text{N} \\ \diagdown \\ \text{Me} \end{array}$	C—H stretch	c.2,800	c.3.57
—C—CH₃	C—H def.	c.1,375	c.7.27
Methylene			
paraffins	C—H stretch	2,930 and 2,853	3.413 and 3.?
	C—H def.	c.1,467	c.6.82
olefines	CH₂ stretch	3,080 and 2,980	3.247 and 3.?
cyclopentanes	C—H stretch	2,952 and 2,866	3.388 and 3.?
	C—H def.	c.1,455	c.6.87
cyclohexanes	C—H stretch	2,927 and 2,854	3.414 and 3.?
	C—H def.	c.1,452	c.6.89
Nitrates	N=O stretch (anti.)	1,620–1,650	6.17–6.06
(covalent)	N=O stretch (sym.)	1,260–1,290	7.93–7.75
Nitriles			
aliphatic	C≡N stretch	2,240–2,260	4.664–4.425
unsaturated	C≡N stretch	2,221–2,235	4.503–4.474
aromatic	C≡N stretch	2,225–2,240	4.495–4.464

(Continued)

Intensity	Remarks	References
		52
strong		
strong		
strong		
strong		
strong		
weak	Liquid or gas state. Easily missed	53, 54
medium	Not very outstanding	
		55, 56
medium	Usually 3 bands. 2,960 cm⁻¹ most useful	
medium		
medium		
medium		
medium	Exact position indicates type of compound	
		57, 58
strong		
strong		
strong		
strong		
strong		
strong		
strong		
strong		128
strong		
		59, 60, 61
weak	Particularly weak with oxygenated compounds	
medium		
variable	Strength very much dependent on the substituent	

TABLE 2

Class of compound	Type of vibration	Wave-number range	Wavelength range
Nitrites	N=O stretch	1,681–1,652 and 1,625–1,613	5.95–6.06 6.15–6.20
	N—O stretch	c. 800	c. 12.5
	? NO₂ def.	c. 600	c. 16.7
Nitro			
aliphatic	N=O stretch (anti.)	1,550–1,570	6.45–6.37
	N=O stretch (sym.)	1,335–1,360	7.49–7.35
	C—N stretch	832–868	12.0–11.5
aromatic	N=O stretch (anti.)	1,490–1,565	6.71–6.39
	N=O stretch (sym.)	1,335–1,360	7.49–7.35
	C—N stretch	832–868	12.0–11.5
Nitroso	N—O stretch	1,550–1,500	6.45–6.67
	N—O stretch	c. 1,320	c. 7.6
Olefines	C—H stretch	3,040–3,010	3.289–3.322
vinyl hydrocarbons	overtone	1,969–1,984	5.078–5.040
	overtone	1,805–1,832	5.541–5.458
	C=C stretch	1,639–1,645	6.102–6.080
	C—H def.	991–1,004	10.09–9.96
	C—H def.	909–916	11.00–10.92
vinyl ethers	C=C stretch	1,631–1,637	6.131–6.126
	C=C stretch	1,607–1,615	6.224–6.193
	C—H def.	960–964	10.42–10.37
	C—H def.	940–944	10.64–10.59
vinyl esters	C=C stretch	c. 1,647	c. 6.07
	C—H def.	947–949	10.56–10.54
	C—H def.	868–870	11.52–11.47
vinyl ketones	C=C stretch	1,618–1,620	6.182–6.173
	C—H def.	982–984	10.18–10.16
	C—H def.	953–955	10.49–10.47
propenyl —CH=CH— (trans)	C=C stretch	c. 1,667	c. 6.00
	C—H def.	964–979	10.37–10.21
propenyl —CH=CH— (cis)	C=C stretch	1,631–1,661	6.13–6.02
	uncertain	1,397–1,429	7.156–7.00
	C—H def.	675–729	14.8–13.7

(Continued)

Intensity	Remarks	References
strong	Due to *cis* and *trans* forms	62
strong		
strong		
strong		
		63, 64
strong	Very useful	
strong	Very useful	
medium	Much less useful	
strong	Weakened by amino groups	
strong	Very useful	
much weaker		
strong	Refers to monomers in dilute solution	65
strong	Refers to dimers in solids	
medium	All these correlations are very useful in diagnosis	29, 66, 67
weak		
weak		
medium		
strong		
strong		
strong		
strong		
strong		
medium		
strong		
strong		
strong		
strong		
strong		
strong		
very weak	Conjugation with C=O lowers the wave-number and intensifies the band	
strong	Little affected by conjugation	
weak	Not as well characterised as the trans type	
weak		
variable		

TABLE 2

Class of compound	Type of vibration	Wave-number range	Waveleng range
isopropenyl hydrocarbons	overtone	1,783–1,792	5.608–5.58
/	C=C stretch	1,639–1,661	6.102–6.02
(CH₂=C)	C—H def.	892–887	11.21–11.27
\			
isopropenyl ketones	C=C stretch	c.1,630	c.6.135
	C—H def.	c.930	c.10.75
isopropenyl esters	C=C stretch	1,672–1,676	5.98–5.97
	C—H def.	879–867	11.38–11.53
tri-subst. olefines	C=C stretch	1,667–1,692	6.00–5.91
	C—H def.	808–833	12.38–12.0
Oximes	O—H stretch	3,602–3,590	2.776–2.785
	O—H stretch	3,100–3,250	3.21–3.08
aliphatic	C=N stretch	1,665–1,680	6.006–5.952
aromatic	C=N stretch	1,620–1,630	6.17–6.14
	uncertain	c.1,300 and	c.7.69
		c.920	c.10.9
Ozonides	O—O stretch	1,064–1,042	9.40–9.60
Peroxides	O—O stretch	1,000–833	10–12
diacyl, aliphatic	C=O stretch	1,811–1,820 and	5.52–5.49
		1,798–1,808	5.56–5.53
diacyl, aromatic	C=O stretch	1,780–1,805 and	5.62–5.54
		1,760–1,780	5.88–5.62
Phenols	O—H stretch	3,605–3,615	2.774–2.766
	O—H stretch	c.3,640	c.2.747
	O—H stretch	c.3,550	c.2.817
	O—H stretch	c.3,320	c.3.01
	O—H stretch	c.3,200	c.3.12
	? O—H def.	1,100–1,200	9.09–8.33
Phosphorus organic	P—H stretch	2,440–2,280	4.10–4.39
	P—O—H stretch	2,650–2,700	3.77–3.70
	P—O—P stretch	870–970	11.5–10.3
aliphatic	P—O—C stretch	980–1,050	10.2–9.52
aromatic	P—O—C stretch	1,190–1,240	8.40–8.07

(Continued)

Intensity	Remarks	References
weak		
medium		
strong		
medium		
strong		
strong		
strong		
weak		
medium	Not very useful except in hydrocarbons	
strong	Dilute carbon tetrachloride solution	18, 69
strong	Solids	
weak		
medium	Ring bands interfere	
variable		
strong	Useful in diagnosis	70
rather weak	Not very characteristic	
strong		
strong		
strong	In dilute carbon tetrachloride solution	18, 71
strong	Dilute CCl_4. Compounds with bulky ortho substituents	
strong	Dilute CCl_4. Internal bonding to $C=O$	
strong	Liquid state. Bulky ortho substituents raise the wave-number	
strong	Solids. Broad band	
strong	Not very useful	
medium	Sharp band	72, 73, 74
strong	Very broad band	
strong		
very strong		
strong		

TABLE 2:

Class of compound	Type of vibration	Wave-number range	Wavelength range
$(RO)_3 \cdot P{=}O$	P=O stretch	1,250–1,300	8.00–7.69
$R_3P{=}O$	P=O stretch	1,170–1,190	8.55–8.40
	P=S stretch	600–750	16.7–13.3
Proteins and polypeptides	N—H stretch	c. 3,280	c. 3.05
	? N—H stretch	c. 3,060	c. 3.27
	C=O stretch	c. 1,630	c. 6.135
	C=O stretch	c. 1,660	c. 6.02
	N—H def.	c. 1,550	c. 6.45
	N—H def.	c. 1,530	c. 6.54
Quinones	C=O stretch	1,660–1,685	6.024–5.934
	C=O stretch	1,700–1,720	5.882–5.814
	uncertain	1,200–1,350	8.33–7.41
Silicon derivatives	Si—H stretch	2,270–2,080	4.4–4.8
	$Si{—}CH_3$ def.	1,280–1,250	7.8–8.0
	$Si{—}O{—}CH_3$ stretch	c. 1,190	c. 8.4
	$Si{—}O{—}CH_2$ stretch	1,190–1,140,	8.4–8.8,
		1,100–1,170 and	9.1–9.3 a
		990–945	10.1–10.6
	Si—O—aryl stretch	1,030–1,090	9.71–9.17
	Si—O—Si	1,120–1,010	8.9–9.9
Sulphides			
aliphatic	C—S stretch	600–700	16.7–14.3
aliphatic and aromatic	S—S stretch	430–520	23.3–19.2
Sulphonamides	S=O stretch	1,350–1,310	7.4–7.65
	S=O stretch	1,180–1,150	8.5–8.7
primary compounds	N—H stretch	3,390–3,330 and	2.95–3.00 a
		3,300–3,250	3.05–3.08
secondary compounds	N—H stretch	3,280–3,250	3.05–3.08
Sulphones	S=O stretch (sym.)	1,130–1,160	8.83–8.62
	S=O stretch (anti.)	1,300–1,350	7.69–7.41

Continued)

Intensity	Remarks	References
very strong		
very strong		
variable		
strong		75, 76
weak		
strong	Chains in β-form	
strong	Chains in α-form	
strong	Chains in α-form	
strong	Chains in β-form. Doubts have recently been cast on correlations with configuration	
strong	Six-ring quinones	77, 78, 79
strong	Five-ring quinones, *e.g.* acenaphthene	
very strong		
medium	Silicon derivatives give outstandingly strong bands	80, 81
very strong		
very strong		
all strong		
very strong		
strong		
		53, 82
rather weak	Broad band	
weak	Ill-defined	
strong	May split into 3 sub-peaks	
strong	Very useful diagnostically	
strong		
strong		
strong		
very strong		83, 84
very strong		

TABLE 2

Class of compound	Type of vibration	Wave-number range	Wavelength range
Sulphonic acids	S=O stretch	1,150–1,250	8.0–8.7
aromatic	S=O stretch	1,040–1,060	9.62–9.43
aliphatic	S=O stretch	1,060–1,080	9.43–9.26
Sulphoxides	S=O stretch	1,030–1,060	9.71–9.43
Thiocyanates	C≡N stretch	2,160–2,175	4.63–4.59
Triazines	C=O stretch	c. 1,740	c. 5.75
	In-plane ring def.	1,520–1,560	6.58–6.41
	Out-of-plane ring def.	c. 816	c. 12.25
Ureas	N—H stretch	c. 3,330	c. 3.0
	C=O stretch	1,661–1,635 and	6.02–6.12
		1,613–1,575	6.20–6.35
Urethans	N—H stretch	c. 3,330	c. 3.0
	C=O stretch	1,690–1,720	5.92–5.81
	uncertain	near 1,540,	near 6.49
		1,300 and 1,230	7.69 and 8.
Uretidiones	C=O stretch	c. 1,770	c. 5.65
Water	O—H stretch	c. 3,300	c. 3.0
	O—H def.	c. 1,667	c. 6.0

(Continued)

Intensity	Remarks	References
very strong	Very broad band	
strong	Much sharper. Both bands unaffected by salt formation	
strong		
very strong		83
medium		50
strong	Hydroxytriazines in the solid state	85
very strong		
medium		
strong		
strong		
strong		
strong		
strong		
strong	Often double	
very strong	May be mistaken for O—H in alcohols	
medium		

The variations from phenol to phenol raise another important point. Since these bands arise from vibrations localised in the O—H link, small variations in its force constant are reflected in the frequency. If therefore a substituent such as the nitro group is introduced, which, via resonance forms such as

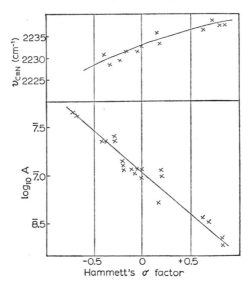

modifies the O—H link, slight frequency changes are to be expected. A parallelism has in fact been found[71], between the O—H frequency of a substituted phenol and the Hammett sigma factor of the substituent. From examination of a large volume of reaction velocity data on benzene derivatives, Hammett[86] was able to assign to many substituents a sigma

Fig. 55. Correlation of Hammett's sigma factor with (a) wave-number, and (b) log (intensity) of —C≡N stretching bands of substituted benzonitriles in carbon tetrachloride solution[91].

factor which measures its average influence on a reaction velocity. These factors are in effect measures of the extent to which the substituent attracts or repels electrons, to or from the ring to which it is attached. Powerfully electron-attracting groups such as nitro have large positive σ values, and electron donators such as the amino group negative values.

Relations have been found between σ and the NH frequencies of substituted anilines and anilides[87], the $C\equiv N$ frequencies of benzonitriles[91], and the carbonyl frequencies of carboxylic acids, ketones and esters[17,21]. Fig. 55 shows a typical plot, that for benzonitriles.

It is therefore clear, not only that characteristic frequencies are useful in detecting groups in unknowns, but also that with compounds of known structure, the precise value may serve to demonstrate electronic shifts within the molecule. Characteristic frequencies may even be used in favourable cases to predict the reactivities of molecules[17].

Absorption in the region 1800 to 1600 cm^{-1} is usually due to stretching of double bonds. Since strong bands between 1680 and 1800 cm^{-1} almost invariably arise from $C=O$ groups, carbonyl compounds are particularly suitable for infra-red studies. Examination of Table 22 shows that the exact carbonyl frequencies of acids, esters, amides, etc. differ enough for it to be possible not only to detect $C=O$ groups in unknowns, but often to specify the class of compound. Inductive and mesomeric effects of neighbouring atoms in the molecule have effects on the force constant of a $C=O$ bond, which determines its frequency. Carbonyl bonds have considerable ionic character arising from resonance of the type $\ce{>C=O <-> >C+-O-}$. An electron attracting atom such as chlorine, in acid chlorides, tends, by its inductive effect to pull the electrons towards the centre of the bond, reducing its single bond ionic character and causing an abnormally high force constant and frequency. In acid chlorides, the opposing tendency to weaken the bond by mesomeric electron transfer involving $\overset{\displaystyle Cl^+}{\underset{\diagdown}{}}$ C—O$^-$ is unimportant,

but with amides electron transfer from the nitrogen to the oxygen atoms via the form H_2N^+

$$\underset{\diagup}{\overset{\diagdown}{}}\ C\!-\!O^-$$

overcomes the inductive effect, increasing the single bond character of the link, and leading to a low force constant and frequency. An intermediate situation holds with acids, esters and ketones.

Conjugation shows clearly in values of double bond frequencies. For example as the degree of conjugation of C=O with C=C increases in the series aliphatic ketones, acetophenones and benzophenones, the carbonyl frequency assumes the approximate values 1715, 1680 and 1650 cm^{-1}. Likewise whilst aliphatic acids normally absorb in the range 1700–1720 cm^{-1}, the values for aromatic ones fall between 1680 and 1700 cm^{-1}. Similar effects are found when two C=C links, or a C=C and a C=N are conjugated, the C=C frequencies of butadiene and polyenes being well below the normal value of 1650 cm^{-1}.

Substituent effects in aromatic systems, when transmitted through the ring, are clearly reflected in carbonyl frequencies. Thus the values for acetophenones in chloroform vary smoothly with the σ factor of the substituent from 1693 cm^{-1} at one end of the scale for the m-nitro compound with an electron attracting substituent, ($\sigma = +0.71$) to 1663 cm^{-1} at the other end for the electron donating p-amino group ($\sigma = -0.66$)[21]. Similar results have been reported for ethyl benzoates, benzoic acids, and benzoyl chlorides[17,21].

Ring strain also affects C=C and C=O frequencies. When the C=C group forms part of a six-membered or larger strain-free ring, its frequency is about the same as in acyclic compounds (1650 cm^{-1}). If however strain is introduced by reducing the ring size, the frequency falls, as shown by the values 1646, 1611 and 1566 cm^{-1} respectively for cyclohexenes, cyclopentenes and cyclobutenes. With exocyclic double bonds, strain factors operate in the opposite direction. Thus methylene cyclobutane absorbs at 1678 cm^{-1}, compared to 1641 cm^{-1} for methylene cyclohexane. Cyclic carbonyl compounds behave similarly, cyclic ketones, lactones and anhydrides with rings of five or less atoms absorbing at abnormally high frequencies.

In addition to skeletal frequencies, the spectrum below 1600 cm^{-1} includes characteristic frequencies associated with bending motions of C—H, O—H and N—H links. Primary amines for example have a strong band of this kind near 1600 cm^{-1}, whilst secondary amides show a highly characteristic peak (the amide II band) near 1550 cm^{-1}, due partly to bending of the N—H link. The bending mode of the methylene group lies near 1460 cm^{-1}, and its precise location may be used diagnostically to distinguish between straight chain and cyclic —CH$_2$— groups. Similarly the exact value of the methyl group frequency near 1375 cm^{-1} depends on how the group is attached to the rest of the molecule. Bending motions of the C—H links of olefines and substituted benzenes give rise to bands whose positions are valuable in distinguishing between mono-, di- and tri-substituted olefines, and between σ-, m- and p-disubstituted benzene derivatives, as shown in the table.

4. Characteristic group intensities

In electronic spectroscopy values of ε_{max} (the molar extinction coefficient) can fairly satisfactorily be associated with chromophores. Assigment of similar intensity coefficients to groups in the infra-red would greatly enhance the value of this spectral region in structural diagnosis, enabling one not only to establish the presence of groups in unknowns, but also to estimate their concentration. Attempts to establish group infra-red ε_{max} values have not proved very successful. Many infra-red bands are so narrow that, unless a grating instrument of very high resolving power is used, the apparent peak intensity depends on the instrumental resolution. This means that even in cases where the group molar extinction coefficient varies little from compound to compound, characteristic ε_{max} values cannot be transferred from one instrument to another.

This difficulty has been partially overcome by using as the measure of intensity the total area underneath the band, a quantity which is much less affected by instrumental factors[127]. The area is given by $\int \log_e (I_0/I) d\nu$ over the frequency range of the band, and a molar quantity A may be defined by the equation

$$A = \frac{1}{Cl} \int \log_e \frac{I_0}{I} \, d\nu,$$

which is analogous to ε_{max}. Clearly A values suffer from the disadvantage of being more difficult to measure than a peak extinction coefficient. Direct measurement of the area under the band by planimeter, or by an integrating device attached to the spectrometer, is the only really satisfactory method, although approximate methods of obtaining the area from the peak density and the width of the band have been described by Ramsay[88].

TABLE 23

VALUES OF A IN CARBON TETRACHLORIDE SOLUTION
(units of moles/l, cm, cm^{-1} and $\log_{10}$)

Group	Class of compound	Approx. wave-number	$A \cdot 10^{-3}$	Reference
O—H	primary alcohol	3,630	2.1–2.4	18, 71
	secondary alcohol	3,620	c. 2.0	
	phenols	3,600	5–6	
	oximes	3,600	5.5–6.5	
	cyanhydrins	3,600	2–3	
N—H	dialkyl amines	3,400	c. 0.04	25, 87
	anilines	3,400	0.8–4.5	
		3,480	1.0–2.5	
	methyl anilines	3,450	1.5–4.3	
	di-arylamines	3,450	c. 2	
	pyrroles, indoles	3,490	4.5–5.5	

TABLE 23 (continued)

Group	Class of compound	Approx. wave-number	$A \cdot 10^{-3}$	References
$—CH_2—$	hydrocarbon	2,900	c. 3.3	89
		1,460	c. 0.2	
	$—CO \cdot CH_2—$	2,900	c. 0.6	
		1,460	c. 1.0	
$—CH_3$	hydrocarbon	2,900	c. 3.8	89
		1,375	c. 0.35	
	$—CO \cdot CH_3$	2,900	c. 0.6	
		1,375	c. 1.7	
$—C≡N$	aliphatic nitrile	2,250	0.38–0.59*	59, 60
			0.22–0.35	
	aromatic nitrile	2,225	0.56–7.40*	
			0.25–4.00	
$—N=C=N—$	carbodiimide	2,130	45–50	33
$—N=C=O$	phenyl isocyanate	2,270	62–74	50
$—S—C≡N$	phenyl thiocyanate	2,170	1.2–2.3	50
$—N=C=S$	alkyl isothiocyanate	2,100	17–52	50
	aromatic isothiocyanate	2,050	65–90	
$C=O$	aliphatic aldehyde	1,730	c. 8	21, 90
	aromatic aldehyde	1,700	8.5–11*	
	dialkyl ketone	1,720	8.1–8.5*	
	unsaturated ketones and			
	acetophenones	1,690	7.5–9.5–	
	benzophenones	1,660	9.0–9.5*	
	aliphatic esters	1,735	12–16*	
			10–14	
	benzoates	1,720	12–16	
$C—O$	esters	1,200	c. 13	37
	alkyl ketones	1,200	c. 2	

* In chloroform solution.

References p. 218

Results to date confirm that characteristic A values can be assigned to certain groups of closely related compounds in a given solvent, as shown in Table 23. Here A is given in practical units of moles/l, wave numbers and logarithms to the base 10. If required they can be converted to absolute units, of molecules/cc, cycles/sec and natural logarithms, as often used in the literature, by multiplication by $1.15 \cdot 10^{-10}$. All alkyl ketones for example have a similar A value, which differs from that of alkyl esters. The N—H links of dialkyl amines, alkyl anilines and diaryl amines[25] have quite different A values, though there is little variation within each group. Francis[89] found that group intensities could be associated with the stretching and bending bands of —CH_3, and —CH_2— groups, provided there is no oxygen atom close to the group, in the molecule. The A value for a O—H group is about three times as great in phenols as in alcohols, and is very susceptible to hydrogen bonding effects[18].

Variations of A, within series of substituted aromatic compounds, have been intensively explored by Thompson's school[91], who have discovered many relationships between band intensities and mesomeric and inductive effects of substituents, as measured by the factors of Hammett and Taft (p. 281). Whereas in ethyl benzoates and acetophenones the intensity of the carbonyl band depends only slightly on the substituents, variations over a factor of ten occur with substituted benzonitriles. In such cases the band intensity obviously cannot be used to measure group concentrations, but with compounds of known structure, its value may throw light on electronic interactions between the substituent and the nitrile group.

C. EXPERIMENTAL METHODS

Before applications of infra-red spectroscopy to organic chemistry are discussed, some indication of the experimental methods must be given. A major reason for the popularity of this technique is the speed and ease with which, using modern infra-red spectrometers, the spectrum of a sample may be obtained, whether it be a gas, a liquid, a crystalline solid, or even an intractable gum, rubber or oil. As a rcsult, a comparatively cheap spectrometer can handle at least four or five samples per hour, so that it is easy to avoid delays in measurement.

1. Modern infra-red spectrometers

For most organic work double-beam spectrometers (or strictly speaking spectrophotometers) are much more suitable than single-beam instruments. By passing the light alternately through the sample and blank beams, both atmospheric water vapour absorption, and, in the case of samples in solution, solvent absorption can be cancelled out, leaving a direct spectrum of wavelength (or wave number) against per cent absorption by the sample.

Since about 1950 several manufacturers, including Grubb-Parsons, Hilger and Watts, and Unicam in Great Britain, and Perkin-Elmer, Beckman and others in the United States have offered large, high performance double-beam instruments. Such instruments, costing around £4,000, offer all that is required in organic applications in respect of resolution, wavelength reproducibility and sample versatility, and, partly by recording on large charts, achieve an accuracy in intensity measurements suitable for accurate quantitative analysis. In the last two or three years much cheaper instruments at £1,000–£1,500 have been marketed, of which the Perkin-Elmer "Infracord" is typical. These scaled down double beam spectrometers are perfectly adequate for the majority of the applications described in the following pages, being unsuitable only in cases where the highest resolving power or accuracy of wavelength or intensity determination is essential.

The same principles are common to all modern infra-red spectrometers. Reflecting mirrors rather than lenses are used, because of the impossibility of obtaining achromatic lenses for the infra-red region. As a light source the Nernst filament is most commonly used. This is a thin rod of rare-earth oxides, which on warming become conducting, and, when incandescent, emits a high proportion of its energy in the infra-red. Light from the source first passes to a beam-splitting device in which the light path is switched alternately at several cycles/sec through the sample and blank beams, which are recombined on the entrance slit of the monochromator. This normally uses as the dispersing element a prism of lithium fluoride, rock-salt or potassium bromide, according to the wavelength range to be covered and the resolving power required. Grating mono-chromators are also available, which give better resolution than prism instruments, but are rather less convenient in operation. As with ultra-violet spectrometers, a spectrum is formed in the plane of the exit slit, and by rotating the prism, or a mirror behind it, any required wavelength may be caused to pass through the exit slit to the detector, usually a vacuum thermo-couple or bolometer.

Fig. 56 shows the optical lay-out of the Grubb-Parsons double-beam prism instrument, in which beam splitting in the double-

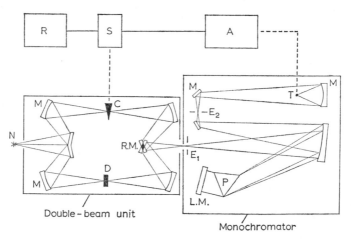

Fig. 56. Grubb-Parsons Double-beam Prism Spectrophotometer (sche-matic). A is the amplifier, C the attenuating comb, D the sample, E_1 and E_2 the entrance and exit slits, LM the Littrow mirror, M a surface reflecting mirror, N the Nernst filament, P the prism, R the recorder, RM the reci-procating mirrors, S the servo-motor, and T the thermocouple.

beam unit is achieved by a pair of mirrors reciprocating at $16^2/_3$ cycles/sec. Whilst a spectrum is being recorded, a motor turns the Littrow mirror, L.M., causing the wavelengths of the range covered to fall successively on the detector. At wavelengths of zero absorption equal signals will reach the detector from both beams. Since the latter is coupled to an amplifier sensitive only to alternating currents of the beam switching frequency, no signal will be generated. When however a band is reached, the beams become unbalanced, and an alternating signal develops in the detector which is amplified and used to drive a servo motor, which in turn drives a comb in to the blank beam, reducing it till balance is again achieved. As the spectrum is scanned, the comb is drawn in and out of the blank beam by the thermocouple signals, which follow intensity variations caused by bands in the sample beam. By coupling this comb to the pen of a recorder which is driven synchronously with the wavelength drive, an automatic record of percentage absorption against wavelength is obtained. Since variations of strength from band to band are much less than in the ultra-violet region, this type of presentation (rather than optical density recording) is usually quite satisfactory.

2. Sample preparation

It is not usually possible to obtain infra-red spectra from very dilute solutions in a solvent, as solvents sufficiently transparent in this region are not available. Even the best infra-red solvents, which are non-polar liquids such as carbon disulphide and carbon tetrachloride (see Fig. 57) cannot normally be used in layers more than a fraction of a millimetre thick. The consequence is that one can obtain infra-red spectra of solutions only if they are rather concentrated (1–5%). Many of the best polar solvents, including water, alcohols, ethers and ketones themselves absorb much too strongly to be useful, except in special cases. Since only a fraction of the samples to be examined are soluble to the required extent in non-polar solvents, various methods have been devised for examining undiluted solids and liquids.

Liquids may be measured in thin cells (0.01 to 0.1 mm), with windows of an infra-red transparent substance, most commonly rock-salt. Both permanent cells, in which the assembly is glued together with a spacer of the required thickness between the

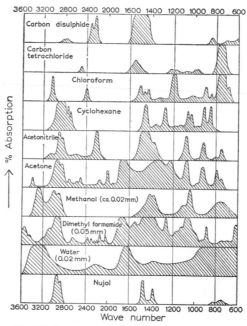

Fig. 57. Spectra of possible infra-red solvents.
Thickness 0.1 mm, unless otherwise stated.

windows, and demountable cells, which are more easily cleaned when using viscous samples, are used. In quantitative work the thicknesses of these very thin cells is best measured from the interference pattern obtained with the empty cell[92]. Very satisfactory variable thickness micrometer cells are available commercially[93], which may be set to any desired width, but these are inevitably more expensive than simple cells.

Several methods are available for dealing with solids. Most of these rely for their success on the progressive reduction of light scattering by particles and surface irregularities as one passes to longer wavelengths. Thus a sample which is almost opaque to visible light may transmit quite highly at 10 μ. The simplest, quickest and more commonly used method with crystalline solids involves mulling them with a relatively transparent oil such as "Nujol", a medicinal paraffin, and pressing the resulting suspension between rock-salt plates. Since the mulling liquid greatly reduces scatter by the solid particles, spectra which are quite adequate for qualitative and even semi-quantitative work are obtained.

A more precise method of dealing with solids, including many amorphous materials and fibres, uses discs of potassium bromide. Weighed amounts, usually about 1 mg of sample and 300 mg of bromide, are thoroughly mixed and ground, transferred to a die, and subjected to a pressure of about 20 tons per square inch in a suitable press, whereupon the bromide forms a transparent disc, carrying in suspension finely dispersed particles of the sample. Provided grinding and pressing conditions are carefully reproduced, the method is fairly satisfactory for quantitative work[94]. Suitable thin films of polymers for infra-red work can often be obtained by solvent casting, melting, or microtome cutting. Low melting solids are sometimes measured above their melting points, in heated liquid-type cells.

D. TYPICAL APPLICATIONS IN ORGANIC CHEMISTRY

This section deals with day-to-day applications, more specialised uses of infra-red spectroscopy being reserved for later sections of the chapter.

1. Identification by comparison

As has already been stressed, the infra-red spectrum provides perhaps the most useful method of finger-printing an organic compound. Its power is illustrated in Fig. 58, which shows the spectra of C_9 alkyl benzenes. Despite the close similarity of most physical properties of these compounds, their infra-red spectra are sufficiently different to be invaluable for their detection and analysis. Clearly infra-red spectra present an attractive method of identifying unknowns.

Within a small field, where spectra of compounds related to the unknown are available, identification is easy and certain. In many cases it may merely involve comparing the unknown spectrum with that of a synthetic sample obtained for com-

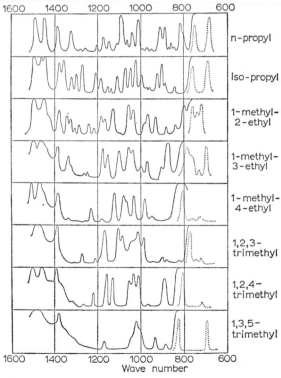

Fig. 58. Infra-red spectra of C_9 alkyl benzenes. ——— 0.1 mm layer; .... 0.01 mm layer.

parison. This technique is particularly valuable with high melting intractable solids, and has the advantage over the X-ray method (p. 360) of being applicable not only to crystalline solids, but also to amorphous materials and liquids. Infra-red identifications have also the important advantage over, for example, melting point determinations, that minor amounts of impurity do not interfere, the band positions of the major component being unaffected.

The broader question of identification in the absence of chemical evidence must now be considered. Clearly an extensive library of spectra is required, together with suitable means of discovering whether or not the unknown spectrum co-incides with one in the collection. Several collections of spectra are available[95-98], of which the Sadtler File of Infra-red Spectra is the most comprehensive, containing at the present time (1960) about sixteen thousand spectra. Two methods are available for matching unknown spectra. A device known as the "Specfinder", sold by the same firm, tabulates the wavelengths of the bands of each spectrum in such a way that, by starting with the strongest band of an unknown spectrum, and working through it band by band, one can rapidly find out whether it occurs in the file. All the data in the Sadtler and other collections has been coded on punched cards by the American Society for Testing Materials, so that unknowns may be identified by machine sorting.

At first sight these methods might appear the complete answer to problems of identification, but there are a number of drawbacks. Firstly the procedure is really satisfactory only when the unknown is a pure compound. Otherwise preliminary separation, for example by chromatography, may be necessary. Given a pure compound, identification depends on rather accurate determination of the band positions both in the unknown spectrum, and in all those of the collection. It is by no means certain that this criterion is always met, particularly when using small spectrometers. Although the spectra of over sixteen thousand compounds have been collected, this number is very small compared to the number of organic compounds which have been described, so that, even if the unknown has already been prepared, the chances of its spectrum being in the collection are not very good. Finally, as described in section B *1*, infra-red spectra are appreciably different in the solid and liquid states and in solution, polymorphs have slightly different spectra, and degree of hydration affects a spectrum. Hence it is essential, that the spectrum of the unknown be determined on a sample in exactly the same form as the sample on which the measurements of the collection were carried out.

The conclusion is that, although infra-red spectroscopy is a powerful method of identification when the chemical nature of the sample is known, there are serious limitations to the identification of completely unknown materials by comparison with known spectra.

2. Impurity detection and quantitative analysis

Since infra-red absorption bands are intrinsically weaker than those in the ultra-violet, detection limits by infra-red spectroscopy often compare unfavourably in cases where ultra-violet spectra can be applied. Infra-red methods compare still less favourably with mass spectroscopy in this respect. The method has, nevertheless, distinct advantages over other techniques in that it may be applied to involatile, insoluble samples, whilst the principle of characteristic frequencies offers a prospect of finding the nature of the impurity.

Definite detection limits cannot be laid down, the sensitivity varying from case to case. Conditions are most favourable when the impurity has strong bands in regions where the main component absorbs little. For example very small amounts (0.1% or less) of a ketone can be detected in a hydrocarbon system, since the latter has practically no absorption near 1720 cm^{-1}, but up to 5% of the same ketone might be missed if the major component were a similar ketone. Likewise whilst very small concentrations of alcohols in non-hydroxylic media can be detected by their —OH stretching band, quite large amounts of one alcohol in another might not show in the spectrum. A fair idea of the chances of impurity detection in a given case can be formed from the data of Table 21. Sharp bands are best for the purpose.

Impurity detection is usually more successful in liquid systems, where relatively thick layers can be used, than with solids, where attempts to use large effective sample thicknesses often lead to excessive light scattering. Considerable improvements in the sensitivity of detection in solids (suspended in potassium bromide or "Nujol"), may result from cooling the sample to the temperature of liquid nitrogen. This often leads to band sharpening and intensification, causing better resolution between the bands of the major component, and the weak impurity peaks and shoulders. Improvements may also be effected by difference methods with the impure sample in one beam, and the corresponding pure material in the blank beam[8,99].

The widespread use of infra-red spectra in quantitative analysis is reflected in the section of each issue of Analytical Chemistry, which is devoted to data on infra-red quantitative analyses of mixtures. Although in many cases less band overlap, and consequently more accurate results are obtainable by gas–liquid chromatography or mass spectroscopy, the infra-red method is often preferred on grounds of convenience, particularly if the highest accuracy is not essential.

When quantitative analysis is contemplated, the spectra of the pure components must first be obtained. The analysis depends on the fact that, as with ultra-violet spectra, the spectrum of the mixture shows the bands of all the components, at intensities proportional to their concentrations. Analyses are most accurate where each component shows at least one strong band which is not significantly overlapped by bands of the other constituents. The optical density of such a band yields the proportion of a compound in a mixture by direct comparison with measurements on the pure compound. More frequently band overlap necessitates more complicated methods of calculation. Solution of simultaneous equations may be applied (p. 104), and other methods, including successive approximations and comparison with synthetic mixtures have been described[100].

Quantitative analyses are often performed on undiluted liquid mixtures, but, if high accuracy is required, solutions in a transparent solvent are preferable, because of the difficulty of reproducing the very small cell thicknesses required with neat liquids. Rather less accurate results can be obtained on solid samples, which cannot be suitably dissolved. With two component mixtures, rough analyses can be made by comparing the strengths of two bands in a "Nujol" mull. Fair accuracy in quantitative analysis can be obtained by the bromide disc method[94].

3. Structural diagnosis

When, as often happens, identification by comparison fails, resource must be had to structural diagnosis by detecting groups from their characteristic frequencies. Although the procedure, using a chart such as Fig. 53, is largely self-evident, care must be taken for several reasons. It must be remembered that many of the bands between 6 and 15 μ are skeletal rather than group frequencies. If then a band is found at, for example, 990 cm^{-1}, this does not necessarily indicate a vinyl group, since the band may arise from a skeletal motion.

Both band position and intensity should be considered in assigning bands to groups. Table 21 includes the data necessary for this to be done. For example a weak band at 1720 cm^{-1} could not indicate carbonyl groups, except as trace impurity, as the band is intrinsically strong, but a weak band near 2250 cm^{-1} might be due to a nitrile group in the molecule. As more quantitative data on group intensities, of the kind given in Table 23 becomes available, intensities will be used increasingly in diagnosis.

In exceptional cases group frequencies may fall outside the limits in the table. Those connected with —OH and —NH— groups are particularly prone to be displaced, if the group is involved in hydrogen bonding. For example, whereas anthraquinone shows a carbonyl band at 1676 cm^{-1}, the corresponding band in its 1.4-dihydroxy derivative falls near 1620 cm^{-1}, as a result of strong internal hydrogen bonding, and no hydroxyl band is found in the normal range[78].

Whenever possible cross-checking of band assignments should be attempted. If for example the 3300–3400 cm^{-1} absorption suggests a primary amine group, confirmation should be sought from the bending band near 1620 cm^{-1}. Similarly an indication of an —OH group from the stretching region should be confirmed by seeking the C—O stretching band between 1000 and 1100 cm^{-1}.

It must be borne in mind that characteristic frequencies are usually associated with small groups of atoms, rather than with large units, and ring structures. With a completely unknown material, the prospects of detecting functional groups are good, but it is seldom possible to deduce much about the overall structure of the molecule. While the above method may thus give leads in the structural determination, the spectrum usually becomes much more useful when sufficient chemical and other physical data has been collected for possible structures to be suggested. Very often these will carry different functional groups, enabling the correct one to be selected from the spectrum. In this connection Table 21 will help in predicting many of the bands in proposed structures. Even if the same groups are present in all the suggested structures, they may occupy different relative positions in the molecule, so that by predicting the precise values of certain characteristic frequencies, a distinction can be made. Simple examples of this occur where two double bonds may or may not be conjugated, or where a carbonyl group may be in a five or a six-membered ring.

4. Study of chemical reactions

Since the majority of chemical reactions involve changes in functional groups rather than more fundamental structural changes, infra-red spectroscopy is particularly suitable for following reactions. It is often sufficient to withdraw a sample from time to time, and use its spectrum to determine how far the reaction has progressed, and whether it is taking the expected course. The speed and ease with which infra-red spectra can be obtained from relatively crude products is invaluable in this connection.

Most common organic reactions can be followed. If, for example, the mechanism of an oxidation is in doubt, spectral studies near 3300, 1720 and 1100 cm^{-1} will indicate the rates of formation of hydroxyl, ketonic and ether groups. Hydrogenations can readily be followed by the disappearance of the well known bands associated with double bonds, benzene rings and nitro groups, and the development of those of $-CH_2-$, $-NH_2$ and similar groups in the product. Many ring closures, including anhydride formation, are accompanied by large

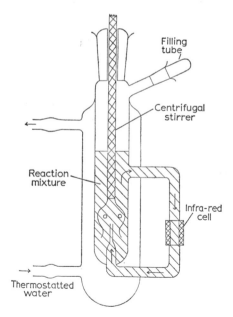

Fig. 59. Apparatus for reaction velocity studies[101].

spectral changes, whilst esterification, hydrolyses of esters, and hydrolyses of nitriles to amides and acids may also readily be followed.

Isocyanate reactions, which are now very important in connection with polyurethane foam production, provide another good example. Not only can the very strong isocyanate band at 4.35 μ be used to determine reaction rates, and as a criterion of completion of the reaction, but the nature of the products can be decided in doubtful cases, since the likely ones, urethans, uretidiones, isocyanurates and ureas all have different characteristic frequencies.

Infra-red spectroscopy has been used not only to follow reactions qualitatively, but also for precise kinetic studies, by placing the reaction mixture in the spectrometer beam, and scanning the appropriate spectral region at frequent intervals. Although results can be obtained simply by placing the mixture in a normal thin cell, this has the disadvantage that adequate stirring and thermostatting cannot be provided. A very satisfactory cell was first described by Higgins[101], and is shown in Fig. 59. In operation thermostatted fluid flows through the outer vessel surrounding the reaction mixture, which is continuously circulated by the centrifugal stirrer through the side arm incorporating the infra-red cell. The only limitation to infra-red spectroscopy for reaction velocity studies is in respect of solvents, since many common reaction media, including water and alcohols, are unsuitable.

E. HYDROGEN BONDING

Of the many methods used in studying hydrogen bonding, infrared spectroscopy is the most direct and sensitive, and has been used consistently for the purpose since the pioneer work described in Pauling's book[102]. The subject has recently been comprehensively reviewed in a book by Pimentel and Mc-Clellan[103].

In the vapour state, or in dilute solution in an inert solvent such as carbon tetrachloride, X–H groups show bands at highly characteristic stretching frequencies. The extent to which the band (or its overtone) is moved to longer wavelengths, intensified and broadened, under conditions where hydrogen bonds are formed, provides an excellent means of detecting them and estimating their strengths. Essentially the same method may be used for both intermolecular bonds, and intramolecular ones, which occur within one molecule.

In early work the frequency shift was the criterion normally used. According to Badger's rule[104], the shift is proportional to the heat of formation of the bond in question, but recent more extensive data have shown this to apply only within restricted groups of similar compounds[103]. The band width (at half its height) also increases roughly in proportion to the bond strength, and the intensity of the fundamental X–H bond behaves similarly. The intensity of the first overtone bands are however decreased by hydrogen bonding. Whenever possible all three quantities should be considered in investigating hydrogen bonds.

1. Intramolecular hydrogen bonds

In the condensed phases it is not usually possible to distinguish between inter- and intramolecular bonds. However in carbon tetrachloride, or a similar solvent, at concentrations below about 0.02 M, one may safely neglect intermolecular associations, and ascribe any perturbations of an X–H band to intramolecular bonding. The most striking cases are provided by O—H . . . O and O—H . . . N bands. Both electronic factors, as discussed by Cannon[105], and steric conditions must be satisfied for a strong bond to be formed. The X–H bond must be partially ionic to facilitate overlap by a lone pair orbital on the nitrogen or oxygen atom. Steric requirements favour five and six-membered rings roughly equally, but there are few reports of strong internal bonds involving larger rings.

In extreme cases, such as 1,4-dihydroxyanthraquinone (I) and 2,2′-dihydroxyazobenzene (II), the hydroxyl absorption is so shifted and broadened that no band is detectable when the compounds are examined under normal conditions.

I   II

Clearly this phenomenon must be guarded against in structural diagnosis. Table 24 lists the frequencies, half widths, and intensities (areas) associated with typical internal bonds in dilute carbon tetrachloride solution. Some of the bands overlap the C—H absorption region, making intensity measurements impossible. Finally it must be stressed that, although such bonds are most readily demonstrated in dilute solution, they persist in the solid and liquid states.

2. Intermolecular hydrogen bonds

Hydrogen bond formation between molecules is a much more widespread and important phenomenon than internal bonding, which is shown by relatively few substances. If dilute solutions of an alcohol in a series of solvents are measured, the frequency, intensity and width, of the O—H stretching band, vary in step with the ability of the solvent to form hydrogen bonds. Attempts have been made to correlate these shifts with the basicity of the solvent[103].

Precise studies of intermolecular bonding are best carried out in an inert solvent, such as carbon tetrachloride. The spectral changes in the region of the —OH stretching band, as the concentration of solutions of n-butanol in chlorobenzene varies (Fig. 60) indicate self-association of the alcohol molecules. In the spectrum of the most dilute solution, the strongest peak, near 3630 cm^{-1}, is due to monomers, whilst the weak one at 3500 cm^{-1} is attributed to dimer species in equilibrium with the

TABLE 24
DATA ON INTERNAL HYDROGEN BONDS (DILUTE CCl₄ SOLUTIONS)

Compound	Structure	Wave-number	Half-width (cm^{-1})	$A \cdot 10^7$ (abs. units)
Ethanol	C_2H_5OH	3,632	39	2.47
Ethyl lactate		3,541	35	3.55
Diacetone alcohol		3,532	56	5.42
Hydracetyl acetone		3,557	90	4.64
1-Diethylamino propan-2-ol		3,468	156	7.37
3-Diethylamino propan-1-ol		3,288	240	25.2
Phenol	C_6H_5OH	3,610	22	7.25
8-Hydroxy quinoline		3,431	57	7.92
2-Nitrophenol		3,243	89	9.51
Disalisal azine		c.3,050	Very broad	—
2-Acetyl-1-naphthol		c.2,700	Very broad	—
1-Dimethylamino-methyl-2-naphthol		c.2,850	Very broad	—

monomers. Proceeding to more concentrated solutions the relative strengths of these bands shows a steady increase in the ratio of associated to monomeric species, as expected from the law of mass action. Moreover the association band moves to

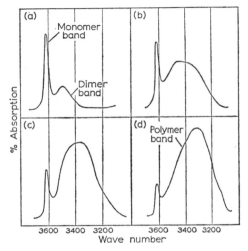

Fig. 60. Spectra of solutions of *n*-butanol in chlorobenzene, in the —OH stretching region: (a) 1.4; (b) 3.4; (c) 7.1; and (d) 14.3 % butanol (wt/wt).

rather longer wavelengths with increasing concentration, showing trimers and higher polymers to be present, in addition to dimers. Many workers[106,107] have attempted from the variations of spectrum with concentration to calculate the equilibrium constants involved. It is normally assumed that only monomers absorb at 3630 cm^{-1}, so that from the optical density at this position the proportion of this species can be deduced. From relatively dilute solutions the dimerisation constant can be obtained. In more concentrated solutions it is sometimes assumed that the same free energy change accompanies each addition of one more unit to the polymer, so that the same equilibrium constant relates concentrations of monomer to dimer, dimer to trimer and so on. On this assumption the single equilibrium constant is given by

$$K = \frac{1}{N_m} (1 - f^{\frac{1}{2}})$$

where N_m is the mole fraction of monomers, and f the fraction of the material in monomeric form. From the equation the proportions of monomers, dimers, etc. may be calculated[106].

Further information about such systems is obtainable by varying the temperature of the system. At a given concentration, a temperature increase reduces the polymer bands relative to the monomer band, showing the equilibrium constant to be reduced. From its variation with temperature the heat of formation of the bond can be calculated from the Van 't Hoff isochore[108].

Hydrogen bonds, in which the two bonding molecules are different, have been studied in the same way[108]. In this work benz-p-toluidide, diphenylamine, phenol and benzyl alcohol were first measured near 3 μ in very dilute carbon tetrachloride solution, under which conditions only a single sharp N—H or O—H band was formed. Solutions of these compounds with increasing concentrations of dioxan, dimethyl formamide, azobenzene and other substances, capable of forming O—H $\cdots$ N, O—H $\cdots$ O, N—H $\cdots$ N or N—H $\cdots$ O bonds were then measured, whereupon the original band decreased, whilst a new, broader band due to the hydrogen bonded complexes developed. Fig. 61 shows some typical results. From the intensity decrease of the monomeric band, equilibrium constants were calculated, from the temperature dependence of which the heats of formation of the hydrogen bonds were deduced.

Hydrogen bonds profoundly affect the spectra of solid and liquid alcohols, phenols, amides and acids, particularly in the short wavelength region. In the condensed states these compounds are normally completely hydrogen bonded, so that condensed state O—H and NII frequencies differ markedly from those in dilute solution. The hydroxyl stretching band of liquid alcohols and phenols usually falls near 3300 cm⁻¹,

Fig. 61. Formation of hydrogen bonded complexes in solution[108]. (a) benzyl alcohol; (b) benzyl alcohol + azobenzene; and (c) benzyl alcohol + dimethyl formamide, all in dilute carbon tetrachloride solution.

compared to 3610–3630 in dilute solution. Exceptions to this may result from steric hindrance. For example in the alcohol

$$CH_3 \diagdown \qquad OH \qquad CH_3$$
$$CH - C - CH \qquad ,$$
$$CH_3 \diagup \qquad C_2H_5 \qquad CH_3$$

the hydroxyl groups are so hindered that association cannot proceed beyond the dimer stage, causing a value of 3510 cm⁻¹ in the liquid[109], whilst the hydroxyl frequency of liquid 2,2,4,4-tetramethyl-3-isopropyl-3-pentanol is 3640 cm⁻¹, since association is virtually impossible.

Similar effects have been found with phenols which are substituted by bulky ortho groups such as *t*-butyl. In this respect liquid phenols fall roughly in to three classes, those without bulky ortho groups (near 3320 cm^{-1}), those with one such substituent (near 3500 cm^{-1}), and those with two (near 3600 cm^{-1}).

F. TAUTOMERISM

Infra-red spectroscopy provides an attractive method of studying tautomeric equilibria. Although less suitable than nuclear resonance spectroscopy for determining quantitatively the proportions of tautomers under given conditions, it has the advantage of being applicable to solids. Each tautomer in most of the common systems, including keto–enol, lactam–lactim, and mercapto–thioamide tautomerism, contains a group such as C=O, OH, NH or C=S with a well-established characteristic frequency, which makes it possible to deduce from the spectrum which form predominates.

Keto–enol systems, —CO—CH$_2$— $\rightleftharpoons$ —C(OH) =CH—, may be characterised by the C=O band of the keto form, near its normal position, and the hydroxyl absorption of the enol. It has been shown[111] that in the solid state, and in chloroform, oxindole and the related compound whose tautomeric possibilities are shown below, both exist entirely in the keto form.

The nature of lactam–lactim systems, —C—NH— $\rightleftharpoons$ —C=N—,
                                      || OH
                                        O
can often be deduced from the presence or absence of a strong

carbonyl band and, in solution, the occurrence of a hydroxyl band near 3600 cm⁻¹. For example solid cyanuric acid shows a strong carbonyl band at 1740 cm⁻¹ and typical NH absorption showing the structure to be

$$\begin{array}{c} NH-CO \\ | \quad \quad | \\ CO \quad \quad NH \\ | \quad \quad | \\ NH-CO \end{array}$$

rather than

$$\begin{array}{c} OH \\ | \\ N-C \\ // \quad \quad \backslash \\ HO-C \quad \quad N \\ \backslash \quad \quad // \\ N=C \\ | \\ OH \end{array}$$

Quite generally, hydroxy triazines as solids, or in neutral solution exist in the keto form.

The 2- and 4-hydroxy derivatives of pyridine and quinoline present similar possibilities, as below

$$\text{(pyridine)}-OH \rightleftharpoons \text{(pyridine)}=O \qquad \text{(pyridine)}-OH \rightleftharpoons \text{(pyridine)}=O$$

Once again infra-red measurements[112] show all these substances in the solid state, and in chloroform to be ketonic. Isatin derivatives and phthalimides provide further examples where the equilibrium is on the keto side.

Equilibria of the type $-N=C- \rightleftharpoons NH-C-$ are well
$\qquad\qquad\qquad\qquad\quad\ \ \overset{|}{SH} \qquad \overset{\|}{S}$
suited to infra-red study. The bands which are available for the study of such systems include the S—H and N—H stretching frequencies, the C=S band near 1140 cm⁻¹, and ring defor-

mation bands between 1600 and 1630 cm^{-1}. An early application was to the rubber accelerator 2-mercaptothiazoline;

In neither the solid state or in solution can any S—H absorption be detected. Solution spectra[113] however show a strong NH band near 3400 cm^{-1} indicating free N—H groups, and a broad absorption centred near 3150 cm^{-1} due presumably to hydrogen bonded N—H groups. Both absence of SH and presence of NH thus indicate the right hand tautomer. Another rubber chemical, normally called 2-mercaptobenzthiazole, has in fact the structure

except in alkaline solutions. Recent studies of 2- and 4-mercapto pyridine[112] indicate that they should be formulated

These, and many other examples, show infra-red spectroscopy to be a very powerful tool, at least for the qualitative study of tautomeric equilibria.

G. APPLICATIONS TO POLYMERS

Although few new principles are involved in applying infra-red spectroscopy in the polymer field to problems of co-polymer analysis, identification and detection of functional groups, brief descriptions will be given of a few cases where the spectrum yields information not obtainable by other means. Most polymers can fairly easily be obtained in thin films suitable for infra-red examination by casting from a volatile solvent, melting between rock-salt plates which are pressed together, or by microtome cutting. Spectra of fibres can often be measured by suitably aligning small bundles of filaments, and moistening with a fluid of comparable refractive index, to reduce scatter.

1. Detection of end-groups and chain-branching in polymers

Spectroscopy is useful in this connection, provided the molecular weight is low enough for the concentration of end groups to be reasonably large, and provided the end-groups or chain-branching units give fairly strong bands at wavelengths where the polymer chains do not absorb strongly.

Since polyethylene (polythene) consists largely of sequences of —CH_2— groups, the polymer chains give rise to few strong bands, so that the sensitivity of detection of end-groups, products of oxidation, and unsaturation is very good. For this reason infra-red spectra have contributed much to our knowledge of the fine structure of this polymer[68], and have enabled certain variations in physical properties from sample to sample to be explained.

It was first reported by Fox and Martin[114] that the infra-red spectrum of polythene indicated methyl groups. More recently a thorough re-examination of the matter[115], during which the spectra of many commercial samples were compared with that of pure polymethylene, (—CH_2—)$_n$, prepared by decomposition of diazomethane, revealed additional bands at 1378 and 891 cm^{-1}, which, by comparison with simpler hydrocarbons, are due to methyl groups. Very careful comparison of the intensities of these bands, in molten polymer samples, with the corresponding hydrocarbon bands, enabled estimates to be made of the numbers of methyl groups per carbon atom, and hence of the degrees of chain-branching. Methyl group concentrations in polythenes made under various conditions show values of between one methyl in fifteen and one methyl in two hundred carbon atoms. The corresponding degrees of branching correlate

References p. 218

well with the crystallinities and other physical properties of the samples.

Whereas the determination of iodine, bromine and hydrogenation numbers gives only the total degree of unsaturation, infra-red spectroscopy is capable of distinguishing the various types of olefinic groups. By comparison with simple olefines, estimates can be made of the concentration of each type in a polythene sample. $RR^1 \cdot C = CH_2$ groups are generally found in direct polymers of ethylene, but $R \cdot CH = CH_2$ units predominate in low molecular weight pyrolysed materials. Weak bands at 1720 and 3360 cm^{-1} in polythene samples indicate respectively aldehydic or ketonic and hydroxyl groups, and their intensities provide an excellent method of following oxidation of the polymer on exposure to light or weather.

A very careful spectroscopic study of the end-groups in polyethylene terephthalate ("Terylene") has been carried out by Ward *et al.*[116,117]. When the spectra of several carefully dried samples of the polymer with various molecular weights were examined, spectral variations between 2800 and 3700 cm^{-1} were found which suggested intensity changes in bands due to end groups. To separate these variable bands from the background absorption of the polymer, samples were deuterated, by prolonged soaking in heavy water, and remeasured. Subtraction of the spectra (on a density scale) before and after deuteration, showed clearly the removal of bands at 3535 and 3240 cm^{-1}, and their replacement by peaks at 2630 and 2460 cm^{-1}. Comparison with model systems proved these bands to be due respectively to —OH, —COOH, —OD and —COOD groups. Satisfactory values for the extinction coefficients of these groups in "Terylene" could not however be obtained from models. Accordingly, after several samples had been deuterated and remeasured, they were combusted and the proportion of H.OD. in the resulting water determined. From this the total numbers of end-groups in the samples were calculated on the very reasonable assumption that only the —OH and —COOH groups were deuterated under the conditions used. It was thus possible to calculate the required extinction coefficients, and the end-group contents of subsequent samples of polymer could be obtained simply by applying the formulae

$$n_{OH} = (218 \pm 35) \, (\text{o.d.})_{OH}$$

and

$$n_{COOH} = (164 \pm 20) \, (\text{o.d.})_{COOH}$$

n_{OH} and n_{COOH} being respectively the numbers of gram equivalents of —OH and —COOH groups per 10^6 grams of polymer, and the optical densities referring to films 0.012 cm thick. This procedure gave for the first time reliable measures of the end-group concentrations and molecular weights of samples of "Terylene".

A final example refers to end-groups in polyisobutene[118]. The spectra of several low polymers made with titanium tetrachloride as catalyst, and water, or an organic acid, as co-catalyst were measured. With water additional bands at 1642, 895 and 825 cm^{-1}, relative to high molecular weight polyisobutene indicate that both $\diagdown \!\!\!\! \diagup \!\! C\!\!=\!\!CH_2$ and $\diagdown \!\!\!\! \diagup \!\! C\!\!=\!\!C\diagup^{R}_{\diagdown H}$ groups are formed. This assignment was confirmed by the disappearance of the 895 cm^{-1} band and part of the 1642 cm^{-1} band on bromine treatment, since the second type of bond is known to be much less reactive toward bromine. Polymers made with trichloracetic acid as co-catalyst showed these double-bond bands, and in addition peaks at 1775 cm^{-1} and 600–900 cm^{-1}, whose disappearance on alkali treatment showed them to be due to trichloracetate end-groups.

2. Crystallinity in polymers

The subjects of this section and the next have recently been admirably reviewed by Elliott[119]. It is generally agreed that solid polymers are often inhomogeneous, consisting of regions known as crystallites where the polymer chains are regularly aligned, as in a crystalline solid, separated by amorphous regions where they intertwine randomly. Fig. 109 (p. 374) illustrates this conception, which, though undoubtedly an oversimplification provides a useful basis for correlating many of the physical properties of polymers. Clearly the crystalline-amorphous ratio is important in determining such properties as hardness, extensibility and softening point of a polymer. For many years this ratio has been estimated by X-ray methods (p. 374) and density measurements, and recently several authors have measured it by infra-red spectroscopy. It must not be expected that in every case identical values will be obtained by infra-red and X-ray techniques since infra-red bands typical of oriented chains may be obtained in cases where the crystalline regions are too small or imperfect to diffract X-rays.

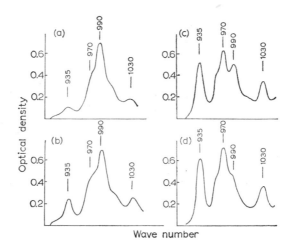

Fig. 62. Spectrum of a 6-nylon film[126]: (a) quenched sample; (b) heated 5 h at 160°C; (c) heated 5 h at 180°C; (d) heated 3 h at 205°C.

Investigations of crystallinity in polymers depend on the fact that, just as the infra-red spectrum of the same compound in the solid and liquid states is slightly different, certain bands of polymer chains in the crystalline and amorphous regions have rather different positions and intensities. In Fig. 62, which illustrates the effect of crystallinity on the spectrum of 6-Nylon, (a) shows the spectrum of an amorphous film. The various heat treatments cause partial crystallisation, which can be followed by the growth of bands at 935, 970 and 1030 cm^{-1}, due to crystallites, whilst the initially strong amorphous band at 990 cm^{-1} diminishes. Provided a highly crystalline sample can be obtained from which one can deduce the extinction coefficient of a band due entirely to crystalline material, such a band may be used to measure crystalline-amorphous ratios, as was done in the case of polychloroprene by Maynard et al.[120].

It is usually more satisfactory to base the determination on the strength of a band due entirely to the amorphous material, since a purely amorphous sample from which one may obtain the extinction coefficient can usually be prepared easily, for example by quenching molten polymer in liquid nitrogen. Miller and Willis[121] for example used amorphous bands respectively at 1305 and 770 cm^{-1} to determine the crystallinities of polythene and polytetrafluoroethylene samples, obtaining results in good agreement with X-ray findings.

3. Use of polarised infra-red radiation

To obtain a full understanding of the properties of synthetic and naturally occurring polymers, it is necessary to know not only the sequence of atoms in the chain but also the distribution of those chains in space. The stretching of rubber, for example, corresponds to uncoiling of the polymer chains.

Such information may sometimes be inferred by examining fibres and oriented films of polymers with polarised infra-red light. If the plane of polarisation is rotated with respect to the fibre axis, or direction of alignment of the crystallites, the intensities of bands associated with groups such as C=O and N—H reach maxima when the direction of the group in question co-incides with the electric vector of the light. By this means the angles which certain groups make with the fibre axes can sometimes be deduced. This technique has been applied extensively by Elliott and his co-workers[119] to polypeptides and proteins. For example they measured the spectra of films of the α and β forms of poly-L-alanine[122], with the plane of polarisation parallel and perpendicular to the axis of orientation. The observed dichroisms of the C=O and N—H stretching bands confirmed an earlier suggestion that the β-form contains fully extended chains of —CO—NH—CHR— units, whereas in the α-form the chains are folded in helices. Polarised infra-red measurements also provide a possible method of distinguishing between folded and extended forms of fibrous proteins.

Some light has been thrown on the structure of cellulose, using similar methods[123]. A number of bands were found near 3μ, and associated with different types of hydrogen bond. These bands show different behaviours with polarised radiation, from which the authors conclude that, in addition to hydrogen bonds between the chains, there are intramolecular bonds along the chain direction, linking oxygen atoms in adjacent glucose residues.

REFERENCES

[1] G. HERZBERG, *Infra-red and Raman Spectra of Polyatomic Molecules*, Van Nostrand, New York, 1945.

[2] C. K. INGOLD *et al.*, *J. Chem. Soc.*, (1936) 966 and 971; (1946) 222.

[3] J. W. LINNETT, *Quart. Revs. London*, 1 (1947) 73.

[4] W. GORDY, *J. Chem. Phys.*, 14 (1946) 305.

[5] H. S. TAYLOR AND S. GLASSTONE, *A Treatise on Physical Chemistry*, Vol. I, Macmillan, London, 1942. Appendix I.

[6] K. S. PITZER, *Chem. Revs.*, 27 (1940) 39.

[7] W. KAYE, *Spectrochim. Acta*, 6 (1954) 257; 7 (1955) 181.

[8] R. G. J. MILLER AND H. A. WILLIS, *J. Appl. Chem. London*, 6 (1956) 385.

[9] J. L. LAUER AND E. J. ROSENBAUM, *Appl. Spectroscopy*, 6 (1952) 29.

[10] L. J. BELLAMY, *The Infra-red Spectra of Complex Molecules*, 2nd ed., Methuen, London, 1958.

[11] R. N. JONES AND C. SANDORFY in: *Chemical Applications of Spectroscopy*, Interscience, New York, 1956.

[12] N. B. COLTHUP, *J. Opt. Soc. Am.*, 40 (1950) 397.

[13] H. W. THOMPSON, *J. Chem. Soc.*, (1948), 328.

[14] J. H. WOTIZ AND F. A. MILLER, *J. Am. Chem. Soc.*, 71 (1949) 3441.

[15] J. H. WOTIZ, *J. Am. Chem. Soc.*, 72 (1950) 5055.

[16] J. L. H. ALLAN, G. D. MEAKINS AND M. C. WHITING, *J. Chem. Soc.*, (1955) 1874.

17 M. St. C. Flett, *Trans. Faraday Soc.*, 44 (1948) 767.

18 M. St. C. Flett, *Spectrochim. Acta*, 10 (1957) 21.

19 H. H. Zeiss and M. Tsutsui, *J. Am. Chem. Soc.*, 75 (1953) 897.

20 S. Pinchas, *Anal. Chem.*, 29 (1957) 334.

21 H. W. Thompson, R. W. Needham and D. Jameson, *Spectrochim. Acta*, 9 (1957) 208.

22 J. H. Wotiz and D. E. Mancuso, *J. Org. Chem.*, 22 (1957) 207.

23 H. W. Thompson and R. E. Richards, *J. Chem. Soc.*, (1947) 1248.

24 M. Beer, H. B. Kessler and G. B. B. M. Sutherland, *J. Chem. Phys.*, 29 (1958) 1097.

25 R. A. Russell and H. W. Thompson, *J. Chem. Soc.*, (1955) 483.

26 J. E. Stewart, *J. Chem. Phys.*, 30 (1959) 1259.

27 B. Chenon and C. Sandorfy, *Can. J. Chem.*, 36 (1958) 1181.

28 H. W. Thompson, D. L. Nicholson and L. N. Short, *Discussions Faraday Soc.*, 9 (1950) 222.

29 H. L. McMurry and V. Thornton, *Anal. Chem.*, 24 (1952) 318.

30 M. St. C. Flett, *J. Chem. Soc.*, (1951) 962.

31 D. Hadži and N. Sheppard, *Proc. Roy. Soc. London, A*, 216 (1953) 247.

32 R. A. Meiklejohn *et al.*, *Anal. Chem.*, 29 (1957) 329.

33 G. D. Meakins and R. J. Moss, *J. Chem. Soc.*, (1957) 993.

34 W. A. Patterson, *Anal. Chem.*, 26 (1954) 823.

35 O. D. Shreve, M. R. Heether, H. B. Knight and D. Swern, *Anal. Chem.*, 23 (1951) 277.

36 H. W. Thompson and P. Torkington, *J. Chem. Soc.*, (1945) 640.

37 R. A. Russell and H. W. Thompson, *J. Chem. Soc.*, (1955) 479.

38 L. H. Briggs, L. D. Colebrook, H. M. Fales and W. C. Wildman, *Anal. Chem.*, 29 (1957) 904.

39 H. Tschamler and R. Leutner, *Monatsh.*, 83 (1952) 1502.

40 A. R. Katritzky, *Quart. Revs. London*, 13 (1959) 353.

41 J. Derfer, C. E. Boord and E. E. Pickett, *J. Am. Chem. Soc.*, 71 (1949) 2482.

42 L. W. Marrison, *J. Chem. Soc.*, (1951) 1614.

43 N. Sheppard and D. M. Simpson, *Quart. Revs. London*, 7 (1953) 19.

44 C. G. Cannon and G. B. B. M. Sutherland, *Spectrochim. Acta*, 4 (1951) 373.

45 J. G. Hawkins, E. R. Ward and D. H. Whiffen, *Spectrochim. Acta*, 10 (1957) 105.

46 H. W. Thompson and S. F. D. Orr, *J. Chem. Soc.*, (1950) 218.

47 J. D. Burnett, R. G. J. Miller and H. A. Willis, *J. Polymer Sci.*, 15 (1955) 592.

48 G. J. Minkoff, *Proc. Roy. Soc. London, A* 224 (1954) 176.

49 W. H. T. Davison, *J. Chem. Soc.*, (1953) 3712.

50 G. L. Caldow and H. W. Thompson, *Spectrochim. Acta*, 13 (1958) 212.

51 G. B. B. M. Sutherland and N. Sheppard, *J. Chem. Soc.*, (1947) 453.

[52] J. F. GROVE AND H. A. WILLIS, *J. Chem. Soc.*, (1951) 877.
[53] H. W. THOMPSON AND I. F. TROTTER, *J. Chem. Soc.*, (1946) 481.
[54] A. MENEFEE, D. O. ALFORD AND C. B. SCOTT, *J. Org. Chem.*, 22 (1957) 792.
[55] R. D. HILL AND G. D. MEAKINS, *J. Chem. Soc.*, (1958) 760.
[56] N. SHEPPARD, *Trans. Faraday Soc.*, 51 (1955) 1465.
[57] E. K. PLYLER AND N. ACQUISTA, *J. Research Natl. Bur. Standards*, 43 (1949) 37.
[58] J. J. FOX AND A. E. MARTIN, *Proc. Roy. Soc. London*, *A*, 175 (1940) 208.
[59] J. P. JESSON AND H. W. THOMPSON, *Spectrochim. Acta*, 13 (1958) 217.
[60] M. R. MANDER AND H. W. THOMPSON, *Trans. Faraday Soc.*, 53 (1957) 1402.
[61] R. HEILMANN AND J. M. BONNIER, *Compt. rend.*, 248 (1959) 2595.
[62] P. TARTE, *J. Chem. Phys.*, 20 (1952) 1570.
[63] R. R. RANDLE AND D. H. WHIFFEN, *J. Chem. Soc.*, (1952) 4153.
[64] B. FRANCK, H. HÖRMANN AND S. SCHEIBE, *Chem. Ber.*, 90 (1957) 330.
[65] W. LÜTTKE, *Z. Elektrochem.*, 61 (1957) 976.
[66] J. A. ANDERSON AND W. D. SEYFRIED, *Anal. Chem.*, 20 (1948) 998.
[67] W. H. T. DAVISON AND G. R. BATES, *J. Chem. Soc.*, (1953) 2607.
[68] J. P. LUORIGO AND D. L. WOOD, *Mod. Plastics*, (1961) 132.
[69] A. PALM AND H. WERBIN, *Can. J. Chem.*, 31 (1953) 1004.
[70] R. CRIEGEE, *Chem. Ber.*, 88 (1955) 1878.
[71] P. J. STONE AND H. W. THOMPSON, *Spectrochim. Acta*, 10 (1957) 17.
[72] D. E. C. CORBRIDGE, *J. Appl. Chem.*, 6 (1956) 456.
[73] L. W. DAASCH AND D. C. SMITH, *Anal. Chem.*, 23 (1951) 853.
[74] L. J. BELLAMY AND L. BEECHER, *J. Chem. Soc.*, (1953) 728.
[75] E. J. AMBROSE AND A. ELLIOT, *Proc. Roy. Soc. London*, *A* 205 (1951) 47.
[76] G. B. B. M. SUTHERLAND, M. BEER, K. N. TANNER AND D. L. WOOD, *Proc. Roy. Soc. London*, *A* 249 (1959) 147.
[77] D. HADŽI AND N. SHEPPARD, *J. Am. Chem. Soc.*, 73 (1951) 5460.
[78] M. ST. C. FLETT, *J. Chem. Soc.*, (1948) 1441.
[79] R. A. DURIE, R. E. LACK AND J. S. SHANNON, *Australian J. Chem.*, 10 (1957) 429.
[80] A. LEE-SMITH AND J. A. MCHARD, *Anal. Chem.*, 31 (1959) 1174.
[81] R. N. KNISELEY, V. A. FASSEL AND E. E. CONRAD, *Spectrochim. Acta*, 15 (1959) 651.
[82] N. SHEPPARD, *Trans. Faraday Soc.*, 46 (1950) 429.
[83] D. BARNARD, J. M. FABIAN AND H. P. KOCH, *J. Chem. Soc.*, (1949) 2442.
[84] K. C. SCHREIBER, *Anal. Chem.*, 21 (1949) 1168.
[85] W. M. PADGETT, II AND W. F. HAMNER, *J. Am. Chem. Soc.*, 80 (1958) 803.
[86] L. P. HAMMETT, *Physical Organic Chemistry*, McGraw-Hill, New York, 1940.
[87] P. J. KRUEGER AND H. W. THOMPSON, *Proc. Roy. Soc. London*, *A* 243 (1957) 143.

88 D. A. RAMSAY, *J. Am. Chem. Soc.*, 74 (1952) 72.

89 S. A. FRANCIS, *J. Chem. Phys.*, 18 (1950) 861; 19 (1951) 942.

90 G. M. BARROW, *J. Chem. Phys.*, 21 (1953) 2008.

91 P. J. KRUEGER AND H. W. THOMPSON, *Proc. Roy. Soc. London*, A 250 (1959) 22.

92 H. A. WILLIS AND G. B. B. M. SUTHERLAND, *Trans. Faraday Soc.*, 41 (1945) 181.

93 Research and Industrial Instruments Co., London.

94 J. J. KIRKLAND, *Anal. Chem.*, 29 (1957) 1127.

95 *The Sadtler Catalogue of Standard Spectra*, Samuel P. Sadtler and Son, Inc., Philadelphia, Pa.

96 *Documentation of Molecular Spectroscopy – The DMS System* (Punched Cards), Butterworths, London.

97 The American Petroleum Institute Spectra.

98 The National Research Council – National Bureau of Standards File of Spectrograms.

99 H. A. WILLIS AND R. G. J. MILLER in: *Molecular Spectroscopy*, (Eds. E. THORNTON AND H. W. THOMPSON), Pergamon, London, 1959.

100 C. R. N. STROUTS, J. H. GILFILLAN AND H. N. WILSON, *Analytical Chemistry*, Vol. II, Oxford University Press, 1955.

101 G. HIGGINS, Private communication.

102 L. PAULING, *The Nature of the Chemical Bond*, 2nd ed., Oxford University Press, 1940.

103 G. C. PIMENTEL AND A. L. McCLELLAN, *The Hydrogen Bond*, Freeman, San Francisco, 1960.

104 R. M. BADGER AND S. H. BAUER, *J. Chem. Phys.*, 5 (1937) 839.

105 C. G. CANNON, *Mikrochim. Acta*, (1955) 555.

106 R. MECKE, *Discussions Faraday Soc.*, 9 (1950) 161.

107 N. D. COGGESHALL AND E. L. SAIER, *J. Am. Chem. Soc.*, 73 (1951) 5414.

108 M. ST. C. FLETT, *J. Soc. Dyers Colourists*, 68 (1952) 59.

109 F. A. SMITH AND E. C. CREITZ, *J. Research Natl. Bur. Standards*, 46 (1951) 145.

110 R. A. FRIEDEL, *J. Am. Chem. Soc.*, 73 (1951) 2881.

111 A. E. KELLIE, D. G. O'SULLIVAN AND P. W. SADLER, *J. Chem. Soc.*, (1956) 2202, 3809.

112 E. SPINNER, *J. Chem. Soc.*, (1960) 1221, 1237.

113 M. ST. C. FLETT, *J. Chem. Soc.*, (1953) 347.

114 J. J. FOX AND A. E. MARTIN, *Proc. Roy. Soc. London*, A 175 (1940) 208.

115 L. H. CROSS, R. B. RICHARDS AND H. A. WILLIS, *Discussions Faraday Soc.*, 9 (1950) 235.

116 D. PATTERSON AND I. M. WARD, *Trans. Faraday Soc.*, 53 (1957) 291.

117 I. M. WARD, *Trans. Faraday Soc.*, 53 (1957) 1406.

118 M. ST. C. FLETT AND P. H. PLESCH, *J. Chem. Soc.*, (1952) 3355.

119 A. ELLIOTT, *Advances in Spectroscopy*, 1 (1959) 214.

[120] J. T. MAYNARD AND W. E. MOCHEL, *J. Polymer Sci.*, 13 (1954) 235.
[121] R. G. J. MILLER AND H. A. WILLIS, *J. Polymer Sci.*, 19 (1956) 485.
[122] A. ELLIOTT AND E. J. AMBROSE, *Nature*, 165 (1950) 921.
[123] J. MANN AND H. J. MARRINAN, *Trans. Faraday Soc.*, 52 (1956) 481, 487, 492.
[124] A. D. CROSS, *An Introduction to Practical Infra-red Spectroscopy* Butterworths, London, 1960.
[125] J. K. BROWN AND N. SHEPPARD, *Discussions Faraday Soc.*, 9 (1950) 144.
[126] I. SANDEMAN AND A. KELLER, *J. Polymer Sci.* 19 (1956) 401.
[127] H. W. THOMPSON in: *Molecular Spectroscopy*, Pergamon, London, 1958, p. 165.
[128] R. A. G. CARRINGTON, *Spectrochim. Acta*, 16 (1960) 1297.

SELECTED BIBLIOGRAPHY TO CHAPTER 6

BEAVAN, G. H., E.A. JOHNSON, H. A. WILLIS AND R. G. J. MILLER, *Molecular Spectroscopy; Methods and Applications in Chemistry*, Heywood, London, 1961, 336 pp.

BELLAMY, L. J., *The Infra-red Spectra of Complex Molecules*, Methuen, London, 1958, 425 pp. This book deals comprehensively with the characteristic frequencies of the various classes of organic compound. It is therefore an essential handbook for any organic chemist who wishes to interpret his own spectra.

CROSS, A. D., *An Introduction to Practical Infra-red Spectroscopy*, Butterworths, London, 1960, 80 pp. Brief descriptions are given of the experimental methods and, largely in tabular form, of the frequencies of organic molecules.

Trans. Faraday Soc., 41 (1945) 296 and *Discussions Faraday Soc.*, Vol. 9. These contain many papers illustrating chemical applications of infra-red spectroscopy.

JONES, R. N., AND C. SANDORFY in: *Chemical Applications of Spectroscopy*, (Ed. W. WEST), Interscience, New York, 1956. The applied infra-red section of this book (pp. 247–580) describes how frequencies and intensities are derived from the instrumental records, lists sources of spectra, and discusses characteristic frequencies. Like Bellamy's book, it is an essential reference work wherever the spectra of organic materials must be interpreted.

HERSHENSON, H. M., *Infra-red Absorption Spectra*, Academic Press London, 1959. In this book, compounds whose infra-red spectra appeared in the literature between 1945 and 1957 are arranged alphabetically, with the appropriate references.

HERZBERG, G., *Infra-red and Raman Spectra of Polyatomic Molecules*, Van Nostrand, New York, 1945, 632 pp. The fundamental principles by which force constants, bond lengths, etc. are derived from the spectra of simple molecules are discussed in this book. Data on large numbers of such molecules are listed.

STROUTS, C. R. N., J. H. GILFILLAN AND H. N. WILSON, *Analytical Chemistry*, Vol. II, Oxford University Press, 1955. Chapter 23 of this book (pp. 749–854) gives a good all-round summary of chemical applications of infra-red spectroscopy, including details of methods of quantitative analysis.

(a) THORNTON, E. AND H. W. THOMPSON (Eds.), *Molecular Spectroscopy*, Pergamon, London, 1959, 352 pp.

(b) THOMPSON, H. W., *Molecular Spectroscopy*, Institute of Petroleum, London, 1955.

These reports of Institute of Petroleum meetings include many papers dealing with recent applications of infra-red spectroscopy.

Ministry of Aviation, *An Index of Published Infra-red Spectra*, H.M. Stationery Office, London, 1960. This consists of a collection of 10,000 references to infra-red spectra of compounds, in the literature up to 1957. These compounds are arranged according to their molecular formulae.

CHAPTER 7

ELECTRON SPIN RESONANCE SPECTROSCOPY

As described in Chapter 5, the electrons of the molecules of the majority of stable organic compounds occupy molecular orbitals in pairs. The two electrons in an orbital differ from one another only in that their spin quantum numbers have the values $+\frac{1}{2}$ and $-\frac{1}{2}$. Every electron in these molecules is thus spin paired, so that there is no net electron spin.

Nevertheless molecules with unpaired electrons are by no means uncommon or unimportant. The first example of a free radical, or molecule with one unpaired electron was discovered by Gomberg nearly fifty years ago. From the chemical properties of hexaphenyl ethane he inferred that in solution it dissociates partly into triphenyl methyl radicals

$$\ddot{\text{O}} \quad \ddot{\text{O}} \qquad \qquad \ddot{\text{O}} \qquad \ddot{\text{O}}$$
$$\text{Ø} : \text{C} : \text{C} : \text{Ø} \;\rightarrow\; \text{Ø} : \text{C} \cdot \;+\; \cdot \text{C} : \text{Ø}$$
$$\ddot{\text{O}} \quad \ddot{\text{O}} \qquad \qquad \ddot{\text{O}} \qquad \ddot{\text{O}}$$

Many similar cases of relatively stable free radicals have subsequently been found. For example solid 1,1-diphenyl-2′-picryl hydrazyl, $(C_6H_5)_2N — \dot{N} — C_6H_2(NO_2)_3$, exists entirely in the radical form.

Stable free radicals are not however of great practical importance. Much more interesting to the chemist are those less stable radicals which are intermediates in many chemical reactions. Quite generally chemical reactions have been divided into two classes, heterolytic, where breakage of a bond into ionic fragments is involved, and homolytic where the initial step generates radicals

$$A : B \rightarrow A \cdot + B \cdot$$

For example the reduction of quinones involves radical intermediates. Potentiometric titration shows that this reduction proceeds in two distinct steps, each corresponding to addition of one electron

According to the pH the intermediate radical may be either an uncharged molecule or a negative ion. Clearly the properties of these substances, the semiquinones, are of commercial importance in the reduction of vat dyes.

Polystyrene, polyvinyl acetate, and poly(methyl methacrylate) are commonly manufactured by a radical process. To the vinyl monomer is added an initiator such as benzoyl peroxide or azobisisobutyronitrile, which fairly readily yields radicals R·. These attack the monomer, forming new radicals which again react, building up the chain, which terminates only when two growing chain ends meet and react by addition or disproportionation (4 and 5).

$$R· + CH_2{=}CHX \rightarrow R·CH_2·\dot{C}HX \quad \ldots \ldots \ldots \ldots \ldots \ldots \quad 1$$

$$R·CH_2·\dot{C}HX + CH_2{=}CHX \rightarrow R·CH_2·CHX·CH_2·\dot{C}HX \quad \ldots \ldots \quad 2$$

$$R(CH_2·CHX)·_n + CH_2{=}CHX \rightarrow R(CH_2·CHX)_n·CH_2·\dot{C}HX. \quad \ldots \ldots \quad 3$$

$$R·(CH_2·CHX)·_n + R·(CH_2·CHX)·_m \rightarrow$$
$$R(CH_2CHX)_{n-1}·CH_2·CHX·CHX·CH_2(CH_2·CHX)_{m-1}·R \quad 4$$

References p. 253

$$R \cdot (CH_2CHX)_{n-1} \cdot CH_2 \cdot \dot{C}HX + R(CH_2 \cdot CHX)_{m-1} \cdot CH_2 \cdot \dot{C}HX \rightarrow$$
$$R \cdot (CH_2 \cdot CHX)_{n-1} \cdot CH_2 \cdot CH_2 X + R \cdot (CH_2 \cdot CHX)_{m-1} \cdot CH = CHX \quad 5$$

Free radicals also play an important part in biochemistry. It is well established that there are quite large concentrations in living tissue. Many enzyme processes are probably chain reactions with free radical intermediates.

Molecules with two unpaired electrons are also known. The 4,4'-polymethylenebistriphenylmethyls,

are typical biradicals. Closely related to these are triplet state molecules (see p. 128) which differ from them in that their two unpaired electrons are closely coupled together, rather than behaving as two separate entities.

Final examples of molecules with unpaired electrons are provided by haemoglobin and such enzymes as catalase and peroxidase, which contain transition metal atoms. In these atoms the higher energy electrons do not always fall into successive energy layers in pairs. 3d levels may remain singly occupied, whilst electrons go into the 4-levels.

From the examples quoted it is clear that unpaired electrons play an important part in organic chemistry. Methods are therefore necessary for their detection, and to determine their concentrations both when constant and when varying during a reaction. In addition the molecular structure of the radicals responsible for phenomena must often be elucidated.

A. METHODS OF STUDYING FREE RADICALS

Basically there are two approaches to the problem. The first makes use of their relative instability and consequent high reactivity. An example of this is Paneth's classical mirror technique[1]. For example the presence of methyl radicals was demonstrated by passing gas suspected of containing them over a thin lead mirror. The lead disappeared and could be redeposited farther down the tube by local heating. Reaction with methyl radicals in the gas, forming volatile lead tetramethyl was the only plausible explanation. Chemical methods of detection are however impracticable in many cases, for example where radicals are formed in a solid, since they are then inaccessible to species with which they might react.

Physical methods offer a second approach. These depend on the property of the electron that, being a spinning charged body, it has associated with it a magnetic moment. The moments of all the spin paired electrons in a molecule cancel out, but the unpaired electrons of free radicals and related molecules, cause a residual magnetic moment.

Magnetic susceptibility measurements provide the most direct method of using this property. The presence of free radicals and hence of magnetic moments renders a substance paramagnetic, so that it is pulled into a region of high magnetic field. From the strength of this pull, the concentration of radicals may be calculated. The method has been applied extensively[2,3] but has serious limitations. If the concentration of paramagnetic centres is small it may be difficult to allow for the diamagnetism of the other atoms of the molecule. Serious errors may be caused

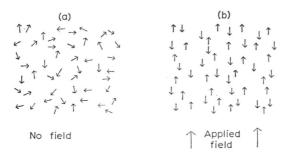

Fig. 63. Effect of an applied field on the magnetic axes of electrons.

by traces of ferromagnetic impurities. Also magnetic susceptibility measurements give no indication of the structure of the
radical in question. The electron spin resonance method, the
basis of which will now be described, suffers from none of these
defects, and therefore provides by far the most powerful tool at
present available for the study of free radicals.

B. THE PRINCIPLES OF ELECTRON SPIN RESONANCE SPECTROSCOPY

Let us regard a system with unpaired electrons as an assemblage
of randomly arranged magnets (Fig. 63a). On application of a
magnetic field (Fig. 63b), these magnets, in obedience to the
quantum laws, line up with their axes either parallel or anti-
parallel to the field direction. A similar phenomenon involving
atomic nuclei forms the basis of nuclear spin resonance spectroscopy. Intermediate positions, as would be expected on a
classical basis are forbidden. A magnet of moment μ which
makes an angle θ with a field H has potential energy

$$E = \mu H \cos \theta$$

For these molecular magnets which are parallel to the field,
$\theta = 0$, so $E = \mu H$, whereas for those which are aligned anti-
parallel $\theta = 180°$ and $E = -\mu H$. The two classes of electron
then differ in energy by $\Delta E = 2\,\mu H$. By the Boltzmann distribution law there will therefore be rather fewer of the higher
energy variety, the relative numbers in the upper and lower
states being given by

$$n_1/n_2 = \mathrm{e}^{-\Delta E/kT} = \mathrm{e}^{-2\mu H/kT} \qquad \ldots \ldots \ldots \; 6$$

There is therefore the possibility of spectroscopic measurements
in which electrons of the lower energy group absorb electromagnetic radiation, and are raised to the upper level, their
magnetic axes being turned through $180°$ in the process. The
frequency of absorption is given by the usual quantum condition

$$h\nu = \Delta E = 2\mu H$$

as shown in Fig. 64. This branch of spectroscopy is remarkable in that the frequency is dependent on the applied field. It therefore appears at first sight that by a suitable choice of H the measurements could be made in any convenient spectral region. Equation 6 however shows that the absorption probability and hence the sensitivity of the measurements, which reach their maximum with small values of n_1/n_2, increase steeply with H. It is therefore essential to use the maximum possible magnetic

Fig. 64. Energy levels of an electron in a magnetic field H.

field. Considerations of magnet construction however limit the field to about 10,000 gauss, which corresponds to absorption in the microwave region, with wavelengths of 1 to 3 cm. Electron spin resonance spectroscopy is therefore normally carried out with microwave sources, receivers etc.

C. MEASUREMENT OF ELECTRON SPIN RESONANCE SPECTRA

During the development of radar, valves called klystrons were discovered which are powerful sources of microwave radiation. These normally emit at a fixed wavelength, which cannot readily be varied. It is not therefore convenient to obtain the spectrum as a graph of wavelength against absorption as in for example ultra-violet or infra-red work. The spectrum is in fact measured by varying the magnetic field. A record is obtained of magnetic field against microwave absorption in which peaks appear where the condition

$$hv = 2\mu H$$

is satisfied. Fig. 65a and b show typical electron spin resonance spectra. (a) has only a single peak and (b) consists of a pattern of lines, due to hyperfine splitting (see p. 238). Microwaves cannot be directed by mirrors, prisms etc. as in shorter wavelength spectroscopy, but can readily be led along rectangular metal tubes known as waveguides.

Fig. 65. (a) **Absorption** spectrum of solid diphenylpicrylhydrazyl; (b) **Absorption** of a dilute solution of *p*-benzosemiquinone.

Fig. 66. Electron spin resonance spectrometer, with crystal-video detection.

The basis arrangement of an electron spin resonance spectrometer is indicated in Fig. 66. Part of the output from the klystron, which is normally operated at 3 cm in free radical studies, is fed to a cavity resonator, whose dimensions are a simple function of the wavelength. Accordingly standing waves are set up, so that the cavity serves as a very long path length cell in which the waves are reflected to and fro thousands of times. The cavity is placed between the pole pieces of a magnet, whose field can be varied over a small range. Provision is made to introduce the sample at the point of maximum microwave power in the cavity. It may be in the form of a single crystal, solid powder, liquid or solution, and is usually contained in a tube about 5 mm in diameter.

The detector is usually a silicon-tungsten crystal rectifier which converts the microwave power to a direct current output. To avoid the difficulty inherent in measuring a small change in a high power level on introducing the sample, a balancing unit is often used, so that with no sample absorption only a small signal reaches the detector. Sample absorption in the presence of the magnetic field then changes the output, which is amplified and recorded by an oscilloscope or pen recorder.

Several variants of the basic spectrometer have been described, with different sensitivities and resolving powers. The design is governed by the type of work to be undertaken. If the main purpose of the experiments is the study of very small concentrations of radicals, for example in a reacting system, the most sensitive available means of detection must be used. Other problems may require measurement of the spacings and widths of the narrow components of a fine structure pattern (*e.g.* Fig. 71). High resolution rather than extreme sensitivity would then be the main target, and a highly homogeneous magnetic field would be required. Brief descriptions of typical spectrometers follow.

1. Simple spectrometers with crystal-video detection

This type of spectrometer, which is shown schematically in

Fig. 66, can be built for about £1000, and is suitable for studying fairly high concentrations of radicals, particularly in the solid state. Here the natural widths of the lines is often so great that little is gained by the use of a more refined spectrometer. A relatively cheap permanent or electromagnet is used. Provision is made to modulate the magnetic field by a low frequency alternating component, which produces a fluctuation of the field, whose amplitude is larger than the width of the spectrum to be scanned. The whole spectrum is thus swept through twice during each cycle. Consequently the detector output varies during each cycle in accordance with the spectrum of the sample. If this output is then amplified and fed to the plates of an oscilloscope, the X plates of which are fed in synchronisation with the field modulation, the spectrum appears on the screen. This type of spectrometer is easy to construct and operate, but is limited in sensitivity by its high signal to noise ratio.

2. More sensitive spectrometers – high frequency modulation and superhet detection

The above simple spectrometer is inherently insensitive because of the high noise level associated with the output from a crystal detector, modulated at a low frequency. It also has the disadvantage that pen records cannot be obtained. These difficulties can be overcome by modulating the magnetic field at a much higher frequency, about 100 kilocycles/sec being the upper limit in practice. Such modulation cannot be satisfactorily transmitted to the sample by varying the magnet current, and must be produced by a small coil inside the cavity. In this case the field modulation amplitude is small compared to the line widths in the spectrum. If then the main magnetic field is swept slowly through resonance over a period of several minutes the output signal will vary as shown in Fig. 67, tracing out the slope or derivative of the absorption spectrum. It is therefore a characteristic of high performance electron resonance spectrometers that they yield the derivative rather than the direct spectrum. Spectrometers of this type employ what is known as phase-sensitive detection, a device which eliminates all noise which is out-of-phase with the signal. A pen recorder is used, but provision may be made for switching to crystal-video detection for preliminary examination of the spectrum.

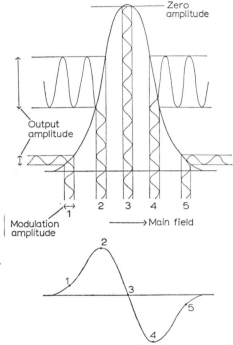

Fig. 67. Derivative signal with high-frequency modulation.

High frequency modulation spectrometers can be made very sensitive, but are not entirely suitable for the study of very narrow lines. As stated above, high frequency modulation was adopted to reduce the noise output of the detector. Additional improvement in this direction could be obtained if the modulation frequency were raised far beyond the practical limit of 100 kilocycles/sec. This can be done in effect with a superhet arrangement. Power from a second microwave source, of frequency about 50 megacycles/sec different from the first is fed into the detector arm. Beats are formed with the main signal at 50 megacycles/sec, which thus becomes the effective output modulation frequency, leading to a low noise level, and subsequent high sensitivity.

Superhet detection has an even more important advantage when very narrow lines must be studied. With frequency modulation, the apparent width of a line is increased above its true value by the presence of side-bands at frequencies equal to the sum and difference of the main oscillation frequency and the modulation frequency. Using superhet detection the side-bands are so close to the main line that broadening from this source is negligible.

It is essential for work on narrow lines that the magnetic field should be homogeneous to about a milligauss over the volume of the sample. This necessitates a precision engineered magnet costing about £5000. For many radical studies a field homogeneity of about 0.1 gauss, which can be obtained with a simple magnet costing about £300, will however be found adequate. The additional complexities of superhet detection would not normally be undertaken, unless a high performance magnet was available.

D. INTERPRETATION OF ELECTRON RESONANCE SPECTRA

There are four features of an electron resonance spectrum to be considered in obtaining the maximum information from it. These are:

(a) the magnetic field at the centre of the absorption, (b) the area enclosed by the curve, (c) the width of the peak at half its height, and (d) the presence of hyperfine splitting if any (Fig. 65b).

In the following sub-sections they are considered in turn.

1. Field value at resonance. g-factor measurements

The derivation of the resonance condition led to the equation

$$hv = 2\mu H$$

on the assumption that unpaired electrons in molecules behaved as free electrons. In practice the assumption is not always justified, as an electron bound to an atom has two distinct motions associated with it. Spin about its own axis has the same value, and gives rise to the same magnetic moment as for a free electron, but a bound electron has in addition an orbital motion about a nucleus, which itself contributes to the magnetic moment. Consequently the quantity μ of the equation is not a true constant. The condition is better expressed by

$$hv = g\beta H$$

where β, the Bohr magneton, is a true constant, and g is variable and is known as the spectroscopic splitting factor. In free radicals and biradicals, little or no coupling between spin and orbital motion occurs. Hence for such species g has almost the same value as for a free electron, namely 2.0023.

When unpaired electrons occur in the d or f shells of transition metal atoms, the situation is very different. Here strong spin-orbit coupling often occurs, so wide g-value variations are shown by transition metals, according to their valence state, and whether the bands formed by the metal to neighbouring atoms are predominantly covalent or ionic.

2. Area under the band – concentration of unpaired electrons

Since the widths of electron resonance bands vary greatly, the peak height does not have much significance. However the total area enclosed by the curve is proportional to the number of unpaired electrons in the sample. An absolute calculation of the number of electrons from the area is difficult, since instrumental factors are involved. A direct comparison is therefore usually made by substituting for the sample a standard containing a known number of radicals, without altering the conditions. The ratio of the two areas then yields the required result. High radical concentrations can be measured by comparison with diphenylpicrylhydrazyl which is completely in the free radical state, and can therefore be shown by a simple calculation to contain $1.53 \cdot 10^{21}$ unpaired electrons per gram. Ingram's school (Ref.[4], p. 98) have found it convenient to prepare a series of substandards, by taking a carbon black sample of known radical content, and diluting it with inert solid so as to obtain a series of mixtures with radical contents varying from 10^{16} to 10^{12} radicals per gram.

As explained above, high performance spectrometers yield the derivative of the spectrum. The record must therefore be integrated before the area can be measured. Unfortunately this may cause considerable errors. For example Whiffen *et al.*[6] estimate that for radicals formed during polymerisation, errors up to 50% of the absolute concentration may arise. There is one other common source of error in quantitative measurements. It was assumed in discussing the theory of the absorption that the ratio of low and high energy electrons, and hence the power absorbed is independent of time. This presupposes that return from the upper to the lower state is extremely rapid, a condition not always realised in practice. In such cases the ratio of high to low energy electrons in a high microwave power flux becomes less than the equilibrium value, so that the power absorption falls. This effect, known as "saturation" reduces the area of the peak, and yields too small a value for the radical concentration.

3. Band-widths

The next feature to be considered is the width of the absorption band at half its height. Although less information is obtainable from this than from the other quantities of this section, a brief explanation must be given of why band-widths vary from hundreds of gauss to a few milligauss.

The width of a band is inversely proportional to the lifetime of the absorbing species in its excited state. If then there are highly efficient modes of deactivating the excited states, the band will be correspondingly broad. Three mechanisms contribute to the deactivation in the case of electron resonance spectroscopy, which are known as

(a) spin-lattice interaction, (b) dipolar spin-spin interaction, and (c) exchange interaction.

Spin-lattice interaction leads to loss of its excess energy by the electron to the rest of the molecule, or to the crystal lattice as a whole in the case of a solid. This loss usually takes place via spin-orbit coupling, which, as mentioned above (p. 235), is very small in the case of free radicals. This form of broadening is therefore unimportant in the majority of organic applications. Spin-spin broadening results when the excited electron is deactivated by the magnetic field of a neighbouring free electron, or spinning atomic nucleus. It can be shown that the nuclear effect is averaged out in liquids or solutions, by the Brownian tumbling motion of the molecules. Spin-spin interactions between electrons may be minimised by working in dilute solution, where on average the electrons are far apart.

The third factor, "exchange narrowing", occurs only in the solid state. It arises from the ability of two electrons with equal energies in neighbouring molecules to exchange their spin orientations. The effect is to reduce dipolar spin-spin broadening and hence to narrow the line.

These three factors may be used to account for the approximate band widths found with solids, liquids, and dilute solutions. Although in the solid state the width may be 100 gauss or more, exchange narrowing sometimes reduces this to the order of 1–10 gauss. In liquids or concentrated solutions, exchange narrowing is absent, and dipolar broadening very strong. Hence lines as wide as or wider than in the corresponding solid may be expected. However in sufficiently dilute solution, all forms of broadening reach a minimum, and widths down to a few milligauss may be observed. For this reason when fine-structure studies are undertaken, dilute solutions should be used where possible.

In addition to these factors, instrumental influences on the apparent width of a line cannot be neglected. If for example a narrow-line spectrum is scanned by a spectrometer whose resolution is limited to a low value by inhomogeneity of its field, apparent widths far in excess of the true values will be observed.

4. *Hyperfine splitting – determination of radical structure*

Since the *g*-value of free radicals is always close to 2.0023, some other feature of the spectrum must be studied if the structure of the radical responsible for the absorption is in question. Many radicals, particularly in dilute solution, show hyperfine splitting, yielding a pattern of several sharp lines, rather than a single peak. From the number and relative intensities of these components, the structure can often be inferred.

The origin of this splitting is the magnetic moment associated with certain atomic nuclei. Like the electron, certain nuclei spin

Fig. 68. Interaction of an electron with protons.

about their axes, and therefore have a magnetic moment. Table 28 (p. 258) shows that of the common nuclei of organic chemistry, the proton, and the nitrogen and halogen nuclei have this property. They therefore assume definite orientations in an applied magnetic field, since their magnetic axes can assume only a limited number of directions relative to the field. Since in most free radicals the unpaired electron is not rigidly attached to a particular atom, but occupies an orbital embracing several atoms, it interacts to a greater or lesser extent with these atoms. The effective field seen by the electron is not therefore identical

TABLE 25

ELECTRON RESONANCE SPECTRA OF BENZOSEMIQUINONES

Parent quinone	No. of lines	Intensity ratio
	1	—
	2	1:1
	3	1:2:1
	4	1:3:3:1
	5	1:4:6:4:1

with the applied field, but is modified by the small magnets associated with the nuclei.

Suppose, in the simplest case, that the electron interacts with one hydrogen atom (Fig. 68a). The effective field is then $H + \Delta H$, or $H - \Delta H$, the ΔH term coming from the proton whose moment may be oriented either parallel or antiparallel to the main field, and therefore adds or subtracts a small component. Viewed statistically, one half of the unpaired electrons when undergoing their transition will happen to be in a field $H + \Delta H$ and the other half in a field $H - \Delta H$. Instead, therefore, of a single absorption line at a position governed by the equation $h\nu = g\beta H$, two lines of equal intensity will occur at frequencies determined by $h\nu = g\beta(H \pm \Delta H)$.

The value of ΔH is governed by the strength of the interaction between the electron and proton. If the electron interacts with two protons, then, as shown in Fig. 68b the second proton causes a second splitting, so that the absorbing electron may be in one of four possible magnetic fields. The magnitudes of the two splittings indicate the degrees of interaction with the two protons. The symbols ↑ and ↓ are used to show the orientations of the protons. Fig. 68c shows how a simplification occurs when the electrons interact equally with two protons. The number of possible fields and absorption lines reduces to three, with intensity distribution $1:2:1$, since the middle level has twice the electron population. Quite generally, if n protons are involved equally, $n + 1$ lines result, whose intensity distribution equals that of the binomial coefficients of the nth order.

The chlorinated benzosemiquinones, where the only important interaction is between the electron and the protons, provide an excellent illustration of this theory. Table 25 shows that the observed number of lines, and their relative intensities agree perfectly with theoretical predictions, assuming equal interaction of the electron with all the protons.

Another interesting case is provided by diphenylpicrylhydrazyl and related molecules. The relevant data is shown in Fig. 69. In this case the electron interacts strongly only with the two central nitrogen atoms, which therefore determine the form of the spectrum. The situation here is more complicated since the nitrogen nucleus has a spin of 3/2 and may assume 3 different orientations in the field, as indicated in the figure by ↑, ↓, and →. The sulphonated compound shows a nine-line spectrum, in agreement with the general case of unequal interaction with the two nuclei. The carbazyl shows only seven lines, which is explained by supposing that the electron interacts exactly twice as strongly with one nitrogen atom as with the other, leading to a partially collapsed energy diagram. Diphenylpicrylhydrazyl gives a five line spectrum with intensity distribution 1:2:3:2:1 which suggests equal interaction with the two nuclei, giving a still simpler energy diagram. This is a rather surprising con-

Fig. 69. Interaction of an electron with two nitrogen atoms.

References p. 253

clusion since the two nitrogen atoms are in quite different environments chemically. The matter has recently been further discussed[14].

The excellent agreement between theory and experiment in these cases enables one, when dealing with unknowns, to deduce with confidence from the observed pattern, the number of nuclei with which the unpaired electron interacts. Possible radical structures can thus be accepted or rejected according to whether they predict interaction with the correct number of nuclei. In favourable cases it is possible not only to deduce the structure of a radical but also, from the various values of ΔH, to determine the strength of the interaction of the electron with the various nuclei in the molecule. An example of this is given in section E4.

E. TYPICAL APPLICATIONS OF ELECTRON SPIN RESONANCE IN ORGANIC CHEMISTRY

The applications of electron resonance are now so widespread that only a few typical examples can be given. For an excellent detailed account, the reader is referred to chapters 5 to 9 of Ingram's book[4], and to the Varian series of advertisements in *Analytical Chemistry*[5].

1. The study of organo-metallic compounds

Since the unpaired electrons of the d or f shells of transition metal atoms give a signal, electron resonance provides a powerful method of determining electron distributions in the immediate vicinity of the atom. In contrast to most other types of spectra, the electron resonance spectrum is not interfered with by bands originating in the organic ligand.

The simplest applications arise in cases where, only in one of its two or more valency states, an atom such as copper has unpaired electrons in its valence shell. Electron resonance may then be used to determine the valence state in cases where this is not obvious on chemical grounds. For example there is some doubt about the mode of action in biology of the copper-protein complex known as Fungal Laccase. A strong signal is obtained from a solution of the substance[7], showing that in its normal state the copper is divalent. However, in a substrate containing catechol, under conditions where the substance is biologically active, the signal is greatly reduced, showing that substantial reduction of the copper to its monovalent state has taken place. Biological activity can therefore be associated in this case with monovalent copper.

The method has been used to demonstrate unusual valency states of certain metals[8]. Divalent copper, silver and gold have nine electrons in their $3d$, $4d$, and $5d$ shells respectively, one of which must be unpaired. Copper forms dithiocarbamates whose structure has been shown by X-ray work to be

When a solution of the normal dithiocarbamate of silver,

is added in benzene to a benzene solution of the corresponding thiuram disulphide, a strong electron resonance signal develops, showing that a divalent silver compound has been formed, according to the equation

This is one of the very few proved cases of divalency in silver. Even more remarkable is the development of a signal when solutions of the dithiocarbamate of monovalent gold, and of the thiuram disulphide are mixed. Since independent experiments show that trivalent gold compounds are not normally paramagnetic, this can only mean that a divalent gold compound is present. This is the first reported instance of gold exhibiting divalency.

With such molecules as phthalocyanines, chlorophylls, and haemoglobins, electron spin resonance spectroscopy provides a possible method of studying the binding of the metal atom to the surrounding nitrogen atoms. For example several phthalocyanines have been studied by Ingram *et al*[9]. Copper phthalocyanine crystals yield *g* values of 2.045 to 2.165 according to the orientation of the crystal, compared to 2.14 to 2.45 for typical ionic copper compounds. Hence the bonds must be partly covalent. Fairly strong covalent bonding was also found for cobalt phthalocyanine. Surprising results were obtained with haemin and related compounds where an iron atom is bound to a ring system similar to phthalocyanine. Magnetic susceptibility measurements indicate an effective moment corresponding to five unpaired electrons, as in normal ionically bound iron. This would give resonance at $g = 2.0$, but in practice a strong absorption was found near $g = 6$. The idea of essentially ionic bonds in such compounds must therefore be revised[16].

2. Reaction velocities and mechanisms

Many organic reactions are known to proceed by a radical mechanism. A direct measure of how radical concentrations vary with time during these reactions would be an invaluable aid in determining their mechanisms. Unfortunately with present day techniques, the radical concentrations in most solution reactions are just below the electron resonance detection limit. However, in certain special cases the method can be applied.

In polymerisations where the viscosity of the medium becomes large, the rate of diffusion of radicals attached to the ends of chains is so slow that mutual interaction is unlikely, and fairly large radical concentrations build up, which can be accurately measured. This effect was utilised by Atherton, Melville and Whiffen[6] to study the copolymerisation of methyl methacrylate and glycol dimethacrylate, where cross-linking leads to the necessary high viscosity during the reaction. The polymerisations were carried out in sealed, evacuated Pyrex tubes placed in the resonant cavity, and were initiated by 2,2'-azo bis(isobutyronitrile), which, when irradiated by a mercury lamp, is a convenient source of free radicals. Fig. 70 shows the variation of radical concentration with time, with 0.40 mole fraction of glycol dimethacrylate at 23°C and 0°C. The maximum in the 23°C curve is explained by supposing that during part of the reaction,

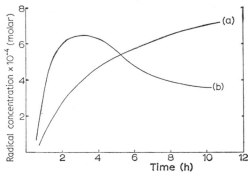

Fig. 70. Copolymerisation of methyl methacrylate and glycol dimethacrylate[6]. Volume ratio 3:2. (a) 0°C; (b) 23°C.

decay of radicals by mutual interaction is faster than photochemical production of new ones. This explanation was confirmed by stopping the reaction at various points by cutting off the irradiation, and following the rate of decay of the signals. The radical concentration levels off at the end of the experiment, showing that some of the radicals have essentially infinite lifetimes probably because the limited volume through which they can diffuse does not overlap the corresponding volume for any neighbouring radical. At 0°C mutual interaction of chain ends is very improbable, so the radical concentration grows steadily, and a rough comparison of rates of initiation and subsequent chain growth is possible.

Band widths may occasionally be used to measure reaction velocities. If equivalent amounts of naphthalene and metallic sodium are dissolved in tetrahydrofuran, a well resolved hyperfine structure develops, corresponding to the formation of negative radical ions

$$C_{10}H_8 + Na\cdot \rightarrow Na^+ + (C_{10}H_8\cdot)^-$$

If a large excess of naphthalene is added, the absorption is greatly broadened. As explained above, broadening corresponds to shortening of the life-time of the radical in the upper energy state. In this case the shortening must be due to the ability of the radical to exchange by the reaction

$$(C_{10}H_8\cdot)^- + C_{10}H_8 \rightarrow C_{10}H_8 + (C_{10}H_8\cdot)^-$$

before it would be deactivated by normal means. From the degree of broadening the rate of this reaction can therefore be calculated.

3. The effect of ionising radiation on matter

A fuller understanding of the chemical reactions which ensue when matter is irradiated with X-rays or γ-rays, or by streams of electrons, α-particles or neutrons is important for two main reasons. In the first place the properties of many polymers can be profoundly altered, rendering them more suitable for some purposes. This happens because free radicals are formed during the initial breakage of bonds by the radiation, which subsequently react with one another, forming links between the chains. For example the softening point of polythene is somewhat lowered by X-irradiation, but as a result of cross-linking it does not flow on softening and therefore becomes more suitable as a cable insulator at high temperatures. Similarly relatively small doses of radiation serve to cross-link silicone polymers, leading to products with properties superior to those of chemically cross-linked materials. Rubber can be vulcanised by high energy irradiation rather than by sulphur treatment, though at present economic factors are still in favour of the latter method.

Under irradiation direct links between the carbon atoms of the chains occur, instead of links via sulphur atoms. Since all these processes involve free radicals, electron resonance measurements of the effects of radiation on polymers are clearly worthwhile.

A typical study of this kind was recently carried out by Abraham and Whiffen[10], who examined various polymers after irradiation *in vacuo* with γ-rays from a ^{60}Co source. All their polymers developed electron resonance signals, because the rigidity of the materials prevented rapid diffusion and mutual interaction of the radicals formed. In some cases the authors were able to decide the structure of the radicals from hyperfine splitting of the spectrum, using the principle (explained on p. 240) that if an electron interacts equally with n protons, $n + 1$ hyperfine lines result. For example polythene yields a seven line pattern, which can plausibly be attributed to the radical $-CH_2 - C\cdot - CH_2-$, the electron interacting equally with the

$$CH_2$$
$$|$$

six protons. The formation of these radicals by attack at the points of chain branching is not unreasonable. Polystyrene shows only three lines. Although this may be due to $-CH(C_6H_5)$ $-CH_2\cdot$ radicals, these are rather unlikely on chemical grounds, so more probably the species responsible is $-CH_2 - C\cdot -CH_2-$

$$|$$
$$C_6H_5$$

only three lines resulting because for steric reasons only one proton of each methylene group interacts strongly. An eight line spectrum has been reported for Teflon (polytetrafluoroethylene), which could be due to $-CF_2 - C\cdot - CF_2-$.

$$|$$
$$CF_3$$

Poly(methylmethacrylate) is an unusually interesting case (Ref.[4], p. 197). A spectrum consisting of two superimposed patterns of four and five lines is observed. At first it was thought that two distinct radicals were responsible, but when precisely the same spectrum was obtained with several different types of radiation, and also from irradiated poly(methacrylic acid) and poly(ethylmethacrylate) it became clear that both sets of lines originated from the same radical, whose structure is probably

$$-CH_2-\underset{\underset{CH_3}{|}}{\overset{\overset{COOR}{|}}{C}}\cdot$$

. It must therefore be assumed that the electron

TABLE 26

ELECTRON RESONANCE SPECTRA OF IRRADIATED AMINO ACIDS

Amino acid	Structure	Nature of spectrum
Glycine	$H-\underset{\underset{NH_2}{|}}{\overset{\overset{H}{|}}{C}}-C\overset{\nearrow O}{\searrow_{OH}}$	Three lines
Alanine	$CH_3-\underset{\underset{NH_2}{|}}{\overset{\overset{H}{|}}{C}}-C\overset{\nearrow O}{\searrow_{OH}}$	Five lines
Valine	$CH_3-\underset{\underset{CH_3}{|}}{\overset{\overset{H}{|}}{C}}-\underset{\underset{NH_2}{|}}{\overset{\overset{H}{|}}{C}}-C\overset{\nearrow O}{\searrow_{OH}}$	2 sets of seven lines
Cystine	$\left(-S\cdot CH_2-\underset{\underset{NH_2}{|}}{\overset{\overset{H}{|}}{C}}-C\overset{\nearrow O}{\searrow_{OH}}\right)_2$	Asymmetric spectrum of four components
Glycylglycine	$HN{=}\underset{\underset{NH_2}{|}}{C}-\underset{\underset{H}{|}}{N}-CH_2-C\overset{\nearrow O}{\searrow_{OH}}$	Doublet

interacts sometimes with three and sometimes with four of the available protons, probably because the stereochemical distribution of the two —CH_2— protons, and the methyl group around the central carbon atom, varies from point to point along the chains.

The study of irradiated biological materials is of particular importance, because of their known susceptibility to destruction or deleterious mutations. Free radical formation may be one of the factors responsible for abnormal cell development, as in cancer. Electron resonance provides the most sensitive and direct method of following these effects. The most obvious use is the quantitative measurement of the concentrations of free radicals formed under various conditions, with different types of radiation. In addition it is sometimes possible from the splitting of the spectrum to learn something of the structure of the radicals. With a view to doing this in the case of irradiated proteins, Gordy, Ard and Shields[11] first measured several irradiated amino acids. Some of their results are given in Table 26. The observed number of lines can often be accounted for by supposing that the unpaired electron interacts equally with all the protons in its vicinity. For example the glycine triplet could be due to a $(CH_2{}^{\cdot})^+$ radical*, whereas if the alanine molecule splits off ammonia and carbon dioxide when irradiated, the remaining carbon and hydrogen atoms may rearrange to $(H_2C\overset{\cdot}{-}CH_2)^+$, which would explain the five line pattern.

On passing to proteins, well defined hyperfine structures are not normally found, and interpretation depends on comparison with the results from simpler compounds. For example it was found[11] that hair, nails and feathers all yield a spectrum very similar to that of cystine. It has been suggested that in each case the unpaired electron is localised in the sulphur–sulphur bond of the cystine unit. If an electron is ejected from some other part of the molecule, the resulting electron deficiency may move along the chain to the sulphur–sulphur bond, which then acts as an electron reservoir. This mechanism probably reduces the likelihood of molecular breakdown in these proteins.

---

* See also Reference 15.

References p. 253

Irradiated silk, cattle hide and fish scale all give a doublet very similar to that of glycylglycine. This has been explained by supposing that the unpaired electron is localised on an oxygen atom hydrogen bonded to another chain, and that the splitting is caused by the hydrogen atom of the bond.

4. Electron resonance in rubber technology

Carbon blacks are used extensively in rubber technology to reinforce natural rubber so as to endow it with the properties required in, for example, motor-car tyres. It was discovered about five years ago by electron resonance studies, that when almost any organic material is charred, large numbers of free radicals are formed. Because of the rigidity of the medium, mutual interaction of these radicals is so unlikely that their lifetimes at room temperature are virtually infinite. By using electron resonance to follow the variation of radical concentration with carbon content during charring, it was found that the concentration increased rapidly at the point where, from X-ray measurements it was known that fairly large clusters of carbon rings were being formed. It therefore appears that when an edge bond is broken during the extension of a ring system, an electron may be liberated, which is then stabilised by its ability to resonate among the ring carbon atoms. Since these free electrons are relatively loosely attached to the ring clusters, they are liable to play an important part in rubber reinforcement, and study of them during the milling of rubber with carbon is a promising line.

It is well established that one of the mechanisms by which rubber and other materials with long hydrocarbon chains are oxidised involves free radicals. The process may be written as follows[12].

$$I \rightarrow X\cdot$$
$$X\cdot + RH \rightarrow R\cdot + XH$$
$$\left.\begin{array}{l} R\cdot + O_2 \rightarrow RO_2\cdot \\ RO_2\cdot + RH \rightarrow RO_2H + R\cdot \end{array}\right\} \text{Chain propagation}$$

I is an initiator, probably present by accident, which produces radicals X· which in turn abstract hydrogen atoms from some point on the chain, whereupon oxidation by a chain reaction takes place. To counteract this, antioxidants (AH) are added, which break the chains by removing RO₂· radicals

$$RO_2 \cdot + AH \rightarrow RO_2H + A \cdot$$

The success of these agents depends on A· being stable enough not to initiate further chains. Clearly unless the mode of action

Fig. 71. Spectra of radicals initially formed by oxidation of phenols[13].

of particular antioxidants is properly understood, the invention of new ones must proceed by trial and error. To obtain this understanding the structure of A· must be known, and since commercial antioxidants often contain several —O—H, C—H

References p. 253

and N—H groups this is not by any means always obvious. Here again electron resonance can often solve the problem.

TABLE 27

ELECTRON SPIN RESONANCE SPECTRA OF PHENOLIC RADICALS

Suggested structure of radicals	Nature of initial spectrum	Hydrogen interaction constants (gauss)		
		ortho alkyl group	para alkyl group	ring hydrogen
tBu, tBu, CH$_3$	quartet of triplets	—	10.7	1.8
tBu, tBu, CH$_2$CH$_3$	triplet of triplets	—	9.0	1.8
tBu, tBu, CH$_2$N(CH$_3$)$_2$	triplet of quintets	—	10.4	1.9*
tBu, tBu, tBu	triplet	—	—	1.3
tBu, CH$_3$, tBu	quartet of triplets	6.9	—	1.9
CH$_3$, CH$_3$, tBu	septet of triplets	6.1	—	1.8

* Also involves interaction with the nitrogen atom.

The structures of the radicals initially formed when various substituted phenols were oxidised in cyclohexane by lead dioxide, emerge very clearly from the work of Becconsall *et al.*[13]. Fig. 71 shows some typical spectra, whilst Table 27 summarises the findings on some of the phenols.

In the spectrum of the first compound, 2,6-di-*t*-butyl-4-methylphenol, the primary quartet splitting clearly stems from the three protons of the 4-methyl group, and the closely spaced triplets result from weaker interactions of the electron with the two meta hydrogen atoms. Similarly the primary triplets in the second compound are connected with the two methylene protons and the further splitting with the ring protons. The quintets of the third spectrum are explained by postulating approximately equal coupling of the nitrogen nucleus and the ring protons. From the observed splittings measures of the degree of interaction between the electron and various protons in the molecule were obtained, as shown in the table.

By observing the spectra over a period of time, the subsequent transformations undergone by the primary radicals were followed. After ten minutes the spectrum from 2,6-di-*t*-butyl-4-methylphenol reduced to a triplet, probably as a result of oxidation of the methyl group to —CHO. Several days later this spectrum was found in turn to have been replaced by a doublet of quintets, thought to arise from the radical

REFERENCES

[1] F. PANETH AND W. HOFEDITZ, *Chem. Ber.*, 62 B (1929) 1335.

[2] F. G. BADDAR, O. M. M. HILAL AND S. SUGDEN, *J. Chem. Soc.*, (1949) 132.

[3] D. F. EVANS, *Nature*, 176 (1955) 777.

[4] D. J. E. INGRAM, *Free Radicals as Studied by Electron Spin Resonance*, Butterworths, London, 1959, 274 pp..

[5] Varian Associates, *This is E.P.R. at work* (series of advertisements in *Anal. Chem.*)

[6] N. M. ATHERTON, H. W. MELVILLE AND D. H. WHIFFEN, *Trans. Faraday Soc.*, 54 (1958) 1300.

[7] B. G. MALMSTRÖM, R. MOSBACH AND T. VÄNNGARD, *Nature*, 183 (1959) 321.

[8] T. VÄNNGARD AND S. ÅKERSTRÖM, *Nature*, 184 (1959) 183.

[9] D. J. E. INGRAM AND J. E. BENNETT, *Discussions Faraday Soc.*, 19 (1955) 140.

[10] R. J. ABRAHAM AND D. H. WHIFFEN, *Trans. Faraday Soc.*, 54 (1958) 1291.

[11] W. GORDY, W. B. ARD AND H. SHIELDS, *Proc. Natl. Acad. Sci. U.S.*, 41 (1955) 983.

[12] D. S. DAVIES, H. L. GOLDSMITH, A. K. GUPTA AND G. R. LESTER, *J. Chem. Soc.*, (1956) 4926.

[13] J. K. BECCONSALL, S. CLOUGH AND G. SCOTT, *Trans. Faraday Soc.*, 56 (1960) 359.

[14] R. M. DEAL AND W. S. KOSKI, *J. Chem. Phys.*, 31 (1959) 1138.

[15] D. K. GHOSH AND D. H. WHIFFEN, *Mol. Phys.*, 2 (1959) 285.

[16] J. E. BENNETT, J. F. GIBSON AND D. J. E. INGRAM, *Proc. Roy. Soc. London, A* 240 (1957) 67.

SELECTED BIBLIOGRAPHY TO CHAPTER 7

GORDY, W., in: *Chemical Applications of Spectroscopy*, (Ed. W. WEST), Interscience, New York, 1956. pp. 71–184.

INGRAM, D. J. E., *Free Radicals as Studied by Electron Spin Resonance*, Butterworths, London, 1959. This is the most useful source available from the viewpoint of an organic chemist.

WERTZ, J. E., *Chem. Revs.*, 55 (1955) 829. A clear discussion is given of the principles underlying electron and nuclear spin resonance spectroscopy.

WHIFFEN, D. H., *Quart. Revs. London*, 12 (1958) 250. This provides an excellent short account of chemical applications.

CHAPTER 8

NUCLEAR SPIN RESONANCE SPECTROSCOPY

The last chapter described a form of spectroscopy in which, as a result of the magnetic properties of an electron arising from its axial spin, microwave radiation was absorbed in a magnetic field, corresponding to rotation through 180° of the magnetic axis of the electron. Many atomic nuclei also spin about their axes, so there is a very similar branch of spectroscopy where the directions of the axes of the nuclear magnets change in a magnetic field, the process being accompanied by absorption of electromagnetic energy. Since the energy differences are much smaller than in the case of the electron, the absorption falls in the radio frequency region. There are two important chemical consequences of this phenomenon. If the same nucleus is studied in a series of compounds, the precise frequency of its absorption gives valuable information about how it is bound to neighbouring atoms. Also each nucleus of a given kind contributes one unit of intensity to the resonance signal, so the number of nuclei of a given type in an unknown molecule can be determined. Nuclear spin resonance spectroscopy (NSR), or nuclear magnetic resonance spectroscopy (NMR) as it is sometimes known, is therefore a powerful tool in elucidating the structures of unknowns, and investigating the finer details of molecular shape and electronic distribution, in cases where the structural formula is known.

A. BASIC PRINCIPLES OF NSR

The object of this section is to outline the principles and types of application. The more important aspects are farther developed in the later sections.

1. Magnetic properties of nuclei

The nuclei of the majority of the isotopes of the periodic table spin about their axes. Where the magnitude of this spin differs from zero, it may assume any of the values $\frac{1}{2}$, 1 3/2, 2, 5/2 etc. in units of $h/2\pi$. As a result these nuclei possess magnetic moments and behave as spinning magnets which tend to orient themselves in an applied magnetic field. In the simplest case, where $I = \frac{1}{2}$, as in the case of the electron, only two directions, parallel and anti-parallel to the direction of the field are possible for the axes. If I is greater than $\frac{1}{2}$, other orientations are possible. Since work must be done to turn a magnet against a magnetic field, each of these directions corresponds to a different energy state of the nucleus. These are obtained by defining a quantum number m, which can take any of the values

$$I, I-1, I-2, \ldots\ldots -I+1, -I.$$

If μ is the magnetic moment of a nucleus, then the possible energy levels in a field H_0 are given by $-m\mu H_0/I$. For the values $\frac{1}{2}$, 1 and 3/2 of I, Fig. 72 shows the resulting energy levels. In all cases the separation between adjacent levels is $\mu H/I$. As in the other forms of spectroscopy, absorption is governed by the basic equation

$$h\nu = \Delta E$$

The position is simplified by a selection rule which permits only transitions between adjacent levels to take place. Hence the equation becomes

$$h\nu = \frac{\mu H_0}{I} \quad \text{or} \quad \nu = \frac{\mu H_0}{hI}$$

In practice, as with electron resonance spectroscopy, it is much easier to vary the magnetic field than the frequency. An NSR spectrum is therefore usually a record of signal intensity against magnetic field at a fixed frequency. Intervals between resonances may be measured in frequency or magnetic field units, irrespective of the method of scanning the spectrum, the two quantities being linearly related by the above equation.

The strength of the signal depends on the ability of the

sample to absorb by promotion of nuclei from the lower to the
higher energy level, and is therefore proportional to

$$\frac{n_{\text{lower}}}{n_{\text{upper}}} - 1 = e^{\mu H_0/IkT} - 1,$$

Therefore large values of H_0 and μ lead to a large population
difference and a strong signal. As strong a field as possible
should therefore be used, and the best results are to be expected
with nuclei of large moment.

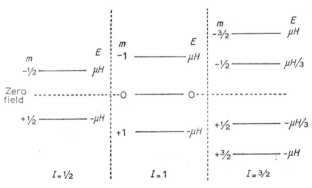

Fig. 72. Energy levels of nuclei in a magnetic field.

Table 28 lists I and μ for the nuclei normally met in organic
chemistry, together with their natural abundances and relative
sensitivities in NSR. The moment of the electron, which is
included for comparison, is of a different order of magnitude
from the others, which explains why electron resonance involves
micro rather than radio waves. Several common nuclei, including
^{12}C and ^{16}O have no spin and cannot therefore be studied. The
proton however has one of the largest moments and is particularly suitable for NSR studies. The common isotope of fluorine
^{19}F, is also outstandingly suitable, as is ^{31}P. Nitrogen has a
much smaller moment, so is much more difficult to study, and
although ^{13}C and ^{17}O have moments, their relative abundances

TABLE 28
PROPERTIES OF NUCLEI

Particle	Natural abundance %	Relative sensitivity for equal number of nuclei (constant field)	Magnetic moment (nuclear magnetons)*	Spin (units of $h/2\pi$)
electron	—	—	1840	$\frac{1}{2}$
^{1}H	99.98	1.000	2.793	$\frac{1}{2}$
^{2}H (D)	0.016	$9.6 \cdot 10^{-3}$	0.857	1
^{12}C	99	0	0	0
^{13}C	1.11	$1.59 \cdot 10^{-2}$	0.702	$\frac{1}{2}$
^{14}N	99.6	$1.01 \cdot 10^{-3}$	0.404	1
^{16}O	99.996	0	0	0
^{17}O	$3.7 \cdot 10^{-2}$	$2.91 \cdot 10^{-2}$	-1.893	5/2
^{19}F	100	0.834	2.627	$\frac{1}{2}$
^{32}S	99.3	0	0	0
^{31}P	100	$6.6 \cdot 10^{-2}$	1.130	$\frac{1}{2}$
^{35}Cl	75.4	$4.7 \cdot 10^{-3}$	0.821	3/2
^{37}Cl	24.6	$2.7 \cdot 10^{-3}$	0.683	3/2

* 1 Nuclear magneton $= 5.049 \times 10^{-24}$ erg/gauss.

are so small that these elements are less suitable, except in artificially enriched samples.

The large differences between the magnetic moments of different nuclei ensure that frequencies of resonance of the isotopes are widely separated, and no overlapping of signals from different nuclei occurs. Measurements can therefore be concentrated solely on the atoms in which one is interested.

2. Effect of state on NSR spectra

The arguments so far suggest that free nuclei should give single sharp absorption lines, with frequencies governed by the equation of the last section. In practice the absorption is however modified by the environment of the nucleus. Consider first the solid state. Any nucleus, X, in a solid will be surrounded by several others of its own and other kinds, within a few Ångstroms of it. From elementary magnetic theory, a magnet of moment μ causes a field at a point P, distant r from its centre, varying between $\pm 2\mu/r^3$, according to the direction of the axis of the magnet, relative to the line joining its centre to P. When, therefore, an external field H_0 is applied to a solid, the net field experienced by nucleus X will be the algebraic sum of H_0 and the small contributions from each of the neighbouring nuclei. Since each of these may assume any of two or more orientations in the field, their contributions are variable. There will therefore be a large number of possible values for the net field at nucleus X so the various X nuclei throughout the solid will experience slightly different fields. If then a spectrum is obtained by varying the frequency at fixed field, or, as is usual in practice, by varying the field at constant frequency, a broad band rather than a sharp line will result. As explained on p. 272, information about the geometry of simple molecules, and molecular rotation in crystals can be obtained from solid state spectra, but the range of applications is much more restricted than with the fluid states of matter. In view of the wide bands, the term "low resolution NSR" is sometimes used to describe solid state studies, since there is no point in using techniques capable of resolving narrow lines.

In liquids, solutions, and gases the nuclei surrounding the one under consideration are in continual motion, as a result of molecular tumbling and rotation. Under these conditions the above magnetic effects which cause band widening average out, so that all identical nuclei in the sample experience the same field. Therefore very sharp lines are to be expected, and to extract all the possible information from these sharp line spectra requires a spectrometer of high resolution.

A single very sharp line is indeed obtained from liquids in whose molecules all the nuclei, whose signals are being studied, are in equivalent positions. For example the proton resonance spectra of chloroform, benzene, methylene chloride, dioxan and cylcohexane are of this type. The physicists who discovered NSR hoped that measurements on fluids would provide a very accurate method of determining nuclear magnetic moments. However, if spectra of field strength against signal are obtained from several liquids containing the same nucleus, small variation of the resonant field is found. While invalidating NSR as an ultra-accurate method of finding magnetic moments, this opens up a whole range of chemical applications. These field differences arise because the protons (or other nuclei) in various liquids are screened to different extents from the applied field, and therefore experience slightly different effective fields. There are two main causes of this screening. In the first place the applied field is attenuated as a result of the bulk magnetic susceptibility of the medium. For this reason the same nucleus in different liquids, or the same substance in different solvents, yield signals at slightly different field values. The effect should be allowed for in comparing spectra measured in different solvents.

3. Effect of molecular environment on spectra – chemical shifts – fine structure

Of much greater importance than the above bulk screening, is screening by electrons within the same molecule. Since the electrons in molecules occupy orbitals which may cover a large part of the molecule, the nuclei may be crudely thought of as being enveloped in an electron cloud. They will therefore be screened from the applied field by this cloud, to an extent depending on the electronic distribution in their vicinity. For example in a series of diatomic hydrides, one would expect the proton screening (and hence the resonant frequency) to depend on the electronegativity of the other atom, which determines the extent to which electrons are pulled from the proton. Clearly it is possible conversely to deduce from signal positions in an unknown case, something about the environment of the nucleus.

The term "chemical shift" is used to describe shifts of resonant field values, due to differing degrees of screening. Clearly it is not practicable directly to compare the field for a nucleus in a given environment with the corresponding value for the completely bare nucleus. Chemical shifts must therefore be measured relative to some suitable standard, usually a pure liquid, containing the nucleus in question. For example water, benzene and cyclohexane, are commonly used as reference liquids in proton measurements. The shift may be expressed in gauss or cycles/sec, but it is much more satisfactory to use δ, a dimensionless quantity, defined by the equation

$$\delta = \frac{H_{\text{sample}} - H_{\text{reference}}}{H_{\text{reference}}}$$

where H with the appropriate suffix represents the field at resonance corresponding to a fixed frequency. δ is independent of the field and frequency used. In practice its value for proton resonances is usually only a few parts per million, but, because of the high precision of modern NSR spectrometers, these small separations can be accurately measured. By an arbitrary convention, if $H_{\text{sample}} > H_{\text{reference}}$, δ is positive. A positive δ then corresponds to a greater degree of screening than in the reference compound.

Fig. 73 shows the NSR spectrum of ethyl alcohol, under rather low resolution. Three distinct signals are obtained corresponding to the different chemical shifts of the three kinds of proton. Since the two methylene protons lie in identical

References p. 307

positions, they absorb at the same field, but give twice as strong a line as the hydroxyl proton. Similarly the three methyl protons give one line, three times as strong as the hydroxyl line. As will be elaborated in section D, the ability to associate particular chemical shifts with groups such as —OH, —CH₂—,

Fig. 73. Proton resonance spectrum of ethyl alcohol, under fairly low resolution.

and —CH₃ makes NSR a powerful tool in structural diagnosis. Just as in infra-red spectroscopy, the occurrence of absorptions at definite positions can be associated in unknowns with particular groups. Also the signal intensity indicates the number of groups.

When the technique of NSR reached the point where very close lines could be resolved, it was often found with both inorganic and organic compounds that more lines appeared than could be accounted for by chemical shift considerations. To take the simplest possible example, one would expect gaseous HD to give two lines, one in the region of proton resonance, and another in the deuterium region. In fact, three and two lines are found respectively for the two nuclei. Since the degree of splitting in each multiplet is found to be independent of the applied field, an explanation must be sought in terms of nuclear interaction within the molecule. As seen above the effects of surrounding nuclei in other molecules cancel out in the gas or liquid state because of random tumbling. However, there sometimes remains a measure of interaction between nuclei which lie close together in the same molecule. In the above example the deuteron has a spin of one unit, and the proton one half. Hence in a given molecule of HD, the axis of the deutron may assume one of three orientations in an applied field, each having a slightly different effect on the proton. In a measurement of proton resonance, therefore, there will be three groups of equal numbers of protons in slightly different states, which explains the observed pattern of three equally intense lines. Similarly, equal numbers of deuterons will be under the influence of protons whose axes are parallel and anti-parallel to the field. Hence there will be two slightly separated deuteron resonances, which explains the observed doublet. This phenomenon causes widespread splitting of lines, especially in more complex molecules, and the resulting fine structure is particularly valuable in structural work, in enabling one to obtain information about the relative positions of various nuclei close to the one the resonance of which is being studied.

B. THE MEASUREMENT OF NSR SPECTRA

The object of this section is to describe spectrometers and methods of sample treatment, and to indicate how chemical shifts and fine structure data are obtained from the records. In solids the bands are intrinsically wide, so that spectrometers of low resolution are adequate. The term high resolution NSR is used to describe work where close lines, arising from the same nucleus in slightly different surroundings must be resolved. As has already been pointed out, it is easier to vary the magnetic field than the frequency. In practice therefore NSR spectrometers are devices in which the field on the sample is varied at a fixed frequency v_0, and signals are obtained at the points where the fundamental equation $v_0 = \mu H/hI$ is satisfied, so that absorption and re-emission of energy takes place.

1. Single-coil spectrometers

The simplest experimental arrangement for measuring NSR spectra is shown in Fig. 74. The sample is placed between the poles of a powerful magnet. Around the sample fits a coil C, which is included in a tuned circuit of a radio frequency generator. If protons are to be studied, and if the largest field readily available is about 7000 gauss, a frequency of about 30 megacycles/sec will be required for resonance.

A second coil is wound on to the pole pieces of the magnet, so that by varying the current through it, the field at the sample

Fig. 74. Single-coil nuclear spin resonance spectrometer.

can be made to cover a range of roughly 7000 ± 15 gauss. If now the current in the magnet (or sweep) coil is varied at 50 cycles/sec, then at the resonance points during each cycle, the equation will be satisfied, and absorption of radio frequency energy will occur. During each cycle the absorption will follow the shape of the spectrum. This 50-cycle signal is separated by the detector from the accompanying radio frequency component, amplified, and fed to the X plates of a cathode ray oscilloscope. If the Y plates are fed by the same source which supplies the sweep current, the required spectrum will be traced on the screen. This simple arrangement suffers from the inherent defect then one must separate a small 50-cycle component from a radio-frequency output of much greater amplitude, which leads to a poor signal to noise ratio. Practical single coil spectrometers therefore place the signal coil in one arm of a bridge, the other arm of which carries an identical dummy coil. The absorption unbalances the bridge, and the out-of-balance signal serves to produce the spectrum.

2. Crossed-coil spectrometers

Many practical NSR spectrometers employ a different method of signal detection from that described above. Two distinct coils

Fig. 75. Crossed-coil nuclear spin resonance spectrometer.

(see Fig. 75) are placed between the magnet pole-pieces, which transmit and receive at the radio-frequency. If the axes of these are almost at right angles, there will be very little coupling between them. Instead of cancelling out most of the radio-frequency signal by using a bridge, double-coil spectrometers achieve this by the geometrical arrangement of the two coils. Only a weak radio frequency signal reaches the receiver coil to

References p. 307

serve as a carrier for the nuclear resonance signal. Just as in the other spectrometer the 50-cycle component of the output is separated, amplified, and led to an oscilloscope, where the spectrum is displayed.

3. High-resolution refinements

Low resolution measurements can be made with a spectrometer of either of the above types, using fairly simple electronic circuits, and a comparatively cheap magnet. However, the fundamental requirement for high-resolution work is a much more elaborate magnet. If one wishes to resolve lines only a few milligauss apart, it is essential that the magnetic field over the whole sample is homogeneous to at least this order, and the more uniform the magnetic field, the better will be the resolution of the equipment. Modern spectrometers have a resolving power of about 1 part in 10^8. This can be achieved only with a precision engineered magnet, which must necessarily be very expensive. In resolving close lines, or if pen recording rather than cathode ray tube presentation is to be used, the field can no longer be swept at 50 cycles, but must pass through the resonance point over a much longer period, which may extend to several minutes. Therefore the main field must be highly homogeneous not only in space but also in time. Both permanent and electromagnets have been used in high resolution work. Because of the time stability requirement, elaborate current stabilisation of an electromagnet is required. The use of permanent magnets simplifies this problem, and they are therefore rather cheaper to build to a given homogeneity, but have certain disadvantages. Changes of field strength are sometimes required in order to distinguish between chemical shifts and spin-spin coupling, and to study different nuclei. These are readily effected with an electromagnet, but are not possible with a permanent magnet. The signal strength in nuclear spin spectroscopy is roughly proportional to the square of the magnetic field. Hence electromagnets, which can be operated at up to 14,000 gauss have an advantage over the permanent type, whose field is limited to about 10,000 gauss. Nevertheless both types of magnet have been used successfully in high resolution NSR.

To take full advantage of the magnet, a transmitter of very high frequency stability must be used. The electronic circuitry throughout, from the receiver coil to the final D.C. output and recorder must be of the highest quality. This ensures a sufficiently high signal to noise ratio in the final spectrum for weak components of fine structures to stand out above the noise level. In practice it is beyond the means of most laboratories to construct a high resolution spectrometer. Such instruments must normally be bought at about £15,000 from specialist manufacturers. The majority are at present supplied by Varian Associates of California, whose design is based on the crossed-coil principle. In Great Britain a single-coil instrument of comparable performance has recently been marketed by Associated Electrical Industries. Varian have announced their intention to market a much cheaper, simplified version of their spectrometer, the performance of which may be adequate for the solution of many chemical problems. A cheap spectrometer has also been made by the Fairey Aviation Company. This offers for about £3000, resolution good enough to resolve most chemical shifts, but often insufficient to split fine structures. Since some chemical problems can be solved by chemical shift data alone, this instrument would seem to provide a happy solution for laboratories who are unable to justify the expense of genuine high resolution equipment.

4. Sample arrangements

It is vital in high resolution NSR studies that the sample be in suitable form, and placed in the most homogeneous part of the field. An important part of the spectrometer is the so-called probe, which usually carries the transmitter and receiver coils, the sample tube, and a preamplifier, to minimise pickup by leads before the first amplification stage. Provision is made for small movements of this assembly in the field, to find the most homogeneous region, and hence obtain the best resolution. The sample is usually held in a cylindrical glass tube 5–8 mm in outside diameter. Field variations over the sample can be still further ironed out if the sample is spun about its axis, at above ten revolutions per second. This averaging of fluctuations of course takes place only in coaxial circles around the axis of the tube, so that field variations along the axis remain.

For high resolution work the sample must be in the liquid state or in solution. Low viscosities ensure the random tumbling which removes the causes of line broadening. For this reason satisfactory results cannot usually be obtained with solutions of polymers or other very large molecules which cannot tumble freely. For solids a solvent should be sought which does not contain nuclei of the kind to be studied. In proton studies carbon tetrachloride, carbon disulphide and heavy water are ideal. It is also often possible to use an aliphatic solvent to study aromatic compounds and vice versa, since aliphatic and aromatic proton signals are well separated. Since NSR signals are intrinsically weak, strong solutions ($> 5\%$) are usually required. The method is not suitable for the detection of small amounts of impurity.

Alternatively solid samples may be studied above their melting point. It will be appreciated that it is not easy to control the temperature of a complicated probe, which already carries two crossed coils, and means of spinning the sample. The problem has been solved by Varian Associates, who offer a probe, where, by blowing hot or cold air over the sample, its temperature can be held at any value between —60°C and +200°C. Temperature control can be achieved much more easily with a single-coil spectrometer such as that of A.E.I.

A compromise must be effected in respect of sample size. The smaller the sample volume, the more homogeneous the field over it is likely to be, and the better the resolution. Against this, the signal strength increases with sample size, so, particularly with dilute solutions it may be necessary to use 1 c.c. or more, although 1/20 c.c. is a typical quantity for pure liquids. As seen from Table 28 larger volumes will be required with nuclei other than hydrogen and fluorine.

Subject to the above factors, the actual recording of NSR spectra with modern equipment is a simple matter, taking only a few minutes.

5. Measurement of chemical shifts

Having obtained a NSR spectrum, as a record of magnetic field against signal intensity, the next step is to determine the field strength corresponding to each line. The chemical shift can then be obtained from the equation

$$\delta = \frac{H_{\text{sample}} - H_{\text{reference}}}{H_{\text{reference}}}$$

Since it is impossible to measure the magnetic field at each line with the necessary accuracy, their positions are determined relative to standard lines by the following method. To illustrate

Fig. 76. Measurement of the separation between lines A and B in the spectrum of toluene. A' and B' are side-bands.

the measurement of line separations, consider Fig. 76a, which shows two lines in the spectrum of toluene, measured at 40 megacycles/sec. If this spectrum is re-run, the oscillator being on the second occasion modulated at a relatively low frequency, 80.4 cycles/sec in the present case, new peaks, termed side-bands, appear (A′ and B′ in Fig. 76b) 80.4 cycles/sec above and below the signal frequencies. If the spectrum has been recorded on a chart driven synchronously with the field variation, then the distance x on the chart corresponds to a separation of 160.8 cycles/sec, which at 40 megacycles/sec equals 4.09 p.p.m. By simple proportion, the separation of A and B is obtained.

The method can be made more accurate if required, and possible errors due to lack of linearity in the chart eliminated, by varying the modulation frequency. In the present example it was found that at 98.2 cycles/sec, side-bands from A and B coincided (Fig. 76c), showing the separation of A and B to be 2×98.2 or 196.4 cycles/sec, that is 4.91 p.p.m.

So far only line separations have been considered. All the lines of a spectrum are usually measured relative to some line of a reference substance R. This might for example be liquid water in the case of proton spectra. On introducing R, either internally in solution in the sample, or externally in a separate compartment of the sample tube, its line appears in the spectrum, and serves as a reference from which the other lines can be measured by the above method. Hence the chemical shift of each line is obtained relative to R. An external standard is usually the more satisfactory, since the line position of an internal standard may vary considerably with the solvent. The best reference liquids are those which give a single sharp line, well away from those of the sample. For proton spectra, suitable external standards, each giving only a single resonance line, include benzene, cyclohexane, chloroform, acetone and tetramethylsilane. For very accurate work water has the disadvantage that its resonance position is temperature dependent. Internal standards should be chemically inert, and not prone to hydrogen bonding. On these grounds tetramethylsilane and cyclohexane are preferred.

As mentioned on p. 261, δ, in parts per million is the most satisfactory measure of a chemical shift. Spin–spin coupling intervals are however commonly expressed in cycles/sec, as in this form they are independent of field and frequency changes. It has recently been recommended by the Chemical Society that chemical shifts should be published as τ values, τ being the shift in parts per million relative to a zero which is arbitrarily defined by taking $\tau = 10$ for tetramethylsilane.

6. Signal intensities

The intensity of a line is proportional to the number of the corresponding nuclei in the sample. For example it might be possible to identify an alkylated benzene from the relative strength of the lines due to aliphatic and aromatic protons. In principle the property may also be used for quantitative analysis of any mixture, where the components give reasonably well resolved signals.

For such applications the area under the peak is normally preferred to the peak height as the intensity measure. This corrects to some extent for band-width differences. It must however be admitted that the accuracy possible in intensity measurements is not comparable with that of signal separations. In general the observed value, even with strong signals, is not better than plus or minus five percent. Also, in quantitative analysis, the signals due to compounds at below about 5% concentration are often undetectable. As in electron resonance spectroscopy, care must be taken in measuring signal intensities to avoid "saturation" effects. Under intense radiation the ratio of excited to ground state molecules may become so great that the probability of transition, and hence the signal strength fall markedly.

C. SOLID STATE STUDIES. LOW RESOLUTION NSR

Liquids and gases give sharp lines, which, if resolved by high resolution techniques, enable chemical shifts and fine structure splittings to be measured, leading to valuable applications in structural diagnosis. In solids on the contrary, the magnetic effects of neighbouring nuclei broaden the lines. Before proceeding to describe applications of the much more important high resolution NSR, it is proposed here to consider the information obtainable from solid state spectra.

1. Structures of simple molecules

As mentioned in section A2, a nucleus in a solid experiences not only the applied field, but also a large number of small fields due to neighbouring nuclei acting as magnets. Calculation of all these contributions is not possible except in simple cases. The field due to a magnet at any point is proportional to the inverse cube of its distance from the centre of the magnet. Some simplifications can therefore be made, as only close neighbours will have large effects. In favourable cases two quantities can be calculated for a given distribution of nuclei. These are the shape of the curve of absorption against magnetic field and the so-called second moment, defined by

$$\Delta H_2 = \frac{\int_{-\infty}^{+\infty} f(H)(H - H^*)^2 \, dH}{\int_{-\infty}^{+\infty} f(H) \, dH},$$

where $f(H)$ is the intensity of absorption as a function of magnetic field strength, and H^* is the resonant field for the isolated nucleus at the given frequency. Its value depends on the width of the absorption, and can readily be obtained from the observed spectrum. In solids with small molecules of uncertain structure one can calculate for various likely distributions of nuclei the curve shape and the second moment, and compare these with experiment.

A good example is provided by the work of Richards and Smith[1], who applied proton resonance to the problem of the structures of the solid hydrates of nitric, perchloric and sulphuric acids. With nitric acid for example the two likely structures are the hydrate $HNO_3 \cdot H_2O$, and the oxonium salt $H_3O^+ \, NO_3^-$. Since the magnetic effects of the nitrogen and oxygen nuclei are small, the first structure approximates to a collection of close pairs of protons in the water molecules, plus relatively distant ones in the nitric acid. From this model it was calculated that the spectrum should include a doublet with peaks 2.5 μ/d^3 apart, d being the separation of the water protons. Interpretation of the spectrum on this basis yields a distance of 1.38 Å, too short a value to be correct. Also the calculated second moment of 36.5 gauss^2 does not agree with the observed value of 29.8.

Fig. 77. Spectrum of hydrate of nitric acid[1].

If the oxonium nitrate structure is correct, the protons would lie in groups of three, at the apices of an equilateral triangle. The authors also calculated the spectrum shape in this case, taking 1.72 Å for the side of the triangle. As shown in Fig. 77, excellent agreement was obtained between the observed points and the theoretical line. This structure also leads to a value of 29.9 gauss^2 for the second moment, in close agreement with experiment. Hence it was concluded that the solid hydrates of nitric and the other acids are oxonium salts.

2. Molecular motions in crystalline solids

In a solid the centres of gravity of the molecules are normally fixed in the crystal lattice. However, particularly near the melting point, rotations of the molecule (or a part of it such as a methyl group) about some axis, often becomes possible. This is clearly a step in the direction of the random tumbling of liquids, and should be reflected in a narrowing of the nuclear resonance spectrum. Fig. 78 illustrates the case of benzene[2], whose second moment falls from 9.7 gauss[2] below $100°K$, to 1.6 gauss[2] above $120°K$. Presumably the high value corresponds to a rigid assembly of molecules. As the temperature increases, so does the fre-

Fig. 78. Variation of line width with temperature for benzene[2].

Fig. 79. Variation of line width with temperature for cyclohexane[2].

quency with which a molecule rotates through 60° about an axis perpendicular to its plane, until, above 120°K, all the molecules are rotating with a frequency comparable to that of molecular rotations in fluids.

Cyclohexane (Fig. 79) is a more interesting case. Between 150 and 180°K, rotation of the molecules about the three-fold symmetry axis increases steadily. At the latter temperature a polymorphic change occurs leading to a large drop in the second moment. This indicates that above the transition point rotation about another axis also becomes possible. Finally between 240°K and the melting point of the solid an even more striking spectral narrowing takes place, reaching a value similar to that of liquids. The interpretation is that not only can the molecules now rotate about their centre of gravity, but can also change position in the lattice. This probably happens when, on nearing the melting point, "holes" appear in the lattice, into which adjacent molecules can move, the "hole" passing through the crystal. These and other examples are discussed in greater detail in Andrew's book[3].

3. Applications to polymers

Most polymers show striking changes of various physical properties with temperature. This is due in part to varying degrees of crystallinity but even non-crystalline polymers show so-called second order transitions. These take the form of a change with increasing temperature, from a rigid "glassy" state to a soft "rubbery" state. NSR is a possible method for investigating the molecular mechanism of these changes.

When natural rubber is heated[4], the width of its proton resonance falls, with two discontinuities (Fig. 80). Below 150°K, the structure is rigid, giving a wide line. From this temperature up to about 225°K, the width falls steadily, indicating the onset of rotation of methyl groups. Above 225°K, the width falls more steeply, probably because the structure has now expanded somewhat, and rotations of whole segments of a polymer chain about its axis become possible. This must not be thought to imply free rotation of the segments, but rather that the segments rotate from one equilibrium position to another at a frequency greater than that corresponding to the line width (p. 300). At 250°K and above, the line width approaches that of a liquid, showing that this "quasi-rotation" is widespread in the polymer chains. In other polymers, such as polyethylene terephthalate[5], no sharp transitions are found. There is however a steady narrowing with increasing temperature, showing a gradually increasing degree of methylene group rotation.

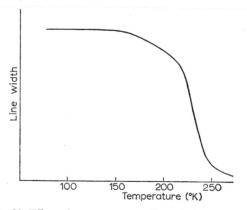

Fig. 80. Effect of temperature on line width in rubber[4].

Nuclear resonance has also been suggested[6] as a means of determining crystalline-amorphous ratios in polymers (p. 374). For example in some samples of polythene and polytetrafluoroethylene, the spectrum consists of two superimposed peaks, one associated with the crystalline regions, and the other, a much sharper peak, due to amorphous polymer. To determine the ratio one is faced with the difficult task of resolving the peaks graphically into two components, so that their individual strengths can be compared. For this reason the method has not been widely used.

This section, and the rest of the chapter, is devoted to high resolution nuclear spin resonance studies of fluids, as opposed to low resolution work on solids.

The chemical shift is the most important quantity obtainable from a NSR spectrum, in connection with problems of chemical structure. As was seen in section A2, the field strength at which the resonance of a nucleus occurs depends somewhat on the chemical compound in which it is combined. This happens because nuclei are always shielded to some extent from the applied magnetic field, both by surrounding molecules and, to a much greater extent, by the electrons within their own molecule. Their resonance is therefore shifted from that of the corresponding bare nucleus. Shielding by external molecules (bulk susceptibility effects) can be largely allowed for by comparing substances in the same solvent at comparable concentrations. There remains the internal shielding which of course varies from point to point within a molecule and accounts, for example, for the three separate peaks in the spectrum of ethyl alcohol, arising from the hydroxyl, methyl and methylene protons.

Brief descriptions will be given in the first part of this section of attempts to explain chemical shifts in terms of theories of electronic distribution in molecules. A summary follows of the many empirical correlations between chemical shifts of protons in organic compounds, and their molecular environments. Finally chemical shifts in nuclei other than protons are briefly described.

1. Theory of the chemical shift – correlation with acidity, electronegativity, and the Hammett sigma factor

Let us consider in rather more detail the mechanism of shielding of nuclei by electrons in the molecule. In a magnetic field the electrons around a nucleus tend to circulate in a plane perpendicular to the field direction. In effect a nucleus has an electric current flowing round it. By the laws of electrodynamics this current causes a secondary magnetic field, in the opposite direction to the applied one. This reduces the net field at the nucleus. To a first approximation one would expect the degree of shielding of a nucleus, and hence the chemical shift, to depend on the electron density in its vicinity. This simple picture however breaks down for molecules with delocalised electrons, in orbitals which cover the whole molecule. For example in benzene the π electron system causes rings of electron density above and below the carbon atom plane. In a field these are equivalent to circular currents giving a secondary field

TABLE 29

CORRELATION OF CHEMICAL SHIFT WITH ACID STRENGTH

Acid	pK (acid)	Chemical shift of —OH protons (p.p.m. relative to water)	Acid	pK (acid)	Chemical shift of —OH protons (p.p.m. relative to water)
sulphonic acids	v. strong	—6.7 ± 0.3	water	14	0
carboxylic acids	4–5	—3 ± 1	acetylenes	rather weak	+2.4 ± 0.4
phenols	c. 10	—2.3 ± 0.3	alcohols	16–18	—0.1 ± 0.7

perpendicular to the plane of the ring. The chemical shifts of the benzene protons are therefore governed both by local circulations of σ electrons and by the contribution from the π electron system. This effect has been put on a sound theoretical basis by Pople[7], and extended to other aromatic ring systems.

Acidic properties are shown by compounds where, because of partial withdrawal of electrons from the vicinity of the acid proton, it tends readily to be lost to a base. Since this electron withdrawal also affects the chemical shift one might expect the properties to run parallel through a series of compounds. Table 29 shows that this is roughly the case in practice. There are however anomalies. For example acetylene falls out of line, presumably because the shift arises both from the electrons circulating round the triple bond, and from local circulations in the hydrogen atoms.

The electronegativity of the atom X in a series of compounds —CH_2—X— measures the extent to which electrons are pushed or pulled to or from the protons. A correlation of this property with chemical shift is to be expected. With compounds CH_3–X–, a general correlation was found by Allred and Rochow[8] between the methyl proton shift and the electronegativity of X. A similar study was made by Dailey and Shoolery[9] of the —CH_2— and —CH_3 proton resonances of compounds of the type CH_3—CH_2—X. Neither signal correlated satisfactorily with the

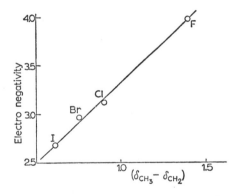

Fig. 81. Parallelism of $(\delta_{CH_3} - \delta_{CH_2})$ and electronegativity in ethyl compounds.

electronegativity value, probably because the idea that chemical shift depends on electron density is an oversimplification. However, as shown in Fig. 81, a linear plot of $\delta_{CH_3} - \delta_{CH_2}$ against the electronegativity of X was obtained. Presumably the factors which prevent correlation with the —CH_2— and —CH_3 signals individually have the same effect on both types of proton.

In monosubstituted benzenes it is sometimes possible to

distinguish signals due to the protons situated *ortho*, *meta*, and *para* to the substituent. Dailey and Corio[10] have tried to relate the location of these signals to the known ability of substituents to transmit electronic effects through the ring to the three positions. They were able to divide substituents into three classes. The first comprised meta directing groups such as —NO₂, —CHO and —COCl, which are known to withdraw electrons from the ring. These produce large negative chemical shifts for all three positions, relative to the value for benzene, the orders of magnitude being $o > p > m$. This clearly shows reduced shielding of the protons. Electron donating groups such as —NH₂, —NHCH₃, and —N(CH₃)₂, have the opposite effect, with large positive shifts. With less powerful substituents, such as —CH₃, —C₂H₅ and —CH₂Cl, separate signals for the three protons could no longer be detected, suggesting that the electronic effects are much smaller, and roughly equal in the *ortho*, *meta* and *para* positions.

A more detailed analysis was undertaken by Taft[11], who used data on the fluorine chemical shifts of a large number of fluoro-benzenes. As mentioned in Chapter 6 (p. 184) the Hammett σ factor provides an excellent overall measure of the effect of an substituent on the benzene ring. Both electromeric (or resonance) and inductive effects are concerned. For example the electromeric effect predominates in aniline where resonance involving such forms as

is important. With chlorine on the other hand, there is an electromeric effect involving such forms as

causing the group to be *ortho-para* directing, but electron withdrawal by the inductive mechanism also takes place, since the ring as a whole is deactivated relative to benzene. Taft has succeeded in splitting the σ factor into two parts, σ_R and σ_I which give quantitative measures of the resonance and inductive effects of a substituent. As shown by Fig. 82b, the fluorine chemical shifts of para substituents, where, because of the distance factor, inductive effects are unimportant, correlate

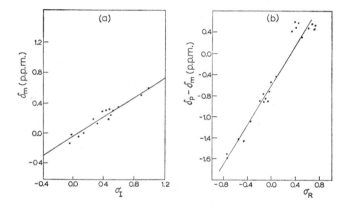

Fig. 82. Fluorine chemical shifts of substituted fluorobenzenes and Taft's sigma factors. (a) meta substituents; (b) para substituents[11].

well with σ_R. With *meta* substituents where no resonance contribution is possible, an equally close parallelism with σ_I is found (Fig. 82a). This work shows strikingly how closely chemical shifts follow electron distributions in a series of compounds where other factors remain constant.

2. Empirical correlations of chemical shift and proton environments

In the case of ethyl alcohol (p. 262) three signals are found corresponding to the three kinds of proton bonding. If several alcohols are measured they are all found to show a shift near zero p.p.m. relative to water. One therefore associates this value with an alcoholic hydroxyl group. Similarly all hydrocarbons and other compounds with the $-CH_2 \cdot CH_3$ group give a methyl group shift near 3.5 p.p.m. The situation is therefore similar to that in infra-red spectroscopy, where frequencies can be associated with chemical groups. Figs. 83 and 84 show some well established correlations between shift (relative to water as standard) and structure. Although, as indicated in the next section, NSR is by no means confined to protons, it must be admitted that the range of groups covered is nothing like as wide as that for infra-red spectroscopy. For this reason it is doubtful whether NSR will become as widely useful an aid to

Fig. 83. Chemical shifts of C—H groups, in p.p.m. relative to liquid water.

the organic chemist. Nevertheless, as the section on typical applications will show, there are many cases where NSR is the more powerful weapon. For example the paraffinic, olefinic, and aromatic C—H signals are much better separated than the corresponding infra-red bands. The O—H and N—H signals from aliphatic and aromatic compounds are likewise in very different spectral regions, whereas in infra-red spectroscopy, OH and NH bands are difficult to distinguish.

There are two possible ways of using the data of Figs. 83 and 84. Given an unknown substance, one can determine its chemical shifts, and try to predict from them the groups present. The chances of success by this method are however clearly limited. If for example a signal near zero p.p.m. is found, at least half a dozen groups may possibly be present. A much more fruitful

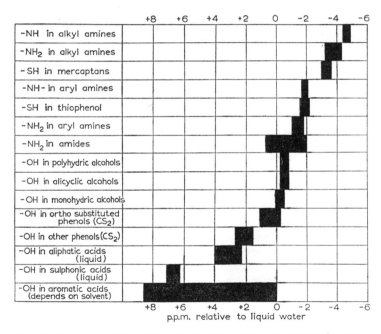

Fig. 84. Chemical shifts of O—H, N—H and S—H groups, in p.p.m. relative to liquid water.

approach is to make all possible use of other chemical and physical data on the unknown. It is often possible to construct two or three possible formulae. From known correlations the chemical shifts of each of these can be predicted, and these predictions compared with experiment. A large volume of NSR data has been collected by Chamberlain[25], and arranged in a very suitable form for this purpose. Charts are given which summarise the NSR spectra of paraffins, olefines, naphthenes, benzene derivatives, multi-ring aromatics, acids, esters, alcohols, ethers, ketones, phenols, amines, amides and other compounds.

TABLE 30

CHEMICAL SHIFTS OF COMMON STANDARDS, RELATIVE TO CYCLOHEXANE

Standard	Relative shift (p.p.m.)	Standard	Relative shift (p.p.m.)
Chloroform	—6.1	Dioxan	—2.2
Benzene	—5.3	Acetone	—0.8
Methylene chloride	—4.2	Cyclohexane	0
Water	—3.6	Tetramethylsilane	1.5

One practical point is important in making comparisons with literature data. Different workers use different solvents and dilutions which may cause quite large variations in a group shift. Also several standards are in use, but measurements may readily be converted from one to another provided the shift of each standard is known on a common basis. The shifts of some common liquid standards, relative to cyclohexane are listed in Table 30.

3. Chemical shifts of nuclei other than protons

Problems sometimes arise in organic chemistry where more direct information can be obtained by studying the resonance of nuclei other than protons. As seen from Table 28, only ^{19}F, on account of its large magnetic moment and 100% abundance, is as satisfactory for NSR measurements as the proton. However ^{31}P, ^{14}N and ^{13}C have also been used with some success. The disadvantages of these nuclei are to some extent offset by their large chemical shifts compared to the proton. Resolution of the lines due to different environments therefore presents no problem, and larger samples can be used to increase the signal strength.

(a) Fluorine. NSR has proved a powerful tool in solving structural problems in fluorine chemistry. Just as with protons, different chemical shifts can be associated with different fluorine groupings. A few are listed in Table 31, which is compiled from data in Ref. [12] (p. 317). Comparison with Figs. 83 and 84 shows that much larger shifts occur.

TABLE 31

CHEMICAL SHIFTS IN FLUORINE COMPOUNDS

Compound type	Chemical shift (p.p.m. relative to CF_3COOH)	Compound type	Chemical shift (p.p.m. relative to CF_3COOH)
$-CH_2-CH_2-F$	149.5–145.5	CF_3-CH_2-	11.9–3.2
$\diagdown C-CF_2-C \diagup$	57.8–21.9	all other CF_3-C	0.0–(−19.7)
$\diagdown C-CF_2-N \diagup$	51.1–8.6	$\diagdown C=CF-O-$	−9.4–(−11.8)
$\diagdown C-CF_2-O-$	14.9–(−6.2)	$CF_3-N \diagup$	−18.8–(−36.2)

(b) Phosphorus. Although, because of its small moment the NSR sensitivity of ^{31}P is only 7% that of the proton, it gives sharp signals with large chemical shifts, and is therefore sometimes quite suitable for study by the technique. Not only do esters of the various phosphoric and thiophosphoric acids occur in natural products, but they have also commercial applications, for example as insecticides. A typical problem involves the equilibria between $(RO)_3P{=}S$ and $\begin{smallmatrix} RS \\ RO \\ RO \end{smallmatrix}\!\!>\!\!P{=}O$. Table 32 lists the shifts for a few typical cases, and, particularly with the

trivalent compounds, shows that large differences in the shift may be caused by small structural changes.

TABLE 32

CHEMICAL SHIFTS IN PHOSPHORUS COMPOUNDS

Compound	Chemical shift (p.p.m. relative to 85% H_3PO_4)	Compound	Chemical shift (p.p.m. relative to 85% H_3PO_4)
PH_3	238	$PO \cdot (OC_6H_5)_3$	17.3
$PH_2 \cdot CH_3$	163.5	$PO \cdot (OC_2H_5)_3$	0.9
$P(CH_3)_3$	61	H_3PO_4	0
$P \cdot (C_6H_5)_3$	5.9	H_3PO_3	—4.5
$P(OC_6H_5)_3$	—127	$PO(CH_3)(OH)_2$	—31.1
$P(OCH_3)_3$	—14.1	$PO(C_2H_5)_3$	—48.3
$PH(OCH_3)_2$	—181	$PO(SC_2H_5)_3$	—61.3
PCl_3	—215	$PS(OC_2H_5)_3$	—68.1

(c) Carbon. The study of carbon nuclei is an attractive prospect. ^{12}C has no magnetic moment, but ^{13}C, at 1.1% abundance, has a relatively large one. Because of its low abundance, the experimental technique is more difficult than with the nuclei so far discussed. Special methods, involving extensive modifications of a commercial instrument are necessary. Lauterbur[13], however, has successfully measured many carbon compounds at natural abundance, and it seems likely that, with advances in technique, day-to-day measurements of carbon resonance will ultimately become possible. Relative to the carbon atoms of benzene, those of paraffins give a shift of +100 p.p.m. On the other hand those of the C=O group in acids, esters, amides, lactones etc. fall at different values between 30 and 90 p.p.m. below that of benzene. Owing to the large shifts carbon resonance studies may be one of the major future developments of NSR.

(d) Nitrogen. Although several measurements of ^{14}N resonances in aqueous solutions of nitrogen compounds have been made, there have been few applications in organic chemistry. The main reason is that, because of its quadrupole moment, arising from its having a spin of 1 rather than 1/2 as with ^{1}H, ^{19}F, ^{31}P and ^{13}C, the resonance lines of nitrogen are intrinsically broad, causing the overlap of signals from nuclei in slightly different environments.

E. NUCLEAR SPIN-SPIN INTERACTIONS – FINE STRUCTURE OF LINES

It was seen in Chapter 7, that the interaction of an unpaired electron in a free radical with nuclei in the same molecule sometimes caused hyperfine splitting of its electron resonance line, which could be used to deduce the structure of the radical. A rather similar internuclear effect is found in NSR spectra, which is likewise useful in structural determinations.

1. Theory of spin–spin interactions

Let us return to the example of HD which was briefly discussed in section A3. Suppose that at a given instant, one of the electrons, e_H, is associated with the proton, and the other, e_D, with the deuteron. If then the axis of the proton happens to lie parallel to the field, in an attempt to minimise the energy of H and e_H, the axis of the latter is rather more likely to lie anti-parallel to the field. e_D must by Pauli's Exclusion Principle tend to lie parallel to the field, and in turn will induce the axis of the deuteron to lie antiparallel rather than parallel. The net result is that an effect has been transmitted through the electrons from the proton to the deuteron. It follows that the transmitted effect on the deuteron will be slightly different according to whether the proton axis lies parallel or anti-parallel, giving rise to two slightly different energy states for the deuteron in HD. This accounts for the double peak in its resonance spectrum. Similarly since the magnetic axis of the deuteron may adopt one of three possible orientations, the proton resonance is a triplet. The magnitude of the interaction between two nuclei is usually described by a coupling constant J, expressed in cycles/second.

Spin-spin splitting occurs widely in the spectra of organic compounds. Consider for example the methyl and methylene proton resonances in ethyl chloride. Since the carbon nuclei have no spin and that of chlorine is small, one is concerned essentially with inter-proton effects. Fig. 85 shows that the spectrum under high resolution consists of a triplet with

Fig. 85. High-resolution spectrum of $CH_3 \cdot CH_2 \cdot Cl$.

intensity ratio 1:2:1, associated with the methyl group, and four lines in the ratios 1:3:3:1 arising from the methylene group. These assignments to —CH_3 and —CH_2— are from chemical shift data. Since any proton in the system may have one of two possible orientations in the applied field, one finds, as in the figure, various combinations of orientations for the three methyl and two methylene protons. Each combination will transmit a slightly different effect to a proton in the other group, explaining the observed numbers of lines. Moreover as a net spin of 3/2 can be made up in only one way, whereas 1/2 can be built up in three ways, and so on, the intensities of the fine structure components are also accounted for. The above simple theory applies only in cases where the spin-spin splitting is small compared to the chemical shift differences of the nuclei. If these quantities are comparable a much more complex spectrum results.

It will have been noticed that Fig. 85 shows no evidence of interaction between the three methyl protons, or the methylene pair. Quite generally no splitting is found involving two nuclei in equivalent positions in a molecule, which is a valuable simplifying factor.

2. The use of fine structure in structural diagnosis

The first problem is the practical one of distinguishing fine structure lines from those due to chemical shifts. With experience this can usually be done by inspection, but in doubtful cases it is advisable to measure the spectrum at more than one field strength. Whereas the separation of lines due to chemical shifts increases in proportion to the field, fine structure separations remain constant, so a distinction can be made.

Suppose that the chemical shifts and signal intensities of the spectrum of an unknown show it to contain one methyl and one methylene group. It may nevertheless be impossible from the

Fig. 86. High-resolution spectrum of pure, dry ethanol.

chemical shifts to say whether the structure is $X—CH_2—CH_3$ or $—CH_2—X—CH_3$, where X represents another part of the molecule. If the first structure is correct, the methyl and methylene groups under high resolution should show fine structures of respectively three and four components. Absence of splitting would indicate the second type of structure.

Applications of this kind clearly depend on ability to predict whether or not two given nuclei will interact, so that the observed splittings can be compared with those predicted on the

References p. 307

basis of possible structures of an unknown. Although prediction is not always possible, empirical correlations have been found, from which it can often be seen whether a signal should be split.

TABLE 33

INTER-NUCLEAR COUPLING CONSTANTS

Structure	Coupling constant (cycle/sec)	Structure	Coupling constant (cycle/sec)
$CH_3—CH_2—$*	6–8		<1
	1–2		10–12
	5–11	$X—\underset{F}{\overset{F}{C}}—CHYZ$	158
	12–18		115–124
	5–8.5		20
	1–3	$^{14}NH_3$**	46

* Between one methyl and one methylene proton.
** Between ^{14}N and H.

The most important of these concerns the rapid fall off of coupling constants with increasing numbers of chemical bonds between the nuclei. For example whereas in pure, dry ethyl alcohol, splitting of the OH resonance by the $-CH_2-$ group, and of the $-CH_2-$ and $-CH_3$ signals by one another is observed (Fig. 86), no interaction can be detected between the hydroxyl and methyl protons, because of the two intervening bonds. Table 33 collects together some coupling constants. With large values of J marked splitting is to be expected. For example in an olefine of the type

$$\begin{array}{cc} H & X \\ \diagdown & \diagup \\ C = C \\ \diagup & \diagdown \\ Y & H \end{array}$$

, the coupling is large (12–18), so a doublet proton signal would be expected. In

$$\begin{array}{cc} X & H \\ \diagdown & \diagup \\ C = C \\ \diagup & \diagdown \\ Y & H \end{array}$$

on the contrary, the splitting might well be too small to be observed. In benzene derivatives, where only with *ortho* protons does strong coupling occur, the effect of distance is clearly shown. In addition to data on protons, a few figures for other nuclei are included. As with chemical shifts, the values for fluorine and ^{14}N are substantially greater than for protons.

F. EXAMPLES OF STRUCTURAL DIAGNOSES BY NSR

As has been seen in the earlier sections several principles may be used in deciding whether the NSR spectrum of an unknown is consistent with a proposed formula. They may be summarised as follows.

(1) The number of main peaks should equal the number of groups of equivalent protons (or other nuclei) in the proposed structure.

(2) These peaks should have chemical shifts consistent with the indications of Figs. 83 and 84.

(3) Since every proton makes the same contribution to peak intensity, the intensities, as measured by the areas under the peaks, should be proportional to the numbers of protons of various kinds.

(4) Where fine structure is observed, the number of lines resulting and their separations should be in accordance with the indications of the last section.

1. Spectra of known compounds

Before quoting examples of structural problems which have been solved, it may be useful to consider the spectra of a few known compounds (Fig. 87), to illustrate how one may often correlate completely a NSR spectrum with a chemical structure.

The spectrum of α-methyl styrene shows excellent separation of the peaks due to the three proton types. As expected, the ring proton signal is much stronger than the others, and the methyl peak about three times as strong as those due to the olefinic protons. There is only slight splitting of the H_A and H_B signals, since interaction between gem protons is small.

The essential oil, eugenol, provides a second example. When the total area under all the sub-peaks is included, the strongest signals are those due to the methyl and ring protons, and the methyl signal is three times as strong as those from the olefinic protons. Interactions between H_C and the —CH_2— group cause doubling of the methylene signal, and a much more complex fine structure in the H_C peak than in those of H_A and H_B. The closely related compound isoeugenol has a considerably different spectrum, the most striking changes being due to replacement of methylene by methyl.

Although the molecular weight of methyl linoleate is 276, the spectrum in Fig. 87d[14] is excellently resolved. This has become possible through recent improvements in Varian magnets, which allow measurements at a field of 14,000 gauss with as good homogeneity as was formerly obtainable at 9,600 gauss. Increased separation of the signals due to the different proton groups results from the increased chemical shifts, while the

Fig. 87. Typical NSR spectra of organic compounds.

coupling constants remain unchanged. All the signals from olefinic protons are split into triplets as expected. Similarly the C_{18} methyl signal is split by the C_{17} methylene protons.

Fluorine chemistry provides the final example in the set. Rotation about the double bond in trifluorochloroethylene being restricted, the three fluorine nuclei are non-equivalent, and the spectrum[15] has three main peaks of equal intensity. Quadruplet fine structures are found since each fluorine signal is split by each of the other two fluorine nuclei.

2. Determination of unknown structures from NSR spectra

Applications to typical structural problems will now be described.

(a) Diketene. There are five plausible structures for this compound:

Previous attempts by chemical and physical methods to decide among these were unsuccessful. For example, Whiffen and Thompson[17] from infra-red spectra, were able to eliminate I and II, but could not decide between the others. The proton resonance spectrum (Fig. 88a) of the liquid provides an immediate solution, since it shows two signals, of equal intensity[26]. Only structure V is consistent with this.

(b) Feist's acid (Fig. 88b). Chemical evidence suggests structure I or II:

It proved rather difficult to obtain a satisfactory resonance spectrum, since the acid is high melting and insoluble in non-polar solvents. Eventually the spectrum of the sodium salt of the acid in D_2O was measured[16], so as to avoid strong interfering signals from H_2O and the carboxyl protons. Two peaks of equal strength were found, whose chemical shifts showed them to be

Fig. 88. Spectra of compounds of uncertain structure.

due to ethylenic and cyclopropyl protons. Structure II is therefore correct.

(c) *Sterulic acid.* This acid provides another example involving a 3-membered ring. The likely formulae are:

$$CH_3(CH_2)_7-C = C-(CH_2)_7 \cdot COOH$$
$$\diagdown \diagup$$
$$CH_2$$
$$I$$

$$CH_2$$
$$\diagup \diagdown$$
$$CH_3 \cdot (CH_2)_5 \cdot CH - CH \cdot CH = CH \cdot (CH_2)_7 \cdot COOH$$
$$II$$

$$\begin{array}{ccc} CH_2 & & CH \\ \diagup \diagdown & & \diagup \diagdown \\ R \cdot CH = C - CHR' & R - CH - C - R' \\ III & & IV \end{array}$$

Since no signal due to ethylenic protons was found[18], I is the probable structure.

(d) *Thujic acid.* I and II are the most probable structures:

I   II

As the ratio of ethylenic protons to methyl ester protons is 5:3 in I and 3:3 in II, a distinction can be made by comparing the areas under the corresponding signals. When this was done[19] (Fig. 88c), a result of 355 units to 210 units was obtained, clearly indicating formula I.

(e) Fig. 86d shows the spectrum of a compound believed to have either the structure I or II.

I   II

A decision on chemical grounds is very difficult, and the results of infra-red measurements are unlikely to be conclusive, since the bands associated with cis-disubstituted olefines are not well defined. Three lines of equal intensity in the middle of the spectrum support II, as only two proton signals would be expected from I in this region. Further confirmation is provided by the main splitting of the olefinic proton signals into doublets, separated by 8–9 cycles/sec.

(f) A rather similar problem is presented by the alkaloid *myosmine*, for which the structures below have been suggested:

By comparison with simple derivatives, the left hand part of the spectrum, which is shown in Fig. 89a (Ref. 12, p. 281), can be associated with the pyridine ring. Three peaks of equal intensity are found at higher fields, each having twice the intensity of the individual pyridine proton signals. This is entirely consistent with formula I, which has three methylene groups, and rules out II.

(g) A striking example is provided by methyl *photosantionate*, for which three very similar structures are possible[20]:

A strong signal was found, with triplet splitting probably caused by an adjacent —CH_2— group, at the chemical shift corre-

Fig. 89. Spectra of compounds of uncertain structure.

sponding to an olefinic proton. Hence of these three structures only I can be correct.

(h) Addition of *methyl dichlorosilane* to *vinyl acetate* gives an adduct whose likely structures[27] are:

$$
\begin{array}{ccc}
\underset{\underset{\underset{Cl}{|}}{|}}{\overset{\overset{Cl}{|}}{CH_3-Si}}-CH_2-CH_2-O-\overset{\overset{O}{\|}}{C}-CH_3
& \text{and} &
\underset{\underset{\underset{Cl}{|}}{|}}{\overset{\overset{Cl\ \ CH_3}{|\ \ \ \ |}}{CH_3-Si}}-CH-O-\overset{\overset{O}{\|}}{C}-CH_3
\\
\text{I} & & \text{II}
\end{array}
$$

The significant feature of the spectrum (Fig. 89c) is the presence of two bands, A and B, with clearly resolved triplet splitting. This is precisely what would be expected from two adjacent methylene groups as in I, whereas the splitting cannot be plausibly accounted for on the basis of II.

*(i)** The most probable structures[30] for a *bis-spiroindane* were

A band at the expected position for —CH_2— (Fig. 89b) strongly indicates structure I. Considering the numbers of protons of the types —CH_3, —CH_2—, aliphatic C—H and aromatic C—H, one predicts a band area ratio of $12:4:0:6$ for I and $15:0:1:8$ for II. The observed ratios provide further confirmation of the first structure.

(j) This example illustrates the power of NSR in distinguishing isomers. A compound was known to be one of the six isomeric *ethyl propanetetracarboxylates*, which may be formulated as follows, where X represents —$COOC_2H_5$.

---

* This example and the following two were provided by Dr. J. K. Becconsall.

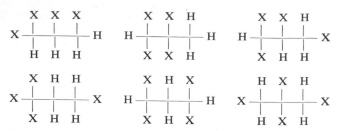

In this case, the spectrum (Fig. 89d) permits of an unequivocal decision among the possibilities. A doublet —CH₂— resonance is observed, which can arise only from a structure in which the —CH₂— group is adjacent to a C—H group. Only

satisfies the conditions.

(k) The final example shows that NSR can sometimes yield the structure of an impurity. An impure sample of diethyl malonate showed a well-defined impurity peak at a position typical of the —O—CH₃ group (Fig. 89e). Intensity considerations indicated either 14% of methyl ethyl malonate or 7% of dimethyl malonate.

G. THE APPLICATION OF NSR TO RATE PROCESSES

In the compounds so far considered, the nuclei have been fixed in a definite chemical structure. Some of the most useful applications however arise when the nuclei under examination can take part in a chemical reaction during the measurement. Consider proton resonance in an equilibrium system

$$X + AH \rightleftharpoons BH + Y$$

In spectroscopic measurements in the ultra-violet and infra-red regions, the time associated with the transition is so short that effectively one measures the spectra of AH and BH simultaneously. An NSR transition however involves re-orientation of the nucleus in the field, a process which takes appreciable time. The mean lifetime of a proton, in AH before it passes to BH (or vice-versa) may therefore be much greater than, equal to or less than the time taken by the transition. In the first case two distinct signals appear in the spectrum at frequencies ν_A and ν_B, corresponding to AH and BH. At the other extreme the lifetime is so short that the proton is transferred many times during the time required for the spin re-orientation. In these circumstances all the protons are equivalent as far as NSR absorption is concerned, and only a single line is observed at $\frac{1}{2}(\nu_A + \nu_B)$,

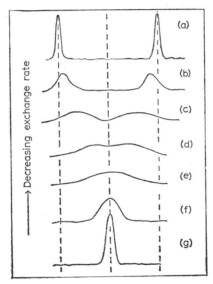

Fig. 90. Effect of exchange rate on a spectrum.

representing the time-averaged state of the proton. If $\Delta\nu_{AB}$ is the difference between ν_A and ν_B, and if t_0 is the mean lifetime, the criterion determining the type of spectrum observed is whether t_0 is much greater than, approximately equal to, or much less than $1/\Delta\nu_{AB}$.

References p. 307

Fig. 90 shows how the spectrum changes as the rate of proton exchange increases. Should the rate of interchange between AH and BH be very slow, there are two distinct signals, as in Fig. 90a. If now, by adding increasing amounts of a catalyst, or by progressively raising the temperature, the rate of exchange is increased steadily, the lines move closer together, and finally coalesce to a single broad signal (Fig. 90e), when the proton exchange frequency becomes comparable to $\Delta \nu_{AB}$. Further increase of the exchange rate causes narrowing of the line, as in (f) and (g). The following sections give examples where the exchange rate is much greater than, roughly equal to, and much less than the frequency difference.

1. Lifetime much greater than $1/\Delta \nu_{AB}$ – keto-enol tautomerism
This is the most straightforward case, in which one finds two distinct sets of signals, corresponding to the species AH and BH. Keto-enol tautomerism provides a good example of this behaviour. Since not only can qualitative evidence of the forms be obtained from chemical shifts, but also the proportions of the two forms at equilibrium from the relative signal intensities, NSR is perhaps the most powerful physical method for studying this phenomenon. Fig. 91 shows the spectrum of liquid acetyl acetone[21], where the equilibrium

$$CH_3—CO—CH_2—CO—CH_3 \rightleftharpoons CH_3—C{=}CH—CO—CH_3$$
$$\overset{|}{\underset{OH}{}}$$

is set up. Peaks are assigned to the —OH, =CH—, and —CH$_3$ groups of the enol form, and to the —CH$_2$— and —CH$_3$ groups of the keto form. By careful measurement of the areas under the —CH$_2$— and =CH— peaks it was deduced[21] that liquid acetylacetone at 25°C, contains $18.6 \pm 0.6\%$ keto form, a value probably much more accurate than the figure of 24% by bromine titration.

Such measurements are clearly capable of extension to other temperatures, as a means of determining the heat content change of the process. Certain solvents may alter the proportions at equilibrium, for example by preferential hydrogen bonding with one of the tautomers. In triethylamine for example, acetylacetone

Fig. 91. Spectrum of acetyl acetone.

exists entirely in the enol form, presumably because of its stabilisation through — $\overset{\diagdown}{\underset{\diagup}{N}}$ ... H — O — bonds.

2. Lifetime comparable to $1/\Delta\nu_{AB}$ — determination of reaction velocities — hindered rotation

Mixtures of pure ethyl alcohol and water provide an example of this. If a small amount, say 5%, of water is added to ethyl alcohol, two distinct peaks are found, separated by 32 cycles/sec in a certain field. They are assigned to the water and ethanol hydroxyl protons. There is however a possibility of exchange:

$$EtOH_1 + H \cdot OH_2 \rightleftharpoons EtOH_2 + H \cdot OH_1$$

As the proportion of water is increased, the lines move together and finally coalesce at about 27% water. Mixtures with more water show only a single line in this region of the spectrum. The explanation is that, as the amount of water is increased, so are the rates of the forward and reverse proton transfer reactions, until, at 27%, the frequency of transfer equals the frequency difference between the alcohol and water lines. In this example, the average time spent by a given proton in water and in ethanol molecules is equal (say t_0). Gutowsky[22] has shown that in these circumstances, if the two individual lines are separated by $\Delta\nu_{AB}$, then at the point where the lines coalesce,

$$t_0 = \frac{\sqrt{2}}{\pi \times \Delta\nu_{AB}}.$$

In the ethanol–water case at 27% water, t_0 equals $\sqrt{2}/\pi \times 32$ or 0.014 seconds, from which value, and the known concentrations, the rate constant of the process can easily be evaluated.

A detailed study of proton exchange in ethanol, methanol, and their mixtures with water, with and without acidic and basic catalysts, has been made by Luz *et al.*[23].

Molecules with hindered internal rotation present a rather similar problem. For example in dimethylacetamide, partly because of the resonance contribution from the ionic form,

the C—N bond has some double bond character, and rotation about it is restricted. Therefore the protons of the two nitrogen methyl groups are in slightly different environments, according to whether they are adjacent to the oxygen atom or the third methyl group. At low temperatures, the potential barrier makes rotation an infrequent process, so the spectrum shows two distinct nitrogen methyl proton signals. With rising temperature, the rate of rotation increases, and the two peaks move together[22]. Finally at about 50°C, they coalesce, the rotation frequency having become comparable to the frequency separation of the separate signals. Further temperature increases sharpen this single line. From the theory of the effect one can, by plotting a function of the peak separation against the inverse of the absolute temperature, determine the height of the potential barrier. The value 12 ± 2 kcals was obtained for dimethyl acetamide.

Similar studies have been made on hindered rotation in other amides, nitrosamines, alkyl nitrites, aldoximes, and many ethanes with bulky substituents.

3. Rapid exchange rates. Hydrogen bonding

Hydrogen bonding in fluids may conveniently be discussed at this point, since the equilibria concerned, such as

$$X - O - H + Y \rightleftharpoons X - O - H \dots Y$$

involve very rapid proton exchange. As a result hydrogen bonded systems of that kind show only a single absorption line in the —OH region, the frequency of which throws light on the time-averaged state of a proton. The effect of hydrogen bonding on the chemical shifts of protons has been clearly shown for simple hydrides by Schneider *et al.*[28]. As seen from Table 34, whilst no change results with non-polar substances on passing from the gas to the liquid state, a shift to low field results in all cases where the liquid is associated through hydrogen bonds. These shifts to low field indicate that hydrogen bond formation reduces the electron shielding of the proton. This accords with current views on the hydrogen bond, which regard it as essentially an ionic interaction with a charge distribution of the type $-\overset{\delta_-}{O} \dots \overset{\delta_+}{H} \dots \overset{\delta_-}{O}-$, in which the proton is electron deficient.

TABLE 34

EFFECT OF HYDROGEN BONDING ON PROTON CHEMICAL SHIFTS

Compound	Chemical shift relative to CH_4 (gas), p.p.m.		Change of shift due to bonding, p.p.m.
	Liquid state	Gas	
CH_4	0	0	0
C_2H_6	—0.73	—0.75	0.02
NH_3	—1.00	0.05	1.05
H_2O	—5.18	—0.60	4.58
HF	—9.15	—2.50	6.65
HCl	—1.60	0.45	2.05
H_2S	—1.58	—0.08	1.50
HCN	—4.48	—2.83	1.65

In organic systems NSR is clearly a possible method of detecting hydrogen bonds. For example the proton shift of chloroform in several solvents has been measured[29], and attempts made to correlate them with the strengths of the corresponding hydrogen bonds. Although no quantitative relationship between magnitudes of low field shifts and hydrogen bond strengths has yet been established, such shifts appear at least to give qualitative indications of bond strengths.

NSR is one of the techniques which have been applied to study association in solution through hydrogen bonding. In general an alcohol in a non-polar solvent like carbon tetrachloride forms a mixture of complexes in equilibrium:

$$\text{ROH} + \text{ROH} \underset{}{\overset{K_2}{\rightleftharpoons}} (\text{ROH})_2 + \text{ROH} \underset{}{\overset{K_3}{\rightleftharpoons}} (\text{ROH})_3 + \text{ROH} \underset{}{\overset{K_4}{\rightleftharpoons}} \ldots$$

The exchange of protons is so rapid that individual signals due to monomers, dimers, trimers etc. cannot be observed. NSR is at a disadvantage in this respect to infra-red spectroscopy, where some of the species give separate bands. Since a proton contributes the same intensity to the signal irrespective of its environment, the observed frequency is a weighted average for the various species, given by the equation

$$\nu = \frac{\nu_1 M_1 + 2\nu_2 K_2 M_1{}^2 + 3\nu_3 K_3 M_1{}^3 \ldots}{M_1 + 2K_2 M_1{}^2 \ldots}$$

where M_1, M_2 etc. are the mole fractions of the various polymers, the K's are the equilibrium constants, and ν_1, ν_2 etc. refer to monomers, dimers etc. As the concentration is increased, the proportion of higher polymers increases, and the signal moves to lower fields. Although there are far too many unknowns in the above equation for it to be solved in terms of the equilibrium constants, attempts have been made to carry out the reverse process. That is, by making assumptions about the values of the equilibrium constants, and neglecting many of them the dependence of signal frequency on concentration can be calculated for various models, and the results compared with experiment.

For example, Saunders and Hyne[24] calculate that for *t*-butanol and phenol in carbon tetrachloride the main equilibrium is between monomers and trimers, whereas methanol forms mainly tetramers. It must however be stressed that even if some model fits the experimental results well, there is no guarantee that other equally good models have not been overlooked.

REFERENCES

1 R. E. RICHARDS AND J. A. S. SMITH, *Trans. Faraday Soc.*, 47 (1951) 1261.
2 E. R. ANDREW, *J. Chem. Phys.*, 18 (1950) 607.
3 E. R. ANDREW, *Nuclear Magnetic Resonance*, Cambridge University Press, New York, 1955.
4 H. S. GUTOWSKY AND L. H. MEYER, *J. Chem. Phys.*, 21 (1953) 2122.
5 R. LAND, R. E. RICHARDS AND I. M. WARD, *Trans. Faraday Soc.*, 55 (1959) 225.
6 C. W. WILSON, III AND G. E. PAKE, *J. Polymer Sci.*, 10 (1953) 503.
7 J. A. POPLE, *J. Chem. Phys.*, 24 (1956) 1111.
8 A. L. ALLRED AND E. G. ROCHOW, *J. Am. Chem. Soc.*, 79 (1957) 5363.
9 B. P. DAILEY AND J. N. SHOOLERY, *J. Am. Chem. Soc.*, 77 (1955) 3977.
10 P. L. CORIO AND B. P. DAILEY, *J. Am. Chem. Soc.*, 78 (1956) 3043.
11 R. W. TAFT, Jr., *J. Am. Chem. Soc.*, 79 (1957) 1045.
12 J. A. POPLE, W. G. SCHNEIDER AND H. J. BERNSTEIN, *High-resolution Nuclear Magnetic Resonance*, McGraw-Hill, New York, 1959.
13 P. C. LAUTERBUR, *J. Chem. Phys.*, 26 (1957) 217.
14 Varian Associates, *This is N.M.R. at work*, No. 54.
15 Varian Associates, *This is N.M.R. at work*, No. 5.
16 A. F. BOTTINI AND J. D. ROBERTS, *J. Org. Chem.*, 21 (1956) 1169.
17 D. H. WHIFFEN AND H. W. THOMPSON, *J. Chem. Soc.*, (1946) 1005.
18 K. L. RINEHART, Jr., W. A. NILSSON AND H. A. WHALEY, *J. Am. Chem. Soc.*, 80 (1958) 503.
19 J. GRIPENBERG, *Acta Chem. Scand.*, 10 (1956) 487.
20 E. E. VAN TAMELEN, S. H. LEVIN, G. BRENNER, J. WOLINSKY AND P. ALDRICH, *J. Am. Chem. Soc.*, 80 (1958) 501.
21 L. W. REEVES, *Can. J. Chem.*, 35 (1957) 1351.
22 H. S. GUTOWSKY AND C. H. HOLM, *J. Chem. Phys.*, 25 (1957) 1228.
23 Z. LUZ, D. GILL AND S. MEIBOOM, *J. Chem. Phys.*, 30 (1959) 1540.
24 M. SAUNDERS AND J. B. HYNE, *J. Chem. Phys.*, 29 (1958) 1319.
25 N. F. CHAMBERLAIN, *Anal. Chem.*, 31 (1959) 56.
26 A. R. BADER, H. S. GUTOWSKY, G. A. WILLIAMS AND P. E. YANKWICH, *J. Am. Chem. Soc.*, 78 (1956) 2385.
27 L. GOODMAN, R. M. SILVERSTEIN AND J. N. SHOOLERY, *J. Am. Chem. Soc.*, 78 (1956) 4493.

[28] W. G. Schneider, H. J. Bernstein and J. A. Pople, *J. Chem. Phys.*, 28 (1958) 601.

[29] C. M. Huggins, G. C. Pimentel and J. N. Shoolery, *J. Chem. Phys.*, 23 (1955) 1244.

[30] R. F. Curtis, *Chem. & Ind. London*, (1960) 928.

SELECTED BIBLIOGRAPHY TO CHAPTER 8

Andrew, E. R., *Nuclear Magnetic Resonance*, Cambridge University Press, New York, 1955, 265 pp. This book describes fully the application of low-resolution NSR to solid-state problems.

Gutowsky, H. S., in: *Technique of Organic Chemistry* (Ed. A. Weissberger), Vol. I, *Physical Methods of Organic Chemistry*, Part IV, pp. 2664–2799, Interscience, New York, 1961. Although much of this article deals with theory and experimental methods, chemical applications are also discussed.

Jackman, L. M., *Applications of Nuclear Magnetic Resonance Spectroscopy in Organic Chemistry*, Pergamon, London, 1959, 134 pp. This book has been written specifically for the use of organic chemists, and stresses applications rather than theory.

Pople, J. A., W. G. Schneider and H. J. Bernstein, *High-resolution Nuclear Magnetic Resonance*, McGraw-Hill, New York, 1959, 501 pp. Clear, detailed descriptions are given of the underlying theory, experimental methods and chemical applications of the subject. The book is likely to remain a standard reference work for some time.

Roberts, J. D., *Nuclear Magnetic Resonance*, McGraw-Hill, New York, 1959, 115 pp. The main emphasis is on organic chemical applications. A good account of reaction velocity studies is included, and the book concludes with a most interesting collection of spectra, which the reader is invited to interpret.

Varian Associates, *NMR and EPR Spectroscopy*, Pergamon, London, 1960. This book collects together the papers presented by the Varian staff at the 1960 Varian "workshop", the object of which was to instruct users of Varian equipment. Theoretical, experimental and chemical aspects of NMR and EPR are discussed by experts in the field.

Varian Associates, *This is NMR at work*. This series of advertisements includes many excellent examples of chemical applications of NSR.

CHAPTER 9

MASS SPECTROMETRY

Mass spectroscopy made a great contribution to chemical science in 1911 when, in the hands of J. J. Thompson, it provided the first conclusive proof of the existence of isotopes. Between that time and 1940, the mass of nearly every isotope was measured accurately, mainly by Aston and Dempster, and mass spectroscopy was also used to study the energetics of ionisation of many gases. During and since the last war, partly as a result of rapid advances in instrumental design, the technique has been extended from essentially physical applications to the study of chemical problems of analysis, impurity detection and structural diagnosis.

A. INTRODUCTION

Suppose that a volatile compound flows through a tube, under pressure sufficiently low for intermolecular collisions to be very infrequent, and that a beam of electrons, the energy of which can be varied, is shot across the gas stream. Collisions between electrons and molecules will then occur, but, provided the energy of the electrons is less than about 10 eV in the case of most organic compounds, these collisions will be elastic and no permanent changes in the molecules will result. When however the electron energy is increased to a critical value, the ionisation potential of the compound in question, removal of electrons by the process

$$m + e \rightarrow m^+ + 2\,e$$

becomes possible, so that the issuing gas will contain positive ions in addition to uncharged molecules. If the energy of the bombarding electrons is increased still further, these positive ions are no longer formed in their ground state, but have excess

References p. 350

energy distributed among their electronic and vibrational levels. This excess energy is not localised at any point of the molecule, but surges randomly through it. There is therefore a possibility that after a short time interval (about 10^{-6} seconds) the excess energy may collect in some particular bond. Should the excess energy be sufficient, it will break the bond, yielding a "fragment ion" plus an uncharged particle.

$$m^+ \rightarrow m_1^+ + m_2$$

TABLE 35

MASS SPECTRUM OF n-BUTANE

Mass-charge ratio	Type of peak	Relative height	Ion	Mass-charge ratio	Type of peak	Relative height	Ion
59	i	0.54		31.9	m	0.20	
58	p	12.3	$C_4H_{10}^+$	30.4	m	0.14	
57		2.46	$C_4H_9^+$	30	i	0.98	
56		0.72	$C_4H_8^+$	29		44.2	$C_2H_5^+$
55		0.93	$C_4H_7^+$	28		32.6	$C_2H_4^+$
54		0.19	$C_4H_6^+$	27.5	d	0.05	$C_4H_7^{++}$
53		0.74	$C_4H_5^+$	27		37.1	$C_2H_3^+$
52		0.26	$C_4H_4^+$	26.5	d	0.08	$C_4H_5^{++}$
51		1.05	$C_4H_3^+$	26		6.17	$C_2H_2^+$
50		1.29	$C_4H_2^+$	25.5	d	0.36	$C_4H_3^{++}$
49		0.40	C_4H^+	25.1	m	0.11	
48		0.06	C_4^+	25		0.46	C_2H^+
45	i	0.05		24.1	m	0.01	
44	i	3.33		24		0.03	C_2^+
43		100	$C_3H_7^+$	20	d	0.02	$C_3H_4^{++}$
42		12.2	$C_3H_6^+$	19.5	d	0.01	$C_3H_3^{++}$
41		27.8	$C_3H_5^+$	19	d	0.04	$C_3H_2^{++}$
40		1.63	$C_3H_4^+$	16	i	0.12	
39.2	m	0.46		15		5.30	CH_3^+
39		12.5	$C_3H_3^+$	14		0.96	CH_2^+
38		1.86	$C_3H_2^+$	13		0.26	CH^+
37.1	m	0.06		12		0.13	C^+
37		1.01	C_3H^+	2		0.10	H_2^+
36		0.08	C_3^+	1		1.11	H^+
35.1	m	0.02					

i indicates isotope peak, p parent peak, m metastable ion peak, and d a peak due to a doubly-charged ion.

In practice an electron energy of 50–70 V is normally used, so that sufficient energy is available for any bond in the molecule to be broken. The fragment ions so formed may in turn break down further. In addition to those ions to be expected from simple bond breakage, others occur in which atomic rearrangements accompany the breakdown process. Bombardment with high energy electrons thus breaks up an organic molecule, yielding a complex mixture of positive ions and uncharged particles. The basic function of a mass spectrometer is to separate this ion mixture and determine the abundance of each constituent ion. For example if n-butane is bombarded with electrons of 70 volts energy, the ions formed, and their abundances relative to that of the commonest species, $C_3H_7^+$, are as listed in Table 35. All the ionic masses are due to ions of the type described above, except those marked i, m and d, which are discussed on p. 320.

Mass spectrometers normally yield data in the form of a so-called mass spectrum, in which ion abundance is plotted against atomic mass. Fig. 95 shows some typical mass spectra of organic compounds, consisting of large numbers of very sharp peaks. Generally speaking, two compounds, even if chemically very similar, yield quite different breakdown patterns, or mass spectra, which immediately suggests the following applications.

1. The unique nature of mass spectra leads to their use in problems of identification, and quantitative analysis of mixtures.

2. As seen from Fig. 93, some of the peaks are extremely sharp and intense, enabling the compound to be detected at very low levels when present as an impurity.

3. The case of n-butane suggests that, to a considerable extent the breakdown pattern of a molecule can be predicted. Conversely it is sometimes possible from the fragment ions of an unknown to reconstruct the molecule, and thus determine its structure.

In addition, mass spectrometry is an essential adjunct to the use of stable isotopes such as ^{15}N and ^{18}O in investigating reaction mechanisms, and in biological tracer work. It also provides valuable data about bond energies.

B. THE ANALYSIS OF POSITIVE IONS

Since mass spectrometry is basically a means of analysing mixtures of positive ions, this brief section deals with the appropriate physical principles. Magnetic analysers of the type commonly used in commercial instruments stem ultimately from the apparatus built by Dempster in 1920 for isotope analysis. The mode of operation is roughly as follows. After their formation in the ionisation chamber, the ions are driven by a small positive potential through a slit, in to the space between B and C (Fig. 92) where several thousand volts (E) are applied. Here they are accelerated, and ions of masses m_0, m_1, m_2 etc. emerge from the slit at C with velocities and kinetic energies given by

$$E = \tfrac{1}{2}m_0 v_0^2 = \tfrac{1}{2}m_1 v_1^2 = \tfrac{1}{2}m_2 v_2^2 = \text{etc.} \quad . \quad . \quad . \quad . \quad (1).$$

Beyond the slit they enter a magnetic field, H, at right angles to the plane of the paper. By a fundamental electromagnetic law, they now experience a force Hev at right angles to their path, and are constrained, like particles attached to a string, to describe circles in which the magnetic force is balanced by the centrifugal force. Hence, they describe a radius r given by:

$$Hev = \frac{mv^2}{r} . \quad . \quad . \quad . \quad . \quad . \quad . \quad . \quad . \quad . \quad (2)$$

Eliminating the velocity between (1) and (2), one finds that the radius for mass m_0 is given by

$$r_0^2 = (m_0/e) \cdot 2E/H^2$$

All particles of mass m_0 thus follow a common circle, but other masses have different radii, as shown in the figure.

In practice the ion stream entering the field will diverge slightly because of the finite slit width. However, as can readily be seen geometrically, the corresponding circular paths very nearly meet in a point when the ions have turned through 180°. In other words the magnetic field, in addition to separating the ions has a focussing effect on them, so that all ions of the appropriate mass (m_0) which pass through C reach D.

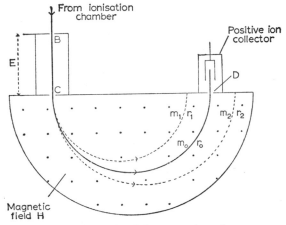

Fig. 92. Principle of the magnetic analyser.

There is another slit at D, behind which lies an electrometer valve or other device for measuring concentrations of positive ions. If the strength of the accelerating electric field, or the magnetic field is varied continuously, each ionic mass in turn will describe a circle of radius r_0, and reach the detector. The mass spectrum may thus be scanned and recorded.

With this arrangement a mass resolution of about 1 in 200 can be obtained with careful technique; that is, peaks of masses 200 and 201 are just separated. For applications (p. 336) where much higher resolving power is required, a magnetic analyser alone is inadequate, largely because the above theory depends on the slightly inaccurate assumption that all the ions are formed with zero kinetic energy, and therefore enter the magnetic field with identical energies. This difficulty is overcome in so-called double-focussing mass spectrometers, by interspersing an

References p. 350

electrostatic analyser between the ion accelerating chamber and the magnetic field. This analyser, in which the ions pass through the field between the plates of a cylindrical condenser, has the property that if ions of slightly variable kinetic energy enter through a slit at one end, only those within a very much narrower energy range emerge from an axial slit at the other end. Double-focussing instruments of this kind readily give resolving powers of 1 in 10,000[1].

Positive ion analysers have also been described which do not depend on a magnetic field[4]. These use the fact that after acceleration, the ions of different masses achieve the same energy and therefore different velocities. Such instruments are sometimes described by the term "time of flight". An instrument of this kind has been described by Harrington[2], which is particularly suitable for following rapid phenomena. It operates on a cycle which is repeated 10,000 times per second. A pulse of ionising electrons is passed for 0.25 microseconds, after which the ions formed are accelerated, and simply pass down a 100 cm field-free tube to the ion detector. Having different speeds, ions of different masses reach this detector, a special electron multiplier, in groups at slightly different times. So rapid is the response of this detector that it signals the arrival of each group separately, during the 1/10,000 second of each cycle. By synchronising the electron bursts with the time base of a cathode ray oscillograph which is coupled to the output, a continuous mass spectrum is displayed on the screen, which is only slightly inferior in resolution to those given by conventional mass spectrometers.

C. EXPERIMENTAL METHODS

For reasons which will become apparent, the accurate measurement of mass spectra requires rather elaborate apparatus, which is inevitably expensive, and is best maintained and operated by a physicist. Various single and double-focussing instruments are available in Great Britain from A.E.I. Ltd., a general purpose machine costing about £10,000. There is no prospect that in the near future cheap simple instruments designed for operation by organic chemists will become available, as in the infra-red field. Nevertheless from the point of view of a large organisation, dealing with organic chemistry, these disadvantages are out-

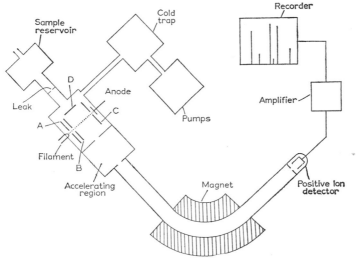

Fig. 93. Arrangement of the components of a mass spectrometer.

weighed by the ability of the mass spectrometer to solve many problems which cannot be tackled by any other technique. Fig. 93 shows the arrangement of the parts in a typical single-focussing mass spectrometer, and the following sub-sections describe these components.

1. Sample handling equipment

An excellent account of this topic has been given by Beynon[5]. As was previously explained the sample should enter the ionisation chamber at very low pressure, about 10^{-5} mm of mercury, so that intermolecular collisions do not interfere. Whenever possible this is done by sucking the sample from a reservoir where it is held in the gas state at $10^{-1} — 10^{-2}$ mm,

References p. 350

through a fine leak, such as a pin-hole in a thin diaphragm, or a sintered disc. If this leak is sufficiently short and wide, flow conditions will be such that the rate of transfer of a component of a mixture to the ionisation chamber will not be affected by

Fig. 94. Sample handling equipment: (a) for gases; (b) for liquids[5].

the other components. Gases are easily handled, being transferred to the reservoir by an arrangement such as that of Fig. 94a. Liquids are often introduced from a micro-burette via a sinter, which is fine enough to be impervious to mercury, but passes most liquids (Fig. 94b). A measured drop of liquid when deposited on the top of the sinter is rapidly sucked through and should volatilise completely in the reservoir. With a mixture of variable volatility, incomplete vaporisation of some components may cause difficulty.

The above methods are applicable only to substances with appreciable vapour pressures at room temperature. Heated sample handling systems greatly extend the range, enabling materials of which the vapour pressure is as little as a millimetre at 300°C to be examined, provided that a lower limit is not set by thermal decomposition. Care must be taken in the design of such systems to minimise exposure of the hot vapour to metal surfaces, which may catalyse their decomposition. In difficult cases a mass spectrum may sometimes be obtained by direct volatilisation from a micro-furnace into the ionisation chamber.

2. The ionisation chamber

Successful and reproducible analyses of positive ion mixtures depends on careful control of the ionising conditions. It is essential, that a narrow stream of electrons be used. After emission from a hot filament, usually of tungsten, they are accelerated by 50–70 V between A and B (Fig. 93), then "coast" with constant energy between B and C, before being collected by an anode. Another electrode D, with a small positive potential, pushes the ions formed through a slit into the ion accelerating region. In practice, to ensure uniformity, ionisation chambers have additional electrodes and also use a magnetic field further to control the width of the electron beam.

3. Spectrometer tube

The heart of the apparatus is this tube, surrounded by a strong magnetic field in which the ion separation takes place. Since this field must be uniform over a large volume, an electromagnet controlled by electronic circuits is normally used. Scanning of the spectrum is conveniently achieved by varying the magnet current.

As was first demonstrated in practice by Nier[7], resolution as good as that of a 180° Dempster type instrument can be obtained with a field in the form of 60° or 90° section. This principle is used in most commercial instruments to reduce the cost of the magnet, but leads to other complications. Both metal and glass tubes are used, each having merits and demerits[4].

4. Pumping system

It is vital that the system be attached to a highly efficient pump, both to ensure that ions can traverse the entire system without collisions with residual gas molecules, and for rapid removal of molecules adsorbed on the walls. In view of the low pressure required (*ca.* 10^{-7} mm), high standards of vacuum technique are essential. Either mercury or oil diffusion pumps may be used, and a liquid nitrogen trap should be placed between the pumps and the apparatus. The pumps are operated continuously, 24 hours per day.

Molecular adsorption on to the walls is a constant possible source of error, since strongly adsorbed polar substances may continue to be desorbed over a period of hours or even days, giving false peaks. For this reason provision is usually made for heating as much as possible of the assembly at 200°C overnight, to remove traces of sample adsorbed during the day.

5. *Detectors and recorders*

The first modern electrical device for the measurement of positive ion currents was the electrometer valve. After collection, the ions flow through a resistance, developing a D.C. potential, which is applied to the grid of this valve, acting as a first stage of a D.C. amplifier. Inherent difficulties in D.C. amplification led to a search for means of obtaining an alternating signal. The electrometer valve may be replaced by a vibrating reed electrometer, the essential part of which is a condenser whose capacity varies periodically, thus converting to an A.C. signal, more suitable for subsequent amplification. An A.C. output can more easily be obtained by modulating the potential of the repeller plate in the ionisation chamber, or by varying the electron output of the filament.

Electron multipliers have recently been developed as positive ion detectors, the ion beam impinging directly on the first plate, or cathode. They are much more sensitive than the above devices, and their rapid response is an advantage if spectra must be scanned frequently.

After amplification the signal is normally fed to a high speed pen recorder. Because of the wide intensity variations from peak to peak, the recorder must include a device which automatically cuts down the stronger peaks by a fixed factor, so as to keep them on scale.

D. THE MASS SPECTRA OF ORGANIC COMPOUNDS

1. Types of ion

Before the mass spectra of various classes of organic compound are described, the different kinds of ion which give rise to the peaks must be considered.

(a) Parent ions. Parent or molecular ion peaks, arising from removal of an electron only from the molecule, are perhaps the most important in dealing with unknown structures, since they lead to both the molecular weight, and, if the mass is measured accurately enough, to the molecular formula (p. 336). Unfortunately parent ion peaks are sometimes rather weak and difficult to locate. As a rule the parent peak intensity decreases as a homologous series is ascended, and branched molecules show weaker peaks than straight chain or cyclic structures of the same molecular weight.

(b) Fragment ions. These are of two main types, the first being those to be expected from bond breakage in the molecule. Typical ions of this kind are listed in the spectrum of *n*-butane, in Table 35. In addition so-called rearrangement peaks are quite common, where the bond breakage is accompanied by transfer of hydrogen atoms. A simple example is afforded by iso-butane, which shows a quite strong peak at mass 29, due to the process

$$(CH_3)_2CH\overset{+}{\text{—}}CH_3 \rightarrow CH_3\overset{+}{C}H_2 + C_2H_5$$

Similarly 2,2-dimethylbutane, 3-ethylpentane and 3,3-dimethyl pentane all show a strong peak at mass 43, due to $CH_3 \cdot CH_2 \cdot CH_2^+$ ions. The phenomenon is also common in oxygenated compounds, all primary alcohols for example rearranging to give $CH_3OH_2^+$ ions. Although such ions are of great interest to

References p. 350

theoretical chemists, their presence adds greatly to the difficulty of structural diagnosis by building up an unknown molecule from its fragments.

(c) Isotope ions. Since carbon contains about 1 part per 100 of ^{13}C, nitrogen 4 parts per thousand of ^{15}N, oxygen two parts per thousand of ^{18}O and small proportions of ^{17}O, and hydrogen two parts per ten thousand of deuterium, most peaks of organic compounds show weak satellites one or two units higher in mass. For example the methylene ion may be $^{12}CH_2^+$, $^{12}CHD^+$, $^{12}CD_2^+$, $^{13}CH_2^+$, ^{13}CHD or $^{13}CD_2$. It can be shown statistically that this leads to peaks at masses 14, 15 and 16, of relative heights 100 : 1.11 : 0.004. Considering a rather more complicated case, Table 36 lists the formulae of some ions of mass 45, together with the percentage strengths of the satellites at mass 46 and 47, relative to mass 45, and their ratio. In dealing with unknowns such ratios clearly provide a possible method of deciding the molecular formulae of ions.

TABLE 36

ISOTOPE PEAKS OF IONS OF MASS 45

Ion	% Height of peak 46	% Height of peak 47	46/47
HN_2O	0.818	0.202	4.04
CHO_2	1.175	0.402	2.92
CH_3NO	1.549	0.206	7.52
CH_5N_2	1.924	0.0112	171.7
C_2H_5O	2.280	0.215	10.62
C_2H_7N	2.655	0.0228	116.3

Chlorine- and bromine-containing compounds show much more spectacular isotope effects, since these elements are composed respectively of 3 parts ^{35}Cl to one of ^{37}Cl, and equal parts of ^{79}Br and ^{81}Br. Ions containing these elements may often be identified simply by observing characteristic groups of peaks. For example an ion of mass m (based on Cl = 35) containing three chlorine atoms gives a group in which the relative intensities at m, $m+2$, $m+4$ and $m+6$ are 0.428, 0.419, 0.137 and

0.015. Referring again to the mass spectrum of *n*-butane, there are several peaks marked *i*, arising from ions containing D or ^{13}C.

(d) Double-charged ions. Since the masses of all isotopes very nearly equal integers, all the above ions give peaks at almost integral masses. One cause of peaks at non-integral masses is the occasional formation in the ionisation chamber of a doubly charged ion, two electrons being removed by the collision. From the equation of section B such an ion appears at half its true mass, and, if this mass is odd, the peak can easily be recognised.

(e) Meta-stable ions. The time spent by an ion in the ionisation chamber after its formation is comparable to the time taken for the subsequent stages. It is therefore rare, but quite possible for fragmentation to take place during or immediately after passage through the ion accelerator. If an ion of mass m_0 dissociates at this stage, according to the equation

$$m_0^+ \rightarrow m^+ + (m_0 - m),$$

the ion m^+ will enter the magnetic analyser with energy $m/m_0 \times eE$, and it can easily be shown that a peak will result at the position of a normal ion of mass m^2/m_0. Peaks due to these meta-stable ions are usually diffuse, and at non-integral mass numbers. Examples are the peaks at 31.8 (or $43^2/58$) and at 39.2 (or $41^2/43$) in the *n*-butane spectrum, arising from the processes

$$C_4H_{10}^+ (58) \rightarrow C_3H_7^+ (43) + CH_3 \quad \text{and} \quad C_3H_7^+ (43) \rightarrow C_3H_5^+ (41) + H_2$$

Although meta-stable ions have only nuisance value in quantitative analysis, and instruments intended primarily for this purpose are designed to minimise their formation, these ions have definite uses in structural diagnosis, giving the masses not only of the final positive ions but also of the neutral fragments lost in the fragmentation stage.

(f) Ion-molecule complexes. Despite the low pressure inside a mass spectrometer, ion-molecule collisions occasionally occur in the ionisation chamber, yielding unexpected ions, which cause sharp but usually weak peaks. Thus several esters and nitriles show peaks one mass unit above the parent, arising from

References p. 350

collisions in which the parent ion abstracts a hydrogen atom. *n*-Butyl acetate (M.W. 116) shows in addition a peak at 159, corresponding to the molecule plus CH_3CO^+, and adiponitrile similarly adds the CH_3CN^+ ion to its molecule.

Such peaks are liable to cause confusion since, being the highest masses in a spectrum they may be mistaken for parent ions. Their nature can if necessary be established by increasing the pressure of the system, which will increase the collision frequency, and intensify these peaks relative to the rest of the spectrum. If their nature can be established, the compound giving rise to them can be classified as belonging to one of the few types in which such peaks occur.

2. The mass spectra of various classes of compound

Although strong peaks at certain masses in the spectrum of an unknown may suggest the chemical class to which it belongs, the determination of structure usually depends ultimately on building up the molecule for the masses and intensities of the fragment peaks. Because of the frequent occurrence of re-arrangement peaks, this is not a straightforward process, and usually depends on an ability to predict the breakdown pattern of various possible structures. The mass spectra of some two thousand compounds have now been published, from which generalisations have been made about the spectra of most classes of organic compound.

Before some typical spectra are described, a few fairly general rules may be stated.

(1) The most abundant ions are often parent ions, or those formed from the parent ion by breaking one single bond. Although carbon-carbon bonds break more readily than the stronger carbon-hydrogen bonds, and double bonds seldom break, there is no exact parallelism between ion abundances and bond strengths, since all bonds are greatly modified in the molecular ion.

(2) In a branched, single bonded structure breakage is much more probable at the bond adjacent to the branch than at those

remote from it. For example by far the strongest peaks in the spectra of the trimethyl pentanes I and II are at mass 57, arising from fragmentation as shown below, at the most highly branched carbon atom. Similarly III loses one or three carbon atoms much more readily than two.

(3) With a double bond, or a nitrogen or oxygen atom, the most likely bond to break is that β to this unit. For example the most abundant ion from most alkyl benzenes is at mass 91 ($C_7H_7^+$) rather than at 77 ($C_6H_5^+$), and alcohols and amines show the same tendency.

(4) Rings frequently retain their identity during fragmentation. Cyclopentanes for example usually show strong peaks at mass 69 ($C_5H_9^+$) and at the mass 69 units less than the parent peak. Ring compounds usually show strong parent peaks.

(5) For reasons which are not completely understood, certain ions are peculiarly stable, and contribute strong peaks even if rearrangement is required for their formation. Because of the great stability of the $C_3H_7^+$ and $C_4H_9^+$ ions, 43 and 57 are the strongest peaks in the spectra of most paraffins above C_4. Of the 18 isomeric octanes, all but five have their strongest, or base peak at mass 43. The $C_7H_7^+$ ion previously mentioned provides another example, being extremely prominent in the spectra of most alkyl aromatics.

(6) Parent ions containing oxygen and nitrogen often eliminate stable molecules such as H_2O, CO, NO and HCN. Phenol for example splits off CO, probably from the form

whilst anthraquinone shows a very strong peak due to loss of CO from the parent ion, giving the fluorenone ion, which in turn eliminates another CO molecule yielding the *ortho* diphenylene ion. Further examples are the loss of H_2O from alcohols, and HCN from amines and alkyl indoles.

(7) Rules (3) and (5) often work together, the initial product of β-bond fragmentation rearranging by transfer of a hydrogen atom, to give an unusually stable ion. For example the strongest

Fig. 95. Some typical mass spectra.

peak in the spectra of many carboxylic acids is due to the ion CH_3COOH^+.

The operation of these rules can be seen in the subsequent brief descriptions of spectra. For an authoritative account of this topic the reader is referred to Beynon's book[4], where all the available data on organic compounds is collected and discussed. Fig. 95 shows a few typical mass spectra.

Aliphatic hydrocarbons. The parent peak of straight chain paraffins decreases in intensity with increasing chain length, but is still detectable at C_{40}. Branching leads to easier fragmentation and diminishes the parent peak strength. Elimination of CH_3, C_2H_5 etc. from the parent ion gives peaks at masses C_nH_{2n+1}, including that at 43 due to the peculiarly stable propyl ion, which is usually the strongest in the spectrum, and peaks due to higher homologues at 57, 71, 85 etc. of decreasing intensity. This series and another at masses C_nH_{2n-1} in which splitting of the radical is accompanied by elimination of a hydrogen molecule, characterise the spectra of straight chain paraffins. As already mentioned the spectra of branched compounds are determined by the tendency for breakage at the branches. Paraffins also show weak peaks due to loss of one, two or more hydrogen atoms from the stable ions. Alicyclic compounds yield much more abundant parent ions, partly because removal of carbon atoms from the ring requires breakage of two carbon–carbon bonds.

Aromatic hydrocarbons. These have strong parent peaks, from which the molecular weights of unknowns can be deduced. The most probable mode of breakdown of many alkyl benzenes yields the $C_7H_7^+$ ion, making 91 the strongest peak in the spectrum. This ion is also formed by rearrangement from many polyalkyl benzenes. Fairly strong peaks also arise at mass 77 from splitting α to the ring, together with 78 and 79 from the $C_6H_6^+$ and $C_6H_7^+$ ions, formed by transfer of hydrogen atoms during the breakdown. Several of the peaks at lower masses can be attributed to further breakdown of $C_7H_7^+$. These include mass 65, by elimination of C_2H_2, 63, 52, 51 and 50. Another

References p. 350

prominent peak arises from the very stable $C_3H_3^+$ ion (39). The complexity of these spectra naturally increases with the length of the alkyl side-chains. A weakness of mass spectroscopy in dealing with aromatic hydrocarbons is the close similarity of the breakdown patterns of isomeric groups such as the xylenes.

Alcohols. Identification of alcohols from their mass spectra is rendered difficult by the weakness of the parent peak, particularly in secondary and tertiary compounds, and by a tendency to thermal decomposition before ionisation[8]. Breakage of the bond β to the oxygen atom gives a strong peak at mass 31 ($-CH_2OH^+$) in primary alcohol spectra, whilst secondary and tertiary compounds show analogous peaks at 45 [$-CH(CH_3)OH^+$] and 59 [$-C(CH_3)_2 \cdot OH^+$]. Quite generally peaks at 31, 45 and 59 are strongly suggestive of oxygen in an unknown. β-Bond breakage where the charge remains on the hydrocarbon fragment also takes place. Another feature of alcohol spectra is the olefinic ion, formed by loss of H_2O, and its breakdown products. For example the strong peaks of masses 56 and 41 in the spectrum of *n*-butanol arise from the process

$$CH_3 \cdot CH_2 \cdot CH_2 \cdot CH_2 \cdot OH^+ \rightarrow CH_3 \cdot CH_2 \cdot CH=CH_2^+ \rightarrow -CH_2 \cdot CH=CH_2^+$$

Finally the formation of H_3O^+ and $CH_3OH_2^+$ by hydrogen abstraction during splitting accounts for the peaks at masses 19 and 33 in alcohol spectra.

Ketones[9]. Since the $C=O$ group has very nearly the same mass as $-CH_2-CH_2-$, ketones show many peaks in common with hydrocarbons. The C_nH_{2n+1} series, 43, 57, 71 etc. is usually prominent, but accurate mass measurements show some of these ions to contain oxygen. In addition the peaks at 31, 45 and 59 found in alcohol spectra again reveal oxygen in unknown ketones. Further information about unknown ketones follows from their tendency to break at the carbon–carbon bond next to the carbonyl group. For example ethyl ketones usually show a strong peak 29 units below the parent mass. Rearrangement peaks complicate ketone spectra. Most methyl ketones have a strong peak at 58, the molecular weight of acetone, formed by hydrogen addition to $CH_3CO \cdot CH_2^+$, and analogous peaks at masses 72 and 86 have also been reported. It is difficult in unknowns to distinguish such peaks from parents.

Aldehydes[10]. Like most oxygenated compounds, aldehydes show strong peaks at 31 and 45, due to the rearrangement ion —CH_2OH^+, and its higher homologue. Another feature of their spectra is a peak of roughly equal intensity one unit below the parent, reflecting the tendency of the weak aldehydic C—H bond to break. β-Bond breakage, accompanied by hydrogen transfer is again very probable, giving such ions as CH_3CHO^+, at masses of 44, 58, etc. Characteristic peaks also result from elimination by the parent ion of the stable neutral fragments H_2O, CO and acetaldehyde, giving peaks of masses 18, 28 and 44 less than that of the parent.

Ethers[11]. Once again rearrangement peaks at 31, 45, etc. are prominent, and breakage β to the oxygen atom, preferentially in the longest chain, also leads to abundant ions. Rupture of the α carbon–carbon bond is usually accompanied by rearrangement, giving peaks one or two mass units below the corresponding alkyl radicals.

Carboxylic acids[12]. Removal of —OH, H_2O, and —COOH from the parent ion gives characteristic strong peaks in fatty acid spectra. A very stable rearrangement ion of mass 60, the molecular weight of acetic acid, causes the strongest peak in many acid spectra. Carboxylic acids show quite strong parent peaks, the relative intensity increasing from valeric to stearic acid in the fatty series.

Esters. The strongest peaks in the spectra of the lower aliphatic esters, $R \cdot CO \cdot OR'$, are often due to the ions R^+, $(COOR')^+$, $(OR')^+$ and RCO^+. Of these the last usually gives an outstanding peak at 57, 71, 85, etc., which can be distinguished from the corresponding hydrocarbon peaks on intensity grounds, or by accurate mass measurements. Another useful peak arises from fragmentation at the β carbon–carbon bond, followed by hydrogen transfer, giving $R \cdot COOCH_3^+$ or higher homologues. In long chain esters these peaks are not easy to distinguish from the many fragments formed by chain breakage, and the spectrum of the ester resembles that of the corresponding acid, from which it differs mainly in that the typical acid peak at mass 60 is absent. Esters show only very weak parent peaks, but, if the molecular weight of an unknown ester is required, it can sometimes be obtained from the intermolecular peak one unit above the parent, by working at an unusually high pressure. Aromatic esters show strong parent peaks, and even stronger ones arising from loss of $(OR')^+$.

Amines[13]. Amines show a powerful tendency to break β to the nitrogen atom, so that the ion $—CH_2NH_2^+$ (30) often causes the strongest peak in the spectra of primary amines. This mass is not however characteristic of primary compounds, since the ion is formed from other amines by rearrangements such as

$$\begin{array}{ccc} C_2H_5 & —CH_2 & \\ \diagdown & \diagdown & \\ NH^+ \rightarrow & NH^+ \rightarrow —CH_2NH_2^+ + C_2H_4 \\ \diagup & \diagup & \\ C_2H_5 & C_2H_5 & \end{array}$$

With secondary and tertiary amines β bond breakage, occurring preferentially in the longest chain, may again be responsible for the base peak, which falls for example as mass 86 in triethylamine. If the primary carbon atom is substituted, the base peak may arise from a more complicated breakdown, in which both α and β bonds are broken, together with hydrogen transfer, as follows

$$R \cdot CH(CH_3) \cdot NHR^+ \rightarrow —CH(CH_3) \cdot NH—^+ \rightarrow —CH(CH_3) \cdot NH_2^+ \ (44)$$

Amine spectra show a highly characteristic peak at mass 18, (NH_4^+), analagous to the H_3O^+ peak in alcohol spectra. Rearrangement peaks are also found at masses 31, 45, 59 etc., equal to those of lower amines.

Amides[14]. Amides show strong parent peaks, and their breakdown patterns resemble those of the corresponding acids. The strongest peak often arises from breakage of the carbon–carbon bond β to the amide group, accompanied by hydrogen transfer, yielding the ion of a lower amide.

Nitriles[15]. Nitriles provide yet another example of the same process, the base peak in the lower aliphatic compounds being due to CH_3CN^+. In long chain nitriles a series of peaks due to the ions $—(CH_2)_n \cdot CN^+$ are prominent. Because of weakness of the parent peaks in this class of compound, the intermolecular peaks at 1 and 41 units above the parent are sometimes useful.

Nitro compounds. Nitromethane shows strong peaks at masses 46 and 30, due to the NO_2^+ and NO^+ ions, but the strongest peaks in the spectra of higher aliphatics are derived from breakage of carbon–carbon bonds. More characteristic nitro group peaks are shown by aromatic compounds, both the NO^+ peak and one 30 units below the parent mass being prominent. Another typical peak is found 28 units below the last one, as a result of further elimination of a CO molecule. Further confirmation of the structure of an unknown nitro compound can often be derived from a peak 16 units below the parent.

Sulphur compounds. Because of the large proportion of ^{34}S in sulphur, this atom causes groups of isotopic peaks in a mass spectrum which can readily be recognised. Mercaptans show

Fig. 96. Part of the mass spectrum of octachloro-1,3,5-hexatriene, showing the effect of isotopes.

large parent peaks, and break most readily β and γ to the sulphur atom, giving ions of masses 47 and 61 in primary compounds. As with amines, should the α carbon atom be substituted, the longest chain is most likely to be broken. Peaks due to loss of H_2S and SH from the parent ion can usually by picked out.

Halogenated compounds. The power of mass spectroscopy in detecting chlorine and bromine atoms in parent and fragment ions from their isotopic patterns has already been mentioned. This is illustrated in Fig. 96, which shows part of the spectrum of a compound with eight chlorine atoms[29]. Fluorocarbons show a number of characteristic peaks, of which the most intense is often that due to CF_3^+, whilst CF^+ is also a common ion. Elimination of a fluorine atom often causes an easily recognised peak 19 units below the parent mass.

E. ANALYTICAL APPLICATIONS OF MASS SPECTROMETRY

This section describes various chemical applications where mass spectra are used for finger-printing a molecule, and no detailed interpretation of the spectrum is required.

1. Identification and impurity detection

Although the number of reference mass spectra is not yet as large as for example in the infra-red field, the American Petroleum Institute have published about 2000 spectra, the literature contains collections of spectra of several classes of compound, and many laboratories have large numbers of spectra of the compounds they are likely to meet. No satisfactory way of card-indexing mass spectra has yet been devised, so that rapid identification by comparison depends partly on the skill of the operator in recognising the salient features of a spectrum. Mass spectrometry has two main advantages over other methods of identification. Since the spectra are always measured in the gas state, complications due to change of state and solvents do not arise. Also, particularly with gas samples, the amount required is much less than with most other techniques. Against this, if a sample is very impure, the spectrum may be so complicated that the peaks of the major component cannot readily be distinguished. In such cases preliminary separation by gas chromatography may solve the problem. The scope is also limited by the need for a measure of volatility. Successful identifications of quite involatile substances have nevertheless been reported in a few cases. If for example polystyrene is flash-pyrolysed above 1000°C, the product is pure styrene, which can be collected in the sample-handling system. Similarly co-polymers often split into their various monomers which can be identified.

The great power of mass spectrometry in impurity detection has already been mentioned. When the structure of the impurity differs considerably from that of the major component, and perhaps contains different atoms, parts per million of it can often be detected. Detection of high molecular weight impurities is particularly favourable, since their higher mass peaks are quite free from overlap by those of the major component. On the contrary relatively large amounts of a lower homologue may be overlooked.

It frequently happens that, although the infra-red, ultra-violet and nuclear resonance spectra of several samples of a compound are identical, the mass spectrum clearly shows one or more impurities. This is extremely useful in the chemical industry, where very small amounts of impurity may render a product unsatisfactory, for example by poisoning a catalyst, or by imparting to a compound an objectionable smell or colour. The sharpness of mass spectral peaks compared to those of other spectra often permits the detection of more impurities in a sample than is possible by any other technique.

Another industrial application is the determination of the route by which a competitor's product has been manufactured. By using the method to detect traces of solvents and intermediates, the manufacturing process can sometimes be deduced.

Impurity detection is by no means confined to volatile samples; with volatile impurities, involatility of the major component may even be an advantage, since no interference from it occurs.

A fairly large quantity of finely powdered sample is placed in a vessel attached to the sample-handling system, and first evacuated at a low temperature. As it warms up, volatile impurities pass directly to the spectrometer for measurement. If necessary the heating can be continued above room temperature.

2. Quantitative analysis

Mass spectroscopy was originally applied in the chemical industry for the quantitative analysis of the complex mixtures of hydrocarbons which constitute petrols, fuel oils, and lubricating oils. It remains the most powerful technique available, where frequent rapid analyses of complex hydrocarbon mixtures are required on a control basis. In certain oil refineries gas streams carrying thirty or forty compounds are sampled at frequent intervals, their mass spectra measured, and the results fed automatically by the spectrometer to computing equipment, which prints out the proportion of each component. Very rapid warning of any change in composition is thus provided, and the necessary adjustments can be made before large quantities of unsatisfactory material have passed through. This process is of course expensive, so that, once conditions are sufficiently standard for less detailed analyses to be adequate, a cheaper, but less sensitive, method of analysis, such as gas chromatography, may be adopted.

To obtain accurate quantitative analyses, steps must be taken to ensure that three basic conditions are satisfied.

(a) The conditions of measurement must be sufficiently constant for variations in the breakdown pattern to be insignificant over the time required for the examination of the mixtures and pure reference components.

(b) The intensities of the peaks due to a compound must be proportional to its partial pressure in the reservoir. Careful consideration of the geometry of the leak connecting the sample reservoir and the ionisation chamber is necessary to ensure this.

(c) The spectrum of a given component must be unaffected by the others. If, for example, one component were strongly absorbed on to the filament, reducing its emission, this would affect the spectra of the others.

If these conditions are satisfied, a series of equations of the type

$$h_{11}p_1 + h_{12}p_2 \ldots h_{1n}p_n = H_1 \quad \text{and} \quad h_{21}p_1 + h_{22}p_2 \ldots h_{2n}p_n = H_2$$

and so on, may be written, the H's being the observed peak heights in the mixture, the p's the partial pressures in the reservoir of the components in this mixture, and the h's the peak intensities for the pure components at unit pressure. As in other branches of spectroscopy, this set of equations may be solved for the partial pressures. There will normally be many more peaks than components, so that more equations are available than is strictly necessary. If an electronic computer is available all the peaks may be used, and the best least squares solution obtained. Otherwise as many peaks as there are components are selected, in such a way as to minimise the arithmetical labour involved.

Consider, as a very simple example, a mixture of n-butane, iso-butane, propane, ethane and methane. Only the butanes show peaks at masses 58 and 57 (due to $C_4H_{10}^+$ and $C_4H_9^+$), which yield two equations from which the amounts of these components may be calculated. Passing now to mass 44, the parent peak of propane, the contributions of the butanes can be allowed for, and, since there is of course no interference from ethane and methane, the propane content can be deduced. Finally the peaks at masses 30 and 16, corrected for contribution from the higher homologues, serve to determine ethane and methane.

With hydrocarbon mixtures too complicated for precise quantitative analysis, it may still be possible to determine the proportions of various classes of compound. For example the sum of the peak intensities at the characteristic paraffin peaks 43, 57, 71, 85, etc. gives an indication of the paraffin content of a gasoline, whilst the sum of the series, 77, 99 ... 133 indicates the proportion of aromatics. Quayle[17] has analysed gasolines with respect to the groups paraffins, naphthenes, olefines,

References p. 350

cyclenes plus dienes, and aromatics. Further development of such methods by O'Neal[3,16] has yielded data on the overall compositions of lubricating oils and paraffin waxes, where, because of the high molecular weights and numbers of components, an analysis for each one is quite impossible. Fig. 97 illustrates the case of a paraffin wax[16].

Fig. 97. Composition of a paraffin wax[16].

3. Isotope dilution analysis

The measurement of isotope ratios occasionally provides the best method of estimating one component in a complicated mixture, from which it cannot be separated quantitatively. Suppose for example that the weight of glycine, x, is required in an aqueous solution containing a mixture of 20 or 30 amino acids, obtained from a protein hydrolysis. This glycine will contain ^{14}N and ^{15}N atoms in their normal ratio, R_1. If now a known weight, y, is added of a synthetic sample of glycine, enriched in ^{15}N, in which the ratio, R_2, is known, the isotope ratio in the solution will assume a new value, R. By expressing the condition that the weights of the two separate portions of ^{15}N containing glycine equal its weight in the final mixture, one obtains the equation

$$\frac{x}{R_1 + 1} + \frac{y}{R_2 + 1} = \frac{x + y}{R + 1}$$

Finally suppose that a sample of glycine is separated from the mixtures, for example by chromatography. The essential feature of the method is that it is quite unnecessary for the isolation to be quantitative. If R is now determined experimentally, all the quantities in the equation except x become known, enabling the required weight to be calculated.

The basic problem of isotope dilution analysis is determination of isotope ratios. This can be done very easily with a Geiger counter for such elements as sulphur, which have a radio-active isotope of convenient half-life. Nitrogen and oxygen however have no such isotopes, so the stable ^{15}N and ^{18}O species must be used. The mass spectrometer is then the only method of finding the isotope ratio. Compared to the radio-active method, this introduces the complication that the sample must be converted to a suitable form, usually nitrogen gas or carbon dioxide for measurement.

In addition to the amino acid case, the method has been used for example to measure the gibberelic acid contents of fermentation broths, and the amount of caffeine in coffee.

F. STRUCTURAL DIAGNOSIS

1. Determination of the molecular formulae of ions

Although as described in section D, peaks at certain masses indicate particular classes of compound, a detailed determination of an unknown structure usually requires a knowledge of its molecular formula, and those of several of its fragments.

The first step in this direction is to consult a compilation such as that of Appendix 1 of Beynon's book[4], where all the likely ions containing C, H, N and O, of a given mass are listed. Table 36 is a typical extract from this table. The number of such formulae increases steeply with the mass, reaching 18 at mass 100 and 60 at mass 250, and is further increased by the presence of other atoms. An immediate reduction in the number of possibilities can often be effected if the absence of some atoms can be established chemically. For example if only C, H and O are present, only two formulae remain at mass 45.

In favourable cases a further distinction may be possible by considering the ratio of the strengths of isotope peaks at $m+1$ and $m+2$, but this is of limited usefulness, since one can never be certain that the ratio has not been grossly falsified by contributions at one or both masses from other ions.

A much more powerful method of molecular formula determination depends on accurate mass measurement. Reference to Table 36 shows that the true masses of the ions all nominally of

Fig. 98. Mass separations with high resolution[4].

mass 45, relative to the standard $^{16}O = 16$ atomic mass units, vary between 45.0120 and 45.0723. Although masses cannot be read to this accuracy from the spectral records, it is quite possible to introduce together with the unknown, a compound known to yield say the ion C_2H_5O, and to measure the difference between this mass and the unknown. This procedure requires a mass spectrometer capable of resolving peaks differing in mass by 1 part in 1000 or less. Only in rather favourable cases is this possible with single focussing instruments, so that the double-focussing type has great advantages in this kind of work. Typical separations achieved with the A.E.I. company's M.S. 8 instrument[1] are shown in Fig. 98.

2. Determination of unknown structures

Because of the great sensitivity of mass spectra to impurities, one problem in investigating an unknown is the association of groups of peaks with components. Where possible a preliminary purification, for example by gas chromatography should be undertaken. Even after a rough separation, it may prove that many of the peaks are little affected, whilst the intensities of others vary enormously, showing them to be due to minor components.

Usually the most important information obtainable by mass spectrometry is the molecular formula of the unknown. This involves identification of the parent peak, followed by determination of its formula by the methods of the last section. As indicated in section D, the location of parent peaks is by no means always easy, since, particularly with branched compounds, they may be very weak. It may then be uncertain whether the highest mass in the spectrum is in fact a parent, an impurity peak, or an intermolecular peak. Any likely parent peak must therefore be subjected to various tests before its molecular formula is assumed to be that of the unknown.

It must first be confirmed that the formula of the ion in fact corresponds to a structure in which all the atomic valencies are satisfied. Formulae not in Beilstein should be suspect. A very valuable rule states that all organic compounds of even molecular weight, containing only carbon, hydrogen, nitrogen, oxygen, sulphur and the halogens, must contain an even number (including zero) of nitrogen atoms. Similarly those of odd molecular weight have an odd number of nitrogens. This rule stems from the fact that, of the above elements, only nitrogen has an odd valency and an even atomic weight. From the rule one can immediately say that an ion containing an odd number of nitrogen atoms, at an even mass, or an even number at an odd mass, cannot be a parent.

When examined under high resolution, the parent peak should of course be a singlet; an asymetric peak should be viewed with suspicion when the highest resolution is not available. The distance below the suspected parent of the next strong peak may also be significant. Intervals such as 15(—CH₃) or 17(—OH) lend support to the assignment.

One final powerful test for parent peaks must be mentioned. As explained in the introduction, if the energy of the ionising electrons only just exceeds that of the ionisation potential, the molecular ions are formed with little excess energy and are unlikely to fragment. On dropping the ionising voltage from say 50 to 10 eV, one therefore expects the parent peak to become much more prominent.

Even when the molecular formula is established, a great many structures may be possible. Beilstein for example lists 129 compounds of formula $C_{10}H_{16}O_4$. It will usually be possible to exclude many of these on chemical grounds, volatility, etc., and to make a choice among the remainder by considering the breakdown pattern. This usually involves predicting how the various structures are likely to fragment, and comparing these predictions with experiment. By far the most powerful weapon in tackling this problem is a comprehensive knowledge of how various classes of compound break down. This can be acquired only after considerable practice, since, as shown in section D, even simple compounds may give quite unexpected ions. Clearly the task will be aided by determination of the molecular formulae of as many of the fragment ions as possible.

3. Examples of structural determination

(a) A simple example from hydrocarbon analysis was given by Powell and Ross[18]. Although the infra-red spectrum of a sample of 1,3-dimethylcyclopentane showed no abnormality, the freezing point was lower than expected. The mass spectrum revealed an impurity whose molecular weight was two units lower than that of the major component. Since on chemical grounds unsaturated hydrocarbons and non-hydrocarbons could be ruled out, the only likely structure for the impurity was bicyclo[1.2.2.]heptane. This was later confirmed by its isolation.

(b) In view of the great current interest in the composition of cigarette smoke, one of the less volatile fractions of the smoke was led into a mass spectrometer sample-handling system[20]. By gradually raising its temperature, a rough fractionation was carried out, and a great many peaks were thus found, including several shown to be parents. These included a series at masses 90, 107, 122, 136 etc., the molecular weights of phenol, the cresols, the xylenols and higher homologues. A second series at 124, 138 and 152 were due to molecules with two oxygen atoms, probably methoxy phenols. Yet another series of compounds had molecular weights of 134, 148 etc., two units less than the corresponding alkyl phenols, suggesting that they were I, II and higher homologues.

I   II   III

Finally a peak at 272 was shown by accurate mass measurements to be due to a compound with the formula $C_{19}H_{12}O_2$, possibly a dihydroxy derivative of structure III. This example shows the large number of compounds which can be detected by means of a mass spectrum.

(c) The next example, which is due to Beynon[6], illustrates the power of mass spectroscopy in the identification of reaction products, where chemical speculation can be combined with spectroscopic interpretation. During investigations of the thermal decomposition of nylon, cyclopentanone was reacted with *n*-butylamine in the gas phase at 300–360°C, and mass spectroscopy was among the methods used to identify the products. On chemical grounds, the most likely reactions at this temperature involve elimination of water or ammonia.

Of the many parent peaks observed, one at 150 must be due to a compound with an even number, or zero nitrogen atoms. A likely structure is IV, formed by elimination of a water molecule from two of cyclopentanone ($2 \times 84 - 18 = 150$). Similarly, structure V can plausibly be assigned to the molecule causing a peak at 198, three water molecules being eliminated from three molecules of cyclopentanone ($3 \times 84 - 3 \times 18 = 198$). Further, even masses at 140 and 196 were shown by accurate mass measurements to arise from the formulae $C_9H_{16}O$ and $C_{13}H_{24}O$. Since these cannot be formed by self-condensation of cyclopentanone, the most probable structures are VI and VII, formed by the equations

$$C_5H_8O + C_4H_{11}N \rightarrow C_9H_{16}O + NH_3$$

and

$$C_5H_8O + 2C_4H_{11}N \rightarrow C_{13}H_{24}O + 2NH_3$$

IV   V   VI

VII   VIII   IX

Finally the structures of two nitrogen-containing compounds, causing peaks at 139 and 201 were deduced. The former can be attributed to elimination of water between one molecule of each reactant, giving VIII ($84 + 73 = 139 + 18$). Mass 201 cannot be accounted for by a simple elimination reaction of the above kind. However, elimination of two water molecules between two of cyclopentanone and one of the amine, gives a structure with the elements of IV and VII; this by ring closure and removal of two hydrogen atoms could yield the pyridine derivative IX, with the required mass of 201.

(d)* There was, until recently, some doubt about the structure of a white, crystalline solid, obtained by polymerising HCN. An ebullioscopic molecular weight determination indicated a tetramer, probably

$$\begin{array}{c} H_2N\text{---}C\text{---}CN \\ \parallel \\ H_2N\text{---}C\text{---}CN \end{array}$$

but certain X-ray measurements suggested a dimer. The mass spectrum[30] conclusively ruled out the dimeric structure. Peaks at 108, due to $(HCN)_4^+$, at 81, due to $(HCN)_3^+$, and the presence of various other fragment ions, leave no doubt that a tetramer is the only species present in the vapour state. Infra-red and Raman spectroscopy further substantiated the above structure.

(e) In the course of organic chemistry aimed at preparing derivatives of cyclobutadiene, the mass spectrum of tetraphenyl cyclopentadienone was measured. Strong peaks were found at masses 384 and 356, indicating the process

The fact that tetraphenylbutadiene is stable enough for its ion to be formed, encourages attempts to prepare it chemically.

(f) An unknown reduction product of glutarimide showed

---

* This example, and the following two, were suggested by Mr. A. E. Williams.

parent peaks at 141 and 155. The strongest peak in the spectrum was, however, at mass 98, suggesting one or other of the ions

From the known behaviour of caprolactam, one would expect the former ion readily to split off masses 28 (CO) and 29. The corresponding ions being, in the present case, extremely weak, the second structure is more likely for the 98 ion, and is further supported by other peaks at 84, 70, 55 and 42, which are found in the spectra of N-alkyl piperidines. It was therefore concluded that the unknown consisted of N-*n*-butyl piperidine (141) and the corresponding *n*-pentyl compound.

G. APPLICATIONS BEARING ON CHEMICAL REACTIVITY

Most of the applications so far discussed are used on a day-to-day basis in solving organic chemical problems. There are several other less obvious ways in which mass spectrometry is applied in chemistry, some of which are described in this section.

1. Bond strengths: stabilities of ions

Consider the process

$$RX + e \rightarrow R^+ + X + 2e,$$

taking place in a mass spectrometer. Suppose the spectrometer is set to detect only ions with the mass of R^+, and that the electron energy is increased steadily. No positive ion current will be detected until the electrons reach the critical energy necessary to cause the above fission, after which the current will increase steadily as in Fig. 99. Using a normal ionisation chamber the plot will curve near the axis, as a result of small kinetic energy variations among the electrons, causing uncertainty as to where the curve cuts the axis. With special apparatus[21], using additional electrodes, this difficulty can be largely overcome, an almost linear plot being obtained. The point P (or P') is known as the appearance potential, $V(R^+)$, of the ion R^+,

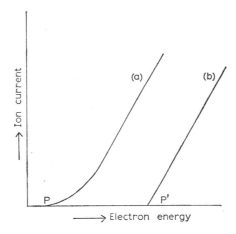

Fig. 99. Ionisation curves (a) with conventional ion sources, (b) by the method of Fox *et al.*[21].

and equals the energy, or heat content change of the reaction

$$RX \rightarrow R^+ + X + e$$

provided that, as is normally assumed, the kinetic energies of the particles are negligible.

Valuable information may be deduced from these appearance potentials. One may write

$$V(R^+) = I(R) + D(RX) \quad . . . . (1)$$

where $D(RX)$ is the dissociation energy of the R–X link, and $I(R)$ the ionisation potential of the radical R. If the radical can be obtained in sufficient concentration in the ionisation chamber, a separate experiment may be carried out in which this potential, the energy of the process

$$R + e \rightarrow R^+ + 2e$$

References p. 350

is measured directly. $D(RX)$ may then be obtained from equation (1). For example measurements of the appearance potentials of mass 15 in the processes

$$CH_4 + e \rightarrow CH_3^+ + H + 2e$$

and

$$CH_3 + e \rightarrow CH_3^+ + 2e$$

yields a value of 4.44 ± 0.2 eV (or 102 kcal/mole) for the dissociation energy of the H_3C-H bond of methane.

Direct determinations of bond energies in this way is often prevented by the difficulty of obtaining the uncharged radicals. The required bond energy may nevertheless be obtained by finding the appearance potentials of the ion in question, in two separate processes. For the C—H bond one could for example take the reactions

$$C_2H_6 + e \rightarrow C_2H_5^+ + H + 2e$$

and

$$C_3H_8 + e \rightarrow C_2H_5^+ + CH_3 + 2e$$

and, by subtracting the two appearance potentials of the ethyl ion, eliminate the inaccessible quantity $I(C_2H_5)$ between two equations of type (1). Excellent agreement between the results of the direct and indirect methods for the C—H link is described by Barnard[22].

One of the main sub-divisions of organic reactions comprises those with ionic intermediates. Although strictly speaking a full understanding of such reactions requires the stabilities (or heats of formation) of the ions in solution, it is sometimes possible to predict the course of a reaction where one of two possible ions may be formed, from considerations of ion stabilities in the gas phase. These heats of formation can be obtained from appearance potentials. If equation (1) is rewritten in terms of heats of formation, one obtains for the process

$$RX + e \rightarrow R^+ + X + 2e$$

the equation

$$V(R) = \Delta H(R^+) + \Delta H(X) - \Delta H(RX) \quad \ldots \ldots \quad (2)$$

The last quantity will normally be available from thermo-chemical data, and, if $\Delta H(X)$ is unknown it may sometimes be eliminated between the two equations obtained when the ion is formed in two different ways. This method has for example been applied to the ethyl ion, using its appearance potentials from ethane and propane. Table 37 gives some ΔH values calculated by Field and Franklin[24].

TABLE 37

HEATS OF FORMATION OF IONS

Ion	CH_3^+	$C_2H_5^+$	$n.C_3H_7^+$	$sec.C_3H_7^+$	$n.C_4H_9^+$	$sec.C_4H_9^+$	$isoC_4H_9^+$	$tert.C_4H_9^+$
ΔH	261	224	216	190	207	181	211	166

Consider for example the addition of HCl to propylene. The rate determining step, addition of a proton, can in principle occur in two ways:

$$CH_3 \cdot CH_2 - CH_2^+ + Cl^- \rightarrow nC_3H_7Cl$$
$$\nearrow$$
$$H^+ + CH_3 \cdot CH{=}CH_2$$
$$\searrow$$
$$CH_3CH^+ - CH_3 + Cl^- \rightarrow isoC_3H_7Cl$$

From the table the isopropyl ion is about 26 kcal/mole the more stable, so that one would expect its formation almost exclusively, leading to isopropyl chloride, as is indeed found in practice. Similarly with acid catalysed hydration of isobutylene, there are two possibilities,

$$(CH_3)_2C^+ - CH_3 + OH^- \rightarrow tert.C_4H_9OH$$
$$\nearrow$$
$$H^+ + (CH_3)_2C{=}CH_2$$
$$\searrow$$
$$(CH_3)_2CH - CH_2^+ + OH^- \rightarrow sec.C_4H_9OH$$

Of the two ions *tert.*-butyl is about 45 kcal/mole more stable, which accounts for the exclusive formation of *t*-butyl alcohol. The well known reaction of neo-pentylchloride $(CH_3)_3C \cdot CH_2Cl$, to give 2-Me-2-Cl-butene and methyl butenes, which must involve the ion $(CH_3)_2C^+—CH_2CH_3$ as an intermediate, becomes understandable in terms of ion energies. This ion has been calculated to be some 35 kcal/mole more stable than the neo-pentyl ion, $(CH_3)_3C—^+CH_2$.

2. The study of free radicals

The importance of free radicals in organic chemistry was indicated in Chapter 7. Although electron resonance spectroscopy provides an excellent method for their study in solids, liquids, and solutions, it cannot be applied so readily to gases. Many gas phase reactions, including combustion, involve free radical intermediates, and mass spectrometry provides a good method for their detection and estimation.

The reaction vessel containing the radicals normally adjoins the ionisation chamber, from which it is separated by a very fine pinhole in a quartz thimble. Careful design is necessary to minimise collisions with walls and electrodes, leading to recombination of the radicals before ionisation.

Two distinct methods of detecting the radicals have been used, the relative merits of which depend on the concentrations involved. In a case such as mercury dimethyl above 650°C, where the degree of dissociation is considerable, the normal ionisation energy of about 50 V may be used. Methyl ions are formed by the reaction

$$CH_3 + e \rightarrow CH_3^+ + 2 e,$$

which causes an ion current at mass 15, the strength of which is proportional to the partial pressure of radicals in the ionisation chamber. Methyl radicals will simultaneously be formed directly from mercury dimethyl.

$$Hg(CH_3)_2 + e \rightarrow CH_3^+ + HgCH_3 + 2 e,$$

but this can be allowed for by determining the ratio of the $HgCH_3^+$ and CH_3^+ peaks in a spectrum obtained under conditions which preclude dissociation.

This correction procedure is only feasible if the radicals

constitute 1 % or more of the whole mixture. For the detection of small concentrations, it is better to select a low ionisation energy, sufficient to ionise the radicals, but insufficient to break up the molecules. Robertson[25] calculates that, using this method, the minimum detectable radical concentration should lie between 1 part in 10^4 and 1 in 10^6.

Lossing *et al.*[19] give some typical examples of radical detection. Methyl radicals were obtained in almost 100 % yield in the thermal decomposition of, among other compounds, azomethane (at 700–800°C), mercury dimethyl (at 650–750°C), 1-butene (at 1000°C), and *n*-propyl iodide (at 650–850°C). Smaller yields were obtained from anisole, dimethyl ether, ethylene oxide, methyl iodide and ethane. Moderate concentrations of ethyl resulted from decomposition of azoethane at 690°C, but, as the temperature was increased, the ratio of ethyl to ethylene fell steeply, indicating further decomposition of the radicals.

No evidence of the *n*-propyl radical was found, probably because it is thermally unstable, but azoisopropane at 660°C yielded fair amounts of isopropyl. The allyl and vinyl radicals were also found to be fairly stable, and benzyl was obtained almost quantitatively from benzyl iodide at 670°C. No good source of phenyl radicals could be found.

The same authors describe a determination of the rate of recombination of methyl radicals. Mercury dimethyl, in a stream of helium, flowed through a furnace in which it was completely dissociated, and thence to the pinhole leading to the ionisation chamber. By varying the distance of the furnace from the pinhole, the degree of recombination during the various times taken for the gas to flow this distance was obtained, leading to the rate of the reaction.

3. Labelled atoms in reaction mechanism studies

Whilst it is relatively easy to discover the end-products and rate of a reaction, the elucidation of its mechanism, which may involve intermediates, is a much more difficult task. The

References p. 350

mechanism may nevertheless be of great importance in understanding the dependence of a reaction rate on changes in reagent concentration, medium and temperature. One method of deciding between alternative mechanisms is by labelling a particular atom in a starting material by replacing it by an isotope, and subsequently locating this atom in one of the products. As in the isotope dilution technique, radioactive isotopes are the most convenient labelling agents, but since oxygen and nitrogen have no such isotopes of convenient lifetime, the stable isotopes ^{15}N and ^{18}O must be used, in conjunction with a mass spectrometer to perform the isotopes analyses.

The saponification of esters by alkali illustrates the method. There are two possible mechanisms, according to which of the C—O links in the ester molecule is broken; these are

$$R \cdot C \overset{O}{\underset{O-R'}{\diagup}} + {}^{18}O-H^- \rightarrow R \cdot C \overset{O}{\underset{O^-}{\diagup}} + R' - {}^{18}O - H \quad . . \quad (1)$$

and

$$R \cdot C \overset{O}{\underset{O-R'}{\diagup}} + {}^{18}O-H^- \rightarrow R \cdot C \overset{O}{\underset{{}^{18}O^-}{\diagup}} + R' - O - H \quad . . \quad (2)$$

A decision between them was made by Polanyi et al.[26], who hydrolysed n-amyl acetate in $H_2{}^{18}O$. Of the products only the acetic acid contained ^{18}O, showing that the second mechanism operates. Similarly it was shown[27] that during esterification using ^{18}O methanol, the ^{18}O collected in the ester, showing the reaction to be

$$R \cdot C \overset{O}{\underset{O-H}{\diagup}} + CH_3{}^{18}O-H \rightarrow R \cdot C \overset{O}{\underset{{}^{18}OCH_3}{\diagup}} + H \cdot OH$$

Many applications of this kind have been made in biochemistry and biology. They are well summarised in Barnard's book[23]. Clearly the possibility of feeding labelled compounds to a plant or animal, and subsequently finding how it becomes distributed through the organism, opens up vast fields of biological research. The most striking discovery in this connection is that some of the proteins in a living animal are in a continuous state of formation and degradation. For example 10% of the rat liver proteins are daily degraded and re-synthesised, whilst the life span of a red blood cell in man is about 120 days.

Several biological applications are described by Bentley[28]. The method was applied to discover whether the bacterial metabolite acetyl dihydrogen phosphate,

$$\begin{array}{c} O \\ \diagdown\diagdown \\ HO-P-O-COCH_3 \\ \diagup \\ HO \\ 12 \end{array}$$

behaves as an acetylating agent, by breakage of bond 1, or as a phosphorylating agent by breaking bond 2. Hydrolysis in alkaline $H_2^{18}O$ yielded acetic acid whose ^{18}O content showed that the C—O bond had been split:

$$H_2O_3P - O-COCH_3 + H-^{18}OH \rightarrow CH_3CO^{18}OH + H_2O_3P - OH$$

In acid solution on the contrary, practically no ^{18}O was found in the acetic acid, showing that the P—O bond had broken. It seems therefore that, according to the conditions *in vitro*, either phosphorylation or acetylation could take place.

In the oxidation of glucose to gluconic acid and hydrogen peroxide by molecular oxygen in aqueous solution, catalysed by the specific enzyme notatin, it is important to find out whether the O—O bond is broken as in (3) or whether the oxygen molecule removes hydrogen atoms, as in (4).

References p. 350

$$C_5H_{11}O_5CH^{16}O + H_2{}^{18}O + {}^{16}O_2 \rightarrow C_5H_{11}O_5C^{16}O^{16}OH + H_2{}^{16}O^{18}O \quad (3)$$

$$C_5H_{11}O_5CH^{16}O + H_2{}^{18}O + {}^{16}O_2 \rightarrow C_5H_{11}O_5C^{16}O^{18}OH + H_2{}^{16}O^{16}O \quad (4)$$

On decomposing the hydrogen peroxide formed, when the reaction was performed in $H_2{}^{18}O$, with catalase, no ^{18}O was found in the resulting oxygen gas, showing that the oxidation in fact follows equation (4).

REFERENCES

[1] R. D. CRAIG AND G. A. ERROCK in: *Advances in Mass Spectrometry*, (Ed. J. D. WALDRON), Pergamon, London, 1959, p. 66.

[2] D. B. HARRINGTON, *ibid.*, p. 249.

[3] A. HOOD AND M. J. O'NEAL, *ibid.*, p. 175.

[4] J. H. BEYNON, *Mass Spectrometry and its Applications to Organic Chemistry*, Elsevier, Amsterdam, 1960.

[5] J. H. BEYNON, *ibid.*, Chapter 5.

[6] J. H. BEYNON, *ibid.*, p. 432.

[7] A. O. NIER, *Rev. Sci. Inst.*, 11 (1940) 212.

[8] R. A. FRIEDEL, J. L. SHULTZ AND A. G. SHARKEY, *Anal. Chem.*, 28 (1956) 926.

[9] A. G. SHARKEY, J. L. SHULTZ AND R. A. FRIEDEL, *Anal. Chem.*, 28 (1956) 934.

[10] J. A. GILPIN AND F. W. MCLAFFERTY, *Anal. Chem.*, 29 (1957) 990.

[11] F. W. MCLAFFERTY, *Anal. Chem.*, 29 (1957) 1782.

[12] G. P. HAPP AND D. W. STEWART, *J. Am. Chem. Soc.*, 74 (1952) 4404.

[13] J. COLLIN, *Bull. soc. sci. Liège*, 21 (1952) 446.

[14] J. A. GILPIN, *Anal. Chem.*, 31 (1959) 935.

[15] F. W. MCLAFFERTY, *4th Annual Meeting, A.S.T.M. Committee E-14*, Cincinnatti, 1956.

[16] M. J. O'NEAL in: *Applied Mass Spectrometry*, Institute of Petroleum London, 1954, p. 27.

[17] A. QUAYLE, *ibid.*, p. 63.

[18] H. POWELL AND G. N. ROSS, *ibid.*, p. 6.

[19] F. P. LOSSING, K. U. INGOLD AND I. H. S. HENDERSON, *ibid.*, p. 102.

[20] G. R. CLEMO, *Tetrahedron*, 3 (1958) 168.

[21] R. E. FOX, W. M. HICKAM, T. KJELDAAS AND D. J. GROVE, *Rev. Sci. Instr.*, 26 (1955) 1101; *Phys. Rev.*, 84 (1951) 859.

[22] G. P. BARNARD, *Modern Mass Spectrometry*, The Institute of Physics, London, 1953, p. 232.

[23] G. P. BARNARD, *ibid.*, p. 255.

[24] F. H. FIELD AND J. L. FRANKLIN, *Electron Impact Phenomena*, Academic Press, New York, 1957, p. 226.

[25] A. J. B. ROBERTSON, *Mass Spectrometry*, Methuen, London, 1954.
[26] M. POLANYI AND A. L. SZABO, *Trans. Faraday Soc.*, 30 (1934) 508.
[27] I. ROBERTS AND H. C. UREY, *J. Am. Chem. Soc.*, 60 (1939) 2391.
[28] R. BENTLEY in *Mass Spectrometry*, Institute of Petroleum, London, 1952, p. 117.
[29] F. W. MCLAFFERTY, *Anal. Chem.*, 28 (1956) 306.
[30] D. A. LONG, W. O. GEORGE AND A. E. WILLIAMS, *Proc. Chem. Soc.*, (1960) 285.

SELECTED BIBLIOGRAPHY TO CHAPTER 9

BARNARD, G. P., *Modern Mass Spectrometry*, The Institute of Physics, London, 1953, 326 pp. This book provides an excellent description of the experimental side of the subject up to 1952. Chemical applications are also considered, the sections on hydrocarbon analysis and biochemical applications being particularly valuable.

BEYNON, J. H., *Mass Spectrometry and its Applications to Organic Chemistry*, Elsevier, Amsterdam, 1960, 583 pp. This book, being the only one written specifically for organic chemists who wish to use mass spectrometry in solving their problems, is an essential tool. Both experimental methods and chemical applications are fully described.

DUNNING, W. J., *Quart. Revs. (London)*, 9 (1955) 23.

FIELD, F. H., AND J. L. FRANKLIN, *Electron Impact Phenomena*, Academic Press, New York, 1957, 349 pp. The energies of gaseous ions are discussed, particularly in relation to chemical problems.

Mass Spectrometry, The Institute of Petroleum, London, 1952, 205 pp. *Applied Mass Spectrometry*, The Institute of Petroleum, London, 1954, 333 pp. Both these volumes are collections of papers presented at conferences arranged by the Institute of Petroleum. They cover all branches of the subject, and demonstrate the wide applicability of the technique to chemistry.

ROBERTSON, A. J. B., *Mass Spectrometry*, Methuen, London, 1954, 135 pp. This book provides a general introduction to the subject. There are particularly valuable chapters on the energetics of ionisation, and on free radicals.

WALDRON, J. D., (Ed.), *Advances in Mass Spectrometry*, Pergamon, London, 1959, 704 pp. This is another collection of papers on all aspects of mass spectrometry. A valuable feature is the comprehensive collection of references at the end of the book.

STEWART, D. W., in: *Technique of Organic Chemistry*, (Ed. WEISSBERGER), Vol. 1, Part 4, pp. 3449–3539, Interscience, New York, 1961. All types of application are considered.

CHAPTER 10

X-RAY CRYSTALLOGRAPHY

In recent years X-ray crystallography has scored many major triumphs in the field of organic structure determination. For example it was the first method to reveal the structure of penicillin, at a time when evidence from purely chemical methods was conflicting. More recently the structures of much more complicated substances, such as vitamin B_{12} have been deduced. The object of this chapter is not only to explain what is involved in these major investigations, but also to show how X-ray methods can be used in less spectacular ways in the day-to-day work of the organic chemist. The method makes use of the geometrical properties of crystals and is therefore fully applicable only to crystalline solids, and those polymers which are made up partly of crystalline regions where the chains are lined up in an orderly array.

A. THE NATURE OF CRYSTALS

Before applications can be discussed the nature of crystals must be briefly considered. All chemists must at some time or other have been struck by the beauty and perfection of form of crystals, when they first separate from a solvent. When several crystals from the same crop are examined, it is found that their faces are plane, and that all the angles between corresponding faces are identical. This external regularity is the outward manifestation of an equally regular arrangement of the molecules within the crystal.

Examination of any wall paper, or floor covering designed to cover an indefinite area, will reveal a unit of pattern from which the whole can be built up by repetition in two dimensions. Fig. 100 shows a typical pattern, on which dotted lines indicate the repeat units or unit cells as they are called in crystallography.

By repetition of this unit any required area can be covered. The unit cell concept applies also to distribution of atoms in crystals. Fig. 101 shows a plane layer of carbon atoms, arranged as in a graphite crystal, the area being symmetrically divided up by the carbon–carbon bonds. A graphite crystal is built up by superimposing such layers, which are held together by Van der

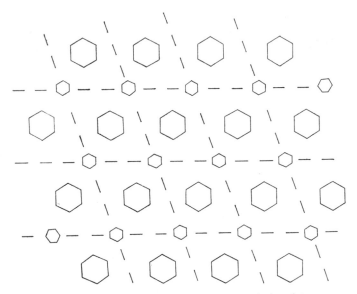

Fig. 100. Repeat units, or unit cells, in a pattern designed to cover an indefinite area.

Waals forces. Quite generally the space occupied by the crystal of any pure substance can be divided into three-dimensional unit cells, just as the area covered by a wall-paper can be split into two-dimensional repeat units. Clearly this fact greatly simplifies the determination of the distribution of atoms in a crystal. Once the structure of a single unit cell has been worked out, that of the whole crystal becomes known.

In general unit cells are unsymmetrical parallelpipeds, but

often two adjoining sides may be equal, or one of the angles may be a right angle. The unit cell may contain only one molecule, but more frequently two or more molecules are

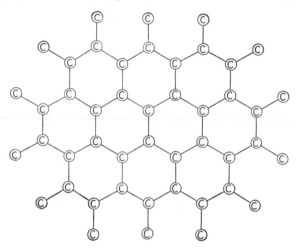

Fig. 101. Layer of carbon atoms in a graphite crystal.

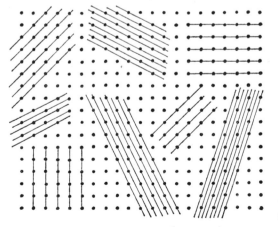

Fig. 102. Parallel rows of points in an array.

present. Nevertheless if any molecule is selected it is repeated in exactly the same position in each of the adjoining unit cells. The crystal therefore contains planes of atoms parallel to the unit cell axes, sets of identical planes being separated by distances a, b and c, the dimensions of the unit cell. There are many other atomic planes running through the crystal in directions other than those of the unit cell surfaces. The reason for this can be seen in two dimensions by observing the groups of lines which can be drawn through a planar array of points, as in Fig. 102.

B. THE DIFFRACTION OF X-RAYS BY CRYSTALS

The phenomena of interference and diffraction of light have long been known to physicists, and explained in terms of wave-theory. Everyday examples of interference by thin films are provided by the coloured patterns provided by a thin oil film on a water surface, and by the iridescence of certain birds' wings, whilst diffraction gratings are being increasingly used in spectroscopy.

Fig. 103 illustrates the elementary theory of a transmission diffraction grating, consisting of alternate opaque and transparent lines, the spacing being of the same order as the wavelength of light. When a monochromatic light beam is directed normally on to the grating each transparent line becomes a secondary source of waves which diverge in all directions. At certain angles however (case A) the peaks and troughs of adjacent wave trains fall opposite each other. This occurs throughout the grating, so that the net amplitude of the light transmitted in this direction is zero. At other angles (as in case B) reinforcement of the wave trains from adjacent lines takes place. The net effect is that strong transmission occurs only at certain definite angles where the path difference between two adjacent wave trains equals an even number of wavelengths. By elementary geometry the angles are given by

$$n\lambda = c \cos \phi$$

λ being the wavelength, c the line spacing, and n an integer.

References p. 377

Since a crystal is made up of units which repeat at definite distances, the possibility arises that it might behave as a three-dimensional grating for radiation of suitable wavelength. The atomic planes in a crystal are much too close together to show such effects with visible light. Reference to Fig. 28 (p. 74), shows however that the wavelength of X-rays, being only of the order of one thousandth that of visible light is roughly equal to the spacings of crystal planes. For example if a copper target is bombarded with high energy electrons, transitions involving the inner K-shell atomic electrons occur.

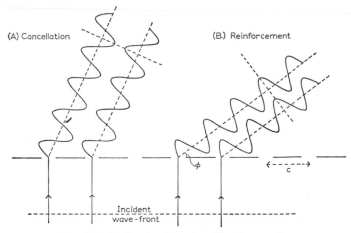

(A) Cancellation   (B.) Reinforcement

Incident wave-front

Fig. 103. Mode of action of a diffraction grating.

On dropping back to their ground state, these electrons emit high energy X-rays, which, by the equation

$$\Delta E = h\nu$$

are of very high frequency and short wavelength. In this case a beam of wavelength about 1.54 Å may be isolated.

An excellent elementary account of the diffraction of X-rays by a crystal has been given by Bunn. It is found that each plane of atoms partially reflects an X-ray beam, the angles of incidence and reflection being equal. When the action of a parallel set of

planes is considered (Fig. 104), there is the additional complication that waves reflected from successive planes may either
reinforce or cancel each other, as with the grating of Fig. 103.
In this case the condition for reinforcement is that the path
difference AB + BC must equal an integral number of wavelengths. It is readily shown that the condition is that

$$n\lambda = 2d \sin \theta$$

d being the spacing between the planes, λ the wavelength and θ
the angle of incidence (and reflectance) of the X-ray beam.

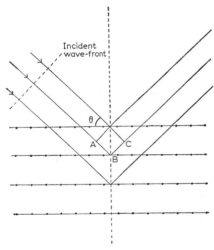

Fig. 104. "Reflection" of X-rays by a crystal lattice.

This relationship, known as the Bragg equation, is the basis
of most chemical applications of crystallography. If a single
crystal is suitably rotated in a monochromatic X-ray beam, it
is possible photographically, or with a Geiger counter to determine the angles at which reflections occur, and hence to deduce
the directions and spacings of all the atomic planes in the
crystal. By measuring also the intensities of the various reflected
beams, it is in principle possible to calculate the positions of
every atom in the unit cell.

C. X-RAY POWDER PHOTOGRAPHS

This section deals with the simplest type of X-ray experiment, in which the sample is reduced to a fine powder before examination. Although the information obtainable from powder photographs is limited, the method is rapid, and can be applied to any crystalline substance without special sample preparation.

1. Experimental methods

X-rays are normally produced by a tube in which electrons emitted by an electrically heated tungsten filament are accelerated *in vacuo* by a potential of the order of ten thousand V, and impinge on a metal target. Under these conditions the inner electrons of the target atoms are excited, and X-rays are emitted. Sealed, evacuated tubes are usually satisfactory, but

Fig. 105. Method of taking X-ray powder photographs.

for certain applications it is necessary frequently to change the target material, and hence the wavelength of the X-rays. In this event a demountable tube which is continuously pumped is sometimes preferred to a series of permanently evacuated tubes.

Copper is the target metal most commonly used. Its K X-ray emission spectrum consists of two lines (α and β) of which β may be filtered out if required by nickel foil, leaving a very close doublet at 1.544 and 1.541 Å, which behaves effectively as a monochromatic source. Various cameras have been described for the determination of X-ray powder diagrams, of which the cylindrical type, shown diagramatically in Fig. 105 will serve in explaining the principles of the method. The beam passes directly from the tube into the camera, where the sample is located at the centre of a cylindrical strip of suitable X-ray sensitive photographic film. Sample preparation is relatively simple. The sample, which may be any crystalline substance is finely ground, made coherent with a trace of adhesive, and suspended at the centre of the camera, in the path of the X-ray beam, by a hair or glass fibre. To understand the resulting photograph, consider some particular set of planes in the crystal, say that containing the a and b axes of the unit cell. In the random mass of tiny crystals, there will be some so oriented that these planes make with the incident beam the critical angle θ for first order reflection. However the crystals in which these planes reflect will be distributed through a complete circle. The reflected beams will therefore fall on the surface of a cone, with apex at the sample. As a narrow film strip is used only two arcs from this cone appear on it, together with a similar pair of arcs corresponding to every set of planes in the crystal.

After a suitable exposure which may take up to several hours, depending on the strength of the X-ray beam and the type of sample, the film is removed from the camera, developed and straightened out for examination. The general appearance of such photographs is indicated by Fig. 105.

Apparatus is also available in which the camera is replaced by a Geiger counter. As the counter is moved across the reflection pattern, signals are obtained from each line, which if required may be recorded automatically. Fig. 106 shows the type of record obtained.

References p. 377

2. Use in identification

Since the position of the arcs depends only on the spacing of the planes in the crystal, a powder photograph provides an excellent method of identification, both for inorganic and organic compounds. Identifications are best made by direct comparison with photographs taken in the same camera. When this is impossible, comparison with published data should be tried. Before this can be done, the corresponding values of *d* must be

Fig. 106. Geiger-counter records of the X-ray diffraction of pigments[1].

calculated, using the known dimensions of the camera, the wavelength of the X-rays and the Bragg equation. Data on many substances are published by the American Society of Testing Materials in such a way that identification of unknowns can be carried out, based on the strongest three arcs of the photograph. Fig. 106[1] illustrates the power of the method. Geiger counter records are shown from several pigments, which have only minor structural differences. The tracings are highly characteristic of the individual compounds.

In the case of mixtures, unless mixed crystals are involved, the diffraction patterns of the components all appear on the film. This fact can be used for detecting and characterising impurities, and for quantitative analysis, provided a calibration is constructed, based on mixtures of known composition. The method has for example been used to demonstrate that bleaching powder is a mixture of $Ca(OCl)_2$, and the basic chloride $CaCl_2 \cdot Ca(OH)_2 \cdot H_2O$[2].

3. Study of polymorphism

Powder photographs provide one of the most powerful available methods of studying polymorphism. Both inorganic and organic compounds often exist in two or more polymorphic forms, with different arrangements of the molecules in the crystals. The spacings of the atomic planes in two such polymorphs are different, so they give different X-ray patterns. Catalysts for chemical reactions are often efficient only if the correct substances are present in the correct polymorphic forms. X-ray examination may often therefore provide an explanation of catalyst failure. Polymorphism is also an important factor in determining the properties of pigments such as copper phthalocyanine, for use in paints. The presence of an undesirable polymorph may lead to growth of relatively large crystals in a paint, with resultant loss of covering power.

Crude copper phthalocyanine, which is manufactured in the undesirable β form must therefore be subjected to salt milling, acid pasting or solvent treatment to convert it to the α polymorph, which has the desired pigmentary properties. X-ray methods are valuable in comparing the efficiencies of these methods, and in ensuring that the final product is entirely in the α form.

Manufacturing difficulties may arise from the formation of a product in a physical state unsuitable for rapid filtration. In such cases X-ray methods are invaluable in checking whether the trouble is due to failure of the material to crystallise from an amorphous form, or to formation of an unexpected polymorph.

If a sample contains very small crystals ($<10^{-5}$ cm side) there may not be sufficient planes of atoms available for satisfactory reflection. This leads to broadening of the arcs, and provides a possible method of estimating crystal sizes in the range 10^{-5}–10^{-7} cm. In favourable cases the size of the crystalline units in polymers may also be deduced.

D. SINGLE CRYSTAL X-RAY CRYSTALLOGRAPHY

Powder photographs are quickly and easily obtained, but the information obtainable from them is limited. In particular it is difficult to obtain the dimensions of the unit cell if the crystal symmetry is low, or any information about the distribution of atoms and molecules within it. If such information is required, a different experimental arrangement must be used, based on a single crystal of the substance, rather than a micro-crystalline powder.

1. Experimental technique. Unit cell dimensions

A suitable single crystal is not always easy to obtain. The crystal must be perfectly formed and its dimensions should be of the order of a few tenths of a millimetre, so that the crystallographer can readily mount it in the camera. Too large a crystal may cause excessive absorption of the X-ray beam. Sometimes a fair amount of experimenting with different solvents and conditions of isolation may be needed to obtain a satisfactory crystal.

For the determination of the lengths of the unit cell sides, and the angles between them, so-called single crystal rotation photographs are required, which are obtained with various types of camera, one of which is shown diagrammatically in Fig. 107. It is cylindrical, and carries a film rolled to the same shape. The crystal is mounted on arcs at the centre of the cylinder, in such a way that the direction of one edge of the unit cell (say the c axis) is along the cylinder axis. While the photograph is being taken, the crystal is irradiated by a monochromatic X-ray beam at right angles to the camera axis, and rotated slowly about this axis.

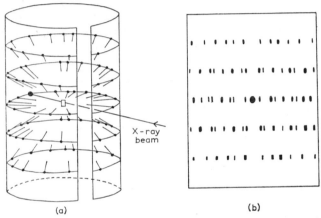

(a)   (b)

Fig. 107. (a) Arrangement for taking single crystal rotation photographs on a cylindrical film; (b) Photograph after flattening out.

During the rotation various sets of crystal planes at some moment make the critical angle of the Bragg equation and reflect momentarily, each causing a spot on the photograph. Fig. 107 shows the type of photograph obtained, which consists of spots of different intensities distributed along layer lines. The spacing of the repeat units at right angles to the beam being c, an extension of the treatment of a line grating to a net-work of points shows that all the scattered beams fall on the surfaces of cones with axes along that of the cylinder, and half angles given by

$$n\lambda = c \cos \phi$$

The layer lines represent the intersections of these cones with the photographic film. From the dimensions of the camera, and the distances between the layer lines, ϕ may be determined, and c deduced from the above equation. Repetition of the experiment with the other two crystal axes parallel to that of the camera yields a and b.

2. Molecular weight determinations

The volume of the unit cell can readily be calculated from its dimensions. If the density of the crystal is also determined (usually by a flotation method), the weight of one c.c. of it becomes known, from which, by simple proportion, the weight of material in the unit cell can be found. If the cell contains only one molecule, this obviously equals the molecular weight. Although the number of molecules per unit cell is not always easy to discover, the method invariably yields a simple multiple of the molecular weight. If therefore the molecular weight is known from some other source to within a factor of two, a much more precise value can be obtained. The method is capable of an accuracy of 2–3%, provided sufficient care is taken in measuring the density. Occasionally the unit cell dimensions yield information about the shapes of the molecules of an unknown. When two or more structures have been suggested, it may be possible to eliminate some of them on the grounds that their molecules will not pack into the observed unit cell. The sterol framework provides an example. Up to 1932 sterols were thought to be based on structure I. This represents a relatively "thick" molecule, since the union of three rings at one point causes buckling of the structure.

I   II

Unit cell determinations by Bernal[3] of calciferol, egosterol and other sterols, showed that the main part of the molecule must be nearly flat, which is consistent with the revised structure II.

3. Complete structure determinations

The previous sections have indicated how X-ray methods may be used for identification and molecular weight determinations, and to obtain rough ideas about molecular shapes. This information can be obtained relatively easily in a matter of hours or days. Occasionally it is also possible to decide quickly whether or not a molecule has a centre of symmetry. The diphenyl molecule was for example shown to have a centre of symmetry in the solid state, which is possible only if the two rings are coplanar, rather than at right angles.

Single crystal X-ray photographs can however yield much more detailed results. In favourable cases the position of every atom in the unit cell can be deduced. This gives, for an unknown structure, not only the structural formula, but the length of every bond in the molecule and the angles between them. The molecular shape is therefore completely defined. This detailed information cannot be quickly or easily obtained. Complicated calculations are involved, which, even if full use is made of modern calculating machines and electronic computers, may take several months. One difficulty is that these high speed methods of calculation can only be applied when a rough idea of the structure has already been obtained. Nevertheless there are two main situations where these difficult calculations must be undertaken.

The first arises when, as often happens, particularly with natural products, progress in elucidating the structure by purely chemical methods becomes very slow or stops completely. Possibly because of the presence of unknown ring systems, identification of degradation products may prove impossible, or if they are identified, it may be impossible to build up a reasonable structure for the unknown. The chemist may then try such methods as infra-red spectroscopy and nuclear magnetic

References p. 377

resonance. Generally speaking, however, these will only tell him about the small functional groups in the molecule, rather than about its overall structure. An X-ray structural determination must therefore be seriously considered, even though it may take months to complete. Although the X-ray crystallographer cannot say at the outset whether the determination will be possible or not, this can usually be decided fairly quickly. From a knowledge of the unit cell size, the number of molecules in it, and the chances of applying one of the special techniques mentioned below, he should be able to say within a week or so whether the determination is possible, and roughly how long it will take. The chemist must then weigh this information against the

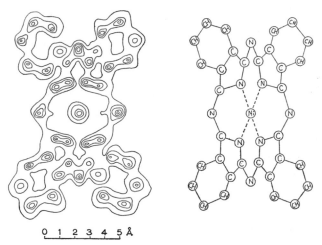

0 1 2 3 4 5 Å

Fig. 108. Electron density projection of nickel phthalocyanin. The contours are at two-electron units.

chances of more rapid success by other methods. In so doing he should bear in mind that the structure obtained by X-rays will be much more detailed than the structural formula, which is the most he can hope for by purely chemical methods.

The second call for complete structure determinations is in the accurate measurement of bond lengths and angles in molecules of known structure, for correlation with chemical properties, or with the results of theoretical calculations.

Since the technique of crystal structure determination is highly specialised, no attempt will be made here to describe how the positions of the atoms in the unit cell are calculated from the positions and intensities of the spots on an X-ray photograph. The calculation is somewhat shortened if a molecule contains heavy atoms such as bromine, or a metal of fairly large atomic number. The process may also be simplified in some cases by considering together two isomorphous derivatives of the unknown, such as a potassium and a rubidium salt. Successful application of these methods depends on the co-operation of chemists in preparing suitable derivatives.

The results can be presented in the form of electron density maps of projections of the unit cell on suitable planes. Fig. 108 gives an example. In these maps the atoms show up as peaks, and from the height of the peak one can infer which atom is responsible. Clearly for a complete structure determination, at least two projections in suitable directions are required.

E. DETERMINATION OF UNKNOWN STRUCTURES

Three examples follow where, despite extensive chemical work, the structure could not be firmly settled. In each case the X-ray method provided a conclusive answer.

1. Penicillin

The importance of the penicillins, the first and best known of the mould anti-biotics was realised during the second world war. At that time their production from mould in the necessary quantities and with reproducible quality proved difficult, so, in view of their military importance, hundreds of organic chemists attempted to find the structure with a view to synthesis. By 1943 many suggestions had been made and rejected, leaving only three for serious consideration, the oxazolone (III), tricyclic (IV) and β-lactam (V) formulae

III   IV   V

Because of the known tendency of such compounds to rearrange on decomposition, no definite decision among those three seemed possible from the degradation products. Two groups therefore undertook X-ray studies[4], one using the isomorphous replacement method with the potassium and rubidium salts of benzyl penicillin. This work showed conclusively that IV is the correct formula.

2. Strychnine

An outstanding feature of the brilliant work of Sir Robert Robinson's school on the structures of alkaloids during the thirties was the suggested formula VI for strychnine. VII and VIII were also thought possible at the time X-ray work on the substance was begun. Clearly a definite decision on chemical grounds is very difficult.

VI   VII   VIII

Two distinct attacks were made by X-ray methods. Robertson et al.[5] studied the hydrobromide, taking advantage of the presence of a heavy atom. The other group based their solution of the problem of the isomorphous sulphate and selenate. Both groups found a structure which shows formula VII to be correct, and also shows the shape of the molecule, which may well be useful in the future in explaining the physiological action of the drug. Rings 1, 2, 7 and 4 form a concave surface, from the edges of which 3, 5 and 6 hang like curtains. The net effect is a compact three dimensional structure from which the benzene ring protrudes.

3. Vitamin B₁₂

One of the most complicated structures so far worked out by a physical method, before there was any detailed chemical knowledge of it, is that of vitamin B_{12}. X-ray work began[6] following the isolation from it of a hexacarboxylic acid of empirical formula $C_{46}H_{60}O_{13}N_6CoCl$. Since, except for the presence of the heavy cobalt atom no short cuts were possible, an enormous volume of calculation was involved. The task was accomplished in a reasonably short time (about 6 months), by making full use of electronic computers. Formula IX was finally assigned to the carboxylic acid.

IX

X

References p. 377

All the interatomic distances and angles which were found were in excellent agreement with known bond lengths and stereochemistry. The work was extended to vitamin B_{12} itself. This determination was greatly simplified by the findings from the acid, and formula X deduced. Again the data yield not only the structural formula but also the molecular architecture. The elements of the B_{12} structure are beautifully disposed in space, leading to an almost spherical molecule. The planes of the central cobalt containing nucleus and the benzimidazole ring fall close together, almost perpendicular to each other, whilst the amide side chains pack round in such a way that the reactive groups lie almost on a spherical surface. Clearly when biochemistry has advanced sufficiently for a full explanation of the biological functions of vitamins to be attempted, information of this kind will be invaluable.

F. APPLICATIONS TO SUBSTANCES OF KNOWN STRUCTURE

Although the structural formula of a substance is well known, X-ray methods may yield a more detailed picture, which may be of the utmost importance in correlating the structure with physical and chemical properties. The following sections give a few examples of this.

1. Molecular architecture

To understand many phenomena such as the affinity of a dye for a fibre, or the physiological action of a drug, one must know not only the structural formula, but also the shape of the molecule, to see how it interacts with the substrate. Three main methods are available for determining molecular shapes, namely spectroscopy, electron diffraction and X-rays. The first two are limited to substances which can be vaporised at reasonably low temperatures, whereas X-rays are most often applied to substances which are solids at room temperature. By the use of special low temperature techniques detailed X-ray studies of, for example, benzene and ammonia have also been carried out. This implies that, except for fairly simple molecules, there is more prospect of the X-ray method being applicable than any other.

From the time of Kekulé up to 1928, the geometry of the benzene ring remained uncertain. This problem was largely solved when Lonsdale[7] determined the crystal structure of hexamethylbenzene, showing that, at least in the solid state, the benzene ring is a plane regular hexagon, with its external valencies symmetrically disposed in the same plane. Subsequently X-ray and other methods have amply confirmed this conclusion, and shown that most condensed ring hydrocarbons are likewise planar. A very interesting situation however arises with polycyclic hydrocarbons such as XI and XII.

more prospect of the X-ray method being applicable than any
XI   XII

Here, if the molecule were planar, points A and B would approach too closely to leave room for the hydrogen atoms. Robertson et al.[8,11] have determined the structures, and find that neither ring system is in fact planar. In XII most of the distortion is taken up by twisting of ring 1, so that the molecule retains much of its aromatic character.

Another ring structure whose shape has aroused interest is cyclo-octatetraene, C_8H_8. At least three possibilities present themselves, a symmetrical plane octagon, analogous to benzene, a "crown" and a "tub". Spectroscopy rapidly showed that the symmetrical octagon was impossible, but could not distinguish between the other two. X-ray measurements by Kaufmann et al.[9] decided in favour of the tub, in agreement with later electron diffraction work.

Much effort has been directed towards determining the distribution in space of the bonds around the metal atom in

References p. 377

metal complexes, a problem which has also attracted many theoretical chemists. Once again X-rays provide the surest method, subject only to the time and effort involved. The subject is reviewed in Martell and Calvin's book[15]. For example X-ray studies by Cox et al.[10] indicated that the Ni, Pt and Pd complexes of salicyl aldoxime (XIII) are trans-planar. Similarly trans-planar structures

have been assigned to the copper complexes of acetylacetone and various analogues (XIV).

A group of metal complexes which have been thoroughly investigated are the phthalocyanines. Since the ring can accommodate several metals, the method of isomorphous replacement is applicable. The dimensions of the ring systems have thus been obtained with great accuracy.

When the remarkable substance ferrocene (cyclopentadienyl iron) was discovered, it was first formulated XV. However its physical properties, particularly its diamagnetism, were inconsistent with this, and led to suggested sandwich type structures such as XVI and XVII.

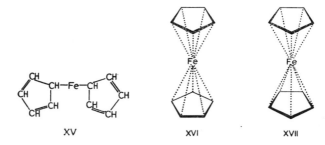

X-ray measurements revealed a centre of symmetry in the molecule, occupied by the iron atom, strongly supporting structure XVI. This was later confirmed by nuclear resonance spectroscopy.

2. Bond lengths

Modern theoretical chemistry has associated with chemical bonds many such properties as bond order, polarity, bond energy and force constant, which cannot usually be measured directly, but must be inferred from measurements involving the molecule as a whole. Bond length has the great advantage that it can be directly measured, and therefore provides something concrete by means of which theoretical deductions concerning the other quantities can be tested. The condensed ring hydro-

TABLE 38

BOND LENGTHS IN ANTHRACENE

Formula	Bond	Length from X-ray measurements (Å)	Calculated length (Å)
	A	1.391	1.396
	B	1.419	1.420
	C	1.364	1.382
	D	1.390	1.408
	E	1.440	1.430

carbons provide good examples of tests of this kind. They are readily treated by the quantum mechanical methods, which enable the lengths of the various bonds to be calculated. Table 38 shows the excellent agreement between X-ray measurements and theoretical calculation in the case of anthracene. The postulated presence of resonance forms can often be checked by bond length measurement.

3. Hydrogen bonds

Many physical methods are used to study hydrogen bonds, of which infra-red spectroscopy is perhaps the most widely

References p. 377

applicable. However in some ways the most fundamental property of a hydrogen bond is the distance between the two atoms bonded by hydrogen. This has been determined for large numbers of hydrogen bonds by X-rays. A good summary is given by Robertson[11]. In some recent work the electron density maps have been sufficiently refined to give an indication also of the hydrogen atom position. This is of the utmost importance in deciding whether such bonds are symmetrical, and whether they are straight or "bent".

4. Applications to high polymers

So far in this chapter we have considered only perfectly crystalline materials. Although many polymers, including waxes and resins, are amorphous and do not lend themselves to X-ray study, others such as carbohydrates, proteins, rubbers and synthetic polymers, are partly crystalline and reflect X-rays. Fig. 109 gives a crude picture of the nature of many fibres and drawn films. The polymer chains are seen to pass through crystalline regions, which hold together the chains and provide tenacity. These regions are roughly aligned, with their length along the fibre axis. From the intensities of reflections associated with the crystalline portions of a substance, the crystalline-amorphous ratio can be deduced.

Fibre axis

Fig. 109. Crystalline and amorphous regions in a polymer.

The X-ray diffraction of fibres can be used quite empirically. For example the effect of various degrees of extension on crystallinity could be found, or the effects on crystallinity of different methods of spinning compared. Crystallinity in a polymer is closely related to its dyeing behaviour, since generally speaking dye molecules can readily permeate the amorphous region, but do not penetrate crystallites. For example Ramie, the most crystalline form of cellulose, is the most difficult to dye.

However more detailed results can often be obtained. Since the crystallites in a fibre are aligned along the fibre axis, the X-ray pattern from a stationary fibre is rather similar to a single crystal rotation photograph, but much less sharp. It is therefore sometimes possible to determine one side at least of the unit cell, and hence the separation of repeat units along the polymer chain. For example nylon yields excellent X-ray photographs showing a chain repeat distance of 17.2 Å, which corresponds exactly with a fully extended —NH—$(CH_2)_6$NH—CO·$(CH_2)_4$·CO— group. Rubber and gutta percha are another interesting case. The repeat patterns indicate that whereas in rubber the polyisoprene chains follow a *trans* pattern, XVIII, those in gutta percha are *cis*, XIX.

XVIII

XIX

X-rays have proved perhaps the most fruitful single method of studying the structure of naturally occurring proteins. The foundations of this knowledge were laid by Astbury's school. It was found that proteins from such different sources as hair, wool, horn and nails all showed the same repeat distances along the chain. The protein with the corresponding amino acid backbone is called α-keratin, and shows a repeat distance of about 5.5 Å. On stretching, these materials transform to β-keratin, with a repeat distance of 7 Å, corresponding to a fully extended chain of the type

The configuration of the α-keratin chain is less certain, but more detailed X-ray studies[12] indicate that the chains form helices, involving internal hydrogen bonds, with about 3.7 amino acid residues per turn, and a repeat pattern along the axis of the helix of 5.5 Å.

The more complicated globular proteins, and even crystalline viruses have also been studied with some success. For example structural determinations of haemoglobin[13] and myoglobin[14] have recently been reported with resolutions of 5 and 2 Å respectively. Although this does not permit exact location of every atom, an excellent overall picture of the structure was obtained. Haemoglobin has a molecular weight of 67,000 and contains 10,000 atoms, four of which are iron atoms. Nevertheless, by using the isomorphous replacement method, a detailed 3-dimensional electron density map of the whole molecule was obtained. As can be seen from the molecular models photographed in the paper, the four iron atoms, surrounded by photoporphrin residues, occupy pockets on the surface of the roughly spherical molecule, the inside of which is occupied by four intertwined polypeptide chains.

REFERENCES

1 I. SCHNOPPER, J. O. BROUSSARD AND C. K. LAFORGIA, *Anal. Chem.*, 31 (1959) 1542.

2 C. W. BUNN, L. M. CLARK AND I. L. CLIFFORD, *Proc. Roy. Soc.*, A 151 (1935) 141.

3 J. D. BERNAL, *Chem. & Ind. London*, 51 (1932) 259, 466.

4 H. T. CLARKE, J. R. JOHNSON AND R. ROBINSON (Eds.), *Chemistry of Pencillin* Princeton University Press, Princeton, 1949, p. 310.

5 J. M. ROBERTSON AND C. A. BEEVERS, *Acta Cryst.*, 4 (1951) 270.

6 D. C. HODGKIN, J. PICKWORTH, J. H. ROBERTSON, K. N. TRUEBLOOD R. J. PROSEN AND J. G. WHITE, *Nature*, 176 (1955) 325.

7 K. LONSDALE, *Proc. Roy. Soc.*, A 123 (1929) 494.

8 A. O. MCINTOSH, J. M. ROBERTSON AND V. VAND, *Nature*, 169 (1952) 322.

9 H. S. KAUFMAN, I. FANKUCHEN AND H. MARK, *Nature*, 161 (1948) 165.

10 E. G. COX, F. W. PINKARD, W. WARDLAW AND K. C. WEBSTER, *J. Chem. Soc.*, (1935) 459.

11 J. M. ROBERTSON, *Organic Crystals and Molecules*, Cornell University Press, Ithaca, 1953, pp. 228–246.

12 L. PAULING AND R. B. COREY, *J. Am. Chem. Soc.*, 72 (1950) 5349.

13 M. F. PERUTZ, M. G. ROSSMANN, A. F. CULLIS, H. MUIRHEAD, G. WILL AND A. C. T. NORTH, *Nature*, 185 (1960) 416.

14 J. C. KENDREW, R. E. DICKERSON, B. E. STRANDBERG, R. G. HART, D. R. DAVIES, D. C. PHILLIPS AND V. C. SHORE, *ibid*, p. 422.

15 A. E. MARTELL AND M. CALVIN, *Chemistry of the Metal Chelate Compounds*, Prentice-Hall, New York, 1952.

SELECTED BIBLIOGRAPHY TO CHAPTER 10

BUNN, C. W., *Chemical Crystallography*, 2nd ed., Oxford University Press, London, 1961, 422 pp. The book, from a chemist's point of view, deals with the theory, experimental methods, and interpretation of the results of powder and single-crystal X-ray crystallography. It is a valuable source of basic information.

NYBURG, S. C., *X-ray Analysis of Organic Structures*, Academic Press, London, 1961, 434 pp. The X-ray structural method is described with a minimum of mathematics, and a survey is made of the organic and biological materials which have so far been examined.

ROBERTSON, J. M., *Organic Crystals and Molecules*, Cornell, New York, 1953, 340 pp. The theory of single-crystal X-ray structure analysis is dealt with, and such applications to organic chemistry as bond length measurements, studies of hydrogen bonding, elucidation of unknown chemical structures, and the study of macromolecules, are discussed.

ROBERTSON, J. M., in *Determination of Organic Structures by Physical Methods*, (Eds. E. A. BRAUDE AND F. C. NACHOD), Academic Press,

New York, 1955, pp. 463–502. The ground covered by the above book by the same author is dealt with more briefly.

STROUTS, C. R. N., J. H. GILFILLAN AND H. N. WILSON, *Analytical Chemistry*, Vol. II, Oxford University Press, London, 1955.

Tables of Interatomic Distances and Configuration in Molecules and Ions, (Ed. SUTTON, L. E.), The Chemical Society, London, 1958. Data on molecular geometry obtained by X-ray and other methods is assembled.

WHEATLEY, P. J., *Determination of Molecular Structure*, Oxford University Press, London, 1959, 263 pp. This book includes a good account of methods of determining crystal structure.

SUBJECT INDEX